HUMAN INFECTION WITH FUNGI, ACTINOMYCETES AND ALGAE

BY

ROGER DENIO BAKER

AND

A. ANGULO O. · C. BARROSO-TOBILA · L. M. CARBONELL
R. CÉSPEDES F. · E. W. CHICK · B. M. CLARK · O. DUQUE
G. M. EDINGTON · B. F. FETTER · J. H. GRAHAM · D. J. GUIDRY
R. W. HUNTINGTON, JR. · H. ICHINOSE · G. K. KLINTWORTH
H. I. LURIE · L. N. MOHAPATRA · J. MORENZ · H. S. NIELSEN, JR.
J. C. PARKER, JR. · C. E. PEÑA · P. PIZZOLATO · L. POLLAK
K. SALFELDER · J. SCHWARZ · J. P. WIERSEMA
H. I. WINNER · D. J. WINSLOW

SPECIAL EDITION OF
HANDBUCH DER SPEZIELLEN PATHOLOGISCHEN
ANATOMIE UND HISTOLOGIE III/5

WITH 796 FIGURES
2 IN COLOR

SPRINGER-VERLAG
NEW YORK · HEIDELBERG · BERLIN
1971

ISBN 0-387-05378-6 Springer-Verlag New York - Heidelberg - Berlin
ISBN 3-540-05378-6 Springer-Verlag Berlin - Heidelberg - New York

Special edition of Handbuch der speziellen pathologischen Anatomie und Histologie, Band III/5
ISBN 3-540-05140-6 Springer-Verlag Berlin-Heidelberg-New York
ISBN 0-387-05140-6 Springer-Verlag New York-Heidelberg-Berlin

Druck: Joh. Roth sel. Ww., München
Buchbinderei: Brühlsche Universitätsdruckerei, Gießen

Preface

Half a century ago our knowledge of mycoses, especially pulmonary mycoses, was rather fragmentary. It was limited to rare case reports as oddities. Accordingly, in the "Handbuch der speziellen pathologischen Anatomie und Histologie" the chapter on lung diseases caused by budding and spore-forming fungi by J. WÄTJEN (Halle) took up as little as 27 pages. Only ARNDT (Göttingen) could report on several cases from which he made his observations on actinomycotic changes of the lungs and pleura.

Since then our knowledge of mycoses has deepened and expanded in an unpredictable manner. This progress was mainly due to research and publications in the USA and South America. In Central Europe the number of cases of mycoses has increased during the last two decades, being reported especially as a second disease in patients with spontaneous or iatrogenic destruction of the bone marrow after treatment of cancer with cytostatic agents.

The number of known types of pathogenic fungi has increased. The knowledge of their types and conditions of growth have given rise to a subspecialty. Therefore, a great need has arisen for a new edition of the chapter on mycoses in the Henke-Lubarsch-Roessle Handbook of Special Pathological Anatomy and Histology.

The publishers as well as the editors had the great fortune to find as author Prof. ROGER D. BAKER, who himself has contributed substantially to the knowledge of human mycoses. It is thanks to Prof. Baker that a large number of eminent scientists could be won as co-authors. Today, under his guidance, a complete handbook on human infection with Fungi, Actinomycetes and Algae has been written. At the present time no other book exists which describes so extensively the fundamentals of human mycology, including taxonomy, clinical aspects, epidemiology, and pathological anatomy.

For all the great progress of the past decades we should not forget that 50 years ago MAX ASKANAZY wrote, for the textbook of General Pathology edited by LUDWIG ASCHOFF, a substantial and thoughtful chapter on fungi as germs. Among his illustrations there is a marvelous colorprint of an aspergilloma of the lungs. This, an early milestone, should not get lost among the abundance of genuine and supposed newer discoveries.

Zürich/Heidelberg 1971   Prof. Dr. E. UEHLINGER

Contents

General Chapters (Chapter I—III)

The Great Endemic Mycoses (Chapter IV—VII)

Infections by Fungi That Are Commonly Primary Pathogens (Chapter VIII—XV)

Unusual and Rare Mycoses (Chapter XXII—XXIII)

Infections with Actinomycetes (Chapter XXIV—XXV)

Infection with Algae (Chapter XXVI)

List of Authors

ALBERTO ANGULO O., M.D.
Profesor Titular, Director del
Instituto de Anatomía Patológica
Facultad de Medicina, Universidad
Central e Instituto National de
Tuberculosis
Correos de Sabana Grande
Apartado 50647
Caracas, Venezuela

ROGER DENIO BAKER, M.D.
Professor of Pathology
Rutgers Medical School
New Brunswick, New Jersey 08903, USA
Formerly Professor of Pathology, Louisiana
State University, School of Medicine
New Orleans, Louisiana, USA

CESAR BARROSO-TOBILA, M.D., Jefe
Dermatología y Dermapathología
Policlinica Maracaibo
Av. 8 (Santa Rita) Esq. Calle 71
Maracaibo, Venezuela

LUIS M. CARBONELL, M.D.
Jefe del Departamento de Micro-
biología, Instituto Venezolano
de Investigaciones Científicas
(I.V.I.C), Apartado 1827
Caracas, Venezuela

RODOLFO CÉSPEDES F., M.D.
Profesor de Anatomía Patológica en
la Facultad de Medicina, Universidad
de Costa Rica, Jefe del Servicio de
Anatomía Patológica del Hospital
San Juan de Díos y Hospital Central
del Seguro Social
Apartado 3275, San José
Costa Rica

ERNEST W. CHICK, M.D., Professor
Department of Community Medicine
Mycology Program, University of
Kentucky, College of Medicine
Lexington, Kentucky 40506, USA
Formerly Professor and Chairman
Division of Preventive Medicine
West Virginia, Medical Center
of Morgantown, West Virginia, USA

BETTY M. CLARK, M.B., M.R.C. Path.
Associate Professor
Department of Medical Microbiology
University College Hospital
Ibadan, Nigeria

OSCAR DUQUE, M.D.
Profesor y Jefe del Departamento
de Patología, Facultad de Medicina
Universidad de Antioquia
Medellín, Colombia

GEORGE M. EDINGTON, C.B.E., M.D.
M.R.C. Path.
Professor and Head of the
Department of Pathology
University College Hospital
Ibadan, Nigeria

BERNARD F. FETTER, M.D.
Professor of Pathology
Duke University, Medical Center
Durham, North Carolina 27706, USA

JAMES H. GRAHAM, M.D.
Professor of Medicine (Dermatology)
Chairman, Division of Dermatology
Professor of Pathology, Department
of Pathology, California College
of Medicine, University of California
Irvine, California, USA
Address at Orange County Medical Center
101 South Manchester Avenue
Orange, California 92668, USA

D.J. GUIDRY, Ph.D.
Associate Professor of Microbiology
Louisiana State University
Medical Center
1542 Tulane Avenue
New Orleans, Louisiana 70112, USA

ROBERT W. HUNTINGTON, JR., M.D.
Clinical Professor of Pathology
University of Southern California
School of Medicine
Los Angeles, California. USA
Address: Pathologist, Kern County
General Hospital
Bakersfield, California 93305, USA

HERBERT ICHINOSE, M.D.
Associate Professor of Pathology
Tulane University, School of Medicine
1430 Tulane Avenue
New Orleans, Louisiana 70112, USA

GORDON K. KLINTWORTH, M.D., Ph.D.
Associate Professor, Department
of Pathology, Duke University
Medical Center
Durham, North Carolina 27706, USA

HARRY I. LURIE, B.Sc., M.B., Ch.B.
M.R.C. Path., Professor of Pathology
Medical College of Virginia
Richmond, Virginia 23219, USA

L.N. MOHAPATRA, M.D., Dip. Bact.
(London), Professor of Microbiology
All-India Institute of Medical Sciences
New Delhi 16, India

J. MORENZ, M.D.
Professor of Medical Microbiology
and Epidemiology
Medizinische Akademie Magdeburg
301 Magdeburg, Leipziger Straße 44, GDR

HARRY S. NIELSEN, JR., Ph.D.
Formerly Assistant Professor of
Microbiology, Duke University
Medical Center. Presently Director
California Allergenics Laboratories
2602 First Avenue, Suite 104
San Diego, California 92103, USA

JOSEPH C. PARKER, JR., M.D., M.S.
Formerly Fellow in Neuropathology
Duke University, Medical Center
Presently at Laboratory of Pathology
New England Deaconess Hospital
185 Pilgrim Road
Boston, Massachusetts 02215, USA

CARLOS E. PEÑA, M.D.
Formerly Assistant Professor of
Pathology, University of
Pittsburg, School of Medicine
Presently Assistant Professor
of Pathology, Georgetown University
Medical School
Washington, D.C. 20007, USA

PHILIP PIZZOLATO, M.D.
Professor of Pathology, Louisiana
State University, Medical Center
Pathologist, Veterans Administration
Hospital. Address at Veterans
Administration Hospital
Perdido Street
New Orleans, Louisiana 70140, USA

LADISLAO POLLAK, M.D.
Profesor Asociado, Jefe de la
Cátedra de Microbiología
Escuela Vargas, Facultad de Medicina
Universidad Central e Instituto
National de Tuberculosis
Correos de Sabana Grande
Apartado 50647
Caracas, Venezuela

K. SALFELDER, M.D. (Prof. Titular)
Jefe del Departamento de Patología
Instituto de Anatomía Patológica
Universidad de los Andes
Hospital "Los Andes"
Apartado No. 75
Mérida, Venezuela

JAN SCHWARZ, M.D.
Associate Professor of Pathology
The University of Cincinnati
School of Medicine
The Jewish Hospital
Cincinnati, Ohio 45229, USA

JAN P. WIERSEMA, M.D.
Formerly Research Pathologist
Leonard Wood Memorial
Special Mycobacterial Diseases
Branch, Geographic Pathology
Division, Armed Forces Institute
of Pathology
Washington, D.C., USA
Presently Pathologist
Good Samaritan Hospital
1425 West Fairview Avenue
Dayton, Ohio 45406, USA

H.I. WINNER, M.D., M.R.C.P.
F.C. Path., Professor of Bacteriology
Charing Cross Hospital
Medical School, University of London
13 William IV Street
London WC2N 4DW, England

DONALD J. WINSLOW, M.D.
Formerly Chief, Infectious
Disease Branch, Geographic
Pathology Division, Armed Forces
Institute of Pathology
Washington, D.C., USA
Presently Chief
Laboratory Service
Veterans Administration Center
Bay Pines, Florida 33504, USA

Introduction

At the First Symposium on Mycotic Diseases of The International Academy of Pathology, meeting in London, Professor Dr. E. A. UEHLINGER of the Institute of Pathology of the University of Zürich, Switzerland, invited me to prepare a volume on the pathologic anatomy of the mycoses. This treatise would be a part of the section on the lung of the "Handbuch der speziellen pathologischen Anatomie und Histologie", now edited by Professor UEHLINGER, and would be published in English. It was my good fortune to persuade pathologists, microbiologists, and epidemiologists the World over to contribute chapters on subjects in which they had long experience and special competence.

The result is this authoritative volume of monographs, a number of which presently represent the most comprehensive exposition of "Infection with Fungi, Actinomycetes, and Algae". The investigation of the literature necessary to write the chapters has lead to new insights and correlations concerning the nature, epidemiology, diagnosis, prevention, and treatment of these increasingly significant diseases. This material is indispensable not only to pathologists, but to microbiologists, research workers, dermatologists and other practising physicians.

I owe a debt of gratitude to the co-authors of this volume, to my wife, ELEANOR USSHER BAKER, who helped in the preparation and editing of the volume, and to Springer-Verlag.

Professor ROGER DENIO BAKER, M.D.
Senior Author
New Brunswick, N.J., 1971

The Scope and General Pathology of Human Infection with Fungi, Actinomycetes, and Algae

ROGER D. BAKER, New Brunswick/New Jersey, USA

The Causative Organisms

Infections of man by fungi, actinomycetes, and algae constitute a large group, with fungi responsible for the great majority of cases, and actinomycetes and algae for the small minority.

In books on medical mycology the infections due to true fungi and actinomycetes are treated simply as fungi (CONANT et al., EMMONS et al., BADER) but the actinomycete organisms are so different from the true fungi that actinomycetic infections must be placed in a separate group. The actinomycete organisms of human infections are much thinner than the fungi proper and are quite like the bacilli of bacterial organisms except that they branch.

SKINNER et al. suggest a need for further division by the title of their book, "Molds, Yeasts and Actinomycetes." In the present volume, molds and yeasts are designated as fungi.

Infections due to algae are also included because the tissue appearance of the organism is similar to that of fungi, because there is a kinship between fungi and algae, and because the field of medical algology is limited and does not warrant a separate volume.

How are algae and fungi related? They are both among the Thallophyta, one of the four divisions of the plant kingdom.

The Thallophyta are characterized by their growth in irregular plant masses not differentiated into roots, stems, and leaves like higher plants (SKINNER et al.). Such a mass of plant tissue is called a thallus, hence the name Thallophyta for algae and fungi. The algae, being provided with chlorophyll, are capable of synthesizing their food from inorganic compounds by the energy of sunlight. The fungi, being devoid of chlorophyl, must depend for their food upon organic matter synthesized by other organisms, growing as either saprophytes or parasites. The reader is referred to Chapter XXVI for an example of infection by an alga. The lichens (Lichenes) have been considered a third subdivision of the Thallophyta, because they are peculiar plants composed of algae and fungi growing together in symbiosis. Most authors classify them with the fungi. The lichens have not been reported as pathogenic for human beings.

Yeasts are true fungi whose usual and dominant growth form is unicellular (SKINNER et al.). The organisms causing cryptococcosis and candidosis are examples of yeasts. The other pathogenic fungi are multicellular, are molds, and have a mycelium, though they often have a yeast phase in tissue.

The fungi are widely distributed in nature and only a few are pathogenic for healthy man. Others become pathogenic when man's resistance is lowered. About the same occurrence of fungous infections is found in animals as in man, but fungi are exceedingly important and common pathogens in plant pathology.

Fungus Diseases

Some fungous diseases are deep infections resembling tuberculosis or bacterial pyemias, whereas others are superficial infections of the skin and are regarded simply as nuisances. Fungi are vegetable parasites, larger and more complicated in structure than bacteria. The true fungi have thick filaments or hyphae which branch and often produce rounded bodies or spores, though some remain as yeasts. Pleomorphism of growth is often exhibited so that the organism grows largely in a filamentous form on blood agar at room temperature but in a rounded form at body temperature. Deep fungus infections involve subcutaneous, bony or visceral tissues, whereas the superficial infections occur on the surface of the skin or of mucous membranes.

Fungus *diseases* comprise more than is covered in this volume, which is limited to fungus *infections*. As an example, mushroom poisoning is a fungus disease and will not be discussed because it is an intoxication rather than an infection. However, a discussion of aflatoxins will be found in the chapter on aspergillosis.

Infection by fungi implies that the fungus enters the tissues and incites a characteristic inflammatory response. If the organisms are seen in microscopic sections of tissue in giant cells or in microabscesses, infection seems valid. *Care must be taken to exclude from the category of fungus infections cases in which a fungus is grown in culture from a lesion but which cannot be seen in section or in direct smear.* Organisms in culture may come from the normal flora of nonpathogenic fungi existing on the skin or mucous membranes. However, if a pathogenic fungus not commonly an inhabitant of a body region or an ordinarily nonpathogenic fungus in a debilitated person is repeatedly cultured from a lesion, the probability is increased that it may be the causative agent. *Clinical diagnoses* of bronchopulmonary candidosis must be made, on occasion, because of repeated, heavy growth of the organism in cultures of sputum. It may be impractical to obtain biopsy material to demonstrate the fungus in tissue in relation to a characteristic inflammatory response.

The Distribution and Epidemiology of Fungus Diseases

The soil is the usual source of fungus infections. The fungi live in the soil or on vegetation and propagate there, infecting man only occasionally through the inhalation of dust or through puncture wounds. Candidosis may be endogenous in origin, inhabiting the digestive tract and entering the mucous membrane of the esophagus or intestine.

Two of the great endemic mycoses, coccidioidomycosis and histoplasmosis, have large but limited geographical origin. *Coccidioidomycosis* originates in California and in the Southwest of the United States, in bordering Mexico, and in regions of Central and South America. The fungus requires a special environment of temperature, moisture and type of soil. Man contracts the disease by breathing in the dust of these areas. The occurrence of histoplasmosis is similarly based on the presence of *Histoplasma capsulatum* in the soil of the regions adjacent to the Mississippi and Ohio Rivers of the United States, and of many scattered regions in North and South America.

The third great endemic mycosis, *dermatophytosis* (athlete's foot and ringworm), is apparently different in origin. Dermatophytosis in the form of tinea pedis will be found where persons wear shoes and where the moisture between the toes provides a favorable place for the fungus to grow. Ringworm of the scalp is a contagious disease, being contracted from other children with the condition or from animal pets with the disease.

Mycetoma is an occupational hazard. The barefoot farmer or the wood carrier is infected from a fungus in the soil or in wood, via a puncture wound on a leg or on the back.

The remainder of the mycoses come from the soil or vegetable material, namely cryptococcosis, North and South American blastomycosis, Lobo's disease, sporotrichosis, rhinosporidiosis (perhaps from water), the phycomycoses (mucormycosis, subcutaneous phycomycosis, rhinoentomophthoromycosis), the mycoses caused by the dematiaceous brown fungi (chromoblastomycosis, cladosporiosis and brown-fungus infections of the lungs and subcutaneous tissues), aspergillosis, and several of the rare or doubtful mycoses. Geotrichosis may be endogenous or exogenous in origin.

The mycoses are therefore generally noncontagious, in striking contrast to many of the viral and bacterial diseases. The cutaneous tineas, especially ringworm of the scalp, are probably the only contagious mycoses.

Pathologists have, however, contracted North American blastomycosis and perhaps other mycoses as cutaneous infections of the hands as a result of performing postmortem examinations. This is an example of contagion from a dead body to a living one. There are also examples in which coccidioidomycosis may have been contracted by nursing personnel apparently as the result of organisms derived from the mycelial phase from the sinuses of patients who have infected the bedlinen or plaster casts. This occurrence may be questioned, as the nursing personnel was in an endemic region for coccidioidomycosis, and may have contracted the disease while off duty.

One form of environmental or occupational infection is the *laboratory*. Many cases of coccidioidomycosis and histoplasmosis have been reported because physicians, medical students and laboratory workers handled or inhaled cultures of the causative fungi in the mycelial form.

How Pathogenic Fungi Infect Man

Potentially pathogenic fungus organisms are numerous in the soil of many regions, and healthy individuals are frequently infected. For example, in the Cincinnati region there is evidence from histoplasmin skin tests and from autopsy demonstration of dead organisms in lesions that 85% of the population has been infected and has coped successfully with the infection, causing it to be calcified and inactive. The great majority of these infections occur in healthy persons and a decreased host resistance plays no part in favoring the infection. The fungus is aspirated deeply into the lung and there finds an environment of temperature and other factors which permit it to multiply. It lives in macrophages for a time, then forms tubercles in the lung, in the draining lymph nodes and in half of these cases in the spleen as well. For a fungus organism to be pathogenic, it must find in the tissues an environment suitable for continued existence and multiplication. Innumerable nonpathogenic organisms must enter the tissues of normal individuals during their lifetime, through wounds and abrasions, and then perish because the conditions are not favorable for continued growth.

Once histoplasmosis has developed to the stage of a primary complex, immunity and hypersensitivity show themselves. The infection usually fails to spread further. Also it is apparently more difficult to reinfect the individual from exogenous sources than it was the first time. The factors of hypersensitivity and immunity are similar to those of tuberculosis, except that the residual histoplasmic lesion is less prone to reactivation than is the residual tuberculous lesion.

Reduced host resistance plays a minor, but definite role in the original infection, and in the spread within the body, of some primary fungal pathogens. (Symposium on Opportunistic Fungus Infections, 1962.)

Mycoses Associated with Lowered Host Resistance, and Caused by Fungi Which are Usually Nonpathogenic and "Opportunistic"

There are three well known mycoses, candidosis, aspergillosis and mucormycosis, which are encountered in individuals with lowered bodily resistance. The causative species of *Candida*, *Aspergillus*, and *Rhizopus* (or *Mucor* or *Absidia*) rarely infect healthy human beings. These organisms are "opportunistic" or "facultatively pathogenic."

An antifungal factor is present in the tissues of the normal body and can be demonstrated in the serum of normal individuals by its inhibiting effect on the growth of the fungus on culture media made up with varying proportions of normal sera (OWENS et al.). This factor is reduced in persons who are suffering some of the conditions which predispose to infection by these facultatively pathogenic organisms.

The factor of lowered host resistance to *Rhizopus* has been extensively studied in mucormycosis, both by observation of human cases and by research with animals (see Chapter XXI). These factors may also relate to the other two "opportunistic" mycoses and to two other infections which are occasionally opportunistic, namely cryptococcosis and nocardiosis.

Mucormycosis develops in persons in diabetic acidosis or suffering from leukemia, and especially when the leukemia is accompanied by neutropenia and when corticosteroids have been administered. Lowered host resistance to nonpathogenic organisms and to some of the usually pathogenic fungi is based upon metabolic disturbances, blood dyscrasias and drug therapy, especially the immunosuppressants (BAKER, 1964). The unifying underlying factor common to these conditions is not yet understood. These factors have been operative in the production of several of the rare and unusual mycoses (see Chapter XXIII) and it is probable that new mycoses will continue to appear.

Fungi as Inflammatory Irritants

In general fungi are indolent as inflammatory irritants in comparison with many of the bacteria (BAKER, 1961, 1966). Some fungi compare with the tubercle bacillus or leprosy bacillus in this respect. For example, we find apparently viable *Histoplasma capsulatum* in macrophages and viable *Blastomyces dermatitidis* in giant cells. Frequently, living or disintegrating fungi are seen in giant cells or in minute abscesses. This is well exemplified in North American blastomycosis. In skin lesions which have persisted for many months, with the patient's general health unaffected, we expect the biopsy to show organisms in micro-abscesses or in giant cells (BAKER, 1961, 1966). The organisms appear to be acting much as foreign bodies do. A splinter of wood or other foreign substance in the tissues is often found surrounded by pus or by giant cells. It is not clear that variations in chemical composition of different organisms has much affect on these basic responses. The role of developing allergy or hypersensitivity is difficult to assess in studying human tissue, but the acute inflammatory response is more rapid than it was at the primary contact with the organism and the body exerts a more necrotizing effect.

Tissue Changes in Fungus Diseases

No one tissue change seems to be entirely characteristic or pathognomonic of fungus disease (BAKER, 1947, 1968; SYMMERS).

If the microscopic appearances of fungus lesions are tabulated with respect to the degree of suppuration, macrophages, giant cells, caseous necrosis and fibrosis, the following is observed:

1. Several of the deep fungous infections, such as blastomycosis (North and South American), coccidioidomycosis and sporotrichosis, show all of these tissue changes.

2. Others of the deep infections, such as mycetoma and chromoblastomycosis, show all of these changes except caseous necrosis.

3. Mucormycosis may run its entire course with only infarction due to vascular thrombosis and with minimal acute inflammation.

4. Suppuration is absent or minimal in many lesions of histoplasmosis and cryptococcosis. Animal experimental studies indicate, however, that the initial response of the body to *Cryptococcus neoformans* is the neutrophil. This stage has usually disappeared at the time tissue is examined by biopsy or at autopsy.

5. The superficial fungus diseases often appear to have no inflammatory response. For example, microspores of tinea capitis occur in the hair shaft and hair follicle with no inflammatory reaction. In some instances giant cells and lymphocytes are noted outside the hair follicle. However, in active phases of dermatophytosis all forms of acute and chronic inflammation may be encountered, even inflammatory edema in the form of vesicles and bullae.

Chronic suppuration with fibrosis is the most general tissue change in deep fungous infections and the neutrophil is usually the primary reacting cell. In some instances the macrophage or giant cell may be the primary reacting cell. Factors responsible for the tissue changes of fungous infections are the following: (1) the large size of the organism acting as a foreign body, (2) the location of the fungus as to whether it is superficial or deep in the body, (3) endotoxins and the chemical constitution of the organism, (4) the development of hypersensitivity to the fungus, and (5) chronicity of the process.

The term *granulomatous inflammation* should *not* be too broadly used in characterizing the mycotic infections. If granulomatous inflammation is defined chiefly on the basis of participation of clusters of macrophages and giant cells, it is clear that other features, such as suppuration and fibrosis, are more characteristic of many fungus infections. If one thinks of granulomatous tissue as characterized by a focal type of reaction, such as the tubercle, then some of the fungous infections are of this type; but the tubercles of fungous disease tend to have purulent centers in contrast to those of tuberculosis and are abscesses.

One of the most interesting responses to fungus infection is that of calcification. This is most conspicuous in the inactive histoplasmic lesions of the lung, mediastinal lymph nodes and spleen. The primary lesions of coccidioidomycosis often calcify. The remainder of the mycoses calcify rarely, if at all. I have observed calcification in only one case of cryptococcosis and one of North American blastomycosis. In histoplasmosis and coccidioidomycosis the calcification occurs probably because the lesions undergo a stage of caseous necrosis and the calcium salts are deposited in the necrotic tissue. It is not reasonable to expect that calcification would develop in lesions which are predominantly suppurative as in many of the deep mycoses.

The macrophage is active in many mycoses by itself or as part of a giant cell. The essence of histoplasmosis is macrophagic phagocytosis of *Histoplasma capsu-*

latum. This is seen on a grand scale in acute disseminated histoplasmosis in which the macrophages of the reticuloendothelial system of the spleen, liver, lymph nodes and bone marrow are stuffed with parasites and the spleen and liver become greatly enlarged, while the bone marrow is destroyed to the point that secondary purpura develops.

Vascular thrombosis is found in mucormycosis, and occasionally in aspergillosis and candidosis as a result of the organisms penetrating blood vessels.

Morbidity and Mortality in Mycotic Disease

The total number of persons affected with fungus infections is large when one considers histoplasmosis, coccidioidomycosis and dermatophytosis. More than 30,000,000 persons in the United States of America have been infected with *Histoplasma capsulatum.* There may be 400,000 new cases of coccidioidomycosis annually. Most of the cases are in an inactive stage and the disability is not great in comparison with tuberculosis. Sporadic cases of severe and prolonged disability are encountered in the form of cryptococcal meningitis, coccidioidal meningitis, histoplasmic chronic pulmonary disease and mycetoma.

The mortality of fungus infections is not great in comparison with the total number of persons infected. Worldwide there might be 40 deaths per year from coccidioidomycosis, perhaps the same number from histoplasmosis and cryptococcosis, 10 cases of mucormycosis and about the same number of systemic candidosis and aspergillosis. There are small numbers of deaths from North and South American blastomycosis, cladosporiosis, and from the rare mycoses.

The Demonstration of Fungi in Tissues

The demonstration of fungi in human tissues is usually a simple matter. Blocks of tissue are taken from autopsy material or from surgically removed organs or biopsies, embedded in paraffin and sections cut from the blocks are stained with hematoxylin and eosin (BAKER, 1957, 1967; EMMONS et al.). Examination of these routine slides may make possible the diagnosis of histoplasmosis, African histoplasmosis, coccidioidomycosis, some of the tineas, such as tinea capitis and tinea versicolor, cryptococcosis, North American blastomycosis, South American blastomycosis, Lobo's disease, mycetoma, rhinosporidiosis, subcutaneous phycomycosis and rhinoentomophthoromycosis, chromoblastomycosis, cladosporiosis, brown-fungus subcutaneous abscesses, candidosis, aspergillosis, mucormycosis and otomycosis.

This list includes all of the fungus diseases considered in this book with the exception of sporotrichosis, geotrichosis and several of the rare mycoses.

Sporotrichosis can be diagnosed histologically under certain conditions, but the organisms are often not obvious in hematoxylin and eosin stained slides, and culture demonstration is highly desirable. Refer to chapter XIII.

In nocardiosis the hematoxylin and eosin stain is not effective in coloring the organisms. The gram stain must be applied.

The various kinds of grains in mycetoma can often be differentiated one from another on histologic study.

Occasionally there is confusion between spherules of calcium and fungus organisms. The problem may be solved by remembering that a fungus occurs in relation to a characteristic inflammatory response, and not just anywhere in cerebral or connective tissue.

In most instances special stains are not superior to the hematoxylin and eosin stain for the identification of the fungus in tissues, but they often show the fungus with increased clarity, and make a beautiful preparation (BAKER, 1957). The most helpful special stains for fungi are: (1) the Grocott-Gomori methenamine-silver nitrate technique (GMS), (2) the Gram stain, (3) the periodic-acid Schiff stain with a hematoxylin counterstain (PASH), and (4) the mucicarmine stain.

STAINING PROCEDURES

1. A Stain for Fungi in Tissue Sections and Smears, Using Gomori's Methenamine - Silver Nitrate Technique, G.M.S. or Grocott-Gomori Stain — Cut paraffin sections at 6 μ from any well-fixed tissue.

SOLUTIONS

1. Five per cent aqueous chromic acid (chromium trioxide, CrO_3).
2. Stock methenamine-silver nitrate solution: Add 5 ml of 5% silver nitrate to 100 ml of 3% methenamine, U.S.P. grade $(CH_2)_6N_4$. A white precipitate forms but immediately dissolves on shaking. The clear solution remains usable for months at refrigerator temperature.
3. One per cent aqueous sodium bisulfite ($NaHSO_3$).
4. Five per cent aqueous borax, U.S.P. grade ($Na_2B_4O_7.10H_2O$).
5. One-tenth per cent aqueous gold chloride ($AuCl_3.HCl.3H_2O$). May be used repeatedly.
6. Two per cent aqueous sodium thiosulfate ($Na_2S_2O_35H_2O$).

TECHNIQUE

1. Deparaffinize sections and bring to distilled water as usual. Smears are prepared on albumin-treated slides and fixed in 95% alcohol.
2. Hydrated sections and smears are oxidized in 5% chromic acid for 1 hour, washed in running tap water for 10 min, and then treated in sodium bisulfite for 1 min to remove any residual chromic acid. They are then washed in tap water for 5 min and finally in 3 changes of distilled water.
3. Silver at 45—50° C in a working solution prepared by adding 25 ml of stock methenamine-silver nitrate to an equal portion of distilled water containing 1—2 ml of 5% borax. Fungi and mucin will begin to stain at the end of 25—30 min and will be adequately stained at the end of an hour. Slides are then rinsed in distilled water 2 or 3 times.
4. Tone in 0.1% gold chloride for 5 min. This will also bleach the background. Rinse in distilled water.
5. Remove unreduced silver by treating with 2% sodium thiosulfate for 1 or 2 min and, after washing thoroughly, counterstain if desired; using safranin if a red nuclear stain is desired, or a light hematoxylin-eosin combination if tissue detail is important.
6. Dehydrate, clear, and mount as usual.

RESULTS

Fungi are sharply delineated in black with the inner parts of mycelia and hyphae staining an old rose as a result of toning in gold. Mucin also assumes a rose-red color as a result of toning.

2. MacCallum-Goodpasture Stain for Gram-Positive and Gram-Negative Bacteria in Tissues. Any well-fixed tissue may be used. Cut thin paraffin sections.

SOLUTIONS

Goodpasture's Stain

Basic fuchsin	0.59 g
Aniline	1.00 c.c.
Phenol crystals (melted)	1.00 c.c.
Alcohol, 30%	100.00 c.c.

Gram's Iodine

Iodine	1.00 g
Potassium iodide	2.00 g
Distilled water	300.00 c.c.

Sterling's Gentian Violet Stain

Gentian violet (crystal violet)	5.00 g
Absolute alcohol	10.00 c.c.
Aniline	2.00 c.c.
Distilled water	88.00 c.c.

Picric Acid Solution

A saturated aqueous solution of picric acid.

TECHNIQUE

1. Deparaffinize to distilled water.
2. Place in Goodpasture's stain for 15 min.
3. Wash in distilled water.
4. Differentiate in full strength formalin for a few min until section becomes pink.
5. Wash in distilled water.
6. Counterstain in saturated aqueous picric acid for 3—5 min.
7. Wash in water.
8. Differentiate in 95% alcohol for 3—5 min.
9. Wash in water.
10. Stain in Sterling's gentian violet solution for 3 min.
11. Wash in water.
12. Place in Gram's iodine solution for 1 min.
13. Blot dry.
14. Place in a solution of equal parts of aniline and xylene, 2 changes.
15. Xylene, 2 changes.
16. Mount in Permount or Clarite.

RESULTS

Gram-positive organisms will be blue; gram-negative organisms, red; background, purplish.

3. *Periodic Acid-Schiff Reaction (P.A.S.H. Stain)*. — Cut paraffin sections at 6 μ from formalin or Zenker-fixed tissue.

SOLUTIONS

Periodic Acid Solution

Periodic acid crystals	0.5 g
Distilled water	100.0 c.c.

Schiff's Leucofuchsin Solution

Dissolve 1 g of basic fuchsin in 200 c.c. of distilled water. Bring to boil. Cool to 50° C. Filter and add 20 c.c. of normal hydrochloric acid. Cool further and add 1 g of anhydrous sodium bisulfite. Keep in the dark. The fluid may take two days to become straw-colored; then it is ready for use. Store in refrigerator.

Normal Hydrochloric Acid

Hydrochloric acid, concentrated, sp. gr. 1.19	83.5 c.c.
Distilled water	916.5 c.c.

Sulfurous Acid Rinse

10% sodium bisulfite ($NaHSO_3$)	6.0 c.c.
Normal hydrochloric acid	5.0 c.c.
Distilled water	100.0 c.c.

TECHNIQUE

1. Bring sections to distilled water in the usual way.
2. Periodic acid solution for 5 min.
3. Rinse in distilled water.
4. Place in Schiff's leucofuchsin solution for 15 min.
5. Rinse in 3 changes of sulfurous acid rinse for 2 min each.
6. Wash in running tap water for 10 min.
7. Counterstain with Harris hematoxylin for 1 min.
8. Differentiate in acid alcohol (2 or 3 quick dips).
9. Wash in running tap water until nuclei are clear blue.
10. Dehydrate in graduated alcohols, clear in xylene, and mount in Permount.

4. Mayer's Mucicarmine Stain. — Cut paraffin sections at 6 μ from any well-fixed tissue. Use control slide.

SOLUTIONS

Picric Acid Solution

Picric acid, saturated solution	100.0 c.c.
Glacial acetic acid	5.0 c.c.

Weigert's Iron Hematoxylin
Solution A
1% hematoxylin in 95% alcohol

Solution B

Ferric chloride, 29% aqueous	4.0 c.c.
Distilled water	95.0 c.c.
Hydrochloric acid	1.0 c.c.

Working Solution
Equal parts of solutions A and B. Prepare fresh

Metanil Yellow Solution

Metanil yellow	0.25 g
Distilled water	100.00 c.c.
Glacial acetic acid	0.25 c.c.

Mucicarmine Stain

Carmine (alum lake)	1.0 g
Anhydrous aluminium chloride	0.5 g
Distilled water	20.0 c.c.

Mix stain in a small flask and heat over small flame until solution becomes deep red (approximately 2 min). Add 80 c.c. of 50% alcohol. Filter each time before use. (Stain is usable immediately and is good for several days, giving best results at 24—48 hours.)

TECHNIQUE

1. Deparaffinize and bring sections to water as usual.
2. Treat sections for 30 min in saturated aqueous picric acid solution.
3. Wash in running water until clear.
4. Place slides on rack and pour on freshly prepared Weigert's hematoxylin for 4 min.
5. Wash in tap water.
6. Stain in metanil yellow solution for 1 min.
7. Rinse in distilled water.
8. Place in mucicarmine stain for 30 min to 1 hour or longer, check control slide microscopically for staining time.
9. Rinse quickly in 95% alcohol.
10. Dehydrate in absolute alcohol, clear in xylene, mount in Permount.

RESULTS
Mucin will be deep rose to red; nuclei, black; other tissue elements, yellow.

Examination for Fungi at Postmortem Examination and in Surgical Specimens

Make direct examination of the tissues of the lung or meninges or other organs, or of pus, other fluids, or exudates from ulcers (BAKER, 1967). Scrape the cut surface of the tissue with a scalpel and secure fluid and tissue. Place this on a slide, put a cover glass over the material, and examine the preparation with the microscope, cutting down the light to make the walls of the fungus organisms prominent. A definitive diagnosis can often be made by this direct method in the autopsy room or in the surgical pathology laboratory before the tissue is fixed. It is important to make it before fixation, so as to obtain cultures.

If cryptococcosis is suspected, place a drop of the sediment in a drop of India ink on a slide, cover with a coverslip, and examine under the microscope. If you suspect *Nocardia*, make a smear and stain by Grams' method.

Culture for fungi if fungi are found on direct examination or if there is suspicion of mycotic infection. Streak blood agar plates and incubate at 37° C. Streak Sabourauds' glucose agar slants and keep them at room temperature. Also inoculate media that contain antibiotics to suppress bacterial growth. To recover the organisms of mucormycosis take material on a swab and plant on glucose agar to which has been added sterilized white bread.

Infection by Actinomycetes

Infection of man by actinomycetes is relatively rare in comparison with infections by the true fungi. An actinomycete is defined as any organism belonging to the order Actinomycetales, composed of filamentous or rod-shaped bacteria tending strongly to the development of branches and true mycelium and lacking photosynthetic pigment. The Actinomycetaceae are a family of filamentous bacteria of the order Actinomycetales, often branching, sometimes forming a mycelium that readily breaks up into bacillary elements, and sometimes producing conidia.

There are three infections well known to pathologists and clinicians caused by actinomycetes, namely actinomycosis, nocardiosis and nocardial mycetoma. These are described in chapters XII, XXIV and XXV.

These infections are of world wide occurrence. Nocardiosis and nocardial mycetoma are exogenous infections, derived from organisms in the soil, but actinomycosis is an endogenous infection, the organisms inhabiting the gum margins and the tonsillar crypts and entering the tissues when a tooth is extracted. In the abdominal form of actinomycosis, organisms apparently escape from the appendix in connection with a rupture or ulceration as part of an ordinary appendicitis, and develop in the periappendiceal region.

All three are suppurative infections. The Gram stain is indispensable in demonstrating the branching organisms in the pus of nocardiosis and in the granules in nocardial mycetoma and actinomycosis. The G.M.S. stain is also helpful.

Infection by Algae

Protothecosis is the rare disease in this category. The organisms are frequently found in giant cells, and the G.M.S. stain is useful in demonstrating them clearly. See chapter XXVI for a full account.

References

BADER, G.: Die visceralen Mykosen. Pathologie, Klinik und Therapie. Jena: VEB Gustav Fischer 1965. — BAKER, R. D.: Tissue changes in fungous disease. Arch. Path. **44**, 459 (1947). ~ The diagnosis of fungus diseases by biopsy. J. chron. Dis. **5**, 552 (1957). ~ Essential Pathology (p. 204). Baltimore: Williams & Wilkins Co. 1961. ~ Drug-induced mycoses (p. 50). In: Excerpta Medica International Congress Series No. 85. Proc. 2nd Symposium on Drug-Induced Diseases, State University of Leyden, 1964. ~ Fungus Infections. Chapter 12. In: ANDERSON, W. A. D., Pathology, 5th ed. St. Louis: C.V. Mosby Co. 1966. ~ Postmortem Examination (p. 158, Examination for Fungi). Philadelphia and London: W. B. Saunders Co. 1967. ~ Organ distribution and pathogenesis in the deep mycoses (p. 9). In: Systemic Mycoses. A Ciba Foundation Symposium. London: J. and A. Churchill Ltd. 1968. — BRASS, K.: Zur histologischen Diagnostik der Pilzerkrankungen. Schweiz. med. Wschr. **1954**, 1273—1275. ~ Fortschritte in der histologischen Diagnostik der Pilzerkrankungen. Verh. dtsch. Ges. Path. **1955**, 260—269. — CABANNE, F., KLEPPING, C., MICHIELS, R., DUSSERRE, P.: Septicémie fungique terminale d'une leucose aigue traitée par antibiotiques et corticoides. Arch. Anat. path. **11**, 83—90 (1963). — CONANT, N. F., SMITH, D. T., BAKER, R. D., CALLAWAY, J. L., MARTIN, D. S.:

Manual of Clinical Mycology. 2nd ed. Philadelphia and London: W.B. Saunders Co. 1954. — COURTOIS, G., DE LOOF, C., THYS, A., VANBREUSEGHEM, R., BURETTE: Neuf cas de pier de madura congolais, par allescheria boydii, monosporium apiospermum et nocardia maduroe. Ann. Soc. belge Méd. trop. **34**, 371—405 (1954). — EMMONS, C.W., BINFORD, C.H., UTZ, J.P.: Medical Mycology. Philadelphia: Lea & Febiger 1963. — FORS, B., SÄÄF, J.: Localized pulmonary mycosis. A problem of diagnosis. Acta chir. scand. **119**, 212—229 (1960). — FRÉOUR, P.: Données recentes sur quelques grandes mycoses pulmonaires: Histoplasmose et coccidioidose. Rev. Praticien **1951**, 335—342. — HASHIMOTO, T., YOSHIDA, N., FUJIMOTO, M.: Osmium tetroxide fixation for the structural studies of fungi. J. Electronmicr. **15**, 99—101 (1966). — OWENS, A.W., SHACKLETTE, M.H., BAKER, R.D.: An antifungal factor in human serum. I. Studies of *Rhizopus rhizopodiformis*. Sabouraudia **4**, 179—186 (1965). — SKINNER, C.E., EMMONS, C.W., TSUCHIYA, H.M.: Henrici's Molds, Yeasts, and Actinomycetes. 2nd Ed. New York: John Wiley & Sons Inc. 1947. — *Sporotrichosis*. Infection on Mines of the Witwatersrand. A. Symposium, 1947. Johannesburg, Transval Chamber of Mines. — SYMMERS, W.: Deep-seated fungal infections currently seen in the histopathologic service of a medical school laboratory in Britain. Amer. J. clin. Path. **46**, 514—537 (1966). — SYMMERS, W.ST.C.: Aspects of the contribution of histopathology to the study of deep-seated fungal infections. In: Systemic Mycoses (p. 26), a Ciba Foundation Symposium. London: J. and A. Churchill Ltd. 1968. — TVETEN, L.: Cerebral mycosis. A clinico-pathological report of four cases. Acta neurol. scand. **41**, 19—33 (1965). — WUNDERLICH, CH.: Beitrag zum Problem der endogenen Mykosen. Dtsch. med. Wschr. **1953**, 1736—1738. — ZETTERGREN, L., SJÖSTRÖM, B.: Disseminated mycosis after treatment with antibiotics. Report of two cases reaching autopsy. Acta med. scand. **147**, 203—212 (1953).

Mycology of the Agents Producing
Deep Mycoses

Jan Schwarz, Cincinnati/Ohio, USA

With 21 Figures

Fungi are plant organisms; they lack chlorophyl but often contain specialized organs of reproduction (spores). For the medical mycologist, spores are of decisive importance in the identification of species. Certain medically important fungi are dimorphic, appearing in tissues as yeasts of different sizes and shapes, whereas cultures on artificial media and at room temperature render molds. Specifically and universally accepted as such dimorphic (biphasic) organisms are *Blastomyces dermatitidis* (Gilchrist and Stokes, 1898), *Blastomyces (Paracoccidioides) brasiliensis* (Splendore) (Almeida, 1930), *Histoplasma capsulatum* (Darling, 1906), *Histoplasma duboisii* (Vanbreuseghem, 1952) and *Sporotrichum schenckii* (Hektoen and Perkins) (Matruchot, 1910). Reports on dimorphism in *Cryptococcus neoformans* have been exceptional (Shadomy and Utz) and in *Candida albicans* controversial.

The term *dimorphism* is often restricted to the above five fungi causing systemic disease in man and lower animals. The parasitic (yeast) forms reproducing by budding are seen in the animal tissues and *in vitro* at 37° C and/or under certain nutritional conditions. The saprophytic (mycelial) phase presents hyphae in nature and *in vitro* at 20° C and develops asexual and sexual spores. The yeast form is labile and reverts easily into the mycelial form when, *in vitro*, temperature is lowered or other conditions change. The mycelial form is stable and if left alone has no tendency to change into the yeast form.

Romano, applying a broader concept to the definition of dimorphism, speaks of dimorphism as an environmentally controlled, reversible interconversion of yeast and mycelial forms, denoted as M $\rightleftharpoons$ Y.

The mechanism leading to formation of yeast forms *in vitro* varies in the five fungi discussed in this chapter.

Different Mechanisms of Conversion from M to Y Phase

In *Blastomyces dermatitidis* and *B. brasiliensis*, the yeast phase develops by simple change of temperature from 20—37° C (actually conversion already takes place at about 34° C), but can be more easily induced — in some strains — at higher temperatures, e.g. 40—42° C. No special media are necessary for the conversion in either fungus (Nickerson and Edwards, Salvin), to which Nickerson and Edwards apply the term "thermal dimorphism." The conversion of *Sporotrichum schenckii* to the yeast form is accomplished either (at 37° C) by gas mixtures with 5% CO_2 or by increase of the tension CO_2 in media from decarboxylation of certain amino acids (Drouhet and Mariat).

Induction of the yeast phase of *Histoplasma capsulatum* is far more complex. The conditions for de facto conversion are: heavy inoculum; availability of SH groups in amino acids in media; temperature of 37° C, though selected experiments have obtained conversion at 30° C (PINE). Chelation of metal ions by serum albumin conceivably could be involved in the conversion taking place in the animal body, since, experimentally, such agents as citric acid, magnesium, and calcium can be shown contributing to or inhibiting the conversion. The discussion of the involved issues is beyond the scope of this chapter (PINE and PEACOCK).

Speculation on why this important group of fungi invades tissues under the disguise of "yeast cells" points to the greater energy potential of yeasts, which absorb 5—6 times more oxygen than mycelial elements. BAKER et al. have mentioned that yeast forms represent the greatest possible number of new cells with the least synthesis of protoplasm, conceivably assuring in this manner survival in the abnormal (hostile) animal tissue.

Table 1. *Dimorphic, pathogenic, yeast-like fungi*

Stable, mycelial (saprophytic) form. 20° C	Labile, yeast, unicellular (parasitic) form. 37° C
1. *Blastomyces dermatitidis*	
Septate (racquet) hyphae. Oval or spherical conidia on short stalks or terminal (2—4—10 μ)	Round, multinucleated yeast with single, broad based, well-adherent buds (2—8—30 μ)
2. *Blastomyces (Paracoccidioides) brasiliensis*	
Septate hyphae with some chlamydospores; sessile conidia similar to *B. dermatitidis* (fewer)	Large round multinucleated yeast cells (1—30—60 μ), sometimes with numerous buds covering the entire surface
3. *Histoplasma capsulatum*	
Septate (racquet) hyphae, numerous small conidia (2—4 μ). Smooth and crenated or tuberculate spores (8—15 μ)	Ovoid yeast cells (2—5 μ), seldom larger; single bud with narrow neck; single nucleus
4. *Histoplasma duboisii*	
Identical — cannot be differentiated in mycelial form from *H. capsulatum*	Large, spherical yeast cells (10—20 μ) with single buds ("duboisii forms"); in young culture also small ovoid yeasts ("capsulatum forms"); single nucleus
5. *Sporotrichum schenckii*	
Delicate, thin, septate hyphae with conidiosphores bearing terminal pyriform conidia arranged like daisies	Small ovoid yeast forms with single or multiple buds (2—4 μ); rod-like "cigar bodies" with pointed ends; larger round yeast cells (5—8 μ)

Mechanism of induction of yeast phase *in vitro*:
1 and 2 = thermal; 3 and 4 = thermal, plus nutritional (SH groups in amino acids); 5 = thermal plus CO_2 tension.

Blastomyces Dermatitidis (GILCHRIST and STOKES, 1898)

Blastomyces dermatitidis presents in tissues as ovoid to round yeast cell, generally with a thick wall and, if budding, with single buds which communicate broadly with the mother cell (Fig. 1). This wide porus in *B. dermatitidis* is characteristic enough to permit morphologic identification in most cases. The organism varies considerably in size, especially if one includes the "microforms," which are only about 2 μ in size, ranging all the way to such "giants" as yeast cells of 25 μ to 30 μ; however, an average *B. dermatitidis* would probably fall within a range

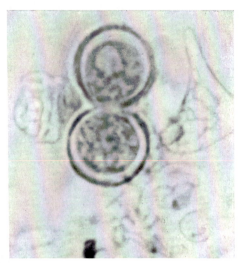

Fig. 1. *B. dermatitidis* in sputum suspended in 10% KOH. Budding yeast with broad pore between mother and daughter cell. The latter is almost as large as the mother cell. × 1500

from 8—24 μ. Within lung tissue or in abscesses in other tissues, the variation in size may be quite bewildering and may tax the observer's judgement as to whether he is dealing with a single or more than one species of yeast organisms. If *B. dermatitidis* is present in large amount in a lesion, culture on blood agar at 37° C may result in a warty, sometimes slightly brownish colony within 2—3 days, which on subculture may grow even more rapidly. However, the commonly associated bacterial contaminants make recovery of *B. dermatitidis* from "open" lesions rather difficult; hence animal inoculation may have to be used in order to supress the bacterial contaminants. Attempts to come to such results can be also made by incorporating chloramphenicol into the media, but it will take care only of a moderate contaminating flora and will not necessarily inhibit saprophytic fungi that were present in the material.

Culture mounts from such yeast form cultures reveal round yeast cells of 8—15 μ. Many budding cells are found in young cultures, all characteristically with a broad pore between the mother and daughter cells (Fig. 2). The attachment of the daughter cells is of long duration and the two generations can become of equal size and remain conjoined. Multiple buds, mentioned especially by Emmons, are distinctly exceptional rather than the rule. Lipoid bubbles are easily recognized within the cytoplasm of the cell. After proper fixation or with the electron microscope, *B. dermatitidis* is seen to have multiple nuclei, a very useful point for differentiation from yeasts of similar size and shape (Fig. 3). Specifically, *Histoplasma duboisii* and *Cryptococcus neoformans* have only one nucleus. Induction of the yeast phase is especially easy on Weeks' cotton-seed agar.

At room temperature *B. dermatitidis* develops as white mold, sometimes only after several weeks duration. Some strains turn brownish in back, others develop very little pigment. The aerial mycelium forming the colony is seldom very long; sometimes the surface is almost waxy, with spiny projections extending from the level of the vegetative portion of hyphal growth. Culture mounts reveal segmented hyphae, often with racquet-like swellings at the point of segmentation. Conidia, born laterally or terminally, measure 2—4 μ, but in some strains reach up to 10 μ. The superficial resemblance of the conidia with yeast cells can lead to confusion,

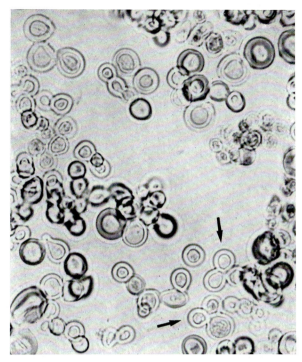

Fig. 2. Culture mount of *B. dermatitidis* grown on blood-agar at 37° C after 4 days. Large, thick-walled spherical yeast cells. Budding cells (arrow) form the figure "8." When buds do not separate, short chains are seen. Considerable difference in cellular size. Cotton-blue mount × 1300

especially in cultures which are in transitional stage between yeast and mold forms. Bizarre forms are seen in such cultures when chains of coherent buds are formed or large, extended yeast forms, having little resemblance to the classical size and shape of *B. dermatitidis*, are seen. Crenated or tuberculate spores, so characteristic for Histoplasma, are never seen in *B. dermatitidis*.

A possible explanation for the puzzling difficulty of recovery of *B. dermatitidis* from soil is given by McDONOUGH et al., who demonstrated lysis of *B. dermatitidis* in unsterilized soil, whereas sterilized soil was inactive. The mechanism of the lytic process is not understood. McDONOUGH and LEWIS were successful in growing *B. dermatitidis* in the ascigerous form, which they named *Ajellomyces dermatitidis*. The mature cleistothecium of *Ajellomyces dermatitidis* is 200—350 μ in diameter and exhibits tightly coiled spirals when young. The ascogenous hyphae are especially frequent near the central origin of the coils. The asci contain 8 smooth, spherical uninucleate spores from 1.5—2 μ in diameter. Ascospores from such cultures, removed by micromanipulator give, on the one hand, origin to characteristic mold colonies of *B. dermatitidis* and, on the other hand, produce typical tissue forms after animal inoculation.

Ajellomyces dermatitidis is assumed to be heterothallic, since cleistothecia form only after pairing of cultures. McDONOUGH and LEWIS induced the formation of fertile cleistothecia on yeast extract agar with steamed bone meal (Armour) added in the midline of a petri dish. When strains are inoculated 2 cm distant on each side from the midline, fruiting bodies become visible grossly after $2^{1}/_{2}$—5 weeks.

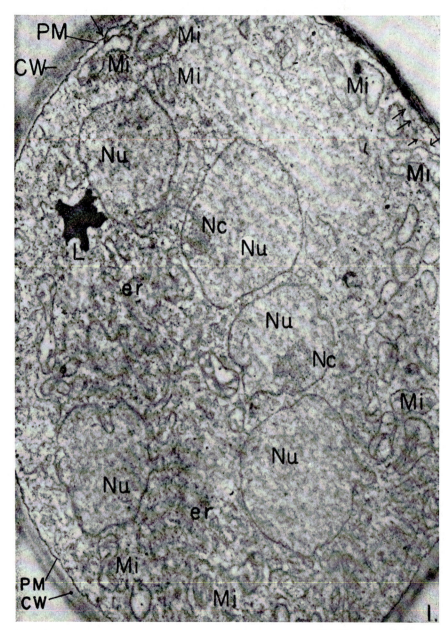

Fig. 3. Yeast cell of *B. dermatitidis*. This complex, unicellular organism has a fairly thick cell wall (CW) averaging 190 mμ. The plasma membrane (PM) appears wavy and averages 9 mμ in thickness. The organism is multinucleated (NU), an essential difference from the yeast cell of *H. capsulatum* and *H. duboisii*, both of which have only one nucleus. The nuclei have a slightly irregular outline and measure 1.1 × 1.7 μ. Numerous mitochondria (Mi), vesicles and tubules of the endoplasmic reticulum (er) and lipid (L) deposits are seen. Nucleoli (Nc) are present in 2 of the 5 nuclei. × 32,000.
From Edwards, G.A., Edwards, M.R.: Amer. J. Botany, *47*, 622 (1960)

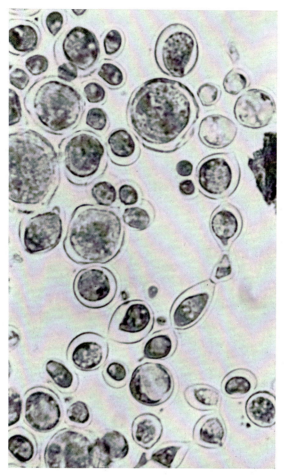

Fig. 4. Culture mount from yeast phase of *B. brasiliensis* grown for 48 hours on blood agar at 37° C. Yeast cells with thick walls and marked variation in diameter. Single large buds are seen, multiple small ones and chains of budding cells, that have not separated. The differential diagnosis with *B. dermatitidis* is fairly easy in view of the large size of some cells and the multiple buds. Lactophenol-cotton blue × 1300

Blastomyces (Paracoccidioides) Brasiliensis (Splendore, 1912)

Almeida, 1930 is in tissue and exudates a round yeast cell varying in size from 1—40 or even 60 μ (Fig. 4), often seen with multiple buds. Generally present in large numbers in the lesions it produces, it has a thick wall quite similar to *B. dermatitidis*. The buds are either few in number and large in size or can surround the mother cell in form of innumerable small "diverticula." After clearing pus for 20 minutes in 10% potassium hydroxide, very satisfactory preparations for the study of the cell structure are obtained. It should not be forgotten that obviously single buds can occur which should not lead to confusion with *B. dermatitidis*, considering the greater (average) size of *B. brasiliensis*, the geographic history, the presence of organisms with the typical multitude of small spores, some of which are hardly 1—2 μ in size (Fig. 5). On the other hand, mother cells producing but one

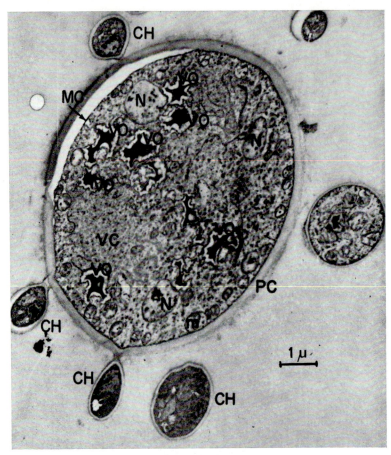

Fig. 5. Budding yeast cell of *B. brasiliensis*. The multiple buds (CH) are obvious, as are the multiple nuclei (N). The cytoplasmic membrane (MC), the cell wall (PC), the osmiophilic vacuoles (VO), central vacuole (VC), and mitochondria (M) are well defined. Note the osmiophilia of most daughter cells (buds). × 10,000.
Courtesy of Dr. Luis M. Carbonell, Caracas, Venezuela

or just a few buds can have daughter cells of 10—15 *μ* in diameter. The buds seem to separate quite easily from the mother cell in some instances, which explains the presence of very small abortive forms of the organism; on the other hand, it is not unusual to find short chains of spores if the primary bud starts reproducing before it becomes separated from the maternal cell.

Culture on Sabouraud's glucose agar at room temperature gives a slow growing organism; the primary isolation from infectious material may take several weeks to develop and is not necessarily positive in every case where organisms are demonstrable in the clinical material. This difficulty of growing the organism is significant, especially in cases of the keloidal form (Lobo's disease). The mycelial growth may first be glabrous or waxy, covering itself slowly with a white cottony aerial mycelium; older cultures may turn tan to brown. Some colonies have a powdery appearance; the length of the aerial hyphae changes from strain to strain and even on subculture of the same strain. Mounts from the cultures are indistinguishable from the mycelial growth of *B. dermatitidis*. Septate hyphae, sometimes with racquet swellings on the point of septation, bear a few sessile conidia of oval to round shape, 2—4 μ in size, seldom larger.

Transfer into the yeast phase is easily accomplished at 37° C on any media supporting the growth of the organism. Blood agar and Kurung's egg medium are very satisfactory for this purpose. The resulting colonies are small, smooth at first, developing into whitish to tan waxy, soft, sometimes cerebriform colonies. The culture mount permits immediate differentiation from *B. dermatitidis*, since it shows the large yeast cells with multiple buds described under "microscopy of the infectious clinical material." Mice, hamsters, and guinea pigs are susceptible to infective material, but the spread of the lesions is generally restricted and the development of pathologic changes is slow. *Proechimys guayanesis* is considered more susceptible than the standard laboratory animals (BORELLI).

A culture mount of the yeast phase shows enormous variability in size of the yeast cells, from 1—60 μ. Some of the larger yeast cells which are budding have a dozen or more very tiny buds connected with the mother cell by thin but elongated bridges. Other yeast cells may have one, two, or more fairly large buds or chains of buds consisting of three or even more cells clinging together. Germination of isolated cells can be seen here and there. Whereas the majority of mature cells are round, the larger buds frequently are elongated or almost fusiform.

Histoplasma Capsulatum (DARLING, 1906)

At room temperature, *Histoplasma capsulatum* develops from clinical material as white mold, generally after 10—14 days, seldom after longer intervals. Some strains stay white and cottony, others acquire slightly brownish pigment, visible especially in the back. Exceptionally, one sees granular and glabrous colonies. If the source material is animal tissue (planted on the media), the colony frequently is outspokenly glabrous or even waxy and covers itself after several weeks with a fine cotton, generally starting as patches in the periphery of the colony.

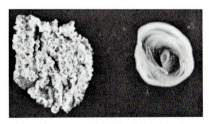

Fig. 6. Growth pattern of *Histoplasma capsulatum* on blood agar: on the right growth of a pure yeast phase; the appearance is smooth, moist, yeast- to bacteria-like. The left illustrates growth of an intermediate phase with numerous yeast cells but with many hyphal forms remaining. The growth is wrinkled, dry, and does not emulsify as readily as the yeast form. Growth after 72 hours on blood-agar

The yeast form of *H. capsulatum* can be easily induced in most strains on Kurung's medium, where after 10 days the strains change to a creamy, soft colony which, on subculture on blood agar, develops white to creamy colonies. Fast reproduction on solid media results if frequent subcultures are made. Optimal smoothness of the colony is obtained if subcultures are made on blood agar every 48 hours (Fig. 6). Heart-brain infusion agar is quite satisfactory as solid media for recovery of large amounts for antigen production. Thick agar plates give better growth than thin layers of agar. Occasionally, strains can be found which remain coarse and

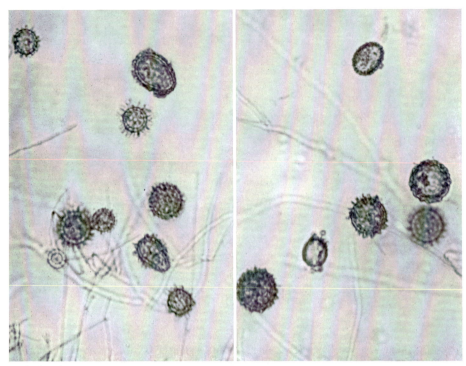

Fig. 7. "Tuberculate spores" of *Histoplasma capsulatum* and *H. duboisii* grown at 20° C on Sabouraud's glucose agar. Some projections are needle-like and comparatively long, others give the surface of the spore a crenated appearance. Round and pyriform spores are visible. Some strains have more pyriform than round spores, but may lose the pyriform cells on subculture. Other strains permanently produce a majority of pyriform spores. Cotton-blue mount × 1300

warty for prolonged periods or cannot be changed at all into a smooth yeast phase, but in the great majority of cases, repeated subculture, strict adherence to the temperature ceiling, and abundance of medium provide for satisfactory development of the yeast form of *H. capsulatum*. If mounts are made from such growth, a uniform ovoid yeast cell of 2 to 4 μ is found, with large numbers of budding cells. The bud is connected by a narrow neck with the mother cell, from which it separates easily.

Mounts from mycelial colonies reveal segmented hyphae, frequently with racquet-like swellings at the point of segmentation, with variable amounts but often numerous microconidia, 2 to 4 μ in size and usually spherical in shape. The majority of these microconidia are smooth but occasionally the surface is somewhat irregular to spiny. It has been shown that the small spores are representing the great majority of the total spore count and are decisive for spontaneous infection, but the larger tuberculate spores are more important for diagnosis (Fig. 7). After approximately 2 weeks, large (8 to 15 to 20 μ) spores are found in the culture mount, many of which are round, smooth, and seem to have no tendency to form crenations of the surface. Other colonies develop numerous crenated or tuberculate spores from the start. The exact structure of the warty projections representing strictly formations of the wall without cytoplasmic implications has been elucidated by electron microscopy and has made obsolete previous speculative interpretations (Figs. 8, 9). Certain strains have pyriform tuberculate spores more

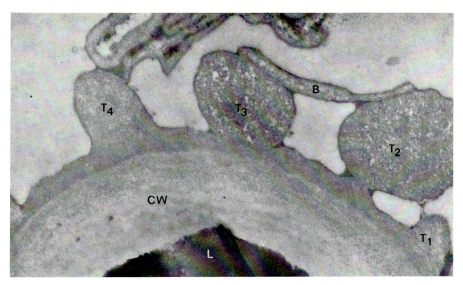

Fig. 8. Tuberculate spore of *H. capsulatum:* A newly-formed tubercle (T1) containing fine radial filaments and an older tubercle (T2) in which the fine filaments are clumped by apposition to each other. The basal constriction in T2 is evident. The tubercle (T3) has a less advanced basal constriction. The 2 latter tubercles (T2 and 3) are connected by an appendage (B). The structure is similar to T3. T4 is a maturing tubercle. — The heavy cell wall (CW) and the large lipid bubble (L) of the mature spore are obvious. × 44,000.
From EDWARDS, M. R., HAZEN, E. L., EDWARDS, G. A.: Canad. J. Microbiol. *6*, 65 (1960)

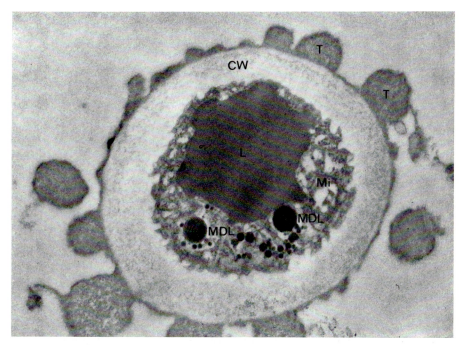

Fig. 9. Maturing tuberculate spore of *H. capsulatum*. Details of cell wall (CW) and its relation to the tubercles (T). Mitochondria (Mi), lipid clumps (L), and membrane-contained microdroplets (MDL) of lipid material can be seen. × 50,000.
From EDWARDS, M. R., HAZEN, E. L., EDWARDS, G. A.: Canad. J. Microbiol. *6*, 65 (1960)

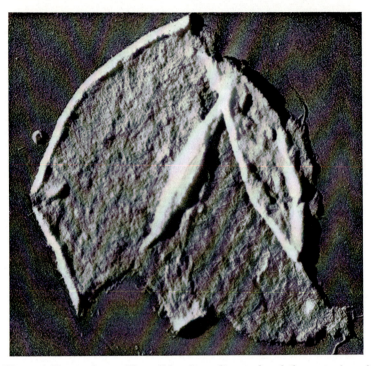

Fig. 10. Yeast of *H. capsulatum*. The cell has been disrupted and the protoplasm has been removed. The outer layer of the collapsed cell wall is granular; the internal layer shows an interlacing fibrillar architecture. No capsular material can be identified. × 90,000.
From Ribi, E., Salvin, S. B.: Exp. Cell Res. *10*, 394 (1956)

or less permanently, and in variable number; other strains develop pyriform spores initially, only to change to round forms with aging of the colony or on subculture. The tuberculate spore, while not unique for *H. capsulatum*, is diagnostic for *H. capsulatum* and *H. duboisii* in the context of the history and the geographic location, due to the fact that in tissues, yeastlike cells are or could be found and also that the mold can be induced *in vitro*, or changed back *in vivo* into the unicellular form (yeast phase) (Fig. 10). However, the experienced worker, from the slow development of the cottony colony, from the presence of numerous microconidia, and from the slow development of large smooth and later on crenated or tuberculate spores, will conclude that he is dealing with *Histoplasma*. If initially, as sometimes happens, only large, smooth spores are found, extensive search and numerous mounts may be necessary before a single or a very few tuberculate spores are found. In intermediate cultures (yeast form cultures changing into mycelial forms), elongated yeast cells may be seen which do not fit any of the classical descriptions.

The difference between *H. capsulatum* and *H. duboisii* cannot be established from the growth at room temperature.

Apparently, the inoculum need not contain many spores in order to give rise to the development of a colony, but sometimes growth cannot be obtained in spite of the presence of organisms in the source; an explanation for such negative results is extremely difficult and entirely hypothetical.

The apparent ascigerous form of *H. capsulatum* was named *Gymnoascus demonbreunii* by Ajello and Cheng (1967). Inocula of what were believed to be pure cultures of *H. capsulatum* on soil plates with chicken feathers or horsehair produced globose cleistothecia of 230—400 μ. Thin-walled hyaline asci of 6.6—8.8 μ, containing 8 elliptical golden-tinted ascospores of $2.7 \times 3.8 \mu$, developed within 4—6 weeks. The homothallic nature of the apparent perfect form of *H. capsulatum* was assumed by the development of fertile cleistothecia from single ascospores. KWON-CHUNG from Hasenclever's laboratory and BERLINER have demonstrated, that the ascigerous cultures obtained by AJELLO and CHENG were coming from a mixed culture and represent the ascigerous form of *Gymnoascus demonbreunii* and not *of Histoplasma capsulatum*.

Histoplasma Duboisii (VANBREUSEGHEM, 1952)

Histoplasma duboisii is a dinstinct species and can be differentiated from *H. capsulatum* by its geographic limitation (to Africa), by its large size in tissues and in the yeast phase *in vitro* (Fig. 11a, b), by its considerably lesser invasiveness in laboratory animals, and, to some degree, by biochemical (COREMANS) and immunofluorescent tests (PINE et al., 1964).

The mold growth is in every respect comparable to *H. capsulatum* except for the particularly slow growth of many strains of *H. duboisii*, but this is a relatively minor difference and certainly cannot be used for classification purposes. Mounts from the mold phase are indistinguishable from *H. capsulatum*, hence the description is not repeated here.

Originally, VANBREUSEGHEM observed low response to *H. duboisii* in experiments with guinea pigs, hamsters, rabbits and rats, but animal inoculation is of considerable help in differentiation of the species, since *H. duboisii* forms unusually large giant cells in most animals, especially the hamster, and presents with small, middle-sized, and large yeast cells, with increase in the number of large yeast cells with time, and with occasional production of Schaumann bodies even in mice.

In contrast, the classical *H. capsulatum* is mostly invasive and lethal for hamsters, mice, and, to lesser degree, for the other animals. It produces almost exclusively small yeast cells which are found especially in histiocytes; giant cells, if at all present, are not prominent. In mice, Schaumann bodies are never produced; in hamsters, they are formed in both species.

The demonstration by TASCHDJIAN of anastomosis between hyphae of *H. capsulatum* and *H. duboisii* underlines the close (and obvious) relationship but does not prove genetic identity.

The yeast cells of *H. duboisii* show *in vitro* considerable variation, both from strain to strain and from day to day, with considerable influence upon cell size by frequency of subculturing, choice of media, etc. PINE et al. (1964) believed this variation to be more prominent in strains of *H. duboisii* than in *H. capsulatum*. The cells of *H. duboisii* are oval and thick-walled. Thin-walled large, round cells, often without protoplasm, occur in old cultures both in the classical *H. capsulatum* and in *H. duboisii* and can be artificially induced on tissue explants (SCHWARZ) from either. PINE et al. interpreted such cells as spheroplasts and found them occasionally in high numbers. Particularly confusing are the transitional forms seen when yeasts revert to mycelial growth or, on the contrary, at a time when the yeast phase is being induced but the hyphae have not yet completely converted into yeast. The buds of the typical duboisii cell have a broad base and originate on one pole of the mother cell.

PINE et al. (1964) concluded that the "capsulatum forms" seen in early *in vitro* or *in vivo* studies are transitional forms, and that later "duboisii forms" become

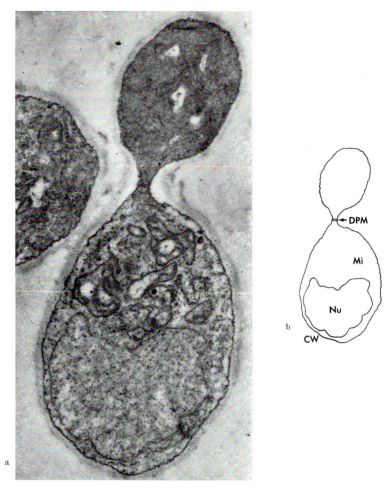

Fig. 11. *H. duboisii.* The bud has a high electron density and its mitochondria are large with parallel cristae. Note the double plasma membrane (DPM) formed in the splitting zone (arrow) of the neck of the bud. Nucleus (Nu), mitochondria (Mi), and cell wall (CW) are recognizable. × 35,000.

From Edwards, M.R., Hazen, E.L., Edwards, G.A.: J. Gen. Microbiol. *20,* 495 (1959)

the exclusive cells, even if some are formed that reach only the size ordinarily associated with "capsulatum forms."

A recent review by Ajello (1968) would relegate *H. duboisii* to a variety of *H. capsulatum,* rather than accepting it as distinct species. This is at present certainly a minority opinion.

Sporotrichum Schenckii (Hektoen and Perkins), Matruchot (1910)

On primary isolation of *Sporotrichum schenckii* from clinical material, creamy, waxy colonies with slightly fuzzy spreading borders can be seen as early as 48—72 hours after inoculation of Sabouraud's glucose agar, especially if the original material contains large numbers of spores. The colony enlarges, adjacent colonies merge, keeping a glabrous character and turning darker within a week, to become often completely black, occasionally with segmental distribution of the pigment (Fig. 12). Strains without pigment have been observed, and sometimes the intensity of pigmentation decreases on multiple subcultures. No valid reason appears to exist for recognizing species other than *S. schenckii* as the cause of human or animal sporotrichosis. Complete change to yeast forms often takes several subcultures but is more easily and more dependably obtained than in any of the other dimorphic organisms.

Mounts from the mycelial (parasitic) form show a delicate septate hypha with prompt development of conidiophores and characteristic formation of terminal daisy-like rosettes, consisting of groups of 6—10 or more conidia. The conidia separate easily from the conidiophores; hence slide cultures may be necessary to show the daisies in full beauty. Conidia are sometimes found arising laterally from the hyphae but the diagnostic feature is certainly the conidiophore with the terminal grouping of conidia.

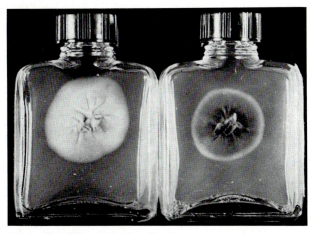

Fig. 12. *Sporotrichum schenckii* on Sabouraud's glucose agar at room temperature with and without blackish pigment. Both cultures were obtained at the same time from mouse injected with one single strain

The hyphae are delicate, generally 1—2 μ in diameter, and septation is visible (Fig. 13). Conidiophores generally take their origin from short hyphal segments. The length of conidiophores varies. Some are very short when they develop conidia; others are quite long (60—80 μ), and may in turn give origin to lateral conidiophores. It is sometimes dificult to establish whether these are in reality lateral branches of hyphae with spore formation at the end of the hyphae, in which case the lateral conidiophores arise from a hyphal branch rather than from a "primary" conidiophore. Isolated conidia are also found either on very short stalks or connected laterally to the hyphae by a very thin sterigma. In slide cultures (Fig. 13), it is quite common to see the development of parallel hyphae separated only by a few microns of free space, giving the impression that mechanical support is obtained by this relationship. Occasionally, one sees very young but long conidiophores with just 1 or 2 conidia on the tip but, as a rule, the bouquet of spores surrounding the tip of conidiophores is well developed. Most conidia are pyriform, with the tips pointing toward the sterigma. Variations from pyriform to ovoid to globose are seen in one and the same culture at any given time. If stained with aniline dye, a band-like structure crossing the spore transversely can be easily demonstrated and is found most commonly in the center of the spore, but occasionally in the rounded end of the spore. This is especially true if the spores are more oval or globose; this dark-staining spot is then always in the periphery of the spore. When conidia fall to the surface of rich media, budding has been observed even at room temperature (Emmons). Conidiophores are seldom segmented except for one transverse septum which is generally found close to its hyphal origin.

Triangular conidia have been described in the South African epidemic by Brown et al.; the authors mention the spores as biconvex, since they appear pear-shaped when seen from the side. This is easily seen in fresh culture mounts, where the spores still move and turn about. The length of the triangular spores is sometimes more than 5 μ. The oridinary conidia, usually seen as variations of oblong structures, measure about 2—4 μ.

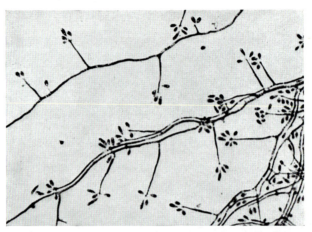

Fig. 13. Delicate hyphae of *Sporotrichum schenckii*. Conidiophores with daisy-like bouquets of pyriform conidia. Some conidia arise on short stalks laterally from the hyphae. Slide culture at room temperature after 5 days. Methylene blue stain × 1300

After intraperitoneal injection of the mycelial or yeast phase in mice (Emmons), rats (Simson et al.), and hamsters (Schwarz), testicular lesions regularly develop. Twelve to 15 days after injection of spore suspensions into rats, Norden observed swelling of cigar bodies, which became round (ring forms). In liver and spleen, these round formations acquired a double outline (cryptococcal forms). Radially arranged acidophilic projections appeared around the organism (asteroid bodies). Norden considers the cigar bodies direct descendants of microconidia.

In mice, ulcerative lesions on the tail, feet, and scrotum developed after intraperitoneal injection after 3—5 months. Asteroid bodies in humans were first described by Talice in 1935. The number and the presence of asteroid bodies vary from strain to strain. In the South African epidemic, asteroid bodies were consistently present in human lesions (Simson et al., Lurie). Howard observed in slide cultures secondary conidia (1 or 2), apparently formed on top of the first row of conidia, arising on extremely delicate sterigmata.

Cigar bodies predominate in mice after intraperitoneal injection in the first 2—3 weeks; ring forms appear after 4—5 weeks (Fig. 14). When many organisms are found in peritoneal granulation tissues, cigar bodies prevail; when few organisms are detected, ring forms are relatively more common. Three distinct ring forms are seen: 1) round bodies staining homogenously with PAS; 2) round cells with homo·

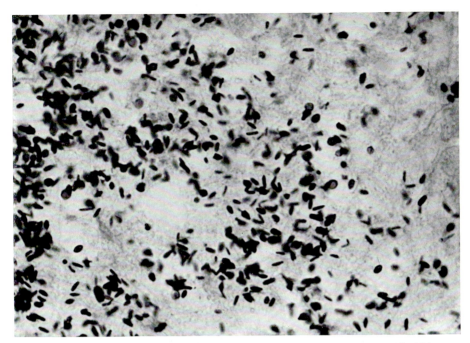

Fig. 14. The cigar bodies and ring forms of *S. schenckii*, rarely seen in man outside Africa, are plentiful in experimental animals after a great variety of routes of inoculation. Scrotal fat tissue after intraperitoneal inoculation. Grocott × 900

geneous central mass ("cryptococcal forms") and 3) thin-walled round cells without demonstrable staining cytoplasm (OKUDAIRA et al.). The same authors found organisms commonly intracellular — in the liver in the Kupffer cells and in periportal histiocytes — in the spleen in the follicular reticulum (but no in the sinusoidal endothelial cells); hyphal elements in tissues were not completely exceptional in our experiments. If and when organisms are demonstrable in human disease, cigar bodies predominate in widely disseminated cases, whereas the presence of asteroid bodies is interpreted as an immunoreaction in slowly progressing or self-limited infections (LURIE).

Cryptococcus Neoformans (SANFELICE), VUILLEMIN (1901)

Cryptococcus neoformans is a round to slightly ovoid yeast organism which varies from 4 to 20 μ in size and which is surrounded by a mucopolysaccharide capsule, the width of which shows variations similar to the diameter of the cell proper (Fig. 15). The smallest diameters of the yeast cell are, in part, due to the frequently abortive separation of small buds from the mother cell; the width of the capsule differs with various strains and nutritional availability. Ordinarily, *Cryptococcus neoformans* can be identified easily in India ink preparations where the colloidal silver particles are prevented from penetrating the capsular material, giving a large, white contrast. In the center of the white hole, the yeast cell proper is recognized; it is important to find budding yeast cells, to eliminate any doubt about the nature of the organism. In spinal fluid, white cells, less frequently red cells, may be surrounded by an irregular and hazy halo,

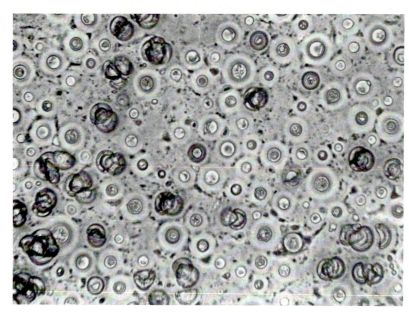

Fig. 15. *Cryptococcus neoformans* can be neatly visualized in polarized light. This method is
used with advantage for different fungi but has never found widespread use. × 200.
Photograph courtesy Dr. A. Fingerland, Hradec Králové, Czechoslovakia

which frequently leads to confusion of such cells with *C. neoformans*. Therefore, the
microscopist should try to identify lipid bubbles characteristic of the yeast cell, or
budding, which is even more conclusive, whereas obviously in polymorphonuclear
leukocytes or lymphocytes the nuclei can be recognized by proper use of the diaphragm and lowering of the condensor, even before staining with Giemsa's or
similar methods.

On culture, the organism grows with considerable variability in reference to the
velocity of development. Sometimes colonies can be recognized overnight. In other
cases, it takes several days before colonies are seen. The colonies at first are very
similar to bacterial or *Candida* colonies. They are white to creamy but they remain
round for a much longer time than *Candida* colonies. According to the amount of
capsular material, the colony looks waxy and almost dry on the one hand, whereas
on the other end — the extreme capsular development, a honey-like, "runny"
colony develops, with the accumulation of a large amount of mucoid-appearing
material in the bottom of the flask or tube. Mounts from culture growths sometimes show disappointingly few capsulated organisms, but it has been our experience that even one or two well encapsulated organisms are admissible as positive
evidence of the cryptococcal character of the organism under scrutiny. The culture
can be speedily identified as belonging to the genus *Cryptococcus* by the positive
urease test (Seeliger); the inhibition by actidione also favors definition of the
cryptococcal nature of the organism. Growth at 37° C will be, for all practical purposes, conclusive for *C. neoformans*. Assimilation tests (auxanograms) proving that
potassium nitrate and lactose are not assimilated are conclusive for identification.

After intracerebral injection into young white mice, the organisms produces
meningoencephalitis, which may be lethal in a few days to several weeks. Intraperitoneal or intravenous injection into mice also can produce general dissemination.

It has been our experience that inhibition by actidione, growth at 37° C, positive urease test, and lack of assimilation of lactose and potassium nitrate are sufficient for all practical purposes and, for clinical diagnosis, more conclusive than animal inoculation in view of the long duration of asymptomatic infection and in view of the fact that sometimes of as many as 8 animals, only 1 or 2 will develop conclusive and lethal meningoencephalitis or septicemia (KAO and SCHWARZ).

EMMONS has mentioned the occasional presence of pseudohyphae in tissues and SHADOMY and UTZ have recently published the description of a strain which seems regularly to produce such pseudohyphae *in vitro*. However, compared with *Candida*, where the development of hyphal structures is customary, the development of hyphae in *Cryptococcus* can be described as totally exceptional. The identification with fluorescent antibody stain is quite satisfactory in *C. neoformans*.

Most of the usual laboratory animals are susceptible to cryptococcosis, particularly mice, hamsters, and rats, whereas dogs, rabbits, and monkeys are less susceptible. Recently, infection of pigeons has been accomplished by intracerebral (LITTMAN) and intraocular routes (SETHI and SCHWARZ). Similar to the behavior in man, either violent reaction, tubercle formation, or simple "colony formation" is found in pigeons, where innumerable organisms are seen compressing and displacing normal tissue without inflammatory response on the part of the invaded organism. In tissues, the specific affinity of *C. neoformans* to the mucicarmine stain gives a welcome "specific" staining reaction which is extremely helpful if only a few organisms are present. However, it should be pointed out that even in typical culturally proven cryptococcosis, only a few cells may sometimes stain with the mucicarmine procedure; yet, on other occasions, the intensity of stain in all cells will be surprising. In tissues, *C. neoformans* can be demonstrated with other fungus stains and may be confused with *Blastomyces dermatitidis*, *Histoplasma duboisii* and *Candida albicans*, from all of which it can be easily differentiated by a positive mucicarmine stain.

Budding in cryptococcus is always through a narrow pore and generally one, seldom more, buds can be seen per mother cell. Great disparity in size can exist between maternal and daughter cells.

Candida Albicans (ROBIN), BERKHOUT (1923)

Candida albicans is a yeast-like, egg-shaped organism which ordinarily measures from 2 to 4 μ but can reach extreme sizes of 8×14 μ. The organism is easily identified in exudates or tissues, in the former by suspension in 10% potassium hydroxide, in the latter on hemotoxylin-eosin stain or with any of the numerous available fungus stains; probably the most impressive for *Candida* is the Gridley procedure. In material from membranes, urine, or pus, the Gram stain is very useful, since the egg-shaped yeast cell and the heavy pseudomycelia are clearly visible.

Whether in *Candida* pseudohyphae are exclusively formed or whether true hyphae with septation occur is controversial, despite a large volume of information in the literature. Pseudohyphae, which are considered to be stretched out yeast cells, develop constrictions which give origin to budding yeast cells and secondary pseudohyphal formation (Fig. 16).

Both fermentation and assimilation tests are useful in recognizing *Candida albicans*, revealing both lack of fermentation of and inability to assimilate lactose and sucrose. However, the assimilation test is preferable, since interference of contaminants is more easily recognized and prevented. To differentiate *Candida* from the genus *Cryptococcus*, the (negative) urease test for *Candida* is most helpful.

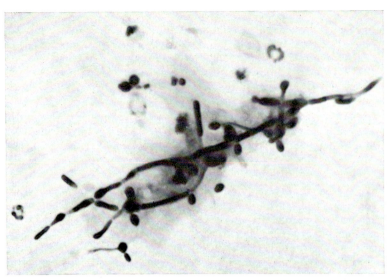

Fig. 16. *Candida albicans*: Budding yeast cells and pseudohyphae in smear from blood clot within intravenous catheter. Gram × 700

The organism grows on simple media, available in every bacteriology laboratory, producing overnight white to creamy colonies, which enlarge and end with irregular borders with clearly recognizable finger-like projections after several weeks of observation. Mounts from *C. albicans* kept overnight at room temperature show exclusively yeast cells with buds, exceptionally with short chains of yeast cells where the bud has failed to separate from the mother cell.

Identification of *C. albicans* is easily accomplished by inoculation of human serum or plasma; within 1 to 4 hours, germination occurs which is specific for *C. albicans* (Table 2). Likewise, cultures on cornmeal agar give, after a few days, the typical round chlamydospores which frequently arise from a "hyphal" growth, from which it is suspended by short segments of elongated yeast cells. The organism is pathogenic for most rodents; after intravenous injection in mice and rabbits, and intracardiac injection in guinea pigs or hamsters, hematogenous dissemination occurs, with renal and cerebral abscesses heading the list of complications. Myocarditis and involvement of other organs is likewise observed.

Due to the variation in size of *C. albicans*, it can be confused in smears and tissues with several other organisms, but the simultaneous presence of yeast cells and hyphae appears to be most pathognomonic for recognition of the organism. Remarks can be found in the literature that morphologic differences between *C. albicans* and other *Candida* species are sufficient to make a tentative identification. We feel that this is hazardous and unrealistic and that only proper cultures with sugar assimilation are a reasonable base for identification of the species (Table 2). The organism is selectively susceptible to nystatin and amphotericin B and seems not to be inhibited by actidione, whereas other candida species are.

The concept that only *C. albicans* is pathogenic cannot be maintained, even though it seems to be the most frequently identified in pathologic conditions. However, with no other fungus is interpretation of positive culture results more difficult than with *Candida*. In view of its common occurrence in the oral cavity and upper respiratory tract of healthy persons, its cultural recovery from sputum cannot be interpreted as indicative of pulmonary moniliasis. The only way to establish with

Table 2. *Rapid identification of candida**

Species	Results in 4 hours Serum + yeast 37° (filamentation = +)	Media: Cornmeal** (chlamydospores = +)	Media: Sabouraud + actidione (growth = + inhibition = 0)	glucose	maltose	lactote	saccharose	galactose	raffinose	nitrate
C. albicans	+	+	+	+	+	0	+	+	0	0
C. stellatoidea	±	0	+	+	+	0	0	+	0	0
C. tropicalis	0	0	0	+	+	0	+	+	0	0
C. pseudotropicalis	0	0	+	+	0	+	+	+	+	0
C. guillermondii	0	0	+	+	+	0	+	+	+	0
C. krusei	0	0	0	+	0	0	0	0	0	0
C. parakrusei	0	0	0	+	+	0	+	+	0	0
C. zeylanoides	0	0	+	+	0	0	0	0	0	0
C. pulcherrima	0	0	0	+	+	0	+	+	0	0
C. pelliculosa	0	0	0	+	+	0	+	±	±	+

The header above the auxanogram columns reads: Results in 24 hours — Auxanogram (Carbohydrate / Nitrogen).

* Adapted from E. Drouhet: Candidoses.
** Sometimes only after 48—72 hours.

certainty the presence of pulmonary candidiasis is by open thoracic biopsy or, in lieu of this, by needle biopsy of the lung through the chest cage. The repetitious discovery of *Candida* or its recovery by bronchoscopy do not, in our opinion, contribute to clarification, since the former is only repetition of an obvious error and the latter puts the organism potentially straight into the instrument during its introduction through the oral cavity.

Fluorescent antibody staining seems to be quite specific for identification of *C. albicans* and its differentiation from other species, but the difficulty of obtaining specific and well-absorbed antiserum must be recognized (Gordon et al.).

Coccidioides Immitis (Rixford and Gilchrist, 1896)

This organism is seen as sporangium (spherule) measuring from 10 to 80, rarely up to 240 μ, in tissues and exudate from patients (Fig. 17). Initially, the spherule is a round, unicellular structure, with subsequent septation occurring within the cytoplasm and leaving round, thin-walled endospores as a final result. The number of endospores varies from a few to hundreds, their size being in reverse relation to their number. On maturation the spherule ruptures, releasing the endospores into tissues or exudates, where repetition of the cycle of development continues, until immunologic or therapeutic balances interrupt the process. The endosporulating spherule (sporangium) is pathognomonic for coccidioidomycosis; in view of its size, spherules can be easily recognized with and without staining procedures. Occasionally, hyphae and arthrospores are seen in pulmonary cavities and granulomas (Puckett). Isolation of *C. immitis* from clinical material is quite feasible on Sabouraud's dextrose agar, where, after a few days to a week, a grayish membranous colony develops, which is covered rapidly by aerial mycelium, often appearing first in the center of the colony, surrounded by a zone of lesser growth of aerial mycelium, with subsequent rings of cottony growth. The light gray color becomes darker with time and yellow, tan, and brownish in some strains. It should be stressed that both pigment and development of aerial mycelium vary a great deal and, as in other mycoses, a large number of strains must be studied to acquire the "feel" for acceptance as "typical" within the extremes of natural variation.

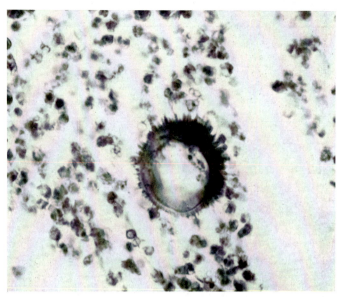

Fig. 17. *Coccidioidis immitis* with asteroid projections surrounding spherule in lung tissue.
H and E × 900

Arthrospores introduced into the animal body become round spherules. In turn, spherules observed in culture develop germ tubes from one or several endospores (Figs. 18, 19). A few strains can be induced to produce spherules *in vitro*.

Germ tubes develop from endospores within or outside the spherules within a few hours; these can be seen in a most chamber or in a slide culture. Germination from arthrospores takes place also on subculture of the hyphal growth.

In serum or plasma, some strains develop "culture spherules" temporarily or constantly when incubated at 37° C and slowly rotated in a roller apparatus (SCHLUMBERGER). Numerous methods using complex media or various gas tensions result likewise in spherule formation *in vitro*, but only certain strains behave in this fashion. The culture spherules are generally only about 10 μ in size and are often arranged in chains.

Hyphae have been induced to grow in animal tissue in air pouches in rats (WRIGHT et al.). In view of the extreme danger of pulmonary infection for laboratory workers because of the great volatility of the arthrospores, cultures should neither be kept, nor opened, in nonspecialized laboratories.

In general, the injection of clinical material into the guinea pig testis is the safest and fastest form of diagnosis, since spherules can be found in the testis within 3 days by needle aspiration or biopsy. The injection of culture material into guinea pigs may also be necessary for final identification. Mounts from the aerial mycelium reveal septate hyphae with numerous racquet swellings at the point of septation. Chains of rectangular arthrospores develop within a week or two, each arthrospore separated from its neighbor by a clear space — "empty cells" — marking the shell of cell-wall material. The interspace seems to be particularly fragile, and arthrospores become airborn with great ease and regularity. The arthrospores become either separated as single cells or in short chains; change to barrel or elliptic shape is the rule when, and even before, arthrospores lose the hyphal connection.

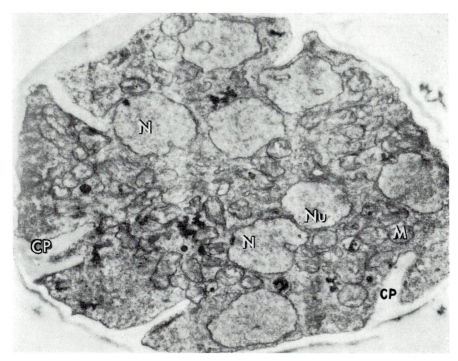

Fig. 18. Culture spherule of *C. immitis* in the cleavage stage. The cytoplasmic membrane shows invaginations (CP) representing the initial step of cleavage wall material. Little structural detail is defined in the future septa. Mitochondria (M) and multiple nuclei (N), some with nucleoli (nu), are seen. × 11,500.
From Breslau *et al.*: J. Biophys. and Biochem. Cytology *9*, 627 (1961)

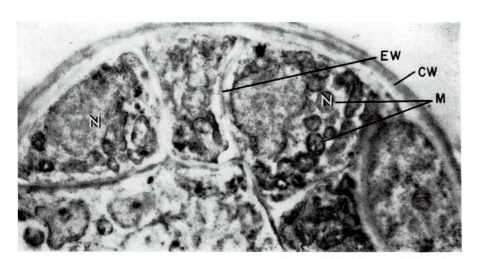

Fig. 19. Culture spherule of *C. immitis*. The cleavage is accomplished with septa clearly surrounding the individual endospores, just before rounding up of the newly formed elements. The cell wall (CW) has a lamellar structure and there is some osmiophilic substance in the septa. × 8600. From Breslau *et al.*: J. Biophys. and Biochem. Cytology *9*, 627 (1961)

Table 3. *Gross and microscopic appearances of fungi producing chromoblastomycosis*

1	2	3	4	5
Gross colony elevated dark gray fur-like colony. Short aerial hyphae	dark greenish gray elevated; short aerial hyphae	scanty brownish aerial hyphae on brittle olive colony	black moist shiny on sub-culture (or late) aerial hyphae	flat, green-brown-gray short hyphae
Hormodendrum type predominant short chains	rare to exceptional	rare short chains		long branching chains of spores
Acrotheca type variable	rare	—	rare	none
Compactum type —	—	predominant	—	—
Phialophora type rare	predominant	small ≠ on cornmeal agar	rare	none
Conidia elliptical-elongated $3—6 \times 1.5—3\,\mu$	elliptical $1.5—3 \times 2.5—4\mu$	cask-shaped to subspherical $1.5—2 \times 2—3\,\mu$	—	—
Budding yeast cells —	—	—	in young cultures oval to spherical cells	—

Dematiaceous Fungi

1. *Phialophora pedrosoi* (Brumpt, 1922) Emmons (1944)
2. *Phialophora verrucosa* Medlar (1915)
3. *Phialophora compactum* (Carrion, 1935) Emmons (1944) *
4. *Phialophora dermatitidis* (Kano, 1937) Emmons comb. nov.
5. *Cladosporium carionii* Trejos (1954).

The foregoing are the most commonly accepted species responsible for the disease chromoblastomycosis. Many authors prefer the generic names "*Hormodendrum*" or "*Fonsecaea*" instead of *Phialophora*, but little in the way of a positive contribution could be made by spreading the arguments on these pages. The variations acceptable within one species can be considerable, extending to the presence or absence of specific sporulation. The hyphae of the fungi are dark brown in culture mounts, with sharp, almost black septa.

The brown bodies recognizable in the skin lesions are known as "sclerotic cells" and are round or sometimes almost polyhedric. Septa are often seen and the cells seem to break open like the shell of an oyster (Fig. 20). The diameter of the sclerotic cells is about 10 μ in tissues and about 30 μ in exudates. Most frequently, small groups of the cells are seen (2 to 4 cells) in or outside of giant cells. Asteroid bodies surrounding the sclerotic cells have been described (Lavalle). Culture on Sabouraud's glucose agar reveals extremely slow-growing blackish colonies after 10 days or even later. Most species have elevated, "furry" colonies. Three types of sporulation are found in this group of fungi, with considerable variation in the frequency

---

* This group of fungi is seemingly as confusing for the specialist as it is for the "general" medical mycologist, even to the point where the wrong ending P. compact*um* instead of the correct compact*a* is accepted.

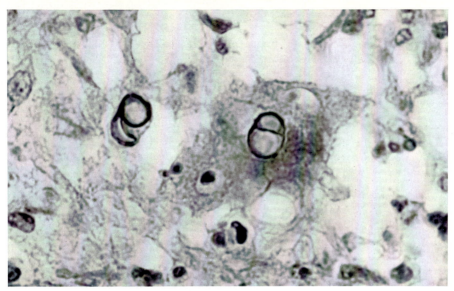

Fig. 20. Sclerotic spores in chromoblastomycosis. Notice equatorial split. H and E × 900

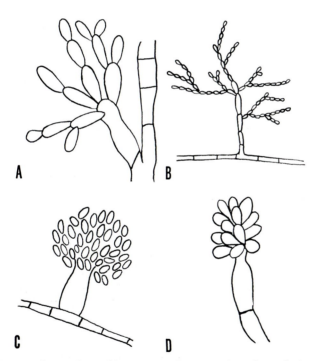

Fig. 21. The fungi producing chromoblastomycosis have a variety of sporulations. The different forms occur singly or in combination (see Table 3). Schematic drawings of the different types of sporulation: A. (left upper corner) Hormodendrum type of sporulation; conidiophore with terminal, short, branching chains of conidia. — B. (right upper corner) Cladosporium type of sporulation; long, branching chains of conidia, developing on lateral or terminal conidiophores. C. (left lower corner) Phialophora type of sporulation; mature phialide with globose accumulation of smooth spores formed within the basal part of the flask-shaped conidiophore. — D. (right lower corner) Acrotheca type of sporulation; somewhat swollen terminal conidiophore with conidia produced on all sides of its surface. Short chains of spores are sometimes formed

3*

or predominance of one particular sporulation per culture. Much of the argument and confusion about the dematiaceous fungi actually emanates from the fact that patient observers, after long search in multiple culture mounts, will find types of sporulation that are easily overlooked on superficial examination.

The *Hormodendrum* type — found in pathogenic and saprophytic members of the genus — is an acrogenous catenate sporulation (Fig. 21A). (Conidiophores bear branching chains of conidia.) The inidividual spore is separated from its neighbor by black, sharply accentuated disjunctors.

The acrothecal type is an acropleurogenous sporulation (Fig. 21D). Conidiophores are both terminal and lateral on the hyphae.) From the swollen conidiophores, conidia arise on short tubercles, covering laterally part or the entire surface of the conidiophore.

The *Phialophora* type is a semiendogenous form of spore formation. Few to many flaskshaped conidiophores form laterally or terminally on both aerial and vegetative hyphae and produce spores from a peripheral cup by a process of budding (Fig. 21C). The spores are held together by a water-soluble adhesive.

In addition, in *P. compactum*, conidia surround the terminal or lateral conidiophore in solid masses formed by conidial chains of variable length. The conidia are subspherical, in contrast to the oblong-shaped conidia of the acrotheca type.

References

AJELLO, L.: Comparative morphology and immunology of members of the genus *Histoplasma*. Mykosen **11**, 507 (1968). — AJELLO, L., CHENG, S.: Sexual reproduction in *Histoplasma capsulatum*. Mycologia **59**, 689 (1967). — AJELLO, L., GEORGE, L. K., KAPLAN, W., KAUFMAN, L.: Laboratory Manual for Medical Mycology. U.S. Dept. Health, Education and Welfare. Public Health Service Publication No. 994, Washington 1963. — AZULAY, R. D.: Die südamerikanische Blastomykose (Lutz-Mykose). In: JADASSOHN, Handbuch der Haut- und Geschlechtskrankheiten. Ergänzungswerk Bd. IV/4, S. 120 (1963). — BAKER, E. E., MRAK, E. M., SMITH, C. E.: The morphology, taxonomy, and distribution of *Coccidioides immitis*, Rixford and Gilchrist, 1896. Farlowia **1** (2), 199 (1943). — BERGMAN, F.: Pathology of experimental cryptococcosis. Acta path. microbiol. scand. Suppl. **147**, Vol. 1 (1961). — BERLINER, M. D.: On *Gymnoascus demonbreunii*-letter to the editor. Sabouraudia **6**, 272 (1968). — BORELLI, D.: Modelos isotermicos para la parasitologia experimental: paracoccidioidosis en Echimys, Proechimys y Heteromys. Derm. Venez. **3**, 98 (1962). — BROWN, R., WEINTROUB, D., SIMPSON, M. W.: Timber as a source of sporotrichosis infection in sporotrichosis. Infection in mines of the Witwatersrand. A symposium. Transvaal Chamber of Mines. Johannesburg 1947. — CHICK, E. W., PETERS, H. J., DENTON, J. F., BORING, W. D.: Die Nordamerikanische Blastomykose. Ergebn. allg. Path. path. Anat. **40**, 34 (1964). — CONANT, N. F., SMITH, D. T., BAKER, R. D., CALLAWAY, J. L., MARTIN, D. S.: Manual of clinical mycology. Philadelphia: W. B. Saunders Co. 1954. — COREMANS, J.: Un test biochimique de différenciation de *Histoplasma duboisii* Vanbreuseghem 1952 d'avec *Histoplasma capsulatum* Darling 1906. C.R. Soc. Biol. (Paris) **157**, 1130 (1963). — DENTON, J. F., McDONOUGH, E. S., AJELLO, L., AUSCHERMAN, R. J.: Isolation of *Blastomyces dermatitidis* from soil. Science **133**, 1126 (1961). — DENTON, J. F., DI SALVO, A.: Isolation of Blastomyces dermatitidis from natural sites at Augusta, Georgia. Amer. J. trop. Med. Hyg. **13**, 716 (1964). — DROUHET, E., MARIAT, F.: Etude des facteurs déterminant le développement de la phase levure de Sporotrichum schenckii. Ann. Inst. Pasteur **83**, 506 (1952). — EMMONS, C. W., MURRAY, I. G., LURIE, H. I., KING, M. H., TULLOCH, J. A., CONNOR, D. H.: North American blastomycosis; two autochthonous cases from Africa. Sabouraudia **3**, 306 (1964). — EMMONS, C. W., BINFORD, C. H., UTZ, J. P.: Medical Mycology. Philadelphia: Lea & Febiger 1963. — FIESE, M. J.: Coccidioidomycosis. Springfield/Ill.: Charles C Thomas 1958. — GOLDMAN, J. N., SCHWARZ, J.: Cytology of four yeastlike organisms in tissue explants. Mycopathologia (Den Haag) **29**, 161 (1966). — GORDON, M. A., ELLIOT, J. C., HAWKINS, T. W.: Identification of *Candida albicans*, other *Candida* species and *Torulopsis glabrata* by means of immunofluorescence. Sabouraudia **5**, 323 (1967). — GROCOTT, R. G.: A stain for fungi in tissue sections and smears. Amer. J. clin. Path. **25**, 975 (1955). — HOWARD, D. H.: Dimorphism of *Sporotrichum schenckii*. J. Bact. **81**, 464 (1961). — HOWARD, D. H., HERNDON, R. L.: Tissue cultures of mouse peritoneal exudates inoculated with *Blastomyces dermatitidis*. J. Bact. **80**, 522 (1960). — HUPPERT, M.: The laboratory aspects of pulmonary mycotic disease. In: J. D. STEELE, The treatment of mycotic and parasitic diseases of the chest, pp. 148. Springfield/Ill.: Charles C Thomas 1964. — KADEN, R.: Die Sporotrichose. In: JADASSOHN, Hand-

Ultrastructure of Human Pathogenic Fungi and Their Mycoses

L. M. CARBONELL, Caracas, Venezuela

With 25 Figures

Introduction

Fine structural research is adding a new dimension to mycology in animal and plant pathology. Ultrastructural investigation of human pathogenic fungi and their mycoses was neglected until the last decade when studies on the Dermatophytes and the fungi which cause the systemic mycoses began to appear. The main attention has been focussed on the organism and not on its cellular reaction in the tissues. In addition, isolation of the cell wall of human pathogenic fungi has been accomplished only incidentally as part of biochemical and immunological studies.

The same organelles that have been described in human pathogenic fungi are found in nonpathogens. However, some structures characterize species, as in the cell envelope of *Cryptococcus neoformans*.

Most human pathogenic fungi and most fungal contaminants in cultures, belong to the order of the Moniliales of the Fungi Imperfecti.

Actinomyces, Nocardia and *Streptomyces* which belong to the Actinomycetes have long been considered a transitional group in the phylogenetic scale, and intermediate between bacteria and fungi (MacLennan, 1961). They are included in this review.

The action of drugs on fungi, especially on the Dermatophytes, has been studied with the electron microscope. However, attention has been focussed on the action of drugs on organisms in culture rather than on the parasites infecting the host. The study of the fine structure of fungi has been essentially descriptive, and little attention has been paid to the function of the structures described. Interpretations of the morphological findings have been numerous, but clear experimental explanations of these findings have been few. Only studies of this kind will elicit further knowledge of some of the pathogenic characteristics of these fungi.

Methods

The techniques used in the investigation of human pathogenic fungi are similar to those employed in ultrastructural studies. The culture media used for growing microorganisms are the same as those used in other mycologic studies. Embedding in agar after fixation (CARBONELL, 1967) has been widely used by some authors to consolidate the material. Fixation can be achieved with the following: in osmium tetroxide with suitable buffer (BLANK, 1960; EDWARDS et al., 1959; EDWARDS and EDWARDS, 1960; EDWARDS, 1966; EDWARDS et al., 1967; FURTADO et al., 1967a, b; GALE, 1963; GALE and McLAIN, 1964; O'HERN and HENRY, 1950; TSUKAHARA et al., 1964; WERNER et al., 1966), in potassium permanganate (ADAMS et al., 1963; ITO et al., 1967; LADEN and ERICKSON, 1958; MONTES et al., 1965; TSUKAHARA et al., 1964; WERNER et al., 1967) and in osmium and potassium permanganate (MOORE and McALEAR, 1961a, b, 1962, 1963). Glutaraldehyde (SABATINI et al., 1963) has been recently introduced as a prefixative before the use of osmium tetroxide, or permanganate (EDWARDS et al., 1967; CARBONELL, 1967). The prevalence of permanganate fixation is due to the clear cut figures of

buch der Haut- und Geschlechtskrankheiten, Ergänzungswerk Bd. IV/4, S. 240. Berlin-Göttingen-Heidelberg: Springer 1963. — KAO, C.J., SCHWARZ, J.: The isolation of *Cryptococcus neoformans* from pigeon nests. Amer. J. clin. Path. **27**, 652 (1957). — KAPLAN, W., IVENS, M.S.: Fluorescent antibody staining in *Sporotrichum schenckii* in cultures and clinical materials. J. invest. Derm. **35**, 151 (1960). — KURUNG, J.M., YEGIAN, D.: Medium from maintenance and conversion of *Histoplasma capsulatum* to yeastlike phase. Amer. J. clin. Path. **24**, 505 (1954). — KWON-CHUNG, K.J.: *Gymnoascus demonbreunii* Ajello and Cheng evidence that it is not the perfect state of *Histoplasma capsulatum* Darling. Sabouraudia **6**, 168 (1968). — LACAZ, C.S.: South American Blastomycosis. An. Fac. Med. Univ. S. Paulo **29**, 1 (1956). — LAVALLE, P.: Chromomykose. In: JADASSOHN, Handbuch der Haut- und Geschlechtskrankheiten, Ergänzungswerk Bd. IV/4, S. 267 (1963). — LITTMAN, M.L., BOROK, R., DALTON, T.J.: Experimental avian cryptococcosis. Amer. J. Epidem. **82**, 197 (1965). — LITTMAN, M.L., ZIMMERMAN, L.E.: Cryptococcosis. New York: Grune & Stratton 1956. — LURIE, H.I.: Sporotrichosis. The significance of variations in morphology of spores in the tissue. Med. Coll. Virginia, Quart. **3**, 13 (1967). — McDONOUGH, E.S., LEWIS, A.L.: *Blastomyces dermatitidis:* production of the sexual stage. Science **156** (1967). — McDONOUGH, E.S., VAN PROOIEN, R., LEWIS, A.L.: Lysis of *Blastomyces dermatitidis* yeast-phase cells in natural soil. Amer. J. Epidem. **81**, 86 (1965). — NICKERSON, W.J., EDWARDS, G.A.: Studies on the physiological bases of morphogenesis in fungi. I. The respiratory metabolism of dimorphic pathogenic fungi. J. gen. Physiol. **33**, 41 (1949). — NORDEN, A.: Sporotrichosis. Clinical and laboratory features and a serologic study in experimental animals and humans. Acta path. microbiol. scand. **89**, 1 (1951). — OKUDAIRA, M., TSUBURA, E., SCHWARZ, J.: A histopathological study of experimental murine sporotrichosis. Mycopathologia (Den Haag) **14**, 284 (1961). — OKUDAIRA, M., SCHWARZ, J.: Infection with *Histoplasma duboisii* in different experimental animals. Mycologia **53**, 53 (1961). — PINE, L.: Morphological and physiological characteristics of *Histoplasma capsulatum*. In: H.C. SWEANY, Histoplasmosis, pp. 40. Springfield/Ill.: Charles C Thomas 1960. — PINE, L., DROUHET, E., REYNOLDS, G.: A comparative morphological study of the yeast phases of *H. capsulatum* and *H. duboisii*. Sabouraudia **3**, 211 (1964). — PINE, L., KAUFMAN, L., BOONE, C.J.: Comparative fluorescent antibody staining of *Histoplasma capsulatum* and *H. duboisii* with a specific anti-yeast phase *H. capsulatum* conjugate. Mycopathologia (Den Haag) **24**, 315 (1964). — PINE, L., PEACOCK, C.L.: Studies on the growth of *Histoplasma capsulatum*. IV. Factors influencing conversion of the mycelial phase to the yeast phase. J. Bact. **74**, 167 (1958). — PUCKETT, T.F.: Hyphae of *Coccidioides immitis* in tissues of the human host. Amer. Rev. Tuberc. **70**, 320 (1954). — ROMANO, A.H.: Dimorphism. In: G.C. AINSWORTH and A.S. SUSSMAN: The fungi. II, pp. 181. New York: Academic Press 1966. — SALVIN, S.B.: Phase-determining factors in *Blastomyces dermatitidis*. Mycologia **41**, 311 (1949). — SCHLUMBERGER, H.G.: A fatal case of cerebral coccidioidomycosis with cultural studies. Amer. J. med. Sci. **209**, 483 (1945). — SCHWARZ, J.: Giant forms of *Histoplasma capsulatum* in tissue explants. Amer. J. clin. Path. **23**, 898 (1953). — SEELIGER, H.P.R.: Use of urease test for the screening and identification of cryptococci. J. Bact. **72**, 127 (1956). — SEELIGER, H.P.R., WERNER, H.: Erzeugung von Krankheitszuständen durch Sproßpilze und Schimmelpilze. Handbuch experimentelle Pharmakologie, Infektionen III, S. 1—290. Berlin-Heidelberg-New York: Springer 1967. — SETHI, K.K., SCHWARZ, J.: Experimental ocular cryptococcosis in pigeons. Amer. J. Ophthal. **62**, 95 (1966). — SHADOMY, H.J., UTZ, J.P.: Preliminary studies on a hypha forming mutant of *Cryptococcus neoformans*. Mycologia **98**, 383 (1966). — SHIELDS, A.B., AJELLO, L.: Medium for selective isolation of *Cryptococcus neoformans*. Science **151**, 208 (1966). — SILVA, M.: Growth characteristics of the fungi of chromoblastomycosis. Ann. N.Y. Acad. Sci. **89**, 17 (1960). — SIMSON, F.W., HELM, M.A., BOWEN, J.W., BRANDT, F.A.: The pathology of sporotrichosis in man and experimental animals. In: Sporotrichosis. A symposium. Transvaal Chamber of Mines. Johannesburg 1947. — STAIB, F.: New concepts in the occurrence and identification of *Cryptococcus neoformans*. Mycopathologia (Den Haag) **19**, 143 (1963). — SUTTHILL, L.C.: Feathers as substrate for *Histoplasma capsulatum* in its filamentous phase of growth. Sabouraudia **4**, 1 (1965). — TALICE, R.V., McKINNON, J.E.: The asteroides form of Splendore in spontaneous and experimental sporotrichosis. Proc. 3rd Int. Congr. Microbiol. 1945, p. 510. — TASCHDJIAN, C.L.: Hyphal fusion studies on *Histoplasma capsulatum* and *Histoplasma duboisii* Vanbreuseghem 1952. Mykosen **2**, 1 (1959). — TEWARI, R.P., CAMPBELL, C.C.: Isolation of *Histoplasma capsulatum* from feathers of chickens inoculated intravenously and subcutaneously with the yeast phase of the organism. Sabouraudia **9**, 17 (1965). — VANBREUSEGHEM, R.: L'histoplasmosis africaine ou histoplasmose causée par *Histoplasma duboisii* Vanbreuseghem 1952. Bull. Acad. roy. Méd. Belg. **4**, 543 (1964). — WEEKS, R.J.: A rapid, simplified medium for converting the mycelial phase of *Blastomyces dermatitidis* to the yeast phase. Mycopathologia (Den Haag) **22**, 153 (1964). — WINNER, H.I., HURLEY, R.: *Candida albicans*. London: Churchill Ltd. 1964. — WRIGHT, E.T., NEWCOMER, V.D., STERNBERG, T.H.: The growth of *Coccidioides immitis* in the granuloma pouch of the rat with the development of hyphae and other forms. J. invest. Derm. **26**, 217 (1956).

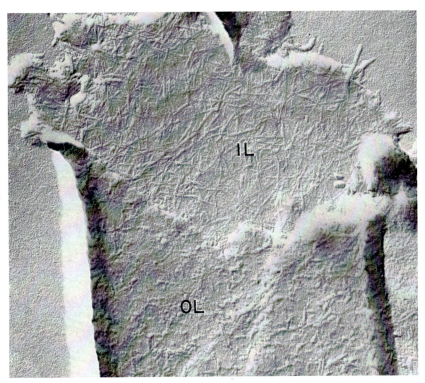

Fig. 1. Shadowed isolated cell wall of a hyphae of *Blastomyces dermatitidis*. The inner layer (IL) is fibrillar, while the outer layer (OL) is less fibrillar and has a bark-like appearance. × 20,000

mitochondria, endoplasmic reticulum and nuclear membranes, but it obscures details in the interior of the nuclei and destroys the ribosomes. Since all human pathogenic fungi have a cell wall, penetration of the fixatives, especially osmium tetroxide, is difficult, and this results in poor preservation of the fungi. Their preservation and contrast are better when glutaraldehyde is used as a prefixative. Intracytoplasmic membrane systems are also clearly observed when this method is employed. Fixation with lithium permanganate is better than with potassium permanganate when studying the fine structure of *Candida albicans* (MIZUNO and MONTES, 1966; MONTES et al., 1965). A detergent (alkane sulfonate) was used together with osmium tetroxide and/or permanganate in the study of *Microsporum gypseum* and *Epidermophyton floccosum* (WERNER et al., 1964; WERNER et al., 1967).

Methacrilate is widely used as an embedding material (BLANK, 1960; EDWARDS et al., 1959; EDWARDS and EDWARDS, 1960; LADEN and ERICKSON, 1958; O'HERN and HENRY, 1950), but better results are obtained with Epon (EDWARDS and EDWARDS, 1960; MEINHOF, 1967a, b, c), Araldita (MIZUNO and MONTES, 1966; MONTES et al., 1965) and Maraglas (CARBONELL, 1967).

Staining with either uranyl acetate or different preparations of lead (REYNOLD, 1963; WATSON, 1958a, b) are used to enhance contrast. The simultaneous use of uranyl and lead give very contrasty preparations (CARBONELL, 1967; FURTADO et al., 1967a, b).

Shadowed preparations are used to study the inner and outer layers of the cell wall of some pathogenic fungi (CARBONELL, 1967; RIBI et al., 1955; RIBI and SALVIN, 1956) (Fig. 1). The freezing-etching technique has been employed to study the organelles in *Saccharomyces cerevisiae* (MOORE and MÜHLETHALER, 1963) and recently in *Paracoccidioides brasiliensis* (GIL, personal communication) (Fig. 2).

Cell Wall

The fungal cell can be divided into two types, the yeast cell and the filamentous fungus. Pathogenic fungi have either one, or both of these forms, and their organel-

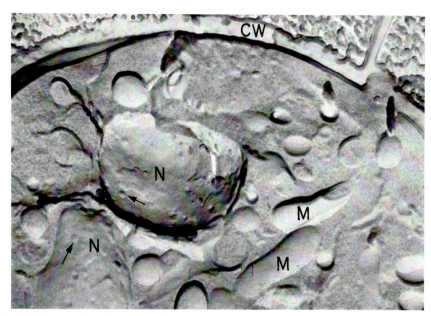

Fig. 2. Freezing-etching of a yeast of *Paracoccidioides brasiliensis*. With this technique a fracture of the material is made at low temperature, and later, etching and shadowing of the fractured surface. Two nuclei (N) with nuclear pores (arrow) are observed. M, mitochondria.
CW, cell wall. × 22,500. (Courtesy of Mr. F. GIL)

les are the same as those found in non-pathogenic fungi. However, there are some
details worth mentioning because they may be of value for the elucidation of the
physiological features of these fungi.

Outer Wall. Since the first studies on the fine structure of fungi were published,
there has been much discussion of the outer cell wall which gives the fungus its
form and rigidity. Most of these controversies arise from the different materials
employed, the techniques used for prefixation, fixation and embedding, and from
the sectioning angles and the age of the cells under observation. The cell walls of
human pathogenic fungi differ slightly in the yeast form from those of the mycelial
form. There is a general agreement that in the latter phase the cell wall is composed
of an outer, thin, electron-dense layer and an inner, broad, electron-lucid layer
(BLANK, 1960; ITO et al., 1967; MEINHOF, 1967a, b, c; TSUKAHARA et al., 1964;
WERNER et al., 1966; WERNER et al., 1967). In the yeast the cell wall is somewhat
thicker, and in *P. brasiliensis* and *Blastomyces dermatitidis* different layers are
observed depending on the sectioning angle (CARBONELL, 1967) i.e. homogenous
electron density throughout the cell wall, outer thin electron-dense layer with inner
broad electron light layer and lamellated cell walls. The thickness of the cell wall
varies from one fungus to the other. It ranges from 50—100 mμ in *C. albicans*
(ADAMS et al., 1963) to 60—300 mμ in the hyphae of *Trichophyton violaceum* (ITO
et al., 1967).

In *C. neoformans* (EDWARDS et al., 1967; TSUKAHARA, 1963) the cell wall proper
is included with the plasma membrane and the capsule in the so-called cell envelope. The capsule is the outermost structure of the cell envelope and it is composed of densely packed microfibrils (30—40 Å in diameter) which, apparently, are
long and coiled. It seems that there is a relationship between the age of the cell and
the capsular material; cells with the least capsular material display better pre-

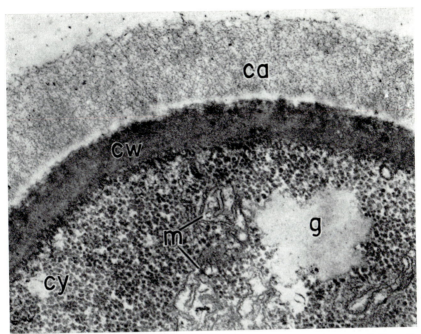

Fig. 3. Cell envelope of *Cryptococcus neoformans*. Observe the capsule (ca) and the cell wall (cw). A halo is seen between these structures. In the granular cytoplasm (cy), mitochondria (m) and storage granules (g) are present. Osmium in Sorensen's buffer. × 60,000
(From EDWARDS et al., 1967)

servation of intracytoplasmic structures (Fig. 3). The interpretation of the difference in structure of the cell wall must be made cautiously. It might be that these changes correspond to gross variations in the composition of the cell wall, or to minor physical or chemical changes of a particular wall component.

Shadowing techniques are used to study the outer and inner surface of isolated cell walls, and the outer surface of whole cells. In *Histoplasma capsulatum* both the outer and inner layers are fibrillar (RIBI et al., 1955). Isolated cell walls of the mycelia of *P. brasiliensis* and *B. dermatitidis* show a bark-like or slightly fibrillar outer layer, while the inner layer displays a delicate network of fibrils.

These techniques failed to show a capsule or thin layer in whole cells of *H. capsulatum* (RIBI and SALVIN, 1956). However, when applied to *C. neoformans* a distinct capsule was observed.

Biochemistry and Ultrastructure. HOUWINK and KREGER (1953) studied the cell wall of several different nonpathogenic fungi by combining the use of the electron microscope and X-ray diffraction, as well as by treating the cells chemically with alkali and acids. With the electron microscope, they differentiated and identified chitin as granules or fibrils, and hidro-glucan fibrils. X-ray diffraction and diluted mineral acids indicated that a major portion of the cell wall of *H. capsulatum* is composed of chitin (RIBI et al., 1955). Using X-ray diffraction, BLANK (1954) found that the skeleton of the mycelial and yeast phase of *B. dermatitidis*, *P. brasiliensis*, *H. capsulatum*, *Sporotrichum schenckii* as well as of several dermatophytes (BLANK, 1953) consist of chitin. Using a combination of digestion with chitinase, X-ray diffraction and the electron microscope on isolated cell walls of the yeast phase of *P. brasiliensis* and *B. dermatitidis*, chitin was identified as fibrils 80 Å in diameter.

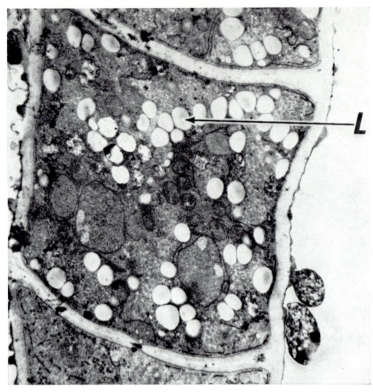

Fig. 4. *Microsporum gypseum.* Longitudinal section of a hypha. The cell wall displays an outer electron dense layer and an inner broad and electron clear layer. L, lipid inclusions. × 18,720 (From WERNER, H.J., et al., 1966b)

The remnants obtained after digestion with chitinase have a fibrilar appearance and biochemically are identified as glucan. The importance of the immunologic properties of the cell wall of pathogenic fungi makes it advisable to perform more studies on the macromolecular structure of cell walls and their morphological counterpart.

Peeling of the Outer Cell Wall. The loose fragments or fibrils that peel off of the external surface of the outer cell wall of fungi have been largely overlooked. Because these fibrils have immunologic properties and because the cell wall is the first structure of fungi to come in contact with the host, it is advisable to investigate this subject in greater depth.

In the yeast phase of *P. brasiliensis,* the cell wall peels off in distinct fibrils, whereas, in *B. dermatitidis,* it does so in bundles of fibrils, making it difficult to identify them (CARBONELL, 1967). In the mycelial phase of both fungi, the peeling process is also fibrillar, but very moderate compared with the yeast phase. The outer coating described in *T. violaceum* (ITO et al., 1967) and the material that sticks to the outer surface of the cell wall of *M. gypseum* (WERNER et al., 1967) may be a special type of peeling of these fungi (Fig. 4). In some fungal cells, clear fibrils are identified, in others, there is an amorphous material, i.e. in *Microsporum canis* (WERNER et al., 1966) in *C. albicans* (GALE, 1963) and in other fungi. These fibrils and the amorphous material may be a kind of peeling process of these cells.

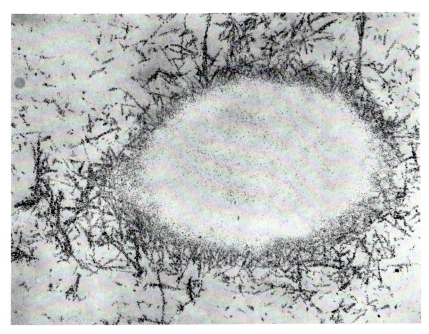

Fig. 5. Cytochemical demonstration of polysaccharides of the cell wall of *Paracoccidioides brasiliensis*. Silver granules are deposited in the fibrillar network of the cell wall. Glutaraldehyde and hexa-methylen-tetramine reaction. × 15,000

Ultrastructural Cytochemistry. The modification of Gomori's silver methenamine staining (GROCOTT, 1955) is widely used for the identification of fungi in tissues and in cultures. Since metallic silver, which is produced in the reaction, causes the electron beam to become opaque, this reaction has been modified for use with the electron microscope (RAMBOURG, 1967). The deposit of metallic silver is supposed to be specific, in a wide sense, for polysaccharides. This technique applied to the yeast phase of *P. brasiliensis* and *B. dermatitidis* shows a clear positivity of the peeling fibers and of the outer layer of the cell wall of *P. brasiliensis* (Fig. 5) and of the amorphous material which sticks to the outer wall of *B. dermatitidis*. The production of osmium black as a terminal product to demonstrate polysaccharides (SELIGMAN et al., 1965) with the electron microscope is very poor in *P. brasiliensis* and *B. dermatitidis* while in the cell wall of *Saccharomyces cerevisiae* a very strong reaction is observed. The interpretation of these results depends on the different types of polysaccharides in the cell wall (chitin, β-glucan, etc.).

Formation and Ultrastructure of Septa. It is evident that several types of septa exist in fungi. The range includes complete septa, those with perforations, and partial septa that are little more than thickening of lateral walls (BRACKER, 1967). The septa described in human pathogenic fungi are simple plates with a central pore. These types of septa have been described in Ascomycetes and in Fungi Imperfecti with ascomycetous affinities (ITO et al., 1967; LADEN and ERICKSON, 1958; O'HERN and HENRY, 1956; TAPLIN and BLANK, 1961; TSUKAHARA et al., 1964; WERNER et al., 1966). *Geotrichum candidum* presents plasmodesmata or septal micropores, but the septa are otherwise complete (HASHIMOTO et al., 1964; KIRK and SINCLAIR, 1966; WILSENACH, 1965b) (Fig. 6).

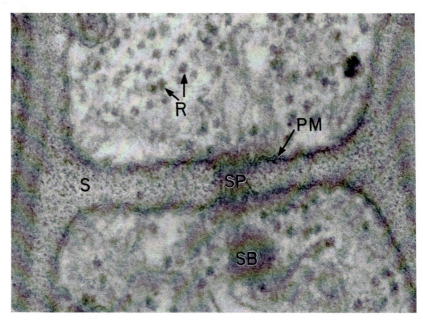

Fig. 6. Septum in *Blastomyces dermatitidis*: The septum (S) is formed by the less electron dense layer of the outer cell wall. A septal plug (SP) and a septal body (Woronin's bodies) are seen. R, ribosomes. PM, plasma membrane. Glutaraldehyde-osmium fixation. × 102,000

The septum may be considered a sort of deep invagination of the innermost layer of the cell wall (Tsukahara et al., 1964). In *C. immitis* (O'Hern and Henry, 1956) formation of the septum appears to begin with the division of the cytoplasm by the invagination of the plasma membrane, then the membrane splits and newly formed cell wall material lies between the two resulting membranes. At the site of the septum implantation, there is an increase in the diameter of the hyphae caused by bulging of the cell wall at this point. The developing septal wall is at all stages surrounded by the invaginated plasma membrane even when the septum reaches maturity. In *T. violaceum* (Ito et al., 1967) the septum's thickness diminishes towards the septal pore where the cytoplasm of adjoining segments of a hypha flow together. In the fungi under study no organelles have been seen passing through the septal pore as was observed in *Rhizoctonia solani* (Bracker and Butler, 1964). In *P. brasiliensis* and *B. dermatitidis*, the septum appears to be continuous and one or two layers are visualized when the sectioning angle is not made at the level of the pore, but they are never as clearly outlined as in other nonpathogenic fungi (Bracker and Butler, 1964). *Epidermophyton floccosum* (Laden and Erickson, 1958) exhibits a broad electron dense line running through the center of the septum.

Woronin bodies or septal bodies are round and/or elongated, granular, electron-dense structures which are found lying near the septum, or closing the pore. In this latter case they are called septal plugs. They have been found in all hyphae of human pathogenic fungi. Blurring of the plasma membrane is observed at the site in which the septal plug comes in contact with the pore. Septal plugs have been found in degenerated hyphae, in hyphae undergoing degeneration, or in hyphae which have been damaged (Reichle and Alexander, 1965).

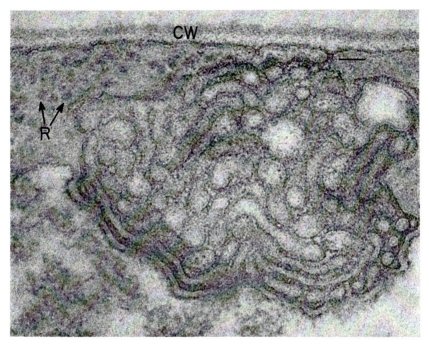

Fig. 7. Intracytoplasmic membrane system in *Blastomyces dermatitidis*. Observe the invagination and continuity of the plasma membrane (arrow) with a structure formed by successive invaginations of the same. CW, cell wall. R, ribosomes. Glutaraldehyde-osmium fixation. × 110,000

The Cell Contents

Plasma Membrane. The cell membrane proper (plasma membrane) has a higher electron density than the cell wall (ADAMS et al., 1963) and depending on the sectioning angle it appears either as an electron dense layer closely attached to the cell wall on one side and on the other to the cytoplasm, or as a clear three layered structure. Two of these layers which are electron dense and measure about 30 Å each are separated by an electron-lucid layer measuring approximately 30 Å (EDWARDS et al., 1959; EDWARDS and EDWARDS, 1960; EDWARDS et al., 1967). In the mycelial phase of *P. brasiliensis* and *B. dermatitidis* granules with light cores and dark rims are found attached to the outer surface of the two electron dense layers. The plasma membrane is convoluted and undulating, with invaginations. In *C. albicans* (GALE, 1963) the depth of the invaginations measures up to 150 mμ. MONTES et al. (1965) demonstrated these invaginations particularly well in material fixed with lithium permanganate. In these small invaginations, blurring of the plasma membrane is observed at the site in which cell wall material adheres to the plasma membrane. It is also observed at the tip of the hypha. It seems that this blurring of the plasma membrane is related to an increase in metabolic activity. Continuity of the plasma membrane with the nuclear envelope, endoplasmic reticulum and mitochondria has been reported in several fungi (ADAMS et al., 1963; EDWARDS and EDWARDS, 1960; O'HERN and HENRY, 1956).

MOORE and McALEAR (1961) demonstrated continuity of the nuclear envelope with the plasma membrane using serial sections of a Deuteromycete.

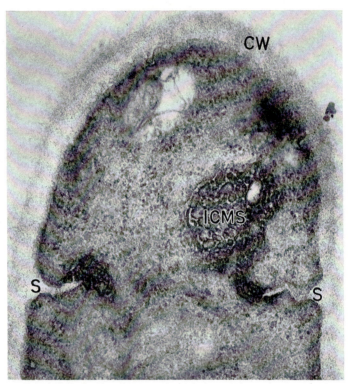

Fig. 8. Intracytoplasmic membrane system and septum formation in *Blastomyces dermatitidis*. Observe the forming septum (S) with ICMS attached to the tip of the same. Serial sections of this material were obtained in order to be sure of the relationship between the ICMS and the septum. CW, cell wall. Glutaraldehyde-osmium fixation. × 30,000

In *H. capsulatum* and *H. duboisii*, the plasma membrane exhibits considerable vesiculation which is indicative of pinocytotic activities (Edwards et al., 1959).

Intracytoplasmic Membrane System (ICMS). The ICMS comprises the lomasomes (Moore and McAlear, 1961) and the mesosome-like structures described in *C. neoformans* (Edwards et al., 1967; Hashimoto, 1966), *P. brasiliensis* and *B. dermatitidis* (Carbonell, 1967).

The term lomasomes was introduced by Moore and McAlear (1961) to describe the "spongy-like structures contiguous with the cell wall and whose interior limits are defined by variously sharp, dark lines of the plasma membrane." These structures were found between the plasma membrane and the cell wall and were named on the basis of their location at the cell peripheries. Lomasomes have been described in a number of pathogenic (Ikeda, 1964; Iwata and Irata, 1963) and nonpathogenic fungi (Moore and McAlear, 1961; Wilsenach and Kessel, 1965). The invaginations of the plasma membrane are interpreted as the beginning of the ICMS. Serial sections show that this membranous system undergoes additional invaginations which form multivesicular or lamellar structures that are interpreted as tubular infoldings of the plasma membrane seen in different sectioning angles (Fig. 7). The term mesosome is applied in bacteria to a membranous structure that originates as an invagination of the plasma membrane which subsequently expands into the cytoplasm (Imaeda and Ogura, 1963; Ellar et al., 1967). The main features of mesosomes are their vesicular structures and their role in cell division

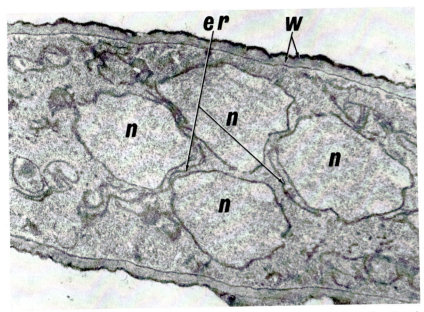

Fig. 9. *Microsporum audouini.* Longitudinal view of a hypha. Observe the cell wall and the multiple nuclei (n). The cell wall (w) has two clear distinct layers. Membranes identified as endoplasmic reticulum (er) are observed in the cytoplasm. (Courtesy of Dr. H.J. WERNER)

and septum formation. A clear relationship between septum formation and the ICMS has been observed in serial sections of pathogenic fungi (Fig. 8). The role of lomasomes has been much discussed. Evidence of their participation in wall formation (WILSENACH and KESSEL, 1965), secretion (MOORE and McALEAR, 1961), and glycogen synthesis (HASHIMOTO, 1966) is mostly circumstantial. BRACKER (1967) questioned the reality of lomasomes on the basis that they had not been identified in living cells, nor had they been demonstrated in cells prepared other than by chemical fixation. Many experimental studies like isolation, genesis and the, conditions that favor their formation, must be done in order to clarify their significance. The same can be said for the mesosome-like structures observed in pathogenic fungi.

   Nucleus. The general morphology of the nucleus in fungi is not different from that described in higher animals (Fig. 9). Some of the fungi under study are multinucleated, such as the yeast and mycelial forms of *P. brasiliensis* and *B. dermatitidis* (CARBONELL, 1967; EDWARDS and EDWARDS, 1960) and the mycelia of *C. immitis* (BRESLAU et al., 1961). Others are uninucleated such as *C. neoformans* (EDWARDS et al., 1967), *C. albicans* (Fig. 10) (ADAMS et al., 1963), *T. rubrum* (BLANK et al., 1960), *H. capsulatum* and *H. duboisii* (EDWARDS et al., 1959), *T. violaceum* (ITO et al., 1967). The nucleoplasm is enveloped by the nuclear membrane which is composed of two electron dense layers, separated by a less electron dense layer 10 mμ thick. In *H. capsulatum* and *H. duboisii* a perinuclear cisterna of approximately 28 mμ in diameter is described, contiguous with the endoplasmic reticulum. The nuclear membranes have pores about 700 Å wide (MONTES et al., 1965) which show very clearly with permanganate fixation. In the yeast form of *B. dermatitidis* the nuclear membranes are contiguous from one nucleus to the other as happens with the perinuclear cisterna (EDWARDS and EDWARDS, 1959). The matrix of the nucleus is

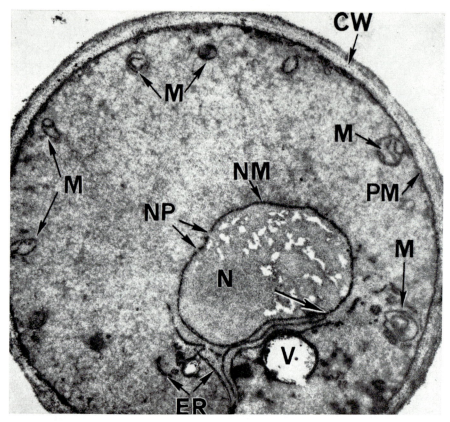

Fig. 10. Cultures of *Candida albicans*. Mitochondria (M) in close proximity to the plasma membrane (PM). Observe the nuclear pore (NP). The endoplasmic reticulum (ER) at one point (arrow) is continuous with the nuclear membrane (NM). CW, cell wall. V, cytoplasmic vacuole. (From MIZUNO, N., and MONTES, L. F., 1966)

finely granular and the nucleoli are identified by their increased density relative to the nuclear matrix and by their usually coarse granularity. The nucleoli can be single or multiple. The above description refers to the nucleus at the interphase. Chromosomes have not been observed in human pathogenic fungi.

Other Cytoplasmic Components. The term endoplasmic reticulum is generally used to describe the endoplasmic membranous system in fungal cells (HAWKER, 1965). This endoplasmic reticulum is scanty and usually appears as a single double-stranded membrane with or without ribosomes attached to them. It must not be mistaken with the ICMS which has no relation with ribosomes and until now has not shown continuity of the nuclear membranes, or mitochondria. In addition, permangantate fixation clearly evidences the membranes of the endoplasmic reticulum while the ICMS is poorly seen. Scanty, smooth and rough surfaced endoplasmic reticulum are observed in all human pathogenic fungi. In some of these fungi (EDWARDS and EDWARDS, 1960; EDWARDS et al., 1967) ribosomes are identified as electron dense particles of 140—170 Å in diameter scattered throughout the cytoplasm. Because ribosomes disappear with permanganate fixation, their identification has been poor due to the fact that this fixative has been employed in most of the studies of human pathogenic fungi.

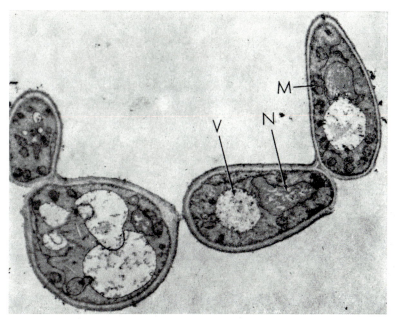

Fig. 11. Culture of *Candida albicans*. These cells show numerous mitochondria (M) and one or several vacuoles (V) located close to the nuclei (N). Fixed in 15% LiMnO$_4$. × 9,100 (From MONTES, L. F., et al., 1965)

Mitochondria similar to the ones described in higher plants and animals are found in all fungi (THYAGARAJAN et al., 1961). The number of cristae seems to be lower in fungi than in plants and animals. In the hyphae of some dimorphic pathogenic fungi, mitochondria are elongated and their long axes are parallel to the main axis of the hypha. In *C. neoformans*, they are oval or ring-shaped (EDWARDS et al., 1967). In *M. gypseum* (MEINHOF, 1967), tubular and lamellated structures are observed in the mitochondria. There is a possibility that tubular mitochondria may be converted into cristated mitochondria. In the mycelial and yeast phase of *P. brasiliensis*, electron-dense bodies and membrane-like structures are also observed in mitochondria (CARBONELL and POLLAK, 1963). In *C. neoformans*, mitochondria may enclose particles similar to ribosomes (EDWARDS et al., 1967). The origin of mitochondria has been much discussed; in *B. dermatitidis* they seem to be related to the endoplasmic reticulum (EDWARDS and EDWARDS, 1960).

Glycogen is the primary storage polysaccharide in fungi (KANETSUNA and CARBONELL, 1965, 1966). Its identification in thin sections of pathogenic fungi depends upon the age, type of culture and preservation of the fungi during the embedding process. For instance, neither EDWARDS et al. (1967) nor TSUKAHARA (1963) were able to find glycogen in *C. neoformans*, but HASHIMOTO and YOSHIDA (1966) and other authors (CARBONELL and POLLAK, 1963; CARBONELL, 1967; WERNER et al., 1967) have found this polysaccharide in other fungi. Glycogen has a tendency to cluster in rosette-like structures instead of spreading throughout the cytoplasm. It is abundant in young yeast and hypha, but not at the tip. Glycogen is also found, sometimes abundantly, in hyphae in which organelles are not recognized and in the dead hyphae of intra-hyphal hyphae.

Lipid inclusions are considered as reservoirs of energy-rich material and potential sources of carbon compounds (FAWCET, 1966). Lipid droplets have been described in several pathogenic fungi (ADAMS et al., 1963; BLANK et al., 1960; TSUKAHARA, 1964; WERNER et al., 1966). A well fixed lipid droplet is not surrounded by a membranous structure, but when the fixative does not penetrate completely, a dark cortical zone that resembles, superficially, a membrane, is observed. Lipid inclusions are seen in mature yeasts and hyphae (CARBONELL and POLLAK, 1962; CARBONELL, 1967). In *C. neoformans* (EDWARDS et al., 1967) lipidic vacuoles are similar to poly-β-hidroxibutirate bodies of bacteria.

Large and small vacuoles with irregular contours are observed in mature fungi (Fig. 11). Some of these vacuoles are filled with electron-dense particles while others are empty. Frequently, the ICMS invaginates into a vacuole, or a vacuole invaginates into another vacuole giving the appearance of a double membrane.

In *C. albicans* MONTES et al. (1965) demonstrated with the electron microscope, electron-dense bodies of approximately the same size of mitochondria. They were identified as lisosomes since when observed with the light microscope they were found to be granules and acid phosphatase-positive.

The Golgi apparatus has not been truly identified in human pathogenic fungi. Although the cytoplasmic ground substance seems to be granular, caution must be exercized in this interpretation since these granules may be artifacts caused by fixatives.

Developmental Studies

Bud Formation in Yeast. Bud formation in yeast forms of pathogenic fungi has been studied in *H. capsulatum, H. duboisii* (EDWARDS et al., 1959), *P. brasiliensis* (Fig. 12) and *B. dermatitidis* (CARBONELL, 1967) and only mentioned in *C. neoformans* (EDWARDS et al., 1967) and *C. albicans* (ADAMS et al., 1963). The earliest indication of the budding process seems to be a thickening of the cell wall around a small nipple-like invagination of the cytoplasm. In *P. brasiliensis* all the layers of the cell wall increase their optical density at the site where the budding begins; at the same time the cytoplasm starts to bulge takes on a convex appearance. The bulging of the cytoplasm occurs when the hydrogen is transferred by the enzyme protein disulfide reductase to the S—S-linkage in the polysaccharide-protein complex of the yeast of the cell wall (NICKERSON and FALCONE, 1956). At the site of the bulging of the cytoplasm, extreme vesiculation, accumulation of mitochondria and blurring of the plasma membrane are observed. When a thumb-like process is formed, only cytoplasm with few ribosomes is observed. In *P. brasiliensis*, the bud is attached to the mother cell by a narrow neck which shows increase of the optical density of the cell wall. In *H. capsulatum* the neck is also narrow compared with that of *B. dermatitidis*, which is broad, allowing free communication between the two cells. Mitochondria, ribosomes, glycogen and nuclei are observed passing through the neck. A clear division of the nucleus between the daughter and mother cell has not been reported in pathogenic fungi. In *P. brasiliensis* and *B. dermatitidis*, several nuclei can be seen in the mother and daughter cell. The nuclei diminish in number with the age of the cell until few or none are observed. One nucleus is always seen in the mother and daughter cell of the uninuclear yeast pathogenic fungi. The cleavage starts with a furrow in the cytoplasmic membrane which is later occupied by an annular centripetal growth of the inner layer. At this moment, increased amounts of ICMS are seen on both sides of the infolded cell wall. The bud scar has been extensively studied in *Schizosaccharomyces pombe* (STREIBLOVA and BERAU, 1963; STREIBLOVA et al., 1966) and in other non-pathogenic fungi (AGAR and DOUGLAS, 1955; BARTHOLOMEW and MITTWER, 1953). In *B. dermatitidis*, the bud scar is recognized only at the end of the division exhibiting a flat surface. In

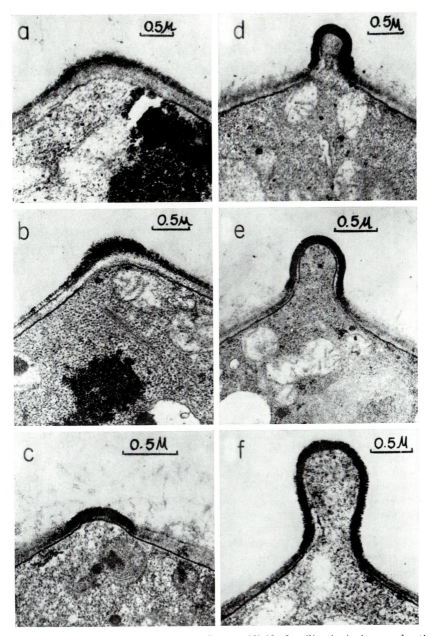

Fig. 12. Beginning of the budding process in *Paracoccidioides brasiliensis*. An increased optical density of the middle layer of the cell wall is observed (1b). The outer layer has a fibrillar structure (1c) and tends to disappear during the budding process. Fig. 1f shows ribosomes in the daughter cell. (From CARBONELL, L. M., 1967)

P. brasiliensis it takes on a truncated cone form, caused by a bulging cytoplasm, covered at the sides by the optically dense cell wall. In shadowed isolated cell walls, the bud scar appears as a circular raised rim made up of fibrils arranged in a swirl.

4*

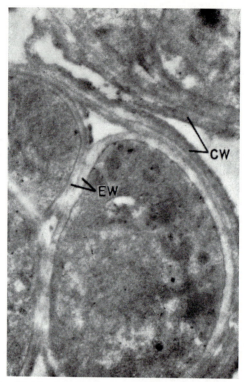

Fig. 13. Culture of *Coccidioides immitis*. Section through the sporangial wall (CW) and two adjacent endospores. Each endospore has its own cell membrane and relatively thin wall (EW). Note the lamellation of the outer sporangial wall. × 16,800. (From Breslau, A. M., 1961)

It seems that shortly after the division is accomplished the bud scar disappears since it is not found in the old cells.

Most of the fungal hyphal growth takes place by apical extension (Aronson, 1965). The cell wall increases its thickness and its optical density at the tip of the hyphae at which time blurring of the plasma membrane, increased ICMS, accumulation of mitochondria and ribosomes are always observed. Glycogen is only occasionally identified. All these structural details point to an increased metabolic activity at the tip of the hypha. Further structural, metabolic and experimental studies are necessary to clarify the mechanisms involved in hyphal growth.

Ultrastructure of Dimorphism. The term "dimorphism" has been applied to certain pathogenic fungi which have two distinct morphological forms: a parasitic form that exists in tissues of a host, and a saprophytic form that occurs in nature or in ordinary media at room temperature (Wilson and Plunkett, 1965).

Ultrastructure of the changes from mycelium to spherules and later to endospore formation has been described in the dimorphic fungus *C. immitis* (Breslau et al., 1961; Erickson and Breslau, 1960; O'Hern and Henry, 1956) (Fig. 13). The mycelium begins to transform into spherules when the hyphal cell rounds up. The individual spherule's wall develops beneath the hyphal wall. The spherules become independent before cleavage begins. They have a cell wall thickness of 200 to 600 mμ. They have multiple nuclei and the organelles described above. Formation of endospores starts with cleavage furrows originating in the cell wall. The septum formation has the same characteristics as those described above except that no

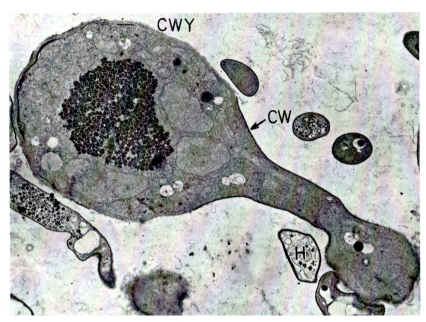

Fig. 14. Transformation of mycelium to yeast in *Paracoccidioides brasiliensis*: Observe the swelling of the apical portion of the hypha. The electron dense layer of the cell wall (CW) of the hyphae disappears when the new cell wall of the yeast (CWY) is formed. Dead hyphae (H) are seen. Glutaraldehyde-osmium fixation. × 20,000

granules (Woronin bodies) comparable to those associated with septum formation have been seen in cleaving spherules. The separation of the endospores occurs between two layers of the cell wall prior to the release of spores.

The transformation of mycelium and yeast of *P. brasiliensis* in cultures and experimental inoculations has been investigated by means of the light microscope (CARBONELL and RODRIGUEZ, 1965; MALFATI and ZAPATA, 1954). In the transformation from yeast to mycelium in *P. brasiliensis* and *B. dermatitidis* a germ tube is formed which shows a cell wall characteristic of hyphae. This tube elongates at the tip. Later, septa appear inside the hypha with all the characteristics already mentioned.

The transformation of mycelium to yeast phase in *P. brasiliensis* (Fig. 14) starts by rounding up of the space between two septa. The cell wall thickens and at the end of the transformation the cell wall has the same characteristics as in the yeast. Later, these yeasts have buds.

Intra-Hyphal Hyphae. Cultures of *P. brasiliensis* and *B. dermatitidis* grown in liquid media always show dead hyphae with the penetration and subsequent growth of live hyphae within them. These structures which are also called intrahyphal mycelium, endohyphae (LOWRY and SUSSMAN, 1966) and self-parasitism (DODGE, 1920) have been observed in Basidiomycetes and Ascomycetes (DODGE, 1920) (Fig. 15).

The live hyphae found inside the dead hyphae are indistinguishable from the hyphae that are outside. The space between the live hypha and the cell wall of the dead hypha is filled with mitochondrial ghosts, remnants of ICMS and glycogen, but never nuclei and seldom ribosomes. SUSSMAN et al. (1965) suggested that intrahyphal hyphae are probably induced by wounds or intoxications with subsequent

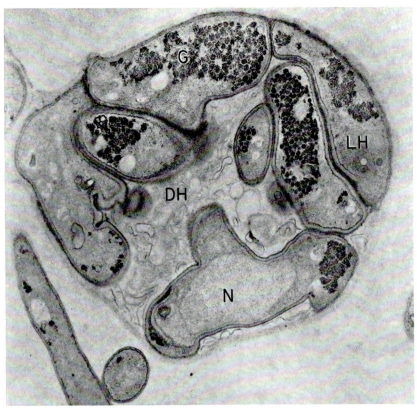

Fig. 15. Intra-hyphal hyphae in *Blastomyces dermatitidis*. Observe the live hyphae (LH) surrounded by the cell wall. The dead hypha (DH) does not show organelles that may be recognizable. G, glycogen. N, nucleus. Glutaraldehyde-osmium fixation. × 30,000

death of the hyphae, accompanied by blockage of the septal pore. The mechanism by which the live hyphae is attracted towards the dead one or *vice versa* remains obscure.

Action of Drugs on Fine Structure of Pathogenic Fungi

Biochemical studies of the action of drugs on fungi have been extensive. However, the ultrastructural changes in pathogenic fungi are few. The following alterations were observed in *T. rubrum* (Blank et al., 1960) and in *T. mentagrophytes* var. asteroides (Tomomatsu, 1960) while under the action of griseofulvin: the tip of the hypha becomes swollen and rounded, the hyphal cell may be completely filled with large lipid granules, the electron dense outer layer of the cell wall becomes granular, the organelles are no longer recognizable, but there is persistence of the plasma membrane.

Gale (1963) used benzalkonium chloride, amphotericin B and filipin on cultures of *C. albicans*. The benzalkonium-treated cells showed a less dense cytoplasm. Nuclei, mitochondria and intracytoplasmic membranes could not be demonstrated. With amphotericin B and filipin there is reduction of the cytoplasmic density but no action on nuclei or mitochondria. The decrease in density of the cell is apparently due to loss of material through the cytoplasmic membrane which has lost its selective permeability.

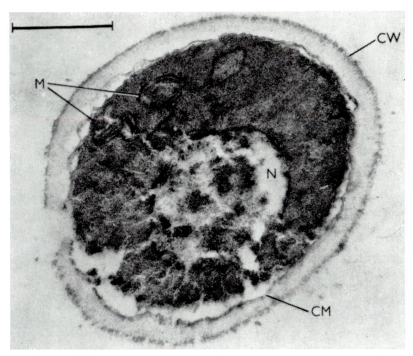

Fig. 16. *Candida albicans* under the action of thiobenzoate. Exposure after 3 hours. Canaliculi radiate from the nucleus to the periphery of the cell. Cytoplasm has partially retracted while the cytoplasmic membrane appears to remain associated with the cell wall. M, mitochondrion. CW, cell wall. CM, cytoplasmic membrane. (From GALE, G.R., and McLAIN, H.H., 1964)

The effect of thiobenzoate has been studied on *C. albicans* (Fig. 16) (GALE and McLAIN, 1964) by observing lessened electron density of the nucleus, formation of canaliculi that radiate from the nucleus to the periphery of the cell, and greater electron density of the cytoplasm.

ADAMS et al. (1963) and WATT et al. (1962) studied the effect of sodium caprylate on *C. albicans*. Budding was inhibited with 2.5×10^{-3}M of sodium caprylate. There were changes in the size and number of mitochondria, and these lacked lamellar structure and presented abnormal cristae.

In order that these studies be fruitful, biochemical observations must be made simultaneously.

Action of Ultrasound on Pathogenic Fungi

REISS and LEONARD (1958) studied the fine structure of *T. mentagrophytes* under the action of ultrasonic irradiation. In comparison with the non-irradiated fungi, the changes consisted mainly of a mechanical damage caused by the microwaves. Besides breakage of mycelia, swelling and bursting of microconidia and damaged cell walls, cavity formation was a common feature.

Fine Structure of Mycoses

The information available on the ultrastructure of pathogenic fungi infecting tissue is scanty. More attention is placed on the parasite itself and less to the reac-

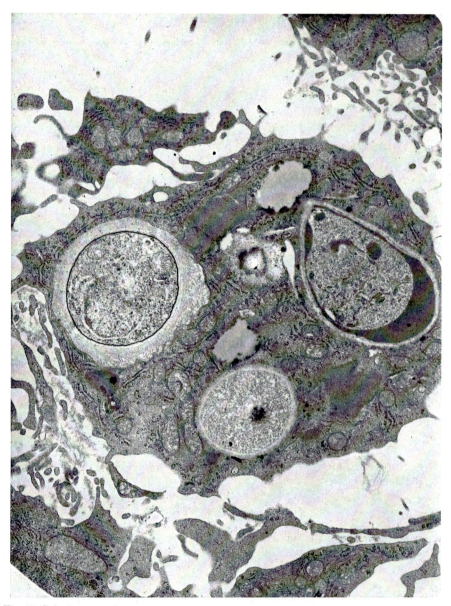

Fig. 17. Splenic macrophage parasitized by three cells of *Histoplasma capsulatum*. The macrophage show mitochondria (M₂), pallid granules, and a considerable ergatoplasm. The fungus cell at lower right has a large granular nucleus (NU), dense mitochondria, endoplasmic reticulum, and a plasma membrane (PM₂). The upper fungus cell shows a cell wall (CW) distinct from the surrounding tissue debris comprising the zonal ring. A small portion of the third fungus cell may be seen at upper left. Osmium fixation. × 24,600
(From Edwards, G. E., et al., 1959)

tion of the host to the parasite. Edwards et al. (1959) studied the spleens of mice infected with *H. capsulatum* and *H. duboisii* (Fig. 17). She found that the fungal cell has all the structural details observed in cultures. *Histoplasma* organisms are localized

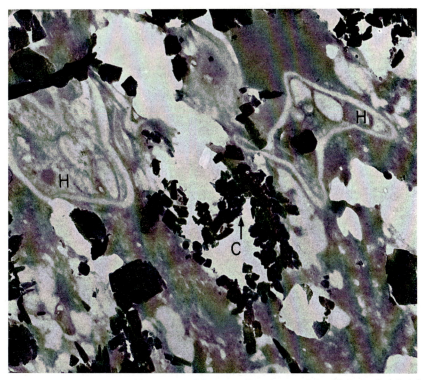

Fig. 18. *Histoplasma capsulatum* in calcified human pulmonary nodule. Observe the abundant electron dense material, identified as calcium (C). Two fungal cells (H) are seen. Both cells show some debris and cytoplasmic organelles which can not be identified. Osmium fixation. × 40,000

in large mononuclear cells (reticuloendothelial cells) and vary in number from one to five. A characteristic feature is a zonal ring between the cell wall of the fungus and the cytoplasm of the host cell. In this space and with high magnification, fragments of the cytoplasm of the host cell are found. In *P. brasiliensis* and *Paracoccidioides loboi* (FURTADO et al., 1967a, b) the same space is found. The reacting edge in *H. capsulatum* is essentially microrugose suggesting that the host cells react in rhythmic fashion to a toxin segregated also rhythmically by the fungus. Near the vicinity of the parasite, dense homogeneous bodies are observed and identified as modified mitochondria. Lipid accumulation, granular cytoplasm and calcifications in the host cells are also found. CARBONELL and ANGULO (1961) studied one coin lesion produced by *H. capsulatum* and found mostly calcified parasites (Fig. 18). However, in a few of them mitochondrial ghosts, plasma membranes and structures resembling nuclei were observed. Outside the parasite, electron dense granules were found; they were identified as calcium.

FURTADO et al. (1967a, b) studied *P. brasiliensis* and *P. loboi* (Figs. 19, 20) in human skin lesions. In *P. brasiliensis* the structures found in cultures are the same as the ones found in tissue. The authors described two types of reproduction in the fungus; formation of catenular series and the well known multiple sporulation. Blastopores have a high content of RNA-protein. In cells with multiple sporulation a large central vacuole is seen pushing the cytoplasm and the other components. *P. loboi* shows the same structures as *P. brasiliensis* and an invagination of the old

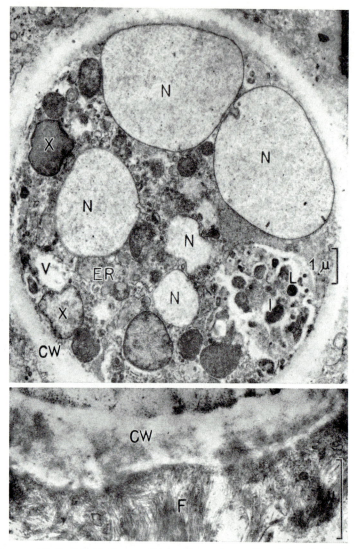

Fig. 19. *Paracoccidioides loboi* in human tissue. Upper figure. Complete cell showing the well preserved wall (CW), vacuoles (V), endoplasmic reticulum (ER), droplets of lipid (L), the various nuclei (N), and unidentified structures (X). Lower figure. Details of the cell wall (CW) showing a poorly osmiophilic inner layer and fibrillar (F), strongly osmiophilic outer layer
(From FURTADO, J.S., et al., 1967)

fungal cell caused by the cytoplasm of the host cell. In *P. brasiliensis* (Figs. 21, 22, 23), in addition to this phenomenon, fibrils from the cell wall can be seen free in the cytoplasm or enclosed in a vacuole. It would be interesting to know the fate of these fibrils since the cell wall may have antigenic properties.

Actinomyces, Nocardia and Streptomyces

Although the *Actinomyces*, *Nocardia* and *Streptomyces* pathogenic for man are not fungi, they are considered as such in this review because they have a mycelium,

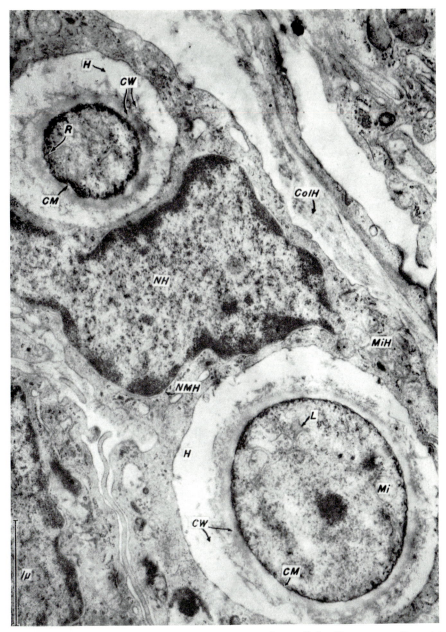

Fig. 20. *Paracoccidioides brasiliensis* in human tissue. Intracellular blastospore adjacent to nucleus of the host (NH). A halo of host reaction (H) with abundant peeling of the cell wall of the fungi (CW). CM, cell membrane. NMH, nuclear membrane of host. MiH, mitochondria of the host. Mi, mitochondria of the fungi. L, lipid. ColH, collagen of host. R, ribonuclein particles. (From Furtado, J.S., et al., 1967)

produce septa and have tip growth. However, they do not have nuclei or mito-chondria which are characteristic features of fungi. Other differences are related to

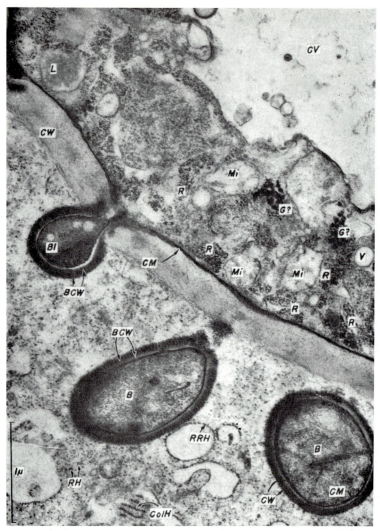

Fig. 21. *Paracoccidioides brasiliensis* in human tissue. Multiple sporulation. BCW, blastopore cell wall. BI, blastopore initial. RH, ribonuclein particle of the host. RRH, rough endoplasmic reticulum of the host. CV, central vacuole. (From Furtado, J.S., et al., 1967)

the composition of the cell wall (Avery and Blank, 1954), ultrastructure (Imaeda, 1965) and phage infections (Bradley et al., 1961). These organisms are classified as Actinomycetes to which Mycobacteriacea, Actinomycetacea and Streptomycetacea belong. Glucosamine, alanine, muramic acid and glutamic acid are the main components of the cell wall of *Actinomycetes*. In comparison, the cell wall of fungi has different types of sugars and their amino derivatives. Phage infections of *Streptomyces* and *Nocardia* definitively suggest their bacterial nature.

Nocardia. There are some reports on the ultrastructure of the genus *Nocardia* (Hagedorn, 1959; Arai et al., 1960) but few that describe *Nocardia asteroides* (Farshtchi and Mc Clung, 1967; Kawata and Inoue, 1965) which produces disease in humans. The cell wall appears as a single electron-dense layer (Kawata

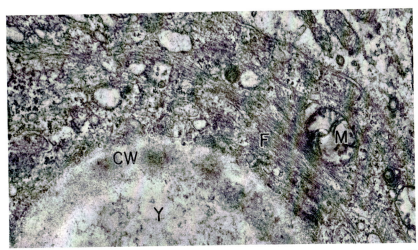

Fig. 22. *Paracoccidioides brasiliensis* in testis of guinea-pig. Observed an empty yeast (Y) in which only an altered cell wall (CW) is identified. Fibrils (F) of the cell wall of the fungi are identified in the cytoplasm. M, mitochondria. Osmium fixation. × 48,000

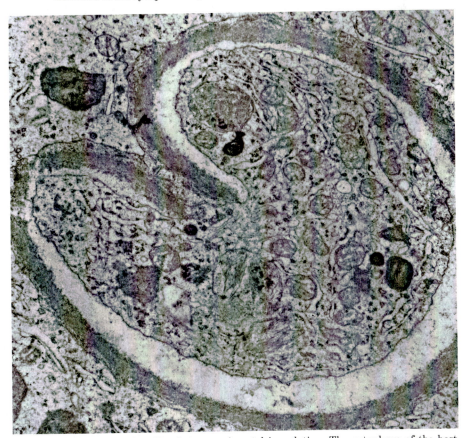

Fig. 23. *Paracoccidioides brasiliensis* in experimental inoculation. The cytoplasm of the host invading an empty cell of the fungus, Osmium fixation. × 44,000

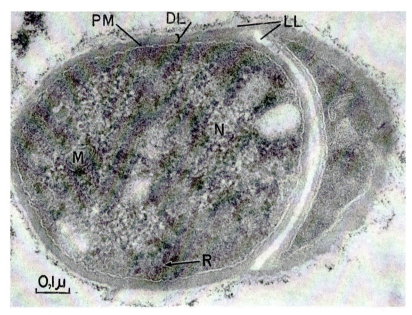

Fig. 24. *Nocardia asteroides*. Late stage of cellular division. The cell to the right is cut obliquely. Outer low density layer (LL), inner moderately dense layer (DL) adherent to the outer plasma membrane (PM), the low density layer can be seen at the septum. Note the ribosomes (R) and nuclear substance (N) in the cytoplasm. Osmium fixation. × 120,000 (Courtesy of Dr. J. A. SERRANO and T. I. IMAEDA)

and INOUE, 1965) or as a triple layered membrane (FARSHTCHI and MC CLUNG, 1967). This difference seems to be related to the age of the organism. Negative staining and shadowing technics reveal on the surface of *N. asteroides*, fibrillar structures similar to the ones described in Mycobacteria (SERRANO and IMAEDA, personal communication). The plasma membrane exhibits two electron dense layers separated by a less electron-dense layer measuring approximately 30 Å each. In the cytoplasmic matrix, electron-dense granules about 150 Å in diameter are identified as ribosomes. The nuclear area is an electron-transparent area located in the center of the organism. The bacterial DNA is represented by fibrils measuring 30 Å, which are observed in this area. These fibrils are interwoven without any definite arrangement. Lipid inclusions are also observed.

Division of *Nocardia* (Figs. 24, 25) begins with the formation of septa similar to the ones described in fungi. In *N. asteroides* a special kind of branching reproduction is described. It begins with a lateral bulging of the cell wall, along any part of the organism, which subsequently develops into a complete filamentous hypha. Mesosomes have also been observed by several authors (FARSHTCHI and MC CLUNG, 1967; KAWATA and INOUE, 1965; SERRANO and IMAEDA, personal communication; SILVA, 1966).

Actinomyces. There are few reports on the fine structure of Actinomycetacea pathogenic to man (EDWARDS and GORDON, 1962; GORDON and EDWARDS, 1963; OVERMAN and PINE, 1963). OVERMAN and PINE (1963) studied the cytoplasmic structures of several *Actinomyces* and found that the cell wall of *Actinomyces bovis* is thinner than that of *Actinomyces israelii*; thus this criteria was advanced for differentiating these two species. Another difference observed in fine structural

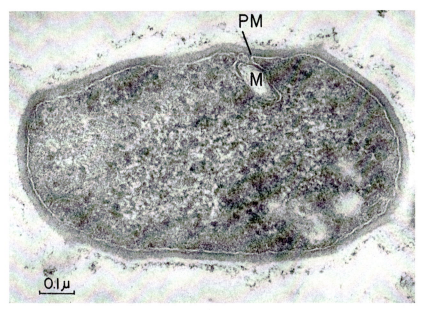

Fig. 25. *Nocardia asteroides*. Early stage of cellular division. Note the connection between the mesosome (M) and the plasma membrane (PM). Osmium fixation. × 120,000 (Courtesy of Drs. J. A. SERRANO and T. I. IMAEDA)

studies is the general morphology: *A. bovis* shows conically shaped cells with budding tips and total absence of the cytoplasmic figures which readily separates it from the rod-like branching form of *A. israelii* containing cytoplasmic figures. In addition, *A. bovis* contains rhamnose and fructose in the cell wall, whereas *A. israelii* has only galactose as its major sugar component (MacLENNAN, 1961).

Dermatophilus congolensis (GORDON and EDWARDS, 1963) is a holocarpic actinomycete which has been found to be transmissible from deer to man (DEAN et al., 1961). This actinomycete has a peculiar developmental morphology: the motile spores form septate hyphae. These proceed by means of perpendicular branching, continued transverse septation, and longitudinal segmentation in two or more planes. At the end of the process, branched, distally tapering filaments, comprising a series of coccal packets resembling those of *Sarcina*, are observed.

A clear cell wall is defined in coccal forms and young filaments. Abundant intracytoplasmic membranes (onion bodies) connected with the plasma membrane are observed. Ribosomes are free in the cytoplasm. A nuclear apparatus, like the one described in bacteria, is observed.

Concluding Remarks

Studies on the ultrastructure of human pathogenic fungi have just begun. The accumulated data show that pathogens are not different from nonpathogens with respect to fine structure. The ultrastructure of lesions caused by fungi is still an unexplored field of research.

Moreover, ultrastructural studies alone have a limited scope; and only the use of the electron microscope combined with histochemical, immunological and biochemical technics will enlarge our knowledge of these mycoses.

References

ADAMS, J.N., PAINTER, B.G., PAYNE, W.J.: Effect of sodium caprylate on *Candida albicans*. I. Influence of concentration on ultrastructure. J. Bact. **86**, 548 (1963). — AGAR, H.D., DOUGLAS, H.C.: Studies of budding and cell wall structure of yeast; electron microscopy of thin sections. J. Bact. **70**, 427 (1955). — ARAI, T., KURODE, S., SUENAZA, T.: Cytological studies on *Streptomyces* and *Nocardia*. Ann. Rep. Inst. Food Microbiol. Ciba Univ. **13**, 32 (1960). — ARONSON, J.M.: The cell wall. In: G.C. AINSWORTH, and A.S. SUSSMAN, Eds. The Fungi, Vol. 1, New York: Academic Press 1965. — AVERY, R.J., BLANK, F.: On the chemical composition of the cell wall of the Actinomycetales and its relation to their systematic position. Canad. J. Microbiol. **1**, 140 (1954). — BARTHOLOMEW, J.W., MITTWER, T.: Demonstration of yeast bud scars with the electron microscope. J. Bact. **65**, 272 (1953). — BLANK, F.: The chemical composition of the cell walls of Dermatophytes. Biochim. biophys. Acta (Amst.) **10**, 110 (1953). ~ On the cell walls of dimorphic fungi causing systemic infections. Canad. J. Microbiol. **1**, 1 (1954). — BLANK, H., TAPLIN, D., ROTH, F.J., Jr.: Electron microscopic observation of the effects of griseofulvin on Dermatophytes. Arch. Derm. **81**, 667 (1960). — BRACKER, C.E., BUTLER, E.E.: Function of the septal pores apparatus in *Rhizoctonia solani* during protoplasmic streaming. J. Cell Biol. **27**, 152 (1964). — BRACKER, C.E.: Ultrastructure of fungi. Ann. Rev. Phytopathol. **5**, 343 (1967). — BRADLEY, S.G., ANDERSON, D.L., JONES, L.A.: Phylogeny of Actinomycetes as revealed by actinophage susceptibility. Develop. Ind. Microbiol. **2**, 223 (1961). — BRESLAU, A.M., HENSLEY, T.J., ERICKSON, J.O.: Electron microscopy of cultured spherules of *Coccidioides immitis*. J. biophys. biochem. Cytol. **9**, 627 (1961). — CARBONELL, L.M., ANGULO, O.A.: Ultraestructura del *Histoplasma capsulatum* en histoplasmomas. Rev. lat.-amer. Anat. pat. **5**, 26 (1961a). — CARBONELL, L.M., POLLAK, L.: Ultraestructura del *Paracoccidioides brasiliensis* en cultivos. Rev. lat.-amer. Anat. pat. **5**, 26 (1961b). ~ "Myelin figures" in yeast cultures of *Paracoccidioides brasiliensis*. J. Bact. **83**, 1356 (1962). ~ Ultraestructura del *Paracoccidioides brasiliensis* en cultivos de la fase levaduriforme. Mycopathologia (Den Haag) **19**, 184 (1963a). ~ Ultraestructura de los hongos especialmente los patógenos. Acta cient. venez. **1**, 174 (1963b). — CARBONELL, L.M., RODRIGUEZ, J.: Transformation of mycelial and yeast forms of *Paracoccidioides brasiliensis* in cultures and in experimental inoculation. J. Bact. **90**, 504 (1965). — CARBONELL, L.M.: Cell wall changes during the budding process of *Paracoccidioides brasiliensis* and *Blastomyces dermatitidis*. J. Bact. **94**, 213 (1967a). ~ Ultraestructura y gemación comparativa del *Paracoccidioides brasiliensis* y del *Blastomyces dermatitidis*. Acta cient. venez. **3**, 277 (1967b). — DEAN, D.J., GORDON, M.A., SEVERINGHAUS, C.W., KROLL, E.T., REILLY, J.R.: Streptothricosis: a new zoonotic disease. N.Y. St. J. Med. **61**, 1283 (1961). — DODGE, B.O.: The life history of *Ascobolus magnificus*: origin of the ascocarp from two strains. Mycologia **12**, 115 (1920). — EDWARDS, G.A, EDWARDS, M.R., HAZEN, E.L.: Electron microscope study of *Histoplasma* in mouse spleen. J. Bact. **77**, 429 (1959). — EDWARDS, G.A., EDWARDS, M.R.: The intracellular membranes of *Blastomyces dermatitidis*. Amer. J. Botany **47**, 622 (1960). — EDWARDS, M.R., HAZEN, E.L., EDWARDS, G.A.: The fine structure of the yeast-like cells of *Histoplasma* in cultures. J. gen. Microbiol. **20**, 496 (1959). — EDWARDS, M.R., GORDON, M.A.: Membrane systems of *Actinomyces bovis*. Fifth Intern. Conf. Electron Microscopy **2**, VV-3 (1962). — EDWARDS, M.R.: Internal and external fine structure of the yeast *Cryptococcus neoformans*. Sixth International Congress for Electron Microscopy Kyoto 783 (1966). — EDWARDS, M.R., GORDON, M.A., LAPA, E.W., GHIORSE, W.C.: Micromorphology of *Cryptococcus neoformans*. J. Bact. **94**, 766 (1967). — ELLAR, D.J., LUNDGREN, D.G., SLEPECKY, R.A.: Fine structure of *Bacillus megaterium* during synchronous growth. J. Bact. **94**, 1189 (1967). — ERICKSON, J.O., BRESLAU, A.M.: Electron microscopy of *Coccidioides immitis*. Fed. Proc. **19**, 243 (1960). — FARSHTCHI, D., McCLUNG, N.M.: Fine structure of *Nocardia asteroides* grown in a chemically defined medium. J. Bact. **94**, 255 (1967). — FAWCET, D.W.: An atlas of fine structure. The cell, its organelles and inclusions, 448 pp. Philadelphia: Saunders 1966. — FURTADO, J.S., DE BRITO, T., FREYMULLER, E.: The fine structure and reproduction of *Paracoccidioides brasiliensis* in human tissue. Sabouraudia **5**, 226 (1967a). ~ Structure and reproduction of *Paracoccidioides loboi*. Mycologia **59**, 286 (1967b). — GALE, G.R.: Cytology of *Candida albicans* as influenced by drugs acting on the cytoplasmic membrane. J. Bact. **86**, 151 (1963). — GALE, G.R., McLAIN, H.H.: Effect of thiobenzoate on cytology of *Candida albicans*. J. gen. Microbiol. **36**, 297 (1964). — GORDON, M.A., EDWARDS, M.R.: Micromorphology of *Dermatophylus congolensis*. J. Bact. **86**, 1101 (1963). — GROCOTT, R.G.: A stain for fungi in tissue sections and smears using Gomori's methenamine silver nitrate technic. Amer. J. clin. Path. **25**, 975 (1955). — HAGEDORN, H.: Licht- und elektronenmikroskopische Untersuchungen an *Nocardia corallina* (BERGEY et al., 1923). Zbl. Bakt., II. Abt. **112**, 214 (1959). — HASHIMOTO, T., KISHI, T., YOSHIDA, N.: Demonstration of micropore in fungal cross-wall. Nature (Lond.) **202**, 1353 (1964). — HASHIMOTO, T., YOSHIDA, N.: Unique membranous system associated with glycogen synthesis in an imperfect fungus, *Geotrichum candidum*. In electron microscopy. Proc. 6th

Intern. Congr. Electron Microscopy Kyoto 1966, **11**, 305 (Maruzen Co., Tokyo). — HAWKER, L. E.: Fine structure of fungi as revealed by electron microscopy. Biol. Rev. **40**, 52 (1965). — HOUWINK, A. L., KREGER, D. R.: Observations on the cell wall of yeast. An electron microscope and X-ray diffraction study. Antonie v. Leeuwenhoek **19**, 1 (1953). — IMAEDA, T., OGURA, M.: Formation of intracytoplasmic membrane system of mycobacteria related to cell division. J. Bact. **85**, 150 (1963). — IMAEDA, T.: Electron microscopy. Approach to leprosy research. Int. J. Leprosy **33**, 669 (1965). — IKEDA, H.: An electron microscopic study of *Trichophyton rubrum*. Jap. J. Derm. **74**, 269 (1964). — ITO, Y., SETOGUTI, T., NOZAWA, Y., SAKURAI, S.: An electron microscopic observation of *Trichophyton violaceum*. J. invest. Derm. **48**, 124 (1967). — IWATA, K., IRATA, T.: Studies on the fine structures of the cell of pathogenic fungi by electron microscope. I. On the fine structure of *Candida albicans*. Jap. J. Bact. **18**, 393 (1963). — KANETSUNA, F., CARBONELL, L. M.: Glycogen in yeast form of *Paracoccidioides brasiliensis*. Nature (Lond.) **208**, 686 (1965). ∼ Enzymes in glycolysis and the citric acid cycle in the yeast and mycelial forms of *Paracoccidioides brasiliensis*. J. Bact. **92**, 1315 (1966). — KAWATA, T., INOUE, T.: Ultrastructure of *Nocardia asteroides* as revealed by electron microscopy. Jap. J. Microbiol. **9**, 101 (1965). — KIRK, B. T., SINCLAIR, J. B.: Plasmodesmata between hyphal cell of *Geotrichum candidum*. Science **153**, 1646 (1966). — LADEN, E. L., ERICKSON, J. O.: Electron microscope study of *Epidermophyton floccosum*. J. invest. Derm. **31**, 55 (1958). — LOWRY, R. J., SUSSMAN, S.: Intra-hyphal hyphae in "clock" mutants of *Neurospora*. Mycologia **43**, 541 (1966). — MAC LENNAN, A. P.: Composition of the cell wall of *Actinomyces bovis*, the isolation of 6-deoxy-L-talose. Biochim. biophys. Acta (Amst.) **48**, 600 (1961). — MALFATI, M. G., ZAPATA, R. C.: El dimorfismo de algunos hongos patógenos observados a travéz del microscopio el ectrónico. Pren. méd. argent. **41**, 3869 (1954). — MEINHOF, W.: Untersuchungen zur Ultrastruktur von *Microsporum* von *Keratinomyces Ajelloi* Vanbreuseghem 1952. Arch. klin. exp. Derm. **226**, 33 (1966). ∼ Untersuchungen zur Ultrastruktur von *Microsporum gypseum* (BODIN, 1907), Guiart et Grigoraki, 1928. I. Aufbau der Zellwand der Septen und der cytoplasmatischen Membran. Arch. klin. exp. Derm. **228**, 111 (1967a). ∼ Untersuchungen zur Ultrastruktur von *Microsporum gypseum* (BODIN, 1907), Guiart et Grigoraki, 1928. II. Aufbau und Vermehrung der Mitochondrien. Arch. klin. exp. Derm. **228**, 122 (1967b). ∼ Untersuchungen zur Ultrastruktur von *Trichophyton verrucosum* (BODIN, 1902) und *Trichophyton schönleinii* (LEBERT, LANGERON et MILOCHEVITCH, 1930). Arch. klin. exp. Derm. **229**, 265 (1967c). — MIZUNO, N., MONTEZ, L. F.: Oxidative enzyme activity in *Candida albicans*. Sabouraudia **5**, 46 (1966). — MONTES, L. F., PATRICK, T. A., MARTIN, S. A., SMITH, M. S.: Ultrastructure of blastospore of *Candida albicans* after permanganate fixation. J. invest. Derm. **45**, 227 (1965). — MOORE, H., MUHLETHALER, H.: Fine structure in frozenetched yeast cell. J. Cell Biol. **17**, 609 (1963). — MOORE, R. T., McALEAR, J. H.: Fine structure of mycota. 5 Lomasomes previously uncharacterized hyphal structures. Mycologia **53**, 194 (1961a). ∼ Fine structure of mycota. Reconstruction from skipped serial sections of the nuclear envelope and its continuity with the plasma membrane. Exp. Cell Res. **24**, 588 (1961b). ∼ Fine structure of mycota. 7. Observation on septa of Ascomycetes and Basidiomycetes. Amer. J. Botany **49**, 86 (1962). ∼ Fine structure of mycota. 9. Fungal mitochondria. J. Ultrastruct. Res. **8**, 144 (1963). — NICKERSON, W. J., FALCONE, G.: Identification of protein disulfide reductase as a cellular division enzyme in yeast. Science **124**, 722 (1956). — O'HERN, E. M., HENRY, B. S.: A cytological study of *Coccidioides immitis* by electron microscopy. J. Bact. **72**, 632 (1956). — OVERMAN, J. R., PINE, L.: Electron microscopy of cytoplasmic structures in facultative and anaerobic *Actinomyces*. J. Bact. **86**, 656 (1963). — RAMBOURG, A.: An improved silver methenamine technique for the detection of periodic acid-reactive complex carbohydrates with the electron microscope. J. Histochem. Cytochem. **15**, 409 (1967). — REICHLE, R. E., ALEXANDER, J. V.: Multiperforate septations, Woronin bodies, and septal plugs in *Fusarium*. J. Cell Biol. **24**, 489 (1965). — REISS, F., LEONARD, L.: Electron microscopic studies of ultrasonic irradiated *Trichophyton mentagrophytes*. Dermatologica (Basel) **117**, 401 (1958). — REYNOLDS, E. S.: The use of lead citrate at high pH as an electron-opaque stain in electron microscopy. J. Cell Biol. **17**, 208 (1963). — RIBI, E., HOYER, B. H., GOODE, G.: The fine structure of the cell wall of *Histoplasma capsulatum* as revealed by electron microscopy and X-ray diffraction studies. Fed. Proc. **15**, 105 (1956). — RIBI, E., SALVIN, S. B.: Antigens from the yeast phase of *Histoplasma capsulatum*. I. Morphology of the cell as revealed by the electron microscope. Exp. Cell Res. **10**, 394 (1956). — SABATINI, D. D., BENSCH, K., BARNETT, R. J.: Cytochemistry and electron microscopy. The preservation of cellular ultrastructure and enzymatic activity by aldehyde fixation. J. Cell Biol. **17**, 19 (1963). — SELIGMAN, A. M., HAUKER, J., WASSERKRUG, H., DMOCHOWSKI, H., KATZOFF, L.: Histochemical demonstration of some oxidized macromolecules with thiocarbohydrazide (TCH) or thiosemicarbazide (TSC) and osmium tetroxide. J. Histochem. Cytochem. **13**, 629 (1965). — SERRANO, J. A., IMAEDA, T.: Mecanismo de la transformación a "Formas L" de Actinomycetales (Personal communication). — SILVA, M. T.: Studies on the fixation of the mesosomes of some gram-positive bacteria for electron microscopy. Proc. 6th Int. Congress for Electron Microscopy, 1966. **11**, 275 (Maruzen Co., Ltd.,

Japan). — Streiblova, E., Beran, K.: Demonstration of yeast scars by fluorescence microscopy. Exp. Cell Res. **30**, 603 (1963). — Streiblova, E., Malek, I., Beran, K.: Structural changes in the cell wall of *Schizosaccharomyces pombe* during cell division. J. Bact. **91**, 428 (1966). — Sussman, A. S., Durkee, T. L., Lowry, R. J.: A model for rhythmic and temperature-independent growth in "clock" mutants of *Neurospora*. Mycopathologia (Den Haag) **25**, 381 (1965). — Taplin, D., Blank, H.: Microscopic morphology of *Trichophyton rubrum*. J. invest. Derm. **37**, 523 (1961). — Thyagarajan, T. R., Conti, S. F., Naylor, H. B.: Electron microscopy of yeast mitochondria. Exp. Cell Res. **25**, 216 (1961). — Tomomatsu, S.: A study on griseofulvin. I. Comparison of electron microscopic observations of effects of griseofulvin with that of fungicidal drugs. Bull. pharm. Res. Inst. **26**, 11 (1960). — Tsukahara, T.: Cytological structures of *Cryptococcus neoformans*. Jap. J. Microbiol. **7**, 53 (1963). — Tsukahara, T., Sato, A., Okada, R.: Electron microscopic studies on the cytological structure of *Trichophyton mentagrophytes*. Jap. J. Microbiol. **8**, 83 (1964). — Watson, M. L.: Staining of tissue section for electron microscopy with heavy metals. J. biophys. biochem. Cytol. **4**, 475 (1958a). ~ Staining of tissue sections for electron microscopy with heavy metals. II. Application of solution containing lead and barium. J. biophys. biochem. Cytol. **4**, 727 (1958b). — Watt, L. S., Adams, J. N., Payne, W. J.: Cytological and physiological effects of sodium caprylate on *Candida albicans*. Antibiot. and Chemother. **12**, 173 (1962). — Werner, H. J.. Jolly, H. W., Lee, J. H.: Electron microscopic observations of *Epidermophyton floccosum*. J. invest. Derm. **43**, 139 (1964). — Werner, H. J., Jolly, H. W., Spurlock, B. O.: Electron microscope observations of the fine structure of *Microsporum canis*. J. invest. Derm. **46**, 130 (1966). — Werner, H. J., Catsulis, C., Jolly, H. W., Carpenter, C. L.: Electron microscope observations of the fine structure of *Microsporum gypseum*. J. invest. Derm. **48**, 481 (1967). — Wilsenach, R., Kessel, M.: The role of lomasomes in wall formation in *Penicillium vermiculatum*. J. gen. Microbiol. **40**, 401 (1965a). ~ Micropores in the cross-wall of *Geotrichum candidum*. Nature (Lond.) **207**, 545 (1965b). — Wilson, W. J., Plunkett, O. A.: The fungous diseases of man. University of Calif. Press, Berkeley, Los Angeles, 1965.

Histoplasmosis

JAN SCHWARZ, Cincinnati/Ohio, USA

With 35 Figures

Definition

Histoplasmosis is a disease apparently almost world-wide in distribution, with great variations of incidence in different localities. Histoplasmosis is generally caused by *Histoplasma capsulatum* Darling, and rarely (in Africa) by *Histoplasma duboisii* Vanbreuseghem.

The portal of entrance in natural disease is the lung, where a primary focus is formed which commonly becomes arrested and calcified. Probably more than 95% of all primary infections are benign and self-limited, or even subclinical. The frequency of infection in lower animals, specifically mice, rats, dogs, cattle, and horses, is similar to that in man (EMMONS, 1950; FURCOLOW and MENGES). The rare disseminated form of the disease is especially dangerous in infants, causing hepatosplenomegaly, fever, anemia, leukopenia, and enteric ulcerations. A so-called "epidemic" type occurs after inhalation of heavy concentrations of spores in such places as silos, abandoned chicken houses, storm cellars, and caves infested with bats or birds. In man, chronic pulmonary cavitary disease is seen most often in middle age. "Solitary" tumor-like lesions, "histoplasmomas," occur in all age groups, but are rare in children. They are most often 2 to 3 cm in size when detected. Other important complications are adrenal caseation, meningoencephalitis, endocarditis, pericarditis, and a questionable, but possibly common, eye involvement.

History

Histoplasmosis was discovered in 1905 by the young pathologist, DARLING, in Panama. The discovery, like many before and after, illustrates the fact that an able and intuitive observer at the right time and place can make discoveries of things that should have been obvious to many before him and to contemporaries. Under the influence of the then recent findings by LEISHMAN and DONOVAN, DARLING mistook the organism for a protozoan. In 1912, DA ROCHA-LIMA first ventured the opinion that *H. capsulatum* was a yeast and not a protozoan organism. In 1906, STRONG, an American, described organisms he had observed in the Phillipine Islands, which could have been *H. capsulatum*, but there is no way to verify this assumption.

The first culture of *H. capsulatum* was obtained in 1933 by DEMONBREUN at Vanderbilt University in Nashville, Tennessee. DEMONBREUN had been advised by the clinicians of the imminent death of a child with histoplasmosis, diagnosed during life from blood smears. He prepared numerous culture media and did not discard the mold which was growing from the organs of the child, although it was unexpectedly and completely different from the yeast seen in the tissues. Thus almost 30 years elapsed between recognition of the dimorphic character of *H. capsulatum* and its culture, and one can only guess how many investigators must have, in these 30 years, cultured the mold form of this organism and discarded it, believing it to be a contaminant.

Around 1940 it became increasingly apparent that in the United States many children and adults had intrathoracic calcifications not associated with positive tuberculin skin tests. It was therefore only a question of time until someone would use antigens other than tuberculin for skin testing: CHRISTIE and PETERSON, again at Vanderbilt University, were the first to use *histoplasmin* in an epidemiologic survey. In 1944, CHRISTIE reported: "It was clear to me shortly after I came here and learned about histoplasmosis and its similarity to tuberculosis

5*

and coccidioidomycosis, that the proper lead was to try and find the benign form of the infection to explain the pulmonary calcification in tuberculin negative people in the area." Palmer, Furcolow, and many others in subsequent series confirmed the existence of subclinical cases of histoplasmosis which reacted positively to the skin test.

Epidemiology

The possibility that the disease is airborn was at first clinically suspected and expressed after investigators observed epidemic outbreaks occurring after brief stays of persons in storm cellars (Cain et al.), chicken coops (Adriano et al.), caves (Ajello et al., 1962; Dean); the disease could often be traced to the presence of *H. capsulatum* in the soil of areas containing feces from chickens, other birds, and bats. Lately, successful cultures of *H. capsulatum* from bat tissues and intestines have been reported (Klite and Diercks) but the exact role of birds and bats in the epidemiology of histoplasmosis is not yet clear. The recent report of Tewari and Campbell on the affinity of *H. capsulatum* to chicken feathers could open new leads about the significance of chickens at sites of heavy concentration of *H. capsulatum* in the soil. The proven susceptibility of chickens and pigeons to intraocular and intracerebral inoculation with *H. capsulatum* (Sethi and Schwarz, 1965 and 1966) highlights the potential importance of birds in the epidemiology of the disease.

The anatomic proof that the lung is the portal of entrance was brought into focus by Straub and Schwarz (1960); in persons dying of diseases other than histoplasmosis in Cincinnati, located in the center of the endemic area, we found calcified pulmonary lesions, products of infection with *H. capsulatum*, in 84% of consecutive unselected autopsies. The organisms were demonstrated in every instance by the Gridley or Grocott (Straub and Schwarz) procedures, and subsequently by fluorescent antibody stains (Yamaguchi et al.).

Geographic Pathology

Histoplasmosis occurs very commonly in an area comprising the Ohio-Mississippi Valley in the USA, where up to 90% of the population tested react positively to the histoplasmin skin test. However, outside this "endemic" area, histoplasmosis is by no means a rarity (Edwards and Palmer); focal outbreaks have been seen in many parts of the world, and endemicity, measured by positive skin tests, of 30—50% is quite common in many parts of Central and South America, Africa, Indonesia, and other areas (Edwards and Klaer). When more data become available from Asia, very likely more endemic areas will be identified. Isolated cultures from soil have been obtained in Italy (Sotgiu et al.; Mantovani et al.), and intensified research along these lines should reveal new sources of the disease in Europe and elsewhere (Ajello, 1967).

H. capsulatum has been repeatedly isolated from the bowel mucosa of several species of bats (Klite and Diercks). Whether the bat is *the* animal reservoir or an accidental carrier of the organism is at present not decided. The bat defecates 60 times or more *per diem*, and in view of its habit of roosting in caves, trees, and attics, must constitute a prime source of dissemination of the organism in nature. Numerous epidemics related to visits in caves are on record (Ajello, Campins, Gonzalez-Ochoa, Dean, Jackson, Murray et al.), and conceivably epidemics arising from soil excavation or transport may be also related to bat droppings rather than to starlings and other birds, which have been incriminated in the past. The bat is a proven carrier of the organisms; the birds, so far, are *not*. The connection with inhalation of spore-containing soil is overwhelmingly convincing from numerous outbreaks, and the presence and prolonged survival of *H. capsulatum* in soil is beyond any question.

The epidemiology of *Histoplasma duboisii* is less well established and definite statements in regard to this organism will have to be left to the future.

The transmission in natural infection in man is therefore from soil to man, and no proof exists of transmission from man to man or of animal to man or *vice versa*. However, in view of the overwhelmingly benign character of the primary infection, which commonly is asymptomatic, transmission from man to man has not been

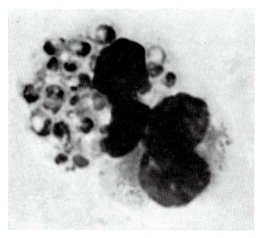

Fig. 1. *Histoplasma capsulatum* in a macrophage. Tissue press with simple Wright stain shows the organisms excellently; this is the fastest and best method of diagnosis of superficial erosions, shallow mucosal ulcers, cut surfaces from organs at autopsy, or in experimental pathology. Wright stain × 1600

eliminated on exact clinical grounds at least as an occasional *possibility*, especially considering the abundance of organisms in the sputum of cavitary cases. Such patients may eliminate so many organisms that they can be recovered in culture from every sputum or can even be recognized microscopically in the sputum by a simple Wright stain (Fig. 1) or by the more sophisticated fluorescent antibody procedure (CARSKI et al.). We recently recovered *H. capsulatum* from 10 consecutive sputa of a cavitary case; this is the rule rather than the exception in chronic pulmonary cavitary disease.

Mycology

Histoplasma capsulatum, first cultured from a patient by DEMONBREUN in 1933, and first isolated from soil by EMMONS in 1948, is a dimorphic organism, presenting in the animal body and at 37° C as a yeast of 2 to 5 μ in size. The yeast form grows on blood agar or Kurung's egg medium as a moist white "yeast" colony. Colonies in the yeast form become visible on subculture as soon as 18 hours after inoculation of media. In contrast, the mycelial form found in nature (outside the animal body) and in the laboratory at room temperature (24—28° C), appears as a slow-growing white cottony colony after 2 weeks or more. Mounts after 2 weeks or more reveal septate hyphae, often with racquet-hyphae, numerous small conidia of about 2 to 3 μ, and variable amounts of large spores, smooth or with tuberculate projections, the latter pathognomonic for the species.

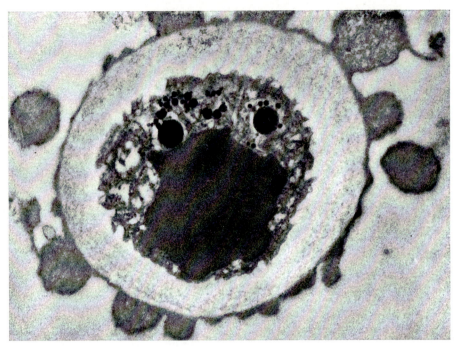

Fig. 2. Electromicrograph of tuberculate spore (courtesy, M. R. EDWARDS et al.). Tuberculation is shown to be a warty formation of the cell without a connection with the cytoplasm of the spore. The large black spot represents lipid; two sharply outlined black dots surrounded by smaller ones are microdroplets of the same

The circumspect mycologist who has isolated the mold will always insist upon the induction of the yeast phase in order to clinch the diagnosis. The organisms, when *injected into mice* or hamsters (the two most susceptible species of laboratory animals), will produce progressive disease and death when given intravenously or intracerebrally and in large numbers. Intraperitoneal or subcutaneous infection may not always lead to widespread dissemination, especially with a small inoculum. Sometimes the yeast phase can be induced *in vitro* only after repeated transfers on protein-containing media, and the yeast culture (labile form) always has the tendency to revert to the mycelial (stable) form. Intermediate forms can therefore be seen on culture mounts, containing yeast cells which sometimes form chains of budding yeast and hyphae. Sabouraud's glucose agar quite adequately supports the growth of the organism in the mycelial form.

When organ particles in primary isolates from animal or human sources are placed on the surface of the *agar*, waxy colonies frequently are produced at room temperature. This smooth surface can persist for 2 or more weeks and is only slowly covered by white cottony mold growth from the periphery of the colony. Both the change of phase (depending on temperature and media), and the waxy character on primary culture in the presence of blood or tissue particles is confusing to the neophyte.

The number of large spores, about 10 μ in diameter, is only 4% of the spore total (COZAD and FURCOLOW), but in view of their size and shape they are prominent and outshine the inconspicuous small conidia. However, it is the small conidia which are the true sources of infection, since the size of the large spores pre-

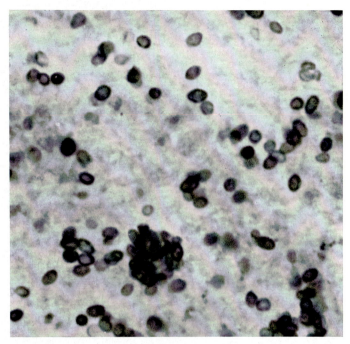

Fig. 3. Large numbers of *H. capsulatum* organisms are frequently found in the center of a primary focus, irrespective of the age of the lesion. Even completely petrified foci preserve the organisms well. The organism is prevented from disintegration by a chitinous envelope. Grocott × 1300

vents their entering the lung in most instances (HATCH). Again, only about 22% of the large spores show tuberculated surfaces (COZAD and FURCOLOW), but the tuberculate macroconidium is a *conditio sine qua non* for laboratory diagnosis. The fine structure of the organism in both the yeast and mycelial forms has been studied by EDWARDS et al. (1959, 1960) in electron photomicrographs (Fig. 2).

Staining of Histoplasma Capsulatum in Tissues

Without the benefit of special stains *H. capsulatum* will often be overlooked in tissue sections, particularly in necrotic and calcified materials. Calcific particles, nuclear fragments and red cells are frequently mistaken for yeast cells in H & E stain. It is our conviction that search for *H. capsulatum* in H & E sections is, especially in necrotic or calcific areas, unproductive of correct results, wasteful in time and effort, and downright wrong. The stain of choice for the demonstration of *H. capsulatum* is the *Grocott-Gomori methenamine silver stain* (Figs. 3, 4). The method is technically simple (when clean glassware is used and the temperature requirements fulfilled), gives excellent contrast, both for search and photography, and produces a constant image with easily demonstrated constant size and shape of the organism. Controls from human or experimental animal sources must be available for every group of stained sections.

In decalcified material we found great improvement of the staining of the yeast cells by shortening the prescribed 45 min oxidation in chromic acid to 10 min. We recommend as counter-stain a short dip of the sections into hematoxylin (10 sec), which facilitates orientation for the examiner with the recognition of the landmarks of histology. The superiority of the

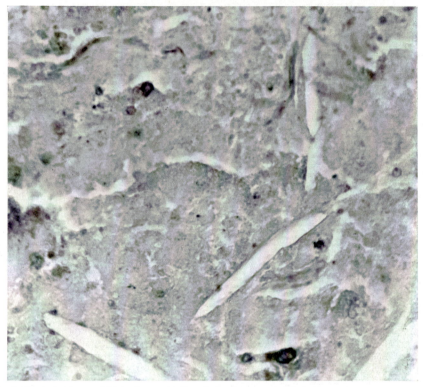

Fig. 4. Necrotic tissue of histoplasmosis. Search for *H. capsulatum* in H & E sections of necrotic
tissue is misleading. Calcific particles mimic *H. capsulatum*. H & E × 500

Grocott procedure is so self-evident that it would seem unnecessary to document this fact. But
almost daily experience teaches that many institutions have started with the PAS stain, never
to abandon it.

Of 122 histoplasmomas in Steele's paper, 118 showed organisms with the Grocott, 32 with
the Gridley stain, and only 24 with PAS. Of 84 granulomas submitted as "unidentified etiology,"
83 were stained with the Grocott procedure: 53 were positive (*H. capsulatum*); 70, when stained
with the Gridley stain, gave only 9 positives, and 60 PAS gave 17 positives. The Grocott procedure gives excellent results according to Schulz et al. (1958), Greendyke and Emerson,
Straub and Schwarz (1960), and others.

The Gridley stain of the yeast cells is frequently lacking in intensity, varying from deep
lavender to very pale red, which makes difficult the finding of isolated cells. However, good
contrast will be found in some instances, and we have occasionally seen yeast cells with the
Gridley stain when none were recognized in the Grocott. Therefore, in our laboratory — where
staining for fungi is done several times a week — Grocott and Gridley stains are examined in
the search for an etiologic diagnosis in a granuloma. Since elastic, and to a slight degree collagen, fibers take the color of Schiff's reagent, transverse sections of such fibers are sometimes
mistaken for yeast cells (Schulz et al., 1958).

The lack of contrast and weak staining of yeast cells with PAS stain is very noticeable, and
while the PAS method signified great progress, and was later improved by Gridley, it was
not as satisfactory as Grocott's method. A comparative paper in 1955 by Kade and Kaplan
discusses the Hotchkiss-McManus, Bauer, and Gridley stains, but does not include the Grocott
stain; it should, however, be consulted for a list of Schiff-reagent positive substances and useful
suggestions of slight modifications in using the 3 procedures.

Fluorochrome stains, while not specific, can lead to recognition of yeast cells in sputum, in
tissues, and in blood smears (Holland and Holland). On the other hand, the *fluorescent antibody stain*, highly specific on theoretic grounds, can be quite disappointing, unless high titer
and absorbed antiserum is available, and unless sets of controls are used. In tissues, fluorescent

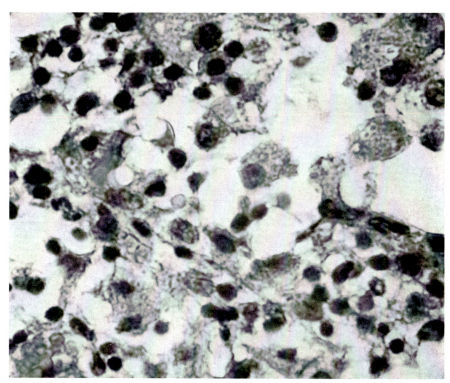

Fig. 5. *Penicillium marneffei* isolated from a bamboo-rat (Segretain) has a superficial resemblance to, and the same intracellular location as, *H. capsulatum*. Experimental infection of mouse 80 days after intraperitoneal injection. H & E × 700

antibody stains are of limited value, especially if formalin, Zenker, and other fixed material must be used. The reaction in tissues is unpredictable and is at best capricious. This is indeed not meant as criticism of an outstanding method in principle, but as a confession of often frustrating impotence when culturally proven cases, with morphologically consistent yeast forms, do not stain with the fluorescent antibody method. Only two reports on the use of the fluorescent antibody stain in histologic preparations come to mind (Procknow et al., Yamaguchi et al.). whereas extensive and successful use has been made in sputum and culture material (Carski et al., Kaufman and Kaplan, Lynch and Plexico, Rezai and Haberman).

Morphologic Variations of *H. capsulatum*: Variations in the morphology of *H. capsulatum* are not frequent but are important. Ordinarily, the organism is seen in its yeast form in animal tissues. The usual size is 1 to 5 μ with an average of about 3 μ, the shape varying from round to oval. However, in necrotic tissue, larger yeast cells are found (Silverman et al.) and exceptionally short filaments have been seen in endocarditis (Binford) and in meningitis (Gerber et al.), which can be recognized as *H. capsulatum* only with the help of positive culture and from the presence of typical yeast cells in addition to the atypical forms.

Unusually large cells of *H. capsulatum* are differentiated from small yeasts of *Blastomyces dermatitidis* in well-fixed material by demonstrating the uninuclear nature of *H. capsulatum* as opposed to *B. dermatitidis*, which exhibits several nuclei. The organism *Leishmania donovani* has a rodlike parabasal body (kinetoplast), best seen on Giemsa or Wright stain, which is absent in *H. capsulatum*; but while *H. capsulatum* stains readily with the PAS and similar procedures, Leishmania bodies do not stain. However, in tissues, the differentiation on HE can be

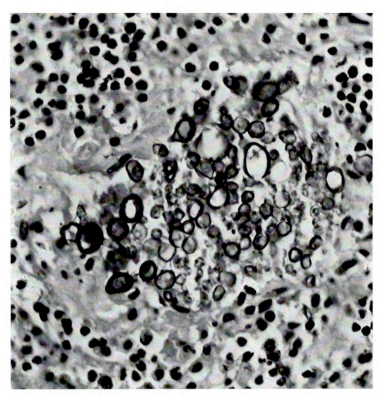

Fig. 6. *H. capsulatum* shows irregular huge yeast forms in necrotic lesions, sometimes on heart valves and in tissue slides left for several days on the surface of agar in the incubator. The large forms represent spheroplasts of organisms and must be considered moribund nonreproductive cells. H & E × 650

close to impossible, and confusion has occurred on attempts of morphologic diagnosis (Woo and Reimann). Both organisms are indeed selectively found in phagocytic cells.

Rare organisms appearing similar to *H. capsulatum* are *Penicillium marneffei* (Fig. 5) (Segretain) and *Paecilomyces viridis* (Segretain et al.).

The differentiation of individual (single) cells of *Pneumocystis carinii* from *H. capsulatum* can be quite difficult unless some beanlike or dishlike (Napfform) bodies are seen within the Pneumocystis. If many organisms are present, the intra-alveolar location of *P. carinii* will be decisive in the differentiation from *H. capsulatum*, which will be found in confluent caseated lesions or nodular granulomas but hardly ever — and certainly not in large amounts — in the alveolar content. The similar size and shape of *Candida albicans* can present a considerable problem unless the pseudohyphae of Candida suggest the nature of the organism. Other yeasts (e.g., Hansenula, Saccharomyces) can be quite confusing when found in leukocytes (Wang and Schwarz). M. Moore mentions that small forms of *Blastomyces brasiliensis* may possibly be confused with *H. capsulatum*.

The morphology on silver stain of *Coniosporium (Cryptostroma) corticale*, the agent producing maple bark disease, is surprisingly similar to *H. capsulatum*, but the unstained spores of *Cryptostroma* have a brown to black color (Towey et al.; Emanuel et al.).

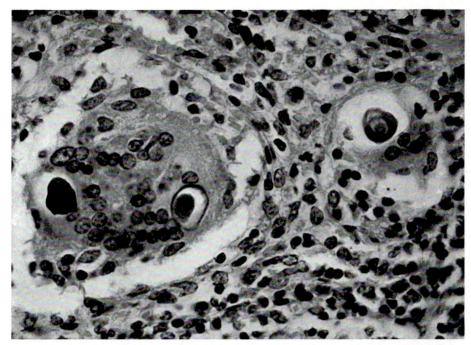

Fig. 7. Experimental histoplasmosis. In many organs of the hamster, crustaceous envelopes, comparable to the Schaumann bodies of "sarcoid" and other disorders of man are found surrounding yeast cells. H & E × 650

Giant forms of *H. capsulatum* have been seen in necrotic tissue and old cultures, but can also be induced at will in tissue particles kept on agar plates in the incubator at 37° C (Fig. 6). Forms up to 20 μ were produced on such explants (SCHWARZ, 1953), which was essentially confirmed by PINE et al. in liquid media. PINE et al. interpreted the huge, odd-shaped cells as spheroplasts — cells in the terminal phase of growth, incapable of further development. According to PINE et al., the large forms, rarely seen in human and animal tissue, and the large forms obtained in tissue explants (SCHWARZ) can be considered as spheroplasts.

Still other bewildering morphologic images are obtained after injection of culture material into the golden hamster (Fig. 7). This species (*Cricetus auratus*) reacts to the introduction of numerous heterogenous microorganisms, including *H. capsulatum*, with the formation of concentric structures: Schaumann bodies (OKUDAIRA et al.). The mechanism of this extraordinary reaction is unknown; the chemical composition of the bodies seems to be hydroxyapatite (RASMUSSEN and CAULFIELD). FRENKEL interprets the Schaumann bodies in the hamster as an expression of cellular immunity which results in isolation of the fungus by incrustation either intra- or extracellularly.

Pathogenesis

Histoplasma capsulatum produces a variety of tissue reactions in the human body. The overwhelming infection commonly observed in infants, but rarely in later life, is characterized by almost exclusive and intense *proliferation of histiocytes* (each the carrier of several to numerous yeast cells). The number and size of such

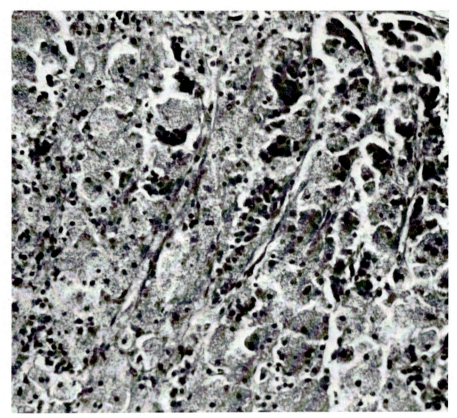

Fig. 8. Histoplasmosis of adrenal gland. Huge macrophages have replaced cortical cells of the adrenal gland. Fine granularity of their cytoplasm denotes the presence of yeast cells. H & E
× 300

histiocytes often leads to complete obliteration of the normal architecture of organs; this is especially true in the spleen, bone marrow, lymph nodes, and liver, but is also seen in the intestinal mucosa, the lung, and in other organs (Fig. 8). Frequently, the histiocytic foci are so overwhelming that it becomes impossible to determine whether foci of necrosis are occurring in the "normal tissue" or in the histiocytic infiltrates. Specialized entities like the Kupffer cells of the liver swell greatly in such instances and are completely filled with yeast cells. Such widely disseminated cases — while impressive — are rare and are not at all typical or representative of the disease histoplasmosis.

In addition to the "cytomycosis" variety, a gamut of lesions can be observed, from nodular histiocytic formations with few organisms to epithelioid cell ("tubercles" with Langhans giant cells, the latter indistinguishable from tuberculous lesions or — if not caseated — from sarcoid (Fig. 9). The demonstration of organisms in epithelioid-cell tubercles without caseation is one of the most tedious of searches, and perfect special stains (Grocott, Gridley) are unconditional prerequisites. When caseation ensues, yeast cells are generally more numerous, but the use of special stains is again indispensable for recognition of the organisms. The most misleading conclusions will be made on inspection of H & E sections, since cell debris, calcium particles, and other fragments can simulate *H. capsulatum*.

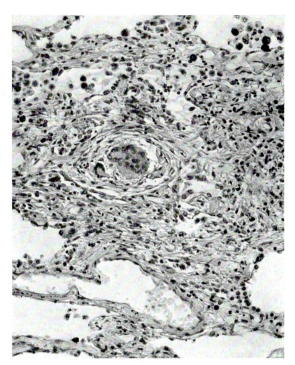

Fig. 9. Histoplasmic tubercle of lung. Interstitial "tubercular" lesions are indistinguishable from similar lesions produced by other agents (bacterial, fungal, inorganic). Small scars result from healing lesions of undisclosed etiology. H & E × 160

The degree of tissue destruction increases with the size of the individual focus but is seldom complete, for instance, in reference to the elastic tissue in the lung. Special mention must be made of subendothelial proliferative processes in small and medium-sized arterial and venous vessels (AGRESS and GRAY; BEAMER et al.; FISCHER et al.; SCHULZ). Such lesions undoubtedly decrease circulatory volume and may well contribute to the production of necrotic alterations (Fig. 10). The subintimal proliferative lesions are quite frequent and can be seen in most organs. In the lung and brain (in cases of meningitis) the vascular lesions seem to be most conspicuous but are frequent also in branches of the portal vein (SCHULZ). Mononuclear cells are found in addition to yeast-containing histiocytes. HARTUNG and SALFELDER described a case of laboratory infection with granulomatous arteritis in the wall of mediumsized branches of the pulmonary artery.

From the above, it should be quite obvious that histoplasmosis mimics in every aspect other *infectious granulomata of mycobacterial and fungal origin. The absolute need for demonstration of the organism by culture or special stains cannot be over-emphasized.* PUCKETT was the first to unravel the etiology of solitary pulmonary granulomas by the use of special stains; STRAUB and SCHWARZ demonstrated with the Gridley procedure the frequency of the healed primary lesion, and SCHWARZ et al. the high incidence of splenic and hepatic histoplasmic foci. The search for organisms in suspected lesions can be very time consuming and — if negative — most frustrating. When only isolated organisms are found, the diagnosis should be made with extreme caution. If many typical yeast cells of 2 to 5 μ are visible, the diagnosis is quite simple.

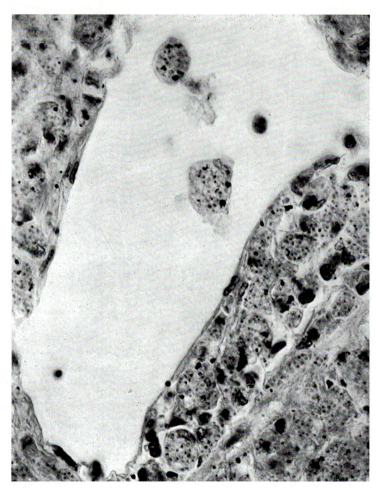

Fig. 10. Pulmonary vein in disseminated histoplasmosis in a teenager. Dissemination of *H. capsulatum* by the bloodstream is morphologically more easily demonstrable than bacterial septicemia, because of the larger size and better visibility of yeast cells. Macrophages filled with organisms are seen in the wall and lumen of the vein. Whether the presence of the two phagocytes in the lumen is artifactual or not, it shows how cells find their way into the lumen. H & E × 650

Table 1. *Influence of staining methods on diagnosis of pulmonary nodules*
(Modified from Hutcheson and Waldorf)

	Only AF stain 1946—1948	AF + PAS + Gridley 1954—1957	AF + Crocott 1958—1959
Tuberculosis	6	15	6
Histoplasmosis	0	0	14
Undiagnosed	18	50*	8

* When restained with Grocott, 21 showed *Histoplasma capsulatum*.

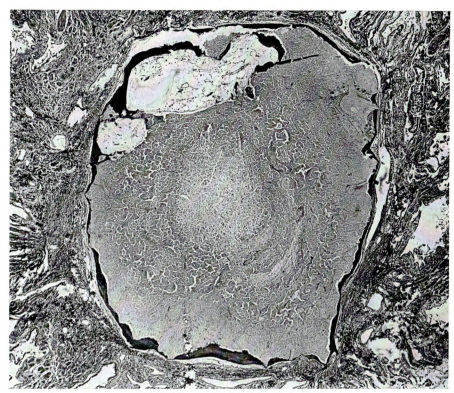

Fig. 11. Healed primary focus of histoplasmosis. Center shows complete liquefaction necrosis, the spot where yeast cells abound. The focus, as usual, is surrounded by a thin bony rim, with an area of bonemarrow. Van Gieson × 27

The Primary Lesion in the Lung

The primary focus in histoplasmosis can be best described as similar to the Ghon-focus in tuberculosis, but larger, as a rule. SCHULZ (1954) published excellent descriptions and pictures of three active primary complexes (lung focus plus satellite lymph nodes). The foci in two infants (3 and 4 months of age, respectively) already showed calcified deposits. The central caseated mass was surrounded by a fibrous capsule which was in turn infiltrated by mononuclear cells, giant cells, and macrophages with organisms. It has been our experience that a small area of pneumonia develops in response to inhalation of microconidia or fragments of mycelium. In this focus, central caseation occurs regularly after a few weeks. *The change from a negative skin reaction to histoplasmin to a positive one seems to coincide with this delay of a few to 6 weeks.* The regional lymph nodes enlarge markedly, become similarly involved, with progression from macrophages through necrosis to scarring and calcification.

In man, early hematogenous spread is the rule, with seeding especially in the spleen and liver. The primary complex and the splenic and hepatic foci heal in uncomplicated cases, probably in 99 of 100 infections (STRAUB and SCHWARZ, 1962) (Fig. 11). In a series of 55 unselected necropsies of adults, 47 primary complexes could be identified as histoplasmic (Fig. 12). None of the patients died of or had active histoplasmosis. In this series (STRAUB and SCHWARZ, 1960) the primary focus was multiple in 4 instances and the largest number of primary foci was 5. The importance of unbiased examination was evident from an autopsy series of 53 cases from California: 20 of 39 calcified lesions revealed *H. capsulatum* and only 6 *Coccidioides immitis*, pointing to the migratory habits of our population. This material

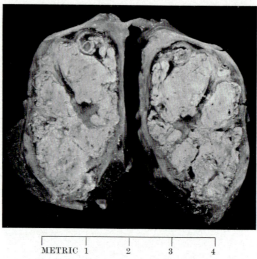

METRIC 1   2   3   4

Fig. 12. Lymph node histoplasmosis. Huge "chalky" type of calcification of a lymph node, of the primary complex of histoplasmosis

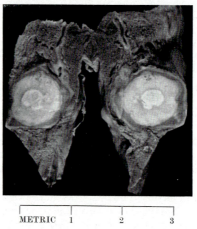

METRIC 1   2   3

Fig. 13. Large primary semiactive histoplasmic focus with liquefied center, which is yellowish and ready to sequestrate. The subpleural location and the presence of regional lymph nodes in the same state of development make this clearly a primary focus, even if the gross appearance makes differentiation from a histoplasmoma difficult and arbitrary. Such foci acquired in adulthood may be indistinguishable from histoplasmomas in surgical specimens, when lymph nodes are not submitted

collected in the endemic area of coccidioidomycosis highlights also the need for special (Grocott) staining methods (Straub et al.). The primary foci of histoplasmosis and tuberculosis are comparable, representing expanding caseous pneumonia, leading to encapsulation, frequently with liquefaction (and after healing, chalky deposits) in the center of the histoplasmic lesion (Fig. 13). In contrast, the primary focus of coccidioidomycosis has a capsule as the result of healing of a granulomatous perifocal infiltrate (STRAUB and SCHWARZ, 1962).

The activity of the capsule of the primary histoplasmic lesion can vary greatly. Sometimes a few scattered epithelioid cell tubercles with an occasional giant cell are seen in the external layers of the capsule. More often only connective tissue, with scarce lymphocytic infiltrates, is seen. The primary focus acquires calcium salts, often in the form of stippled foci rather than as a solid mass. The center often is chalky and the periphery develops a narrow osseous ring and a surrounding thin fibrous capsule. The bone often shows a cavity filled with bone marrow. From the active lesion, lymphangitic streaks lead in the interstitium toward the pleura. Later, the interstitium is somewhat thickened, with a few extra strands of collagen. Large foci often have small satellite nodules in the pleura, each about 1 to 3 mm in size. Rarely, there are many nodules, which then form small confluent plaques.

The lymph nodes swell early in the formation of the complex, and occasionally there already is necrosis in the lymph node before it becomes recognizable in the pneumonitis. More often, however, focus and lymph node go through the different stages of inflammation in parallel fashion. The caseated foci in the lymph nodes are generally discrete, leading after healing to the stippled calcification that is a hallmark of histoplasmosis.

In the caseated lesions of lung and lymph nodes the organisms are numerous, but demonstrable only with a perfect stain (GROCOTT, GRIDLEY). To look for *H. capsulatum* in H & E stained caseated or decalcified lesions must be compared with a search for tubercle bacilli in sections stained also with H & E. Occasionally small corpuscles can be seen in H & E preparations, but most small particles are calcium flecks, nuclear debris, and such matter. Most workers consider it both a waste of time and a sign of inexperience to examine H & E sections of caseated or calcified foci for Histoplasma.

With the Grocott stain, sharply outlined black rings of round or ovoid shape are seen, often in clusters. The clusters represent accumulations of yeast cells in phagocytes; long after the phagocyte has been lysed, the groups of yeast cells remain together and stainable since no chitinase is available to break down the yeast cell. In very old calcified lesions, the yeast cells may stain paler (shades of grey), but short oxidation of about 10 min with chromic acid will often give more intense staining.

Budding is never very numerous in tissues in the case of *H. capsulatum*. The size of the yeast cells is quite uniform in most foci and only seldom, especially in necrotic lesions, larger yeast cells up to 8 μ in size are seen. With the Gridley stain, a purple-lavender color graces the wall of the yeast cells but fewer organisms are captured with this procedure, which needs a great degree of technical perfection to give results comparable to the Grocott methenamine-silver stain. For quick review, for cases with few organisms, and for good contrast for photomicrography, the Grocott stain is far superior to any other available method. The counterstain in the Grocott procedure is of little importance; as mentioned earlier, we dip the slides for about 10 sec into hematoxylin, which gives added orientation, since nuclei become stained and a faint tissue background appears, and necrotic foci can be differentiated from histiocytic infiltrates and other matter.

MASHBURN et al. confirmed, in all but details, the presence of calcified primary lesions in 111 autopsies (likewise in the endemic area), with 71 lung foci with *H. capsulatum* demonstrable in the calcified areas. Even outside the endemic area, histoplasmic foci can be found, in part at least due to the influx of migratory segments in a hospital population. BAKER found 12 such cases in Durham, N.C., and

22 in New Orleans, in 100 autopsies each; Straub et al. demonstrated 20 histo-plasmic foci in 53 autopsies in Los Angeles, California. In Merida, Venezuela, Salfelder and Liscano found, in 244 autopsies, 60 healed lesions of histoplas-mosis, a proportion corresponding to the histoplasmin skin reactivity of the area.

The presence of necrosis and liquefaction in the center of so many primary foci in human lungs was interpreted in 1962 as the result of attraction of mononuclear cells. The frequency of hypersensitivity illustrated by erythematous skin eruptions (Leznoff et al.; Medeiros et al.; Sellers et al.) during primary infection was not known at that time; in the light of present knowledge, the interpretation of the necrosis in the primary focus may need revision, leaning toward sensitivity reaction as an important factor.

The time necessary for the development of a recognizable circumscribed primary lesion varies. It may be very short, as seen in the example of a child autopsied by Schlumberger and Service.

This infant was only 9 weeks old at death. The first 2 weeks of his life were spent in the hospital; five weeks later, he was hospitalized with disseminated histoplasmosis, and had apparently multiple primary foci of 3—8 mm, appearing in the photomicrographs like active primary foci. In contrast, a girl less than 4 months of age at the time of death had nonspecific pneumonitis without strict focalization and without necrosis (Salfelder and Capretti), but regional lymph nodes of the infant already showed epithelioid cell granulomas with necrosis.

The lymph node involvement of the primary complex varies with the age of the individual at which the primary infection takes place. In adult infection, less calci-fication results than in childhood complexes and only 1 or 2 lymph nodes show lesions as opposed to the childhood complexes with about five nodes involved (Straub and Schwarz, 1962). We also have the distinct impression that the focus acquired in adult life stays active for a long time, is very large, and cannot always be differentiated from a histoplasmoma.

The primary lesion is substantially larger in histoplasmosis than in tuberculosis (Straub and Schwarz, 1955).

Table 2. *Size of primary complex*
(Modified from Straub and Schwarz, 1955)

	Histoplasmosis	Tuberculosis
Lung focus:		
1—4 mm	23	27
5—10 mm	42	7
greater than 10 mm	2	2
Lymph nodes:		
1—10 mm	48	21
greater than 10 mm	22	3

The microscopic architecture of the primary focus has been described with sur-prising accuracy in single instances (Colvin et al.) and in larger series has been found to depend on such factors as the stage, size, and age of the patient (Straub and Schwarz, 1960).

The lung/tissue reaction of early infection is a nonspecific bronchopneumonia with polymorphonuclear infiltrate which slowly changes with time. Histiocytes become prominent, the phagocytized yeast cells multiply, and necrosis develops. The focus becomes more circumscribed and a fairly sharply outlined caseous lesion is visible. Generally, the focus is subpleural with little reaction of the pleura. Bands connecting visceral and parietal pleura, so commonly seen in tuberculosis, are not seen in histoplasmosis; neither are major scars in the visceral pleura. In the active

primary infection, the pleura shows, grossly, very delicate fibrinous reaction covering the primary focus, which becomes organized to a slight pleural fibrosis. We have
only rarely seen heavy pleural plaques, and these have been only a few millimeters
in thickness. Calcium deposits in pleural scars are rarely seen. Calcium deposits
precipitate with variable velocity in the primary focus, sometimes as soon as a few
weeks, more often, after several months. Exceptionally, such foci remain without
calcification for years.

Ordinarily, the histoplasmic primary focus is larger than the Ghon focus of
tuberculosis, and this is one of the most striking gross differences. While thorough
examination, preferably with roentgenography of the lung after removal from the
thorax and palpation of the thin slices of lung parenchyma, is necessary to find the
minute active or residual tuberculous focus, in the case of histoplasmic infection
the focus protrudes quite prominently from the surrounding lung tissue. The
primary focus is generally subpleural and may be seen in all lobes of the lung. There
is at present no large accumulation of information on the distribution of the primary focus which could numerically compare with the extensive statistics about the
localization of the primary tuberculous focus. But if small numbers can be at all
an indication of the distribution, our figures indicate that no lobe has a particular
status. We found healed primary foci in the right upper lobe in 11 cases, in the right
middle lobe in 7, the right lower lobe in 15, the left upper lobe in 14, and the left
lower lobe in 21. The astute morphologist observes also that the calcification in
histoplasmosis is a composite of small foci rather than a solid chunk of calcium; this
stippled appearance is especially prominent in the lymph nodes and can be recognized also radiologically.

The involvement of vascular structures in the active primary lesion must be
common and must determine the dissemination to spleen and liver which is extremely common, as will be documented later. In the vicinity of the caseated primary focus it is easy to demonstrate *H. capsulatum* in capillaries and small veins and
sometimes even in veins with muscular wall. More often than not, the yeast cells
are within histiocytes and when found "free", suggest possible mechanical rupture
of macrophages during dehydration. However, a small number of yeast cells can
be seen outside of histiocytes in cases of active lung lesions. Since yeast cells are
not difficult to stain and can be recognized with greater ease than isolated bacilli,
including acid-fast organisms, the active proof of vascular invasion is demonstrable
in histoplasmosis, while it can often be only postulated in other diseases. In part,
the intravascular dissemination originates in subintimal pillows which secondarily
open into the lumen, shedding phagocytes loaded with yeast cells. The subintimal
histiocytic nodule sometimes forms a completely round granuloma but more often
one sees just a bulging "pillow," pushing the endothelium into the venous lumen.
It can be assumed that the "pillows" form either from the outside through *vasa
vasorum* or even finer preformed channels, or else (and this is less likely) from the
lumen. These germ-spitting formations occur in the lung in chronic disease also
(after the primary sensitizing focus has healed), and can be seen with lesser frequency in other organs, especially in overwhelming infection with myriads of
organisms in all tissue clefts. In the center of the caseated primary lesion, necrotic
(and thrombosed) vessels are indeed always demonstrable, but the process of destruction is far too advanced, preventing recognition of the presence of organisms
in the lumen. However, there can be little doubt that vascular channels within the
focus must be exposed to the same subintimal infiltration, forming sources of dissemination as in the vessels in the vicinity of active foci. The thrombosis associated
with the vascular necrosis in the center of the caseated lesion seals off this source
of dissemination, but no doubt "after the horse has been stolen."

In phagocytes, dozens of yeast cells are sometimes present. This simple fact, which is also demonstrable *in vitro*, in itself proves that multiplication occurs within the phagocytic cell. The conclusion must then be that the intracellular environment at certain times is not damaging to the Histoplasma organism. It may be permissible to assume that the intracellular environment gives some protection from the circulating antibodies. These pathogenetic speculations are necessary to explain why *H. capsulatum* is carried with such frequency to the spleen, and to a lesser degree to other organs.

In all likelihood, similar disseminations occur also in other infections but for several reasons are not as regularly documented as in histoplasmosis. *H. capsulatum* is fairly easily demonstrable with modern staining methods: the splenic calcifications, if not unique, are so prominent in histoplasmosis that it takes special skill to overlook them!. Similarly, foci in the liver, even if necrotic or calcified, reveal their true nature by the presence of innumerable yeast cells. Much effort has gone into the verification of this fact; the morphologic identity of the yeast cells in experimental animals, with the appearance in human tissue, both with active and healed lesions, has been a strong argument which in experienced hands will be conclusive in 99 out of 100 cases. The fluorescent antibody technique has produced additional proof of the safety with which morphologic methods can be used to elucidate the pathogenesis of most lesions (Yamaguchi et al.).

Histoplasmoma

Puckett was the first to call attention to the true nature of pulmonary nodules, called arbitrarily "tuberculomas." Sophisticated observers in the USA had noticed the frequent absence of acid-fast bacilli, creating the category of "granuloma — etiology undetermined." The X-ray image of the corresponding generally solitary lesion was labeled "coin lesion," which term only serves as description without attempting etiologic classification. Little purpose would be served by enumerating all diagnostic potentialities of nodules appearing in the lung. The only important nongranulomatous nodular lesion is carcinoma; the only frequent nonhistoplasmic granulomata are tuberculosis, and in the southwest of the USA, coccidioidomycosis. A tomogram showing the presence of laminated rings of calcium within the lesion may eliminate considerably but not entirely the fear of neoplasm. For very rarely, carcinoma may develop around a pre-existing calcified nodule and the X-ray may become misleading. Calcium in tumors is exceedingly infrequent.

In 1953 Puckett reported 22 cases of surgically removed lesions of the lung (Fig. 14), only one of which gave a positive culture of *H. capsulatum*. With the PAS procedure, organisms were demonstrated in tissue sections and the impossibility of their recognition in H & E stains was stressed. The material contained focal encapsulated pneumonic foci with or without daughter lesions and cavitary histoplasmosis. The round foci were always subpleural with a visible focal thickening of the pleura on top of the lesion. A central yellow focus of 2—5 mm was present; this is the spot where yeast cells are most abundant. This was also the only area with complete tissue destruction, whereas outside the central area, alveolar patterns remained visible, best seen with special stains. The foci with daughter lesions probably represented primary foci, but since generally only wedge resections were made, no lymph nodes were available for examination; in 2 cases, where lymph nodes were available, they participated in the inflammation.

A year later, Zimmerman (1954) found in 35 lesions submitted as "tuberculomas," acid-fast bacilli only 6 times, but *H. capsulatum* 19 times, and *Coccidioides immitis* 3 times. The same author found, in 1957, of 40 cases diagnosed as

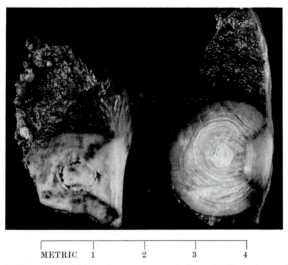

METRIC 1 2 3 4

Fig. 14. Two surgically removed histoplasmomas, each 2 cm in diameter and subpleural. The lesion on the right shows characteristic concentric rings, and a trapezoid contribution from the pleura, demarcated by a narrow band of pigment. A collaborative effort of the pleura and the lung is evident in this case from the continuation of the rings into the scar formed principally by the pleura.
The lesion on the left shows another typical finding: a hairline demarcation of the central liquefaction necrosis from the peripheral part of the granuloma. If a connection with a bronchus exists, the liquefied center may be expelled and a small cavity may form. There is little to indicate that this is the origin of chronic cavitary lung disease. Radiologic followup indicates that such "microcavities" fill in within a few months

histoplasmomas at the Armed Forces Institute of Pathology, Washington, D.C., only 9 submitted as such by the contributors. STARR et al. were successful in demonstrating Histoplasma with the PAS stain only once in 22 solitary lung lesions. GREENDYKE and EMERSON were able to demonstrate the superiority of the Grocott stain over the PAS procedure by finding *H. capsulatum* in 20 of 26 granulomas removed at surgery. Of the 20, 2 were children (9 and 11 years), 16 were between 40 and 60 years of age. Thirteen had been completely asymptomatic, 5 had cough, 2 dyspnea, and 2 hemoptysis. All nodules were subpleural, evenly distributed in all lobes of the lung, and none had free fluid in the pleural space at the time of surgery. The lesions had concentrically layered greyish rings around a soft, pale yellow, "mushy" center of 5—10 mm. Daughter lesions of 1—3 mm diameter in the vicinity of the main nodule were common and sometimes numerous (2—30). In view of the common presence of satellite lesions, it is surprising that in this, as in other series, subsegmental or segmental resection proved prognostically sufficient.

STEELE reported the results of collected cases in man: of 887 solitary asymptomatic nodules, 316 were cancers and 474 were granulomas. Of the latter, 164 were due to *H. capsulatum*, 98 to *C. immitis*, 122 to *M. tuberculosis*, and 82 remained unidentified. In this series, of 280 cancers, 10 (3.6%) showed calcification; of 164 histoplasmomas, 15 (9.1%), which was a much higher percentage than in tuberculosis and coccidioidomycosis (both 5%). The histoplasmomas were fairly equally distributed in upper (52%) and lower (48%) lobes, in contrast to tuberculomas favoring the upper (73%) over the lower lobes (27%). This discrepancy was even more marked when the segments of the upper lobe were compared. In the apical and posterior segments, histoplasmomas appeared 15 times, in the anterior segments

14 times. In contrast, the corresponding features in tuberculosis were 52 and 8, respectively. Hutcheson and Waldorf found of 35 histoplasmomas only 40% in the upper lobes.

Baum et al. found radiologic evidence of increase in size of 4 histoplasmomas followed over a considerable time. When the lesions were removed, they were found to be inactive, with a broad, fibrous capsule, and seemingly incapable of recent growth. This discrepancy between apparent growth in X-ray examination and an encapsulated lesion without signs of activity was explained as follows: the lesions did not grow in size, but the periphery developed greater radiodensity with progress of time, simulating absolute increase in size, and in this way inducing need for removal through fear of a growing neoplasm.

In the endemic area the histoplasmoma is the predominant granulomatous lesion and can be found in teenagers and very old persons. Often the lesion is discovered in an incidental X-ray film, or is recognized in X-ray films taken years earlier, when searched catamnestically. When the lesion is attacked surgically, the overlaying pleura will show slight thickening, and the absence of diffuse or bandlike adhesions between the two pleural coverings is constant.

The histoplasmoma is almost without exception subpleural and the foci vary in size from about 10—40 mm or even larger. Most foci are solitary, but rarely 6 or more lesions are seen in one lobe or scattered through the lungs. On the cut surface a concentric pattern is almost always prominent. In the center, especially of larger lesions, a soft spot a few millimeters in size is found which, as in the large primary focus, represents liquefaction necrosis with complete destruction of the anatomical structures, including elastic fibers. Here organisms will be found in large numbers, a point of great diagnostic importance: if this central nidus is not examined, the presence of organisms may remain undetected, even with numerous and adequately stained Grocott sections.

In the periphery outside the liquefied area the alveolar pattern can be demonstrated with an elastic tissue and Van Gieson stain. The structure of a histoplasmoma changes with age from caseous, with occasional mineral deposits, to rocklike lesions with abundant calcification in concentric fashion. The concentric rings are seen in splenic and hepatic lesions as well, and we believe that the rings of necrosis and subsequent mineral deposits are due to immunologic processes rather than to fungal proliferation. This belief is based on the paucity or absence of yeast cells outside the central spot. On the other hand, if there is more than one "central" liquefied focus — a common finding in histoplasmomas — organisms are found in each of the necrotic areas, but still strictly limited and without spread to the peripheral layers. The fresh lesion shows small epithelioid-cell tubercles in the fibrous capsule of the histoplasmoma, sometimes on the inner aspect of the wall, sometimes seemingly incorporating discrete lesions just outside the fibrous capsule. In older histoplasmomas the fibrous capsule is completely inactive, without any granulomatous nodularity, and with few lymphocytes.

From the pleura a trapezoid contribution is added which enters between the orderly concentric rings of the histoplasmoma for as much as 4 or 5 mm. The "keystone" part is often shiny-white, and microscopically hyalinized. Rarely the orderly process of progressive calcification and arrest of the histoplasmoma is interrupted by extension of the central necrotic area, leading to cavitation. Such cavities are small, irregular, and fragments of caseated material are seen hanging into the liquid content of the cavity. Clinical experience indicates that such small excavations within a histoplasmoma fill in over the years and in all likelihood do not represent the source of chronic cavitary histoplasmosis. But much more work needs to be done to decide this question definitively.

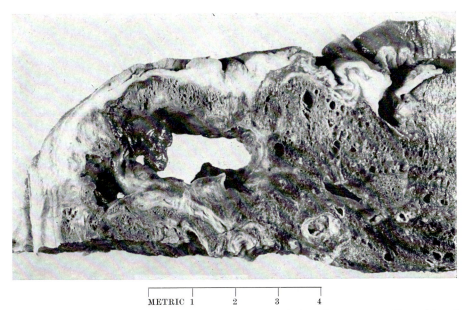

METRIC 1   2   3   4

Fig. 15. Chronic histoplasmic cavity with pachypleuritis, thick walls, remnants of bronchi, and vessels crossing the lumen and subdividing it into several chambers. The surrounding lung tissue is scarred, emphysematous, and distorted

Not infrequently, small epithelioid-cell "tubercles" are found in the vicinity of the histoplasmoma, but distinctly outside the capsule and without connection with the histoplasmoma. These satellite lesions are remarkable for two reasons. First, they may represent a source of growth of the histoplasmoma — if they become incorporated in the main lesion, as they often do. Second, simple wedge resection must often cut through such small satellite lesions, but the surgical results of even very narrow segmental resections are excellent. In spite of apparently completely successful removal, it would seem advisable to resect such lesions with somewhat wider margins to avoid the possibility of postoperative spread. When left alone, the histoplasmoma may change in density over the years, or may remain without alteration. The follow-up by X-ray study of such patients saved from thoracotomy is one of the satisfactions of the conservative physician.

Cavitary Histoplasmosis

Chronic progressive cavitary histoplasmosis is seen in older men and represents the breakdown of pneumonic infiltrates in the apical and subapical regions of the lung. The small acute cavity with an irregular wall can progress to a thick-walled lesion, 2—3 cm in diameter (SWEANY et al.). FURCOLOW and BRASHER (1956) reviewed chronic progressive cavitary histoplasmosis. The existence of this entity has been slowly accepted, especially in endemic areas. The observation that chronic cavitary histoplasmosis is seen more frequently in middle-aged men than in younger persons suggested reinfection as a probable cause. Anatomic evidence for reinfection was presented in 5 cases from Cincinnati by SCHWARZ and BAUM (1963), when they reported the presence of caseous or cavitary lesions distant from, or even contralateral to, calcified and inactive primary complexes (Fig. 15).

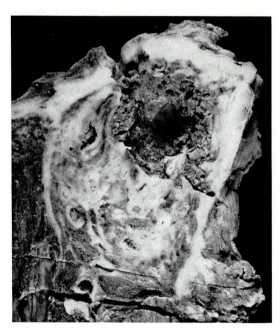

Fig. 16. Old histoplasmic pulmonary cavity, kept open by the presence of a fungus ball in the subapical region. Intense fibrosis in the lower part of the cavity and loose crumbly appearance of the contents are conspicuous. *Aspergillus* species are most frequently isolated

A much larger series would be necessary to decide whether reinfection is exogenous or endogenous. However, the anatomic proof for its existence has been established. We favored the exogenous route based on epidemiologic considerations: the frequency of sources of infection related to soil. Sweany et al. considered reepithelialization an infrequent event, but this opinion was based on only occasional random sections. The knowledge of the origin, development, and healing of histoplasmic cavities is limited and cannot compare with the abundant information available in tuberculosis, derived from a wealth of material and the work of numerous investigators in phthisiology. According to Beatty et al., the histoplasmic cavities are frequently open, communicating with one or more bronchi, and are in his experience commonly seen in the posterior-superior portion of the lung. Bronchiectases in connection with cavities are frequently mentioned, but the claim is easier made than proven. Sinus tracts are less common than in tuberculosis (Beatty et al.). It has been claimed that emphysematous blebs can become infected with *H. capsulatum* (Ramirez and Levy), but on the other hand Sweany et al. claim that about one third of cavities progress to cyst formation. Our limited experience with cavitary histoplasmosis seemed to indicate a tendency to develop heavy-walled structures, often divided by residual bronchi and vessels into subdivisions, in every aspect comparable to tuberculous cavitations. (The great frequency of combination forms with dual infection, *M. tuberculosis* plus *H. capsulatum*, has been covered in the chapter on concurrent diseases.)

Demonstration of only one agent in dual infection can have disastrous therapeutic results. Fortunately, in cavitary histoplasmosis, the organisms are plentiful in the sputum and can be demonstrated by culture, fluorescent antibody stain (Carski et al., Lynch and Plexico) or simple Wright stain (Woods et al.).

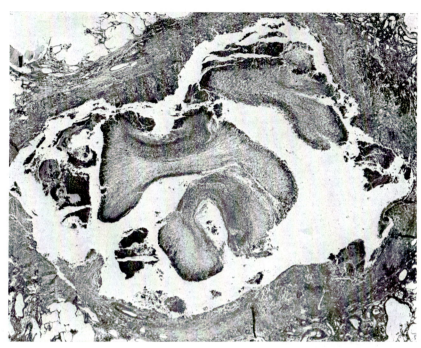

Fig. 17. Small cavity of histoplasmic origin. Organisms were demonstrated in the necrotic tissue of the wall. The cavity is filled by a "fungus ball," the result of proliferating Aspergilli. H & E × 12

The presence of fungus balls in histoplasmic cavities (PROCKNOW and LOEWEN; SCHWARZ et al., 1961) has become a prestige diagnosis in endemic areas (Fig. 16). The development of fungus balls, generally composed of Aspergillus species, in cavities of variable etiology, has been recognized for some time. The simultaneous presence of Histoplasma in the wall and Aspergillus in the lumen of a cavity was not demonstrated until 1960—1961. It is not known why *Aspergillus* develops so prolifically in pulmonary cavities. Once the cavity is nearly filled by the Aspergillus, bronchial obstruction may occur and lead to death of the Aspergillus possibly by asphyxia. The macerated swollen hyphae can be seen years later, but viability leading to positive culture will seldom be found. A crescent-shaped air space shown in X-ray picture over the fungus ball floating in the exudate of the cavity can be easily dislodged by the patient's change of posture, proof of the floating nature of the foreign object in the cavity. On opening a cavity containing a fungus ball, a brownish, moist-to-dry substance is found, parts of which may be adherent to the wall of the cavity (Fig. 17). So inconspicuous is this substance that we have sometimes mistaken it for a blood clot. Some fungus balls reach or surpass the size of

Table 3. *Morphologic demonstration of H. capsulatum in sputum of cavitary cases*

Culture	Stain Pos.	Author
25 positive	18 PAS	LYNCH and PLEXICO
59 negative	8 PAS	LYNCH and PLEXICO
38 positive	27 Wright	WOODS et al.

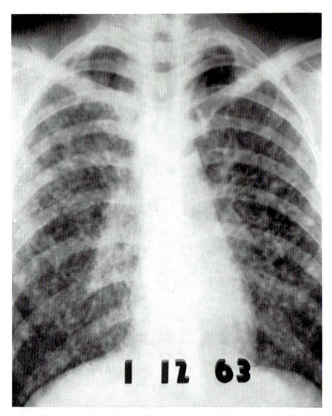

Fig. 18. Comparatively recent "epidemic histoplasmosis." Innumerable foci of equal size are seen in both lung fields, many already calcified. The patient was exposed to heavily contaminated dust 2 months prior to photographing

golf balls. The importance of the fungus ball is mostly mechanical, preventing closure of the cavity. Aspergillus from the cavity is seldom and sporadically found in the sputum, apparently only when the draining bronchus is open. We have occasionally found one out of a dozen cultures from the contents of the cavity positive for Aspergillus.

This histoplasmic cavity is exposed to the same dangers and complications as the tuberculous cavity: hemorrhage, perforation with empyema, or bronchopleural fistula. Of 19 cavitary cases, Furcolow and Brasher found 12 bilateral and 3 multiple. Diveley and McCracken reported only 3 bilateral cavities in a group of 29 surgical resections.

"Epidemic" Histoplasmosis

Furcolow and Grayston, Loosli et al., and others are responsible for the development of the concept of "epidemic histoplasmosis." This entity refers to infection of small or large groups of people by spore-laden dust at a point source. Such infections have developed in groups of persons who entered a silo on a farm (Loosli et al.), a storm cellar (Cain et al.), a cave (Murray et al.; Gonzalez-Ochoa), or who cleaned water towers, bridges, or attics, or who explored a hollow tree (Feldman and Sabin; Englert and Phillips; Furcolow and Grayston).

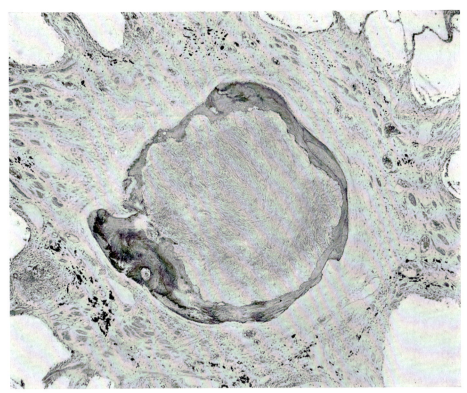

Fig. 19. Primary focus (one of many) in "epidemic histoplasmosis." The patient had hundreds of similar foci, each of the same size and stage of development. Most had bony rings filled with bone marrow. Except for its small size, a focus of "epidemic histoplasmosis" mimics the solitary classical primary focus. H & E × 35

The common denominator in all outbreaks was the abundant presence of *H. capsulatum* in the soil at the source of infection, frequently proved by means of culture or by experimental exposure of lower animals to the same environment. The clinical picture varied from an asymptomatic to a severe septic course. The prognosis was good in most outbreaks in the United States (ADRIANO et al.; LEHAN and FURCOLOW), but greater fatality rates occurred in other countries, especially in Mexico (GONZALEZ-OCHOA). In asymptomatic, as in clinically ill patients, the X-ray has often showed multiple pulmonary lesions which in due course have appeared as multiple calcific nodules, interpreted as multiple primary foci (Fig. 18). From a purely logical point of view, therefore, it would seem more nearly correct to speak of "infection with multiple primary foci" rather than of "epidemic histoplasmosis," since the former is based on anatomic findings and the latter does not represent an accurate representation of facts, as many patients with multiple primary foci acquire the disease "privately" and do not necessarily form part of a group-infection.

The multiple foci, in both the acute and healed forms, resemble the solitary primary focus. The multiple foci are smaller then the average solitary focus and are generally fairly uniformly about 5 mm in diameter (Fig. 19). There may be from a few dozens to many hundreds of foci in a single case. The lymph nodes participate, but in view of the multitude of lung foci, it is impossible to trace the individual lung lesion to a particular lymph node or even to a lymph node group; they all participate. However, the lymph node involvement is not necessarily prominent or larger than in a solitary infection of a lower lobe, where most of the homolateral lymph nodes are seen to be caseated and where, in some cases, the infection even crosses over at the level of the carina, affecting also the contralateral paratracheal nodes.

In dogs, multiple primary pulmonary foci are much more frequent than in man (Straub and Schwarz, 1960); we believe that this has to do with the tendency of dogs to dig and snuffle in the soil. In addition to the simple mechanical closeness of the dog to infected soil, species differences may also play a role.

Multiple primary foci have been seen also in reinfection; in 1947, several men cleaning a water tower in Cincinnati (Feldman and Sabin; Schwarz and Baum, 1960) developed mild to severe disease. It would be most unlikely to find in the endemic area (with a skin sensitivity rate close to 90%) 12 unselected men who would be free from previous contact with Histoplasma. Therefore, the disease and pathologic confirmation in 2 of the individuals (dead from other causes) must be interpreted as reinfection under the picture of "multiple primary foci." The multiple pulmonary calcifications, a radiologic hallmark of healed "epidemic" histoplasmosis (Silverman, 1950), have to be differentiated from the rare ossified nodules seen with mitral stenosis (Daugavietis and Mautner) and from familial pulmonary microlithiasis (Sosman et al.).

In healed epidemic histoplasmosis each calcified focus represents a minute primary lesion that has healed, often with a rim of bone surrounding the calcified center. It is common to find a bone-marrow space in the bony ring on the periphery of the focus. When such lungs are examined, the uniformity in size and architecture of the dozens to hundreds of foci is astonishing. Clearly the represent simultaneous formation of "primary foci" in an individual who was exposed to a heavy concentration of spores, generally in a dusty environment, as in a silo, storm cellar, cave, an excavation for construction, or a hollow tree. The nodular pulmonary ossifications associated with mitral stenosis are solid bone without evidence of a calcified, necrotic center as in the histoplasmic lesions. The so-called osteomas of the lung, rare in man, but common in dogs, have an architecture similar to the bony lesions seen in mitral stenosis. If widely disseminated miliary tuberculosis ever healed (prior to antibiotic therapy), it must have been so exceptional that we wholeheartedly agree with Sosman et al.: "Most if not all of the cases reported as healed, calcified, miliary tuberculosis have been either calcified histoplasmosis or other fungus disease."

The Spleen

The spleen partakes in histoplasmosis in two different ways: 1. splenomegaly; 2. "miliary lesions." During the rare infantile form, unbelievable numbers of yeast cells become trapped in the splenic phagocytes. Grossly, splenomegaly is seen, the organ is several times normal in size and has a tense capsule. Microscopically, such spleens show huge macrophages uniformly filled with the small yeast cells. The splenic invasion (by phagocytes) leads to complete obliteration of the normal architecture. The phagocytic infiltrates in turn show great propensity to necrosis. The splenic condition is only part of a widely disseminated and generally progressive and fatal disease. In addition to diffuse histiocytic infiltration, discrete nodular lesions of different size and in variable numbers are seen in disseminated histoplasmosis.

The second much more common form of splenic histoplasmosis occurs during primary infection when from the pulmonary primary complex an early, generally

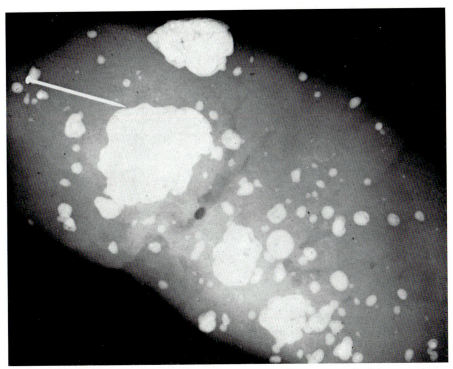

Fig. 20. Splenic calcifications of histoplasmosis, even very large ones as in this unusual case, are in our experience never associated with clinical symptoms. This is remarkable considering the huge size of the calcifications (indicating even larger foci of active necrosis before scarring decreases the size of the lesions)

benign and self-limited, hematogenous dissemination occurs. A few to hundreds of small foci are formed during this early hematogenous spread, and active lesions of this nature can be found in surgically removed spleens and less frequently in autopsy material. In the latter cases, the pulmonary complex is found in a condition similar to that of the spleen, supporting our belief that the foci are formed during the primary phase of infection. The foci, even if extremely numerous — and what is less common, even if very large — tend to heal (Fig. 20). Hence we have concluded that round calcific foci in the spleen are most commonly of histoplasmic origin if:

1) there are 5 or more round foci of 3—5 mm diameter, or

2) if the foci show a central calcification separated by a less dense zone of calcification from one or more heavily calcified peripheral rings (SCHWARZ et al., 1955; OKUDAIRA et al.; MASHBURN et al.; SALFELDER et al.; SERVIANSKY and SCHWARZ).

In 2 autopsy series of patients dead of diseases other than histoplasmosis, calcified foci in the spleen were found in 44% (SCHWARZ et al., 1955) and over 60% (STRAUB and SCHWARZ). These figures were confirmed, albeit with a lower percentage, by MASHBURN et al.

Microscopic examination of the active foci reveals single or confluent groups of epithelioid cells in different stages of caseation. Soon a capsule is formed; fibrosis and calcification follow (Fig. 21). In the debris, cholesterol clefts may form and, as in all histoplasmic mass lesions, organisms are found in the exact center of the lesion. The concentric layering in many foci resembles the (colloid) rings of Liese-

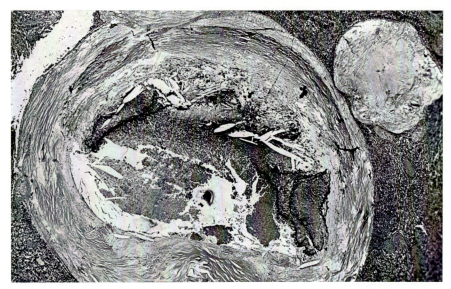

Fig. 21. Healing splenic focus of histoplasmosis. In endemic areas, splenic foci are found in great numbers of patients, generally without a history of disseminated disease. Foci become calcified later, permanent evidence of "benign asymptomatic primary dissemination" (dissemination during primary infection). Even contiguous foci remain separate. H & E × 15

gang and is no doubt responsible for the differences in concentration of calcific deposits within the focus. Such foci may be mistaken for non-specific scars if the fibrous capsule is cut instead of the central core. Frequently the round foci are close to the ubiquitous veins and trabeculae of the spleen. This does not imply a relationship between veins and foci; the multiple calcified splenic lesions are not phleboliths.

In view of the large number of splenic foci, it is surprising that the clinical symptomatology so far has escaped attention. Often such spleens have been found in persons who supposedly had been in good health all their lives and definitely lacked any history of prolonged febrile illness. Similar foci are found in the liver less frequently, and exceptionally in the kidney and other organs. One apparent reason for the frequency of splenic involvement is the ready availability of phagocytes, but circulatory factors may play a role also. Occasionally, foci 2 cm or more in diameter are found, but even such cases have no corresponding history or symptomatology (STRAUB and SCHWARZ, 1962).

Occasionally, large caseous foci are seen, with breakdown of tissue resulting in abscess-like structures. COLVIN et al. described prominent asteroid bodies in splenic giant cells in an autopsy case of disseminated histoplasmosis, without attempting interpretation. Calcific residual lesions of brucellosis were 2—23 mm in diameter, with a solid center and a peripheral snowflake pattern, in one case 25 years after the acute disease occurred (YOW et al.).

Splenic *needle biopsy* is seldom practiced, but a positive result confirmed by culture is on record (ALEXANDER and BAKIR). Recently, we were able to report a series of 12 cases showing the complete development of the calcific lesions, previously postulated from incidental findings (SALFELDER and SCHWARZ, 1967). Over the years, in spleens removed for traumatic rupture or other reasons, unrelated to histoplasmosis, we have found small groups of histiocytes, typical noncaseated "tubercles," and, later, caseated discrete foci, some of which had already become calcified. In none of the patients were symptoms recorded attributable to histoplasmosis (SALFELDER and SCHWARZ, 1967).

The Liver

The liver can become very large in the infantile form of histoplasmosis, the cells of the liver being separated and compressed by swollen phagocytes teeming with organisms, sometimes to the point of necrosis. Kupffer cells participate prominently in the phagocytosis. In infantile hepatomegaly due to histoplasmosis, inflammatory cells of other types than macrophages may be remarkably scarce or even absent. Numerous submiliary or miliary granulomatous infiltrates can occasionally be found on biopsy (ALEXANDER and BAKIR) but the correct pathogenic diagnosis can be extremely difficult to establish unless cultures turn out positively (HOLLAND and HOLLAND). The smallest lesion consists sometimes of a few necrotic cells and polymorphonuclear or mononuclear leukocytes. Nothing points toward a granulomatous lesion and unless cultures are made routinely from liver biopsies, the etiology will never be established in such cases. The number of yeast cells is so small that even the demonstration of a few isolated yeast cells by the Grocott procedure may be inconclusive unless the yeasts are well preserved and located within the microfoci.

Somewhat larger lesions have epithelioid cells with occasional giant cells of the Langhans type and various degrees of caseation. Organisms are scarce even in such foci and culture results will be more rewarding than the attempt at morphologic demonstration of yeast cells.

In the liver, the search for organisms, even in established cases of histoplasmosis, can be most frustrating. In one liver biopsy, we observed acid-fast bacilli and yeast cells of *H. capsulatum* in individual "tubercles" that could not be etiologically differentiated by cellular appearance. Comparatively large foci of an embolic nature, similar to those seen in the spleen, may be observed; the lesions are commonly directly below or involving the capsule of Glisson and measure a few millimeters in diameter (Fig. 22). Calcified lesions, the result of benign self-limited hematogenous dissemination during the primary infection, are somewhat less frequent than similar splenic lesions, and can be confused with calcified liver flukes and other parasites. Such hepatic lesions are sometimes mistaken for metastases during laparotomy for abdominal cancer. The huge number of organisms in such "large" lesions is in sharp contrast to the pauci-cellular infection described under miliary and submiliary foci. The lack of symptoms in patients with such hepatic and splenic foci, even in the presence of dozens to hundreds of lesions, is astonishing (OKUDAIRA et al.).

Bone-Marrow, Bone and Joints

Bone-marrow invasion is common in the infantile type and in hematogenous dissemination in general. Either isolated, more or less well-formed epithelioid cell tubercles, or, secondly, histiocytes packed with yeast cells are found. The latter form of bone-marrow invasion can be discrete or completely diffuse. In the latter form, the reason for depression of the bone-marrow function is self-evident, but it seems that bone marrow, with the discrete form of histiocytic invasion or with widespread "tubercles," can also be associated with pancytopenia. In infantile and other disseminated cases, the bone-marrow aspirate becomes an important substrate for the demonstration of the organism, either by smear, with Wright

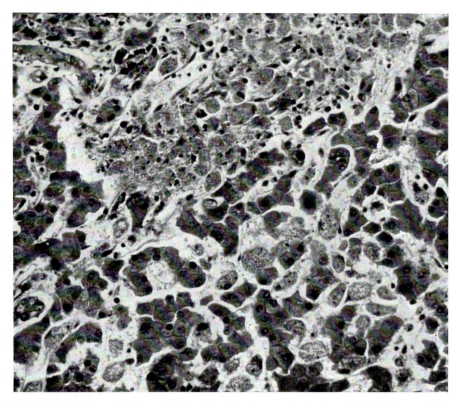

Fig. 22. Histoplasmosis of liver. Massive hepatosplenomegaly is characteristically seen in infantile primary histoplasmosis in the course of hematogenous dissemination from the pulmonary primary complex. The same picture rarely can be seen in adults with late primary infection. The liver cells are separated by huge phagocytes, each stuffed with innumerable yeast
cells. There is a confluent focus of macrophages in the upper central part of the illustration.
H & E × 300

stain or by similar procedure (Cooperberg and Schwartz), or by culture. In the
infantile type of the disease, associated hepatosplenomegaly duplicates the intense
phagocytosis of fungus organisms in the bone marrow. In the marrow, with prominent histiocytic proliferation, organisms are so plentiful that they can be recognized readily in the H & E preparation (Fig. 23). In contrast, the tubercular forms
may have so few yeast cells that their demonstration is beyond possibility even
with special stains. Here again diagnostic recognition may depend on culture.

In view of the common involvement of the bone marrow in disseminated histoplasmosis, it is astonishing how rarely bone and joint lesions are observed. This
problem becomes even more enigmatic when we realize how common bone lesions
are in the closely related disease caused by *H. duboisii*.

In our own material, we have seen only one case of suspected bone lesion. This
was the case of a young man in whom so much granulation tissue was seen around
the tendons of the left wrist that clinically a sarcoma was suspected. The tissue
response in this instance was tubercular, with discrete but complete areas of
necrosis. Organisms were fairly numerous microscopically and their identity was
further verified by a positive culture. No demonstrable bone lesions were evident,
the chest X-ray was read as unrevealing, and the patient had no septic picture at

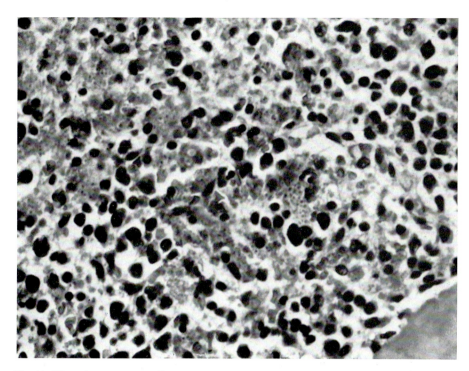

Fig. 23. Histoplasmic yeast cells in macrophages of the bone marrow in infantile progressive disease. Various degrees of infiltration occur sometimes forming solid "sheets" of phagocytes. H & E × 500

any time. The complement fixation in this florid case was only 1:8 positive, and the final diagnosis was tenosynovitis. A similar case, verified by culture, involving the os triquetrum radiologically, with recovery after surgery and amphotericin B therapy, was reported by OMER et al.

It seems almost superfluous to repeat that bone, joint, and tendinous lesions are indeed secondary to pulmonary infection, whether the latter is demonstrable or not.

Osteolytic lesions in skull, clavicle, and femur were described by MARTZ as resembling syphilis in a 3-year-old girl. The knee joint (bone and synovia) was involved in a case reported by KEY and LARGE. ALLEN reported two cases of bone involvement. The first was a 3-month-old Negro boy with disseminated histoplasmosis, in whom subperiosteal thickening of all long bones was seen radiographically. Cortical bone sections were not examined at autopsy. The second case, a 9-month-old Negro boy, had on X-ray patchy destruction of the skull in the frontal and parietal areas, similar to lesions observed in a previous case report (KLINGBERG). Extensive rarefaction was also seen in long and flat bones; the child recovered on amphotericin B therapy. A bone biopsy showed granulomatous lesions with organisms, but the report is essentially limited to these two facts (ALLEN).

Right hip involvement on X-ray, with intact joint space, was mentioned in the case of a 14-year-old boy with a positive histoplasmin skin test (E. SCHWARZ). In another disseminated case, reported by DUBLIN et al., the body of the third lumbar vertebra was filled with granulomatous lesions. POLLAK describes a positive culture from the apical granuloma of an extracted tooth.

The small number of reported osteoarticular cases, and the paucity of descriptive pathology even in those cases, precludes any broader discussion, but it is clear that bone and joint lesions can on occasion be caused by *H. capsulatum* infection.

Lymph Nodes

Lymph-node pathology in histoplasmosis closely resembles the sequence so well documented in tuberculosis. During the primary histoplasmic (pulmonary) infection, the regional lymph nodes become swollen, and develop discrete or confluent epithelioid-cell granulomata. In turn, the granulomatous lesions become centrally or diffusely necrotic. Sometimes, large markedly swollen lymph nodes of a most unusual ochre color are found draining the primary focus; microscopically, innumerable histiocytes and the familiar picture of myriads of yeast cells are seen. The foci of caseation necrosis in histoplasmic lymph nodes draining the primary focus are often discrete and the resulting calcification is likewise spotty ("stippled") (Fig. 24). This, and the large size of the necrotic or, later on, chalky-

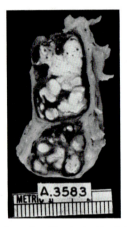

Fig. 24. Histoplasmosis of a lymph node. Classical stippled appearance of calcification in a lymph node draining a primary focus. The lymph nodes are very large, and the number involved is greater in childhood than in adult primary infection

to-calcified lymph nodes pertaining to the primary complex, are the hallmarks of the gross anatomic picture (Straub and Schwarz, 1955). When we examined lungs of American Negroes, in an attempt to find differences in comparison to work previously done elsewhere by Straub, it became obvious that autopsy material in the endemic area of histoplasmosis exhibited unique calcifications. In searching for healed lesions of tuberculosis, it had been often necessary to laminate the lungs and lymph nodes in very thin (3 mm) slices in order to find the small calcific residuals of tuberculous primary infection.

In contrast, in Cincinnati, Ohio, the calcific foci in lung and lymph nodes were of a size that seemed to invite their detection at once. The large size of the lymph-node component produces complications of considerable importance: Compression of trachea or bronchi and vessels; rupture into trachea or bronchi during the acute state, with bronchogenic aspiration and dissemination; or, after healing, erosion and hemorrhage by calcific lymph nodes, with broncholith formation. A less common, but spectacular complication is the formation of tumor-like cystic formations in the mediastinum (Dovenbarger et al.). The cheesy material of the mediastinal cysts has been mistaken for the contents of a dermoid cyst. Such mediastinal masses can be large, 10 cm or more in diameter, and dangerous because of topographic relationships.

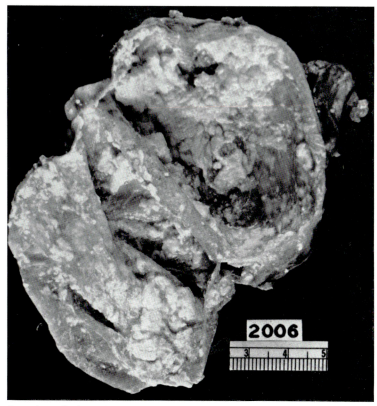

Fig. 25. Lymph node histoplasmosis. Huge sac, the result of a caseated conglomerate of
mediastinal lymph nodes. Such lymph nodes and even larger tumor-like "cysts" compress and
distort structures in the vicinity and can be mistaken for dermoid cysts. Microscopy of selected
areas reveals remnants of lymph-node tissue, and organisms can be demonstrated with the
Grocott procedure

Caseation is seldom seen in lymph nodes beyond the primary infection, and the
morphologic picture of epithelioid cell tubercles found in post-primary infection
can tax the diagnostic acumen even of the most experienced morphologist.
Organisms, either mycobacteria or fungi, can be very scarce in "productive"
tubercles, and numerous slides and even more hours may be necessary to find a
few unquestionable organisms.

The occurrence of the epithelioid-cell tubercle of histoplasmosis leads to confusion with "sarcoid" and other noncaseating granulomata, such as those of
Brucella, beryllium, and other mycoses. Lymph nodes from the hepatic hilus frequently show tubercles which may be interpreted as those of sarcoid, tuberculosis,
or histoplasmosis) (APONTE). The need for convincing demonstration of the causative microorganism in this lymph-node group is possibly greater than that in connection with draining of the lung or corresponding parenchymatous organ exhibiting active histoplasmosis. A case in point, of a 20-year-old student with febrile
illness, is reported by BULLOCK and RAY. Biopsy from the supraclavicular lymph
nodes was first read as "sarcoid," but grew *H. capsulatum* on culture.

Scalene lymph nodes can contribute to the diagnosis of pulmonary histoplasmosis (JOHNSON and MCCURDY; WILCOX et al.), but cultural methods will be of

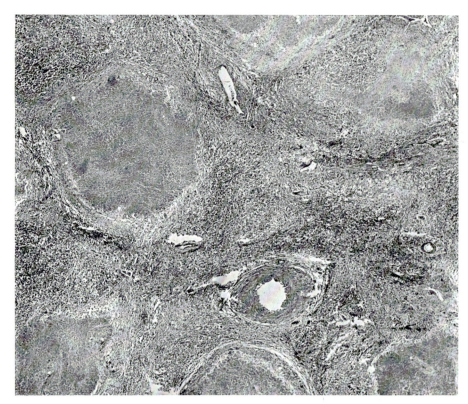

Fig. 26. Discrete foci of caseation in a lymph node of the primary complex of histoplasmosis. This results subsequently, on healing, in stippled calcification typically associated with histoplasmosis. H & E × 36

immeasurable assistance in reaching the diagnosis. Widespread or even generalized lymphadenopathy is sometimes seen in young children during progression of the primary infection. External lymph nodes can protrude in tumor-like fashion, and mesenteric lymph nodes are not only palpable but sometimes even visible through the thin distended abdominal skin cover. Such lymph nodes show invasion by yeast-laden histiocytes to a point where any resemblance to normal lymph-node architecture disappears. Necrosis is not a constant feature of the development, but occasionally may lead even to liquefaction; and perforation, when it occurs in the cervical region, mimics the scrofula of yesteryear.

Isolated lymph nodes which swell up without clinically traceable source can occasionally be seen about the neck, and exceptionally elsewhere, in all age groups. Liquefied mediastinal lymph nodes can compress the airways to a point where life-saving emergency surgery is needed (Friedman et al.). The tissue destruction in such individual lymph nodes, as in the cystic lesions (Dovenbarger et al.) can be so complete that, grossly, the existence of a lymph node can be just suspected from the presence of small anthracotic specks on the capsule (Fig. 25). Microscopically, the evidence for lymph nodes may be equally scarce. In the exceptional cases of true primary mucocutaneous histoplasmic infection, the regional lymph nodes were, as expected, found to be prominently swollen (Spicknall et al.; Tesh and Schneidau; Tosh et al.) but regressed over a period of several months.

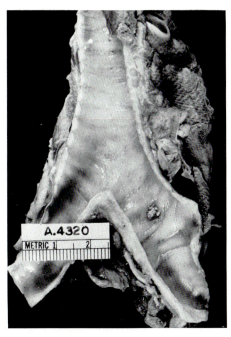

Fig. 27. Complications from healed lymph nodes of histoplasmosis consist largely in perforation into the tracheobronchial tree. Erosion by the sharp fragments of a calcified focus into a right main bronchus is shown here. Spastic cough, hemorrhage, sometimes lethal, and frequent expectoration of numerous broncholiths, represent the clinical picture. Some patients live for years with severe cough, proudly collecting stones, sometimes expelled by frightening attacks of coughing

The prominent enlargement of mesenteric lymph nodes by no means proves intestinal primary infection, since this condition is found with regularity in progressive infantile histoplasmosis in the presence of unquestionable primary pulmonary complexes. However, no demonstrated cases of intestinal ulcers in the absence of pulmonary infection have been reported.

A disturbing report (COLLINS) of almost 53% positivity in 151 mesenteric lymph nodes removed at appendectomy lacks any morphologic, cultural, or epidemiologic basis, and is mentioned only as an example of misleading and unfounded information.

Upper Airways: Broncholithiasis is a serious complication ordinarly associated with the sequelae of primary infection. It has been pointed out by early observers that calcification of the lymph nodes pertaining to the primary complex is a prominent feature of healed histoplasmosis, and it has been shown that radiologically (SERVIANSKY and SCHWARZ) and anatomically (STRAUB and SCHWARZ, 1962) the calcifications in the lymph nodes have characteristics which permit suspicion of the etiologic agent (Fig. 26). The lymph nodes can grow very large and, during the acute stage, become attached to surrounding structures, especially bronchi, trachea, esophagus, and less frequently to the large vessels in the thoracic cage. When the lymph nodes retract after the acute caseating lymphadenitis subsides, they often produce complications.

Errosion of trachea and bronchi is of common occurrence. Demonstration of organisms in calcified particles is easier in histoplasmosis than in tuberculosis, and organisms have been found repeatedly in broncholithis (Baum et al.; Weed and Andersen; MacInnis).

Perforation of caseated histoplasmic lymph nodes into the upper airways is therefore a well-established fact, and in the endemic area such perforations occur frequently; healed pigmented scars in trachea and bronchi with attached calcified lymph nodes are commonplace in our autopsy material (Fig. 27). If the existing

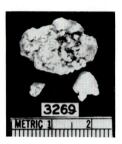

Fig. 28. Multiple histoplasmic broncholiths removed by bronchoscopy (G. Peabody, Washington, D.C.). If strategically located and of proper size, complete obstruction of bronchi and atelectasis can result from stones. After decalcification we have been successful in demonstrating *H. capsulatum* in every instance

fistula between the lymph nodes and airways does not close in time, calcific particles, or sequesters, will wander through the opening, producing spasms of cough and hemoptysis before they find their way into the bronchi and are expectorated (Baum et al.) (Fig. 28). Variable degrees of hemoptysis, including fatal hemorrhage, are seen during the entrance of the irregular calcium particles into the airways.

Lymphoma and Histoplasmosis

The association of lymphoma with complicating disseminated fungus disease is poorly understood but well documented. However, it is useful to remember that bacterial and viral complications in terminal lymphomas are equally or more common than fungus; this puts the fungal infection into its rightful place as "just another complication." *Candida albicans* and *Cryptococcus neoformans* probably are much more often "opportunistic" invaders in lymphomas than any other group of fungi. It has been advocated that the finding of disseminated fungus disease in lymphomas could represent coincidental occurrence, but the relative rarity of either group of disorder rules this out. The thesis that fungus diseases mimic lymphomas is more interesting in view of the common difficulty of precise diagnosis in some lymphomas; we have to confess that at the level of our present knowledge the diagnosis of lymphoma is largely a morphologic one, without the benefit of constant serologic or chemical supporting data. Small wonder that in a few cases lymphoma was diagnosed but at autopsy histoplasmosis was found.

Cases like R. D. Moore's, who found lymphoma at biopsy but at autopsy only histoplasmosis, are hard to accept. The concurrent presence of disseminated histoplasmosis with lymphomas can be rationalized in several ways: the lymphomatous patient is susceptible because of: a) altered immunology; b) destruction of gamma globulin sources; c) destruction of histiocytes (otherwise available for phagocytosis of yeasts); and finally, d) because of therapeutic measures as cytotoxic drugs, corticosteroids, radiation, etc. It should be pointed out again, that *Cryptococcus neoformans* has a much higher incidence rate in lymphomas than *H. capsulatum*. But both are seen mostly in Hodgkin's disease (Bunnel and Furcolow; Casazza et al.; CONRAD et al.; DEL NEGRO et al.; ENDE et al.; PARSONS and ZARAFONETIS; RODGER et al.; SAGLAM, VIVIAN et al.; ZIMMERMAN, 1955).

Histoplasma has been also reported in lymphoblastic lymphomas (NELSON et al.; R.D. MOORE), "malignant lymphoma" (STURIM et al.), reticulum cell sarcoma (MURRAY and SLADDEN), and in cases of leukemic symptomatology (DAVIS and RIPKA), lymphatic leukemia (WILLIAMS and CROMARTIE; REINHARD et al.); and one case (RODGER et al.) had simultaneously tuberculosis and cryptococcosis complicating disseminated Hodgkin's disease and histoplasmosis. Increased numbers of fungal infections in lymphomas are to be expected with prolongation of the life of the lymphomatous patient, but little evidence points to a new alarming trend.

The possible confusion of *H. capsulatum* with *Pneumocystis carinii* must be mentioned, since pneumocystosis is reported in increasing numbers in patients with lymphoma, agammaglobulinemia, etc. With the rarest of exceptions, pneumocystosis has remained restricted to the pulmonary alveoli, which may be a most helpful differential diagnostic point in the presence of scarce organisms. Indeed, the foamy character of the alveolar content is in typical cases most convincing in favor of pneumocystosis. So is the demonstration of "cysts" with 8 inner bodies in Giemsa stain. In view of the great variation of "personally-hued" diagnoses in lymphomas and the lack of uniform diagnostic criteria, it might be safest to rest the case with the statement that the association between lymphomas and histoplasmosis occurs, and is most commonly found in Hodgkin's disease.

Heart and Mediastinum

Heart, Pericardium, Mediastinum and Pleura. In 1966, sixteen documented cases of endocarditis caused by *H. capsulatum* were recognized by GERBER et al. The aortic and, in second place, the mitral valves were most commonly involved and the size and extension of the vegetations varied from case to case (WEAVER et al.). Histoplasmic endocarditis was found on the thickened valves of a previous rheumatic valvulitis (BERMAN, FAWELL et al., KORNS, PALMER et al.) or on previously normal valves (MERCHANT et al.).

Yeast cells were generally abundant in the valvular thrombotic masses, and sometimes blood cultures have yielded *H. capsulatum* (DERBY et al., GERBER et al.). Cultures taken from the vegetations at autopsy have given positive cultures (PALMER et al., MERCHANT et al.). The organisms found on the valves are sometimes larger than 5 μ, up to 16 μ (KORNS) and of atypical round shape (BINFORD, HAUST et al.) and even hyphal elements have been seen (BINFORD, KORNS, MERCHANT et al.). Extension of the endocarditis into the sinus of Valsava (BERMAN) and embolic phenomena have been observed (BERMAN, DERBY et al., FAWELL et al., GERBER et al.). The spleen shows complicating infarcts more frequently than other organs. Necrotizing arteritis in the subcutis (BERMAN) or aorta (HAUST et al.) has been found associated with histoplasmic endocarditis. Experimental endocarditis of the aortic valves has been produced in dogs after the induction of traumatic valvular incompetence. Sometimes, in this experiment, up to 13 consecutive blood cultures were needed before a positive result was obtained (AKBARIAN et al.). Two forms of hemic invasion could be recognized; one had "incidental" positive blood cultures with low colony count, representing occasional and inconsequential escape of organisms into the blood stream. The second group had repeated positive cultures with high colony counts, sometimes several hundred colonies per millilitres of blood. In dogs with the "incidental" blood culture, the positivity had no prognostic implications; in the second modality, it was generally lethal.

In middle-sized vessels of the lung, and also in other organs, a peculiar sub-endothelial proliferation occurs with histiocytes and occasional mononuclear cells separating the intima from the media. Such subintimal "pillows" in arterioles of the lung were recognized as early as 1939 in an infant (Agress and Gray) and in 1942 (Reid et al.). Sometimes, this proliferation is circular; in other instances, pillow-like focal protrusions into the venous, or less frequently, arterial lumina occur. Sometimes organisms are found in the macrophages, representing an excellent source for the introduction of Histoplasma into the blood stream. Actual intimal ulceration with discharge of yeast-laden macrophages can be observed occasionally, and is especially impressive when stains of Gridley or Grocott outline the organisms. The subendothelial swelling is also seen in meningitis, and softened foci of brain tissue could be explained by the decreased flow, similar to the findings in tuber-culous meningitis. In meningitis, there is frequently associated panangiitis with necrosis of the vessel wall, similar to the change noted in coccidioidomycosis or tuberculosis. This massive vascular response must be much more important in its circulatory consequences than the rather discrete subintimal "pillow," even if the latter is prominently protruding into the vascular lumen.

Myocarditis is uncommon in histoplasmosis. Granulomatous involvement was observed by Prior et al. in their case 4 in disseminated histoplasmosis. See also Humphrey's case 1, Schulz (1953) and Weed et al. Lesions without organisms in the heart are described by Pinkerton and Iverson. Myocarditis pericarditis are briefly mentioned by Kneidel and Segall in their case 1. Pinkerton and Iverson show a typical tubercular granuloma in striated skeletal muscle, a finding of some consequence in view of the diagnostic acceptance of sarcoid from muscle biopsies.

Organisms should be searched for by adequate methods. Pericarditis is by no means common, considering the millions of people infected with *H. capsulatum*, but in its clinical manifestations it is so spectacular that many single case reports have appeared, giving the impression of a frequent happening. Riegel and Schriever recently found 17 cases of pericarditis acceptable to them as histo-plasmic in origin. Fox described acute fibrinous pericarditis associated with specific pleuritis in a 17-year-old girl receiving steroid therapy. In other cases massive sero-fibrinous exudate threatened life (Murray and Howard, Owen et al., case 1; Gregoriades et al., Dix and Gurkaynak), and there was need for removal of as much as 1200 ml of exudate. The diagnosis is often tentative even after biopsy. In a young patient whose reactions to the histoplasmin skin test had changed from negative to positive in the presence of a high titer in the complement fixation test, we found epithelioid-cell tubercles in a pericardial biopsy, but were unable to demonstrate organisms on culture and microscopy. Hundreds of sections stained with the Grocott procedure had to be called negative after many long hours of scrutiny. Clinically and by circumstantial evidence, the patient was going through a complication of his primary infection, but we were unable to prove it by direct methods. A similar situation confronted Leedom et al.

Only two successful cultures from pericardial taps are on record (Gregoriades et al., Webb and Herring). Microscopically, in constrictive pericarditis *H. cap-sulatum* is seen more often, especially in the presence of calcific deposits. Apparently major areas of necrosis contain large numbers of organisms that remain stainable even when enshrined in calcium (Friedman et al., Klieger and Fisher, Babbit and Waisbren, Riegel and Schriever, Wooley and Hosier). Less certain cases, basing the etiologic diagnosis on a negative tuberculin skin test and positive histo-plasmin reaction, are published by Billings and Couch, Hurwitz and Pastor, McNerney, Webb and Herring, Owen et al. (case 1). In at least two publications the pericarditis was reported as seeming to be associated with clinical myocarditis (CRAWFORD et al., FRIEDMAN et al.).

Fibrinous and serofibrinous pericarditis can develop quickly and the accumulation of fluid can rapidly produce a dangerous situation. Absorption of exudate can take place either with or without the benefit of therapy. Adhesion formation and constriction, sometimes in the presence of calcified plaques, may be the resulting sequela. Myocarditis has been clinically suspected in association with pericarditis, but endocarditis does not seem to be recognized with pericarditis.

As a sequel of the primary complex, the infection may extend to mediastinal or cervical structures. The inflammation spreads into the perilymphnodal tissue producing cellulitis which, upon healing, becomes "stony hard" and encases the local anatomic structures in a type of fibrous "mediastinitis" (LULL and WINN). It may be impossible to determine the etiology of such cases, since the morphologic picture of a scar almost precludes the finding of organisms in the tissues. The clinical picture of *superior vena cava obstruction*, with the distended cervical and cranial vessels and the massive edema of soft tissues, is too well known to need description in greater detail. Obstruction of the superior vena cava proven to be due to histoplasmosis has been described only a few times. It is "rare in children, in adults a curiosity" (PATE and HAMMON). Most published cases of histoplasmic superior vena caval obstruction are based on circumstantial evidence such as the skin test: case 4 of OWEN et al., two cases of MILLER et al. 1958; (skin test and serology); SALYER et al., two cases of MARSHAL et al., GILLESPIE; or microscopic demonstration of the organism in the mediastinal or adjacent lung (BAUM and SCHWARZ, 1958), PATE and HAMMON, OWEN et al., case 3; or microscopy and culture as in a 2-year-old child reported by GRYBOSKI et al. Reconstructive surgery of vena caval obstruction is not very successful because of the common tendency of transplanted vascular structures to become again blocked.

In most reported cases, the lymph nodes of the primary complex are already calcified and the mechanism of obstruction becomes rather hard to understand. As a rule, caval obstruction is caused by compression of the vein between an expanding mass in the right anterior mediastinum and the sternum. Secondary thrombosis in the vein aggravates the condition or makes the obstruction complete. On the one hand, it would seem that "calcified lymph nodes" have little activity, but X-ray evidence of calcification does not necessarily indicate the extent of the calcification which may only occupy the center or a part of the lymph node. One therefore can visualize inflammatory hyperplasia of partially calcified lymph nodes with resultant compression of the vena cava. On the other hand, such lymph nodes may be shrinking and, in this process, produce distortion or actual kinking of the large but thin-walled blood vessel.

Interpretation of Indirect Diagnostic Methods

This may be the place to discuss our approach to diagnosis in cases where culture and morphologic methods are unsuccessful in demonstrating the organism. If the patient's reaction to histoplasmin changes from negative to positive, the circumstantial evidence is fairly good for recent infection with *H. capsulatum*. But even such a conversion — which is not often observed because of circumstances — is no proof that the disease under scrutiny is caused by *Histoplasma capsulatum*, since two independent processes can be well coexistent in the same body. A positive skin test *per se*, without the information of recent changeover from negative, is diagnostically not significant except in very special circumstances, as in a positive test in a laboratory worker in a nonendemic area where the general incidence

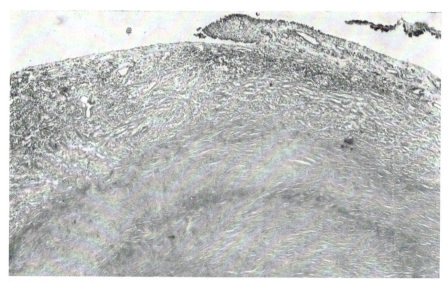

Fig. 29. Caseous subpleural primary focus of histoplasmosis. The overlying pleura shows only a delicate organizing reaction. H & E × 40

of skin-reactors would be fractions of 1%. A positive serologic reaction with rising (or even falling) titer could be used for interpretation of active (albeit subsiding) disease.

One word of caution is needed: the positive skin test elevates in some individuals the complement fixing titer considerably and therefore can ruin the immunologic approach to diagnosis completely. It is therefore advisable to restrict the use of the skin test for diagnostic purposes since little information accrues from its performance and since it, on the contrary, can ruin the value of serologic procedures. But even under optimal circumstances, the positive complement fixation test with rising titer will be only circumstantial evidence and its value cannot be compared with the conclusions drawn from a positive culture or morphologic demonstration of *H. capsulatum* in the lesion. It also should be pointed out that a single serologic test will bear very little weight compared with serial serologic tests; by preference, the complement fixation tests of sequential blood samples should be run simultaneously in order to have strict comparison of the titer.

Closely related to the obstruction of one specialized structure, such as the vena cava, are more widespread instances of posterior fibrous mediastinitis with tracheal compression (Woods) by a large mass, or with involvement of bronchial walls and obstruction of pulmonary veins (Bennett). In this latter case, organisms were finally demonstrated with the Grocott stain; previously, in two independent papers, fibrosis of undetermined origin had been accepted. Dysphagia due to extrinsic pressure upon the esophagus has been attributed to histoplasmic lymph nodes by Fifer et al., in 3 cases based on results of skin tests, serology, and X-ray.

Cynically, the supposedly "increasing incidence of histoplasmic mediastinitis" might be said to exist *in spite* of published reports. Proof is available only in the cases of Baum and Schwarz, Bennett, Gryboski et al., Lull and Winn, Owen et al.

Pleural involvement in histoplasmosis is, in many respects, more discrete than in tuberculosis (Fig. 29). The pleura covering the active primary focus sometimes shows a few histiocytes with or without fibrinous exudate. Later, a slight opalescent thickening remains. On the free surface of the lung, adhesions or bands are rarely formed over the primary focus. If the primary lesion is close to an inter-lobar surface, fine, easily disrupted adhesions may be found between the two sheets of opposing visceral pleura. Major accumulation of exudate — serous or serofibrinous — are uncommon in histoplasmosis (MILLER et al., 1961; Fox), which is somewhat surprising in view of the rather prominent accumulation of fluid in the pericardial sac during the formation of the primary infection. Empyema of the pleura in connection with bronchopulmonary fistula or as a complication of resec-tive surgery is an unusual complication (POLK et al.) and contains a mixed bac-terial flora.

Occasionally, small hard tubercles are seen in the visceral pleura surrounding the primary subpleural focus; these represent lymphogenous satellite spread, which is restricted to the immediate vicinity of the focus. Occasionally, the lymphangitic pleural streaks leading from the focus to the regional lymph nodes become fibrotic or even hyalinized and show, better than any injection of lymph spaces could, the pathways of lymphatic spread. Pleural thickening with tubercular reaction comes to occasional observation in biopsy material and, especially when simultaneous cultures are initiated, the etiology can be established (SCHUB et al.).

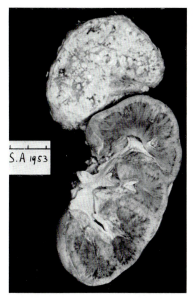

Fig. 30. Adrenal caseation in histoplasmosis. The glands may be discretely or completely caseated, with marked increase in size and with variable impact on the output of hormones. Classical Addisonian symptomatology in the endemic area is probably more often caused by histoplasmic adrenal involvement than by any other granulomatous destructive disease

Adrenals

Adrenal involvement in histoplasmosis is common, and there can be little doubt that there is actual predilection of the yeast cells to settle in this organ. The involvement of the adrenals can vary from isolated, inconspicuous, histiocytic proliferation to miliary tubercles, to focal and finally, to complete caseation (Fig. 30). Cases have been observed in which the adrenal had increased several times in weight and was confused at autopsy with tumor or tuberculosis (EARLE

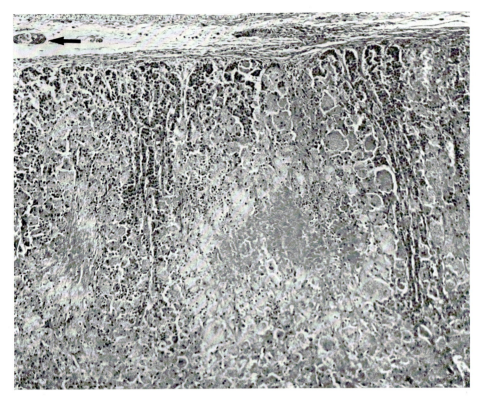

Fig. 31. During primary histoplasmic infection, progressive hematogenous dissemination is rare; when it occurs, the adrenals are seldom spared. Numerous huge macrophages filled with yeast cells are easily recognized with adrenal separating cortical cells. There are two foci of necrosis. Notice the yeast-containing macrophages in a small capsular vein (arrow).
H & E × 110

et al., Gerber et al., Layton et al., Pinkerton and Iverson, Vivian et al.). In the case of Kirsch, the right adrenal weighed 280 g, the left 260 g.

In cases of complete caseation, the clinical symptomatology may be that of Addison's disease, which in the past was frequently associated with tuberculosis. In the caseated adrenal gland numerous organisms are frequently found (Fig. 31). We have observed yeast cells considerably larger than the average yeast cells of *Histoplasma capsulatum* (Silverman et al.). Such large cells occur also in other necrotic tissues and have been induced in artificially autolyzed tissue explants (Schwarz, Goldman and Schwarz).

The true incidence of adrenal involvement in histoplasmosis is not known at present, but it must be high, because in all fatal disseminated cases we have found adrenal involvement of different types. Binford found adrenal involvement in all but one of 22 disseminated cases, Rubin et al. in 14 of 17 fatal cases. Of 18 cases of Addison's disease in Kansas, 6 were due to tuberculosis; 7, to histoplasmosis; 3, to cryptococcosis; 1, to coccidioidomycosis, and 1 was a primary atrophy (Frenkel). It is not surprising that the classical syndrome of Addison's disease does not always develop (Pierce), since this obviously will depend greatly on the rapidity of the destruction and particularly on the extent of the caseation of the adrenal cortex. However, several cases are on record where all criteria for the diagnosis of Addison's disease, both from clinical and laboratory observation, were present (BROOKLER et al.; CRISPELL et al., 4 cases; FITZPATRICK and REUBER; O'DONNELL, 2 cases; RAWSON et al.; RUDNER and BALE). The case of MERCHANT et al. was associated with histoplasmic endocarditis.

In our experience, several cases of adrenal involvement were observed in elderly men who in addition had mucocutaneous histoplasmosis or extensive ulceration of the mucosa of the digestive tract. This has also been noted by WEISS and HASKELL. However, such manifestations are just one more hematogenous localization of the disease (BAUM et al., 1957; HANSMANN and SCHENKEN). The formal pathogenesis of adrenal involvement is most likely arterial and embolic; at least this theory fits the best, generally accepted concept in tuberculosis, in which, during early or late dissemination, isolated or multiple hematogenous metastases occur. These may be found in any organ but rather frequently they localize symmetrically in such structures as the adrenals, the kidneys, the epididymes and the Fallopian tubes.

In view of the common unquestionably hematogenous involvement of the spleen in histoplasmosis, it would seem that the symmetrical adrenal involvement is also hematogenous. The bilateral involvement of organs certainly is governed by factors other than symmetry or simple mechanical distribution. The embolization of organisms into a particular structure is not necessarily productive of metastatic foci. Local and systemic factors determine the development of secondary lesions. FRENKEL believes that the local effect of corticoids in the adrenal influences the character of the tissue response as contrasted with the morphology observed in other organs of the same patient. Retrograde venous invasion and lymphogenous infection are unlikely. Calcification indicates that adrenal histoplasmosis can heal. However, in the course of disseminated histoplasmosis, the adrenal is only one of numerous organs involved, and unless the blood stream can be sterilized and the production of new metastases inhibited, the outcome of the case may be disastrous even if the foci in the adrenal should heal.

In early childhood the adrenal involvement seems to be most frequently the result of multiple small embolic foci which secondarily exhibit confluence until major parts of the adrenal cortex undergo caseation. On the other hand, in similar situations, one may find a healing small tubercle, indicating that the degree of involvement, either progression or arrest, is in direct proportion to the number of embolic organisms on the one hand and immunologic reaction on the other.

The diagnosis of adrenal histoplasmosis is possible during life under certain circumstances: first, when a patient with proven histoplasmosis develops Addisonian symptoms, or second, when an Addisonian syndrome shows a negative skin reaction to tuberculin and a positive skin reaction to histoplasmin, with a high complement-fixation titer. In such cases the diagnosis can be only tentative, since even in a set of circumstances as in the second example, Addison's disease still could be due to primary atrophy of the adrenal glands. *Histoplasma capsulatum* and *Blastomyces dermatitidis* were found side by side in an almost completely necrotic adrenal (LAYTON et al.).

Mucocutaneous Histoplasmosis

Mucocutaneous lesions, while not uncommon, are not as prominent in histoplasmosis as in two other deep fungus diseases, namely North and South American blastomycosis. In chronic and disseminated histoplasmosis, ulcers of the tongue, the palate, and the nasal septum occur, and physicians in the endemic area will do well to consider histoplasmosis in the differential diagnosis of any chronic mucosal defect (BENNETT, 1968).

Erythema Nodosum and Multiforme. During primary infection, erythema nodosum and multiforme may develop, and recent reports have been frequent. The
explanation given is that previously, major epidemics were not defined with such
promptness as in the Greenwood outbreak (Sellers et al.), and that the recently
reported occurrences of such erythematous lesions have been due to better recognition rather than to a change of pattern of histoplasmosis. In three outbreaks
(Leznoff et al., Sellers et al., Medeiros et al.), of 73 females and 11 males, 16
had erythema nodosum, 52 had erythema multiforme, and 16 had both forms.
There was good evidence of the association of these lesions with primary histoplasmosis in most, if not all, of the patients. Isolated cases of erythema nodosum
and multiforme have been recognized in connection with primary histoplasmosis
by Dickie and Murphy, Saslaw and Beman, Salfelder (1964), Nutall-
Smith, Little and Steigman, Heilbrunn and Cain, Murray and Howard.

Exfoliative Dermatitis. Another cutaneous involvement, exfoliative dermatitis,
was present in the case published by Hansmann and Schenken in 1934, and has
been redescribed, in 1953, by Fox.

Primary Accidental Cutaneous Histoplasmosis. The exceptional occurrence of
primary inoculation of *H. capsulatum* into the skin and mucosa is undeniable under
(accidental) "experimental" conditions, when misdirected culture material from
needles finds its way into the skin (Tosh et al., Tesh and Schneidau), or conjunctiva (Spicknall et al.). Spicknall et al. reported (case 2) a 36-year-old male
who sprayed a suspension of *H. capsulatum* into the conjunctival sac of his right
eye while he was injecting the aortic valve of a dog. Six days later he felt soreness
at the angle of the right mandible; after another 4 days there was edeme of the
palpebral conjunctiva and upper lid with profuse lacrimation. The preauricular
and upper anterior cervical lymph nodes were painful, tender, and enlarged. A skin
test, which had been negative for histoplasmosis on the day of admission, was
positive 10 days later. There was a shallow ulcer over the upper border of the tarsal
plate, which healed within 5 days. Culture and complement-fixation tests were at
all times negative.

Such well-defined instances of primary mucocutaneous histoplasmosis should
be clearly separated from the unwarranted implication of cutaneous primary infection in the average clinical case, where no definite source for percutaneous
entrance of the organisms exists. A reported case of assumed primary vulvar histoplasmosis is not acceptable to us for lack of supporting data. The autopsy protocol
is sketchy, and the findings in the lungs are not mentioned (Stankaitis and
McCuskey).

Two cases similar to syphilitic chancre are often cited as histoplasmic primary penile
lesions (Curtis and Cawley), but only the first case is a proven histoplasmosis and it can not
be claimed as an unquestionable primary lesion. Prepucial involvement was apparently of
secondary nature in a widely disseminated case (Palmer et al.).

A primary cutaneous histoplasmosis was diagnosed in a small boy (Barquet et al.) with
an ulcer of the *left* heel with widespread lymph node swelling, of the axiliary, cervical, intra-
abdominal, and especially of the *right* inguinal region. In childhood, peripheral lymph nodes
swell, sometimes to very considerable size, even after proven pulmonary infection (Silverman
et al.) and the lymphadenitis in this boy can therefore not be accepted as proof of a heel-inguinal
primary complex, as 1) the inguinal lymph node swelling was bilateral, but more pronounced
contralateral to the leg ulcer, and 2) the general lymphadenopathy precludes interpretation of
connection with the leg ulcer.

The reasons for insisting upon the rarity of primary cutaneous histoplasmosis,
i.e. spontaneous inoculation from nature, are both obvious and logical. In the case
of a primary focus, the regional lymph nodes swell. This has been observed in the
few cases of accidental infection in the laboratory (Tosh et al., Tesh and Schneidau). Moreover, we were able to reproduce the lymph node swelling in animals

(SALFELDER and SCHWARZ, 1965). Therefore, an ulcer of the skin or mucous membranes will be acceptable as a primary histoplasmic chancre only if the regional lymph nodes show simultaneous involvement. The lung in such a case must be free of lesions in order to make the case acceptable as primary cutaneous histoplasmosis.

Mucocutaneous Histoplasmosis. The laryngeal, lingual, buccal, pharyngeal, or labial erosions and ulcers have one common denominator: they are found together and dependent on chronic pulmonary histoplasmosis which is frequently cavitary (BAUM et al., 1957; DROUHET et al., 1962; GREENDYKE and KALTREIDER; PIERINI; WEED and PARKHILL; BENNETT, 1968). Some, probably the majority, are of hematogenous origin; others may represent an autoinoculation of fungus-containing sputum into superficial wounds and infections of the mouth. We have seen nonspecific-appearing, flat, histoplasmic lesions of the mucosa at the nasal entrance and around the anus. Identification is facilitated by the knowledge that there is disseminated histoplasmosis and by a biopsy of the lesion. Even biopsy may be disappointing, unless special stains are used with regularity, since the morphologic picture sometimes differs from that of nonspecific lesions only by the presence of yeast-containing histiocytes, which are not necessarily numerous or in groups or nodules. Histoplasmic ulcers may occur on the borders of at the base of the tongue, and are often suspected of being luetic. Simple contact smears, made by holding a clean slide against the lesion, give excellent results when stained with the Wright or Giemsa method. They represent the stains of choice in this situation, since they permit differentiation from *Leishmania* organisms, a highly desirable distinction in the mucosa of the oropharynx. The absence of the kinetoplast in *H. capsulatum* was already known to DARLING in 1905.

Leishmania occurs in the skin also and requires differential diagnosis. Leishmaniasis of the chin in an Italian girl was first diagnosed as histoplasmosis but finally recognized for what it was (WOO and REIMANN).

If ulcerations, either of the skin or of the mucosa, exist, smears or contact preparations give rapid information (PLOTNICK and CERRI). Biopsies can expedite diagnosis (WEED and PARKHILL), and cultures should be obtained.

Larynx

The upper respiratory tract is frequently involved in disseminated and chronic cavitary histoplasmosis (BENNETT, 1968). In some instances, massive papillary and ulcerative laryngitis has extended into the pyriform sinuses (HULSE, GAMMEL and BRECKENRIDGE). Other cases extended from the larynx into the trachea and main bronchi (SONES et al., KING and CLINE). Less spectacular cases affecting only parts of the larynx in more discrete form are more frequent (WITHERS et al., FURCOLOW, VAN PERNIS, PARKES and BURTOFF, CHARR, BURTON and WALLENBORN). BEEMAN and CHANG found a bulging mass on X-ray pressing against the larynx, with a small ulcer on the epiglottis. Histoplasmosis of the larynx was erroneously diagnosed in a 42-year-old man, and only after 4 biopsies recognized as leishmaniasis (ZINNEMAN et al.).

It should be unnecessary to emphasize that laryngeal lesions are complications of pulmonary disease and should not be interpreted as primary, even if clinically the hoarseness may be more impressive than the pulmonary lesion. Especially in biopsy specimens, the diagnosis can be difficult to ascertain unless special stains are routinely studied in ulcerative lesions of necrotic or ganulomatous character. In addition to mucosal ulceration in trachea and bronchi, perforation of caseous lymph nodes is found, with a surprisingly high healing rate, to judge from the common finding of pigmented scars in these tubular structures. The obvious differential diagnosis in the larynx includes tuberculosis, leishmaniasis, neoplasm, other fungus diseases and rarer lesions.

Gastrointestinal Tract

The gastrointestinal tract has been found involved frequently in disseminated histoplasmosis ever since Darling's first case. Beginning with erosions or ulcers around the lips and ending with anal lesions, every part of the digestive system has been found infected by histoplasmosis. Whether primary intestinal infection ever occurs is not known; no acceptable case is on record. This seems to indicate that primary intestinal histoplasmosis, if it occurs at all, must be an exceptional rarity. One case (Martz) in a 3-year-old girl was considered to be of intestinal origin, because the lungs seemed negative at autopsy. However, considering our rather rudimentary knowledge of the disease in 1947, we feel that the intestinal origin in this case is not proven beyond reasonable doubt. In order to accept intestinal infection (as well as any other extrapulmonary location) as primary, the point of entry should show an ulcer or scar, with distinct reaction in the regional lymph nodes. The lung should be negative on careful examination, following X-ray taken after removal of the lung from the body. Even experienced eyes and hands can miss a soft (not calcified) lesion in the lung.

A few words must be said about an article by Raftery et al., who reported that 58 of 1173 acutely inflamed and 35 of 768 chronically inflamed appendices were morphologically positive for *H. capsulatum*. Much time and effort had to be spent to disprove this claim. Cultural and morphologic study, by Christopherson et al., of 100 appendices was completely negative, as was the additional search in 512 appendices with the PAS method. Emmons and Mattern (1955) had completely negative results on 500 appendices.

Neither are the claims of Collins substantiated by culture, special stains, or pictures. Collins reported that 3905 (7.8%) of 50,000 appendices, collected in different institutions, were diagnosed as positive for *H. capsulatum* by "scores of pathologists." He gives no data about the way the diagnosis was made. In view of his subsequent statements, considering a "starry sky pattern" as diagnostic for histoplasmosis, the complete lack of confirmatory evidence in material examined by Christopherson et al. and Emmons and Mattern (1955), and the complete absence of histoplasmosis in appendiceal examination, in cases not suffering from disseminated histoplasmosis, in our own thousands of specimens, those claims must be without scientific foundation.

Much confusion to neophytes, who got their introduction to the problem by the rather copious output of Collins, has been wrought by his reports and those of Raftery; however, no confirmation has come from any quarter. Enthusiasm is no substitute for scientific facts!

Prior to 1953 (Gridley) and 1955 (Grocott), Histoplasma was not easily detected in tissues, and if special stains are not used, a diagnosis of histoplasmosis in lymphoreticular tissue cannot, in our opinion, be justified. Hence Collins' continuous emphasis on the frequency of histoplasmosis in a variety of disorders like mesenteric lymphadenitis and anorectal disease cannot be accepted in the light of the more recent studies cited above.

The most spectacular and direct cause of death from gastrointestinal histoplasmosis was a bleeding gastric ulcer (Fitzpatrick and Neiman); sudden death was precipitated by perforation of ulcers. Several cases on record were located in the ileum with resulting abscesses or peritonitis (Fischer et al., Henderson et al., Morgan and Shapiro, Sturim et al.). In the above cases the ileitis was only part of a widespread intestinal and systemic involvement. Perforation in midjejunum was reported by Shull. In turn, esophageal and gastric ulcers are as a rule associated with lesions in the lower intestinal segments (Weed et al., Worgan, Sturim et al.).

Little proof of the etiology is found in a case of a 6-year-old child with recurrent intussusception supposedly associated with histoplasmosis of Peyer's patches (Carmona and Allen). Perforation of esophagus and ileum was found in a case of histoplasmosis of the tongue, but apparently the perforations were the result of tuberculous infection (Peabody and Buechner). A radiologic description of 5 ulcerative intestinal lesions is well documented by culture or examination of the resection specimens. Ulcerative lesions were seen in stomach, small and large bowel, respectively (Perez et al.). Tumor-like gastric lesions were observed in disseminated histoplasmosis by Parsons and Zarafonetis and by Nudelman and Rakatansky.

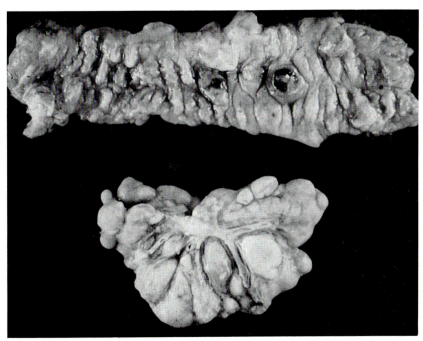

Fig. 32. Multiple colonic ulcers in infantile histoplasmosis. Mesenteric and mesocolic lymph nodes were massively enlarged and necrotic, but so were numerous peripheral groups of lymph-nodes, illustrating the occurence of huge lymphadenopathies in disseminated histoplasmosis. The focal occurrence of large external lymph-node clusters may mislead the investigator toward an apparent primary skin lesion. This child had a classical semiactive pulmonary primary complex

In the latter case constrictive lesions existed also in the jejunum. A small-bowel lesion with giant intestinal villi, which were not only enlarged but also flat-topped, seemed associated with protein-loosing enteropathy (BANK et al.). Much of the increase in volume was due to massive infiltrates of the villi by macrophages.

BERSACK et al. found inflammatory polypous lesions due to histoplasmosis in a 63-year-old man who died with widespread histoplasmosis. Lesions were seen on X-ray throughout the intestinal tract, distal from the duodenum. Again, macrophages filled with yeast cells dominated the morphologic alterations. The polypous tendency was seen in both ureters. The pigmentation almost certainly was related to extensive histoplasmic destruction of the adrenals.

Granulomatous enteritis is reviewed, and a case added by DEIBERT. In chronic disseminated disease the digestive tract participates prominently under a great variety of pathology, from shallow superficial erosions in the oropharyngeal area to deep ulcers in the tongue, ulcers or intramural lesions (HINSHAW and GUILFOIL) in the esophagus, and stomach, with or without associated hemorrhage. In children, intestinal ulcers can be legion, with masses of prominent mesenteric lymphadenitis sometimes reaching diameters of 8—10 cm (Figs. 32, 33). In adults, widespread intestinal ulceration has been observed in all parts of the small and large bowel, including the rectum and anus. In view of evidence in personally examined cases (SILVERMAN et al.), that intestinal lesions are often hematogenous in origin, since tubercular lesions in the submucosa were found to slowly open a path to the lumen, the pathogenesis, at least of disseminated cases, is not by deglutition (Fig. 34). However, such an origin in cases of cavitary pulmonary lesions containing myriads of organisms must also be considered. The impossibility of intestinal "takes" was documented in 3 monkeys by SASLAW et al.

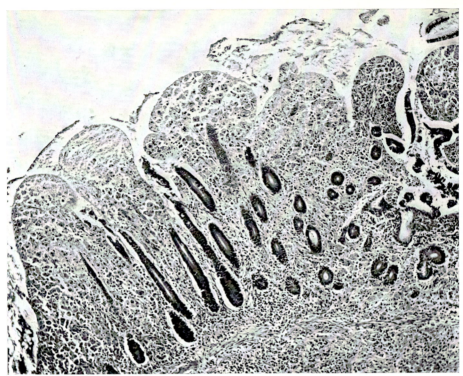

Fig. 33. Massive histoplasmic infiltration by yeast-laden histiocytes of the mucosa of the small bowel in a 10-month-old infant. The folds become flattened, thickened, and eroded. H &E × 70

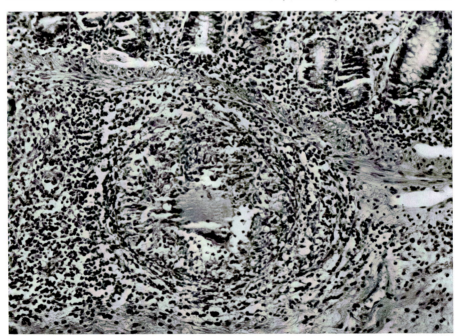

Fig. 34. Histoplasmic intestinal ulcers, frequently present in chronic cases of adults and in disseminated infantile histoplasmosis, are clearly secondary. In this instance, multiple submucosal hematogenous foci were demonstrated, some of which were breaking through the muscularis mucosae and opening into the lumen of the bowel. H & E × 160

Genitourinary System

The kidney shows foci of histoplasmosis of various forms in disseminated disease. Isolated macrophages filled with yeast cells, caught in the capillary tufts of isolated glomeruli (RAMSEY and APPLEBAUM; SCHULZ, 1954; WEED et al.) are found comparatively often. Frequently the macrophages seem recent arrivals, to judge from the absence of inflammatory reaction. Rarely a few leukocytes are found reacting to the intruding yeast cells, and we have seen occasional giant cells trying to engulf the organisms.

A more conspicuous picture is the presence of necrotic interstitial foci with or without associated granulomatous reaction (DAVIS and RIPKA, FITZPATRICK and REUBER, KIRSCH). The hematogenous nature is obvious from the multiplicity of the foci, the presence of similar foci in other organs and the equal (approximate) size of the lesions. Rarely have we seen in such instances metastases in the glomeruli and rupture of interstitial foci into tubules.

A most unusual case from Japan was recently reported by WILL et al. In a 74-year-old native, who had spent many years in Malaysia and India, a destructive papillitis with huge numbers of yeast cells was found. The organisms were quite consistent in size, shape, and staining properties with *H. capsulatum*. Attempts to obtain fluorescent antibody staining were negative in KAPLAN's laboratory (C.D.C. Atlanta) and in ours. However, fluorescent antibody staining is frequently negative on formalin-fixed material. One unusual feature was the overwhelming number of organisms, both intra- and extracellular. The man had a small pulmonary cavity without demonstrable causative agents. Less spectacular but considerable papillitis in widely disseminated disease has been reported repeatedly (BINFORD, 3 examples in a series of 22 disseminated cases; POST et al., VIVIAN et al.).

Iatrogenic, acute disseminated histoplasmosis was induced by the transplantation of kidneys from a cadaver, thought to have only thrombocytic purpura, into a patient with glomerulonephritis (HOOD et al.), and in a second case in the kidney of an unrelated donor (PARK et al.). Donor and recipient in HOOD's case had at autopsy disseminated histoplasmosis, with hepatic phagocytes full of yeast cells in the recipient. The picture of the overwhelming hepatic involvement is reminiscent of the pathology seen in experimental animals a few weeks after massive intravenous infection. Death occurred 14 days after transplantation and the kidneys were so badly damaged that no conclusion from histologic study was possible (HOOD et al.). PARK's patient died with widespread lesions of histoplasmosis.

A quite different, but still iatrogenic renal damage, is a typical complication of amphotericin B therapy of histoplasmosis. This drug, a polyene antifungal antibiotic isolated in 1955 by GOLD et al., has saved many lives and damaged many kidneys.

BUTLER et al., in a review of 81 patients on amphotericin B, noted increase of the blood urea nitrogen (BUN) and 93% and of creatinine in 83%. The increase was in direct proportion to the total dose of drug given. Of 26 patients studied, 24 had tubular damage extending to necrosis and calcium deposits. The authors feel that the functional and anatomic damage is at least in part irreversible. Amphotericin given to dogs resulted in marked renal vasoconstriction, with decrease of renal blood flow, glomerular filtration rate (GFR), and profound depression of inulin clearance (BUTLER et al.). Nephrotoxic tubular damage in 7 patients treated with amphotericin B associated with calcium deposits in proximal and distal convoluted tubules, in the presence of degenerative tubular changes, had progressed

8*

all the way to necrosis of tubular epithelium (see also McCurdy et al.). No inflammation or giant cells around the calcium were seen.

Bell et al., in a well-planned study, showed decrease of renal function with amphotericin B therapy as measured by inulin clearance, para-aminohippurate clearance, concentrating ability, and increase of BUN and creatinine levels. Return to pretreatment levels was the rule and the decrease in GFR was considered to be reversible (1961). It is assumed that the mechanism of increased permeability due to amphotericin affects not only the wall of fungal but also of tissue cells, permitting the escape of sodium, potassium chloride, and thiourea (Lichtenstein and Leaf).

The prostate is sometimes involved in disseminated histoplasmosis of adults (Fitzpatrick and Reuber, Rubin et al., Stiff, Worgan), but the participation is only minor and part of the widespread disease. Sometimes macrophages with organisms are seen filling the prostatic glands, but more often the phagocytes are found in small numbers in the interstitium of the organ. Much the same is true in reference to testis and epididymis. Involvement is rare, inconspicuous, and asymptomatic. Ovary and fallopian tubes escape similarly prominent localization by *H. capsulatum*, in contrast with the common salpingitis in disseminated tuberculosis. We were unable to find reports on uterine histoplasmosis. Winckel et al. have reported 71% of 31 curettings as histoplasmosis in women with menstrual disturbances. In view of the lack of cultural or serologic findings, and of special stains, and of the confirmation by other observers within the endemic area, the report must be put in the same class as the undocumented papers of Collins and of Raftery.

Gass et al. have reported on 2 placentas from a 31-year-old woman who had active cavitary histoplasmosis during both pregnancies. Cultures from the placenta were negative, but complement-fixing antibodies were found in the two infants (Zeidberg et al.).

In massive experimental intratracheal inoculation in two pregnant *Macaca mulatta*, death occurred after 7 days. Cultures were positive from both placentas, but negative from the organs of the foetuses (Saslaw et al.).

Brain, Meninges and Eye

Meningitis is proportionally less prominent in histoplasmosis than in cryptococcosis and coccidioidomycosis, and the available data do not permit conclusive statements about the pathogenesis. Little or no work has been done to elucidate whether underlying nodular lesions (histoplasmomas) are commonly found in the brain substance causing meningitis, in analogy to the convincing findings in tuberculous meningitis (Rich and McCordock, Schwarz). We, therefore, must simply state that the occasional cases of histoplasmic meningitis are commonly associated with disseminated disease and expressions of hematogenous seeding — leaving in the air the question whether this occurs by capillary embolism or from intracerebral histoplasmomas.

Plasma cells and lymphocytes are found in the meninges, and granulomatous arteritis, similar to the well-known lesions in tuberculous meningitis, occurs either focally or in diffuse form (Gerber et al.). Necrosis of part or all of the arterial wall, with a variety of cell infiltrates, has been observed (Fig. 35). In cases of histoplasmic endocarditis, meningitis will be a complication to be anticipated (Gerber et al.). The largest clinical series of 5 cases of histoplasmic meningitis (Tynes et al.) occurred in male adults. Brain involvement at autopsy was as high as 6 of 11

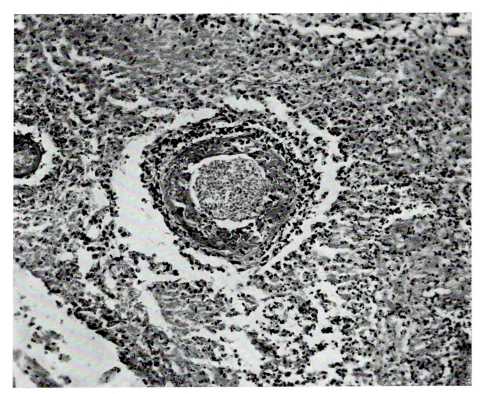

Fig. 35. Histoplasmic meningitis, with perivascular cuffs and necrosis of vascular walls. No information exists as to whether meningitis is always associated with underlaying encephalic granulomas or not. H & E × 160

patients dead of disseminated disease (SHAPIRO et al.), or 5 of 17 patients (RUBIN et al.) and 12 of 120 reviewed autopsies (SCHULZ, 1953). Small granulomata projecting from the tela chorioidea into the fourth ventricle are in every cellular aspect comparable to tuberculous lesions, except for the causative agent. On the other hand, examples of solitary granulomas in the brain are on record, as in the case of GREER et al., in which a 46-year-old man had had surgical removal of a "tumor" 2 cm in diameter, located in the frontal cortex near the Sylvian fissure, that turned out to be a histoplasma by cultural and morphological identification.

Multiple, histoplasmomas in the brain substance have also been noted (FITZPATRICK and REUBER, VOST and MOORE, WHITE and FRITZLEN), and in the cerebellum by BRIDGES and ECHOLS. Two cases of histoplasmoma were described by COOPER and GOLDSTEIN. They also tabulated a review of the literature up to 1963 of 20 cases of central nervous system involvement in persons of 4 months to 75 years of age. SNYDER and WHITE observed a 5-year-old boy with meningitic paralysis of both legs; whether, as assumed, the neurologic findings were primarily or exclusively due to intrathecal amphotericin therapy seems open to question. A case report of myelin degeneration after therapy falls into the same dubious category (HABER and JOSEPH). The cell count is seldom above 200—300, the majority lymphocytes; the pressure and protein are generally elevated, glucose only occasionally decreased. Cultures from spinal fluid are not always positive in histoplasmic meningitis, in view of the small number of organisms. This same reason explains the appearance of colonies as late as 50 or more days after inoculation of media (Gerber et al.).

Changes of intense arteritis of the meningeal vessels resemble in their entirety the findings in tuberculosis; the smaller arteries are predominantly involved (Sprofkin et al.). Adventitia and media show polymorphonuclear leucocytes, macrophages, and fibrinoid necrosis. Subendothelial infiltrates and endothelial proliferation are commonplace. Perineuritic inflammation extends from the cerebrospinal leptomeninges for variable stretches along the cranial nerves. Granulomatous, sometimes necrotic, lesions are found also in the large basal cisterns. The exudate in the leptomeninges and the cisterns varies from polymorphonuclear to mononuclear, apparently in relation to the age of the meningeal involvement. Large macrophages with numerous yeast cells help to establish the diagnosis. Sometimes the meninges can be grossly deceivingly transparent or only slightly turbid, only to show on microscopy scattered single or groups of histiocytes with yeast cells. Lymphocates in such minimal meningitis may be scarce.

A complicated case of mixed infection with *H. capsulatum* and *Cryptococcus neoformans* was reported by Morris et al. Cryptococcus was cultured 6 times from the spinal fluid during life, but at autopsy only pulmonary cryptococcosis was found. The brain had a necrotic focus in the region of one putamen with *H. capsulatum* in the lesion.

Meningoencephalitis with perivascular, often eccentrically arranged cuffs, has been seen in the brain stem and base of the brain of a 14-year-old boy. Granulomatous lesions in the perivascular cuffs contained phagocytes packed with organisms, mononuclear cells, epithelioid cells, foci of necrosis, but no giant cells (Schulz, 1953). In widely disseminated cases, the pituitary shows a few scattered macrophages with yeast cells. The same can be said of the parathyroid, thyroid (Locket et al.; Schulz, 1953, case 1), and the thymus. Of the endocrine organs, symptomatic disease seems to be located only in the adrenals.

The Eye: Histoplasmic eye involvement is postulated by ophthalmologists in the United States with considerable frequency (Falls and Giles, Jarvis and McCulloch, Krause and Hopkins, Mackley et al., Mann, Schlaegel, Schlaegel and Kenney, Van Metre et al., Van Metre and Maumenee, Walma and Schlaegel, Woods and Wahlen); and several medical centers in the endemic area have special clinics for "histoplasmic eye involvement." This postulate is not borne out up to now by anatomic evidence, although such patients show consistently small chorioretinal foci in the center or periphery of the fundus on ophthalmoscopy.

H. capsulatum has been demonstrated in the eye in spontaneous histoplasmosis of men, only once (Hoefnagels and Pijpers), and the sometimes impressive clinical correlation is based on indirect evidence, specifically a positive skin test, complement fixation, and the occasional observation of petechia in the choroid or retina after histoplasmin is injected intradermally. In dogs, granulomatous lesions have been observed after experimental histoplasmic aortic endocarditis (Salfelder et al.). In pigeons, chickens, and rabbits, histoplasmic ophthalmitis with a great variety of tissue response has been induced with intraocular infection (Sethi and Schwarz, Singer and Smith, Smith and Jones). After sensitization and challenge by dead or living *H. capsulatum* or even histoplasmin, violent reactions could be elicited in rat eyes, which were interpreted as immunogenic ophthalmitis (Okudaira and Schwarz). The experimental response, especially to histoplasmin, would lend support to the clinical hypothesis of immunogenic ophthalmitis in men. Intraperitoneally sensitized rats reacted to the intraocular challenge with histoplasmin, with outpouring of fibrinous and mononuclear exudate into the anterior chamber, nodular iridocyclitis and perivascular infiltrates, and hemorrhages in the optic nerve head (OKUDAIRA and SCHWARZ). The response was both ophthalmoscopically and anatomically compatible with a hypersensitization reaction.

If the clinically postulated histoplasmic *eye syndrome* exists, it would, in all likelihood, be of *immunogenic character*, not infectious, and organisms would not be expected to be present in the eye. The pathogenic relationship will be therefore always hard to establish. The lesions on ophthalmoscopy are generally described as small, scattered yellowish to greyish spots, with or without macular involvement. SCHLAEGEL and KENNY go even so far as to subdivide the macular involvement into diffuse, nodular, mixed, and hemorrhagic. Except for the hemorrhagic cases, little symptomatology was observed in this series. Our knowledge is severely limited by the paucity of available anatomic material, since eyes in this clinical condition are not enucleated; further, in cases of disseminated histoplasmosis, permission for removal of the eyes at autopsy is seldom requested and hard to obtain. Scars considered specific by clinical observers turned out completely nonspecific in one such eye we examined (the patient had such lesions bilaterally), when the eye removed for reasons other than histoplasmosis.

The problem is of great interest Leinfelder and importance in view of impairment of sight or even blindness, which occurs mostly in young patients; but unless anatomic material becomes more abundant, the morphologist will not be able to contribute a decisison. MAKLEY et al., for instance, reported 79 cases with chorioretinitis of presumed histoplasmic origin. Forty-one had bilateral lesions and in 19, both maculas were involved. All 79 had a positive histoplasmin skin test, but only 5 reacted to tuberculin. SPAETH questioned the existence of histoplasmic ureitis from observations on 34 cases of proven histoplasmosis. The pressure on the physician to provide therapy and the unquestionable need for treatment have led to certain polypragmatisms. If the lesions are at all related to histoplasmosis, they would in all likelihood be hypersensitivity reactions rather than true mycotic granulomatous disease. This, then, would preclude results from amphotericin therapy (MAKLEY, SCHLAEGEL, discussion of MAKLEY, GILES).

Associated Diseases

The problem of the association of histoplasmosis with lymphoma is discussed elsewhere. Sarcoid, that melting pot of granulomatous diseases without recognizable etiology, must be often "caused" by *H. capsulatum* (PINKERTON and IVERSON), but indeed such cases are not sarcoid at all, but histoplasmosis under the morphologic appearance of a sarcoid. The more special stains are used and attempts at culture are made in clinical cases of "sarcoid," the more etiologic agents will be unmasked (ISRAEL et al., BULLOCK and RAY, ENGLE, REIMANN and PRICE, SYMMERS).

Special mention should be made of the small forms of *Blastomyces dermatitidis*, which by simple measurements very closely resemble *H. capsulatum* (MANWARING; SCHWARZ, 1953; TOMPKINS and SCHLEIFSTEIN; WEED, 1953). This becomes even more of a problem of differentiation, if one considers the presence of large forms of *H. capsulatum* as occasionally found in necrotic foci or heart valves (BINFORD; SCHWARZ, 1953; SILVERMAN et al.), not to speak of the possible confusion between *H. duboisii* and *B. dermatitidis* in tissues. The fluorescent antibody technique, when applicable in fixed tissues, may be (in the absence of cultures) the safest method of conclusive differentiation. *H. capsulatum* and *H. duboisii* are uninuclear, a fact recognizable in well-fixed tissue. Several poorly defined pulmonary granulomatous diseases: pigeon-breeders lung (REED et al.), farmers lung (DICKIE and RANKIN), mushroom workers disease (BRINHURST et al.), byssinosis (TUFFNELL), feather sorters disease (Plessner), and others, may well have clinical and radiologic pictures suspiciously similar to epidemic acute histoplasmosis. Clarification cannot be expected without thorough cultural, epidemiologic, and morphologic work which is missing in most of the above citations.

Histoplasmosis, at least in part due to its ubiquitousness, is found associated with a host of other diseases, including other deep mycoses. *H. capsulatum* and *Blastomyces dermatitidis* was recovered from the same sputum specimen of one patient by Allison et al., and from 5 patients of Brandsberg et al. Dual infection at autopsy needs specific definition concerning the activity of the histoplasmic lesion, since healed histoplasmic lesions in the presence of active widespread blastomycosis hardly fall into the same category as truly dual disseminated disease (Brandsberg et al.; Layton et al.; Zimmerman, 1957). Tuberculosis in association with histoplasmosis is of considerable clinical importance, since the concomitance of the two diseases will preclude cure if only one organism is attacked by antibiotic therapy. We are far from having established figures on the true incidence of this combination, but numerous reports have been made (Beatty et al.; Conrad et al., 2 cases; Larkin and Phillips; Fitzpatrick and Reuber; Goodwin et al., 14 cases; Meleney; Murray and Brandt, 1951; Orr and Wilson; Peabody and Buechner; Polk et al., 3 cases; Post et al.; Saliba et al.; Schulz, 1954, 4 cases; Sutliff et al., 1953; Sweany et al., 1958; Vivian et al.; Goodwin et al., 24 cases); hence in the endemic area the finding of *H. capsulatum* in a cavity should call for repeated smears and cultures to rule out concomitant tuberculosis.

H. capsulatum and a scotochromogenic mycobacterium were cultured from cervical adenitis in a 2-year-old girl (Hughes). Cryptococcosis and histoplasmosis have been associated (Frenkel, Mider et al., Morris et al., Vivian et al., Zimmerman and Rappaport) and even cryptococcosis, tuberculosis, and histoplasmosis (Rodger et al.). A case was described by Winslow and Hathaway as having a healed primary focus of histoplasmosis, teeming with organisms, next to pulmonary lesions containing a mixture of *Cryptococcus neoformans* and *Pneumocystis carinii*. Histoplasmosis and coccidioidomycosis were found in the same sputum by Perry et al. A peculiar granulomatosis in childhood, which shows morphology consistent with infectious granuloma, has resisted etiologic clarification (Berendes et al.). This suppurative, lethal, lymphadenitis, with necrosis and giant cells, and pulmonary and hepatic lesions must be considered in differential diagnosis of histoplasmosis.

Even under optimal conditions technical difficulties remain mountainous and are hard to overcome. *H. capsulatum* is easily cultured only from biopsy material and from the sputum of cavitary cases; sputum of noncavitary cases will rarely give positive results. Blood and bone-marrow cultures, beyond the infantile form of progressive disease and beyond histoplasmic endocarditis, will be little rewarding. And even in the two pathologic forms, repeated cultures and prolonged search on smears may be necessary before success rewards the effort. It must be stated clearly (and repetitiously) that the granulation tissue produced by *H. capsulatum* is in no way unique or specific (Vivian et al.). The epithelioid-cell tubercles caused by *H. capsulatum* in lung, lymph nodes (especially cervical), liver, and kidney appear identical to the lesions seen in tuberculosis, blastomycosis, berylliosis, and what is called sarcoid. Organisms in noncaseating epithelioid-cell tubercles are scarce or absent, and unless cultures for fungi and bacteria are made systematically at autopsy and from biopsy material, many cases will figure as "granuloma of unknown etiology."

Caseated lesions especially seen in lung and lymph nodes are generally full of organisms, and therefore can be recognized easily with the proper special stains

(GROCOTT, GRIDLEY). The morphologic character of the caseated lesion is not only indistinguishable from that of tuberculosis but also from blastomycosis and coccidioidomycosis. Sometimes the necrosis is combined with suppuration and becomes similar to the pathology seen in cat scratch disease, tularemia, and lymphopathia venereum. It is virtually hopeless to attempt to differentiate these various lesions without positive cultural and staining support. Sometimes history, skin test, and CFT must suffice for a tentative classification. The caseation of the foci of the primary complex, both in lung and lymph nodes, is more discrete in histoplasmosis than in tuberculosis. The large size of the histoplasmic primary complex in comparison to the tuberculous (Ghon) complex has been mentioned repeatedly. The cavitary lesions also are identical to those seen in tuberculosis, coccidioidomycosis, and some of the less-common granulomas.

Small multiple acute excavations can sometimes be seen in what can be described best as "gelatinous pneumonia." Older cavities have thick walls, bronchi, and vessels crossing the cavity, and the exudate found in the lesions is in no way different from that of the "competing" diseases. In coccidioidomycosis even large cavities sometimes have thin walls, but this is by no means constant. Examination of the cavitary wall will show occasional reepithelization or, on the contrary, superficial ulceration with necrotic exudate covering the defect. Organisms may be numerous in this pseudomembrane, but scarce or absent in the wall proper. The etiology of chronic fibrosing or fibrotic lesions is impossible to determine, and we shall have to leave it as "scars are scars." No organisms are ever seen in the common fibrous and fibrohyaline pulmonary, mediastinal, and similar scars; only if calcification is found can organisms be expected to be demonstrable.

Miliary nodules in the leptomeninges are seldom seen in histoplasmosis associated with meningitis, but otherwise the exudate and its localization could pass for tuberculosis. The vasculitis has been referred to repeatedly.

Endocarditis of histoplasmic origin has the morphologic appearance of bacterial endocarditis, and only the demonstration of *H. capsulatum* will lead to recognition of the etiology.

The pathologic anatomy of histoplasmosis historically has been constantly compared with that of tuberculosis, a disease studied for centuries and by the best of pathologists. The knowledge acquired in histoplasmosis has been accelerated by the possibility of analogies and shortcuts available by comparing notes from the studies of tuberculosis. But the detailed knowledge available from the protocols of thousands of autopsies in tuberculosis will quantitatively be never reached, for histoplasmosis, not only because of limitations of material but also because modern trends have switched the spotlight considerably from classical anatomic changes. Yet identification of histoplasmosis offers possibilities that are not available in tuberculosis: specifically, the facility of demonstrating *H. capsulatum* with the Grocott procedure, permitting one to follow the protean metamorphoses of the yeast with much greater precision than was ever possible with *Mycobacterium tuberculosis*.

References

ADRIANO, S., SCHWARZ, J., SILVERMAN, F.N.: Epidemiologic studies in an outbreak of histoplasmosis. J. Lab. clin. Med. **46**, 592 (1955). — AGRESS, H., GRAY, S.H.: Histoplasmosis and reticulo-endothelial hyperplasia. Amer. J. Dis. Child. **57**, 573 (1939). — AJELLO, L.: Comparative ecology of respiratory mycotic disease agents. Bact. Rev. **31**, 6 (1967). — AJELLO, L., GREENHALL, A.M., MOORE, J.C.: Occurrence of Histoplasma capsulatum on the island of Trinidad, B.W.I. II. Survey of chiropteran habitats. Amer. J. trop. Med. Hyg. **11**, 249 (1962). — AKBARIAN, M., SALFELDER, K., SCHWARZ, J.: Cultural and serological studies in experimental canine histoplasmosis. Antimicrob. Agents Chemother. **1964**, 656. ~ Experimental histoplasmic endocarditis. Arch. intern. Med. **114**, 784 (1964). —

ALBRECHT, J.: Neues über Histoplasmose. Med. Mschr. 6, 692 (1952). — ALES-REIN-
LEIN, J.M., RIOS-MOZO, M.: Histoplasmosis. Übersichtsreferat. Rev. clin. esp. 51, 209
(1953). — ALEXANDER, J.T., BAKIR, F.B.: Acute disseminated histoplasmosis. Report of a
case diagnosed by needle biopsy of the spleen and liver. Med. Ann. D.C. 22, 389 (1953). —
ALLEN, J.H., Jr.: Bone involvement with disseminated histoplasmosis. Amer. J. Roentgenol.
82, 250 (1959). — ALLISON, F., LANCASTER, M.G., WHITEHEAD, A.E., WOODBRIDGE, H.B., Jr.:
Simultaneous infection in man by Histoplasma capsulatum and Blastomyces dermatitidis.
Amer. J. Med. 32, 476 (1962). — APONTE, G.E.: A histopathologic study of hepatic lymph
nodes. Amer. J. clin. Path. 34, 57 (1960). — BABBIT, D.P., WAISBREN, B.A.: Epidemic pul-
monary histoplasmosis, roentgenographic findings. Amer. J. Roentgenol. 83, 236 (1960). —
BADER, G.: Die visceralen Mykosen. Jena: Gustav Fischer 1965. — BAKER, R.D.: Histo-
plasmosis in routine autopsies. Amer. J. clin. Path. 41, 457 (1964). — BANK, S., TREY, C.,
GANS, I., MARKS, I.N., GROLL, A.: Histoplasmosis of the small bowel with "giant" intestinal
villi and secondary protein-losing enteropathy. Amer. J. Med. 39, 492 (1965). — BARQUET,
A.C., CHEDIAK, M., MAGRINAT, G.: Histoplasmosis. Resumen de la enfermedad. Presentacion
de un caso diagnosticado por puncion ganglionar. Bol. Col. méd. Habana 2, 365 (1951). —
BAUM, G.L., GREEN, R.A., SCHWARZ, J.: Enlarging pulmonary histoplasmomas. Amer. Rev.
resp. Dis. 82, 721 (1960). — BAUM, G.L., SCHWARZ, J., BRUINS SLOT, W.J., STRAUB, M.: Mucocutaneous histoplasmosis. Arch. Derm. 76, 4 (1957). — BAUM, G.L., BERNSTEIN, I.L., SCHWARZ,
J.: Broncholithiasis produced by histoplasmosis. Amer. Rev. Tuberc. 77, 162 (1958). — BAUM,
G.L., SCHWARZ, J.: Pulmonary histoplasmosis. New Engl. J. Med. 258, 677 (1958). — BEAMER,
P.R., SMITH, W.B., BARNETT, H.L.: Histoplasmosis; report of case in infant and experimental
observations. J. Pediat. 24, 270 (1944). — BEATTY, O.A., SALIBA, A., LEVENE, N.: A study of
cavities and bronchi in pulmonary fungus diseases. Dis. Chest 47, 409 (1965). — BEEMAN,
E.A., CHANG, P.L.: Disseminated histoplasmosis with laryngeal involvement and acquired
hemolytic anemia. Report of a case. Med. Ann. D.C. 34, 275 (1965). — BEHREND, H., HORT, W.,
JANKE, D.: Über das Krankheitsbild der Histoplasmose. Z. klin. Med. 157, 291 (1962). —
BELL, N.H., ANDRIOLE, V.T., SABESIN, S.M., UTZ, J.P.: On the nephrotoxicity of amphotericin B in man. Amer. J. Med. 33, 64 (1962). — BELLIN, E.L., SILVA, M., LAWYER, T., JR.:
Central nervous system histoplasmosis in a Puerto Rican. Neurology (Minneap.) 12, 148
(1962). — BENNETT, D.E.: Histoplasmosis of the oral cavity and larynx. Arch. intern. Med.
120, 417 (1967). — BENNETT, I.L., JR.: CPC. Bull. Johns Hopk. Hosp. 118, 73 (1966). —
BERENDES, H., BRIDGES, R.A., GOOD, R.A.: A fatal granulomatosis of childhood. Minn. Med.
40, 309 (1957). — BERLINER, M.D., RECA, M.E.: Vital staining of Histoplasma capsulatum
with Janus Green B. Sabouraudia 5, 26 (1966). — BERMAN, B.: Histoplasmosis endocarditis.
Sinai Hosp. J. (Baltimore) 9, 4 (1960). — BERSACK, S.R., HOWE, J.S., RABSON, A.S.: Inflammatory pseudo-polyposis of the small and large intestines with the Peutz-Jeghers syndrome in a case of diffuse histoplasmosis. Amer. J. Roentgenol. 80, 73 (1958). — BILLINGS,
F.T., JR., COUCH, O.A., JR.: Pericardial calcification and histoplasmin sensitivity. Ann. intern.
Med. 42, 654 (1955). — BINFORD, C.H.: Histoplasmosis. Tissue reactions and morphologic
variations of the fungus. Amer. J. clin. Path. 25, 25 (1955). — BLANCHARD, A.J., OLIN, J.S.:
Histoplasmosis with sarcoid-like lesions occurring in multiple myeloma. Canad. med. Ass. J.
85, 307 (1961). — BOONE, W.T., ALLISON, F.: Histoplasmosis. Amer. J. Med. 46, 818 (1969). —
BRANDSBERG, J.W., TOSH, T.E., FURCOLOW, M.L.: Concurrent infection with Histoplasma
capsulatum and Blastomyces dermatitidis. New Engl. J. Med. 270, 874 (1964). — BRIDGES,
W.R., ECHOLS, D.H.: Cerebellar histoplasmoma. J. Neurosurg. 26, 261 (1967). — BRINHURST,
L.S., BYRNE, R.N., GERSHON-COHEN, J.: Respiratory disease of mushroom workers: Farmer's
lung. J. Amer. med. Ass. 171, 15 (1959). — BROOKLER, M.I., BAHN, R.C., MARTIN, W.J.,
GASTINEAU, C.F.: Histoplasmosis. Minn. Med. 47, 1460 (1964). — BULLOCK, J.B., RAY, S.E.:
Histoplasmosis simulating sarcoidosis. Virginia med. Mth. 88, 153 (1961). — BUNNEL, I.L.,
FURCOLOW, M.L.: A report of ten proved cases of histoplasmosis. Publ. Hlth Rep. (Wash.) 63,
299 (1948). — BURTON, C.T., WALLENBORN, P.A., JR.: Histoplasmosis of the larynx. Virginia
med. Mth. 80, 665 (1965). — BUTLER, W.T., HILL II, G.J., SZWED, C.F., KNIGHT, V.: Amphotericin B renal toxicity in the dog. J. Pharmacol. exp. Ther. 143, 47 (1964). — BUTLER,
W.T., BENNET, J.E., ALLING, D.W., WERTLAKE, P.T., UTZ, J.P., HILL II, G.J.: Nephrotoxicity of Amphotericin B. Early and late effects in 81 patients. Ann. intern. Med. 61, 175
(1964). — CAIN, J.C., DEVINS, E.J., DOWNING, J.E.: An unusual pulmonary disease. Arch.
intern. Med. 79, 626 (1947). — CAMPINS, H., ZUBILLAGA, C., GOMEZ LOPEZ, L., DORANTE, M.:
An epidemic of histoplasmosis in Venezuela. Amer. J. trop. Med. Hyg. 5, 690 (1956). —
CARMONA, M.G., ALLEN, M.S.: Recurrent intussusception in a 6 year old child with histoplasmosis of Peyer's patches. J. Fla med. Ass. 44, 955 (1958). — CARSKI, T.R., COZAD, G.C.,
LARSH, H.W.: Detection of Histoplasma capsulatum in sputum by means of fluorescent antibody staining. Amer. J. clin. Path. 37, 465 (1962). — CASAZZA, A.R., DUVALL, CH.P., CAR-
BONE, P.P.: Infection in lymphoma. J. Amer. med. Ass. 197, 118 (1966). — CHARR, R.: Histoplasmosis. Report of two cases. Amer. Rev. Tuberc. 67, 376 (1953). — CHEESMAN, R.J.,

HODGSON, C.H., BERNATZ, P.E., WEED, L.A.: Surgical resection in the treatment of pulmonary histoplasmosis: a follow up study. Dis. Chest **37**, 356 (1960). — CHRISTOPHERSON, W.M., MILLER, M.P., KOTCHER, E.: Examination of human appendices for Histoplasma capsulatum. J. Amer. med. Ass. **149**, 1684 (1952). — COCKSHOTT, W.P., LUCAS, A.O.: Histoplasmosis Duboisii. Quart. J. Med. **33**, 223 (1964). — COLLIER, W.A., WINCKEL, W.E.F.: Beiträge zur geographischen Pathologie von Suriname. 6. Histoplasmose bei Säugetieren in Suriname. Antonie von Leeuwenhoek **18**, 349—356 (1952). — COLLINS, D.C.: A study of 50,000 specimens of the human vermiform appendix. Surg. Gynec. Obstet. **101**, 437 (1955). ~ Histoplasma capsulatum: the principal cause of mesenteric lymphadenitis in juveniles. Mississippi V. med. J. **77**, 146 (1955). ~ Histoplasmosis *is* a common disease of the colo-rectum. Amer. J. Proctol. **16**, 219 (1965). — COLVIN, S.H., GORE, I., PETERS, M.: A case of histoplasmosis (Darling) with autopsy. Amer. J. med. Sci. **207**, 378 (1944). — CONRAD, F.G., SASLAW, S., ATWELL, R.J.: Protean manifestations of histoplasmosis as illustrated in 23 cases. Arch. intern. Med. **104**, 692 (1959). — COOPER, R.A., JR., GOLDSTEIN, E.: Histoplasmosis of the central nervous system: report of two cases and review of the literature. Amer. J. Med. **35**, 45 (1963). — COOPERBERG, A.A., SCHWARTZ, J.: Diagnosis of disseminated histoplasmosis from marrow aspiration. Ann. intern. Med. **61**, 289 (1964). — CORTEZ, W.S., LANGELUTTIG, H.V., YATES, J.L., BRASHER, C.A., FURCOLOW, M.L.: Is there a relationship between silicosis and histoplasmosis? Dis. Chest **41**, 645 (1962). — COZAD, G.C., FURCOLOW, M.L.: Laboratory studies of Histoplasma capsulatum. II. Size of the spores. J. infect. Dis. **92**, 77 (1953). — CRAWFORD, S.E., CROOK, W.G., HARRISON, W.M., SOMMERVILL, B.: Histoplasmosis as cause of acute myocarditis and pericarditis: report of occurrence in siblings and review of literature. Pediatrics **28**, 92 (1961). — CRISPELL, K.R., PARSON, W., HAMLIN, J., HOLLIFIELD, G.: Addison's disease associated with histoplasmosis. Amer. J. Med. **20**, 23 (1956). — CURTIS, A.C., CAWLEY, E.P.: Genital histoplasmosis. J. Urol. (Baltimore) **57**, 781 (1947). — CURTIS, A.C., GREKIN, J.N.: Histoplasmosis: Review of cutaneous and adjacent mucous membrane manifestations with report of three cases. J. Amer. med. Ass. **134**, 1217 (1947). — DAELEN, M.: Über das Krankheitsbild der Histoplasmose. Tuberk.-Arzt **3**, 521 (1949). — DA ROCHA-LIMA, H.: Beitrag zur Kenntnis der Blastomykosen, Lymphangitis epizootica und Histoplasmosis. Zbl. Bakt., I. Abt. Orig. **67**, 233 (1912). — DARLING, S.T.: Notes on histoplasmosis — a fatal disorder met with in tropical America. Maryland med. J. **50**, 125 (1907). ~ A protozoan general infection producing pseudotubercles in lungs and focal necrosis in liver, spleen, and lymph nodes. J. Amer. med. Ass. **46**, 1283 (1906). — DAUGAVIETIS, H.E., MAUTNER, L.S.: Disseminated nodular pulmonary ossification with mitral stenosis. Arch. Path. **63**, 7 (1957). — DAVIS, P.L., RIPKA, J.W.: Pancytopenia with leukemia-like picture. Effects of histoplasmosis. J. Amer. med. Ass. **188**, 184 (1964). — DEAN, G.: Cave disease. Centr. Afr. J. Med. **3**, 79 (1957). — DEIBERT, K.R.: Case report. Disseminated histoplasmosis. J. Tenn. med. Ass. **45**, 19 (1952). — DEL NEGRO, G., VERONESI, R., FIGUEIREDO, M. DE A.: Histoplasmose generalizada e molestia de Hodgkin. Rev. paul. Med. **43**, 291 (1953). — DEMONBREUN, W.A.: Cultivation and cultural characteristics of Darling's H. capsulatum. Amer. J. trop. Med. **14**, 93 (1934). ~ The dog as a natural host for H. capsulatum. Amer. J. trop. Med. **19**, 565 (1939). — DERBY, B.M., COOLIDGE, K., ROGERS, D.E.: Histoplasma capsulatum endocarditis with major arterial embolism. Arch. intern. Med. **110**, 63 (1962). — DICKIE, H.A., MURPHY, M.E.: Laboratory infection with Histoplasma capsulatum. Amer. Rev. Tuberc. **72**, 690 (1955). — DICKIE, H.A., RANKIN, J.: Farmer's lung. Acute granulomatous interstitial pneumonitis occurring in agricultural workers. J. Amer. med. Ass. **167**, 1069 (1958). — DIVELEY, W., McCRACKEN, R.: Cavitary pulmonary histoplasmosis treated by pulmonary resection: 13-year experience with 29 cases. Ann. Surg. **163**, 921 (1966). — DIX, J.H., GURKAYNAK, N.: Histoplasmosis with massive pericardial effusion and systemic involvement: Report of a case. J. Amer. med. Ass. **182**, 687 (1962). — DOVENBARGER, W.V., TSUBURA, E., SCHWARZ, J., BAUM, G.L.: Mediastinal cystic granuloma due to Histoplasma capsulatum. J. thorac. cardiovasc. Surg. **42**, 193 (1961). — DOWE, J.B., GRAHAM, C.S., BROWN, S., DURIE, E.B.: A case of histoplasmosis. Med. J. Aust. **1953 I**, 142—144. — DROUHET, E.: Quelques aspects biologiques et mycologiques de l'histoplasmose. Sem. Hôp. Paris, Path. et Biol., Arch. Biol. (Liège) **1957**, 439. ~ Quelques aspects cliniques et biologiques de l'histoplasmose. Sem. Hôp. Paris **1957**, 789. — DROUHET, E., SUREAU, B., DESTOMBES, P., BEROD, J., TAPIE, P.: Histoplasmose bucco-pharyngée chronique recidivante évoluant depuis 8 ans. Activité thérapeutique de l'amphotericin B et de l'antibiotique X-5079 C. Bull. Soc. franç. Derm. Syph. **69**, 46 (1962). — DUBLIN, W.B., CULBERTSON, C.G., FRIEDMAN, H.P.: Histoplasmosis. Amer. Rev. Tuberc. **58**, 562 (1948). — DUBOIS, A., VANBREUSEGHEM, R.: Histoplasmose existe-t-elle en Belgique? Bull. Acad. roy. Méd. Belg., Ser. 6, **1**, 14 (1955). — EARLE, J.H.O., HIGHMAN, J.H., LOCKEY, E.: A case of disseminated histoplasmosis. Brit. med. J. **1**, 607 (1960). — EDWARDS, M.R., HAZEN, E.L., EDWARDS, G.A.: Micromorphology of the tuberculate spores of Histoplasma capsulatum. Canad. J. Microbiol. **6**, 66 (1960). ~ The fine structure of the yeast-like cells of Histoplasma in culture. J. gen. Microbiol. **20**, 496 (1959). — EDWARDS, P.Q., KLAER, J.H.: World-wide distribution of histoplasmosis and histoplasmin sensitivity. Amer. J. trop. Med. Hyg. **5**, 235 (1956). — Edwards, P.Q., Palmer, C.E.: Nationwide histoplasmin sensitivity and histoplasmal infection. Publ. Hlth Rep. (Wash.) **78**, 241 (1963). — Emanuel, D.A., Wenzel, F.J., Lawton, B.R.: Pneumonitis due to Cryptostroma corticale (Maple bark disease). New Engl. J. Med. **274**, 1413 (1966). — Emmons, C.W.: Isolation of Histoplasma capsulatum from soil. Publ. Hlth Rep. (Wash.) **64**, 892 (1949). ~ Histoplasmosis: Animal reservoirs and other sources in nature of the pathogenic fungus, Histoplasma. Amer. J. publ. Hlth **40**, 436 (1950). ~ Histoplasmosis. Bull. N.Y. Acad. Med. **31**, 627 (1955). — Emmons, C.W., Binford, C.H., Utz, J.P.: Medical Mycology. Philadelphia: Lea and Febiger 1963. — Ende, N., Pizzolato, P., Ziskind, J.: Hodgkin's Disease associated with histoplasmosis. Cancer (Philad.) **5**, 763 (1952). — Engle, R.L., Jr.: Sarcoid and sarcoid-like granulomas. A study of 27 post-mortem examinations. Amer. J. Path. **29**, 53 (1953). — Englert, E., Jr., Phillips, A.W.: Acute diffuse pulmonary granulomatosis in bridge workers. Amer. J. Med. **15**, 733 (1953). — Falls, H.F., Giles, C.L.: Use of amphotericin B in selected cases of chorioretinitis. Amer. J. Ophthal. **49**, 1288 (1960). — Farber, S., Craig, J.M.: C.P.C. J. Pediat. **50**, 77 (1957). — Fatorelli, A.: Histoplasmose ocular apresentacao de case. Rev. bras. Oftal. **18**, 349 (1959). — Fawell, W.N., Browns, H.L., Ernstene, A.C.: Vegetative endocarditis due to Histoplasma capsulatum. Cleveland Clin. Quart. **18**, 305 (1951). — Feldman, H.A., Sabin, A.B.: Pneumonitis of unknown etiology in a group of men exposed to pigeon excreta. J. clin. Invest. **27**, 533 (1948). — Fetter, B.F., Klintworth, G.K., Hendry, W.S.: Mycoses of the central nervous system. Baltimore: Williams and Wilkins Co. 1967. — Fifer, W.R., Woellner, R.C., Gordon, S.S.: Mediastinal histoplasmosis. Report of three cases with dysphagia as the presenting complaint. Dis. Chest **47**, 518 (1965). — Fischer, H., Marks, A.R., Wilson, J.E., Hathaway, R.: Histoplasmosis. W. Va med. J. **47**, 114 (1951). — Fitzpatrick, M.J., Reuber, M.D.: Addison's disease associated with disseminated histoplasmosis and pulmonary tuberculosis. Amer. Rev. Tuberc. **72**, 675 (1955). — Fitzpatrick, T.J., Neiman, B.H.: Histoplasma capsulatum infection associated with gastric ulcer and fatal hemorrhage. Arch. intern. Med. **91**, 49 (1953). — Fox, H.: Exfoliative dermatitis complicated by fatal acute disseminated histoplasmosis. Arch. Derm. Syph. (Chic.) **68**, 734 (1953). — Frenkel, J.K.: Role of corticosteroids as predisposing factors in fungal diseases. Lab. Invest. **11**, 1192 (1962). — Friedman, J.L., Baum, G.L., Schwarz, J.: Primary pulmonary histoplasmosis. Amer. J. Dis. Child. **109**, 298 (1965). — Furcolow, M.L.: Further observation on histoplasmosis. Mycology and bacteriology. Publ. Hlth Rep. (Wash.) **65**, 965 (1950). — Furcolow, M.L., Brasher, C.A.: Chronic progressive (cavitary) histoplasmosis as a problem in tuberculosis sanatoriums. Amer. Rev. Tuberc. **73**, 609 (1956). — Furcolow, M.L., Grayston, J.T.: Occurrence of histoplasmosis in epidemics. Etiologic studies. Amer. Rev. Tuberc. **68**, 307 (1953). — Furcolow, M.L., Menges, R.W.: Comparison of histoplasmin sensitivity rates among human beings and animals in Boone County, Missouri. Amer. J. publ. Hlth **42**, 926 (1952). — Furcolow, M.L., Tosh, F.E., Larsh, H.W., Lynch, H.J., Shaw, G.: The emerging pattern of urban histoplasmosis. Studies on the epidemic in Mexico, Missouri. New Engl. J. Med. **264**, 1226 (1961). — Gammel, E.B., Breckenridge, R.L.: Histoplasmosis of the larynx. Ann. Otol. (St. Louis) **58**, 249 (1949). — Gass, R.S., Zeidberg, L.D., Hucheson, R.H.: Chronic pulmonary histoplasmosis complicated by pregnancy and spontaneous pneumothorax. Amer. Rev. Tuberc. **75**, 111 (1957). — Gerber, H.J., Schoonmaker, F.W., Vazquez, M.D.: Chronic meningitis associated with Histoplasma endocarditis. New Engl. J. Med. **275**, 74 (1966). — Giles, C.L., Falls, H.F.: Amphotericin B. Therapy in the treatment of presumed Histoplasma chorioretinitis: a further appraisal. Trans. Amer. ophthal. Soc. **65**, 136 (1967). — Gillespie, J.B.: Superior vena cava obstruction in childhood. J. Pediat. **49**, 320 (1956). — Gold, W., Stout, H.A., Pagano, J.S., Donovick, R.: Amphotericin A and B. Antifungal antibiotics produced by a Streptomycete. I. In vitro studies. Antibiotics Ann. 1955—1956. New York: Med. Encyclop. 1956. — Goldman, J., Schwarz, J.: Cytology of 4 yeast-like organisms in tissue explants. Mycopathologia (Den Haag) **29**, 161 (1966). — Gonzalez-Ochoa, A.: Peculiaridades de la histoplasmosis pulmonar primaria grave en el pais. Gac. méd. Méx. **91**, 5 (1961). — Goodwin, R.A., Snell, J.D., Hubbard, W.W., Terry, R.T.: Early chronic pulmonary histoplasmosis. Amer. Rev. resp. Dis. **93**, 47 (1966). — Goodwin, R.A., Jr., Snell, J.D., Hubbard, W.W., Terry, R.T.: Relationship in combined pulmonary infections with Histoplasma capsulatum and Mycobacterium tuberculosis. Amer. Rev. resp. Dis. **96**, 990 (1967). — Gordon, M.A.: Fluorescent staining of Histoplasma capsulatum. J. Bact. **77**, 678 (1959). — Gray, H.K., Skinner, I.C.: Constrictive occlusion of superior vena cava. Report of three cases in which patients were treated surgically. Surg. Gynec. Obstet. **72**, 923 (1941). — Greendyke, R.M., Emerson, G.L.: Occurrence of Histoplasma in solitary pulmonary nodules in a nonendemic area. Amer. J. clin. Path. **29**, 36 (1958). — Greendyke, R.M., Kaltreider, N.L.: Chronic histoplasmosis. Report of a patient successfully treated with amphotericin B. Amer. J. Med. **26**, 135 (1959). — Greer, H.D., Geraci, J.E., Korbin, K.B., Miller, R.H., Weed, L.A.: Disseminated histoplasmosis presenting as a brain tumor and treated with amphotericin B. Report of a case. Proc. Mayo Clin. **39**, 490

(1964). — GREGORIADES, D.G., LANGELUTTIG, H.V., POLK, J.W.: Pericarditis with massive effusion due to histoplasmosis. Case report. J. Amer. med. Ass. **178**, 331 (1961). — GRIDLEY, M.F.: A stain for fungi in tissue sections. Amer. J. clin. Path. **23**, 303 (1953). — GROCOTT, R.G.: A stain for fungi in tissue sections and smears. Amer. J. clin. Path. **25**, 975 (1955). — GRYBOSKI, W.A., CRUTCHER, R.R., HOLLOWAY, J.B., MAYO, P., SEGNITZ, R.H., EISEMAN, B.: Surgical aspects of histoplasmosis. Arch. Surg. **87**, 590 (1963). — HABER, R.W., JOSEPH, M.: Neurological manifestations after amphotericin B therapy. Brit. med. J. **1**, 230 (1962). — HANSMANN, G.H., SCHENKEN, J.R.: A unique infection in man caused by new yeast-like organism, a pathogenic member of the genus Sepedonium. Amer. J. Path. **10**, 731 (1934). — HATCH, T.F.: Distribution and deposition of inhaled particles in respiratory tract. Bact. Rev. **25**, 237 (1961). — HARTUNG, M., SALFELDER, K.: Histoplasmose mit tödlichem Ausgang als Berufserkrankung bei einem Mykologen. Arch. Gewerbepath. Gewerbehyg. **19**, 270 (1962). — HAUST, M.D., WLODEK, G.K., PARKER, J.O.: Histoplasma endocarditis. Amer. J. Med. **32**, 460 (1962). — HEILBRUNN, I.B., CAIN, A.R.: Mild histoplasmosis clinically resembling atypical pneumonia and accompanied by erythema nodosum and arthritis. J. Mo. med. Ass. **47**, 503 (1950). — HENDERSON, R.G., PINKERTON, H., MOORE, L.T.: Histoplasma capsulatum as a cause of chronic ulcerative enteritis. J. Amer. med. Ass. **118**, 885 (1942). — HILDICK-SMITH, G., BLANK, H., SARKANY, I.: Fungus diseases and their treatment. Boston: Little Brown & Co. 1964. — HILEY, P., HEILBRUNN, C., FIELDS, J.: Histoplasma ulcer of the tongue. J. Amer. med. Ass. **200**, 206 (1967). — HINSHAW, R.J., GUILFOIL, P.H.: Intramural cystic lesion of the esophagus due to Histoplasma capsulatum. Dis. Chest **47**, 555 (1965). — HOEFNAGELS, R.L.J., PIJPERS, P.M.: Histoplasma capsulatum in a human eye. Amer. J. Ophthal. **63**, 715 (1967). — HOKE, A.W.: Histoplasmosis of the tongue. Arch. Derm. **94**, 667 (1966). — HOLLAND, P., HOLLAND, N.H.: Histoplasmosis in early infancy. Amer. J. Dis. Child. **112**, 412 (1966). — HOOD, A.B., INGLIS, F.G., LOWENSTEIN, L., DOSSETOR, J.B., MacLEAN, L.D.: Histoplasmosis and thrombocytopenic purpura: transmission by renal homotransplantation. Canad. med. Ass. J. **93**, 587 (1965). — HUGHES, W.T.: Histoplasma capsulatum and atypical mycobacterium. Amer. J. Dis. Child. **110**, 89 (1965). — HULSE, W.F.: Laryngeal histoplasmosis. Report of a case. Arch. Otolaryng. **54**, 65 (1951). — HUMPHREY, A.A.: Reticuloendothelial cytomycosis (Histoplasmosis of Darling). Arch. intern. Med. **65**, 902 (1940). — HURWITZ, J.K., PASTOR, B.H.: Pericardial calcification associated with histoplasmosis. Amer. J. Med. **260**, 543 (1959). — HUTCHESON, J.B., WALDORF, V.R.: Use of improved microbiologic and histochemical techniques in the pathological study of pulmonary granulomas. Amer. Rev. resp. Dis. **81**, 340 (1960). — HUTCHISON, H.E.: Laryngeal histoplasmosis simulating carcinoma. J. Path. Bact. **64**k, 309 (1952). — INGLIS, J.A., POWELL, R.E.: Histoplasmosis: a review, with report of a fatal Australien case. Med. J. Aust. **1953**I, 138. — ISRAEL, H.L., DeLAMATER, E., SONES, M., WILLIS, W.D., MIRMELSTEIN, A.: Chronic disseminated histoplasmosis. An investigation of its relationship to sarcoidosis. Amer. J. Med. **12**, 252 (1952). — JACKSON, D.: Histoplasmosis: A "spelunker's" risk. Amer. Rev. resp. Dis. **83**, 261 (1961). — JARVIS, G.J., McCULLOCH, C.: Ocular histoplasmosis. Canad. med. Ass. J. **89**, 1270 (1963). — JEAN, R.: Formes curables et formes pulmonaires de l'histoplasmose infantile. Arch. franç. Pédiat. **10**, 995 (1953). — JOHNSON, J.E., JR., MacCURDY, J.M.: Pulmonary histoplasmosis diagnosed by scalene node biopsy. Amer. Rev. Tuberc. **66**, 497 (1952). — JUBA, A.: Über eine seltene Mykose (durch Histoplasma capsulatum verursachte Meningoencephalitis) des Zentralnervensystems. Psychiat. et Neurol. (Basel) **135**, 260—268 (1958). — KADE, H., KAPLAN, L.: Evaluation of staining techniques in the histologic diagnosis of fungi. Arch. Path. **59**, 571 (1955). — KAPLAN, M.M., SHERWOOD, L.M.: Acute pericarditis due to Histoplasma capsulatum. Ann. intern. Med. **58**, 862 (1963). — KARLSON, K.E., TIMMES, J.J.: Granulomata of the mediastinum surgically treated and followed up to nine years. J. thorac. Surg. **35**, 617 (1958). — KARNAUCHOW, P.N., MARCINIAK, J.L.: Fatal disseminated histoplasmosis. Canad. med. Ass. J. **75**, 929—931 (1956). — KAUFMAN, L., KAPLAN, W.: Preparation of a fluorescent antibody specific for the yeast phase of Histoplasma capsulatum. J. Bact. **82**, 729 (1961). — KEY, J.A., LARGE, A.M: Histoplasmosis of the knee. J. Bone Jt Surg. **24**, 281 (1942). — KING, H.C., CLINE, J.F.X.: Histoplasmosis involving the larynx. Arch. Otolaryng. **67**, 649 (1958). — KIRSCH, E.: Beobachtung einer Histoplasmose mit Sektionsbefund. Z. Tropenmed. Parasit. **3**, 86 (1951). ∼ Die Histoplasmose. Eine Übersicht. Z. Tropenmed. Parasit. **1**, 287 (1949). — KLIEGER, H.L., FISHER, E.R.: Fibrocalcific constrictive pericarditis due to Histoplasma capsulatum. New Engl. J. Med. **267**, 593 (1962). — KLINGBERG, W.G.: Generalized histoplasmosis in infants and children; review of ten cases, one with apparent recovery. J. Pediat. **36**, 728 (1950). — KLITE, P.D., DIERCKS, F.H.: Histoplasma capsulatum in fecal contents and organs of bats in the Canal Zone. Amer. J. trop. Med. Hyg. **14**, 433 (1965). — KNEIDEL, J.H., SEGALL, H.: Acute disseminated histoplasmosis in children. Report of three cases. Pediatrics **4**, 596 (1949). — KÖNIGSBAUER, H.: Beitrag zur experimentellen Histoplasmose der Ratte. Arch. Derm. Syph. (Berl.) **195**, 492 (1953). — KOLLER, F., KUHN, H.: Über Histoplasmose. Ein Beitrag zur ätiologischen Differenzierung von Lungenverkalkungen.

Schweiz. med. Wschr. 1948, 1077. — Korns, M.E.: Coincidence of mycotic (Histoplasma capsulatum) vegetative endocarditis of the mitral valve and the Lutembacher syndrome. Circulation 32, 589 (1965). — Krause, A.C., Hopkins, W.G.: Ocular manifestations of histoplasmosis. Amer. J. Ophthal. 34, 564 (1951). — Kurung, J.M., Yegian, D.: Medium for maintenance of H. capsulatum to yeast-like phase. Amer. J. clin. Path. 24, 505 (1954). — Larkin, J.C., Jr., Phillips, S.: Coexistent pulmonary tuberculosis and fungal disease. A review of the literature and three additional cases. Amer. Rev. Tuberc. 72, 667 (1955). — Layton, J.M., McKee, A.P., Stamler, F.W.: Dual infection with Blastomyces dermatitidis and Histoplasma capsulatum. Report of a fatal case in man. Amer. J. clin. Path. 23, 904 (1953). — Lazzari, J.C., Latienda, R.I., Molina, T.R.: Tumor de orbita y tumor de saco lagrimal por histoplasmosis. Arch. Oftal. B. Aires 38, 404 (1964). — Leedom, J.M., Pritchard, J.C., Keer, L.M.: Probable Histoplasma pericarditis with effusion. Report of case with recurrence. Arch. intern. Med. 112, 652 (1963). — Lehan, P.H., Furcolow, M.L.: Epidemic histoplasmosis. J. chron. Dis. 5, 489 (1957). — Lehan, P.H., Brasher, C.A., Larsh, H.W., Furcolow, M.L.: Evaluation of clinical aids to the diagnosis of chronic progressive cavitary histoplasmosis. Amer. Rev. Tuberc. 75, 938 (1957). — Leinfelder, J.T.: Ocular histoplasmosis (A Survey). Survey Ophthal. 12, 103 (1967). — Lerner, P.I., Weinstein, L.: Infective endocarditis in the antibiotic era. New Engl. J. Med. 274, 199 (1966). — Levaditi, J.-C., Drouhet, E., Segretain, G., Mariat, F.: Sur le caractère histiocytaire de l'histoplasmose à petites formes et le caractère gigantocellulaire de l'histoplasmose à grandes formes. Ann. Inst. Pasteur 96, 659 (1959). — Leznoff, A., Frank, H., Telner, P., Rosenzweig, J., Brandt, J.L.: Histoplasmosis in Montreal during the Fall of 1963, with observations on erythema multiforme. Canad. med. Ass. J. 91, 1154 (1964). — Lichtenstein, N.S., Leaf, A.: Effect of amphotericin B on the permeability of the toad bladder. Clin. Invest. 44, 1328 (1965). — Little, J.A., Steigman, A.J.: Erythema nodosum in primary histoplasmosis. J. Amer. med. Ass. 173, 875 (1960). — Locket, S., Atkinson, E.A., Grieve, W.S.M.: Histoplasmosis in Great Britain. Description of a second case of disseminated histoplasmosis: treatment by ethyl vanillate. Brit. Med. J. 2, 857 (1953). — Lull, G.R., Winn, D.F.: Chronic fibrous mediastinitis due to Histoplasma capsulatum. Radiology 73, 367 (1959). — Lunn, H.F.: A case of histoplasmosis of bone in East Africa. J. trop. Med. Hyg. 63, 175 (1960). — Lynch, H.J., Plexico, K.L.: A rapid method for screening sputums for Histoplasma capsulatum employing the fluorescent antibody technic. New Engl. J. Med. 266, 811 (1962). — MacInnis, F.E.: Broncholithiasis and histoplasmin sensitivity. Case report. Missouri Med. 52, 868 (1955). — Makley, T.A., Long, J.W., Suie, T., Stephan, J.D.: Presumed histoplasmic chorioretinitis with special emphasis on present modes of therapy. Trans. Amer. Acad. Ophthal. Otolaryng. May—June 1965, 443. — Mann, W.H.: Chorioretinitis due to histoplasmosis in clinical practice. Amer. J. Ophthal. 55, 999 (1963). — Mantovani, A., Mazzoni, A., Ajello, L.: Histoplasmosis in Italy. I. Isolation of Histoplasma capsulatum from dogs in the province of Bologna. Sabouraudia 6, 163 (1968). — Manwaring, J.H.: Unusual forms of Blastomyces dermatitidis in human tissues. Arch. Path. 48, 421 (1949). — Marshall, R.J., Edmundowicz, A.C., Andrews, C.E.: Chronic obstruction of superior vena cava due to histoplasmosis. Circulation 29, 604 (1964). — Martz, G.: Histoplasmosis. A case report. J. Pediat. 31, 98 (1947). — Mashburn, J.D., Dawson, D.F., Young, J.M.: Pulmonary calcifications and histoplasmosis. Amer. Rev. resp. Dis. 84, 208 (1961). — Medeiros, A.A., et al.: Erythema nodosum and erythema multiforme as clinical manifestations of histoplasmosis in a community outbreak. New Engl. J. Med. 274, 415 (1966). — McClellan, J.T., Scherr, G.H., Hotchkiss, M.: A clinical pathological and mycological study of a fatal case of histoplasmosis in an infant. Mycopathologia (Den Haag) 6, 86 (1951). — McCurdy, D.K., Frederic, M., Elkinton, J.R.: Renal tubular acidosis due to amphotericin B. New Engl. J. Med. 278, 124 (1968). — McNerney, J.J.: Histoplasmin sensitivity associated with pericardial calcification. Amer. Heart J. 52, 609 (1956). — Meleney, H.E.: Pulmonary histoplasmosis. Report of two cases. Amer. Rev. Tuberc. 44, 240 (1941). — Merchant, R.K., Louria, D.B., Geisler, P.H., Edgcomb, J.H., Utz, J.P.: Fungal endocarditis. Review of literature and report of three cases. Ann. intern. Med. 48, 242 (1958). — Methot, Y., Blank, F., Masson, A.M.: Gingivitis caused by Histoplasma capsulatum. Canad. med. Ass. J. 79, 836 (1958). — Mider, G.B., Smith, F.D., Bray, W.E., Jr.: Systemic manifestations with Cryptococcus neoformans (Torula histolytica) and Histoplasma capsulatum in same patient. Arch. Path. 43, 102 (1947). — Miller, A.A., Ramsden, F., Geake, M.R.: Acute disseminated histoplasmosis of pulmonary origin probably contracted in Britain. Thorax 16, 388 (1961). — Miller, D.B., Allen, S.T., Jr., Amidon, E.L.: Obstruction of the superior vena cava presumably due to histoplasmosis. Amer. Rev. Tuberc. 77, 848 (1958). — Miller, H.E., Keddie, F.M., Johnstone, H.G., Bostick, W.L.: Histoplasmosis. Arch. Derm. Syph. (Chic.) 56, 715 (1947). — Mochi, A., Edwards, Ph.Q.: Geographical distribution of histoplasmosis and histoplasmin sensitivity. Bull. Org. mond. Santé 5, 259 (1952). — Moore, M.: Morphologic variation in tissue of the organisms of the blastomycoses and of the histoplasmosis. Amer. J. Path. 31, 1049 (1955). — Moore, R.D.: Case report: Lymphosarcoma. Ohio St. med. J. 49,

512 (1953). — MORGAN, H.J., SHAPIRO, J.: Histoplasmosis of gastrointestinal tract J. Tenn. med. Ass. **45**, 488 (1952). — MORRIS, J.H., MACAULAY, M., POSER, C.M.: Systemic crypto-coccosis and histoplasmosis in the same patient. A case report. Neurology (Minneap.) **14**, 147 (1964). — MURECANU, A.: Zur Frage des Bildes der pathomorphologischen Veränderungen bei Histoplasmosis. Die ersten in der Rumänischen Volksrepublik entdeckten Fälle von Histo-plasmosis. Arkh. Pat. **18**, Heft 7, S. 84—92 (1956) [Russisch]. — MURESAN, A.: Contribution à l'étude morpho-pathologique de l'histoplasmose humaine. A propos de trois cas. Sem. Hôp. Paris, Path. et Biol., Arch. Anat. path. **1956**, 1465. — MURRAY, J.F., BRANDT, F.A.: Histoplasmosis and malignant lymphoma. Amer. J. Path. **27**, 783 (1951). — MURRAY, J.F., HOWARD, D.: Laboratory-acquired histoplasmosis. Amer. Rev. resp. Dis. **89**, 631 (1964). — MURRAY, J.F., LURIE, H.I., KAY, J., KOMINS, C., BOROK, R., WAY, M.: Benign pulmonary histoplasmosis (cave disease) in South Africa. S. Afr. med. J. **31**, 245 (1957). — MURRAY, P.J.S., SLADDEN, R.A.: Disseminated histoplasmosis following long-term steroid therapy for reticulosarcoma. Brit. med. J. **2**, 631 (1965). — NAUCK, E.G.: Zur Histologie der Chromo-blastomykose. Gaz. méd. port. **4**, 809 (1951). — DEL NEGRO, G., VERONESI, R., DE ASSIS, F.M.: Generalisierte Histoplasmose und Hodgkinsche Krankheit. Rev. paul. Med. **43**, 291 (mit englischer Zusammenfassung) (1953) [Portugiesisch]. — NEGRONI, P.: Histoplasmosis. CIC Buenos Aires 1960. ~ Micosis profundas; histoplasmosis. Comision de investigacion cienti-fica, Buenos Aires, Argentina, 1960. — NELSON, J.D., BATES, R., PITCHFORD, A.: Histoplasma meningitis. Recovery following amphotericin B therapy. Amer. J. Dis. Child. **102**, 218 (1961). — NELSON, N.A., GOODMAN, H.L., OSTER, H.L.: The association of histoplasmosis and lym-phoma. Amer. J. Med. **233**, 56 (1957). — NUDELMAN, H.L., RAKATANSKY, H.: Gastric histo-plasmosis. A case report. J. Amer. med. Ass. **195**, 44 (1966). — NUTALL-SMITH, J.: Pulmonary histoplasmosis accompanied by erythema nodosum. Canad. med. Ass. J. **74**, 59 (1956). — O'DONNELL, W.M.: Changing pathogenesis of Addison's disease. Arch. intern. Med. **86**, 266 (1950). — OKUDAIRA, M., STRAUB, M., SCHWARZ, J.: Etiology of discrete splenic and hepatic calcifications in an endemic area of histoplasmosis. Amer. J. Path. **39**, 599 (1961). — OKUDAIRA, M., SCHWARZ, J.: Experimental ocular histoplasmosis in rats. A histopathologic study of immunogenic and hypersensitive ophthalmitis produced in rats by Histoplasma capsulatum and histoplasmin. Amer. J. Ophthal. **54**, 427 (1962). — OMER, G.E., LOCKWOOD, R.S., TRAVIS, L.O.: Histoplasmosis involving the carpal joint. J. Bone Jt Surg. **45**, 1699 (1963). — ORR, T.G., WILSON, S.J.: Some surgical aspects of histoplasmosis. Two cases of splenectomy. Ann. Surg. **18**, 109 (1952). — OWEN, G.E., SCHERR, S.N., SEGRE, E.J.: Histoplasmosis involving the heart and great vessels. Amer. J. Med. **32**, 552 (1962). — PALMER, R.L., GERACI, J.E., THOMAS, B.J.: Histoplasma endocarditis: Report on a patient treated with amphotericin B therapy for histoplasmosis. Arch. intern. Med. **110**, 359 (1962). — PANISSET, M.: Les histoplasmoses ani-males et l'histoplasmose humaine. Canad. J. comp. Med. **14**, 287 (1950). — PARK, R.K., GOLTZ, W.R., CAREY, T.B.: Unusual cutaneous infections associated with immunosuppressive therapy. Arch. Derm. **95**, 345 (1967). — PARKES, M., BURTOFF, S.: Histoplasmosis of the larynx. Report of a case. Med. Ann. D.C. **18**, 641 (1949). — PARSONS, R.M., ZARAFONETIS, C.J.C.: Histoplasmosis in man. Arch. intern. Med. **75**, 1 (1945). — PATE, J.W., HAMMON, J.: Superior vena cava syndrome due to histoplasmosis in children. Ann. Surg. **161**, 778 (1965). — PEA-BODY, J.W., JR., BUECHNER, H.A.: Coexisting histoplasmosis and tuberculosis of the ali-mentary tract. Amer. J. Med. **21**, 143 (1956). — PEREZ, C.A., STURIM, H.S., KOUCHOUKOS, N.T., KAMBERG, S.: Some clinical and radiographic features of gastrointestinal histoplasmosis. Radiology **86**, 482 (1966). — PERRY, L.V., JENKINS, D.E., WHITCOMB, F.C.: Simultaneously occurring pulmonary coccidioidomykosis and histoplasmosis. Amer. Rev. resp. Dis. **92**, 952 (1965). — PIERCE, E.C.: A case report: adrenal insufficiency due to histoplasmosis. J. Indiana med. Ass. **53**, 57 (1960). — PIERINI, D.O.: Histoplasmosis. A proposito de seis observaciones. Arch. argent. Derm. **4**, 337 (1954). — PINE, L., DROUHET, E., REYNOLDS, G.: A comparative morphological study of the yeast phases of Histoplasma capsulatum and Histoplasma duboisii. Sabouraudia **3**, 211 (1964). — PINKERTON, H., IVERSON, L.: Histoplasmosis. Three fatal cases with disseminated sarcoid-like lesions. Arch. intern. Med. **90**, 456 (1952). — PLESSNER, M.: Disease of feather sorters: duck fever. Arch. Mal. prof. **21**, 67 (1960). — PLOTNICK, H., CERRI, S.: Treatment of oral histoplasmosis by local injection with nystatin. J. Amer. med. Ass. **165**, 346 (1957). — POLES, F.C., LAVERTINE, J.D. O'D: Acute disse-minated histoplasmosis with a report of a case occurring in England. Thorax **9**, 233 (1954). — POLK, J.W., CUBILES, J.A., BUCKINGHAM, W.W.: Surgical treatment of chronic progressive histoplasmosis. J. thorac. Surg. **34**, 323 (1957). — POLLAK, L.: Diagnostico de un caso de histoplasmosis por cultivo de H. capsulatum del granuloma dental apical. Rev. Tisiol. Neumonol. **3**, 61 (1961). — POST, G.W., JACKSON, A., GARBER, P.E.: Histoplasmosis on a small tuberculosis service in a General Hospital. Dis. Chest **31**, 688 (1957). — PRIOR, J.A., SASLAW, S., COLE, C.R.: Experiences with histoplasmosis. Ann. intern. Med. **40**, 221 (1954). — PROCK-NOW, J.J., CONNELLY, A.P., RAY, C.G.: Fuorescent antibody technique in histoplasmosis. Arch. Path. **73**, 313 (1962). — PROCKNOW, J.J., LOEWEN, D.F.: Pulmonary aspergillosis with

caviation secondary to histoplasmosis. Amer. Rev. resp. Dis. **82**, 101 (1960). — PUCKETT, T.F.: Pulmonary histoplasmosis. A study of 22 cases with identification of H. capsulatum in resected lesions. Amer. Rev. Tuberc. **67**, 453 (1953). — RAFTERY, A., TRAFAS, P.C., McCLURE, R.D.: Histoplasmosis: a common cause of appendicitis and mesenteric adenitis. Ann. Surg. **132**, 720 (1950). — RAMIREZ, R.J., LEVY, D.A.: Pseudocavitary histoplasmosis: Infection of emphysematous bullae by Histoplasma capsulatum. Dis. Chest **48**, 442 (1965). — RAMSEY, T.L., APPLEBAUM, A.A.: Histoplasmosis "Darling." Amer. J. clin. Path. **12**, 85 (1942). — RASMUSSEN, P., CAULFIELD, J.B.: The ultra-structure of Schaumann Bodies in the golden hamster. Lab. Invest. **9**, 330 (1960). — RAWSON, A.J., COLLINS, L.H., GRANT, J.L.: Histoplasmosis and torulosis as causes of adrenal insufficiency. Amer. J. med. Sci. **215**, 363 (1948). — REED, C.E., SOSMAN, A., BARBEE, A.: Pigeon breeder's lung. J. Amer. med. Ass. **193**, 81 (1965). — REID, J.D., SCHERER, J.H., HERBUT, P.A., IRVING, M.T.: Systemic histoplasmosis. Systemic histoplasmosis diagnosed before death and produced experimentally in guinea pigs. J. Lab. clin. Med. **27**, 419 (1942). — REIMANN, H.A., PRICE, A.H.: Histoplasmosis in Pennsylvania. Confusion with sarcoidosis and experimental therapy with bacillomycin. Penn. med. J. **52**, 367 (1949). — REINHARD, E.H., McALLISTER, W.H., BROWN, E., CHAPLIN, H., GARFINKEL, L., HARFORD, C.G., KOBAYASHI, G., CATE, T.: Chronic lymphocytic leukemia complicated by disseminated histoplasmosis. Amer. J. Med. **43**, 593 (1967). — REZAI, H.R., HABERMAN, S.: The use of immunofluorescence for identification of yeastlike fungi in human infections. Amer. J. clin. Path. **46**, 433 (1966). — RICH, A.R., McCORDOCK, H.A.: The pathogenesis of tuberculous meningitis. Bull. Johns Hopk. Hosp. **52**, 5 (1933). — RIEGEL, N., SCHRIEVER, H.G.: Fatal pericarditis due to histoplasmosis. Amer. Rev. resp. Dis. **95**, 99 (1967). — ROBERTSON, J.W.: Histological survey of human appendices for Histoplasma capsulatum. J. Albert Einstein Med. Center, August 1954, p. 147. — RODGER, R.C., TERRY, L.L., BINFORD, C.H.: Histoplasmosis, cryptococcosis, and tuberculosis complicating Hodgkin's disease. Amer. J. clin. Path. **21**, 153 (1951). — RUBIN, H., FURCOLOW, M.L., YATES, J.L., BRASHER, C.A.: The course and prognosis of histoplasmosis. Amer. J. Med. **27**, 278 (1959). — RUDNER, G.H., JR., BALE, C.F.: Acute Addisonian crisis and death due to histoplasmosis. Sth. med. J. (Bgham, Ala.) **52**, 1491 (1959). — SAGLAM, T.: First case of histoplasmosis in Turkey. J. Amer. med. Ass. **131**, 1239 (1946). — SALFELDER, K.: Zur Differentialdiagnose der Histoplasmose. Z. Tropenmed. Parasit. **11**, 453 (1960). ~ Fatal case of erythema nodosum and histoplasmosis. Mycopathologia (Den Haag) **22**, 315 (1964). — SALFELDER, K., CAPRETTI, C.: Primo-infeccion pulmonar de histoplasmosis en un lactante. Mycopathologia (Den Haag) **15**, 251 (1961). — SALFELDER, K., LISCANO, R. DE: Lesiones histoplasmoticas autopsicas como indice epidemiologico de la enfermedad en Los Andes Venezolanos. Mycopathologia (Den Haag) **26**, 19 (1965). — SALFELDER, K., SCHWARZ, J.: Histoplasmotische Kalkherde in der Milz. Dtsch. med. Wschr. **92**, 1468 (1967). ~ Experimental cutaneous histoplasmosis in hamsters. Arch. Derm. **91**, 645 (1965). — SALFELDER, K., AKBARIAN, M., SCHWARZ, J.: Experimental ocular histoplasmosis in dogs. Amer. J. Ophthal. **59**, 290 (1965). — SALIBA, N.A., ANDERSON, W.H.: Acute disseminated histoplasmosis. Amer. Rev. resp. Dis. **95**, 94 (1967). — SALYER, J.M., HARRISON, H.N., WINN, D.F., TAYLOW, R.R.: Chronic fibrous mediastinitis and superior vena caval obstruction due to histoplasmosis. Dis. Chest **35**, 364 (1959). — SASLAW, S., BEMAN, F.M.: Erythema nodosum as a manifestation of histoplasmosis. J. Amer. med. Ass. **96**, 1178 (1959). — SASLAW, S., CARLISLE, H.N., SPARKS, J.: Experimental histoplasmosis in monkeys. (25512). Proc. Soc. exp. Biol. (N.Y.) **103**, 342 (1960). — SCHLAEGEL, T.J., JR.: Granulomatous uveitis. An etiologic survey of 100 cases. Trans. Amer. Acad. Ophthal. Otolaryng. **72**, 813 (1958). — SCHLAEGEL, T.F., JR., KENNEY, D.: Changes around the optic nerve head: in presumed ocular histoplasmosis. Amer. J. Ophthal. **62**, 454 (1966). — SCHLUMBERGER, H.G., SERVICE, A.C.: A case of histoplasmosis in an infant with autopsy. Amer. J. med. Sci. **207**, 230 (1944). — SCHUB, H.M., SPIVEY, C.G., JR., BAIRD, G.D.: Pleural involvement in histoplasmosis. Amer. Rev. resp. Dis. **94**, 225 (1966). — SCHULZ, D.M.: Histoplasmosis. A statistical morphologic study. Amer. J. clin. Path. **24**, 11 (1954). ~ A partially healed primary lesion in a case of generalized histoplasmosis. Arch. Path. **50**, 457 (1950). ~ Histoplasmosis of the central nervous system. J. Amer. med. Ass. **151**, 549 (1953). — SCHULZ, D.M., TUCKER, E.B., McLOUGHLIN, P.T.: Observations on the laboratory diagnosis of granulomatous inflammation of the lung. Amer. J. clin. Path. **29**, 28 (1958). — SCHWARTZ, ST.O., BARSKY, S.: Report of 193 marrow biopsy specimens cultured for Histoplasma capsulatum. Blood **7**, 545—549 (1952). — SCHWARZ, E.: Regional Roentgen manifestations of histoplasmosis. Amer. J. Roentgenol. **87**, 865 (1962). — SCHWARZ, J.: Tuberculous meningitis. Amer. Rev. Tuberc. **57**, 63 (1948). ~ Giant forms of Histoplasma capsulatum in tissue explants. Amer. J. clin. Path. **23**, 898 (1953). ~ The primary lesion in histoplasmosis. In SWEANY: Histoplasmosis, p. 292. Springfield/Ill.: Charles C Thomas 1960. — SCHWARZ, J., BAUM, G.L: Primary cutaneous mycoses. Arch. Derm. Syph. (Chic.) **71**, 143 (1955). ~ Reinfection in histoplasmosis. Arch. Path. **75**, 475 (1963). — SCHWARZ, J., GOLDMANN, L.: Die Histoplasmose der Haut und Schleimhäute. In: Handbuch der Haut- und Geschlechtskrankheiten, hrsg. von J. JADASSOHN, Bd. 4, Teil 4, S. 224—239. Berlin-

Göttingen-Heidelberg: Springer 1963. — SCHWARZ, J., SILVERMAN, F. N., STRAUB, M., LEVINE, S., ADRIANO, S.: Relation of splenic calcification to histoplasmosis. New Engl. J. Med. **252**, 887 (1955). — SCHWARZ, J., BAUM, G. L., STRAUB, M.: Cavitary histoplasmosis complicated by fungus ball. Amer. J. Med. **31**, 692 (1961). — SEGAL, E. L., WEED, L. A.: Study of surgically excised pulmonary granulomas. J. Amer. med. Ass. **170**, 515 (1959). — SEGRETAIN, G.: Penicillium Marneffei, n. sp., agent d'une mycose du systeme reticulo-endothelial. Mycopathologia (Den Haag) **11**, 327 (1949). — SEGRETAIN, G., et al.: Paecilomyces viridis n. sp., champion dimorphique, agent d'une mycose generalisée de Chameleo lateralis Gray. C.R. Acad. Sci. (Paris) **259**, 258 (1964). — SELLERS, T. F., JR., PRICE, W. N., NEWBERRY, W. M.: An epidemic of erythema multiforme and erythema nodosum caused by histoplasmosis. Ann. intern. Med. **62**, 1244 (1965). — SERVIANSKY, B., SCHWARZ, J.: Calcified intrathoracic lesions caused by histoplasmosis and tuberculosis. Amer. J. Roentgenol. **77**, 1034 (1957). — SETHI, K. K., SCHWARZ, J.: Experimental ocular histoplasmosis in pigeons. Amer. J. Ophthal. **61**, 538 (1966). — SHAPIRO, J. L., LUX, J. J., SPROFKIN, B. E.: Histoplasmosis of the central nervous system. Amer. J. Path. **31**, 319 (1955). — SHULL, H. J.: Human histoplasmosis: a disease with protean manifestations often with digestive system involvement. Gastroenterology **25**, 582 (1953). — SILVERMAN, F. N.: Pulmonary calcifications, tuberculosis? histoplasmosis? Amer. J. Roentgenol. **64**, 747 (1950). — SILVERMAN, F. N., SCHWARZ, J., LAHEY, M. E., CARSON, R. P.: Histoplasmosis. Amer. J. Med. **19**, 410 (1955). — SINGER, J. A., SMITH, J. L.: Experimental corneal histoplasmosis. Brit. J. Ophthal. **48**, 293 (1964). — SMITH, J. L., JONES, D. B.: Experimental avian ocular histoplasmosis. Arch. Ophthal. **67**, 349 (1962). — SNYDER, C. H., WHITE, R. S.: Successful treatment of Histoplasma meningitis with amphotericin B. A case report. J. Pediat. **58**, 554 (1961). — SONES, C. A., ROTKOW, M. J., DUNN, R. C.: Acute disseminated histoplasmosis. Report of a case in an adult. J. Iowa St. med. Soc. **45**, 463 (1955). — SOSMAN, M. C., DODD, G. D., JONES, W. D., PILLMORE, G. U.: Familial occurrence of pulmonary alveolar microlithiasis. Amer. J. Roentgenol. **77**, 947 (1957). — SOTGIU, G., MASSONI, A., MANTOVANI, A., AJELLO, L., PALMER, J.: Histoplasma capsulatum: occurrence in soil from the Emilia-Romagna region of Italy. Science **147**, 624 (1965). — SPAETH, G. L.: Absence of so called Histoplasma uveitis in 134 cases of proven histoplasmosis. Arch. Ophthal. **77**, 41 (1967). — SPICKNALL, C. G., RYAN, R. W., CAIN, A.: Laboratory-acquired histoplasmosis. New Engl. J. Med. **254**, 210 (1956). — SPROFKIN, B. E., SHAPIRO, J. L., LUX, J. J.: Histoplasmosis of the central nervous system. A case report of Histoplasma meningitis. J. Neuropath. exp. Neurol. **14**, 288 (1955). — STANKAITIS, J., MCCUSKEY, M. C.: Fatal lymph-adenopathy type of histoplasmosis. Ohio St. med. J. **51**, 855 (1955). — STARR, G. F., DAWE, C. J., WEED, L. A.: Use of periodic acid Schiff stain in identification of pathogenic fungi in tissues. Amer. J. clin. Path. **25**, 76 (1955). — STEELE, J. D.: The solitary pulmonary nodules. J. thorac. cardiovasc. Surg. **46**, 21 (1963). — STIFF, R. H.: Histoplasmosis. Oral Surg. **16**, 140 (1963). — STRAUB, M.: Die Anatomie der Tuberkulose in Zusammenhang mit der Epidemiologie. Eine geographisch-pathologische Untersuchung. Beitr. Klin. Tuberk. **90**, 1 (1937). — STRAUB, M., FISHKIN, B.G., SCHWARZ, J.: Residual pulmonary lesions of fungal origin in Southern California. Mycopathologia (Den Haag) **20**, 55 (1963). — STRAUB, M., SCHWARZ, J.: General pathology of human and canine histoplasmosis. Amer. Rev. resp. Dis. **82**, 528 (1960). ~ HEALED primary complex in histoplasmosis. Amer. J. clin. Path. **25**, 727 (1955). ~ Histoplasmosis, coccidioidomycosis, and tuberculosis. A comparative pathological study. Path. et Microbiol. (Basel) **25**, 421 (1962). — STRONG, R. P.: A study of some tropical ulcerations of the skin with particular reference to their etiology. Philipp. J. Sci. **1**, 92 (1905). — STURIM, H. S., KOUCHOUKOS, N. T., AHLVIN, R. C.: Gastrointestinal manifestations of disseminated histoplasmosis. Amer. J. Surg. **110**, 435 (1965). — SUTLIFF, W. D., HUGHES, F. A., ULRICH, E., BURKETT, L. L.: Active chronic pulmonary histoplasmosis. Arch. intern. Med. **92**, 571 (1953). — SWEANY, H.C., GORELICK, D., COLLER, F.C., JONES, J.L.: Pathologic and some diagnostic features of histoplasmosis in patients entering a Missouri hospital. Final report. Dis. Chest **42**, 1, 128, 281 (1962). — SYMMERS, W.ST.C.: Histoplasmosis contracted in Britain. A case of histoplasmic lymphadenitis following clinical recovery from sarcoidosis. Brit. med. J. **2**, 786 (1956). ~ Localized cutaneous histoplasmosis. Brit. med. J. **2**, 790 (1956). — TESH, R.B., SCHNEIDAU, J.D.: Primary cutaneous histoplasmosis. New Engl. J. Med. **275**, 597 (1966). — TESH, R.B., SHACKLETTE, M.H., DIERCKS, F.H., HIRSCHL, D.: Histoplasmosis in children. Pediatrics **33**, 894 (1964). — TEWARI, R.P., CAMPBELL, C.C.: Isolation of Histoplasma capsulatum from feathers of chickens inoculated intravenously and subcutaneously with the yeast phase of the organism. Sabouraudia **4**, 17 (1965). — TIECKE, R.W., BARON, H.J., CASEY, D.E.: Localized oral histoplasmosis. Oral Surg. **16**, 441 (1963). — TOMPKINS, V., SCHLEIFSTEIN, J.: Small forms of Blastomyces dermatitidis in human tissues. Arch. Path. **55**, 432 (1953). — TOSH, F.E., BALHUIZEN, J., YATES, J.L., BRASHER, C.A.: Primary cutaneous histoplasmosis. Arch. intern. Med. **114**, 118 (1964). — TOWEY, J.W., SWEANY, H.C., HURON, W.H.: Severe bronchial asthma apparently due to fungus spores found in maple bark. J. Amer. med. Ass. **99**, 453 (1932). — TUFFNELL, P.: Relationship of byssinosis to bacteria and fungi in air of textile mills. Brit. J. industr. Med. **17**,

304 (1960). — Tynes, B.S., Crutcher, J.C., Utz, J.P.: Histoplasma meningitis. Ann. intern. Med. **59**, 615 (1963). — Van Metre, T.E., Jr., Knox, D.L., Maumenee, A.E.: Specific ocular uveal lesions in patients with evidence of histoplasmosis and toxoplasmosis. Sth. med. J. (Bgham, Ala.) **58**, 479 (1965). — Van Metre, T.E., Jr., Maumenee, A.E.: Specific ocular uveal lesions in patients with evidence of histoplasmosis. Arch. Ophthal. **71**, 314 (1964). — Van Pernis, P.A., Benson, M.E., Hollinger, P.H.: Laryngeal and systemic histoplasmosis (Darling). Ann. intern. Med. **18**, 384 (1943). — Vivian, D.N., Weed, L.A., McDonald, J.R., Claggett, O.T., Hodgson, C.H.: Histoplasmosis: clinical and pathological study of 20 cases. Surg. Gynec. Obstet. **99**, 53 (1954). — Vost, A., Moore, S.: Disseminated histoplasmosis in Quebec. Canad. med. Ass. J. **88**, 571 (1963). — Walma, D., Jr., Schlaegel, T.F., Jr.: Presumed histoplasmic choroiditis. A clinical analysis of 43 cases. Amer. J. Ophthal. **57**, 107 (1964). — Wang, C.J.K., Schwarz, J.: Phagocytosis of yeast cells in vitro. Amer. J. Path. **25**, 901 (1959). — Webb, W.R., Herring, J.L.: Pericarditis due to histoplasmosis. Amer. Heart J. **64**, 679 (1962). — Weed, L.A. (Editorial): Large and small forms cf Blastomyces and Histoplasma. Amer. J. clin. Path. **23**, 921 (1953). — Weed, L.A., Andersen, H.A.: Etiology of broncholithiasis. Dis. Chest **37**, 1 (1960). — Weed, L.A., Iams, A.M., Keith, H.M.: Histoplasmosis in infancy. The pathologic picture as seen in one case. Arch. Path. **43**, 155 (1947). — Weed, L.A., Parkhill, E.M.: Diagnosis of histoplasmosis in ulcerative disease of mouth and pharynx. Amer. J. clin. Path. **18**, 130 (1948). — Weiss, E.D., Haskell, B.F.: Anorectal manifestations of histoplasmosis. Amer. J. Surg. **84**, 541 (1952). — Weaver, D.K., Batsakis, J.G., Nishiyama, R.H.: Histoplasma endocarditis. Arch. Surg. **96**, 158 (1968). — Wertlake, P.T., Butler, W.T., Hill, G.J., Utz, J.P.: Nephrotoxic tubular damage and calcium deposition following amphotericin therapy. Amer. J. Path. **43**, 449 (1963). — White, H.H., Fritzlen, T.J.: Cerebral granuloma caused by Histoplasma capsulatum. J. Neurosurg. **19**, 260 (1962). — Wilcox, K.R., Waisbren, B.A., Martin, J.: The Walworth Wisconsin epidemic of histoplasmosis. Ann. intern. Med. **49**, 388 (1958). — Wildervanck, A., Winckel, W.E.F., Collier, W.A.: Tropical eosinophilia combined with histoplasmosis. Docum. Med. geogr. trop. (Amst.) **5**, 67 (1953). — Wildervanck, A., Collier, W.A., Winckel, W.E.F.: Two cases of histoplasmosis on farms near Paramaribo (Surinam); investigations into the epidemiology of the disease. Docum. Med. geogr. trop. (Amst.) **5**, 108 (1953). — Will, D.W., Hasegawa, C.M., Kawauchi, T., Murashima, S.: Histoplasmosis of the kidney. A case report from Japan. Acta path. jap. **14**, 395 (1964). — Williams, R.H., Cromartie, W.J.: Histoplasmosis. Report of a case. Ann. intern. Med. **13**, 2165 (1940). — Winckel, W.E.F., Collier, W.A., Hillers, A.A.: Histoplasma findings in menstrual disturbances. Docum. Med. geogr. trop. (Amst.) **5**, 216 (1953). — Winslow, D.J., Hathaway, B.M.: Pulmonary pneumocystosis and cryptococcosis. Amer. J. clin. Path. **31**, 337 (1959). — Withers, B.T., Pappas, J.J., Erickson, E.E.: Histoplasmosis primary in the larynx. Report of a case. Arch. Otolaryng. **77**, 25 (1963). — Woo, Z.P., Reimann, H.A.: Cutaneous leishmaniasis. Confusion with histoplasmosis. J. Amer. med. Ass. **164**, 1092 (1957). — Woods, A.C., Wahlen, H.E.: Probable role of benign histoplasmosis in etiology of granulomatous uveitis. Amer. J. Ophthal. **49**, 205 (1960). — Woods, L.P.: Mediastinal Histoplasma granuloma causing tracheal compression in a 4-year old child. Surgery **58**, 448 (1965). — Woods, L.P., Tinsley, E.A., Diveley, W.L.: Direct smear for diagnosis of pulmonary histoplasmosis. J. thorac. cardiovasc. Surg. **48**, 761 (1964). — Wooley, C.F., Hosier, D.M.: Constrictive pericarditis due to Histoplasma capsulatum. New Engl. J. Med. **264**, 1230 (1961). — Worgan, D.K.: Histoplasmosis. A summary of the known facts about the disease. Bull. Sch. Med. Maryland **30**, 69 (1945). — Yamaguchi, B.T., Jr., Adriano, S., Braunstein, H.: Histoplasma capsulatum in the pulmonary primary complex. Immunohistochemical demonstration. Amer. J. Path. **43**, 713 (1963). — Young, J.M., Bills, R.J., Ulrich, E.: Discrete splenic calcifications in necropsy material. Amer. J. Path. **33**, 189 (1957). — Yow, E.M., Brennan, J.C., Nathan, M.H., Israel, L.: Calcified granulomata of the spleen in long standing brucellar infection. A report of a case of 25 years duration. Ann. intern. Med. **55**, 307 (1961). — Zeidberg, L.D., Gass, R.S., Hutcheson, R.H.: The placental transmission of histoplasmosis complement-fixing antibodies. J. Dis. Child. **94**, 179 (1957). — Zimmerman, L.E.: Demonstration of Histoplasma and Coccidioides in so-called tuberculomas of lung. Preliminary report on 35 cases. Arch. intern. Med. **94**, 690 (1954). — ∼ Fatal fungus infections complicating other diseases. Amer. J. clin. Path. **25**, 46 (1955). — ∼ Some contributions of the histopathological method to the study of fungus diseases. Trans. N.Y. Acad. Sci. **19**, 538 (1957). — Zimmerman, L.E., Rappaport, H.: Occurrence of cryptococcosis in patients with malignant disease of reticulo-endothelial system. Amer. J. clin. Path. **24**, 1050 (1954). — Zinneman, H.H., Hall, W.H., Wallace, F.G.: Leishmaniasis of the larynx. Report of a case and its confusion with histoplasmosis. Amer. J. Med. **31**, 654 (1961).

African Histoplasmosis (Part 1)

G. M. EDINGTON, Ibadan, Nigeria

With 1 Figure

African histoplasmosis is a mycosis caused by infection with *Histoplasma duboisii*, a species of the genus *Histoplasma*.

Nodular and ulcerative processes in the skin, and osteolytic lesions of bone, either localised or disseminated, are the most common presenting features of African histoplasmosis.

Historical: The first patient suffering from *H. duboisii* infection was described by BLAN-CHARD and LEFROU (1922) in a Congolese. Cases were then described by BRUMPT (1936), CATANEI (1945), CATANEI and KERVRAN (1945) and FRIESS and DELVOYE (1947) in Senegal and the French Sudan. CATANEI and KERVRAN (1945) noted that the guinea pig could be infected by intracardiac inoculation and the large size of the yeast forms (12—15 μ) in the tissues of man in contrast to the small forms seen in *H. capsulatum* (3—4 μ) was commented upon. DUNCAN (1947) also reported these large intracellular yeast forms which he had noted in 1943 in giant cells in tissue obtained from a papulocircinate skin lesion occurring in an Englishman who had been long stationed in Ghana, West Africa. DUNCAN noted that the mycelial phase of this fungus was similar to that of *H. capsulatum* on culture and animal inoculation but suggested that there might be an African type of histoplasmosis which differed histologically in man from that caused by *H. capsulatum*. VANBREUSEGHEM concurred with this view and considered that the fungus was a new species of *Histoplasma* which he named *H. duboisii* (DUBOIS et al., 1952) and the mycological features were elaborated upon in a number of further papers (VANBREUSEGHEM et al., 1953; VANBREUSEGHEM, 1956, 1957). Doubt, however, existed on the taxonomic validity of considering *H. duboisii* as a species distinct from *H. capsulatum* and some considered the fungus as merely a variant of the latter (TASCHJIAN, 1952; DROUHET and SCHWARZ, 1956; CAMAIN et al., 1958).

The clinical features and geographical distribution of African histoplasmosis have been considered by AJELLO et al. (1960), COCKSHOTT and LUCAS (1964a, b), VANBREUSEGHEM (1964) and PELOUX et al. (1965). At a recent CIBA Symposium on the Systematic Mycoses (1967) it was generally considered that *H. duboisii* could be differentiated from *H. capsulatum* by its differing clinical manifestations, its differing geographical distribution, the different tissue responses it evokes in man and laboratory animals and the differing immunological reactions and minor cultural differences which have been described. In this communication, therefore, *H. duboisii* is considered as a separate species.

Mycology: H. duboisii is a dimorphic fungus the mycelial phase of which is indistinguishable morphologically from that of *H. capsulatum*. It can be differentiated on culture on Sabouraud's medium at 25° C, however, by its inability to produce urease in 24—48 hours (COREMANS, 1963; CLARK and GREENWOOD, 1967). It also differs in its yeast phase in man, the yeasts being 8—15 μ in size in contrast to the 2—5 μ of *H. capsulatum*. The cells are round or oval with a thick doubly contoured capsulate containing a variable quantity of lipoid material and occasionally a nucleus may be observed. They reproduce by budding, the base usually being narrow and the bud attaining the size of the parent before separation. The mycelial phase has not been described in man.

Intratesticular guinea pig or intraperitoneal hamster inoculation with yeast phase or mycelial elements of *H. duboisii* produce at first small 'capsulatum' yeast

9*

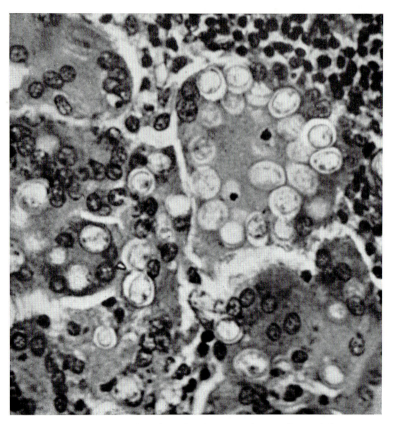

Fig. 1. African histoplasmosis in a lymph node. The cells of *Histoplasma duboisii* are round or oval, 7—15 μ in diameter and limited by a wall 1 μ thick. A single small nucleus and budding may be seen. The fungus cells are within giant cells. Note the resemblance to *Blastomyces dermatitidis*. H & E × 1000

forms and later in 2—5 months giant 'duboisii forms' in contrast to *H. capsulatum* (PINE et al., 1964).

The values of the complement fixation and agar gel precipitin tests in *H. capsulatum* infection have recently been reviewed by KAUFMAN (1966) and SEELIGER (1967), a titre of 1/8 or greater to either mycelial (histoplasmin) or yeast phase antigen in the former test generally being considered presumptive evidence of infection. A lack of response, however, does not exclude infection. Positive responses to *H. duboisii* mycelial and yeast phase antigens with a negative response to *H. capsulatum* antigens have been reported in a Nigerian patient with a pulmonary form of African histoplasmosis (CLARK and GREENWOOD, 1967). Differences in the serum fractions of hyperimmune rabbits against antigens of *H. capsulatum* and *H. duboisii* have also been noted by DROUHET (1963). PINE and his colleagues (1964) studied, by fluorescent antibody techniques, the action of a specific anti-yeast phase *H. capsulatum* conjugate against 13 yeast phase strains of *H. capsulatum* and 9 of *H. duboisii*. The conjugate was specific for the former and no yeast phase of *H. duboisii* obtained *in vitro* or *in vivo* reacted with it. The evidence is, therefore, that these two fungi differ antigenically but further information on the value of serological tests in African histoplasmosis is required.

Epidemiology: African histoplasmosis occurs in all age groups with a peak incidence in the second decade. Males are affected slightly more frequently than females. No significant differences in racial susceptibility are recognised. The greater than random association which has been noted between disseminated *H. capsulatum* infection and lymphoma, leukaemia and Hodgkin's disease (EMMONS et al., 1963) has not been described.

The infection has been widely reported in Africa south of the Sahara and north of Rhodesia in the West, Central and Eastern regions and in both savannah and forest country. The greatest number of cases have naturally been reported in areas where more sophisticated laboratory investigations are available. 56 were reviewed by COCKSHOTT and LUCAS in 1964. It is probable that, with increasing awareness of the condition, African histoplasmosis will be found to be relatively common throughout the tropical belt of Africa. Histoplasmin skin tests have shown positive reactions which vary in incidence from less than 5—21% in different tribes in the Congo (DEVRIESE, 1953; TENRET, 1956). However, *H. capsulatum* infection is also found in Africa and both types of infection have been reported in former French West Africa, Nigeria, the Congo, and East Africa, and, in addition, the histoplasmin skin test is frequently negative in established *H. duboisii* infections. The significance of these findings in relation to duboisii infection is therefore not clear and no assessment of the incidence of this infection in populations is possible until a satisfactory specific antigen becomes available. At the present moment the mode and source of infection are unknown. The presence of isolated skin lesions in the absence of other signs of infection, however, suggest that in some patients infection is acquired through the skin following minor trauma (SYMMERS, 1961; BASSETT et al., 1962). The latter authors reported a skin lesion in a school girl aged 8 years who was in the habit of sweeping out a classroom contaminated with bat droppings which were considered a possible source of infection. Soil contamination of syringes was also suggested as a possible factor in a patient who developed lesions in the buttock within a month of a series of injections at that site (VANDEPITTE et al., 1965). Although lung lesions are not common, CLARK and GREENWOOD (1967) did not consider that the possibility of the portal of entry being via the respiratory passages should be dismissed. On the other hand LANCELY et al. (1961) considered that haematological spread to the lungs was the more likely explanation of the lesions they described. Whatever the portal of entry, both haematological and lymphatic spread occur once the infection is established.

Although the fungus has been cultured in media containing soil and animal faeces (VANBREUSEGHEM and EUGENE, 1958) samples of bat's droppings from caves in East Africa which were a potent source of *H. capsulatum* and from Northern Nigeria and from chicken runs in Southern Nigeria and soil in Senegal have not, on culture, revealed the presence of the fungus (CAMAIN et al., 1958; AJELLO et al., 1960; AJELLO, 1961). It is also of interest that focal outbreaks in association with the cleaning out of chicken houses such as have been reported in *H. capsulatum* infections (EMMONS et al., 1963) have not been recorded. This, however, may be due to less sophisticated methods of poultry farming and, with increasing improvement in these methods such as are taking place in many centres in Africa, it will be interesting to note if such outbreaks occur. Histoplasmin skin testing and a clinical and radiological examination of workers engaged in the poultry farming industry which is rapidly expanding in Africa might be of value in elucidating some aspects of the epidemiology of this condition.

Natural infections in animals have been noted in baboons in French Guinea (COURTOIS et al., 1955; MARIAT and SEGRETAIN, 1956; WALKER and SPOONER, 1960).

From a consideration of the available evidence it would seem most likely that the fungus will eventually be isolated from soil and that minor trauma to the skin will be found to be an important aetiological factor in the infection. The environment of all patients, therefore, should be carefully investigated regarding possible sources of infection but it must be remembered that there may be a latent period of up to 3 years from exposure to signs of infection becoming manifest.

Pathology: African histoplasmosis occurs in a localised or disseminated form and otherwise healthy individuals are usually affected. In the localised form, lesions are usually confined to the skin, regional lymph nodes or bone without evidence of systemic upset. Isolated lesions have however been reported in other viscera including the intestine (Cole et al., 1965).

In the disseminated form almost any organ in the body may be involved, the skin and subcutaneous tissues, the skeletal system, lymphatic glands, the marrow and abdominal viscera, especially the liver and spleen, being most commonly affected. Generalised symptoms include a progressive anaemia, loss of weight, fever and signs of gastrointestinal, hepatic or rarely lung involvement. Dissemination occurs by lymphatic or hematogenous spread. Following a description of the histopathology of the lesions the effect of the infection on various systems is described.

The presence of the yeasts in human tissue in the great majority of instances stimulates the production of histiocytes and giant cells. The *characteristic lesion* consists of a few histiocytes with numerous giant cells of the foreign body or Langhans type containing up to as many as thirty fungal cells. Budding and growth takes place in the giant cells.

On routine haematoxylin and eosin sections the spores are round or oval, 7—15 μ in size and are limited by a well defined thin membrane which is shown to be a cell wall 1 μ thick by periodic-acid schiff and Gomori silver methenamine techniques. The contained eosinophilic protoplasm is usually shrunken either eccentrically or centrally and the impression of a halo may be given. A single small nucleus may be seen. In addition to the giant cells containing spores a variable chronic inflammatory infiltrate of lymphocytes, plasma and epithelioid cells may occur. Epithelioid follicles resembling the tuberculous follicle have been described in the absence of spores but the possible association of the two conditions should be remembered. The giant cell granulomas frequently undergo caseous necrosis and sheets of extracellular yeast forms may be seen in the necrotic material with palisading of epithelioid cells, giant cells and lymphocytes at the periphery. Extensive areas of necrosis with or without spores present are common. Other types of lesions do occur and microabscesses surrounding the fungal elements are not uncommon and an eosinophil response can occur.

With healing, fibroblasts predominate. The absence of calcification is remarkable when the pathology of *H. capsulatum* is considered. The giant cell reaction, extensive areas of necrosis, and microabscesses, may be seen in one individual, and the reasons for these varying tissue responses are unclear.

The Skin and Subcutaneous Tissue: The lesions in the skin have been well described by Lucas (1967) and consist of nodular, ulcerative, circinate, eczematoid or psoriasiform lesions.

They most commonly present as flat slightly raised lesions, become palish papules and lastly shallow ulcers 3—4 mm in diameter. In the pigmented races a well defined hyperpigmented halo surrounds the lesion in its active state and delineates the scar on healing. In the disseminated form the skin lesions are continuously erupting and vary in size and stage of evolution. Ulceration is common. Biopsy reveals the presence of the typical giant cell systems containing spores. Necrosis and an acute inflammatory exudate may be present superficially in this lesion if ulceration has occurred. Pseudoepitheliomatous hyperplasia of the epidermis is not usual. In sinuses and subcutaneous extensions from bone lesions, areas of necrosis containing yeasts are common.

Lesions also occur in the mucosa of the oral cavity, and the gingiva may be affected primarily or secondarily by extension of a mandibular focus.

The Skeletal System: The frequent occurrence of bone lesion in African histoplasmosis has been noted by many authors. A solitary bone lesion may be the sole manifestation of the disease or the lesions may be part of a disseminated and generalized infection. Spontaneous fracture of bone has been noted in a few patients (COCKSHOTT and LUCAS, 1964; PELOUX et al., 1965).

The lesion commences in the medulla, and oval osteolytic lesions are seen radiologically. As a rule the periosteum lays down new bone and the bone may appear to be expanded. The histopathology is characterized by giant cell reaction with extensive areas of necrosis. Yeast forms are numerous. As the lesion expands, the cortex is eroded and extension occurs beneath the periosteum with finally erosion into the soft tissues with the formation of a painful swelling which eventually become a cold abscess. The abscess may rupture externally, with the formation of sinuses or ulcerated lesions with exuberant granulation tissue which may simulate a neoplasm. The flat bones of the skull and the ribs are most frequently affected, to be followed by the sternum, scapulae and jaws. Teeth may be loosened if the mandible is affected. Lesions in the cervical, dorsal or lumbar vertebrae may cause paraplegia by extradural spinal cord compression and large paravertebral abscesses have been described (KERVRAN and ARETAS, 1947; CAMAIN et al., 1958; COCKSHOTT and LUCAS, 1964). There may be single or multiple foci in the long bones, usually diaphyseal in the young child and juxtametaphyseal in older individuals, possibly related to the regression of red marrow towards the metaphyses with advancing age (COCKSHOTT, 1967). Lesions close to the metaphysis may interfere with the maturation of epiphyseal cartilage and ossification and distortion of a growing bone can result (LUNN, 1960). A radiological skeletal survey will often reveal unsuspected lesions in patients with lesions in other systems. Direct spread to joints may occur with evolution of a painful arthritis.

The Reticulo-Endothelial System: Regional lymph nodes may be affected in the localised form of the disease. In the disseminated form the superficial and deep nodes may be widely affected. Widespread lesions may also be present in the marrow with an associated anaemia. Focal lesions in the spleen and splenomegaly are also common. Hepatomegaly is also usual and giant cell granulomas and extensive areas of necrosis containing yeast forms are the usual findings seen on biopsy or at postmortem. It is not known whether the infection originates in the Kupffer cells or by haematogenous spread. There is however no report of the yeast forms being seen in Kupffer cells and the latter method of spread is the more likely.

The Respiratory System: The lungs, in contrast to *H. capsulatum* infection, are not thought to be commonly affected; but CLARK and GREENWOOD (1967) have recently described two patients with lung involvement, in one of whom no extrapulmonary lesions were found, and have discussed a further possible 10 cases in the literature. In a number of these, however, the diagnosis was doubtful, tuberculosis perhaps being responsible for the symptoms in three and in a further three the only evidence of pulmonary involvement was radiological. It is of interest that one of the patients with miliary pulmonary involvement shown as fine nodular opacities on X-ray described by CLARK and GREENWOOD was in the last trimester of pregnancy. Caseating lesions containing spores were noted in the lungs, lymphatic glands, spleen, liver, ileum, bone marrow, kidney, skin and adrenals and it was thought that the extensive caseation might imply a lowered immunity, pregnancy perhaps playing a part. The child, born prematurely, died shortly after birth, with no evidence of a congenital infection. The typical solitary nodule so commonly seen in *H. capsulatum* infections has not been described in duboisii infections nor have miliary calcified opacities been seen.

Gastrointestinal System: Isolated lesions may be found in the intestine (COLE et al., 1965) and a caecal lesion with perforation and peritonitis has been reported (CAMAIN et al., 1958). As previously mentioned, hepatosplenomegaly is common, and liver biopsy may be diagnostic.

Other Organs: The neurological complications of vertebral involvement have already been mentioned. Rarely, soft tissue involvement may also produce clinical evidence of a cord lesion. The central nervous system, however, tends to escape infection, and foci in the skull bones spread externally and do not penetrate the dura mater. Typical granulomas and caseating lesions have been described in the adrenals, kidney, bladder, breast and testicle.

Laboratory Diagnosis: The possibility of infection with *H. duboisii* should always be considered in any patient living in, or coming from, Africa with undiagnosed skin, bone or visceral lesions. The typical yeast forms are usually easily demonstrated on direct microscopic examination of the exudate from skin lesions. Ten per cent potassium hydroxide may be used to clear the specimen prior to direct microscopical examination. The fungus cells can be well demonstrated by any of the routine Romanowsky stains. Occasionally fungus cells may be present in sputum, stool or urine. Unless, however, the possibility of this infection is considered, it is usually first diagnosed on routine histopathological examination of surgical biopsy specimens of skin, bone or liver or in marrow or splenic aspirates. The histopathology is to all intents and purposes diagnostic. The fungi most likely to be confused with *H. duboisii* in tissue sections are *Blastomycosis dermatitidis* and *Cryptococcus neoformans*. The former is rare in Africa and the lungs are usually affected. Budding cells (8—15 μ in diameter) with a broad base and prominent cytoplasm containing several nuclei, and the presence of pseudoepitheliomatous hyperplasia, if the skin is affected, allow of differentiation (EMMONS et al., 1963). The fungus cells of *C. neoformans* are then walled spherical or oval bodies and vary markedly in size. There is frequently a clear surrounding halo 3—5 μ in thickness separating the cell from the cytoplasm of the histiocyte or giant cell in which it is contained. The halo stains positively with Mayer's mucicarmine and allows of differentiation from *H. duboisii*.

Many of our surgical biopsies in Ibadan are subject to phase contrast and imprint examination prior to the preparation of paraffin embedded sections and this has proved of great value in the rapid diagnosis of *H. duboisii* infections.

Although the histopathology of the lesion may be diagnostic, culture and animal inoculation should always be undertaken if laboratory facilities are available. Specimens may be mailed for culture in glycerine containing 1000 units of penicillin and 1000 μg of streptomycin per ml.

The fungus may be cultured at $25°$ C on Sabouraud's or blood agar media. If the original material is infected the addition of 500 units of penicillin and 500 μg of streptomycin per ml of media is advisable.

The colonies are grey, flat and stellate and consist of septate hyphae with small conidia. A profuse growth of tuberculate chlamydospores occurs in two months.

The mycological features on culture are essentially similar to those of *H. capsulatum*. Minor differences (including the lack of urease production) have however been noted (VANBREUSEGHEM, 1956; COREMANS, 1963).

The diagnostic features of *H. duboisii* in laboratory animals have already been discussed. Serological tests have still to be evaluated but it would appear that complement fixation tests to mycelial and yeast phase antigens of *H. duboisii* are of value in diagnosis. Fluorescent antibody techniques may also be employed to enable a specific diagnosis to be made.

As of yet, skin sensitivity testing with available mycelial phase antigens (histoplasmin) are of little value as a diagnostic procedure.

References

AJELLO, L.: Personal communication quoted by COCKSHOTT and LUCAS, 1964a. — AJELLO, L., MANSON-BAHR, P.E.C., MOORE, J.C.: Amboni Caves, Tanganyika. A new endemic area for *Histoplasma capsulatum*. Amer. J. trop. Med. Hyg. **9**, 633—638 (1960). — BASSET, A., Quenum, C., HOCQUET, P., CAMAIN, R., BASSET, M.: Histoplasmose a forme cutaneo-osseuse. Bull. Soc. méd. Afr. noire Langue franç. **7**, 69—70 (1962). — BLANCHARD, M., LEFROU, G.: Presence dans une lesion humaine d'un saccharomycete pathogene pour le cobaye. Bull. Soc. Path. exot. **15**, 915 (1922). — BRUMPT, E.: Precis de Parasitologie, p. 1787. Ed. by Masson, Paris (quoted from DUBOIS et al., 1952). — CAMAIN, R., BUTE, M., KLEFSTAD-SILLONVILLE, F., MAFART, J., VILASCO, J.A., DROUHET, E.: Sept. nouvean cas d'histoplasmose observis en A.O.F. Bull. Soc. Path. exot. **51**, 83—107 (1958). — CATANEI, A.: Resultats de l'etude du pouvoir pathogene d'une souche soudanaise d'*Histoplasma capsulatum*. Arch. Inst. Pasteur Algér. **23**, 260—268 (1945). — CATANEI, A., KERVRAN, P.: Nouvelle mycose humaine observe au Soudan francais. Arch. Inst. Pasteur Algér. **23**, 169—172 (1945). — *Ciba Symposium:* Systemic Mycoses. London: J. & A. Churchill Ltd. 1968. — CLARK, B.M., GREENWOOD, B.M.: Pulmonary lesions in African Histoplasmosis. J. trop. Med. Hyg. **71**, 4 (1968). — COCKSHOTT, W.P.: Radiological patterns of the deep mycoses in "Systemic Mycoses", Ciba Symposium. London: J. & A. Churchill Ltd. 1968. — COCKSHOTT, W.P., LUCAS, A.O.: *Histoplasmosis duboisii*. Quart. J. Med. **33**, 223—238 (1964a). ~ Radiological findings in *Histoplasma duboisii* infections. Brit. J. Radiol. **37**, 653—660 (1964b). — COLE, A.C.E., RIDLEY, D.S., WOLFE, H.R.I.: Bowel infection with *Histoplasma duboisii*. J. trop. Med. Hyg. **68**, 92—96 (1965). — COREMANS, J.: Un test biochemique de differentiation de *Histoplasma duboisii Vanbreuseghem 1952* d'avec *Histoplasma capsulatum Darling 1906*. C.R. Soc. Biol. (Paris) **157**, 1130—1132 (1963). — COURTOIS, G., SEGRETAIN, G., MARIAT, F., LEVADITI, J.C.: Mycose cutanee a corps levuriformes observee chez des signes Africains en captivite. Ann. Inst. Pasteur **89**, 124—127 (1935). — DEVRIESE, J.: Premier resultats due reaction cutanee à l'histoplasmine au Congo belge. Ann. Soc. belge Méd. trop. **33**, 211—213 (1953). — DROUHET, E.: Apropos of 4 strains of *Histoplasma capsulatum* and 7 strains of *Histoplasma duboisii* recently isolated. Arch. Inst. Pasteur Tunis **39**, 291—308 (1962). — DROUHET, E., SCHWARZ, J.: Comparative studies with 18 strains of histoplasma. J. Lab. clin. Med. **47**, 128—144 (1956). — DUBOIS, A., JANSSENS, P.G., BRUTSAERT, P., VANBREUSEGHEM, R.: Un cas d'histoplasmose Africaine. Ann. Soc. belge Méd. trop. **32**, 569—584 (1952). — DUBOIS, A., VANBREUSEGHEM, R.: L'histoplasmose africaine. Bull. Acad. roy. Méd. Belg. Ser. 6, **17**, 551—565 (1952). — DUNCAN, J.T.: A unique form of *Histoplasma*. Trans. roy. Soc. trop. Med. Hyg. **40**, 364—365 (1947). ~ Tropical African histoplasmosis. Trans. roy. Soc. trop. Med. Hyg. **52**, 468—474 (1958). — EMMONS, C.W., BINFORD, C.H., UTZ, J.P.: Medical Mycology. New York: Lea and Febiger 1963. — FRIESS, DELVOUYE: A propos d'un aspect cirurgical d'une mycose rare: Histoplasmose cahiers Med. un l'union francaise Alger. **2**, 419—423 (1947). — JARNIOU, A.P., KERBLAT, G., MOREAU, A.. DUVAL, P., DROUHET, E.: Bull. Soc. méd. Hôp. Paris **74**, 918—927 (1958). — KAUFMAN, L.: Serology of systemic fungus diseases. Publ. Hlth Rep. (Wash.) **81**, 177—185 (1966). — KERVRAN, P., ARETAS, R.: Deux cas d'histoplasmose observes au Soudan francais. Bull. Soc. Path. exot. **40**, 270—276 (1967). — LANCELY, J.L., LUNN, H.F., WILSON, A.M.M.: Histoplasmosis in an African child. J. Pediat. **59**, 756—764 (1961). — LUCAS, A.O.: The clinical features of some of the deep mycoses in West Africa. In: "Systemic Mycoses", Ciba Symposium. London: J. & A. Churchill Ltd. 1968. — LUNN, H.F.: Case of histoplasmosis of bone in East Africa. J. trop. Med. Hyg. **63**, 175—180 (1960). — MARIAT, F., SEGRETAIN, G.: Etude mycologique d'une histoplasmose spontanee du singe africain. Ann. Inst. Pasteur **91**, 874—891 (1956). — PELOUX, Y., THEVENOT, P., ROBERT, H.: L'histoplasmose. Med. trop. (Madr.) **25**, 439—456

(1965). — Pine, L., Kaufman, L., Boone, C.J.: Comparative fluorescent antibody staining of *Histoplasma capsulatum* and *Histoplasma duboisii* with a specific anti-yeast phase. *H. capsulatum* conjugate. Mycopathologia (Den Haag) **24**, 315—326 (1964). — Seeliger, H.P.R.: "Recent applications of immunological techniques in the diagnosis of the deep mycoses". In: "Systematic Mycoses", Ciba Symposium. London: J. & A. Churchill Ltd. 1968. — Symmers, W. St. C.: Further cases of exotic mycoses seen in Britain. Trans. roy. Soc. trop. Med. Hyg. **55**, 201—208 (1961). — Taschdjian, C. L.: Hypha fusion studies on *Histoplasma capsulatum* and *Histoplasma duboisii*. 1959. — Tenret, J.: Étude sur la reaction à l'histoplasmine au Ruanda-Urundi. Ann. Soc. belge Méd. trop. **36**, 859—873 (1956). — Vanbreuseghem, R.: *Histoplasma duboisii* and large forms of *Histoplasma capsulatum*. Mycologia **48**, 264 (1956). ~ Les manifestations cutanees de l'histoplasmose africaine. Ann. Soc. belge Méd. trop. **44**, 1037—1055 (1964). — Vanbreuseghem, R., Eugene, J.: Culture d'*Histoplasma capsulatum* et d'*Histoplasma duboisii* sur un milieu a base de terre et de natieres recales provenant de divers animanx. C.R. Soc. Biol. (Paris) **152**, 1602—1605 (1958). — Vanbreuseghem, R.: Trans. N.Y. Acad. Sci. **19**, 622 (1957). — Vandepitte, J., Gatti, F., Hennebert, P.: *Histoplasmosis duboisii* dans un absces appreas injection. Ann. Soc. belge Méd. trop. **45**, 49—56 (1965). — Walker, J., Spooner, E.T.C.: Natural infection of the African baboon *Papio Papio* with the large-cell form of Histoplasma. J. Path. Bact. **80**, 436—438 (1960).

African Histoplasmosis (Part 2)

JAN SCHWARZ, Cincinnati/Ohio, USA

With 4 Figures

African histoplasmosis is caused by *Histoplasma duboisii* Vanbreuseghem and has, to date, been seen spontaneously only in men and baboons from equatorial Africa.

Geography

The African continent has the doubtful privilege of being the home of infection by both species of *Histoplasma: H. capsulatum*, Darling, and *H. duboisii*, Vanbreuseghem. Only about 60 cases of African histoplasmosis have been observed, and the epidemiology and clinicopathology of this disease need further attention before the final chapter can be written.

The Organism H. Duboisii Vanbreuseghem

Histoplasma duboisii, according to QUENUM-AHINA, was seen by LECENE (1919); BLANCHARD and LEFRON (1922), CATANEI and KERVRAN (1945), and, by DUNCAN who first grew the organisms in May, 1943. *H. duboisii* was described as a distinct species by VANBREUSEGHEM in 1952 (DUBOIS et al.). From all evidence, the organisms seems identical in the mycelial phase to the classical *H. capsulatum*; the slow-growing white mold shows on culture mount tuberculate spores of $\pm$ 10—15 μ, and numerous small microconidia. But in the yeast phase, induced by incubation *in vitro* on protein-containing media or by culture from infected man or animals at 37° C, a large, mostly round to oval, thick walled yeast cell is seen, measuring up to 15 μ, and reproducing as a rule by a single bud, often with a broad base. Both by size and thickness of wall, the yeast cell of *H. duboisii* is more nearly comparable to *Blastomyces dermatitidis* than to *H. capsulatum*.

It may be repeated that *H. duboisii* and *H. capsulatum* are uninucleated, *B. dermatitidis* is multinucleated. This seemingly clear description is somewhat clouded by the fact that both in cultures at 37° C and in tissues in spontaneous and experimental disease, in addition to the large yeast forms ("duboisii forms"), small yeasts are found ("capsulatum forms"). The latter are fairly common in tissues in early experimental infection, but more and more large cells develop, relegating the "capsulatum forms" to become a dwindling minority after 6 weeks or longer. Fluorescent antibody staining suggested to PINE et al. that *H. duboisii* is a separate species (1964). AJELLO lately questions the position of *H. duboisii* as a separate species (1968).

Epidemiology. H. duboisii has been found up to 1964 in some 50 Negroes, six Caucasians, and one Indian (COCKSHOTT and LUCAS) in Equatorial Africa. Attempts in Africa to recover *H. duboisii* from soil were unsuccessful, until 1967 when isolation from a sample collected in Kenya was reported (AL-DOORY and KALTER). Man and baboon (*Papio papio* and *Papio cynocephalus*) were found to be spontaneously infected. For all practical purposes, recognition of most cases was made in the vicinity of the Medical Schools of Dakar, Loranium, Kampala, and Ibadan (Equatorial West Africa), suggesting that other cases may go undetected for reasons of inferior medical surveillance.

Pathogenesis: The disease is said to spare the lungs, but adequate autopsies can hardly be cited in support of this claim. Until otherwise proven, the temptation to seek analogies in the pathogenesis of histoplasmosis caused by either *H. capsulatum* or *H. duboisii* should be considered a healthy one. One of the patients of Basset et al. developed disease while on "sweeping duty" in a bat-infested school. The fact of exposure to bat droppings carried connotations of inhalation infection, in view of the findings of Klite and others, and does not necessarily point to the suggested percutaneous inoculation at the point of an abrasion. Other patients gave histories of association with fowl, but not too convincingly.

Cutaneous involvement is prominent in African histoplasmosis. The skin and subcutaneous tissues of inhabitants of Equatorial Africa show a peculiar reaction to certain Mycobacteria also (Buruli ulceration — Connor and Lunn), supposedly also in the absence of a demonstrable pulmonary lesion. Osteoarticular lesions, so exceptional in classical histoplasmosis, are commonplace in African histoplasmosis. In the 56 cases listed by Cockshott and Lucas, 30 had skin lesions and 29 bone lesions, often both localizations in the same case. Only 8 patients died, but the followup of at least 20 is not available. Most patients were young; 33 were under age 40 and 20 were under age 20, but without data about the age of the population seeking medical advice, these figures lose impressiveness.

Skull lesions were reported in 12 instances by Cockshott and Lucas. One case developing under the eyes of these observers appeared as a small area of diploic destruction, followed by necrosis of the inner and outer tables of the skull. The osteolytic lesions are discrete, remaining visible also in the stage of repair. The overlying "cold abscesses" in the soft tissues are comparable to tuberculous lesions. Most skull lesions were multiple, as generally were rib lesions found in ten patients (Cockshott and Lucas). Expansion of the rib and fistula formation were common.

Scapulae and jaws figured four times and the sternum twice, in the above review. In 3 patients, involvement of the spine led to the fearful complication of paraplegia. Long-bone lesions, when found in children, were mostly diaphyseal; in teenagers and adults they were juxta-metaphyseal. The severity of the osteomyelitis has been seen to lead even to spontaneous fracture. Humerus, femur, tibia, ulna, radius, the bones of the fingers and the clavicle were all involved in some cases. Numerous cases had multiple osteolytic lesions.

Single or multiple caseous lesions have only one pathogenetic source: the blood stream. The blood in turn can distribute organisms only from a source in contact with the external world: skin, some mucosae, and specifically the airways. Following well-established pathogenetic principles, bones can be secondarily involved only from a primary lesion elsewhere (in our opinion, most often the lung).

We have avoided discussing multiple skin lesions, since cutaneous primary infection is, after all, within the realm of possibility. But if one studies the case histories of African histoplasmosis, with one subcutaneous abscess or one ulcer appearing on the head and the next on completely distant parts of the body, once more the possibility of hematogenous spread should be considered, remembering that a fairly similar clinical behavior (multiple cutaneous ulcers and granulomas in North American blastomycosis) has been established and pretty universally accepted as originating from a primary lung lesion (Schwarz and Baum). The fact that cutaneous lesions can be primary is obvious, but they prove to be only most exceptionally primary in North American blastomycosis, classical histoplasmosis, and coccidioidomycosis.

The requirements for accepting a cutaneous primary lesion have been clearly established: 1) a primary chancre with regional lymphadenitis must be present, 2) a pulmonary lesion must be absent (a fact conclusively demonstrated only by competent autopsy), 3) traumatic inoculation of the skin remains hypothetical, unless the instrument producing the wound can be shown to be contaminated with the fungus.

Subcutaneous abscesses are common in African histoplasmosis, both with and without underlying osteomyelitis and osteitis. Skin lesions, from pustular to ulcerous, from eczema to fungating granuloma, are infinitely more prominent in African histoplasmosis than in the classical variety (VANBREUSEGHEM, 1964). No lesions of erythema nodosum seem to be recorded in African histoplasmosis. Mucosal lesions in the oral cavity were seen independently or secondary to mandibular osteitis. Hepatosplenomegaly has been recorded 4 times in the COCKSHOTT and LUCAS review, with liver biopsies helpful in establishing the diagnosis.

Only half a dozen cases were brought to autopsy, and it would be premature to accept the statements made frequently that the *lung* does not show lesion in African histoplasmosis, especially since 3 cases have reported positive sputa (DUBOIS et al., 1952; VANDEPITTE et al., 1957, and JARNIOU et al., 1958). The patient of JARNIOU et al. also had radiologic evidence of pulmonary involvement. LANCELY et al. reported lung lesions on X-ray; VANDEPITTE et al. demonstrated pleural reaction and found post-mortem lung lesions to be caseous and attributed to mycobacterial disease, even when numerous yeast cells of *H. duboisii* were present in the lung.

A 63-year-old patient from whom DUNCAN had isolated *H. duboisii* in 1943, showed clinical and radiologic evidence of lung disease with relapse, and, while only conjectural, is assumed by DUNCAN to have had pulmonary histoplasmosis, possibly combined with tuberculosis. Janke's patient had bronchopneumonia for about 3 months before the skin lesions were manifest; no attempts to culture *Histoplasma* were made in this case.

DEVREESE et al., at autopsy of an African woman, found a $3 \times 3 \times 4$ cm. focus in the lung, with huge mediastinal lymph nodes. RESSELER et al. insist on "normal lungs" in two patients, even when the second patient did not have the benefit of an X-ray. A case reported by QUERE et al. showed massive involvement of the lungs on X-ray. CLARK and GREENWORD report two cases with proven pulmonary involvement, tabulate 10 cases from the literature and conclude that the lung may well be the portal of entry also in African histoplasmosis, as it is in the "classical histoplasmosis" and several other deep mycoses.

The apparent tropism of *H. duboisii* to skin and bone may not prove to stand the test of time and enlightenment any better than the initial claim that Darling's disease was characterized by hepatosplenomegaly and is always fatal. It also should be clear that inhalation of spores or mycelial fragments is unquestionably the route of infection in coccidioidomycosis, North American blastomycosis, and histoplasmosis of the classical type. There is little reason to believe that an organism so similar to *H. capsulatum* as *H. duboisii* is, should invade the human body differently. Good evidence exists that pulmonary lesions can be found in African histoplasmosis if searched for with proper knowledge and open mind. Few performers of autopsies can be trusted to rule out small primary lesions in the lung; even the most experienced pathologists prefer the help of X-rays of lungs removed from the body in order to locate small calcified foci.

Lymphadenopathy is very prominent in African histoplasmosis to judge from available illustrations. Many lymphadenitides are reported local to skin or bone lesions; others do not reveal the source of drainage. Bowel involvement was demonstrated from a sigmoid biopsy and culture in a 33-year-old male who suffered from severe diarrhea and weight loss. Distinct ileocecal pathology on X-ray and the symptomatology improved dramatically after amphotericin B therapy (COLE et al.).

Differential Diagnosis: In view of the recent demonstration of *Blastomyces dermatitidis* in tropical Africa (EMMONS et al.) and the superficial morphologic similarity between *B. dermatitidis* and *H. duboisii*, cultures and careful screening

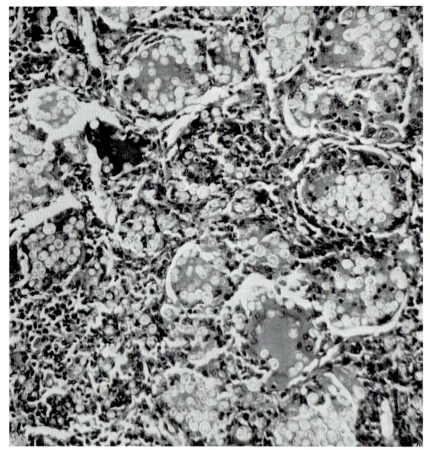

Fig. 1. *Histoplasma duboisii* entices the tissues of man and animals to giant cell formation often of gigantic size. Two months after i.p. injection, the omentum of the hamster shows numerous giant cells filled with round yeast cells, easily recognizable in H & E sections × 320

by cytologic differentiation are mandatory. Individual organisms are also similar to the smaller forms of *B. brasiliensis* and except for greater thickness of the wall and oval shape, resemble *Cryptococcus neoformans*. The latter stains with muci-carmin, *H. duboisii* does not; but not all cells of *C. neoformans* stain uniformly with mucicarmin.

The tissue reaction is very different in *H. duboisii* from the changes seen in classical histoplasmosis. If small yeast cells are present in African histoplasmosis, which, especially in early experimental disease, is often the case, the small yeast cells are taken up by histiocytes exactly as one would expect with *H. capsulatum*. But when only large cells are present, and this is most frequently the case in human spontaneous disease and in long-standing experimental disease, the picture changes completely, and clumps of large yeast cells are seen (Figs. 1, 2). In tissues, these frequently are round or only slightly ovoid, filling enormous giant cells or occupying, in the giant cells, a peripheral rim, resembling the distribution of nuclei in gigantic Langhans cells.

On the other hand, such large yeast cells can also be found in Kupffer cells of the liver or other large phagocytic elements. In view of the great number of such

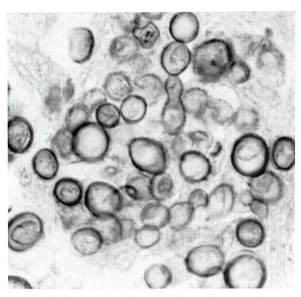

Fig. 2. Closer inspection of the content of giant cell reveals yeast cells to vary considerably in size and shape. Budding is easily recognized. Round and ovoid forms exist. Notice large size of the yeast from magnification given in this and previous photograph. Gridley × 1280

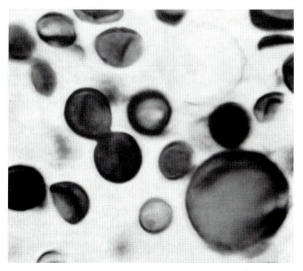

Fig. 3. The variation in size is dramatized in a granuloma from the omentum of a hamster. Budding cell in center of field. Grocott × 2100. (From OKUDAIRA and SCHWARZ: Mycologia **53**, 53, 1961)

yeast cells in individual giant cells, there seems to be little doubt that they multiply within the cytoplasm of the phagocytic cells just as the small cousin of the "classical type" does in similar conditions. Sometimes there is a slight outpouring of polymorphonuclear leukocytes, strictly limited to the immediate vicinity of the organisms in the interstitium of the liver or lung.

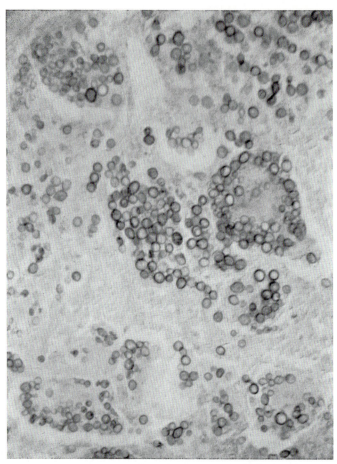

Fig. 4. Intracellular location in giant cells and variation in size is brought out poignantly in Gridley stain of tissue shown in illustration 1. Gridley × 320

In similar locations, one sees occasional histiocytes and epithelioid cells, but little tendency to the formation of true tubercles is ever found. On first glance, the large yeast cells appear uniform in size, but close scrutiny reveals considerable variation in size and shape, with marked differences in the thickness of the wall of the individual cells and great differences in the staining properties of the cyto-plasmic content.

The differential diagnosis of individual yeast cells lies between *Cryptococcus* and the organisms of North and South American blastomycosis. The tendency to conglomeration and giant cell formation is unique, in our experience, for African histoplasmosis and therefore makes differential diagnosis comparatively easy. Occasionally, we found phagocytized polymorphonuclear neutrophils in the same giant cells which harbored numerous yeast cells of the duboisii type. In the spleen, yeast cells seem sometimes to multiply without eliciting much cellular response, but in view of the huge number of such cells, it becomes difficult to decide how many are actually extracellular and which ones are within enormous and very irregular giant cells. In the spleen also, polymorphonuclear leukocytes are fre-quently found within the giant cells. The large number of yeast cells in some organs must at least produce mechanical compression, even if no other toxic or inflammatory reaction were forthcoming.

In view of its large size, the organism can be seen easily with H & E stains, but it literally shines with any of the available special methods, from the PAS through the Gridley to the Grocott (Figs. 3 and 4). With special stains, the presence of "capsulatum" forms surrounding the individual large organisms becomes obvious and is somewhat confusing because at first glance it can be mistaken for *B. brasiliensis* surrounded by numerous buds. Necrosis, both of tissue and of organism, can be seen in long standing disease and in large foci. Soft-tissue lesions most nearly approximate the definition of a granuloma, since they often show a fibrous capsule separating them from surrounding muscle or fat tissue; but close inspection shows once more that these are mostly yeast cells, free and in giant cells, rather than true histiocytic or epithelioid-cell granulomas.

The clinical and pathologic features of African histoplasmosis have a certain resemblance to North American blastomycosis. Both diseases have frequent skin and bone involvement, but the multiple subcutaneous abscesses are distinctly more prominent in African histoplasmosis. The organisms causing the two diseases have a certain resemblance, morphologically and in both growth forms on culture (except for the tuberculate spores of *H. duboisii* in the mycelial phase; such spores are not found in *B. dermatitidis*). The granulation tissue is different. In African histoplasmosis, the large yeast cells, mostly in enormous giant cells, dominate the picture; in blastomycosis a variety of granulation tissue is seen, from the true epithelioid-cell tubercle to forms which are almost suppurative or necrotizing. But if giant cells are found, and they are seldom numerous in North American blastomycosis, they are more often of the Langhans type, with few organisms within the giant cells. Never have we seen the multitude of yeast cells in North American blastomycosis so commonly encountered in African histoplasmosis.

References

AL-DOORY, Y., KALTER, S.S.: The isolation of *Histoplasma duboisii* and keratinophilic fungi from soils of East Africa. Mycopathologia (Den Haag) **31**, 289 (1967). — AJELLO, L.: Comparative morphology and immunology of members of the genus *Histoplasma*. Mykosen **11**, 507 (1968). — ANDRÉ, M., ORIO, J., DEPOUX, R., DROUHET, E.: Histoplasmose africaine à grandes formes à localisations osseuses multiples. Évolution favorable après intervention chirurgicale et amphotéricine B. Bull. Soc. Path. exot. **52**, 345 (1959). — BASSET, A., QUENUM, C., HOCQUET, P., CAMAIN, R., BASSET, M.: Histoplasmose à forme cutaneo-osseuse. Bull. Soc. med. Afr. noire Langue franc. **7**, 69 (1962). — CAMAIN, R., BERTE, M., KLEFSTAD-SILLONVILLE, F., MAFART, J., VILASCO, J.A.: Sept nouveaux cas d'histoplasmose observés en A.O.F. Bull. Soc. Path. exot. **51**, 83 (1958). — CLARK, B.M., GREENWOOD, B.M.: Pulmonary lesions in African histoplasmosis. J. trop. Med. Hyg. **71**, 4 (1968). — CLARKE, G.H.V., WALKER, J., WINSTON, R.M.: African histoplasmosis. J. trop. Med. Hyg. **56**, 277 (1953). — COCKSHOTT, W.P., LUCAS, A.O.: *Histoplasmosis duboisii*. Quart. J. Med. **33**, 223 (1964). ~ Radiological findings in *Histoplasma duboisii* infections. Brit. J. Radiol. **37**, 653 (1964). — COLE, A.C.E., RIDLEY, D.S., WOLFE, H.R.I.: Bowel infection with *Histoplasma duboisii*. J. trop. Med. Hyg. **68**, 92 (1965). — CONNOR, D.H., LUNN, H.F.: Buruli ulceration. Arch. Path. **81**, 183 (1966). — DEVREESE, A., DONKERS, J., NINANE, G., VANBREUSEGHEM, R.: Histoplasmose africaine à formes capsulatum causée par *Histoplasma duboisii* Vanbreuseghem 1952. Ann. Soc. belge Méd. trop. **5**, 403 (1961). — DROUHET, E., SCHWARZ, J., BINGHAM, E.: Evaluation of the action of nystatin on *Histoplasma capsulatum* in vitro and in hamsters and mice. Antibiot. et Chemother. (Basel) **6**, 23 (1956). — DROUHET, E., SCHWARZ, J.: Croissance et morphogénèse d'*Histoplasma*. I.-Etude comparative des phases mycélienne et levure de 18 souches d'*Histoplasma capsulatum* d'origine américaine et africaine. Ann. Inst. Pasteur **90**, 144 (1956). — DUBOIS, A., JANSSENS, P.G., BRUTSAERT, VANBREUSEGHEM, R.: Un cas d'histoplasmose africaine. Avec une note mycologique sur *H. duboisii* n. sp. Ann. Soc. belge Méd. trop. **32**, 569 (1952). — DUNCAN, J.T.: Tropical African histoplasmosis. Trans. roy. Soc. trop. Med. Hyg. **52**, 468 (1958). — EMMONS, C.W., MURRAY, I.G., LURIE, H.I., KING, M.H., TULLOCH, J.A., CONNOR, D.H.: North American blastomycosis: 2 autochthonous cases from

Africa. Sabouraudia **3**, 306 (1964). — Jackson, F.I.: Histoplasmosis in South Africa. S. Afr. med. J. **1952**, 460—461. — Janke, D.: Afrikanische Histoplasmose *(Histoplasma duboisii* Vanbreuseghem 1952*)* der Haut. Hautarzt **12**, 259 (1961). — Jarniou, A.P., Kerbrat, G., Moreau, A., Duval: Histoplasmose pulmonaire africaine avec suppuration diffuse apparue après une année d'évolution. Bull. Soc. med. Hop. Paris **74**, 32 (1958). — Klite, P.D., Diercks, F.H.: *Histoplasma capsulatum* in fecal contents and organs of bats in the Canal Zone. Amer. J. trop. Med. Hyg. **14**, 433 (1965). — Lanceley, J.L., Lunn, H.F., Wilson, A.M.M.: Histoplasmosis in an African child. J. Pediat. **49**, 756 (1961). — Pine, L., Drouhet, E., Reynolds, G.: A comparative morphological study of the yeast phases of *Histoplasma capsulatum* and *Histoplasma duboisii*. Sabouraudia, **3**, 211 (1964). — Pine, L., Kaufman, L., Boone, C.J.: Comparative fluorescent antibody staining of *Histoplasma capsulatum* and *Histoplasma duboisii* with a specific anti-yeast phase *H. capsulatum* conjugate. Mycopathologia (Den Haag) **24**, 315 (1964). — Quenum-Ahina, C.: L'histoplasmose africaine à grandes formes. Paris: Amédée Legrande & Cie. (Editeurs) 1958. — Quéré, M.A., Basset, A., Basset, M., Cave, L.: Histoplasmose generalisée avec localisation orbito-palpébrale et lacunes craniennes. Ann. Oculist. (Paris) **198**, 105 (1965). — Resseler, J.J.C., Farrior, H.L., Vanbreuseghem, R.: Deux nouveaux cas congolais d'histoplasmose par *Histoplasma duboissi* Vanbreuseghem 1952. Ann. Soc. belge Méd. trop. **5**, 801 (1962). — Schwarz, J.: The pathogenesis of histoplasmosis. Ann. N.Y. Acad. Sci. **20**, 541 (1958). ~ Giant forms of *Histoplasma capsulatum* in tissue explants. Amer. J. clin. Path. **23**, 898 (1953). — Schwarz, J., Baum, G.L.: Blastomycosis. Amer. J. clin. Path. **21**, 999 (1951). — Vanbreuseghem, R.: Les manifestations cutanées de l'histoplasmose africaine. Ann. Soc. belge Méd. trop. **44**, 1037 (1964). — Vandepitte, J., Lamote, J., Thys, A., Vanbreuseghem, R.: *Histoplasma duboisii* Vanbreuseghem 1952. Ann. Soc. belge Méd. trop. **37**, 515 (1957). — Walker, J., Spooner, E.T.C.: Natural infection of the African baboon *Papio papio* with the large-cell form of *Histoplasma*. J. Path. Bact. **80**, 436 (1960).

Coccidioidomycosis

Robert W. Huntington, Jr., Bakersfield/California, USA*

With 36 Figures

I. Definition, Synonomy

This review is concerned solely with coccidioidomycosis, defined as infection with the fungus species *Coccidioides immitis*. The initial uncertainty as to the distinction between this agent and that of North American blastomycosis was resolved many years ago through the studies of Ophuls and Moffitt (1900), Ophuls (1905b), Montgomery et al. (1903), Montgomery and Morrow (1904), Evans (1909), Hektoen (1907), Dickson (1915, 1931) and others. Distinction between coccidioides and the agent of South American paracoccidioidomycosis has been clarified by the more recent studies of De Almeida (1930a, b, 1932). Emmons (1967) has recorded decided differences between coccidioides and the agents of European "pseudo-coccidioidomycosis." Of course we shall not deal here with North American blastomycosis; neither shall we take up South American paracoccidioidomycosis nor European pseudococcidioidomycosis.

The salient characteristics of *Coccidioides immitis* have been studied by a number of investigators, among them Ophuls and Moffitt (1900), Ophuls (1905a, 1905b), Wolbach (1904), Baker et al. (1943), Friedman et al. (1953), Hampson (1954), Emmons (1942a, 1942b, 1947), Emmons and Ashburn, Emmons et al. (1945), Ajello (1957, 1967a), Negroni (1967), Huppert et al. (1967), and Spaur (1956). These characteristics include predilection for warm arid regions (see Geographical Pathology), pathogenicity for mice, spherular form in infected tissue with characteristic endosporulative reproduction, and growth on ordinary media, both at room temperature and at $37°$ C as septate mycelium with eventual arthrospore formation (Conant, 1965; Fetter et al., 1967; Fiese, 1958; Lewis et al., 1956; Wilson and Plunkett, 1965).

The strict limitation of our topic to "true" coccidioidomycosis does little to alleviate our vexatious problems in terminology, some of which can only be understood in their historical context. The terminological confusion may be blamed, in accordance with the reader's preferences, either on the conservatively authoritarian character of the nomenclature of biological taxonomy, or on the greater flexibility of clinico-pathologic nomenclature, or perhaps on both. Both Posadas and Wernicke in Argentina and Rixford and Gilchrist in the USA (Rixford, 1894a, b; Rixford and Gilchrist, 1896), who first recognized the organism in infected tissue, believed it to be a protozoan. Although the pioneer studies in Argentina were a few years earlier than those in California, Rixford and Gilchrist were the first to make a formal nomenclatural suggestion. With the counsel of Stiles, they proposed the name *Coccidioides immitis*. This name reflected assurance that the

---

* From the Departments of Pathology, Kern County General Hospital, Bakersfield, California; and the University of Southern California School of Medicine, Los Angeles, California.

organism was a protozoan resembling coccidium. The subsequent suggestion by Posadas' Latin American colleagues of the designation "Coccidium of Posadas" did not have priority (1928). More serious questions were raised by Ophuls' demonstration (Ophuls, 1905a, b; Ophuls and Moffitt, 1900) that the organism was actually a fungus. However, Ophuls' suggestion of a name more consonant with this status was not accepted, and the binomial *Coccidioides immitis* has persisted. Clearly the laws of the Medes and Persians were mere ephemera compared with those of priority in biological nomenclature!

While the organism has retained this singular if implausible title, infection with this organism has gone under a variety of names, each with some claim to rationality. Many of these are names which the student must learn to recognize. It now seems a curious stroke of historical irony that Posadas (1892) and Wernicke (1892) should have spoken of "mycosis fungoides with protozoa (Figs. 1, 2)." This title might suggest to a hasty reviewer some doubt as to the agent's status, or a hint of the possibility of mixed infection. However, the Argentine workers entertained no such notions. The term mycosis fungoides antedates the recognition of minute fungi as agents of human disease (Conant, 1965; Garrison, 1961). It is descriptive, not etiologic, and refers to large rather than to microscopic fungi. Thus it purports not to indicate etiology, but rather to suggest that the lesions look like mushrooms. Mycosis fungoides is now applied to a neoplastic condition of the skin (Allen, 1967; Cawley et al., 1951; Emmons, 1967), entirely unrelated to fungi or for that matter to protozoa. It would now be regarded as an entirely wrong diagnosis in Posadas' and Wernicke's case. Be that as it may, in accepting that diagnosis, Posadas and Wernicke were not anticipating that the "Protozoan" might prove to be a fungus.

It is understandable that Latin American students, unsuccessful in the attempt to apply Posadas' name to the organism, should continue to refer to the infection as Posadas' disease (Campins et al., 1949). North American pioneers spoke of "Protozoic dermatitis" (Rixford, 1894b; Thorne, 1894; Montgomery, 1900), then of "dermatitis coccidioides" (Montgomery et al., 1903, 1904; Wolbach, 1904). After showing that skin lesions were often absent and usually secondary when present, Ophuls (1905a) suggested the term coccidioidal granuloma, which was widely adopted (Beck, 1931a, 1931b; Brown, 1906, 1907; Brown and Cummins, 1914; Cooke, 1914, 1915; Dickson, 1915, 1929, 1931; Evans and Ball, 1929; Greaves, 1934; Ingham, 1936; Rixford, 1931; Ryfkogel, 1913).

For many years the only recognized instances of *C. immitis* infection were in patients whose disease was chronic, disseminated, and progressive. Though Wolbach (1915) reported a case with apparent recovery, Dickson (1915) wrote of an incidental, apparently arrested "coccidioidoma" in the lung of a subject dying of unrelated causes, and Ophuls (1929) continued to suggest the possibility of recovery, coccidioidal granuloma came to imply something dire as well as rare. Then came the demonstration by Dickson (1937a, b, 1939a, b), Dickson and Gifford (1938), Gifford (1936, 1939a, b), and Gifford et al. (1937) that in the southern San Joaquin Valley of California the quite common syndrome of benign pneumonitis with erythema nodosum or multiforme, locally known as "San Joaquin Fever" or "Valley Fever" (Smith, 1939, 1940, 1967) was due to coccidioides.

Since it would hardly have been good cheering bedside medicine to tell a patient with "valley Fever" that he had "coccidioidal granuloma," on practical as well as theoretical grounds a new name for coccidioides infection was called for. Dickson, as his pupil Smith (1967), tells us, was something of a logician as well as an etymological purist. Thus he was unreconciled to the protozooid binomial of the fungus; indeed he had in 1915 seconded Ophuls' suggestion of a new name more suitable

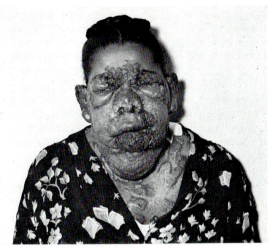

Fig. 1. Coccidioidomycosis. Verrucoid lesions of Posadas. A recent example. The extensive lesions of the skin of the face and upper thorax are elevated, warty, annular, serpigenous, and oozing. Case 1 of this chapter

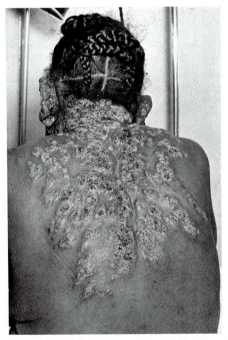

Fig. 2. Coccidioidomycosis. Verrucoid lesions of Posadas, involving the skin of the ears, the neck, and the upper back. Case 1. This is the only case I have ever seen of the verrucoid skin lesions of Posadas (1928). This form of coccidioidomycosis is exceedingly rare

for a fungus. Now that he had justification and opportunity for selecting a new name for the infection, Dickson resolved to include in that name some indication that the agent was in fact a fungus. So he chose the name coccidioidomycosis, using mycosis not in the old descriptive sense of mushroom-like but in the more modern etiologic sense of fungus infection. Coccidioidomycosis may be literally translated as the fungus infection due to the organism which looks like coccidium.

In conversation at least, North American students now tend to dodge both the protozooid name for the fungus and the Dicksonian polysyllable for the infection by using the abbreviation cocci for both. Although no one has suggested an appropriate alternative to Dickson's term, that term does invite complaints to the effect that it is long and awkward and that while it points out some historical errors it doesn't completely correct them. We have had to list a name given to the fungus in the belief that it was a protozoan, and a series of names for infection with that fungus, the last and longest being coccidioidomycosis. It would be futile, we think, to deny that this list has something of an Alice-Through-the-Looking-Glass quality. The reader who wonders whether this quality may have been slightly overemphasized in the present sober review might care to consult the more vivid and perspicuous surveys of Smith (1967) and Emmons (1967). This list does recall the White Knight's recital of what the name of the song was called, what the name was, what the song was called, and (finally) what the song was. In this context the present writer would emphasize that none of the names on the list are his own invention! The problems in terminology reflect our predecessors troubles with observations and concepts. Doubtless our sympathy for those troubles should be quite as vivid as the sympathy expressed in the White Knight's song for the troubles of the aged man!

II. History

Even in defining coccidioidomycosis we become involved in history, and we shall be further involved in discussing biology, distribution, diagnosis, and pathology of the infection. Yet at the risk of a little repetition it seems well to sketch here the development of knowledge of coccidioidomycosis since its first recognition in Argentina, reported in 1892 by Posadas and Wernicke (1892). Additional dates to be remembered include the first California case reports by Rixford and by Thorne in 1894, the naming of the organism by Rixford and Gilchrist in 1896, the demonstration that it was a fungus in the 1900 report of Ophuls and Moffitt, the first report of its isolation from the soil by Stewart and Myer in 1932, and the study of acute benign coccidioidal pneumonia with erythema nodosum between 1936 and 1939 by Dickson and Gifford. One should also take note of the recognition of coccidioidomycosis as an important problem in military medicine at United States Armed Forces installations in world war II. Among the relevant studies are those of Allen (1948), Bass (1945, 1947), Bass et al. (1948, 1949), Cheney and Denenholz (1945), Cherry and Bartlett (1946), Conant (1948), Forbus and Bestebreurtje (1946), Goldstein and Louie (1943), Helper and Watts (1945), Lee et al. (1942), Lee (1944), McLaughlin (1948), Norman and Lawler (1949), Pfanner (1946), Ruhrman (1955), Smith (1943, 1955a, 1958) and Whims (1947). The therapeutic usefulness of amphotericin B was first recorded in 1957 by Fiese and Littman, and Littman et al. in 1958. Subsequent studies have confirmed that usefulness (Einstein, 1967, and personal communication; Einstein et al., 1961; Hunter and Mongan, 1958; Winn, 1959, 1963, 1964, 1967a, b, c). At the same time the dangers from the nephrotoxicity of the drug have become increasingly evident (Beard et al., 1960; Huntington et al., 1967a; Iovine et al., 1963; Reynolds et al., 1963; Sanford et al., 1962; Takacs et al., 1963).

The standard and classic account of the history of coccidioidomycosis is that of Fiese in 1958. Further fascinating bits of lore may be found in Smith (1967) and Emmons (1967). Interesting sideligths on the Argentine pioneers are given by Negroni also in 1967.

Although coccidioidomycosis was first recognized in Argentina (Posadas, 1892; Wernicke, 1892), and endemic foci have been demonstrated in Central America (Mayorga, 1967), in Mexico (Gonzalez-Ochoa, 1948, 1955, 1967) and Venezuela (Campins, 1950, 1961, 1967; Campins et al., 1949), the history of the infection has been largely recorded in the United States. It is convenient to look first at the development of knowledge of clinical and pathologic aspects of the infection, and then at studies of the character and ecology of the organism.

a) Clinical and Pathologic Studies

In Posadas' and Wernicke's case (1892) and in Rixford's first case (1894), the most striking manifestation was a generalized verrucoid skin lesion. A comparable

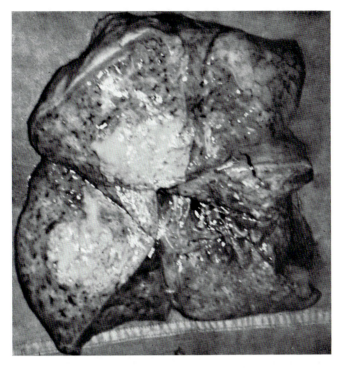

Fig. 3. Pulmonary coccidioidomycosis. There is softening and beginning excavation in a large creamy region of the right upper lobe, and thickening of the right upper lobe pleura. Wet mount from this area of softening showed numerous sporangia (see Fig. 22). Case 9

lesion in a recent case is shown in Figures 1 and 2. In Thorne's case (1894), which was Rixford's second case (RIXFORD and GILCHRIST, 1896) the skin lesions were more nondescript and suppurative. However initial interest centered on skin lesions to such an extent that MONTGOMERY (MONTGOMERY et al., 1903; MONTGOMERY and MORROW, 1904) and WOLBACH (1904) called the infection dermatitis coccidioides. It remained for OPHULS (1905a) to show that the lung was probably the usual portal of entry and that skin lesions were often absent, and usually clearly secondary when present (Fig. 3).

Early studies dealt solely with cases in which there was spread of the infection beyond the lungs (metapulmonary dissemination); it was to this group that the term coccidioidal granuloma was applied (OPHULS, 1905a; BECK, 1931a, b; BROWN, 1906, 1907; COOKE, 1914, 1915; DICKSON, 1915, 1929, 1931; GREAVES, 1934; INGHAM, 1936; RIXFORD, 1931; RYFKOGEL, 1913). All recent students have found it important to distinguish such cases from those in which the infection is confined to the lungs (BEARE, 1945; CHERRY and BARTLETT, 1946; DICKSON, 1937, 1938, 1939; COTTON et al., 1950, 1955, 1959; COX and SMITH, 1939; BUTT and HOFFMAN, 1941, 1945; FABER, SMITH and DICKSON, 1939; FARNESS and MILLS, 1938, 1939; FORSEE and PERKINS, 1954; GIFFORD, 1936, 1939; GIFFORD et al., 1937; GOLDSTEIN and LOUIE, 1943; GOLDSTEIN and McDONALD 1944; GREER et al., 1949a; GREER and CROW, 1949b; HUNTINGTON, 1959a, b; HUNTINGTON et al., 1967b; KRAPIN and LOVELOCK, 1948; MARKS et al., 1967; MELICK, 1949, 1950, 1957; NABARRO, 1948; SCHULZE, 1942; SMITH, 1939 through 1961; WINN, 1941 through 1967).

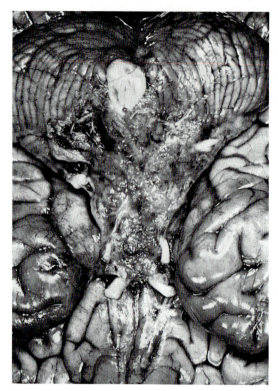

Fig. 4. Coccidioidal meningitis. The abundant inflammatory exudate overlying the brain stem and pons obscures the arteries of the circle of WILLIS

Metapulmonary dissemination may present as widespread miliary involvement of viscera (OPHULS, 1905a; BROWN, 1906, 1907, 1914; DICKSON, 1915, 1929; FORBUS and BESTEBREURTJE, 1946), or as large or small lesions, sometimes single. An early study of coccidioidal bone lesions was that of GARDNER in 1904. More recent studies include those of McMASTER and GILFIAN (1939), BENNINGHOVEN and MILLER (1942), SASHIN (1946, 1947), PILOT (1946), LAMPHIER (1948), MILLER and BIRSNER (1949), BIRSNER and SMART (1956), HIPPS (1953), SCHWARTZMANN (1957), IGER and LARSON (1967). Involvement of synovial tissue was described in 1954 by THIEMEYER and by WALKER and HALL. Lesions in the genital tract have been recorded by McDOUGAL and KLEINMAN (1943), by PAGE and BOYERS (1945), WORMLEY et al. and WEYRAUCH et al. (1950), by ROHN et al. (1951) and by AMROMIN and BLUMENFELD (1953), myocardial lesions by REINGOLD (1950), caseation of the adrenals by MALONEY (1952), and endolaryngeal involvement by SING et al. (1956).

Meningitis, often solitary, i.e. without other metapulmonary lesions, has interested a number of students. Important early studies are those of OPHULS in 1905, of BROWN in 1906 and 1907, of EVANS in 1909, and of RYFKOGEL in 1910. Among more recent studies may be mentioned those of ABBOTT and CUTLER in 1936, of COURVILLE in 1936 and 1938, of CRAIG and DOCKERTY in 1941, of REEVES and BASINGER in 1945, of DANCIS and NUNEMAKER in 1946, of WHIMS in 1947, of Müller and SCHALTENBRAND and FRANK in 1948, of LOWBEER in 1949, of BUSS, GIBSON and GIFFORD in 1950, of JENKINS and POSTLETHWAITE, and ROSEN and BELBER in 1951, and the review of FETTER, KLINTWORTH and HENDRY in 1967. In an autopsy series of 142 cases of fatal coccidioidomycosis (HUNTINGTON et al., 1967b) meningitis was found in 82 (Fig. 4). In 36 the meningitis was the only meta-

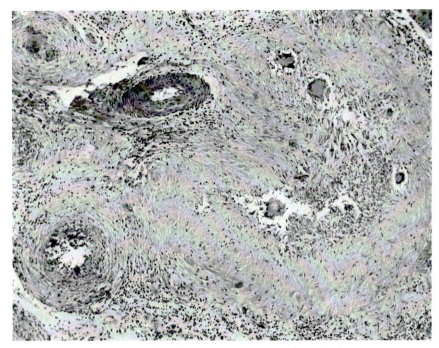

Fig. 5. Coccidioidal meningitis with granulomatous arteritis. Case 3. H & E, × 70

pulmonary lesion demonstrated, while in 46 other metapulmonary lesions were found. In all 82 the meningitis was considered to be the cause of death.

Coccidioidal meningitis may be exceedingly chronic (ROSEN and BELBER, 1951; HUNTINGTON et al., 1967b). It has not been found to resolve spontaneously. It is the most frequent generally accepted indication for amphotericin therapy in coccidioidomycosis (EINSTEIN, 1961; EINSTEIN et al., 1967; WINN, 1964, 1967b). Prolonged treatment is necessary, and the incidence of amphotericin nephropathy has been high (BEARD et al., 1960; IOVINE et al., 1963; SANFORD et al., 1962; REYNOLDS et al., 1963; WERTLAKE et al., 1965; WINN, 1967b; HUNTINGTON et al., 1967a, 1968b; TAKACS et al., 1963). Since diffusion of amphotericin from blood to meninges is poor, and block and hydrocephalus are frequent, neurosurgical collaboration has been called for in the treatment of coccidioidal meningitis (ZEALER and WINN, 1967; CHEU and WALDMAN, 1967b; LOCKS and HAWKINS, 1963; WITORSCH et al., 1965; see Figs. 4, 5, 6, 7, 8).

Although Ophul's study published in 1905 had shown that in disseminated coccidioidomycosis (coccidioidal granuloma) the lung was probably the usual portal of entry, coccidioidal infection confined to the lung, i.e., without metapulmonary dissemination was almost unrecognized until the episode known to coccidioidomycologists as the great Dickson-Gifford breakthrough in the years 1936 to 1939 (FIESE, 1958).

In 1915 DICKSON had reported the incidental autopsy finding of an apparently arrested "coccidiodoma" in the lung of a subject dying of unrelated causes. In 1929 CHOPE, working in Dickson's laboratory accidentally inhaled organisms from a culture of *C. immitis*. When he became ill, coccidioidal spherules were found in his sputum. To the amazement of his physicians he developed nothin more serious

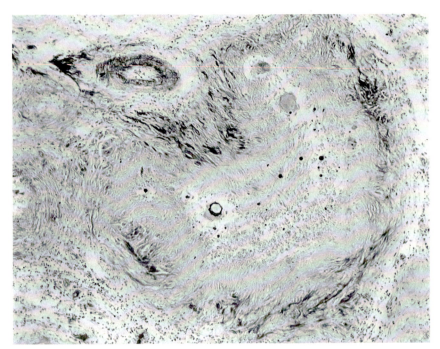

Fig. 6. Coccidioidal meningitis with granulomatous arteritis. From same area as Fig. 5. Grocott-Gomori, × 70

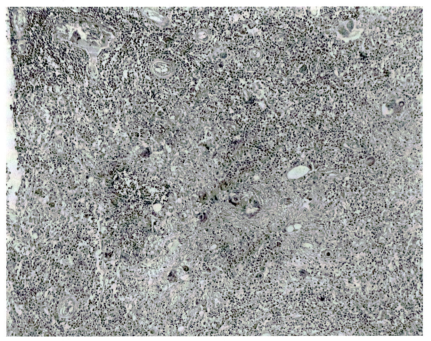

Fig. 7. Coccidioidal meningitis. The reaction is purulent, giant-cell and fibrosing, with some "round cells," i.e., macrophages and lymphocytes. Case 5. H & E, × 70

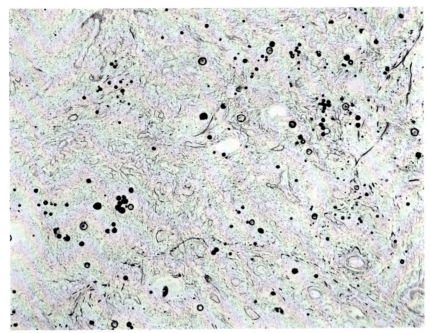

Fig. 8. Coccidioidal meningitis. The area shown in Fig. 7 displays numerous sporangia of various sizes. Case 5. Grocott-Gomori, × 70

than a brisk pneumonia with erythema nodosum and made a rapid recovery (FIESE, 1958; SMITH, 1967).

From these observations ERNEST DICKSON, the august Professor of Public Health at Stanford suspected that it would be well to search for coccidioidal pneumonia without metapulmonary dissemination. He therefore went to Kern County to ask physicians to send him sputum specimens from patients with pneumonia. At his meeting with the County Health Department Staff, Myrnie GIFFORD, assistant health officer, told him of her observations on the "valley fever" syndrome (pneumonia with erythema nodosum or multiforme) and her evidence of its coccidioidal etiology. GIFFORD's first report published in 1936, had chronological priority, but as SMITH (1967) says, "it was immured in the Annual Reports of the Kern County Health Department," while Dickson's paper (1937a) presented at the annual meeting of the California Medical Association was a "clarion call for action." The Dickson-Gifford breakthrough culminated in their superb joint paper (DICKSON and GIFFORD, 1938).

The erythema of "valley fever" unlike the verrucous, granulomatous, or suppurative skin lesions of disseminated coccidioidomycosis, does not represent invasion of the skin by organisms. In fact, in this syndrome the organisms are confined to the lung, and the erythema is a cutaneous reaction to soluble products. Indeed it may be thought of as a giant coccidioidin reaction. Most of the subjects with coccidioidal erythema nodosum or multiforme are very reactive to coccidioidin, and KESSEL's (1939) preparation of coccidioidin played an important part in the studies of DICKSON and GIFFORD (1938).

Just as disseminated coccidioidomycosis had first been recognized in patients with disseminated skin lesions, so localized pulmonary coccidioidomycosis was first recognized in patients with allergic erythema nodosum or multiforme. Just as

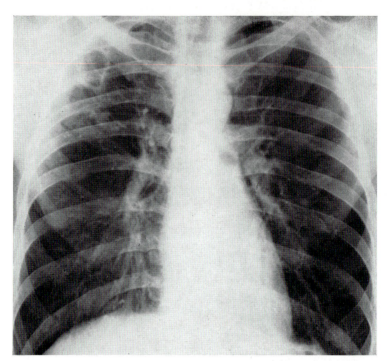

Fig. 9. X-ray showing a thin-walled coccidioidal cavity. (Courtesy of the late Dr. WINN)

it took some time to demonstrate that the majority of patients with disseminated coccidioidomycosis do not have skin lesions (HUNTINGTON et al., 1959b, 1967b), so it took some time to demonstrate that the majority of patients with primary coccidioidal pneumonias do not develop allergic erythemas (SMITH, 1942, 1947; SALKIN, 1967; WINN, 1967).

Yet the recognition of the coccidioidal etiology of the "valley fever" syndrome was a dramatic and significant event, and the two major personages were fully worthy of the drama. The present writer did not have the privilege of acquaintance with DICKSON, but this awesome stature is fully apparent both in his own writings and in those of his successor SMITH (see Ref.). I was fortunate to have begun my studies in Kern County before Gifford's retirement, and it is pleasant privilege and obligation to record her directness, her total devotion to her task, her vivid concern with the unfortunate and downtrodden, the meticulous accuracy of her observations, the rigorous logic of her deductions, her granitic sincerity, and her selflessness with its total lack of either false pride or false modesty.

Studies of coccidioidal infection subsequent to those of GIFFORD and DICKSON have further emphasized its range and diversity. Many infections are asymptomatic, recognizable only by a conversion of skin test (BEADENKOPF et al., 1949; BEAMER, 1955; EDWARDS and PALMER, 1957; JOHNSON et al., 1964; PAPPAGIANIS, 1967; AJELLO, 1967; SMITH et al., 1961; WINN, 1967) and perhaps by stationary calcified pulmonary nodules (ARONSON et al., 1942; BUTT and HOFFMAN, 1941, 1945; COX and SMITH, 1939; STRAUB and SCHWARTZ, 1956). On the other hand overwhelming infection with fungemia (WINN et al., 1967) may cause death with a rapidity undreamed of by the pioneer students who regarded "coccidioidal granuloma" as indolent even though ultimately lethal.

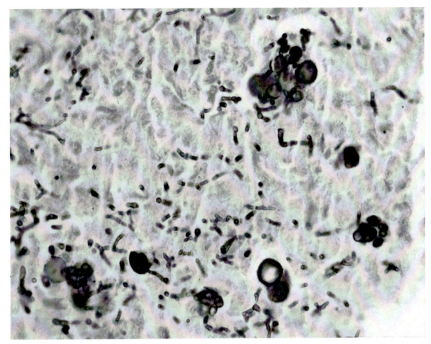

Fig. 10. Hyphae and spherules of *C. immitis* is tissue adjacent to a pulmonary cavity. From case E 1 of Huntington et al. (1967b), Grocott-Gomori, × 500

The coccidioidal pneumonitis with erythema ("Valley Fever"), first recognized by Gifford (1936, 1937, 1939a, b) and Dickson (1937a, b, 1938, 1939a, b), and further studied by Smith (1939, 1940) seemed so thoroughly benign in contrast with the treacherous classic "coccidioidal granuloma" that there was at first an excessive tendency to minimize the seriousness of coccidioidal infection of the lung. Indeed it had been suggested to me by Dr. Smith in a personal communication that coccidioidal infection was never grave unless it extended beyond the lung, that lesions in the lung were invariably self limited, that the lung had a unique ability to handle the fungus while other tissues had none. If this interpretation were correct, it would be difficult to understand both why the lung is actually the usual portal of entry, and why some of the cases of primary extrapulmonary infection (Hagele et al., 1967; Wilson et al., 1953; Levan and Huntington, 1965) have run a benign course, and it would be difficult to interpret the ease with which the mouse may be inoculated either intranasally or intraperitoneally (Tager and Liebow, 1942).

The notion that coccidioidal lung lesions were invariably mild and evanescent was soon disproved by Farness' studies, reported in 1939 and 1940, on coccidioidal pulmonary cavitation (Figs. 9—13). Farness' observations, and those of Winn in 1941 and 1942, of Smith, Beard, and Saito in 1948, of Belanger in 1947, of Bass in the same year, of Waring in 1954, and others, leave no doubt that in endemic areas many pulmonary cavities are coccidioidal. Much of the debate as to the relative gravity of coccidioidal and tuberculous cavitation has been rendered obsolete by the availability of powerful and safe chemotherapy for tuberculosis. There has been spirited argument on surgical versus non-surgical management of coccidioidal cavities. Surgical studies include those of Cotton and

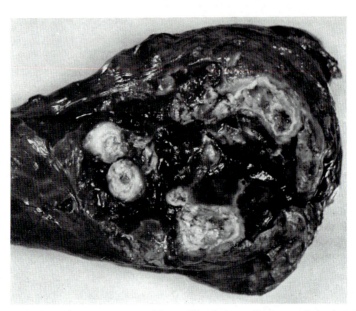

Fig. 11. Coccidioidal pulmonary cavity with satellite lesions. Courtesy of the late Dr. Winn
and University of Arizona Press (Winn, 1967a)

Birsner (1950, 1955, 1959), Findley and Melick (1967), Forsee and Perkins
(1954), Greer (1949a, b), Hughes et al. (1954), Hyde (1955, 1958), Krapin and
Lovelock (1948), Marks et al. (1967), Melick (1950, 1957), Paulsen (1967) and
Weisel and Owen (1949). It is of interest that Winn found it appropriate to
modify within 10 years his original strong antisurgical inclination (Winn, 1942).
The antisurgical argument is based on the undeniable hazard of surgery, and the
undeniable occurrence of spontaneous healing in a few instances of coccidioidal
cavitation. Nevertheless, among the writer's colleagues, both internists and chest
surgeons, there is increasing consensus for resection.

An interesting feature of coccidioidal cavities is the presence in a good many
of them of *C. immitis* in the mycelial phase (Fig. 10) (Fiese et al., 1955; Puckett,
1954; Huntington, 1959a, b, 1967b).

Cavities are by no means the only serious coccidioidal lung lesions. The relationship of coccidioidomycosis to bronchiectasis is sometimes indubitable, and progressive caseating non-cavitary coccidioidomas are sometimes encountered
(O'Leary and Curry, 1956; Helper and Watts, 1945; Alzenauer et al., 1955;
Owens et al., 1960; Salkin, 1967; Huntington, 1959; Huntington et al., 1967b).
Moreover, massive acute coccidioidal pneumonia (Huntington et al., 1967b) can
be fatal with or without metapulmonary dissemination.

Although some students (Baker, 1946; Forbus and Bestebreurtje, 1946;
Winn, 1967) have tended to deprecate comparison of coccidioidomycosis and
tuberculosis, others (Bass, 1945; Dickson, 1929; Yegian and Kegel, 1940;
Moore, 1945; Smith, 1942; Salkin, 1967; Huntington et al., 1959b; Huntington, 1967b) have found it appropriate and inevitable, particularly if the classic
observations on human infection with the bovine tubercle bacillus (Middlebrook,
1965; Rich, 1951) are kept in mind. In coccidioidal regions the consecutive or
simultaneous occurrence of coccidioidomycosis and tuberculosis in the same patient
is not at all rare (Cotton et al., 1954; Kahn, 1950; Rifkin et al., 1947; Stein,

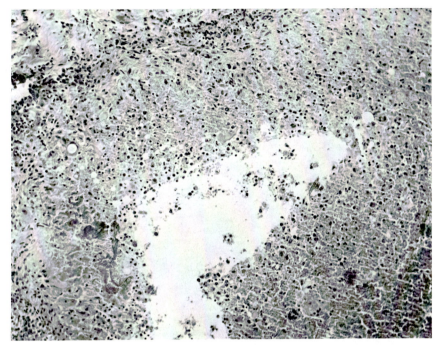

Fig. 12. Minute pulmonary cavity in coccidioidomycosis. The wall is composed of old pus which looks like caseation necrosis. Further out are a few giant cells, granulation tissue and fibrous scar. Case 5. H & E, × 125

1953; STUDY and MORGENSTERN, 1948; HUNTINGTON, 1959b; HUNTINGTON et al., 1967b).

In the cases which first called medical attention to the existence of coccidioidomycosis, the clinical phenomena, especially those in the skin were novel and striking (POSADAS, 1892; WERNICKE, 1892; RIXFORD and GILCHRIST, 1896). Similar cases today would probably offer a minimum of diagnostic difficulty, even though they are actually very unusual compared with those with coccidioidal manifestations of a more prosaic character. Mere clinical inspection of a patient with the Posadas-Wernicke-Rixford type of disease would minimize alternative diagnostic possibilities, and laboratory confirmation of the diagnosis of coccidioidomycosis would be easy, and perhaps hardly needed. Early advances in knowledge of the clinical and pathologic manifestations of the disease indicated that in endemic areas extensive destructive lesions of bone, raised a presumption of coccidioidal etiology (FIESE, 1958). Likewise the observations of DICKSON (1937a, b, 1938, 1939a, b) and GIFFORD (1936, 1937, 1939a, b) revealed that in endemic areas the syndrome of erythema nodosum or multiforme could be presumed to be coccidioidal. Of course no such presumption could apply to individuals without opportunity for exposure to Coccidioides.

Unfortunately in some areas (NEGRONI, 1967), it would seem that the possibility of coccidioidomycosis has seldom been considered in the absence of such striking clinical phenomena. It would, of course, be unfortunate if the diagnosis of coccidioidomycosis were missed in the presence of such distinctive indications. However, in areas where coccidioidomycosis has been extensively studied, only in a small minority of cases has the disease been found to proclaim itself clinically in so blatant a fashion. Much more common and diagnostically much more troublesome, for example, are cases of pulmonary cavitation distinguishable from tuberculous

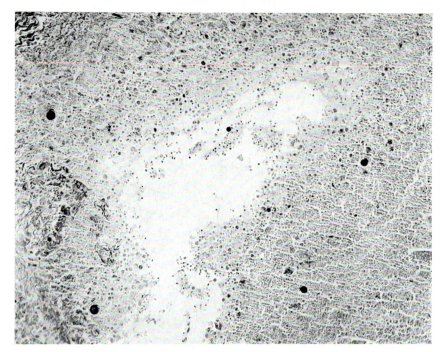

Fig. 13. Minute pulmonary cavity in coccidioidomycosis. In the purulent and necrotic portion of the wall numerous spherules, varying in size, are seen. Same area as Fig. 12. Grocott-Gomori, × 125

cavitation only by successful recovery of coccidioides on culture and failure to demonstrate tubercle bacilli, and cases of low-grade granulomatous meningitis the coccidioidal etiology of which has to be demonstrated by positive spinal fluid complement fixation and perhaps eventually by growth of fungus on spinal fluid culture (Huntington, 1959b).

It has become increasingly clear that coccidioidomycosis is a great "imitator disease" and that its recognition and differential diagnosis require constant clinical alertness and intelligent application of appropriate laboratory tests. The values and limitations of the various laboratory aids will be discussed in the section on diagnosis. We may note here that the coccidioidin skin test most valuable in epidemiologic study (Absher and Cline, 1949; Ajello, 1967a; Aronson et al., 1942; Beadenkopf et al., 1949; Butt and Hoffman, 1941, 1945; Gonzalez-Ochoa, 1948, 1955, 1967; Kessell et al., 1950; Klotz and Biddle, 1967; Loosli et al., 1951; Pappagianis, 1967; Smith et al., 1948b, 1949, 1955), and of great historic usefulness in the demonstration of the coccidioidal etiology of "valley fever" (Smith, 1967), is of limited usefulness in other clinical situations. Serologic study, first suggested by Cooke in 1949 and further purpused by Conant in 1948 and Hazen and Tahler in 1948 has been triumphantly developed by Smith and his colleagues from 1948 through 1967 into something of great value both diagnostically and prognostically.

Chronic pulmonary cavitation and chronic "solitary" granulomatous meningitis have become well recognized in the San Joaquin Valley as manifestations of coccidioidal infection (Figs. 4, 9, 10). In such cases, as well as in the more "classic" cases with skin lesions, bone lesions, and deep abscesses, the diagnosis has been made quite regularly. However in a recent study of fatal autopsied cases from the San

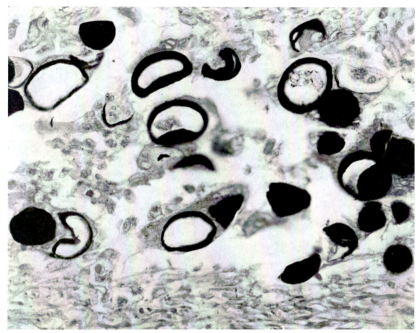

Fig. 14. Spherules without evidence of endosporulation. From the meninges of Case 2, showing fibrous meningitis. Grocott-Gomori, × 500

Joaquin Valley (HUNTINGTON et al., 1967b) it was found that the diagnosis had been missed in many of the cases which did not fall into any of these categories. Evidently even in this hyperendemic area clinicians need to be more flexible in their thinking about coccidioidomycosis. Diagnostic failures were particularly frequent in cases with "fungemia" (WINN et al., 1967), and in those with massive non-cavitary pulmonary lesions.

Something has already been said about the treatment of coccidioidomycosis, and further mention will be made of this topic in subsequent sections. We may note here that a good deal of attention has been given to the possibility of prophylactic immunization (FRIEDMAN and SMITH, 1956, 1957; KONG and LEVINE, 1967; LEVINE and SMITH, 1967; LOWE et al., 1967; PAPPAGIANIS et al., 1967; VOGEL et al., 1954).

b) Character and Ecology of the Organism

As we mentioned earlier, both POSADAS and WERNICKE in their 1892 reports from Argentina, and RIXFORD and GILCHRIST in their study from California which appeared in 1896, regarded the organism as a protozoan. Fortunately their descriptions and illustrations of the organism both in the original human tissues and in inoculated animals were sufficiently vivid, detailed, and meticulous as to leave no doubt whatever that it was the same organism which OPHULS in 1900 and 1905 proved to be a fungus. Unfortunately some later students have been much less aware of the great variability of coccidioides *in vivo*! (Figs. 10, 12—22). In the "preliminary report" of OPHULS and MOFFITT, which appeared in 1900, the authors tell of their dismay at the repeated growth of a "mold" on culture of their lesions and their amazement when the "mold" reverted to the spherular phase on animal inoculation. MONTGOMERY (1900) relates with disarming candor how he, too, kept

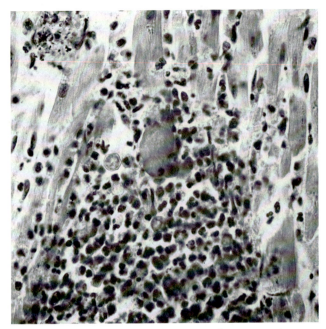

Fig. 15. Coccidioidomycosis of myocardium. A minute abscess contains two clearly visible sporangia. From Case F 30 of Huntington et al. (1967b). H & E, × 660

growing a "mold" but, lacking Ophuls serendipity, threw it out. One wonders with Emmons (1967) how many other students prior to Ophuls grew the mycelial phase and then discarded it.

Ophuls established, once and for all, the extraordinary, perhaps unique biphasic morphology of the organism then and since designated *Coccidioides immitis*. While with especial attention to surface tension and other factors it is possible to maintain spherules *in vitro* (Converse, 1956, 1957, 1959; Lubarsky and Plunkett, 1955b; Breslau and Kubota, 1964), and mycelia are occasionally encountered in infected tissue (Fiese et al., 1955; Puckett, 1954; Huntington et al., 1957, 1959b, 1967b; Levan and Huntington, 1965 — Fig. 10) the consistency of the spherular phase *in vivo* and of the mycelial phase *in vitro*, and the contrast between the two are really very striking (Figs. 15, 23—25). The two phases have been found to differ in their rate of metabolism and reproduction (Pappagianis et al., 1956) and in their antigenic pattern (Landay et al., 1967). Indeed it seems quite clear that the morphologic paradox of coccidioides reflects a biological paradox.

Early studies of "coccidioidal granuloma" failed to reveal evidence of person to person transmission. The question of possible contagiousness has repeatedly been raised (Ajello, 1967a; Kruse et al., 1967; Rosenthal, 1947; Smith, 1958, 1967; Smith et al., 1961; Louria et al., 1957; Bass et al., 1949). However, while coccidioidomycosis is readily transmitted from human to animal or animal to animal with a needle and syringe, direct transmission under more "natural" circumstances appears most unusual. In fact, the writer is aware of only three recorded persuasive instances.

The first, reported by Wilson et al. (1953) is that of an embalmer who jabbed himself with a needle while preparing the body of a victim of disseminated coccidioidomycosis. The second is that of the baby monkey studied by Castleberry et al. (1963); the mother monkey would hold her draining arm lesion against the baby's nose. The third is that of the premature infant

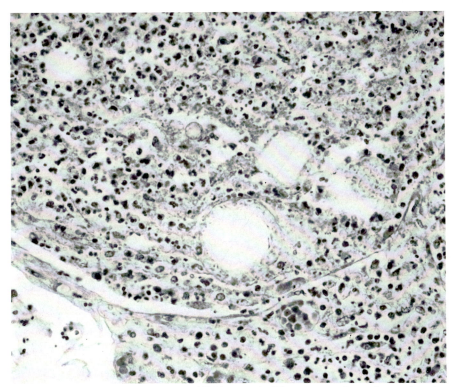

Fig. 16. Suppurative pneumonia in coccidioidomycosis. There are portions of several mature sporangia containing endospores. Note the alveolar wall traversing the lower part of the photograph. From Case D 2 of Huntington et al. (1967b). H & E, × 400

reported by Larwood (1962). Since this infant was taken to the premature nursery right after delivery, fomite transmission, such as was suggested in the case of the infant reported by Christian et al. (1956) seems unlikely. In Larwood's case the mother had a florid coccidioidal endometritis. Unfortunately the placenta had not been examined, but the predominately bronchopulmonary lesions in the infant suggested amniotic-tracheobronchial rather than placental-vascular route of infection. Indirect support for this suggestion is offered by other cases studied by the writer (unpublished observations) in which, though the placenta was massively infected, the foetus escaped infection.

While infection from direct contact with infected humans or animals appears to be most unusual, *infection from contact with cultures* in a laboratory is all too common. Chope's case, mentioned by Smith (1967) is the first of a great many (Nabarro, 1948; Johnson et al., 1964; Kruse, 1962; Symmers, 1967; Smith and Harrell, 1948). The observations by Johnson et al. (1964) were of particular interest since in this large laboratory quite extraordinary precautions were taken to prevent infection of laboratory personnel. Fortunately most of the infections in Johnson's laboratory were asymptomatic, recognized only by conversion of the skin test. However, Smith and Harrell (1948) have reported a laboratory infection with a fatal outcome.

Very early in the California studies the consistent association of coccidioidal infection with the San Joaquin valley was noted by Dickson in 1915. The recovery of the fungus from San Joaquin Valley soil by Stewart and Meyer, reported in 1932, was the result, not of a "shot in the dark," but of a carefully considered and reasonable hypothesis. Subsequent soil isolation studies (Egeberg and Ely, 1956;

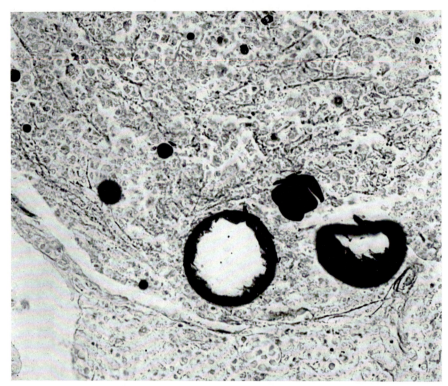

Fig. 17. Suppurative pneumonia of coccidioidomycosis. From the same area as Fig. 16. Note how the special stain sharply demonstrates the various sized spherules. Grocott-Gomori, × 400

Egeberg et al., 1964; Elconim, 1964; Emmons, 1942a; Lubarsky and Plunkett, 1955a; Maddy, 1965; Plunkett and Swatek, 1957; Swatek et al., 1967) have been laborious and at times frustrating, but there have been enough positive results to leave no doubt that coccidioides actually is a soil organism. With the use of fluorescent antibody, Kaplan (1967), in Ajello's laboratory has identified coccidioidal arthrospores in a soil sample. Maddy (1965), simply by adding water, was able to get growth of coccidioidal mycelia in soil samples.

Further evidence of regional endemicity and soil habitat of the fungus has been provided by studies of natural infection in dogs (Ajello et al., 1956; Farness, 1940; Levan and Burger, 1955; Maddy, 1957; Reed, 1956), and in cattle (Giltner, 1918; Prchal, 1948, 1957), and by exposure of dogs and monkeys under "natural" conditions (Converse et al., 1967b; Reed et al., 1967).

Endemic areas have been uniformly characterized by warmth and aridity (Ajello, 1967a). The most thoroughly studied highly endemic areas are the San Joaquin Valley of California and the Salt River Valley of Arizona. However, the endemic area covers much of Southwestern U.S. and adjoining Mexico, and there are endemic areas in Argentina, in Central America and in Venezuela. (Refer to section on Geographical Pathology.)

It has become increasingly clear that infections (other than deliberate experimental infections) are initiated by organisms presumably or certainly in the mycelial phase, either in soil or in laboratory cultures, and very rarely by direct transfer of spherular phase organisms from another host. Further evidence on this point is

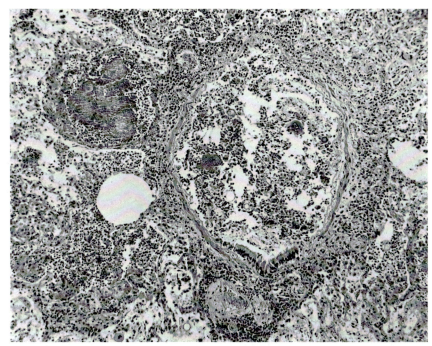

Fig. 18. Coccidioidal bronchiolitis and peribronchiolitis. The bronchopulmonary damage leads to bronchiectasis. Case F 26 of HUNTINGTON et al. (1967b). H & E, × 70

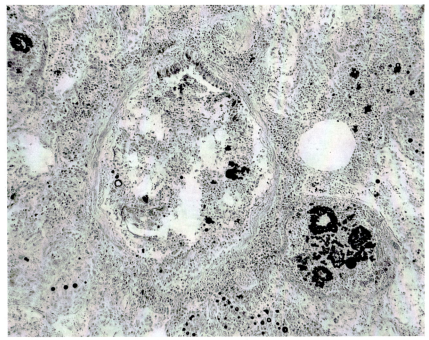

Fig. 19. Bronchopulmonary coccidioidomycosis. Same field as Fig. 18, stained to make the organisms more prominent. Grocott-Gomori, × 70

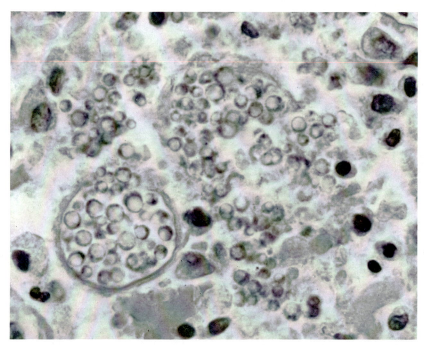

Fig. 20. *C. immitis* in tissue. Two mature sporangia contain endospores. One sporangium has burst through its wall and the endospores are escaping into the tissues. H & E, × 1000

afforded by the interesting experimental studies of Kruse et al. (1967). They infected monkeys by exposure to aerosols containing arthrospores and then caged the experimentally infected monkeys with normal monkeys. If appropriate precautions were taken to eliminate the possibility of secondary arthrospore-containing aerosols from the skins of the original infected monkeys, cross-infections did not occur.

While tissue phase organisms do not die immediately upon extrusion (Louria et al., 1957; Sorensen, 1967) their viability in a simulated natural environment is less than that of mycelial phase organisms. It seems reasonable to assume that if a strain in the spherular phase achieves prolonged survival after ejection from the host, it does so by reconversion to the mycelial phase. In a few instances of ward infection outside endemic areas, there has been substantial evidences of fomite transmission rather than of more direct contagion (Bennett et al., 1954; Eckmann et al., 1964; Albert and Sellers, 1963).

Although the heat and aridity of endemic areas are evidently necessary for maintenance of *C. immitis* in soil, they are not sufficient, for even in areas regarded as hyperendemic the actual distribution of coccidioides is very spotty. This spotty distribution has been known for many years through the frequent occurrence of "point epidemics". An early report of such an epidemic was that of Davis et al. published in 1942. Among similar studies may be mentioned those of Goldstein and Louie (1943), Kritzer et al. (1950), Joffe (1960), Winn et al. (1963) and of Gelman et al. (1965). In recent years soil studies have provided further evidence of the extremely irregular distribution of the fungus.

The fomite — transmitted ward epidemic of Eckmann et al. (1964) suggests the possibility that animal infection might be in part responsible for the irregular

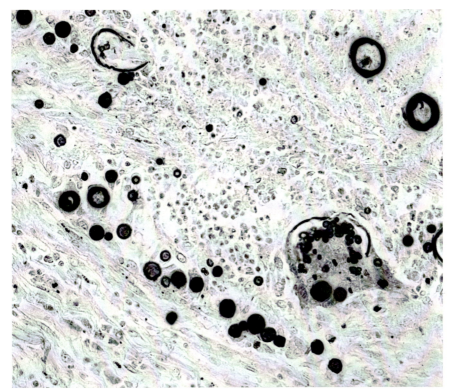

Fig. 21. *C. immitis* in the tissue of a paravertebral abscess. In the lower right corner of the photograph there is a ruptured sporangium with several endospores remaining within. In the upper left corner there is a sporangium with ruptured wall and with three endospores remaining within. The other round dark structures are spherules of various sizes without evidence of endosporulation. Case 6. Grocott-Gomori, × 330

distribution of the fungus in endemic terrain, i.e. that animal infection might have something to do with the maintenance of the fungus in soil. Further support for this suggestion is supplied by the study of MADDY and CRECELIUS (1967) who found that soil areas which previously failed to show coccidioides yielded positive cultures following burial of infected animals and animal tissues. Such a result might perhaps have been anticipated from SORENSEN's observations (1967) on the effect of blood in aiding survival of *C. immitis* in soil. Yet the meticulous and extensive study of SWATEK et al. (1967) yielded no evidence of association between animal activity and the presence of *C. immitis*. Clearly many of the factors which favor the fungus in selected spots are not known. From the studies of the EGEBERG's (1956, 1964) and of ELCONIN, R. and M. EGEBERG (1964) it is obvious that soil salinity and absence of antagonistic organisms are both important. It may be anticipated that further study of the microecology of coccidioides will be laborious but rewarding.

III. Biology

a) The Fungus

SMITH credits K. F. MEYER with the happy phrase characterizing *C. immitis* as a "pathogenic saprophyte." Its biphasic biology is reflected in a biphasic morphology. As a pathogen, it assumes spherular form and characteristically reproduces by endosporulation (Figs. 16, 17, 18, 19, 20, 21, 22). As a saprophyte it grows as aerial septate mycelium with arthrospores (Fig. 23) (Ophuls, 1900, 1905b; Wolbach, 1904; Baker et al., 1943; Kaplan, 1967).

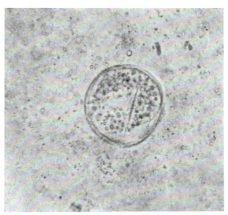

Fig. 22. Mature sporangium of *C. immitis* in a potassium hydroxide wet mount. Case 9. See Fig. 3 for source of this sporangium

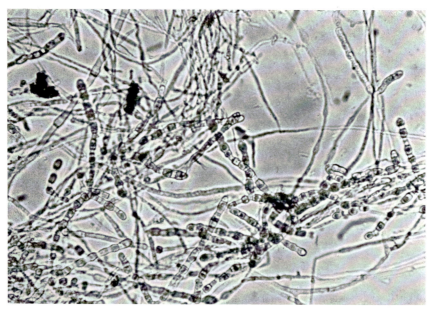

Fig. 23. *C. immitis* from culture, in a wet mount. Note the hyphae, many of which are composed of arthrospores. This photograph illustrates one stage of the life cycle of the fungus

For a saprophyte, coccidioides is extraordinary, perhaps unique, in its pathogenic versatility (Ophuls, 1905; Evans and Ball, 1929; Forbus and Bestebreurtje, 1946; Dickson, 1915—1939; Smith, 1939—1967; Winn, 1967c, d; Winn et al., 1967; Huntington, 1957—1967). As a pathogen, it fails in the important factor of ability to get directly from one host to another (Smith et al.,

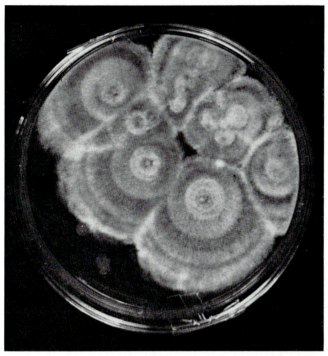

Fig. 24. Culture of *C. immitis*. Courtesy of Dr. Ross Hampson. The photograph is of a culture in a Petri dish. Cultures on slants in test tubes are safer to handle, and preferable

1967). The epidemiology of coccidioidomycosis is rigidly controlled by the ecology of coccidioides as a dry soil saprophyte. Although on culture (Fig. 23) of pus or tissue fragments the active organisms in the spherular phase quickly revert to the mycelial phase (Ophuls, 1900, 1905 b; Ajello, 1957; Conant, 1965; Wilson and Plunkett, 1965; Fetter et al., 1967), and a similar transformation may occur when spherules are extruded into the "natural" environment (Louria et al., 1957; Eckmann et al., 1964; Maddy and Crecelius, 1967), in many, and perhaps in the great majority of instances it would seem that invasion of human or animal tissues represents a "dead end" for the clone of coccidioides in question (Huntington, 1959 b; Swatek et al., 1967). Thus with old stable coccidioidal pulmonary lesions the organism can seldom be recovered on culture, and the actual distribution of coccidioides in desert soil appears unrelated to animal activity.

It might be concluded, therefore, that coccidioides is primarily a soil saprophyte. Yet it can hardly be considered a major biological success in this capacity. It is sharply restricted to hot arid regions, and to specific localities in these regions. The only form which has been directly demonstrated in soil is the resting arthrospore (Kaplan, 1967). The survival of coccidioides in soil appears to require high salinity and absence of competing organisms (Egeberg, 1956, 1964; Elconin et al., 1964).

The more one contemplates this strange organism with its borderline existence and its fantastic dimorphism, the more difficult it becomes to refrain from speculation on its current evolutionary (or devolutionary) status. If parasitic and pathogenic organisms are ultimately derived from free-living forms (and it is difficult to suggest alternative hypothesis), may they not have passed through intermediate

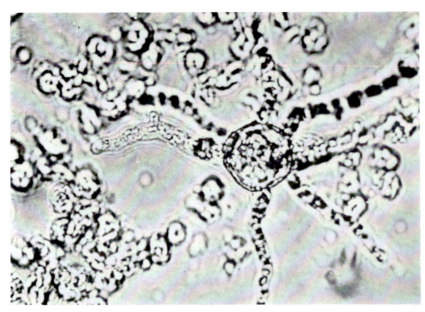

Fig. 25. Spherule of *C. immitis* maintained in pus in saline under a cover slip. Note the sprouting mycelium

stages analogous to that in which the unfortunate coccidioides now finds itself? Is it possible that coccidioides faces the alternative either of extinction or of further evolution towards parasitism? One must grant that such speculations are unsupported, and perhaps risky and even reprehensible; nevertheless it is difficult to suppress them.

While hyphae share with arthrospores the ability to transform into spherules in host tissue (Biddle, personal communication), old cultures with arthrospores are undoubtedly more risky to handle than young cultures without them, and it seems probable that the vast majority of infections result from inhalation of arthrospores (Fig. 23). As previously mentioned, the arthrospore is the only form which has yet been directly demonstrated in soil. This demonstration was the work of Kaplan, who used fluorescent antibodies (Kaplan, 1967).

b) The Infection

Thus there is a vast difference between the epidemiology of coccidioidomycosis and that of tuberculosis (Ajello, 1967). Yet in clinical and pathologic features, and in pathogenesis there are striking parallels between the two infections (Dickson, 1929; Forbus and Bestebreurtje, 1946; Bass, 1945; Smith, 1942; Winn, 1967; Huntington, 1957—1959b; Huntington et al., 1967b; Zimmerman, 1954a, b). In both the usual route of infection is respiratory (Ophuls, 1905a; Fiese, 1958). Asymptomatic infections are frequent (Winn, 1967a, d; Johnson et al., 1964). Clinically recognizable lung infection may be acute and transient (Winn and Johnson, 1942; Dickson, 1939; Dickson and Gifford, 1939; Gifford, 1939; Beare, 1945; Goldstein, 1943, 1944; Schulze, 1942) or it may be acutely fatal (Huntington, unpublished observations; Huntington et al., 1967b). The pneumonic process may disappear entirely, or may leave caseocalcific "coin lesions" (Alznauer et al., 1948; Aronson et al., 1942; Bass et al., 1948; Cox and Smith,

1939; BUTT and HOFFMAN, 1941, 1945; HELPER and WATTS, 1945; HIGGINSON
and HINSHAW, 1955; HUNTINGTON, 1959b; STRAUB and SCHWARZ, 1956, 1962).
On the other hand, cavitation is quite common (FARNESS and MILLS, 1938, 1939;
WINN, 1941—1967d; SMITH et al., 1948; BELANGER, 1947; BASS, 1947; WARING,
1954; COTTON, 1950, 1955, 1959; FINDLEY and MELICK, 1967; FORSEE and PER-
KINS, 1954; GREER et al., 1949a, b; HUGHES et al., 1954; HYDE, 1955, 1958;
KRAPIN and LOVELOCK, 1948; MARKS et al., 1967; MELICK, 1950, 1957; PAULSEN,
1967; WEISEL and OWEN, 1949). The not infrequent occurrence of coccidioidal
hyphae in cavities (FIESE et al., 1955; PUCKETT, 1954; HUNTINGTON, 1957, 1959b;
HUNTINGTON et al., 1967b) raises interesting biological problems. It is probable
that coccidioidal cavities are lesions less grave than tuberculous cavities before the
availability of effective chemotherapy. However, the writer has seen fatal hemorrhage from a coccidioidal cavity and he and his medical and surgical colleagues
share the belief that currently coccidioidal cavities are more difficult to manage
than tuberculous cavities. Less common than cavitation, but not particularly rare,
are large and progressive coccidioidal caseous lesions, and coccidioidal bronchiectasis (O'LEARY and CURRY, 1956; ALZNAUER et al., 1948; HUNTINGTON et al.,
1967b).

Coccidioidal pulmonary lesions may be large or small, indolent or fulminating.
Similarly metapulmonary dissemination may be widespread or restricted, and
metapulmonary lesions range in size from huge to microscopic. Coccidioides differs
from some other fungi which have recently attracted medical attention in being
relatively seldom encountered in patients suffering from debilitation or from obvious immuno-suppression due to other causes (ZIMMERMAN, 1955). Of course such
patients are not immune to coccidioidal infection, though their opportunity for
exposure is perhaps less than that of individuals with a more nearly normal pattern
of activity. However, the usual role of coccidioides is that of a primary pathogen
rather than an opportunistic agonal invader. The factors accounting for the wide
range in severity of coccidioidal infection, from the asymptomatic (WINN, 1967a,
c; JOHNSON et al., 1963) to the rapidly fatal are poorly understood. Although from
general considerations and from experimental data (KONG and LEVINE, 1967), it
would be difficult to disregard the factors of size and even of virulence of the infecting dose, in natural human infections we seldom have any basis for estimation
of either. On the basis of the few cases which have been adequately studied, primary extrapulmonary infection (WILSON et al., 1953; HAGELE et al., 1967; LEVAN
and HUNTINGTON, 1965; WINN, 1965), cannot be said to be definitely more
dangerous than pulmonary infection. Since in general and on the whole a high titre
of complement fixing antibody means massive and aggressive infection, it would
be difficult to conclude that this antibody was a major factor in effective immunity
(SMITH et al., 1950; SMITH et al., 1956; SMITH and SAITO, 1957). It is not clear that
the degree of resistance is correlated with the degree of dermal sensitivity to coccidioidin (LOWE et al., 1967; SALKIN et al., 1967).

A study of a large autopsy series in an endemic area (HUNTINGTON, 1959a) provided definite evidence of differences in racial liability to grave and fatal coccidioidomycosis. Fatal coccidioidomycosis was significantly more common in Negro
and Filipino subjects than in caucasoids and in the largely American Indian group
designated as Mexican. Analogous observations have been made in dogs (MADDY,
1957), a few breeds being peculiarly prone to dissemination.

Grave and mild coccidioidomycosis can occur at any age (TOWNSEND and
McKEY, 1953; HYATT, 1963). The greater frequency of fatal coccidioidomycosis
in males seems attributable to their greater opportunity for exposure (HUNTING-
TON, 1959a, b; HUNTINGTON et al., 1967b). On the other hand, instances of rapidly

fatal disease have been seen in elderly females. In young adult females the coincidence of coccidioidomycosis and pregnancy may be very grave (Mendenhall et al.,
1948; Smale and Birsner, 1949; Vaughn and Ramirez, 1951). In fact Smale
(unpublished observations) has found coccidioidomycosis to be the number one
cause of maternal death in Kern County. Mention has already been made of
Larwood's (1962) case of apparent antenatal transmission to the infant presumably via the amniotic-tracheobronchial route, and of infection of the placenta with
sparing of the fetus in other cases (Huntington et al., 1967b; Huntington, unpublished observations).

One would suspect an endocrine basis for this heightened vulnerability during
pregnancy. Although Einstein (1967) has sometimes found it necessary and
desireable to give steroids along with amphotericin in the treatment of coccidioidomycosis, steroids by themselves do occasionally lead to dissemination of a previously quiescent infection (Lipschultz and Liston, 1964; Farness, 1967).

The series of 142 autopsied fatal cases accumulated over an 18-year-period by
the writer and his colleagues show that in the southern San Joaquin Valley coccidioidomycosis is by no means negligible as a killing disease. The majority of these
deaths (82 in fact) were attributed to meningitis. The meningitis was the only
metapulmonary lesion in 36 of these. Meningitis unfortunately persists when other
lesions, pulmonary and metapulmonary, resolve. Meningitis, never known to have
resolved spontaneously, is sometimes cured, more often checked, by treatment
with amphotericin (Winn, 1967b; Huntington et al., 1967b). "Late" deaths from
coccidioidomycosis are preponderantly meningeal. In 46 of these 142 subjects,
death was attributed primarily to the pulmonary lesion. In 11 of these there was
no evidence of metapulmonary dissemination; while in the remaining 35, though
there was dissemination, the lung lesion was considered the lethal one. While the
decided majority of "late" coccidioidal deaths are meningeal, a good many of the
early deaths are pulmonary. Further details on various modes of fatality will be
given in the section on pathology. It should be emphasized here that of the 131
subjects with dissemination, only 23 showed disseminated skin lesions at the time
of autopsy; in four more there was a history of such lesions.

For many years it was believed that once established, immunity to coccidioidomycosis was much more consistent and reliable than immunity to tuberculosis
(Smith et al., 1948a, 1967, and personal communication) that most of the major
spread and potential damage in coccidioidomycosis occurred early though fatality
might be delayed, and that late spread and clinically significant exogenous reinfection in coccidioidomycosis were most unusual. Some of the chronic disseminators,
who had old abscesses heal and then return, were always a little difficult to fit into
this schematization, and it now appears that the difference between the two
diseases may be less consistent and reliable than we used to believe. Salkin (1967),
while expressing uncertainty about exogenous reinfection, has recorded a number
of instances of late endogenous spread of coccidioidomycosis, and Cheu and Waldmann (1967) have recorded fresh miliary dissemination in patients with chronic
coccidioidal meningitis treated by ventriculo-atriostomy for relief of hydrocephalus.

IV. Geographical Pathology

Despite a great deal of study, much remains to be learned about the actual
distribution of coccidioides in soil and about the factors which control it. While
heat and aridity appear essential to the fungus, too much of either (Maddy, 1957,
1958) had an adverse effect. Endemic areas in Central America (Mayorga, 1967)
have a higher annual rainfall than noted elsewhere, but this is apparently con-

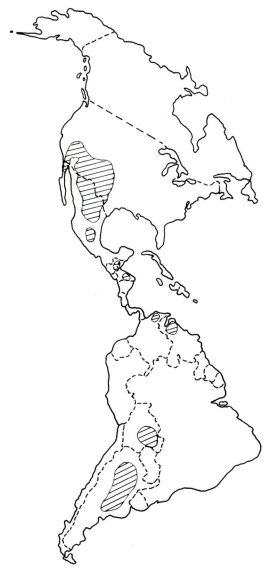

Fig. 26. Map of the Americas showing the endemic areas of coccidioidomycosis

centrated in one season, the remainder of the year being arid. Presently recognized endemic areas are shown on the map. It will be noted that *all* of them are in the Western Hemisphere. For studies in Argentina see NEGRONI (1967); in Venezuela, CAMPINS (1949—1967); in Central America, MAYORGA (1967); in Mexico, GON-ZALEZ-OCHOA (1948, 1955, 1967); in the United States MADDY (1957, 1958) and SCHULZE (1942).

Infections have been recognized by physicians in non-endemic areas. Such infections have resulted from contact with cultures in a laboratory (JOHNSON et al., 1964; NABARRO, 1948; SMITH, 1967; SMITH and HARRELL, 1948), from exposure to material exported from an endemic area (SYMMERS, 1967), and most importantly from travel in endemic areas. Thus many individuals of all levels in the petroleum industry spend some time in the Southern San Joaquin Valley of California; many vacationers of all economic levels winter in the Salt River Valley of Arizona. Hence clinicians and pathologists practising outside of endemic areas have had and will have the opportunity and challenge to recognize coccidioidomycosis. HARRELL and HONEYCUTT (1963) have aptly characterized coccidiodiomycosis as "a travelling fungus disease." It is of interest that in the French case reported by DROUHET (1961) the subject had been in Venezuela and California; in blaming the infection on California DROUHET was apparently unaware of the Venezuelan possibility. FALKINBURG (1952) has recognized a case in New England. Coccidioidomycosis in New York City is reported by REISS et al. (1954), and the case of a German formerly a U.S. prisoner of war by RUHRMANN (1955) (Fig. 26).

Continued search for further endemic areas is doubtless appropriate. Recognition of endemic areas is seldom easy or automatic; intelligence and diligence are required. It may be noted that though the first case to be recognized occurred in Argentina (POSADAS, 1892—1928; WERNICKE, 1892), the second Argentine case to be diagnosed occurred 35 years later (NEGRONI, 1967). In general, recognition of endemic areas has begun with discovery of apparently indigenous infection recognizable clinically or pathologically; this in turn has led to skin test studies of appropriate population samples (NEGRONI, 1967; CAMPINS et al., 1949; CAMPINS 1950, 1961, 1967; MAYORGA, 1967; GONZALEZ-OCHOA, 1948, 1955, 1967). The diagnosis of coccidioidomycosis sometimes can be, and has to be established by demonstration of organisms in tissue sections, after all other opportunities for laboratory confirmation have passed (HUNTINGTON, 1959b). It is therefore desireable that pathologists throughout the world have the oppurtunity to familiarize themselves with the appearance of *Coccidioides* in tissue sections. This will be discussed and illustrated in the concluding sections of this review. Since microphotographs are not an adequate substitute for personal study of sections, the writer will be glad to donate illustrative sections to colleagues who wish them; he will also be happy to review sections which have led colleagues to suspect coccidioidomycosis.

It is encouraging to note that the diligence of SYMMERS (1967) in searching for cases in Great Britain has not led him to suspect the development of endemic foci in that country; all his cases were readily explicable in terms of travel, laboratory contact, or exposure to fomites. At the present time there is no evidence for the development of new endemic areas as a result of travel and commerce. However it might be imprudent categorically to deny such a possibility. Perhaps especial alertness might be appropriate for arid areas, of interest to the petroleum industry.

V. Diagnosis

From extensive opportunity for experience with the disease, the writer has come to realize that coccidioidomycosis is a great imitator and that its recognition and differential diagnosis are often difficult. Among the diagnostic errors which he has had to record as pathologist to the large public and teaching hospital in Kern County, perhaps the world's most hyperendemic coccidioidal area, the two leading categories have been: 1) failure to suspect coccidioidomycosis in cases in which it proved to be the answer and 2) acceptance of coccidioidomycosis as the solution in cases in which the true solution lay elsewhere. It should be added, in all fairness, that in many of these clinical blunders the writer was a full co-blunderer, and indeed that in some of them the correct diagnosis came as a rather shocking surprise upon examination of microscopic sections, having been unsuspected on gross observation at necropsy. In medical school the writer, like most of his generation, was taught that the physician who knew syphilis would know all of medicine. Later it was suggested that tuberculosis was the universal disease, that he who knew it would have to encompass medicine in its entirety. As a result of eighteen years devoted in considerable part to the study of coccidioidomycosis (HUNTINGTON, 1959a, b; HUNTINGTON et al., 1967b) the writer is forced to suspect that any physician who really knew all that was necessary and appropriate to be known about this disease would miss very little of the totality of medical knowledge.

Usually, and in general, the diagnosis of coccidioidomycosis cannot be made simply on the basis of clinical examination or roentgenographic study (CARTER, 1942; POWERS and STARKS, 1941). For that matter, the diagnosis can seldom be made merely from gross morphology or from the microscopic pattern of host response (BAKER, 1946; HUNTINGTON, 1959b). Further evidence pointing specifically to the presence and activity of *Coccidioides* is required. Diagnosis requires alertness in suspecting coccidioidomycosis in a great variety of clinical, roentgenologic, and morphologic patterns, diligence and care in the performance of appropriate laboratory procedures, and judicious evaluation of the results of such procedures. Indirect evidence of the significant presence of the fungus may be provided by tests for dermal sensitivity to coccidioidin (KESSEL, 1939; CHENEY and DENEHOLZ, 1945; SMITH et al., 1948b, 1949; HUNTINGTON, 1959b) and by serologic study (PAPPAGIANIS et al., 1957; SMITH et al., 1950; SMITH et al., 1956; SMITH and SAITO, 1957; SMITH et al., 1957b; SCHUBERT and HAMPSON, 1962). Direct evidence is offered by cultures of the fungus (AJELLO, 1957; BIDDLE, 1953; ALZNAUER et al., 1955; BECK, 1931b; FRIEDMAN et al., 1953; HAMPSON, 1954; HUNTINGTON, 1959b; CONANT, 1965; LEWIS et al., 1956; OPHULS and MOFFITT, 1900; OPHULS, 1905b; SPAUR, 1956; WILSON and PLUNKETT, 1965), or by its morphologic demonstration in wet mount or tissue section (BAKER, 1945, 1966; CONANT, 1965; HUNTINGTON, 1957, 1959b; HUNTINGTON et al., 1967b; JOHNSON, unpublished observations; LEWIS et al., 1956; POSADAS, 1892, 1897, 1898, 1900, 1928; RIXFORD and GILCHRIST, 1896; WERNICKE, 1892; ZIMMERMAN, 1954a, b). The demonstration of *C. immitis* in tissue sections, which may be available and entirely convincing when other opportunities for corroboration of the diagnosis have passed, is of course peculiarly within the province of the pathologic anatomist. This topic is discussed and illustrated in the concluding section of this review. Other procedures, including wet mount, may perhaps be considered outside the realm of pathologic anatomy. Nevertheless it seems well to say something about them here, for the pathologic anatomist who establishes a diagnosis of coccidioidomycosis which his clinical colleagues have missed will probably be expected to give instruction on how the diagnosis might have been made earlier.

a) Skin Tests

Preparation of coccidioidin for *skin testing* has been described by KESSEL (1939), SMITH et al. (1948b), and STEWART and KIMURA (1940). The material, diluted according to directions, is injected intradermally. Although it has been suggested that some reactions which are negative at 48 hours will be significantly positive at 24 hours (SMITH, personal communication), in the absence of suitable 24 hour controls, it seems better to adhere to 48 h readings. The induration and erythema of a positive coccidioidin reaction are similar to those of a positive Mantoux reaction. One of the basic problems in coccidioidin skin-testing is that of cross-reactivity with other fungus antigens (BEADENKOPF et al., 1949; CONANT, 1948; EDWARDS and PALMER, 1957; EMMONS et al., 1945; HUNTINGTON, 1559b; LOURIA, 1967; SCHWARZ and FURCOLOW, 1955; SMITH et al., 1948b, 1949; SMITH, personal communication). Thus it is not practical to use concentrations with which cross-reactivity is frequent and conspicuous. A "conversion" of coccidioidin skin test from negative to positive in association with a clinical episode (if the tests have been performed and read with appropriate care) is, of course, substantial evidence for the coccidioidal etiology of that episode (Salkin et al., 1967). Since dermal coccidioidin reactivity is usually high in coccidioidal erythema nodosum, coccidioidin skin tests were most helpful in the demonstration of the true nature of the "Valley Fever" syndrome (Dickson, 1937a, b; 1938, 1939a, b; Gifford, 1936, 1937, 1939a, b; Faber et al., 1939; Smith, 1940, 1967). On the other hand, skin reactions to appropriate doses of coccidioidin are frequently, indeed usually, negative in the presence of severe and life-threatening dissemination (Huntington, 1959b; Smith, 1967), and are occasionally inexplicable negative with other patterns of coccidioidal infection (Salkin et al., 1967; O'Leary and Curry, 1956). Positive skin tests do not discriminate between infection which is currently active and infection which is old or subclinical (Aronson et al., 1942; Butt and Hofmann, 1941, 1945; Klotz and Biddle, 1967). On the whole, therefore, the skin test has been of greater value in epidemiologic study than in clinical situations. In a situation in which the differential diagnosis lay between coccidioidomycosis and tuberculosis, a positive coccidioidin reaction with a negative second strength Mantoux would have some significance.

b) Serologic Studies

Cross-reactivity among fungi extends to serum antibodies as well as to dermal sensitivity (Landay et al., 1967; Beamer, 1955; Conant, 1965; Hazen and Tahler, 1948; Salvin, 1947, 1949, 1950). Yet this cross-reactivity does not seem to have seriously interfered with the diagnostic usefulness of the precipitin (Smith, 1958, 1955a, 1959b, 1967), complement-fixation (Smith et al., 1956, 1957b, 1961), and immuno-diffusion tests (Hamspon and Larwood, 1967; Schubert and Hampson) in the study of coccidioidomycosis. While cavitary or other localized coccidioidal disease is frequently associated with negative serologic reactions, positive reactions (assuming that technical error can be excluded) have been found to have definite diagnostic significance. A positive precipitin test suggests early infection. A positive complement fixation test suggests active infection. In general, the higher the titre, the greater the activity, and in following patients either untreated or receiving amphotericin, a rise in titre is ominous while a fall is reassuring. Patients with very active disseminated disease commonly have negative coccidioidin skin tests and high coccidioides complement-fixation titres. However, the writer has seen a few cases of very rapidly fatal infection in which the complement-fixation titre remained low (Huntington, unpublished observation).

A low-grade meningitis accompanied by evidence of active coccidioidal infection must be presumed to be coccidioidal. Frequently, though not invariably, this suspicion can be confirmed by the demonstration of complement-fixing antibody in the cerebrospinal fluid. In "solitary" meningitis, i.e., without other metapulmonary foci, antibody is often found in the spinal fluid when the antibody titre in blood serum is low. One cannot deny the possibility that with a very high level of serum antibody, antibody might leak into the spinal fluid in the absence of meningitis. Nevertheless, experience indicates that the presence in the spinal fluid of complement-fixing antibody for coccidioides is extremely ominous; indeed it is practically diagnostic of coccidioidal meningitis (Huntington, 1959b).

Information on the preparation of antigens and the technique of the tests may be found in some of the papers cited. However, it is pertinent to suggest, where local diagnostic facilities are not available, that previous experience with the procedure and centralization of information about results, are alike desireable, that Dr. Ross Hampson of the Kern County Health Department, Bakersfield, Calif., and Miss Margaret Saito of the University of California at Davis, Calif., would be very happy to perform tests which might result in the identification of new "travelling" cases or even of new endemic foci, and that physicians suspecting either possibility might do well to send serum (or spinal fluid) by air mail to either or both of these workers.

c) Wet Mounts

In our experience it has not proved profitable to attempt wet mount studies in material which was not from the center of a lesion. Thus, while wet mounts on sputum are sometimes useful, those from pleural effusions, from urine, or from spinal fluid obtained on lumbar puncture are not. Wet mounts are most apt to be helpful when the material is pus, though they are sometimes worthwhile with material which has to be crumbled. The material is emulsified in 10% KOH, and examined under reduced illumination. In their interpretation one has to learn to disregard fat droplets and other misleading structures. Recently the writer and his microbiologist colleague had the humiliating experience of mistaking an encysted Hartomonella amoeba for a coccidioides spherule in a wet mount! Fortunately that particular problem is unusual. If one is fortunate enough to find a mature or rupturing sporangium with endospores, the diagnosis is unequivocal. Such structures are sometimes readily found. At other times with equally active infection, one may find large numbers of immature spherules while the discovery of mature sporangia is difficult or impossible. Such observations, together with similar observations on tissue sections, make one wonder whether endosporulation is actually the only way in which spherular *C. immitis* can reproduce *in vivo*. Such doubts receive some corroboration from studies in which special techniques have been used to maintain the spherular phase *in vitro* (Breslau and Kubota, 1964; Converse, 1956, 1957, 1959; Lubarsky and Plunkett, 1955b). Evidently it is harder to induce endosporulation then to maintain spherules, and the illustrated chains of culture spherules hardly suggest endosporulation. After a great deal of scowling at spherular *C. immitis* in wet mounts and tissue sections, the writer finds himself loath to dismiss the possibility of reproduction by simple binary fission, and not totally intolerant of other suggested possibilities. The rather mild suggestion by De Lamater and Weed (1946) that *C. immitis* may occasionally bud in tissue has evoked vigorous rebuttal (Ajello). One wonders whether that almost impassioned vigor may be based in part on a fear of blurring the hard-won distinction between *Coccidioides* and the agents of North and South American blastomycoses (Conant, 1965; Fetter et al., 1967; De Almeida, 1930a, 1932). Admittedly there are a number of possible mechanisms for producing something which looks as though it might be a budding pair but actually is not. However, it is important to recognize (and here the writer's experience forces him to be dogmatic) that the appearance of occasional pairs which look as though they might possibly have budded does not prove, or indeed seriously suggest that the fungus in question is not *Coccidioides* (Creitz, 1956).

Technique of Wet Mount (Johnson, unpublished observations)

For a wet mount of pus or tissue, select a specimen of pus, or scrape an abscess wall. Transfer the pus or tissue to saline or 10% KOH on a slide. Make a uniform emulsion. Cover with a cover slip. Scan for spherules (Fig. 22) with a magnification of × 100. Confirm details under high power (× 430).

To prepare a wet mount of a culture, flame a dissecting needle; dip it into plasma; pick up the aerial mycelium on the wet needle, and transfer the fungus to several drops of saline, water, or phenol-cotton-blue on a slide. Cover with cover slip. Scan under low power (as above), and confirm details under high power (Fig. 22).

d) Cultures

The possible risks of handling cultures (AJELLO, 1957; SMITH and HARRELL, 1948; SMITH, 1967; NABARRO, 1948; SYMMERS, 1967; JOHNSON et al., 1964), which have already been emphasized, have led some workers to try to minimize reliance on this diagnostic modality, i.e., not to make cultures. However, in the writer's clinical and pathological laboratory in the center of a hyperendemic area, culturing has been restricted to a few technologists whose dexterity and caution could be trusted, and it is gratifying to record that their skin tests have remained negative. Of course in an area in which "natural" exposure to dust-borne organisms is very likely the additional risk of exposure to laboratory cultures is less than it would be in a non-endemic area. The practice commended by WEED and DAHLIN (1956) of doing microbiologic study on infected tissue to be studied histologically, has seemed to us particularly appropriate here, and we have been eager to corroborate our recognition of C. immitis in wet mounts and tissue sections by attempting to grow the fungus in culture from a portion of the biopsy material. In general, we have found Sabouraud's medium satisfactory (CONANT, 1965), though occasionally blood agar has yielded growth of C. immitis when Sabouraud's did not. Cultures on slants in large test tubes are much safer to handle than cultures on Petri dishes. There is considerable variation in the rate of growth, and we have kept cultures three weeks before discarding them as negative. "Atypical" cultures (HUPPERT et al., 1967; SPAUR, 1956) have been unusual in our experience. Usually the aerial cotton mycelium is readily recognized. If necessary, arthrospores can be looked for in a wet mount (Figs. 23, 24).

Cultures are most likely to be positive when abundant material is obtained from the center of an active lesion. The practice of sending a single dried out swab to the laboratory while pouring a lot of good pus down the drain is therefore to be deplored. Material not from the center of an active lesion will only occasionally yield growth. Thus after extensive trials with gastric washings in cases of acute coccidioidal pneumonia, GIFFORD (unpublished observations) concluded that they were not worth the trouble. With active caseous, cavitary, or bronchiectatic processes, O'LEARY and CURRY (1956) found gastric washings somewhat more worthwhile. Cultures of pleural fluid overlying coccidioidal pneumonias have seldom grown out, in our experience, while cultures of spinal fluid in coccidioidal meningitis have proved singularly frustrating. In many cases it has eventually been possible to get a growth, usually after many negative tries. In others, spinal fluid cultures have been negative right up to the time of death. Not infrequently culture of fluid obtained by cisternal or ventricular tap, or of pus from the base of the brain at autopsy, have yielded growth while repeated samples of lumbar fluid were negative. In our hands the most successful spinal fluid culture technique has been the simple one of drawing at least 5 cc. of fluid into a sterile test tube and then letting the tube stand at room temperature for at least 3 weeks. The fluid itself appears to be a sufficient culture medium, and the more fluid, the greater the likelihood of growth (JOHNSON, unpublished observations).

Such results would suggest that ordinarily the fungus does not diffuse rapidly through the host body. However, WINN et al. (1967) have emphasized a group of promptly fatal cases in which C. immitis grew out on blood culture. Peripheral pockets of pus were present in three of the eleven. The skin tests were consistently negative; in some instances serologic tests were not recorded prior to death, while in others the titres were low or intermediate. Thus in some instances the blood culture was the only clue both to the diagnosis and to the gravity of the situation. Since in two additional cases mentioned by the authors, and one seen subsequently by the present writer, salvage was achieved through prompt amphotericin treatment, diagnostic recognition is clearly an emergency in such situations, and prompt attention to the blood culture may be the only means of recognition.

Demonstration of the coccidioidal etiology of pulmonary cavities often requires culture of the fungus from sputum, bronchial washings, or the contents or wall of the excised cavity. Recognition of the mycelial phase *C. immitis* frequently present in these lesions can often be corroborated by obtaining pure cultures (SMITH et al., 1948a; FIESE et al., 1955; PUCKETT, 1954; HUNTINGTON, 1957, 1959b; HUNTINGTON et al., 1967b) (Fig. 10).

Pus from active disseminated lesions showing *C. immitis* on wet mount or section grows out the fungus quite consistently. So does soft tissue containing miliary granulomata. On the other hand, firm fibrotic-hyaline pulmonary lesions with varying amounts of calcium, even with abundant typical spherules in sections, generally give negative cultures. We have recently seen similarly fibrotic (but not calcified) lesions of the meninges in patients who had had prolonged amphotericin treatment; these, too, have been negative on culture. Both the pulmonary and the meningeal lesions of this pattern are doubtless comparatively inactive. Whether the failure of culture represents non-viability of the organisms or just unmanageability of the tissue is impossible to guess at the present time. Both digestion and animal inoculation techniques might be considered in further study of this important problem. From the practical standpoint it is important to recognize that at present identification of the coccidioidal etiology of such lesions must depend on microscopic rather than on cultural identification.

VI. Pathologic Anatomy

a) Basic Pathologic Processes

Host tissue reactions evoked by *Coccidioides* can be readily compared to those due to the tubercle bacillus (BUTT and HOFFMAN, 1941, 1945; DICKSON, 1929; FORBUS and BESTERBREURTJE, 1946; HUNTINGTON, 1957, 1959b; HUNTINGTON et al., 1967b). In the majority of instances these reactions can be conveniently classified as purulent (Figs. 15—19), granulomatous (Figs. 5—8, 12, 13, 21), or mixed (Figs. 30—34). Purulent reactions start with a polymorphonuclear infiltrate and may go on to liquefaction. While this pattern of abscess is not rare in tuberculosis (RICH, 1951), it is more common in coccidioidomycosis. Granulomatous reactions may exhibit lymphocytes, plasma cells, monocytes, epithelioid cells, giant cells, fibrosis, caseation, and calcification. Mixed reactions are of several types. Thus, the writer would put most coccidioidal pulmonary cavities in the mixed category. Psoas or other abscesses (Figs. 21, 30) often show epitheliod and giant cells on microscopic section of the edges. Microabscess in the midst of miliary tubercle is quite common, and indeed, may be considered characteristic enough to stimulate a particularly vigorous search for spherules. Demarcated coccidioidal lesions come in all sizes from the huge to the microscopic.

There are patterns which do not fit into this scheme of classification. Thus, in the spleens of subjects with "fungemia" (WINN et al., 1967), the writer and his colleagues (1967b) have encountered considerable numbers of organisms with little or nor tissue response. This phenomenon may be attributed to anergy and

agonal dissemination; it reports an interesting exception to Baker's generalization (1945, 1946) that fungi without host reaction are probably post-mortem
contaminants.

In marked contrast to this pattern is the "allergic" response without demonstrable organisms, encountered in coccidioidal erythema nodosum (Winer, 1950;
Allen, 1967). As we have previously mentioned, this lesion is thought to represent
an allergic reaction to soluble products or components of the organism (Dickson,
1937a, b, 1938, 1939a, b; Gifford, 1936, 1939a, b; Gifford et al., 1937; Smith,
1940, 1967; Smith and Baker, 1941). Histologically it is a rather non-descript
panniculitis and angiitis. It is essential not to confuse this lesion with those of
actual dissemination of organisms to the skin. The writer is unaware of histologic
studies of "allergic" coccidioidal arthritis, but would not be surprised if its histology were to resemble that of erythema nodosum. Here again, the lesion must be
carefully kept separate from that of actual coccidioidal invasion of joint tissue
(Winn, 1967a; Rosenberg et al., 1942; Thiemeyer, 1954; Walker and Hall,
1954).

Much more puzzling in its pathogenesis is the nondescript cellular infiltration
of the myocardium discussed by Reingold (1950). While this is something entirely
distinct from the focal granulomas or abscesses seen in that tissue, both occur in
disseminated disease. The writer had disregarded the diffuse myocarditis, partly,
no doubt, because of its nondescript pattern, until Reingold's study came to his
attention. On review, the writer has to agree with Reingold that the association
of this lesion with disseminated coccidioidomycosis is too frequent to be disregarded.
Any guesses the writer might make as to its pathogenesis would be purely speculative. Possibly disseminated coccidiodiomycosis with anergy may still be able to
trigger mechanisms of the variety vaguely termed autoimmune. Thus a 13-year-old
boy recently brought to the writer's attention has a negative coccidioidin skin
test, and complement fixing antibody to *Coccidioides* in rather high titre, and
unequivocal dermatomyositis, which came on with his coccidioidal infection
(Huntington, unpublished observations).

Some lesions not directly due to *Coccidioides* which nevertheless turn up not
infrequently in connection with it merit mention here. These are the nephropathy
due to amphotericin (Fig. 35), and the changes in the parenchyma of the central
nervous system secondary to chronic coccidioidal meningitis. Amphotericin
nephropathy has been studied by Iovine et al. (1963), Sanford et al. (1962),
Wertlake et al. (1965) and by the Brigham Hospital group (Reynolds et al.,
1963; Takacs et al., 1963; Huntington et al., 1967a). Early lesions are predominantly tubular; later on, glomerular lesions become conspicuous. Early stages
appear reversible, but late stages are not. As the Brigham group has shown
(Reynolds et al., 1963; Takacs et al., 1963), amphotericin may remain in the
body for a long time after the last administration, and nephropathy may progress
in that interval. Thus it may be difficult to feel confident that one has not, in fact,
reached the point of no return. In one of Winn's patients with coccidioidal meningitis, renal transplantation did achieve a prolongation of useful life. However,
the writer is informed that the patient eventually died of recurrent coccidioidal
meningitis (Winn, 1967b; Reynolds et al., 1963; Takacs et al., 1963; Huntington, 1968b). An example of fatal amphotericin nephropathy will be summarized in the section on "illustrative cases."

Gross coccidioidal abscesses or granulomas of the brain appear to be distinctly
uncommon. Indeed, the writer has had the opportunity to review but one case in
this category; this case had been admirably reported by his predecessor Rhoden
(1946). Hydrocephalus secondary to chronic coccidioidal meningitis is common,

and focal ischemic lesions attributable to vascular changes induced by meningitis were conspicuous in a recently studied case (HUNTINGTON, unpublished observations). One might anticipate that with continuation of amphotericin therapy, we would see fewer acute deaths and more chronic ones, and that hydrocephalus and focal ischemic encephalomalacia might become more conspicuous.

b) Sources of Material

Organs and tissues with coccidioidal lesions may reach the pathologist either through surgery or through necropsy. Lesions found at surgery may be incidental, or the occasion for the surgery. Lesions found at necropsy may be incidental, of major clinical importance, or lethal. Lesions in fatal cases will be discussed in a later subsection.

Aspirated pus from superficial or deep abscesses is likely to be sent to the microbiology laboratory, rather than to tissue pathology. The possibility of prompt establishment of the diagnosis by a KOH wet mount should be kept in mind.

Disseminated lesions may turn up in surgical specimens of skin (ALLEN, 1967), bone (GARDNER, 1904; McMASTER and GILFILAN, 1939; BENNINGHOVEN and MILLER, 1942; SASHIN, 1947; SASHIN et al., 1946; LAMPHIER, 1948; PILOT, 1946; MILLER and BIRSNER, 1949; BIRSNER and SMART, 1956; HIPPS, 1953; SCHWARTZMANN, 1957; IGER and LARSON, 1967), and other tissues. Thus we have encountered coccidioidomycosis as an unexpected finding in material from thyroid and prostatic surgery, and from lymph nodes (HUNTINGTON et al., 1967b; HUNTINGTON, unpublished observations). At necropsy we have seen widespread disseminated coccidioidomycosis in subjects dying from coronary artery disease, from longstanding chronic glomerulonephritis, and from malignancy. If these subjects had not died of something else first, they might have died a little later of their coccidioidomycosis. We have also seen at necropsy disseminated coccidioidal lesions which are much more obviously incidental, as for example, solitary coccidioidomycosis of the prostate in a subject with plasma cell myeloma and widespread amyloidosis.

In endemic areas, coccidioidal lung lesions will be frequently encountered in both *surgical* and *autopsy material*. The majority of such lesions (other than miliary) may for convenience be classified as pneumonic, cavitary, nodulocaseous, or bronchiectatic. The distribution of such lesions in subjects with fatal coccidioidal infection will be discussed later. Lung resection would hardly be undertaken in the presence of florid coccidioidal pneumonias, and we have not happened to encounter an incidental lesion of this character in a subject whose death was unrelated to coccidioidomycosis. Description and discussion of the process will, therefore, be reserved for the subsection "Lesions in Fatal Coccidioidomycosis."

Coccidioidal bronchiectasis is occasionally encountered in surgical material or as an incidental autopsy finding (Figs. 18, 19). Coccidioidal cavities frequently require surgical resection, and occasionally turn up as incidental findings at necropsy. Nodular-caseous lesions, if large and active, may require therapeutic resection. Small coin lesions may require diagnostic excision and biopsy, since their X-ray shadows may suggest the possibility of malignancy (ARONSON et al., 1942; BASS et al., 1948; BUTT and HOFFMAN, 1941, 1945; COX and SMITH, 1939; BAKER and WASKOW, 1967; COTTON et al., 1955; COTTON and BIRSNER, 1950, 1959; FINDLAY and MELICK, 1967; HELPER and WATTS, 1945; HUGHES et al., 1954; HUNTINGTON, 1959b, 1968b; HUNTINGTON et al., 1967b; HYDE, 1958; MARKS et al., 1967; MELICK, 1949, 1950, 1957; O'LEARY and CURRY, 1956; OWENS et al., 1960; WEISEL and OWEN, 1949; ZIMMERMAN, 1954a, b). Very puzzling situations may result from the coincidence of coccidioidomycosis and pulmonary carcinoma (Hood, 1950; Huntington et al., 1967b). "Coin lesions" of coccidioidomycosis are a very common incidental finding at necropsy. Such lesions, of course, are sometimes found in subjects with active, and indeed lethal, coccidioidal lesions at other sites (Figs. 27—29).

1. Lung Lesions: Coccidioidal Bronchiectasis: Since the causes of bronchiectasis are various, the writer and his colleagues have been exceedingly conservative in the diagnosis of coccidioidal bronchiectasis. They have made this diagnosis only in cases with distinctive coccidioidal lung lesions unequivocally related to the bronchiectasis. They have little doubt that a coccidioidal process which originally triggered a bronchiectasis may sometimes have become unrecognizable by the time that a bronchiectatic lung becomes available for pathologic examination, and would, therefore, suspect that they may have considerably underestimated the actual incidence of coccidioidal bronchiectasis in the Southern San Joaquin Valley. Microphotographs of cases in which they have accepted that diagnosis are shown in the figures. This is one variety of coccidioidal lung disease which may cause "late" coccidioidal deaths (Figs. 18, 19).

Coccidioidal Cavities. The first descriptions of these lesions are those of Farness and Mills (1938, 1939). Additional studies are those of Winn (1941, 1942, 1956, 1967a, c, d), Smith et al. (1948a), Belanger (1947), Bass (1947), Waring (1954), Cotton and Birsner (1950, 1959), Cotton et al. (1955); Findlay and Melick (1967), Forsee and Perkins (1954), Greer et al. (1949a, b), Hughes et al. (1954), Hyde (1955, 1958), Krapin and Lovelock (1948), Marks et al. (1967), Melick (1949, 1950, 1957), O'Leary and Curry (1956), Paulsen (1967), Weisel and Owen (1949). The not uncommon finding of coccidioidal mycelia in cavities (Fiese et al., 1955; Puckett, 1954; Huntington, 1957, 1959b; Huntington et al., 1967b) has already been noted. Coccidioidal cavities have been distressing to the systematiziers in other respects as well. Thus reinfection has been deemed an important factor in the pathogenesis of tuberculosis cavities (Rich, 1951), while most students other than Salkin (1967) have deprecated the importance of reinfection in coccidioidomycosis. Quite naturally, therefore, there has been what the writer would regard as excessive zeal in searching for morphologic and other differences between coccidioidal and tuberculous cavities (Smith et al., 1948a) (Figs. 9—13).

It has been suggested that only *"thin-walled cavities"* should be regarded as typical of coccidioidal cavitation, and that other coccidioidal cavities should be disregarded as far as possible by being cast into the limbo of the atypical. The writer would have to regard this notion as misleading. He finds that coccidioidal cavitation occurs with a great variety and continuous range of patterns, and would be forced to apply the term *coccidioidal cavity* to any coccidioidal lung lesion characterized by conspicuous excavation. It is of incidental interest that since the introduction of modern chemotherapy, "thin-walled" cavities have proved quite common in tuberculosis. The writer finds himself quite unable to distinguish coccidioidal cavities from tuberculous cavities by gross morphology, microscopic pattern of host response, or by any means other than evidence of the presence and activity of *Coccidioides* and the absence of *Mycobacteria*.

Clinically, coccidioidal cavities have been followed by late dissemination to the skin (Levan and Huntington, 1965), and by late development of meningitis (Einstein, personal communication). They have caused death from hemorrhage and from debility, and have been found at autopsy in cases of coccidioidal meningitis (see next section). However, the over-all incidence of dissemination or other fatality with coccidioidal cavitation is low, and some of the cavities close spontaneously (Winn, 1942). Yet the persistent and debilitating character of the majority of those lesions has persuaded the writer's internist and chest surgeon colleagues that most of them should be resected (COTTON and BIRSNER, 1959; EINSTEIN, personal communication; PAULSEN, 1967).

Nodulocaseous Lesions. Such lesions may be large and active; they may be obviously related to bronchiectasis. Much more common are *coin lesions*, thought to represent primary infection which has become quite inactive (ARONSON et al., 1942; BUTT and HOFFMAN, 1941, 1945; COX and SMITH, 1939; STRAUB and SCHWARTZ, 1956, 1962). The latter authors have commented on the irregularity of associated hilar lymphadenopathy with peripheral coccidioidal coin lesions. We, too, have recorded peripheral coin lesions without lymphadenopathy. However, we have also recorded old calcific lesions in hilar nodes in cases in which we failed to find peripheral primary lesions. In coccidioidomycosis in cattle (PRCHAL, 1948, 1957), hilar and mediastinal lymphadenopathy is sometimes the most conspicuous finding. We would feel, therefore, that the interesting and important observation of STRAUB and SCHWARZ requires further systematic study.

Coin lesions due to coccidioidomycosis require differentiation from those due to tuberculosis or histoplasmosis. Multiple lesions, particularly if calcific, suggest histoplasmosis but do not rule out coccidioidomycosis. We have so far failed to identify an endemic focus of histoplasmosis in our own or other areas of California. However, a great many of our subjects are emigrants from areas of endemic histoplasmosis, and histoplasmal coin lesions are currently as common as coccidioidal coin lesions in our autopsy material. Each appears to be currently more common than tuberculous coin lesions. We are particularly grateful to Dr. J. SCHWARZ (personal communication) and to other friends for slides and instruction which have given us confidence in our recognition of *Histoplasma capsulatum* in tissue sections. We would hesitate to make the diagnosis of histoplasmosis merely on the basis of dots of Grocott-positive material, since similar dots occur in tissue which on further study shows large and unmistakeable spherules of *C. immitis*. However, in most cases of histoplasmosis, we have been able to find the yeast-like bodies; these will not be readily confused with the larger, deeper-staining, and more variegated spherules of coccidioides (SCHWARTZ, personal communication).

Although we have seen coccidioidal lesions of the abdominal serosa (GREAVES, 1934; MEIS et al., 1967), we have not seen involvement of the gastro-intestinal mucosa.

c) Lesions in Fatal Coccidioidomycosis

1. Distribution of Lesions: In eleven of our 142 cases of fatal coccidioidomycosis (HUNTINGTON et al., 1967b), there was no evidence of metapulmonary dissemination. The fatal pulmonary lesions in these eleven will be discussed later. In Table 1 the distribution of lesions in our 131 cases of fatal disseminated coccidioidomycosis is compared with that of FORBUS and BESTEBREURTJE's (1946) 50 cases. Some striking differences are at once apparent. Thus the incidence of meningitis was higher in our series, while that of bone and skin lesions was lower. The explanation of these differences is not obvious. It is possible that our series may have been less selective and that it may have covered a greater range of chronicity. Forbus and Bestebreurtje's material was military; one would suspect that the infection might have been acute and recent in the majority of their cases. Moreover, in order to reach the Armed Forces Institute of Pathology, the material might have had to impress the pathologist at the local military installation as unusual and very likely coccidioidal. Unfortunately, even in Bakersfield, the possibility of fatal disseminated coccidioidomycosis has been all too often disregarded if there are no skin or bone lesions (HUNTINGTON et al., 1967b). The important study of BUSS et al. (1950),

Table 1. *Sites of coccidioidal disease in autopsied subjects with fatal dissemination*

	Forbus and Bestebreurtje	Huntington et al.	Excluding Group with Solitary Meningitis	Total
Total	50	131	95	181
Lung	43 = .860	113 = .863	89 = .937	156 = .862
Spleen	35 = .70	67 = .511	67 = .705	102 = .564
Liver	30 = .60	59 = .450	59 = .621	89 = .492
Kidney	30 = .60	46 = .351	46 = .484	76 = .420
Skin and sub-cutaneous	32 = .64	27 = .206	27 = .284	59 = .326
Bone	24 = .480	21 = .160	21 = .221	45 = .249
Leptomeninges . .	18 = .360	82 = .626	46 = .484	100 = .552
Adrenal	16 = .320	22 = .168	22 = .232	38 = .210
Heart	14 (?) = .280	12 (?) = .092	12 = .126	26 = .144
Pancreas	8 = .160	13 = .099	13 = .137	21 = .116
Psoas and retro-peritoneal	5 = .100	13 = .099	13 = .137	18 = .099
Thyroid	4 = .080	9 = .069	9 = .095	13 = .072
Prostate	3 = .060	6 = .046	6 = .063	9 = .050
Larynx	1 = .020	1 = .008	1 = .011	2 = .011
Scrotal contents . .	0 = .000	2 = .016	2 = .021	2 = .011
Optic nerve . . .	1 = .020	1 = .008	1 = .011	2 = .011
Placenta	0 = .000	2 = .016	2 = .021	2 = .011
Bladder	0 = .000	1 = .008	1 = .011	1 = .006

emphasizing *solitary meningitis*, did not appear until four years after Forbus and Bestebreurtje's study, and we were unable to determine whether any cases of this rather chronic category were included in their series. Certain of the differences between our figures and theirs became less marked if our 36 cases of solitary meningitis are excluded. Our uncertainty as to the true figure for heart involvement has already been mentioned, and we were uncertain whether Reingold's (1950) diffuse nondescript myocarditis was recognized and included by Forbus and Bestebreurtje.

Coccidioidal involvement of the *liver, spleen,* and *kidney* is usually microscopic; the lesions may be either microabscesses or miliary granulomata. The pattern of numerous organisms in the spleen with little or no cellular response has already been mentioned. The most common disseminated skin manifestations are abscesses; we have seen but one instance of the generalized verrucoid lesion of Posadas (1892) and Wernicke (1892) (Figs. 1, 2). Bone lesions may be large or microscopic (Iger and Larson, 1967). We have seen massive caseation of the adrenal, but microscopic miliary lesions are more common. Granulomatous pericarditis and focal granulomas and microabscesses of heart muscle are readily recognized and interpreted. Our difficulties with the diffuse myocarditis of Reingold (1950) have already been mentioned. The huge psoas and retroperitoneal abscesses, while not exceedingly common, are not rare; when present, they are quite characteristic. The thyroid lesions which we have encountered have been a surprise on microscopic examination. In one instance we were fascinated by the juxtaposition of microabscesses and miliary granulomata in the thyroid. Laryngeal involvement has been recorded by Singh et al. (1956) and others (Fiese, 1958). Our two cases with placental lesions point out that our civilian series included females, as well as males.

At necropsy in cases of coccidioidomycosis, particular attention should be paid to the *lungs* and the *meninges* (Figs. 16, 17, 27—29). Failure to examine the meninges is regrettable, whether imposed by limitation of consent or attributable to prosectorial inertia (Figs. 4—8, 34). We regret that the meninges were not examined in 27 of our 142 coccidioidal fatalities. Meningitis was found in 82 of the remaining 115 cases, and when found, was considered to be the cause of death. In 36 cases the meningitis was "solitary"; in 46 there were other metapulmonary lesions. Coccidioidal meningitis tends to concentrate in sulci rather than on convex surfaces, and is commonly rather unimpressive to naked eye examination at the autopsy table. In some of our cases it was an unexpected microscopic finding; in all of the cases in which we have recognized coccidioidal meningitis, the process has been diffuse. However, we have recently been told of a case with localized arachnoiditis and symptoms which at first suggested multiple sclerosis (BIDDLE, personal communication). We consider it quite possible that localized meningitis might turn up more frequently if better methods for complete examination of the leptomeninges were available. One sometimes finds groups of polymorphonuclear cells in coccidioidal meningitis, but in general the process is decidedly granulomatous. Coccidioidal meningitis appears to have none of the tendency for spontaneous healing which characterizes coccidioidal lesions of most other tissues. In chronic cases, particularly following amphotericin therapy, the pattern may be strikingly fibrotic. Even in such cases, we have not had difficulty infinding organisms in tissue sections (Fig. 14). Vascular involvement may be striking (Figs. 5, 6). Brain changes secondary to meningitis, viz., hydrocephalus and multifocal encephalomalacia, may be conspicuous. However, gross coccidioidal lesions of brain parenchyma have been most unusual in the writer's experience. In fact, the only one which he has had the opportunity to review is the cerebellar abscess admirably reported by his predecessor, RHODEN (1946). In the same period, there have been several gross cortical tuberculomas in the writer's autopsy service; possibly more ample experience may indicate a genuine difference between the two infections with respect to involvement of the brain cortex. In one instance, the writer has found tiny, microscopic intracortical coccidioidomycosis; meningitis was not demonstrable in this subject.

In some of the writer's cases of fatal dissemination, pulmonary lesions were not found. There was nothing to suggest primary extrapulmonary infection in any of these cases. A similar experience has been noted by FORBUS and BESTEBREURTJE (1946). In several of our cases, the only lung lesions found were those of miliary dissemination. Data on this point are not available from Forbus and Bestebreurtje's material.

More meticulous study, including routine insufflation and roentgenography of excised lungs, might have reduced the number of cases without demonstrable primary lesions. However, we strongly suspect that primary lesions of pulmonary coccidioidomycosis may entirely disappear, both in patients with total arrest of the infection and in those with active dissemination. In our previous study (HUNTINGTON et al., 1967b), we divided our cases of fatal dissemination into several groups. Thus, Group A comprised 36 cases of "solitary meningitis." Group B included 46 cases with meningitis and other metapulmonary coccidioidal lesions. Group C consisted of 18 cases with dissemination in which the meninges were not examined, and Group F, of 31 cases of fatal dissemination without meningitis. On the whole, the most "chronic" fatalities were those of Group A, while the most acute were those of Group F. From general considerations, one might expect to find the highest incidence of active primary pulmonary lesions in Group F, and the highest incidence of "disappeared" primary lesions in Group A.

If we compare the incidence of "disappeared primaries" in the solitary meningitis group (A) with that of the remainder of the series, the figures are 14/36 = .389 and 16/95 = .168. The standard deviation of the difference is .083, and the difference of .221 is thus "probably significant." On the other hand, if we compare the incidence of active primary lung lesions in Group A with that of Group F, we get for "A" 6/36 = .167, and for "F", 25/31 = .806. The standard deviation is .122, and the difference of .639 is, therefore, outstandingly significant. Likewise, if we compare "A" with "B", "C", and "F" together, for the latter we get 61/95 = .642. The standard deviation is .098, and here again the difference of .475 is outstandingly significant.

Analogous differences can be noted in the characters of the lesions considered active. Thus 5 subjects in Group A had cavitary lesions of moderate activity, and the sixth had a coccidioidal pneumonia occupying an area 3—4 cm in diameter. In Group B, nine subjects had moderately active coccidioidal cavitation; four had large areas of active caseation, another had numerous sizable active granulomas, one had granuloma plus diffuse fibrosis, while the remaining three had coccidioidal pneumonias of varying size, pattern and activity. Of the 49 cases in Groups C and F combined (dissemination, but no demonstrated meningitis), 37 had active primary lung lesions, and in 35, these lesions were considered the major factor in the fatality. In one of these 35, the pulmonary lesion was principally bronchiectatic. The 34 others had severe coccidioidal pneumonic processes with variegated gross and microscopic patterns.

At this point it is well to consider the cases of the eleven subjects without evidence of metapulmonary dissemination whose deaths were attributable to their coccidioidal pulmonary disease. Unfortunately, the meninges were examined in but two of the eleven. Five of the subjects had cavitary lesions; in three of the five, death was related to surgery. A fourth, who had refused surgery, died of pulmonary hemorrhage, while the fifth had mixed tuberculous and coccidioidal infection. While the tuberculous component was controlled by appropriate chemotherapy, the coccidioidal infection, not recognized prior to autopsy, had continued to progress. Of the remaining six subjects, one died of acute suppurative coccidioidal pneumonia. Another, who had undergone lobectomy for squamous carcinoma of the lung, developed new shadows on X-ray, which were thought to represent spread or recurrence of the malignancy. Although the patient's cardiovascular status would hardly have encouraged a second look, it was disconcerting to find at autopsy that there was no recurrence of the carcinoma and that the shadows represented caseous pneumonia due to *Coccidioides immitis*. The remaining four subjects all had severe coccidioidal bronchiectasis, associated with peribronchial granulomatous lesions in one and with a coccidioidal pneumonic process in the other.

2. Causes of Death: Thus we regard coccidioidal meningitis as the number one cause of coccidioidal fatality, and coccidioidal pulmonary lesions as the number two. A number of "early" coccidioidal deaths are due to florid coccidioidal pneumonia, with or without metapulmonary dissemination. Late coccidioidal deaths are most commonly due to meningitis, but are sometimes due to coccidioidal pulmonary disease with persistent activity.

After ascribing 82 of our fatalities to meningitis and 46 to coccidioidal pulmonary disease, we have 14 not yet accounted for. One of these was a suicide attributed to the subject's coccidioidal osteomyelitis. Another subject had myocardial coccidioidal lesions, amphotericin nephropathy, and pyelonephritis due to ureteral obstruction by a cystified "burnt out" psoas abscess; the death was attributed to a combination of all these things. Six deaths were associated with the massive tissue destruction of large active psoas abscesses, and six more were attributed in a general way to overwhelming disseminated infection.

Before leaving the subject of fatal coccidioidomycosis, let me write a little more both about the meningeal lesions and about fatal pneumonic lesions. The morphologic resemblance of coccidioidal meningitis to tuberculous meningitis is obvious from the photographs. We have not yet encountered simultaneous infection of the meninges with both *M. tuberculosis* and *C. immitis*. However, we have seen tuberculous meningitis in a patient previously found to have disseminated coccidioidomycosis and treated with amphotericin. Thus in the differential diagnosis between tuberculous and coccidioidal meningitis, even a well-documented history may be misleading. During life, the diagnosis of coccidioidal meningitis may sometimes be established by culture of *C. immitis* from the spinal fluid. The diagnosis of coccidioidal meningitis is very strongly supported by positive spinal fluid complement fixation with coccidioidal antigen (HUNTINGTON, 1959b). At autopsy the diagnosis may be established through demonstration of *C. immitis* in culture, in microscopic sections, or in both. As we mentioned earlier, in chronic meningitis treated with amphotericin, culture may be negative, and definitive diagnosis will require demonstration of the *C. immitis* organism in tissue sections.

While coccidioidal meningitis, like tuberculous meningitis, tends to be rather uniform, even monotonous, in its histology, coccidioidal pneumonia, like tuberculous pneumonia, may be variegated. Granulomatous, histiocytic and caseous pneumonia due to *C. immitis* has to be differentiated from analogous reactions due to *M. tuberculosis*. Organizing and fibrinous pneumonias, and pneumonia with predominantly polymorphonuclear reaction due to *C. immitis* must be distingushed from similar reactions evoked by the tubercle bacillus or by pyogenic bacteria. In subjects with fatal coccidioidomycosis, particularly in those with coccidioidal meningitis, terminal bacterial pneumonia is, of course, quite common. It is important, but usually fairly easy, to distinguish this lesion from coccidioidal pneumonia. Although in the presence of massive polymorphonuclear exudate, the demonstration of *C. immitis* in fixed tissue frequently requires special stains, with appropriate stains such as the Grocott-Gomori (GROCOTT, 1955; HUNTINGTON, 1968a), organisms are readily found in polymorphonuclear pneumonias due to *C. immitis*. On the other hand, the terminal bacterial pneumonias will usually show large clumps of bacteria even in H & E sections. Differentiation between coccidioidal and tuberculous pneumonias is usually clear enough with appropriate cultural and staining techniques. As previously noted, the possibility of mixed infection should be kept in mind.

VII. Categories of Grave and Fatal Coccidioidomycosis

Some Illustrative Cases. In the attempt to impart something of the variegated pathology of coccidioidomycosis, I hope that some case presentations from my experience may prove helpful. I will give clinical and pathologic summaries of eleven cases. In one case (No. 10), the only material available for pathologic study was a surgically resected lung. The others are all necropsy cases. In Case No. 11, there was a long series of coccidioidal abscesses of bone and soft tissue, with eventual death from amphotericin nephropathy. In Case No. 9, death was due to massive florid coccidioidal pneumonia; in Case No. 8, it was due to hemorrhage from a long-standing coccidioidal cavity. Meningitis was present in Cases 1—7; in some, the meningitis was the only metapulmonary lesion, while others had variegated additional dissemination. Case No. 1 is the only instance in my experience of the generalized verrucoid skin lesions of POSADAS (1892).

Case No. 1. (Case B 35 of HUNTINGTON et al., 1967b) (Figs. 1, 2).

This Negro female, born in 1923, came to Kern County General Hospital in August, 1948, with the complaint of swelling of her face. Biopsy confirmed the diagnosis of disseminated coccidioidomycosis. Chest X-ray revealed bilateral hilar adenopathy. She was treated with X-ray and actidione, but the skin lesion continued to spread and the serum complement fixation titre continued to rise. On April 3, 1950, she complained of stiff neck and headache. Lumbar puncture revealed clear fluid with 300 WBC, 92% lymphocytes and a 3+ Pandy's reaction. On a previous lumbar puncture in 1949, spinal fluid had been entirely unremarkable, with a negative complement fixation test. Her condition rapidly deteriorated, and she died April 10, 1950.

At autopsy there were extensive crusted, oozing, annular and serpiginous lesions of the skin of the face, neck, and upper thorax (Figs. 1, 2). Miliary lesions were present in the lung. The hilar lymph nodes were necrotic. The spleen and liver showed miliary granulomata, and there were microabscesses in the myocardium. The meninges were heavily infiltrated with lymphocytes, histiocytes, epithelioid and giant cells, and *C. immitis* spherules were numerous. The skin showed acute and chronic inflammation with giant cells and *C. immitis* spherules.

This case is the only one I have ever seen with the verrucoid skin lesions of Posadas (1928) and Wernicke (1892). Such cases are most unusual.

Case No. 2. (Case F 8 of Huntington et al., 1967b) (Fig. 14).

A Mexican woman, born in 1940, came to the Kern County General Hospital for delivery in 1962. Her premature infant died at 3 weeks of age, and was found to have disseminated coccidioidomycosis, the major lesions being bronchopulmonary. The mother was then found to have coccidioidal meningitis and endometritis. Unfortunately, the placenta had not been examined. However, other cases with placental infection and sparing of the fetus, and the distribution of lesions in this baby, suggested that the route of infection may have been amniotic and tracheobronchial rather than hematogenous and placental.

The mother received intravenous and intrathecal amphotericin B. Hysterectomy was done on March 19, 1963; the endometrium showed granulomata with spherules. In the spring of 1965 a Peckham subgaleal ventricular reservoir was introduced, and she received amphotericin intraventricularly. Between September 21 and October 3, 1965, she was hospitalized with a diagnosis of coccidioidomycosis and grand mal epilepsy. Spinal fluid cultures were negative. The spinal fluid showed a white cell count of 168 with 86% lymphocytes, a sugar of 38 mg/%, a protein of 410 mg/%, increased globulin, and a colloidal gold test of 5555555432.

She was followed in out-patient clinics and readmitted June 19, 1967. Material in the reservoir showed hyphae, which grew *C. immitis* on culture. On July 17 the Peckham reservoir was explored and was replaced with an Ommaya reservoir (Witorsch et al., 1965). She was discharged July 20. Her final admission was on September 19 with a chief complaint of loss of memory. On September 24 she was having Cheyne-Stokes respiration and grand mal seizures. She died on September 29, 1967.

At autopsy, there was an Ommaya reservoir beneath the scalp. There were a few nodular areas of bronchopneumonic consolidation. The hilar lymph nodes were soft. Meticulous search failed to reveal a primary pulmonary coccidioidoma. The free and cut surfaces of the enlarged kidneys showed raised white dots. The brain showed basilar arachnoid thickening, moderate ventricular dilatation, and cystic perivascular softening.

Cultures from the base of the brain yielded no growth on Sabouraud's medium. Microscopic sections showed meningeal and ependymal granulomas with numerous spherules (Fig. 10). Some of the granulomas contained microabscesses; there was much meningeal fibrosis. Areas of cortex showed rarefaction and gliosis.

The terminal pneumonia showed no fungi. Microscopic examination of several sections of kidney showed one small granuloma. Kidney tubules were dilated, and there were focal calcium deposits. Some glomeruli were congested and cellular with thickened capsules, while others showed various stages of hyalinization.

Final Diagnoses: Coccidioidal leptomeningitis and ependymitis; coccidioidomycosis of kidney; amphotericin nephropathy; encephalomalacia due to circulatory disturbance; and terminal bronchopneumonia. *Comment:* This is the first coccidioidal fatality which we have recorded in a Mexican female (Huntington, 1959a; Huntington et al., 1967b). The sparing of this group provides an interesting sidelight on Mexican folkways. Mexican males are less likely to die of coccidioidomycosis than Negro or Filipino males (Huntington, 1959a). Mexican females undergo minimal exposure to *Coccidioides*, for they engage in little outdoor activity, occupational or recreational. From early childhood Mexican girls help their mothers keep house while Mexican boys go to the fields with their fathers. To decorous Mexicans, family picnics would be out of line.

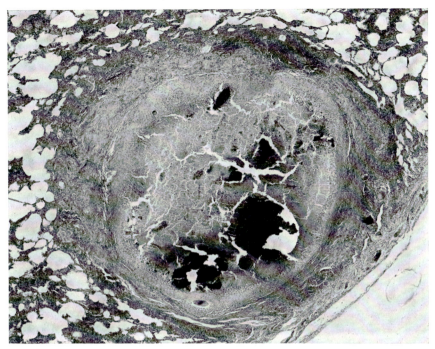

Fig. 27. Caseocalcific primary pulmonary lesion of coccidioidomycosis. Case 3. H & E, × 40

I accept antenatal transmission of infection to this woman's infant. Superficially this case invites comparison with that of CHRISTIAN et al. (1956). In that case the infection of the infant was attributed to fomite contamination by way of the mother's draining sinus. I suggest an alternate mechanism, comparable to that suggested for our case. In our case the absence of draining lesions, the coccidioidal endometritis, and the prompt isolation of the child from the mother make antenatal infection the most reasonable possibility.

This woman did have coccidioidal endometritis during her course. At autopsy the only extrameningeal coccidioidal lesion found was that in the kidney. She would, therefore, be placed in Group B, meningitis with other metapulmonary dissemination, but if the history and surgical pathology findings of the endometritis had not been available, and we had not happened to find the one small renal granuloma at autopsy, we might have put her in Group A, solitary meningitis. Thus this case illustrates the arbitrariness of cassifications. Her infection was certainly chronic, and the disappearance of the primary lung lesion is not surprising.

The ventricular dilatation, and the focal areas of encephalomalacia are doubtless indirect effects of the meningitis, and one might expect that with increasing Amphotericin treatment, and increasing chronicity of meningitis where it is not arrested, we should be seeing more and more effects of this character. It is considerable interest that the concentration of Amphotericin treatment through the intrathecal and intraventricular routes, and the low total dose of the drug did not forestall the development of amphotericin nephropathy in this case (IOVINE et al., 1963; SANFORD et al., 1962; WERTLAKE et al., 1965; REYNOLDS et al., 1963; TAKACS et al., 1963; HUNTINGTON et al., 1967a).

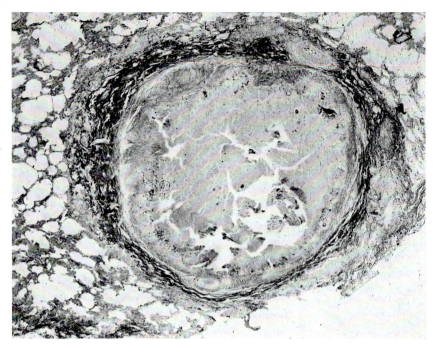

Fig. 28. Caseocalcific primary pulmonary lesion of coccidioidomycosis shown in Fig. 27. Case 3.
Grocott-Gomori, × 40

Case No. 3. (Case B 1 of Huntington et al., 1967b) (Figs. 5, 6, 27—29).

J.L. This white male child, born July 1948, was first admitted to Kern County General Hospital in July, 1949, with high fever, nausea and vomiting. Spinal fluid revealed lymphocytosis. Serum complement fixation was 4 + in 1:16 dilution; spinal fluid showed 3 + complement fixation at 1:2 dilution. He was treated with Actidione. In January 1950 skin tests revealed a 3 + coccidioidin and negative Mantoux. Repeated study of serum and spinal fluid showed rising complement fixation titres. His final admission was on July 13, 1950, with vomiting and opisthotonus. The coccidioidin skin test was now negative. His condition rapidly deteriorated and he died on July 18, 1950.

At *autopsy* a primary chronic granulomatous lesion was found in the right middle lobe (Figs. 27—29). There were small miliary lesions in the lung and the spleen. The brain weighed 1400 g. It was tense and bulging, with extreme flattening of the convolutions and a moderately severe pressure cone. There was much grayish exudate at the base of the brain. There was severe hydrocephalus with thinning of the cortex. Sections of the primary pulmonary lesion are illustrated in Figs. 27—29, while the meningitis and meningeal arteritis are represented in Figs. 5 and 6. Other microscopic findings included miliary granulomata of lung, liver, and spleen.

Case No. 4.

(Case B 45 of Huntington et al., 1967b; Case 10 of Winn et al., 1967).

This 19-year-old daughter of a Filipino father and a Mexican mother, and the wife of a Caucasian, was being attended by a private physician in her second pregnancy. In August 1962, her chest films showed hilar adenopathy. Subsequent films showed a "ground glass" pattern. She had been having headaches for several months, for which she consulted an ophthalmologist in September 1962. On November 12, she noted night blindness in her right eye. The right disc margins were blurred, and there was purulent exudate. The left fundus was unremarkable. Vision improved on steroid administration. When the steroids were "tapered off," vision again

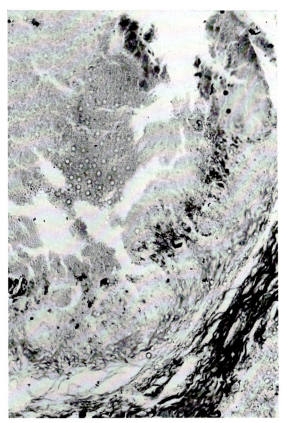

Fig. 29. Caseocalcific primary pulmonary granuloma of coccidioidomycosis. Higher magnification of lesion shown in Fig. 28. Case 3. Grocott-Gomori, × 125

became poor. On January 10, 1963, a coccidioidin skin test was negative. The ophthalmologist referred the patient to a neurosurgeon. Prior to her neurosurgical appointment she fainted, and the neurosurgeon referred her to the hospital.

On arrival at Kern County General Hospital January 15, 1963, her temperature was 104° F, pulse 136, and blood pressure 118/70. She was cooperative, but had intervals of disorientation. The right pupil was larger than the left. The disc margins were obliterated on the right. The left optic fungus was unremarkable. The uterus was obviously gravid. The chest film revealed miliary disease of the lungs. Lumbar puncture revealed turbid fluid with 1,295 cells, 70% polymorphonuclear. Spinal fluid smears showed no acid-fast bacilli.

She was treated with Tetracycline, and beginning on January 17 with Streptomycin and PAS. A few hours after this, some observers thought she looked better. However, she stopped breathing at 3:10 A.M. January 18, 1963. Clinical diagnosis was medullary failure, cause undetermined.

At *autopsy* the body was that of a light-complexioned Filipino-Mexican female, height 63 inches, weight estimated at 120 pounds. The breasts were enlarged and the abdomen was of a size appropriate to an eight month pregnancy. Hilar and peripancreatic nodes showed caseation. The lungs showed edema surrounding miliary nodules. The spleen was studded with light-colored nodules. The uterus revealed the body of a male infant weighing 2400 grams and measuring 46 cm in length. Gross and microscopic examination of the infant's body revealed nothing of significance. The placenta was red and friable, but contained large numbers of nodular caseous areas, 0.5 to 3 cm in diameter. The brain weighed 1300 grams. The meninges of the base of the brain and of the spinal cord were cloudy and edematous. Wet mounts from the lung, the optic chiasm, and the placenta showed numerous typical spherules of *C. immitis*.

Spinal fluid, taken during life but not studied until after death, showed 4+ complement fixation at 1:8 dilution, negative reaction at 1:16. Post-mortem blood serum showed 4+ complement fixation at 1:256, and positive precipitin. Sections showed miliary granulomata of the lung, spleen, kidney, and adrenal, a rather nondescript meningitis, largely round cell, but more frankly granulomatous in the region of the chiasm, perivascular cuffing in the retina, and a small granuloma in the posterior pituitary. Blood culture taken during life grew *C. immitis* after death.

This patient, no doubt, owed her vulnerability to coccidioidomycosis to her Filipino ancestry. Most of the Filipinos in this community are solitary males; pure-blooded Filipino females are scarce. The writer is constantly besieged by inquires from well-qualified Filipino females who wish to come to this hospital for training in medical technology. He finds it his duty to advise them to take their training elsewhere.

The pregnancy was, no doubt, a further factor in this calamity (SMALE, unpublished observations). At the conclusion of his study the writer further noted, "This is the first time that I have encountered optic neuritis as the presenting complaint in coccidioidal meningitis. However, the insidious pattern of coccidioidal meningitis is such that a pattern of this sort, retrospectively, is not at all surprising. The possibility of coccidioidomycosis should in the future in this community be considered both by general physicians and by specialists dealing with optic neuritis. If optic neuritis due to coccidioidomycosis is to be treated with steroids, amphotericin (or a newer, better drug) should be given concomitantly."

Case No. 5. (Case A 17 of HUNTINGTON et al., 1967b) (Figs. 7, 8, 12, 13).

This 14-year-old Mexican male was referred to Kern County General Hospital August 22, 1950, because of a suspicious chest film. There was a history of family contact with tuberculosis. Tuberculin skin test was negative; coccidioidin was positive. X-ray revealed a density in the right upper lung field, and he was sent to Stony Brook Retreat (the County tubercular sanitarium) as "probable minimal active tuberculosis." Acid fast bacilli were never isolated, but he was placed on streptomycin and PAS. He developed signs of meningeal irritation. Lumbar puncture revealed cloudy fluid with 360 WBCs and he was transferred back to Kern County General Hospital in October of 1950. He was continued on streptomycin and was given sodium caprylate and ethyl vanilate. Serum complement fixation was reported as 2 + in 1:128. The course was steadily downhill and he died April 5, 1951, the clinical diagnosis being coccidioidomycosis of the meninges.

At *autopsy* the body was that of a well developed, emaciated Mexican male, length 63 inches, weight estimated at 75 pounds. There was a cavity in the upper lobe of the right lung (Figs. 12, 13), and caseation of the right hilar nodes. Elsewhere the lungs showed patchy bronchopneumonia. The brain weighed 1490 g. The gyri were flattened, and there were dense granulomatous adhesions at the foramen magnum. In the region of the optic chiasm, there was a heavy deposit of organized granulomatous material (Fig. 18). The pituitary was depressed downward and the posterior clinoids were flattened. There was moderate hydrocephalus with uniform dilatation of the ventricular system. No coccidioidal lesions were found outside the lung and the envelopes of the brain. Culture from the base of the brain revealed *C. immitis*.

Case No. 6. (Case B 41 of HUNTINGTON et al., 1967b) (Figs. 21, 30, 31).

This 45-year-old Filipino male came to Kern County General Hospital on December 19, 1956, with a chief complaint of fever. History was unsatisfactory because of language difficulty and the severity of the illness. Apparently he had come from the Philippine Islands in 1929 and had lived in the San Joaquin Valley for two years. He had been ill for 2½ months with fever, malaise, weight loss, cough, and chest pain. Oral temperature was 101.2° F., pulse 110, blood

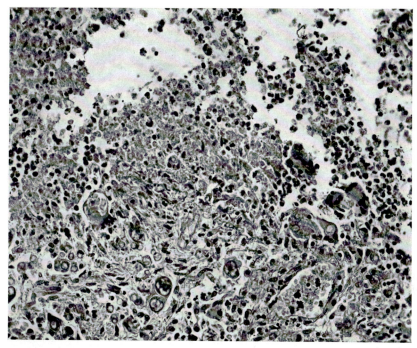

Fig. 30. Mixed reaction. Coccidioidal paravertebral abscess. H & E, × 330. Case 6. Note the pus above and the giant cells, fibroblasts and round cells below. The organisms are readily seen in the giant cells

pressure 120/80. The right pupil did not react to light. There were several dry, crusting lesions of the upper lip, the left cheek, the neck and the arms. At the left lung base, there was dullness to percussion with a few crepitant rales. Lumbar puncture showed slightly cloudy fluid with 234 cells, 80% polymorphonuclear cells, sugar 34 mg/%, protein 274 mg/%. The pus from the face showed *C. immitis* in wet mount and culture. His condition rapidly deteriorated and he died at 1:05 P.M. December 24, 1956.

Autopsy showed several skin lesions similar to those described clinically. Fluid was present in the abdomen, in both pleural cavities, and in the pericardial sac. The right lung weighed 1250 g, the left lung, 1040 g. There was an abscess in the left lower lobe. Both lungs were uniformly studded with small hard nodules. Hilar nodes were enlarged with creamy pus. The spleen showed several light-colored nodules, 0.3—0.5 cm in diameter. The brain weighed 1250 g and was edematous, with thickening of the meninges. There were several paravertebral abscesses (Figs. 21, 30). Sections showed granulomatous meningitis, microabscesses of liver, spleen and kidneys, a granuloma of the pancreas, miliary lesions in the thyroid (Fig. 31), in addition to caseous pneumonia and miliary granuloma-abscess complexes in the lung.

Case No. 7. (Case A 28 of HUNTINGTON et al., 1967b) (Figs. 32—34).

This 63-year-old Negro woman was seen in the Kern County General Hospital Out-patient Clinic on July 8, 1948, with the complaint of chest pain and productive cough. She was admitted to the In-patient-Service on August 20, 1948, with complaints of fever, malaise, and headache. Examination showed nuchal rigidity. Hemogram showed hemoglobin 9.9 g, red cell count 3,100,000, white cell count 6,300, with 64% segmented neutrophiles, 32% lymphocytes, and 4% eosinophiles. Coccidioidin skin test was positive; Mantoux was negative. Sputa failed to reveal either tubercle bacilli or *Coccidioides*. Spinal fluid showed 1,060 white cells, 76%

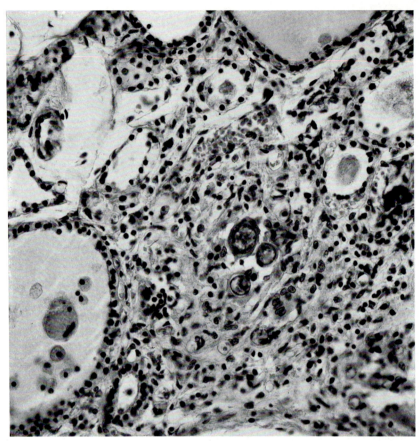

Fig. 31. Focus of coccidioidomycosis in thyroid gland with granulomatous inflammatory response. Case 6. H & E, × 300

lymphocytes, protein 129 mg/%, sugar 55 mg/%, colloidal gold 3344554320. Spinal fluid yielded no growth or culture. On September 13 blood and spinal fluid were sent for coccidioidal serologic studies. Serum precipitin was 4+; serum complement fixation was 4+ in 1:4 dilution, 3+ in 1:8, 2+ in 1:16, 1+ in 1:32, negative in 1:64. Spinal fluid complement fixation showed 3+ fixation in 1:2 dilution, 1+ in 1:4, 0+ in 1:8, negative in 1:16. Further specimens were taken on October 28. The serum still showed 4+ precipitin. Serum complement fixation was 4+ at 1:4 dilution, 3+ at 1:8, 0+ at 1:16, negative at 1:32. Spinal fluid showed 4+ fixation at 1:2 and 1:4 dilutions, 3+ at 1:8, 1+ at 1:16, negative at 1:32. Almost identical results were obtained one month later.

Chest film on July 8, 1948, had shown fibrosis in the right lower lung field.

The patient ran a progressive downhill course. On November 26, she was described as semicomatose; she remained in this state until her death on December 18, 1948.

Autopsy by Dr. J. D. KIRSCHBAUM revealed the body of a cachectic aged Negro female, with numerous decubitus ulcers. The right pleural cavity was obliterated by fibrous adhesions. In the right upper lobe was a firm node, 20 mm in diameter. Hilar lymph nodes were grayish black and mottled. The meninges were thickened and there was a plaque over the pons.

Microscopic examination showed fibrosis and caseation in the lung (Figs. 32, 33), and granulomatous meningitis (Fig. 34).

Case No. 8. (Case D 7 of HUNTINGTON et al., 1967b).

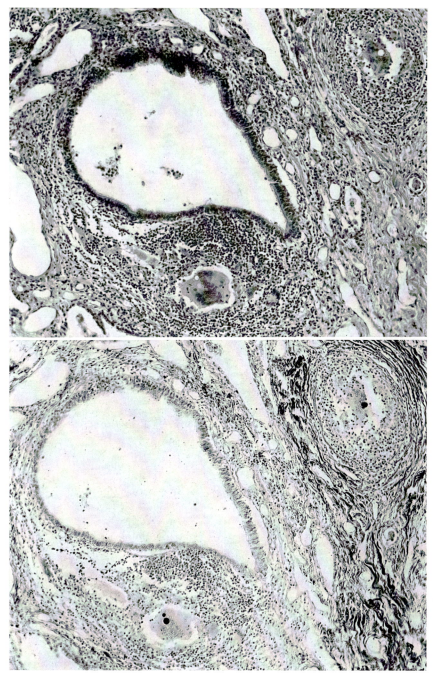

Fig. 32. Peribronchiolar coccidioidomycosis. Above and to the right lies an abscess with an organism of *C. immitis* in a giant cell. Below the bronchiole lies a lymphoid nodule containing two giant cells. Case 7. H & E, × 125

Fig. 33. Peribronchiolar coccidioidomycosis. Same field as in Fig. 32, but stained to display the organisms. Case 7. Grocott-Gomori, × 125

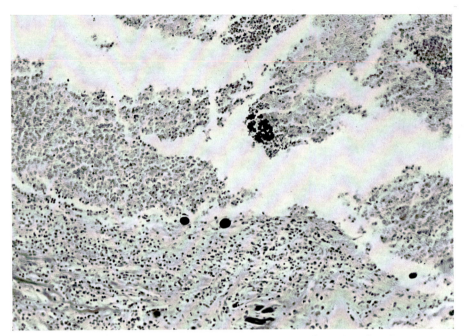

Fig. 34. Case 7. Coccidioidal meningitis. Above it necrotic pus with much nuclear fragmentation of the polymorphonuclear neutrophils and below round cells (lymphocytes and macrophages) and fibrosis. The organisms are present in various regions. Grocott-Gomori, × 125

This Negro woman, born in 1892, had been followed at Kern County General Hospital since 1947 for left upper lung cavity and diabetes. Coccidioidal complement fixation was positive up to 1:32 dilution; repeated sputa had failed to reveal tubercle bacilli. She had several admissions with hemoptysis, but persistently refused surgery. She had massive hemorrhage and died on March 6, 1952.

Autopsy showed a rather obese Negro female, length 62 inches, weight estimated at 170 pounds. The right lung weighed 420 g, and was moderately congested. The left lung weighed 410 g. It had a large cavity in the upper lobe, with considerable blood in the cavity and the bronchial tree. The stomach contained large amounts of blood which was thought to have been swallowed.

Sections showed large pulmonary arteries adjoining the cavity. The reaction at the edge of the cavity was of a nondescript granulomatous pattern. Mycelial forms and spherules were present. Culture showed *C. immitis*, which reverted to spherular form on guinea pig inoculation.

Case No. 9. (Not included in Huntington et al., 1967b) (Figs. 3, 22).

This 57-year-old Filipino male came to Kern County General Hospital November 7, 1967, with a history of fever, cough, and bloody sputum for three days. He had been treated with penicillin. X-ray showed a pneumonic process in the right upper lobe. Serum showed neither coccidioidal precipitin nor coccidioidal complement fixing antibody. Coccidioidin and Mantoux tests were negative. Nine days later, coccidioidal precipitin was present; complement fixation was 4+ in 1:4 dilution, 1+ in 1:8. Spinal fluid was unremarkable. He was given a small amount of amphotericin, but died at 6:55 A.M. November 19. Sputum culture was reported positive for *C. immitis* on the day of death.

At *autopsy* the body was that of an unmistakably Filipino male, length 63 inches, weight estimated at 135 pounds. There were no skin lesions.

The right lung weighed 1200 g and the left lung, 950 g. There was extensive consolidation of both lungs. The consolidation was homogenously light-colored in

some areas; elsewhere there were firm, light-colored nodules, 0.2—0.8 cm in diameter, against a background of reddish, compressible lung. There was softening
and beginning excavation of a large portion of the right upper lobe, approximately
5.0 cm in diameter (Fig. 3), and there was thickening of the right upper lobe pleura.
Wet mount from this area of softening showed numerous sporangia; culture
revealed typical *C. immitis* (Fig. 22). The brain weighed 1480 g; it was diffusely
edematous, without focal lesions and without meningeal thickening.

Microscopic study confirmed the absence of meningitis. The liver showed a few
microabscesses. A single microabscess, surrounded by epithelial cells, was found
in the spleen. The lung sections showed fibrosis, granulomas, and abscesses with
numerous *C. immitis* spherules. Angiitis was striking and there were numerous
eosinophiles.

Although this man did have a few tiny scattered metapulmonary lesions, his
death was due to his fulminant pulmonary coccidioidomycosis. The cutaneous
anergy was to be expected; the low levels of serum antibody were somewhat more
unusual.

Case No. 10. (Not included in HUNTINGTON et al., 1967b).

This case did not end fatally. It is involved in major litigation, both in the area
of industrial compensation (LEVAN, 1954) and in that of medical malpractice. It
presents several points of considerable importance.

This 60-year-old white, heavy equipment operator returned from the Marianas Islands
in the spring of 1965 and went to work on the California Aqueduct Project at Lost Hills, California. On October 6, 1965, he consulted a physician on account of weakness and nausea. He
was told that he had either dust pneumonia or "Valley Fever." After two months he was allowed
to return to work. However, his cough persisted. He was said to have had a negative coccidioidin skin test (dilution not stated) in April of 1966. Shortly thereafter he went to Costa Mesa,
and was admitted to a hospital in Long Beach. On thoracotomy, though on rapid frozen section
the pathologist reported "granuloma," the surgeon felt that the left lung looked neoplastic and
did a total left pneumonectomy.

The writer reviewed the pathologic material at the request of counsel for one
of the industrial compensation carriers. A section marked "left upper lobe"
showed nondescript scarring. Five other sections, including one marked "left lower
lobe," showed small and large aggregates of epithelioid and giant cells, surrounded
by small lymphocytes and fibrous tissue. The large masses had central caseation.
Culture had been reported as positive for *C. immitis*, and numerous typical spherules and sporangia were found on methenamine silver stained sections. There was
encroachment on and damage to bronchi, with beginning diffuse bronchiectasis.
The writer's diagnosis was active progressive coccidioidal infection of the lung,
with a granulomatous pattern, bronchial spread, and beginning bronchiectasis.

The diagnosis of coccidioidomycosis was not at issue, nor was its connection
with the subject's employment at a dusty job in a highly endemic area. He had
worked for several employers, and the question was, whose industrial compensation
carrier was responsible for paying the award. The question of the relation of the
October 1965 episode to subsequent events was of interest, and the date of the
coccidioidal infection. The writer felt that too much attention had been paid to the
negative skin test in April, 1966, and to the alleged clearing of the pneumonitis
in October, 1965, that it was quite likely that the coccidioidal infection had been
present ever since that date, and that the infection could hardly have been less
than two months old at the time of pneumonectomy. The case strikingly illustrates
Salkin's thesis of continued activity.

Case No. 11. (Not included in HUNTINGTON et al., 1967) (Figs. 35, 36).

This man was treated for pulmonary tuberculosis at Kern County General Hospital in
1951 and 1952. In July, 1952, the Mantoux test was 2+, and the coccidioidin negative at both

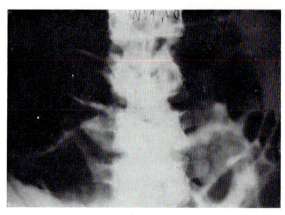

Fig. 35. Coccidioidal osteomyelitis of spine and iliac crests. Case 11

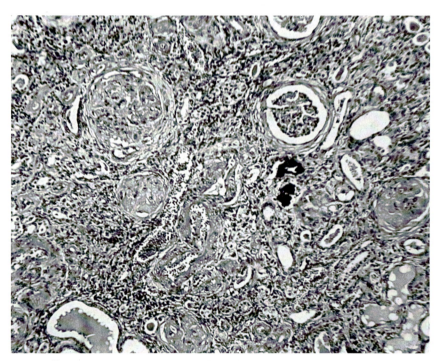

Fig. 36. Chronic interstitial nephritis, evidently due to amphotericin B therapy. Case 11

1:100 and 1:10 dilutions. Coccidioidal serologies were negative. Pleural fluid showed tubercle bacilli on culture. He received PAS and dihydrostreptomycin. A lobectomy (right middle lobe) was performed on June 27, 1953. Reexamination of tissue blocks in 1967 showed a few acid fast bacilli, no spherules. Streptomycin was continued through October, 1954.

On September 18, 1959, he was seen by a thoracic surgeon, who found a fresh pneumonic infiltrate and evidence of disseminated coccidioidomycosis. Since he had moved to Kings County, he was referred to Dr. Winn at Springville. His clinical course was characterized by a series of abscesses. He had destructive lesions of the lumbar vertebrae and the iliac crest (Fig. 36). His serum complement fixation titre remained high. Although he never showed spinal fluid pleocytosis, at one time he did have a positive spinal fluid complement fixation test and an increase in cerebral spinal fluid protein. On May 3, 1965, his total amphotericin was said to have been 11,870 mg. There was progressive evidence of renal failure. In 1967 he shuttled between Springville and Kern County General Hospital, telling neither about what the other was doing. On his last admission at Springville, he had peritoneal dialysis. He was brought to Kern County General Hospital by ambulance on September 20, 1967. At that time he was semicomatose. Blood pressure was 240/120, urine showed 4+ albumen. BUN was 138, creatinine 23.0, uric acid 17.0, calcium 8.5, phosphorus 8.4, potassium 7.9. His condition steadily deteriorated, and he died at 10:15 A.M. September 23, 1967.

At *autopsy* there was no meningitis. An abscess in the groin yielded thick pus, which was negative on wet mount but grew *Coccidioides* on culture. Each kidney weighed 60 g. The pelves and ureters were not dilated. The kidneys were shrunken and pale, with punctate hemorrhages. On microscopic examination the groin lesion was largely granulomatous and caseous, though there were microabscesses. Grocott stain showed moderate numbers of *C. immitis* spherules and a few structures which appeared to be mycelial. Sections of kidney showed extensive interstitial fibrosis with dilatation and distortion of the few remaining tubules (Fig. 35). Some of these tubules had hyaline material in their lumina. Scattered throughout the sections were bits of interstitial and intralobular blue-staining material, presumably calcium. There were very few normal glomeruli. Of the glomeruli present, some were moderately cellular with thickening of Bowman's capsule and often with adhesions or crescents; others showed all stages of hyalinization. The lungs showed fluid and fibrin in the alveoli, with a scattering of polymorphonuclear cells.

In reviewing this case, one wonders whether the subject had ever had coccidioidal meningitis. There was no evidence of meningitis at necropsy. The continued series of abscesses under amphotericin treatment emphasizes that amphotericin is a fungostatic rather than a fungocidal drug. Without some concomitant host resistance, its efficacy is limited. The course and the morphologic changes in the kidney indicate that the fatal nephropathy must be ascribed to amphotericin.

VIII. Demonstration of Coccidioides in Tissue Sections

As the writer has tried to make clear, it is all too easy to miss coccidioidomycosis when it is present, and to proclaim it when it is not. He has recorded many errors of both kinds in this hospital during the past 18 years, and in many instances he has been a full-co-errer. The uses and limitations of the various laboratory aids to the diagnosis of coccidioidomycosis have been discussed in an earlier section. The demonstration of *Coccidioides* in stained sections of fixed tissue has been reserved for this final section. Such emphasis seems appropriate for a number of reasons. While skin tests, antibody determinations, wet mounts and cultures are clinical pathology or clinical microbiology, tissue staining techniques and the study of the stained sections are in the strictest sense pathologic anatomy. Even when the diagnosis of active coccidioidomycosis has already been amply confirmed by the demonstration of serum antibody and by positive culture, the pathologic anatomist who receives relevant tissue will hardly be satisfied until he has completed appropriate attempts to observe and identify the fungus in tissue sections, and to relate it to the cellular response. If the suggestion of coccidioidomycosis has come too late to permit serologic and cultural study and nothing but fixed tissue is left, the pathologic anatomist may still be able to establish the diagnosis by appropriate study of tissue sections. If all the lesions are old and inactive, antibodies will probably not be demonstrable, and cultures will probably be negative, and demonstration of coccidioides in tissue sections will be the only way to identify the etiology of the lesions.

Even when *Coccidioides* is readily recognized in sections stained with hema-toxylin-eosin, or other routine stains, special stains will usually give a much more adequate notion of the number, form, and distribution of the organisms present. If the organisms are scarce or a little atypical, or if there is polymorphonuclear reaction, liquefaction, caseation, or calcification, special stains are not optional but essential. Indeed, one should not accept or record failure to find fungi in tissue sections without study by special stains.

Special stains which have been widely used include the Gridley (Gridley, 1953), the Hotchkiss-McManus periodic acid-Schiff (Kligman et al., 1951) and the Grocott-Gomori methenamine silver (Grocott, 1955). They are basically stains for insoluble but oxidizable polysaccharide (Wheat et al., 1967). Thus they are not specific for fungi in even the limited sense in which the Ziehl-Neelsen stain may be termed specific for *Mycobacteria*. Nevertheless, they are extremely useful. A choice between them is in large part a matter of personal preference. We have found the Grocott-Gomori procedure the most consistently useful, though it lacks the esthetic polychromy of the PAS. The methenamine silver and PAS are less satisfactory than H & E for study of host cellular response, and we have therefore found it desirable to stain the first section with H & E and the next with methen-amine silver (Figs. 5, 6, 12, 13, 16—19, 27, 29, 32, 33).

In searching for fungi in Grocott-Gomori stained sections, one must be familiar with nonfungal tissue structures which take the stain. These include mucus drop-lets, glycogen granules, corpora amylacea of the brain, some fibrillar components of connective tissue and cross striations of voluntary muscle. Unstained anthracotic dust may look a good deal like methenamine silver stained particulate polysac-charide. "Calcospheres" in our experience, have not taken the methenamine silver stain.

It is important to be aware of the morphology of the fungus which one is seek-ing. For specific identification of *Coccidioides*, it is important to search for mature sporangia with endospores. These are sometimes numerous. However, at other times, even with infection of apparently maximal activity, it may be difficult or impossible to find mature sporangia in tissue sections. When scarce, they should be sought in both H & E and methenamine silver stained sections. Endospores which stain too faintly to be recognized with H & E may sometimes be obvious with Grocott-Gomori. On the other hand, sometimes the sporangium stains so deeply and diffusely with Grocott-Gomori that the endospores cannot be distin-guished; at other times, the wall of the old sporangium stains only faintly with methenamine silver. Quite frequently, one observes aggregations of what appear to be very young spherules or endospores with nothing left of the wall of the old sporangium. A hasty observer might confuse a clump of this character with a clump of yeast bodies of *Histoplasma capsulatum*. Endosporulation, therefore, should not be recorded unless at least a portion of the wall of the parent sporan-gium can be identified.

Although *endosporulation*, when found, is characteristic and diagnostic, after a great deal of time spent in the study of *Coccidioides* in infected tissue, the writer is unable to exclude the possibility of binary fission or of other alternative modes of reproduction. His hesitation is reinforced by the reported studies on mainten-ance of the spherular phase of coccidioides *in vitro* (Converse, 1956, 1957; Lubarsky and Plunkett, 1955b; Breslau and Kubota, 1964). In any case, it is essential to recognize that failure to find mature sporangia, or the finding of pairs which look as though they might have budded, or of other odd patterns, are quite common in sections of coccidioidal tissue and do not argue seriously against the identification of a spherular tissue fungus as *C. immitis* (DE LAMATER and WEED, 1946; CREITZ, 1956).

Although Kern County is not endemic terrain for *Histoplasma capsulatum*, it is full of emigrants from histoplasmal areas, and inactive histoplasmal lesions are common on our autopsy service (STRAUB and SCHWARZ, 1956). The writer is particularly grateful to Dr. J. SCHWARZ for guidance with recognition of *Histoplasma capsulatum* (personal communication). He would certainly not diagnose histoplasmosis merely from dots of Grocott-positive material, for similar dots can be found in tissue containing unmistakable *Coccidioides* spherules. However, the typical uniform, small yeast-like bodies of *Histoplasma* are readily recognized. The larger, deeper-staining, more variegated spherules of *C. immitis*, with or without endosporulating sporangia, will not be confused with typical *Histoplasma* bodies. In the North American blastomycosis material supplied by kind friends, the organisms have been more thin-walled than those of *Coccidioides*, and unequivocal budding pairs have been numerous. The writer regrets that he has had no opportunity to study sections of South American blastomycosis. Since this infection was distinguished from coccidioidomycosis only after much work by mycologists (DE ALMEIDA, 1930a, b, 1932), one would suspect that tissue sections of the two diseases might still prove confusing to the casual observer.

Although failure to find endosporulation in tissue sections certainly does not rule out coccidioidomycosis, the complementary question, whether and when, in the absence of other evidence, coccidioidomycosis can safely and assuredly be diagnosed from tissue sections which do not show endosporulation, is a difficult one. In order to begin to formulate a general answer to this question, the writer would need to amplify greatly his experience with other spherular fungi. Perhaps, in any event, the only appropriate answers would be specific and relative. Thus, if the diagnosis of coccidioidomycosis under such circumstances were to involve acceptance of a previously unrecognized endemic area, one would hesitate a good deal. On the other hand, if the subject had known coccidioidal lesions elsewhere in his body, or even a known opportunity for exposure to *Coccidioides*, one would have fewer misgivings.

Mycelial Phase — C. Immitis in Tissue

This has been recognized in the skin in a case of primary cutaneous inoculation (LEVAN and HUNTINGTON, 1965), and in a number of cases of pulmonary cavitation (FIESE et al., 1955; PUCKETT, 1954) (Fig. 10). We have embedded and stained cultures from Sabouraud's medium and have found that while athrospores stained well with the Grocott stain, hyphae stained rather irregularly. *C. immitis* athrospores by themselves would be rather difficult to recognize in tissue sections, and one could hardly deny the possibility that occurrence of mycelial phase *C. immitis in vivo* might be more common than its recognition. In the cases cited, the tissue yielded pure cultures of *C. immitis*. Since opportunistic saprophytes might have been expected to outgrow *Coccidioides*, the results of cultures corroborated the identification of mycelial *C. immitis* in the sections. One of the more critical of the writer's mycologist colleagues (BIDDLE, 1953), believes that she can safely identify mycelial phase *C. immitis* in tissue sections without cultural corroboration. Certainly, the rather frequent juxtaposition with spherular phase organisms (HUNTINGTON et al., 1967b) would be helpful and reassuring.

Acknowledgment to Bibliography: Although coccidioidomycosis is a rather "new disease", its literature is already of staggering bulk. Thus, FIESE's 1958 monograph listed 968 references, while the 1965 edition of CHEU's bibliography consisted of 87 mimeographed pages. A student who wishes the latest edition of that bibliography should write to Dr. Stephen Cheu, Veterans' Administration Hospital, Fresno, California. The preparation of a bibliography for the present chapter necessitated rigorous selection and exclusion.

Those wishing further orientation in the literature on coccidioidomycosis might refer to the references to the clinical studies of Winn, to the variegated studies of Smith, and to the latest symposium on coccidioidomycosis (1967b).

References

Abbott, K., Cutler, O.: Chronic coccidioidal meningitis: Review of the literature and report of seven cases. Arch. Path. **21**, 320 (1936). — Absher, W., Cline, F.: A correlated study of tuberculin, histoplasmin, and coccidioidin sensitivities with pulmonary calcifications in the Rocky Mountain area. Amer. Rev. Tuberc. **59**, 643 (1949). — Ajello, L., Reed, R., Maddy, K., Budurin, A., Moore, J.: Ecological and epizootiological studies on canine coccidioidomycosis. J. Amer. vet. med. Ass. **129**, 485 (1956). — Ajello, L.: *Coccidioides immitis*, isolation procedures and diagnostic criteria. Publ. Hlth Rep. (Wash.) **575**, 47 (1957). ~ Comparative ecology of mycotic respiratory disease agents. Bact. Rev. **31**, 6 (1967a). — Ajello, L., editor: Coccidioidomycosis, Proceedings of the Second Coccidioidomycosis Symposium, 414 pages text, 15 pages references. Tuscon (Arizona): University of Arizona Press 1967b. — Albert, B., Sellers, T.: Coccidioidomycosis from fomites. Report of a case and review of the literature. Arch. intern. Med. **112**, 253 (1963). — Allen, A.: Survey of pathologic studies of cutaneous diseases during World War II. Arch. Derm. Syph. (Chic.) **57**, 19 (1948). ~ The skin: A clinicopathological treatise. 2nd edition. New York and London: Grune & Stratton 1967. — Alznauer, R., Rolle, C., Pierce, W.: Analysis of focalized pulmonary granulomas due to *Coccidioides immitis*. Arch. Path. **59**, 641 (1955). — Amromin, G., Blumenfeld, C.: Coccidioidomycosis of the epididymis: A report of two cases. Calif. Med. **78**, 136 (1953). — Anderson, N.: Coccidioidomycosis. Arch. Derm. Syph. (Chic.) **57**, 562 (1948). — Aronson, J., Saylor, R., Parr, E.: Relationship of coccidioidomycosis to calcified pulmonary nodules. Arch. Path. **34**, 31 (1942). — Ashburn, L., Emmons, C.: Spontaneous coccidioidal granuloma in the lungs of wild rodents. Arch. Path. **34**, 791 (1942). — Baker, E., Mrak, E., Smith, C.: The morphology, taxonomy, and distribution of Coccidioides immitis Rixford and Gilchrist 1896. Farlowia **1**, 199 (1943). — Baker, E., Waskow, E.: The treatment of pulmonary coccidioidomycosis associated with diabetes mellitus. Ajello, L., editor: Coccidioidomycosis (See ref. 6), page 127, 1967. — Baker, R.: The classification of fungus infections according to the form of fungus in tissues. Sth. med. J. (Bgham, Ala.) **38**, 272 (1945). ~ Tissue changes in fungus diseases. Amer. J. Path. **22**, 644 (1946). ~ Coccidioidomycosis. In Pathology, W.A.D. Anderson, ed. 5th ed., vol. **1**, p. 310, 1966. C.V. Mosby Co., St. Louis, Mo. — Bass, H.: Coccidioidomycosis and tuberculosis. A diagnostic problem. Tuberculology **7**, 72 (1945). ~ Pulmonary cavitation in coccidioidomycosis. Tuberculology **9**, 80 (1947). — Bass, H., Schomer, A.: Coccidioidomycosis in veterans of World War II. New York St. J. Med. **48**, 1391 (1948). — Bass, H., Schomer, A., Berke, R.: Coccidioidomycosis, persistence of residual pulmonary lesions. Arch. intern. Med. **82**, 519 (1948). ~ Question of contagion in coccidioidomycosis. Study of contacts. Amer. Rev. Tuberc. **59**, 632 (1949). — Baum, G., Schwarz, J.: Coccidioidomycosis, a review. Amer. J. med. Sci. **230**, 82 (1955). — Beadenkopf, W., Loosli, C., Lack, H., Rice, F., Slattery, R.: Tuberculin, coccidioidin, and histoplasmin sensitivity in relation to pulmonary calcifications; a survey among 6,000 students at the University of Chicago. Publ. Hlth Rep. (Was.) **64**, 17 (1949). — Beamer, P.: Immunology of mycotic infections. Amer. J. clin. Path. **25**, 66 (1955). — Beard, H., Richert, J., Taylor, R.: The treatment of deep mycotic infections with amphotericin B, with particular reference to drug toxicity. Amer. Rev. resp. Dis. **81**, 43 (1960). — Beare, W.: Primary pulmonary coccidioidomycosis. Air Surg. Bull. **2**, 397 (1945). — Beck, M.: Epidemiology, coccidioidal granuloma. Spec. Bull. No. 57, Calif. St. Dep. Pub. Hlth. p. 19 (1931a). ~ Diagnostic laboratory procedure, coccidioidal granuloma. Ibid, p. 16 (1931b). — Belanger, W.: Coccidioidomycosis with special reference to persistent coccidioidal cavitation. Harper Hosp. Bull. **5**, 107 (1947). — Bennett, H., Milder, J., Baker, C.: Coccidioidomycosis, possible fomite transmission. J. Lab. clin. Med. **43**, 633 (1954). — Benninghoven, C., Miller, E.: Coccidioidal infection in bone. Radiology **38**, 663 (1942). — Biddle, M.: Coccidioidomycosis, the diagnosis and epidemiology. Univ. South. Calif. med. Bull. **5**, 12 (1953). ~ Personal communication to R.W.H. — Birsner, J., Smart, S.: Osseous coccidioidomycosis, a chronic form of dissemination. Amer. J. Roentgenol. **76**, 1052 (1956). — Breslau, A., Kubota, M.: Continuous *in vitro* cultivation of spherules of Coccidioides immitis. J. Bact. **87**, 468 (1964). — Brown, P.: Report of the 17th and 18th cases of coccidioidal granuloma. Trans. Ass. Amer.

Phycns. **21**, 651 (1906). ~ Coccidioidal granuloma, review of the eighteen cases and reports of cases fiften and sixteen. J. Amer. med. Ass. **48**, 743 (1907). — BROWN, P., CUMMINS, W.: A differential study of coccidioidal granuloma and blastomycoses. Trans. Ass. Amer. Phycns. **29**, 628 (1914). — BUSS, W., GIBSON, T., GIFFORD, M.: Coccidioidomycosis of the meninges. Calif. Med. **72**, 167 (1950). — BUTT, E., HOFFMAN, A.: A study of latent lesions of coccidio-idomycosis correlated with coccidioidin skin tests. Amer. J. Path. **17**, 579 (1941). ~ Healed or arrested pulmonary coccidioidomycosis, correlation of skin testswith autopsy findings. Amer. J. Path. **21**, 485 (1945). — CAMPBELL, C., BINKLEY, G.: Serologic diagnosis with respect to histoplasmosis, coccidioidomycosis, blastomycosis, and the problem of cross infections. J. Lab. clin. Med. **42**, 896 (1953). — CAMPBELL, C.: Cross reactions of mycotic antigens. Proceedings of the Conference on Histoplasmosis. Publ. Hlth. Serv., Monograph No. 39, p. 144 (1956). — CAMPBELL, C., RECA, M., CONOVER, C.: Reactions of histoplasma capsulatum antigens in sera from mammalian species, including man, infected with Coccidioides immitis. AJELLO, L., editor: Coccidioidomycosis, p. 243 (1967b). — CAMPINS, H., SCHARYJ, M., GLUCK, V.: Coccidioidomycosis (Enfermedad de Posadas); su comprobacion en Venezuela. Arch. venez. Pat. trop. **1**, 215 (1949). — CAMPINS, H.: Coccidioidomycosis, un nuevo problema de salud publica en Venezuela. Rev. Sanid. Asist. soc. **15**, 1 (1950). ~ Coccidioidomycosis, Comentarios sobre la casuistica Venezuela. Mycopathologica (Den Haag) **15**, 306 (1961). ~ Coccidioidomycosis in Venezuela. AJELLO, L., editor: Coccidioidomycosis, p. 279 (1967). — CARTER, R.: The roentgen diagnosis of fungus infections of the lungs with special reference to coccidioidomycosis. Radiology **38**, 649 (1942). — CASTLEBERRY, M., CONVERSE, J., FAVERO DEL J.: Coccidioidomycosis transmission to infant monkey from its mother. A case report. Arch. Path. **75**, 459 (1963). — CAWLEY, E., CURTIS, A., LEACH, J.: Is mycosis fungoides a reticuloendothelial neoplastic entity? Arch. Derm. Syph. (Chic) **64**, 255 (1951). — CHENEY, G., DENENHOLZ, E.: Observations on the coccidioidin skin test. Milit. Surg. **96**, 148 (1945). — CHERRY, C., BARTLETT, A.: The diagnosis of acute coccidioides infections. Bull. U.S. Army med. Dep. **5**, 190 (1946). — CHEU, S.: Coccidioidomycosis bibliography, 1965, edition, 87 mimeographed pages. U.S. Veterans Hospital, Fresno, Calif. — CHEU, S., WALDMANN, W.: Unusual complications of ventriculo-atriostomy for communicating hydrocephalus in coc-cidioidal meningitis, a report of five cases with autopsy findings. AJELLO, L., editor: Coccidio-idomycosis, p. 25 (1967b). — CHRISTIAN, J., SARRE, S., PEERS, J., SALAZAAR, E., ROSARIO DE, J.: Pulmonary coccidioidomycosis in a 21-day old infant; report of a case and review of the literature. Amer. J. Dis. Child. **92**, 66 (1956). — CONANT, N.: The status of immunologic tests in the deep mycoses. 4th International Congress of Tropical Medicine and Malaria **2**, 1263 (1948). ~ Medical mycology, Chapter 36. DUBOS-HIRSCH, editors: Bacterial and Mycotic Infections of Man. 4th ed. Philadelphia: Lippincott 1965. — CONVERSE, J.: Effect of physico-chemical environment on spherulation of Coccidioides immitis in a chemically defined medium. J. Bact. **72**, 784 (1956). ~ Effect of surface acting agents on endosporulation of Coccidioides immitis in a chemically defined medium. Ibid. **74**, 106 (1957). — CONVERSE, J., BESEMER, A.: Nutrition of the parasitic phase coccidioides a chemically defined medium. Ibid. **78**, 231 (1959). — CONVERSE, J., REED, R., KULLER, H., TRAUTMAN, R., SNYDER, E., RAY, J.: Experimental epidemiology of coccidioidomycosis: I. Epizootiology of naturally exposed monkeys and dogs. AJELLO, L., editor: Coccidioidomycosis, p. 397 (1967b). — COOKE, J.: Immunity tests in coccidioidal granuloma. Proc. Soc. exp. Biol. (N.Y) **12**, 35 (1914). ~ Immunity tests in coccidioidal granulomas. Arch. intern. Med. **15**, 479 (1915). — COTTON, B.: Present status of coccidioidomycosis. Ann. West. Med. Surg. **3**, 369 (1949). — COTTON, B., BIRSNER, J.: Surgical treatment in pulmonary coccidioidomycosis, preliminary report of thirty cases. J. thorac. Surg. **20**, 429 (1950). — COTTON, B., PENIDO, J., BIRSNER, J., BABCOCK, C.: Coexistent pulmonary coccidioidomycosis and tuberculosis, a review of twenty-four cases. Amer. Rev. Tuberc. **70**, 109 (1954). — COTTON, B., PAULSEN, G., BIRSNER, J.: Surgical considerations of pulmonary coccidioidomycosis, report of 100 cases. Amer. J. Surg. **90**, 101 (1955). — COTTON, B., BIRSNER, J.: Surgical treatment of pulmonary coccidioidomycosis, a ten year study. J. thorac. cardiovasc. Surg. **38**, 435 (1959). — COURVILLE, C.: Primary chronic coccidioidal meningitis, report of a case with extensive subarachnoid infection at base of brain and about spinal cord. Bull. Los Angeles neurol. Soc. **1**, 116 (1936). — COURVILLE, C., ABBOTT, K.: Pathology of coccidioidal granuloma of the central nervous system and its envelopes. Ibid. **3**, 27 (1938). — COX, A., SMITH, C.: Arrested pulmonary coccidioidal granu-loma. Arch. Path. **27**, 717 (1939). — CRAIG, W., DOCKERTY, M.: Coccidioidal granuloma, a brief review with report of a case of meningeal involvement. Minn. Med. **24**, 150 (1941). — CREITZ, J.: Atypical tissue forms of *Coccidioides immitis* resembling blastomyces. Amer. J. clin. Path. **26**, 1254 (1956). — DANCIS, J., NUNEMAKER, J.: Coccidioidal meningitis. Rocky Mtn. med. J. **43**, 639 (1946). — DAVIS, B., SMITH, R., SMITH, C.: An epidemic of coccidioidal infection (Coccidioidomycosis). J. Amer. med. Ass. **118**, 1182 (1942). — DE ALMEIDA, F.: Differences entre l'agent etiologique du granulome coccidioidique des Etats-unis et celui du Bresil, nouveau genre pur le champignon bresilien. C. R. Soc. Biol. (Paris) **105**, 315 (1930a). ~

Estudos comparativos do granuloma coccidioidico nos Estados Unidos e no Brasil, novo genero para o parsito brasileiro. An. Fac. Med. S. Paulo **5**, 125 (1930 b). ~ Considerations sur les genres Coccidioides immitis et pseudo-coccidioides mazzai. C. R. Soc. Biol. (Paris) **110**, 137 (1932). — DE LAMATER, E., WEED, L.: Budding in the tissue phase of the life cycle of Coccidioides immitis, preliminary report. Proc. Mayo Clin. **21**, 505 (1946). — DICKSON, E.: Oidomycosis in California with especial reference to coccidioidal granuloma. Arch. intern. Med. **16**, 1028 (1915). ~ Mimicry of tuberculosis by coccidioidal granuloma. Trans. Ass. Amer. Phycns. **44**, 284 (1929). ~ The etiology and symptomatology of coccidioidal granuloma. Spec. Bull. No. 57, Calif. St. Dep. Publ. Hlth. **8**, 1931. ~ "Valley Fever" of the San Joaquin Valley and fungus Coccidioides. Calif. West. Med. **47**, 151 (1937 a). ~ Coccidioides infection. Arch. intern. Med. **59**, 1029 (1937 b). — DICKSON, E., GIFFORD, M.: Coccidioides infection (Coccidioidomycosis), the primary type of infection. Arch. intern. Med. **62**, 853 (1938). — DICKSON, E.: Coccidioidomycosis, acute or primary. Pac. Coast Med. **6**, 2 (1939 a). ~ Coccidioidomycosis. Proc. 6th Pac. Sci. Cong. **5**, 785 (1939 b). — DROUHET, E.: Coccidioidomycosis d'importation observee en France. Bull. Soc. Path. exot. **54**, 1002 (1961). — DUEMLING, W. W.: Progessive disseminated coccidioidomycosis. Arch. Derm. **60**, 781—789 (1949). — EDWARDS, P., Palmer, C.: Prevalence of sensitivity to coccidioidin, with special reference to specific and non-specific reactions to coccidioidin and histoplasmin. Dis. Chest **31**, 35 (1957). — EGEBERG, R., ELY, A.: Coccidioides immitis in the soil of the southern San Joaquin Valley. Amer. J. med. Sci. **23**, 151 (1956). — EGEBERG, R., ELCONIN, A., EGEBERG, M.: Effect of salinity and temperature on Coccidioides immitis and three antagonistic soil saprophytes. J. Bact. **88**, 473 (1964). — EGEBERG, R.: Dedication in honor of Charles E. SMITH, M. D. AJELLO, L., editor: Coccidioidomycosis, p. ix (1967). — ECKMANN, B., SHAEFFER, G., HUPPERT, M.: Bedside interhuman transmission of coccidioidomycosis via growth on fomites. Amer. Rev. resp. Dis. **89**, 175 (1964). — EINSTEIN, H., HOLEMAN, C., SANDIDGE, L., HOLDEN, D.: Coccidioidal meningitis, the use of amphotericin in treatment. Calif. Med. **94**, 339 (1961). — EINSTEIN, H.: Some aspects of coccidioidomycosis therapy. AJELLO, L., editor: Coccidioidomycosis, p. 123 (1967). ~ Personal communication to R. W. H. — ELCONIN, A., EGEBERG, R., EGEBERG, M.: Significance of soil salinity in the ecology of Coccidioides immitis. J. Bact. **87**, 500 (1964). — EMMONS, C.: Isolation of Coccidioides from soil and rodents. Publ. Hlth. Rep. (Wash.) **57**, 109 (1942 a). — EMMONS, C., ASHBURN, A.: Isolation of Haplosporangium parvum and Coccidioides immitis from wild rodents. Ibid.: 1715. — EMMONS, C.: Coccidioidomycosis. Mycologia **34**, 452 (1942 b). — EMMONS, C., OLSON, B., ELDRIDGE, W.: Studies of the role of fungi in pulmonary disease, cross reactions of histoplasmin. Publ. Hlth. Rep. (Wash.) **60**, 1383 (1945). — EMMONS, C.: Fungi which resemble Coccidioides immitis. AJELLO, L., editor: Coccidioidomycosis, p. 333 (1967). — EVANS, N.: Coccidioidal granuloma and blastomycosis in the central nervous system. J. infect. Dis. **6**, 523 (1909). — EVANS, N., BALL, H.: Coccidioidal granuloma, analysis of fifty cases. J. Amer. med. Ass. **93**, 1881 (1929). — FABER, H., SMITH, C., DICKSON, E.: Acute coccidioidomycosis with erythema nodosum in children. J. Pediat. **15**, 163 (1939). — FALKINBURG, L.: Disseminated coccidioidomycosis, report of a case in the New England area. J. Amer. med. Ass. **150**, 216 (1952). — FARNESS, O., MILLS, C.: Case of fungus infection primary in lung with cavity formation and healing. Bull. Amer. Acad. Tuberc. Phys. **2**, 39 (1938). ~ Coccidioides infection, a case of primary infection in the lung with cavity formation and healing. Amer. Rev. Tuberc. **39**, 266 (1939). — FARNESS, O.: Coccidioidal infection in a dog. J. Amer. vet. med. Ass. **97**, 263 (1940). ~ Coccidioidomycosis. J. Amer. med. Ass. **116**, 1749 (1941). ~ Some unusual aspects of coccidioidomycosis. AJELLO, L., editor: Coccidioidomycosis, p. 23 (1967). — FETTER, B., KLINTWORTH, G., HENDRY, W.: Mycosis of the central nervous system. Baltimore Md.: Williams & Wilkins, 1967. — FIESE, M., CHEU, S., SORENSEN, R.: Mycelial forms of Coccidioides immitis in sputum and tissues of the human host. Ann. intern. Med. **43**, 255 (1955). — FIESE, M.: Treatment of disseminated coccidioidomycosis with amphotericin B, report of a case. Calif. Med. **86**, 119 (1957). ~ Coccidioidomycosis. 188 page text, 968 references. Springfield, Ill.: Charles C. Thomas, 1958. — FINDLAY, F., MELICK, D.: Treatment of cavitary coccidioidomycosis. AJELLO, L., editor: Coccidioidomycosis, p. 79 (1967). — FISCHER, W.: Über Infektion mit Coccidioides immitis. Zbl. allg. Path. path. Anat. **84**, 273—280 (1948). — FORBUS, W., BESTEBREURTJE, A.: Coccidioidomycosis, a study of 95 cases of the disseminated type with special reference to the pathogenesis of the disease. Milit. Surg. **99**, 653 (1946). — FORSEE, J., PERKINS, R.: Focalized pulmonary coccidioidomycosis, a surgical disease. J. Amer. med. Ass. **155**, 1223 (1954). — FRANK, I.: Chronic coccidioidal meningitis, case history. Arizona Med. **5**, 41 (1948). — FRIEDMAN, L., PAPPAGIANIS, D., BERGMAN, R., SMITH, C.: Studies on Coccidioides immitis, morphology and sporulation capacity of forty-seven strains. J. Lab. clin. Med. **42**, 438 (1953). — FRIEDMAN, L., SMITH, C.: Vaccination of mice against Coccidioides immitis. Amer. Rev. Tuberc. **74**, 245 (1956). — FRIEDMAN, L.: Immunological studies on coccidioidomycosis. U.S. Publ. Hlth. Serv. Publ. **575**, 95 (1957). — GARDNER, S.: An unusual infection in the bones of the foot. Calif. Med. **2**, 386 (1904). — GARRISON, F.:

History of Medicine. 4th ed. (reprinted). Philadelphia and London: W.B. SAUNDERS Co., 1961. — GELMAN, D., WEHRLE, P., COWPER, H.: Coccidioidomycosis, Canoga Park, California. CDC Weekly Morbidity and Mortality Rep. 14, 302 (1965). — GIFFORD, M.: San Joaquin fever. Kern County Hlth. Dep. Ann. Rep. 1935/1936, 22 (1936). — GIFFORD, M., BUSS, W., DOUDS, R.: Data on coccidioides fungus infection, Kern County, 1930—36. Kern County Hlth. Dep. Ann. Rep. 1936/1937, 39 (1937). — GIFFORD, M.: Coccidioidomycosis, Kern County. Kern County Hlth. Dep. Ann. Rep. 1938/1939, 73 (1939a). ~ Coccidioidomycosis in Kern County, California. Proc. 6th Pac. Sci. Cong. 5, 791 (1939b). ~ Unpublished observations. — GILTNER, L.: Occurrence of coccidioidal granuloma (Oidomycosis) in cattle. J. Agri. Res. 14, 533 (1918). — GOLDSTEIN, D., LOUIE, S.: Primary pulmonary coccidioidomycosis, report of an epidemic of 75 cases. War Med. (Chic.) 4, 299 (1943). — GOLDSTEIN, D., McDONALD, J.: Primary pulmonary coccidioidomycosis, followup of 75 cases, with ten more cases from an endemic area. J. Amer. med. Ass. 124, 557 (1944). — GONZALEZ-OCHOA, A., ESQUIVEL-MEDINA, E., CACERES, M.: Investigation de la reactividad cutanea a la histoplasmina, tuberculina y occidioidina relacionada con catastro toracico en Yucatan. Rev. Inst. Salubr. Enferm. trop. (Méx.) 9, 55 (1948). — GONZALEZ-OCHOA, A.: The status of fungus diseases in Mexico. STERNBERG, T., and V. NEWCOMER: Therapy of Fungus Diseases, An International Symposium, p. 66. Boston: Little-Brown, 1955. ~ Coccidioidomycosis in Mexico. AJELLO, L., editor: Coccidioidomycosis, p. 293 (1967). — GREAVES, F.: Coccidioidal granuloma with lesions in the small intestine. U.S. nav. med. Bull. 32, 201 (1934). — GREER, S., FORSEE, J., MAHON, H.: The surgical management of pulmonary coccidioidomycosis in focalized lesions (Discussed by O. ABBOT). J. thorac. Surg. 18, 591 (1949a). — GREER, S., CROW, J.: The surgical lesions of pulmonary coccidioidomycosis. Dis. Chest. 16, 336 (1949b). — GRIDLEY, M.: A stain for fungi in tissue sections. Amer. J. clin. Path. 23, 303 (1953). — GRITTI, E., COOK, F., SPENCER, H.: Coccidioidomycosis granuloma of the prostate, a rare manifestation of the disseminated disease. J. Urol. (Baltimore) 89, 249 (1963). — GROCOTT, R.: A stain for fungi in tissue sections and smears using Gomori's methenamine silver nitrate technique. Amer. J. clin. Path. 25, 975 (1955). — HAGELE, A., EVANS, D., LARWOOD, T.: Primary endophthalmic coccidioidomycosis, report of a case of exogenous primary coccidioidomycosis of the eye diagnosed prior to enucleation. AJELLO, L., editor: Coccidioidomycosis, p. 37 (1967). — HAMPSON, C.: Sporulation capacity of Coccidioides immitus affected by cultural conditions. J. Bact. 67, 739 (1954). — HAMPSON, C., LARWOOD, T.: Observations on coccidioidomycosis immunodiffusion tests with clinical correlations. AJELLO, L., editor: Coccidioidomycasis, p. 211 (1967). — HARRELL, E., HONEYCUTT, W.: Coccidioidomycosis, a travelling fungus disease. Arch. Derm. 87, 188 (1963). — HAZEN, E., TAHLER, E.: Complement-fixation tests in histoplasmosis, blastomycosis, and coccidioidomyosis. N.Y. St. Dep. Hlth., Ann. Rep., Div. Labs Res. p. 79 (1948). — HEKTOEN, L.: Systemic blastomycosis and coccidioidal granuloma. J. Amer. med. Ass. 49, 1071 (1907). — HELPER, M., WATTS, F.: Nodular intrathoracic lesions in coccidioidomyc. Milit. Surg. 96, 524 (1945). — HERRERA, J.M.: Parracoccidioid. brasil. Estudio del primer caso observado en Panamá de Blastomicosis sudameric. en su forma cutánea queloideana o Enfermedad de Lobo y propuesta de una variante técnica para la impregnación argéntica del parásito. Arch. Med. Panama 4, 209 (1955). — HIGGINSON, J., HINSHAW, D.: Pulomnary coin lesion. J. Amer. med. Ass. 157, 1607 (1955). — HIPPS, H.: Bone coccidioidomyc., case report, cured by surgery. Southwest. Med. 34, 416 (1953). — HOOD, R.: Coexisting bronchogenic carcinoma and coccidioidomycosis. J. thorac. Surg. 20, 478 (1950). — HUGHES, F., WHITAKER, H., LOWRY, C., POLK, J., FOLEY, J., FOX, J.: Resection for mycotic pulmonary disease. Dis. Chest 25, 334 (1954). — HUNTER, R., MONGAN, E.: Disseminated coccidioidomycosis, treatment with amphotericin B. U.S. armed Forces med. J. 9, 1474 (1958). — HUNTINGTON, R.: Diagnostic and biological implications of the histopathology of coccidioidomyc. U.S. Publ. Hlth. Serv. Publ. 575, 36 (1957), ~ Morphology and racial distribution of fatal coccidioidomycosis, report of a 10 year autopsy series in an endemic area. J. Amer. med. Ass. 169, 115 (1959a). ~ Pathologic and clinical observations on coccidioidomycosis. Wis. med. J. 58, 471 (1959b). — HUNTINGTON, R., MOE, T., JOSLIN, E., WYBEL, R.: Amphotericin B nephropathy. AJELLO, L., editor: Coccidioidomycosis, p. 135 (1967a). — HUNTINGTON, R., WALDMANN, W., SARGENT, J., O'CONNELL, H., WYBEL, R., CROLL, D.: Pathologic and clinical observations on 142 cases of fatal coccidioidomycosis with necropsy. Ibid: 143 (1967b). — HUNTINGTON, R.: Charles Edward Smith, Coccidioidomycologist. To be published. Dis. Chest. 1968a. — HUNTINGTON, R.: William A. Winn, Reflections about a great clinician and scholar and a good friend. Ibid. 1968b. ~ Unpublished observations. — HUPPERT, M., SUN, S., BAILEY, J.: Natural variability in Coccidioides immitis. AJELLO, L., editor: Coccidioidomycosis, p. 323 (1967). — HYATT, H.: Coccidioidomycosis in a three week old infant. Amer. J. Dis. Child. 105, 93 (1963). — HYDE, L.: Recurrence of coccidioidal cavity following resectional surgery. Amer. Rev. Tuberc. 71, 131 (1955). ~ Coccidioidal pulmonary cavitation. Amer. J. Med. 25, 890 (1958). — IGER, M., LARSON, J.: Coccidioidal osteomyelitis. AJELLO, L., editor: Coccidioidomycosis, p. 89 (1967). — INGHAM,

S.: Coccidioidal granuloma of the spine with compression of the spinal cord. Bull. Los Angeles neurol. Soc. **1**, 41 (1936). — Iovine, G., Berman, L., Halikis, D., Mowrey, F., Chappelle, E., Gierson, H.: Nephrotoxicity of amphotericin B. Arch. intern. Med. **112**, 853 (1963). — Izenstark, J.: Modern travel and coccidioidomycosis. Sth. med. J. (Bgham, Ala.) **56**, 745 (1963). — Jenkins, V., Postlethwaite, J.: Coccidioidal meningitis, report of four cases with necropsy findings in three cases. Ann. intern. Med. **35**, 1068 (1951). — Joffe, B.: An epidemic of coccidioidomycosis probably related to soil. New Engl. J. Med. **262**, 720 (1960). — Johnson, J. (Fort Dietrich), Perry, J., Kekety, F., Kadull, P., Cluff, L.: Laboratory-acquired coccidioidomycosis. A report of 210 cases. Ann. intern. Med. **60**, 941 (1964). — Johnson, J. (Bakersfield): Unpublished observations. — Kaden, R.: Die Coccidioidomykose (Granuloma coccidioides, Granuloma coccidioidale, Talfieber, Wüstenrheumatismus, San Joaquin-Fieber, Posada-Wernicke-Krankheit). Hdb. Haut- und Geschlkrankh. von J. Jadassohn, Bd. 4, Teil 4, S. 285—316. Berlin-Göttingen-Heidelberg: Springer: 1963. — Kahn, M.: Primary coccidioidomycosis and concomitant tuberculosis. Amer. Rev. Tuberc. **61**, 887 (1950). — Kaplan, W.: Application of the fluorescent antibody technique to the diagnosis and study of coccidioidomycosis. Ajello, L., editor: Coccidioidomycosis, p. 227 (1967). — Kessel, J.: The coccidioidin skin test. Amer. J. trop. Med. **19**, 199 (1939). ~ Recent observations on Coccidioides immitis. Ibid. **21**, 447 (1941). — Kessel, J., Biddle, M., Tucker, H., Yeaman, A.: The distribution of coccidioidomycosis in Southern California. Calif. Med. **73**, 317 (1950). — Kirshbaum, J.: Disseminated coccidioidomycosis with severe cutaneous manifestations. Illinois med. J. **97**, 157 (1950). — Kligman, A., Mescon, H.: The periodic acid-Schiff stain for the demonstration of fungi in animal tissues. J. Bact. **60**, 415 (1950). — Kligmann, A., Mescon, H., De Lamater, E.: The Hotchkiss-McManus stain for the histopathologic diagnosis of fungus diseases. Amer. J. clin. Path. **21**, 86 (1951). — Klotz, L., Biddle, M.: Coccidioidal skin test survey of San Fernando Valley State College students over a five year period. Ajello, L., editor: Coccidioidomycosis, p. 251 (1967). — Kong, Y., Levine, H.: Experimental induced immunity in the mycoses. Bact. Rev. **31**, 35 (1967). — Krapin, D., Lovelock, F.: Recurrence of coccidioidal cavities following lobectomy for a bleeding focus. Amer. Rev. Tuberc. **58**, 282 (1948). — Kritzer, M., Biddle, M., Kessel, J.: An outbreak of primary pulmonary coccidioidomycosis in Los Angeles County, California. Ann. intern. Med. **33**, 960 (1950). — Kruse, R.: Potential aerogenic laboratory hazards of Coccidioides immitis. Amer. J. clin. Path. **37**, 150 (1962). — Kruse, R., Green, T., Leeder, W.: Infection of control monkeys with Coccidioides immitis by caging with inoculated monkeys. Ajello, L., editor: Coccidioidomycosis, p. 387 (1967). — Lamphier, T.: Localized coccidioidal osteomyelitis. New Engl. J. Med. **238**, 150 (1948). — Landay, M., Wheat, R., Conant, N., Lowe, E., Converse, J.: Studies on the comparative serology of the spherular and arthrospore growth forms of Coccidioides immitis. Ajello, L., editor: Coccidioidomycosis, p. 233 (1967). — Larson, R., Scherb, R.: Coccidioidal pericarditis. Circulation **7**, 211 (1953). — Larwood, T.: Maternal fetal transmission of coccidioidomycosis. Trans. 7th Ann. VA-Armed Forces Study Group, p. 28 (1962). — Lee, R., Nixon, N., Jamison, H.: Syllabus on coccidioidomycosis. Coccidioidomycosis Control Program for the A.A.F.W. F.T.C. Prepared by Headquarters, Army Air Forces Western Training Command, Office of the Surgeon, Santa Ana, California, 1942 (Various editions, 1942—1944). — Lee, R.: Coccidioidomycosis in the Western Flying Training Command. Calif. west. Med. **61**, 133 (1944). — Levan, N.: Occupational aspects of coccidioidomycosis. Calif. Med. **80**, 294 (1954). — Levan, N., Burger, C.: Coccidioidomycosis in dogs, a report of three cases. Calif. Med. **83**, 379 (1955). — Levan, N., Huntington, R.: Primary cutaneous coccidioidomycosis of agricultural workers. Arch. Derm. **92**, 215 (1965). — Levine, H., Smith, C.: The reactions of eight volunteers injected with Coccidioides immitis spherule vaccine, first human trials. Ajello, L., editor: Coccidioidomycosis, p. 197 (1967). — Lewis, G., Hopper, M., Wilson, J., Plunkett, O.: An introduction to medial mycology. 4th ed., Yearbook Medical Publishers, Chicago, 1956. — Lipschultz, B., Liston, H.: Steroid-induced disseminated coccidioidomycosis, report of two cases. Dis. Chest **46**, 355 (1964). — Littman, M.: Preliminary observations on the use of amphotericin B, an antifungal antibiotic, in the therapy of acute and chronic coccidioidal osteomyelitis. U.S. Publ. Hlth. Serv. Publ. **575**, 85 (1957). — Littman, M., Horowitz, P., Swadey, J.: Coccidioidomycosis and its treatment with amphotericin. Amer. J. Med. **24**, 568 (1958). — Locks, M., Hawkins, J.: Ventriculo-atriostomy in coccidioidal meningitis. Amer. Rev. resp. Dis. **88**, 33 (1963). — Loosli, C., Beadenkopf, W., Rice, F., Savage, L.: Epidemiologic aspects of histoplasmin, tuberculin, and coccidioidin sensitivity. Amer. J. Hyg. **53**, 33 (1951). — Louria, D., Feder, N., Emmons, C.: Viability of tissue phase of Coccidioides immitis. U.S. Publ. Hlth. Serv. Publ. **575**, 25 (1957). — Louria, D.: Deep seated mycotic infections, allergy to fungi and mycotoxins. New Engl. J. Med. **277**, 1065 (1967). — Lowbeer, L.: Report of a case of coccidioidomycotic meningitis. Proc. Hillcrest Mem'l Hosp. **6**, 106 (1949). — Lowe, E., Sinski, J., Huppert, M., Ray, J.: Coccidioidin skin tests and serologic reactions in immunized and reinfected monkeys. Ajello, L., editor:

Coccidioidomycosis, p. 171 (1967). — LUBARSKY, R., Plunkett, O.: Some ecologic studies of coccidioidomycosis in soil. STERNBERG, T., and V. NEWCOMER: Therapy of Fungus Diseases, p. 308. Boston: Little-Brown, 1955a. ~ In vitro production of the spherule phase of *Coccidioides immitis*. J. Bact. **70**, 182 (1955b). — MADDY, K.: A study of one hundred cases of disseminated coccidioidomycosis in the dog. U.S. Publ. Hlth. Serv. Publ. **575**, 107 (1957). ~ Ecological factors possibly related to the geographical distribution of Coccidioides immitis. Ibid. 144. ~ The geographical distribution of Coccidioides immitis and possible ecological implications. Arizona Med. **15**, 178 (1958). ~ Observations on Coccidioides immitis found naturally growing in soil. Ibid. **22**, 281 (1965). — MADDY, K., CRECELIUS, H.: Establishment of Coccidioides immitis in negative soil following burial of infected animals and animal tissues. AJELLO, L., editor: Coccidioidomycosis, p. 309 (1967). — MALONEY, P.: Addison's disease due to chronic disseminated coccidioidomycosis. Arch. intern. Med. **90**, 869 (1952). — MARKS, T., SPENCE, W., BAISCH, B.: Limited resection for pulmonary coccidioidomycosis. AJELLO, L., editor: Coccidioidomycosis, p. 73 (1967). — MAYORGA, R.: Coccidioidomycosis in Central America. Ibid. 287 (1967). — McDOUGAL, T., KLEINMAN, A.: Prostatitis due to Coccidioides immitis. J. Urol. (Baltimore) **49**, 472 (1943). — McLAUGHLIN, F.: Coccidioidal infection. Bull. U.S. Army med. Dep. **8**, 124 (1948). — McMASTER, P., GILFILAN, C.: Coccidioidal osteomyelitis. J. Amer. med. Ass. **112**, 1233 (1939). — MEIS, P., LARWOOD, T., WINN, W.: Coccidioidal peritonitis. AJELLO, L., editor: Coccidioidomycosis, p. 85 (1967). — MELICK, D.: Surgical treatment of pulmonary coccidioidomycosis. Arizona Med. **6**, 24 (1949). ~ Excisional surgery in pulmonary coccidioidomycosis. J. thorac. Surg. **20**. 66 (1950). ~ Treatment of pulmonary coccidioidomycosis from a surgical standpoint. U.S. Publ. Hlth. Serv. Publ. **575**, 69 (1957). — MENDENHALL, J., BLACK, W., POTTZ, G.: Progressive (disseminated) coccidioidomycosis during pregnancy. Rocky Mtn. med. J. **45**, 472 (1948). — MIDDLEBROOK, G.: The mycobacteria. Dubos-Hirsch: Bacterial and Mycotic Infections of Man, chapter 21. 4th ed., Philadelphia: Lippincott, 1965. — MILLER, D., BIRSNER, J.: Coccidioidal granuloma of bone. Amer. J. Roentgenol. **62**, 229 (1949). — MILLS, C., FARNESS, O.: Coccidioides immitis infection in Southern Arizona. Trans. Amer. clin. climat. Ass. **56**, 147 (1941). — MONTGOMERY, D.: A disease caused by a fungus, the Protozoic dermatitis of Rixford and Gilchrist. Brit. J. Derm. **12**, 343 (1900). — MONTGOMERY, D., RYFKOGEL, H., MORROW, H.: Dermatitis coccidioides. J. cutan. Dis. **21**, 5 (1903). — MONTGOMERY, D., MORROW, H.: Reasons for considering dermatitis coccidioides an independent disease. J. cutan. Dis. **22**, 368 (1904). — MOORE, M.: Mycotic granuloma and cutaneous tuberculosis, a comparison of the histopathologic response. J. invest. Derm. **6**, 149 (1945). — MÜLLER, E., SCHALTENBRAND, G.: Coccidioidose der Meningen. Nervenarzt **19**, 327—333 (1948). — NABARRO, J.D.N.: Primary pulmonary coccidioidomycosis. Case of laboratory infection in England. Lancet I: 1948, 982—984. — NEGRONI, P.: The status of fungus diseases in Argentina. STERNBERG, T., and V. NEWCOMER: Therapy of Fungus Diseases, an International Symposium, p. 44. Boston: Little-Brown, 1955. ~ Coccidioidomycosis in Argentina. AJELLO, L., editor: Coccidioidomycosis, p. 273 (1967). — NORMAN, I., LAWLER, A.: Coccidioidomycosis, review of the literature and report of 9 cases. U.S. nav. med. Bull. **49**, 1005 (1949). — O'LEARY, D., CURRY, F.: Coccidioidomycosis, a review and presentation of 100 consecutively hospitalized patients. Amer. Rev. Tuberc. **73**, 501 (1956). — OPHULS, W., MOFFITT, H.: A new pathogenic mould (formerly described as a protozoon: Coccidioides immitis pyogenes), preliminary report. Philad. Med. J. **5**, 1471 (1900). — OPHULS, W.: Coccidioidal granuloma. J. Amer. med. Ass. **45**, 1291 (1905). ~ Further observations on a pathogenetic mould formerly described as a protozoon (Coccidioides immitis, Coccidioides pyogenes). J. exp. Med. **6**, 443 (1905b). ~ In discussion of paper by Evans and Ball (See ref.). J. Amer. med. Ass. **93**, 1885 (1929). — OWENS, C., PAULSEN, G., DYKES, J.: Coccidioidoma. J. thorac. cardiovasc. Surg. **39**, 545 (1960). — PAGE, E., BOYERS, L.: Coccidioidal pelvic inflammatory disease. Amer. J. Obstet. Gynec. **50**, 212 (1945). — PAPPAGIANIS, D., SMITH, C., KOBAYASHI, G.: Relationship of the in vivo form of Coccidioides immitis to virulence. J. infect. Dis. **98**, 312 (1956). — PAPPAGIANIS, D., SMITH, C., SAITO, M., KOBAYASHI, G.: Preparation and property of a complement fixing antigen from mycelia of Coccidioides immitis. U.S. Publ. Hlth. Serv. Publ. **575**, 57 (1957). — PAPPAGIANIS, D., LEVINE, H., SMITH, C.: Further studies on vaccination of human volunteers with killed Coccidioides immitis. AJELLO, L., editor: Coccidioidomycosis, p. 201 (1967). — PAPPAGIANIS, D.: Epidemiological aspects of respiratory mycotic infections. Bact. Rev. **31**, 25 (1967). — PAULSEN, G.: Pulmonary surgery in coccidioidal infection. AJELLO, L., editor: Coccidioidomycosis, p. 69 (1967). — PEERS, R., HOLMAN, E., SMITH, C.: Pulmonary coccidioidal disease. Amer. Rev. Tuberc. **45**, 723 (1942). — PFANNER, E.: Coccidioidomycosis at U.S.M.C. Air Station, Mojave, California. U.S. nav. med. Bull. **46**, 229 (1946). — PILOT, I.: Coccidioidomycosis of bone. Proc. Inst. Med. Chic. **16**, 204 (1946). — PLUNKETT, O., SWATEK, F.: Ecological studies of Coccidioides immitis. U.S. Publ. Hlth. Serv. Publ. **575**, 158 (1957). — POSADAS, A.: Un nuevo caso de micosis fungoides con psorospermias. An. circ. med. Argent. **15**, 585 (1892). ~ Contribucion al estudio de la etiologia de los tumores; psorospermiosis infectante generalizada. Tesis de la Facultad de Medicina de Buenos Aires, 1894. In, POSADAS, A.: Obras Completas, 1928. ~ Ensayo de una neoplasia del hombre producida por un protozoario y transmisible a los animales. An. circ. med. Argent. **20**, 193 (1897). ~ Psorospermiosis infectante generalizada. Comunicacion a la Academia de la Facultad de Medicina de Buenos Aires, 1897 & 1898. In, POSADAS, A.: Obras Completas, 1928. ~ Psorospermias humana y experimental. Trabajos del Primer Conggreso Cientifico Latinoamericano **4**, 703 (1898). ~ Psorosperimiose infectante generalisee. Rev. Chir. Paris **21**, 277 (1900). ~ Obras Completas: Univ. de Buenos Aires, 1928. — POUT, D.D.: Villous atrophy and coccidiosis. Nature (Lond.) **213**, 306—307 (1967). — POWERS, R., STARKS, D.: Acute (primary) coccidioidomycosis; roentgen findings in a group epidemic. Radiology **37**, 448 (1941). — PRCHAL, C.: Coccidioidomycosis of cattle in Arizona. J. Amer. vet. med. Ass. **112**, 461 (1948). ~ Coccidioidomycosis in Arizona cattle. U.S. Publ. Hlth. Serv. Publ. **575**, 105 (1957). — PUCKETT, T.: Hyphae of coccidioides in tissues of the human host. Amer. Rev. Tuberc. **70**, 320 (1954). — RANDOLPH, H., MCMARTIN, H.: Coccidioidomycosis in Phoenix, Arizona. Dis. Chest **13**, 471 (1947). — REED, R.: Diagnosis of disseminated canine coccidioidomycosis. J. Amer. vet. med. Ass. **128**, 196 (1956). — REED, R., SHELDON, J., CONVERSE, J., SEAQUIST, M., DALLDORF, F.: Epidemiology of coccidioidomycosis. II. Pathogenesis of naturally acquired disease in monkeys and dogs. AJELLO, L., editor: Coccidioidomycosis, p. 403 (1967). — REEVES, D., BAISINGER, C.: Primary chronic coccidioidal meningitis, a diagnostic neurosurgical problem. J. Neurosurg. **2**, 269 (1945). — REINGOLD, I.: Myocardial lesions in disseminated coccidioidomycosis. Amer. J. clin. Path. **20**, 1044 (1950). — REISS, F., BUNCKE, C., CAROLINE, L.: Coccidioidomycotic granuloma in New York City. N.Y. J. Med. **54**, 1206 (1954). — REYNOLDS, E., TOMKIEWICA, Z., DAMMIN, G.: The renal lesion related to amphotericin B treatment for coccidioidomycosis. Med. Clin. N. Amer. **47**, 1149 (1963). — RHODEN, A.: Coccidioidal brain abscess. Bull. Los Angeles neurol. Soc. **11**, 80 (1946). — RICH, A.: The pathogenesis of tuberculosis. 2nd ed. Springfield/Ill.: Charles C. Thomas, 1951. — RIFKIN, H., FELDMAN, D., HAWES, L., GORDON, L.: Coexisting tuberculosis and coccidioidomycosis. Arch. intern. Med. **79**, 381 (1947). — RIXFORD, E.: Case for diagnosis presented before the San Francisco Medico-Chirurgical Society, March 5, 1894. Occidental Med. Times **8**, 326 (1894a). ~ A case of protozoic dermatitis. Ibid. 704 (1894b). — RIXFORD, E., GILCHRIST, T.: Two cases of protozoan (coccidioidal) infection of the skin and other organs. Johns Hopk. Hosp. Rep. **1**, 209 (1896). — RIXFORD, E.: Early history of coccidioidal granuloma in California. Calif. St. Dep. Publ. Hlth., Spec. Bull. **57**, 5 (1931). — ROHN, J., DAVILA, J., GIBSON, T.: Urogenital aspects of coccidioidomycosis, review of the literature and report of two cases. J. Urol. (Baltimore) **65**, 660 (1951). — ROSEN, E., BELBER, J.: Coccidioidal meningitis of long duration with necropsy findings. Ann. intern. Med. **34**, 796 (1951). — ROSENBERG, E., DOCKERTY, M., MEYERDING, H.: Coccidioidal arthritis, a report of a case in which the ankles were involved and the condition was unaffected by sulfanilamide and roentgen therapy. Ann. intern. Med. **69**, 238 (1942). — ROSENTHAL, S., ROUTIEN, J.: Contagiousness of coccidioidomycosis. Arch. intern. Med. **80**, 343 (1947). — RUHRMANN, H.: Coccidioidomykose bei einem ehemaligen Kriegsgefangenen der USA. (Coccidioidomycosis in a former prisoner of war in the U.S.A.). Medizinische **39**, 1369 (1955). — RYFKOGEL, H.: Fungus coccidioides. Calif. St. J. Med. **6**, 200 (1908). ~ Coccidioidal meningitis with secondary internal hydrocephalus and death (anaphylactic) following a second injection of Flexner's serum. J. Amer. med. Ass. **55**, 1730 (1910). ~ Coccidioidal granuloma in California. J. Amer. med. Ass. **60**, 308 (1913). — SALKIN, D.: Clinical examples of reinfection in coccidioidomycosis. AJELLO, L., editor: Coccidioidomycosis, p. 11 (1967). — SALKIN, D., BIRSNER, J., TARR, A., JOHNSON, D., BITZER, J.: Roentgen analysis of coccidioidomycosis — pediatric cases in private practice. Ibid., p. 63. — SALVIN, S.: Complement fixation studies in experimental histoplasmosis. Proc. Soc. exp. Biol. (N.Y.) **66**, 342 (1947). ~ The serologic relationships of fungus antigens. J. Lab. clin. Med. **34**, 1096 (1949). ~ Quantitative studies on the serological relationships of fungi. J. Immunol. **65**, 617 (1950). — SANFORD, W., RASCH, J., STONEHILL, R.: A therapeutic dilemma, the treatment of disseminated coccidioidomycosis with amphotericin B. Ann. intern. Med. **56**, 553 (1962). — SASHIN, D., BROWN, G., LAFFER, N., MCDOWELL, H.: Disseminated coccidioidomycosis localized in bone. Amer. J. med. Sci. **212**, 565 (1946). — SASHIN, D.: Coccidioidomycosis with involvement of bone. Bull. Hosp. Jt. Dis. (N.Y.) **8**, 59 (1947). — SCHENKEN, J., PALIK, E.: Coccidioidomycosis in states other than California, with report of a case in Louisiana. Arch. Path. **34**, 484 (1942). — SCHUBERT, J., HAMPSON, C.: An appraisal of serologic tests for coccidioidomycosis. Amer. J. Hyg. **76**, 144 (1962). — SCHULZE, V.: Acute coccidioidomycosis in West Texas. Tex. St. J. Med. **38**, 372 (1942). — SCHWARTZMANN, J.: Coccidioidal bone infection. U.S. Publ. Hlth. Serv. Publ. **575**, 32 (1957). — SCHWARZ, J., MUTH, J.: Coccidioidomycosis, a review. Amer. J. med. Sci. **221**, 89 (1951). — SCHWARZ, J., FURCOLOW, M.: Some epidemiologic factors and diagnostic tests in blastomycosis, coccidioidomycosis, and histoplasmosis. Amer. J. clin. Path. **25**, 261 (1955). — SCHWARZ, J.: Personal communication to R. W. H. — SHELTON, R.: A survey of coccidioidomycosis at Camp Roberts, California.

J. Amer. med. Ass. **118**, 1186 (1942). — SINGH, H., YAST, C., GLADNEY, J.: Coccidioidomycosis with endolaryngeal involvement. Arch. Otolaryng. **63**, 244 (1956). — SMALE, L., BIRSNER, J.: Maternal deaths from coccidioidomycosis. J. Amer. med. Ass. **140**, 1152 (1949). — SMALE, L.: Unpublished observations. — SMITH, C.: An epidemiological study of acute coccidioidomycosis with erythema nodosum. Proc. 6th Pac. Sci. Cong. **5**, 797 (1939). ~ Epidemiology of acute coccidioidomycosis with erythema nodosum ("San Joaquin" or "Valley Fever"). Amer. J. publ. Hlth. **30**, 600 (1940). — SMITH, C., BAKER, E.: A summary of the present status of coccidioidal infection. Calif. St. Dep. Publ. Hlth. Weekly Bull. **20**, 113 and 117 (1941). — SMITH, C.: Parallelism of coccidioidal and tuberculous infections. Radiology **38**, 643 (1942). ~ Coccidiosis -- Coccidioidomycosis. Ibid. **39**, 486 (1942). ~ Coccidioidomycosis. Med. Clin. N. Amer. **27**, 790 (1943). — SMITH, C., BEARD, R., ROSENBERGER, H., WHITING, E.: Effect of season and dust control on coccidioidomycosis. J. Amer. med. Ass. **132**, 833 (1946). — SMITH, C., BEARD. R., WHITING, E., ROSENBERGER, H.: Varieties of coccidioidal infection in relation to the epidemiology and control of the disease. Amer. J. publ. Hlth. **36**, 1394 (1946). — SMITH, C.: Current problems in pulmonary coccidioidomycosis. Surgery **19**, 873 (1946). ~ Recent progress in pulmonary mycotic infections. Calif. Med. **67**, 179 (1947). — SMITH, C., BEARD, R., SAITO, M.: Pathogenesis of coccidioidomycosis with special reference to pulmonary cavitation. Ann. intern. Med. **29**, 623 (1948a). — SMITH, C., WHITING, E., BAKER, E., ROSENBERGER, H., BEARD, R., SAITO, M.: The use of coccidioidin. Amer. Rev. Tuberc. **57**, 330 (1948b). — SMITH, C., SAITO, M., BEARD, R., ROSENBERG, H., WHITING, E.: Histoplasmin sensitivity and coccidioidal infection, occurrence of cross reactions. Amer. J. publ. Hlth. **39**, 722 (1949). — SMITH, C., SAITO, M., BEARD, R., KEPP, R., CLARK, R., EDDIE, B.: Serological tests in the diagnosis and prognosis of coccidioidomycosis. Amer. J. Hyg. **52**, 1 (1950). — SMITH, C.: Diagnosis of pulmonary coccidioidal infections. Calif. Med. **75**, 385 (1951). ~ Coccidioidomycosis, Laboratory Methods U.S. Army, 6th ed., p. 610 (1955a). ~ Coccidioidomycosis. Pediat. Clin. N. Amer. **2**, 109 (1955b). ~ Analogy of coccidioidin and histoplasmin sensitivity. Proc. of Conf. on Histoplasmosis. U.S. Publ. Hlth. Monogr. **39**, 173 (1956). — SMITH, C., SAITO, M., SIMONS, S.: Pattern of 39,500 serologic tests in coccidioidomycosis. J. Amer. med. Ass. **160**, 546 (1956). — SMITH, C., PAPPAGIANIS, D., SAITO, M.: The public health significance of coccidioidomycosis. U.S. Publ. Hlth. Serv. Publ. **575**, 3, CDC Atlanta, 1957a. — SMITH, C., CAMPBELL, C.: Serology of coccidioidomycosis. Ibid. **53** (1957). — SMITH, C., SAITO, M.: Serologic reactions in coccidioidomycosis. J. chron. Dis. **5**, 571 (1957). — SMITH, C., SAITO, M., CAMPBELL, C., HILL, G., SASLOW, S., SPEVIN, S., FENTON, J., KRUPP, M.: Comparison of complement fixation tests for coccidioidomycosis. Publ. Hlth. Rep. (Wash.) **72**, 888 (1957b). — SMITH, C.: Coccidioidomycosis. Vol. 5, Communicable Diseases, Preventive Medicine in World War II. Office of the Surgeon General, Med. Dep., U.S. Army, Washington, 1958. — SMITH, C., PAPPAGIANIS, D., LEVINE, H., SAITO, M.: Human coccidioidomycosis. Bact. Rev. **25**, 310 (1961). — SMITH, C.: Reminiscenses of the flying chlamydospore and its allies. AJELLO, L., editor: Coccidioidomycosis, p. xiii (1967). ~ Personal communications to R.W.H. — SMITH, D., HARRELL, E.: Fatal coccidioidomycosis, a case of laboratory infection. Amer. Rev. Tuberc. **57**, 368 (1948). — SORENSEN, R.:Survival characteristics of diphasic Coccidioides immitis exposed to the rigors of a simulated natural environment. AJELLO, L., editor: Coccidioidomycosis, p. 313 (1967). — SPAUR, C.: Atypical cultures of Coccidioides immitis. Amer. J. clin. Path. **26**, 689 (1956). — STEIN, H.: Coexisting pulmonary coccidioidomycosis and tuberculosis. Amer. Rev. Tuberc. **63**, 477 (1953). — STERNBERG, T., NEWCOMER, V., editors: Therapy of Fungus Diseases, an International Symposium. Boston: Little-Brown, 1955. — STEWART, R., MEYER, K.: Isolation of Coccidioides immitis (Stiles) from the soil. Proc. Soc. exp. Biol. (N.Y.) **29**, 937 (1932). — STEWART, R., KIMURA, F.: Studies in the skin test for coccidioidal infection. I. Preparation and standardization of coccidioidin. J. infect. Dis. **66**, 212 (1940). — STRAUB, M., SCHWARTZ, J.: Primary pulmonary arrested lesions of coccidioidomycosis and histoplasmosis, a study of autopsy material in Tucson, Arizona. Amer. J. clin. Path. **26**, 998 (1956). ~ Histoplasmosis, coccidioidomycosis, and tuberculosis, a comparative pathologic study. Path. et Microbid. (Basel) **25**, 421 (1962). — STUDY, R., MORGENSTERN, P.: Coexisting pulmonary coccidioidomycosis and tuberculosis. New Engl. J. Med. **288**, 837 (1948). — SWATEK, F., OMIECZYNSKI, D., PLUNKETT, O.: Coccidioides immitis in California. AJELLO, L., editor: Coccidioidomycosis, p. 255 (1967). — SYMMERS, W.: Cases of coccidioidomycosis seen in Britain. Ibid.:301 (1967).— TAGER, M., LIEBOW, A.: Intrasal and intraperitoneal infection of the mouse with Coccidioides immitis. Yale J. Biol. Med. **15**, 41 (1942). — TAKACS, F., TOMKIEWICS, Z., MERRILL, J.: Amphotericin B nephrotoxicity with irreversible renal failure. Ann. intern. Med. **59**, 716 (1963). — TARBET, J., BRESLAU, A.: Histochemical investigation of the spherule of Coccidioides immitis in relation to host reaction. J. infect. Dis. **92**, 183 (1953). — THIEMEYER, J.: Monoarticular coccidioidal arthritis, report of a case with apparent cure following synovectomy. J. Bone Jt. Surg. **30-A**, 387 (1954). — THORNE, W.: A case of protozoic skin disease. Occidental Med. Times **8**, 703 (1894). — THORNER, J.: Coccidioidomycosis, relative values of coccidioidin and tuberculin testing among children in the San Joaquin Valley. Calif. west. Med. **54**, 12 (1941). — TOWNSEND, T., MCKEY, R.: Coccidioidomycosis in infants. Amer. J. Dis. Child. **86**, 51 (1953). — TRIMBLE, H.: Coccidioidomycosis, a review. Dis. Chest **20**, 558 (1951). — U.S. Dept. Health, Education & Welfare. Publ. Hlth. Serv. Publ. No. 575: Proceedings of Symposium on Coccidioidomycosis, CDC Atlanta, 1957. — UNIVERSITY OF CALIFORNIA. Publ. Hlth. Alumni Assn. "Highlights", Berkeley/Calif.: Spring 1967. — VAUGHAN, J., RAMIREZ, H.: Coccidioidomycosis as a complication of pregnancy. Calif. Med. **74**, 121 (1951). — VOGEL, R., FETTER, B., CONANT, N., LOWE, E.: Preliminary studies on artificial active immunization of guinea pigs against respiratory challenge with Coccidioides immitis. Amer. Rev. Tuberc. **70**, 498 (1954). — WALKER, O., HALL, R.: Coccidioidal tenosynovitis, report of a case. J. Bone Jt. Surg. **30-A**, 391 (1954). — WARING, J.: Nontuberculous cavities in the lung. Minn. Med. **37**, 565 (1954). — WEED, L., DAHLIN, D.: Bacteriologic examination of tissues removed for biopsy. Amer. J. clin. Path. **20**, 116 (1950). — WEISEL, W., OWEN, G.: Pulmonary resection for coccidioidomycosis. J. thorac. Surg. **18**, 674 (1949). — WERNICKE, R.: Über einen Protozoenbefund bei Mycosis fungoides (?). Zbl. Bakt. **12**, 859 (1892). — WERTLAKE, P., HILL, G., BUTLER, W.: Renal histopathology associated with different degrees of amphotericin toxicity. Proc. Soc. exp. Biol. (N.Y.) **118**, 472 (1965). — WEYRAUCH, H., NORMAN, F., BASSETT, J.: Coccidioidomycosis of the genital tract. Calif. Med. **72**, 465 (1950). — WHEAT, R., TERAI, T., KIYOMOTO, A., CONANT, N., LOWE, E., CONVERSE, J.: Studies on the composition and structure of Coccidioides immitis cell walls. AJELLO, L., editor: Coccidioidomycosis, p. 237 (1967). — WHIMS, C.: Coccidioidal meningitis. Bull. U.S. Army med. Dep. **7**, 466 (1947). — WILLETT, F., WEISS, A.: Coccidioidomycosis in Southern California, report of a new endemic area with a review of 100 cases. Ann. intern. Med. **23**, 349 (1945). — WILLIAMS, J., ELLINGSON, H.: Studies on coccidioidomycosis at air force bases in the Southwestern United States. USAF School of Aviation Med. Unnumbered report, Dec. 1954. — WILSON, J., SMITH, C., PLUNKETT, O.: Primary cutaneous coccidioidomycosis, the criteria for diagnosis and report of a case. Calif. Med. **79**, 233 (1953). — WILSON, J., PLUNKETT, O.: The fungous diseases of man. Berkeley and Los Angeles: Univ. Calif. Press 1965. — WINER, L.: Histopathology of the nodose lesion of acute coccidioidomycosis. Arch. Derm. Syph. (Chic.) **61**, 1010 (1950). — WINN, W.: Pulmonary cavitation associated with coccidioidal infection. Arch. intern. Med. **68**, 1179 (1941). ~ The treatment of pulmonary cavitation due to coccidioidal infection. Calif. west. Med. **57**, 45 (1942). — WINN, W., JOHNSON, G.: Primary coccidioidomycosis a roentgenographic study of 40 cases. Ann. intern. Med. **17**, 407 (1942). — WINN, W.: Pulmonary mycoses, coccidioidomycosis and pulmonary cavitation, a study of 92 cases. Arch. intern. Med. **87**, 541 (1951). ~ Coccidioidomycosis. Trans. Ass. Life Insur. med. Dir. Amer. **36**, 121 (1952). ~ Coccidioidomycosis. Hinshaw-Garland: Diseases of the Chest, p. 592. Philadelphia: Saunders, 1956). ~ The clinical development and management of coccidioidomycosis. U.S. Publ. Hlth. Serv. Publ. **575**, 10, CDC Atlanta, 1957. ~ The use of amphotericin B in the treatment of coccidioidal disease. Amer. J. Med. **27**, 617 (1959). ~ Coccidioidomycosis and amphotericin B. Med. Clin. N. Amer. **47**, 1131 (1963). — WINN, W., LEVINE, H., BRODERICK, J., CRANE, R.: A localized epidemic of coccidioidal infection, primary coccidioidomycosis occurring in a group of 10 children. New Engl. J. Med. **268**, 867 (1963). — WINN, W.: The treatment of coccidioidal meningitis, the use of amphotericin B in a group of 25 patients. Calif. Med. **101**, 78 (1964). ~ Primary cutaneous coccidioidomycosis. Arch. Derm. **92**, 221 (1965). ~ A working classification of coccidioidomycosis and its application to therapy. AJELLO, L., editor: Coccidioidomycosis, p. 3 (1967a). ~ Coccidioidal meningitis, a follow-up report. Ibid.: 55 (1967b). ~ Tuberculosis and coccidioidomycosis, a working classification of coccidioidal disease related to therapy based on differences between the two diseases. Amer. Rev. resp. Dis. **96**, 229 (1967c). ~ Coccidioidomycosis. Tice: Practice of Medicine, Vol. III, Ch. 53, p. 1—14, 1967d (Renewal sheets). Hoeber Med. Div., Harper & Row, Hagerstown, Maryland. — WINN, W., FINEGOLD, S., HUNTINGTON, R.: Coccidioidomycosis with fungemia. AJELLO, L., editor: Coccidioidomycosis, p. 93 (1967). — WITORSCH, P., WILLIAMS, T., OMMAYA, A., UTZ, J.: Intraventricular administration of amphotericin B. J. Amer. med. Ass. **194**, 699 (1965). — WOLBACH, S.: The life cycle of the organism of dermatitis coccidioides. J. Med. Res. **13**, 53 (1904). ~ Recovery from coccidioidal granuloma. Boston med. surg. J. **172**, 94—96, Jan. 21 (1915). — WORMLEY, L., MANOIL, L., ROSENTHAL, M.: Coccidioidomycosis of female adnexa. Amer. J. Surg. **80**, 958 (1950). — YEGIAN, D., KEGEL, R.: Coccidioides immitis infection of the lung, report of a case resembling pulmonary tuberculosis. Amer. Rev. Tuberc. **41**, 393 (1940). — ZEALEAR, D., WINN, W.: The neurosurgical approach in the treatment of coccidioidal meningitis, report of ten cases. AJELLO, L., editor: Coccidioidomycosis, p. 43 (1967). — ZIMMERMAN, L.: Fatal fungus infections complicating other diseases. Amer. J. clin. Path. **25**, 46 (1955). ~ Etiology of socalled pulmonary tuberculoma. Med. Ann. D. C. **23**, 423 (1954a). ~ Demonstration of histoplasma and coccidioides in so-called tuberculomas of the lung, preliminary report on thirty-five cases. Arch. intern. Med. **94**, 690 (1954b).

Dermal Pathology
of Superficial Fungus Infections[1,3]

J. H. Graham[2], Irvine/Calif., USA and **C. Barroso-Tobila**[2], Maracaibo,Venezuela

With 156 Figures

Introduction

During the past three decades there has been a tremendous increase in the search for knowledge of fungus infections of man and animals. Until about two decades ago, only dermatologists and a few pathologists shared the botanist's interest in fungus diseases, but now almost every specialty includes discussions of the mycoses on scientific programs and in publications.

Superficial cutaneous fungus infections primarily involve keratinized tissues of the epidermis, pilosebaceous follicle and nails, and constitute a group of organisms classified as causing dermatophytosis, candidiasis, tinea nigra, tinea versicolor, and piedra. Because of the predilection of superficial fungus infections to involve skin and its appendages, gross hairs and scrapings of keratinized tissue are readily available for direct microscopic examination and culture studies. For this reason, the pathologist is not often called upon to establish the correct diagnosis of the patient's disease. In processing approximately 5000 skin specimens each year at The Skin and Cancer Hospital of Philadelphia, at least once a week a tissue diagnosis of cutaneous fungus disease is made which was not suspected by the clinician. A high index of suspicion for superficial fungus infections is maintained by the dermal pathologists in the section of dermal pathology since the various pathogens cause a spectrum of gross and microscopic tissue reactions which show a striking resemblance to a variety of cutaneous diseases. Generally used textbooks of medical mycology (Lewis et al.; Götz, 1962, 1963; Emmons et al.; Hildick-Smith et al.; Wilson and Plunkett; Conant et al.) contain limited information about the tissue pathology of the superficial fungus infections. Except for Gans and Steigleder, even recognized textbooks of dermal pathology (Percival et al.; Allen; Montgomery; Lever) allot only a limited number of pages to the discussion of tissue changes in superficial fungus diseases. The referenced textbooks of medical mycology adequately cover superficial fungus infections with regard to termino-

1 From the Departments of Dermatology and Pathology, Temple University School of Medicine; and The Skin and Cancer Hospital of Philadelphia, 3322 North Broad Street, Philadelphia, Pennsylvania 19140.

2 Professor of Dermatology and Pathology, Temple University School of Medicine, and Director of Laboratory, The Skin and Cancer Hospital of Philadelphia (Dr. Graham); Fellow in Dermal Pathology, Section of Dermal Pathology, The Skin and Cancer Hospital of Philadelphia (Dr. Barroso-Tobila). Dr. Graham is now located at the University of California, Irvine, California College of Medicine, where he is: Professor of Medicine (Dermatology), Chairman, Division of Dermatology; and Professor of Pathology, Director, Section of Dermal Pathology. Dr. Barroso-Tobila is now located at the "Policlinica Maracaibo", Dermatología Y Dermopatología, Maracaibo, Venezuela.

3 This investigation was supported in part by Research Training Grant CA–05189, National Institutes of Health, United States Public Health Service, Bethesda, Maryland 20014.

logy, etiology, historical data, geographic distribution, epidemiology, incidence, mycology, pathogenesis, allergy, immunology, treatment and clinical description, and the reader is encouraged to utilize these sources and others for additional complete information. As historical references, the pioneer studies of Gruby and Sabouraud on fungus infections of the skin, including their microscopic and histopathologic observations, will always stand as a basis for knowledge of this group of diseases.

Our interest in cutaneous superficial fungus infections has been greatly enhanced in an era made possible through tremendous technical advances, particularly by the application of histochemical methods as an aid for studying these diseases. During the past 20 years, several excellent and practical histochemical stains have been developed which enable tissue pathologists to demonstrate and identify fungi with simplicity not thought possible in the past. Lillie (1947) called attention to the effectiveness of the Bauer stain for detection of fungi in tissues, and the McManus periodic acid-Schiff method was reported in 1951 (Kligman et al.) as an improved technique for demonstration of fungal elements in skin sections. Gridley (1953) reported an additional useful stain for fungi, and Grocott (1955) observed that the methenamine silver nitrate technique was highly sensitive for demonstration of fungal elements in tissue sections.

Because of our knowledge in dermal pathology, the curiosity and desire of explaining tissue reactions on an etiological basis represents a daily challenge in handling all case material. We shall not compare histopathologic and histochemical methods with those generally accepted for establishing the diagnosis of superficial fungus infections. Techniques utilized by the pathologists for diagnosing fungus infections are merely an aid, and should not be competitive, but rather looked upon as complementary and supplementary procedures. Histopathologic and histochemical methods for studying disease can provide knowledge and answers not supplied by other techniques.

The purpose of this paper is to record our clinicopathologic and histochemical observations of tissue from patients with superficial fungus diseases which include dermatophytosis, candidiasis, tinea nigra, tinea versicolor and piedra. In addition, we shall briefly discuss erythrasma because for over a century it was grouped with diseases due to fungus, and also report our observations of a papular, pustular, and follicular eruption which we have classified as *Pityrosporum* folliculitis. Under the various types of dermatophytosis, we will discuss the pathology of infections caused only by those pathogens from which tissue specimens were available for histopathologic and histochemical studies.

Material and Methods

This report is based on 1 or more biopsies from over 300 patients with superficial fungus infections. The causative pathogens were identified by mycologic culture studies except for cases of tinea versicolor and *Pityrosporum* folliculitis. In most of the patients, prior to or after biopsy, the diagnosis was supported by direct microscopic demonstration of fungal elements, and where appropriate, Wood's light examination. The majority of tissue specimens were obtained using a 4 mm cutaneous punch, although some were surgically excised. Tissue specimens were fixed in 10% neutral buffered formalin. Routinely, the tissue was processed for sections cut vertically to the skin surface, but at least half or one entire biopsy specimen from each patient with tinea capitis was embedded on end in paraffin for 5 μ sections cut parallel to the epidermis. Selected specimens obtained from diseased skin tissue on smooth parts of the body were also processed for parallel sectioning. Tissue was oriented in the paraffin-block so that initial parallel sections showed subcutaneous fat, and subsequent ones demonstrated various transverse levels of the pilosebaceous follicle and/or adjacent dermis and epidermis. Gross hairs from patients with piedra were initially fixed in a solution of 10% neutral buffered formalin and 2% lithium bromide for at least 24 hours, then routinely processed through a tissuematon. Following this, the infected hairs were cut in lengths of 3—5 mm so that each separate piece had at least 1 concretion on it, and several fragments of hair were embedded together on end in paraffin for serial sectioning of the block. Multiple transverse paraffin sections through the hairs were mounted on clean, dry glass slides, and every fourth slide was stained with the McManus periodic acid-Schiff (PAS) method or Mallory's phosphotungstic acid hematoxylin (PTAH) stain. After routine deparaffinizing, some of the slides mounted with transverse sections of hairs infected with piedra were dipped in celloidin followed by 80% alcohol, and then stained by a variety of techniques. Dipping the slides in celloidin solution similar to that described for Snook's reticulum stain enhances the opportunity for a greater number of transverse sectioned hairs to remain on the microscopic slide. In examining skin tissue specimens from patients with tinea capitis, parallel sections through the suprapapillary matrix and higher levels were examined polariscopically (LILLIE; PEARSE) utilizing polarizer and analyzer lenses. Birefringence of the upper hair matrix level was considered the critical zone of keratinization with regard to evaluating the depth of follicular penetration by the fungal elements. A previous study on tinea capitis (GRAHAM et al., 1964) included scalp specimens from 53 patients. All tissue blocks were sectioned serially and an average of 6 tissue cuts of 5 μ thickness were mounted on clean, dry glass slides. Every sixth cut represented a series of sections approximately 30 μ distant from each other. Initially, every third slide mounted with multiple tissue sections was stained with hematoxylin and eosin (H & E) for routine study. Subsequently, selected sections of scalp tissue from 25 patients were prepared by a variety of histochemical methods. Since 1964, we have similarly processed tissue from patients with tinea capitis due to *Microsporum (M.) audouinii*, *M. canis*, *M. gypseum*, *Trichophyton (T.) schoenleinii*, *T. mentagrophytes* variety *granulosum*, *T. mentagrophytes* variety *asteroides*, *T. tonsurans*, *T. sulfureum*, and *T. violaceum*. Tissue was studied from patients with various types of dermatophytosis caused by *T. rubrum*, *T. mentagrophytes* variety *interdigitale*, *T. mentagrophytes* variety *granulosum*, *T. mentagrophytes* variety *asteroides*, *T. mentagrophytes* variety *niveum*, *T. verrucosum* variety *discoides*, *T. tonsurans*, *T. sulfureum*, *T. violaceum*, *T. concentricum*, *T. epilans*, *M. audouinii*, *M. canis*, *M. gypseum*, and *Epidermophyton (E.) floccosum*. Specimens from other superficial fungus diseases and erythrasma include those from patients with infections caused by *Candida (C.) albicans*, *Malassezia (M.) furfur*, *Pityrosporum (P.) ovale*, *Cladosporium (C.) werneckii*, *Piedraia (P.) hortai*, *Trichosporon (T.) beigelii*, and *Corynebacterium minutissimum*. Diseased skin tissue was not available for histopathologic and histochemical study from superficial fungus infections caused by *T. simii* (RIPPON et al., 1968), *T. soudanense* (JOHNSON and ROSENTHAL), *T. yaoundei* (GEORG et al., 1963), *T. ajelloi* (HILDICK-SMITH et al.), *T. megninii* (NEVES), *T. ferrugineum* (LEWIS et al.), *M. ferrugineum* (HILDICK-SMITH et al.), *T. equinum* (LEWIS et al.; HILDICK-SMITH et al.); *T. gallinae* (LEWIS et al.; HILDICK-SMITH et al.), *M. nanum* (BROCK), and *M. quinckeanum* (BLANK et al., 1961). The taxonomy of dermatophytes is not a settled issue, since no binding international agreement exists. From the standpoint of uniformity, we have followed the nomenclature and opinions of BLANK (1959) on classification of the dermatophytes, and this practice has been workable based on current isolation techniques and in keeping with observations made by SABOURAUD. Information regarding the dermatophytic flora of isolations from patients seen at The Skin and Cancer Hospital of Philadelphia during a four and one-half year period was recently published (McCaffree et al.).

Multiple sections stained with H & E were prepared and examined from all patients with the various superficial fungus infections including *Pityrosporum* folliculitis and erythrasma, and additional biopsy sections from typical cases of each disease were prepared as follows: PAS, with and without the diastase digestion method; Gridley's method for fungi; Grocott's method for fungi (GMS); Snook's reticulum stain; Fontana-Masson silver method; Brown and Brenn method for Gram positive and Gram negative bacteria (B & B); Gomori's method for iron; PTAH; modification of Mowry's 1958 colloidal iron stain for acid mucopolysaccharides, with and without the hyaluronidase digestion method; Movat's pentachrome method; aldehyde fuchsin pH 1.7 and 0.4 method for mucosubstances (Johnson); alcian blue method for mucosubstances at pH 2.5 or 0.4; Wolbach's Giemsa method; and Ziehl-Neelsen method for acid-fast bacteria. With some exceptions, the procedures were carried out as outlined in the *Manual of Histologic Staining Methods*. Some of the material on tinea nigra was sent to us through the courtesy of Francisco Kerdel-Vegas, M.D. and Jacinto Convit, M.D., Caracas, Venezuela, South America. Dr. Jacinto Convit also supplied 1 case each of gross scalp hairs infected with white and black piedra.

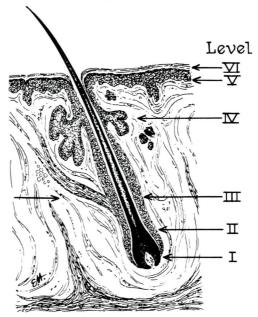

Fig. 1. Diagram of pilary complex showing objective landmarks: Level I, hair bulb (dermal hair papilla and matrix); Level II, keratogenous zone (KZ); Level III, arrectores pilorum muscle (APM); Level IV, sebaceous gland (SG); Level V, stratum Malpighii and acrotrichium (SM-AT); and Level VI, stratum corneum (SC)

Tinea Capitis

1. Introduction

Histopathologic alterations in the hair follicle produced by dermatophytes has been a neglected field of investigation since the pioneer studies of Gruby and Sabouraud. However, recent reports by Kligman (1952, 1955) and Riddell have

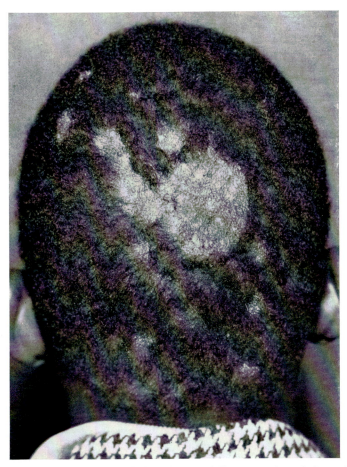

Fig. 2. Tinea capitis caused by *M.audouinii* showing dull gray, circinate lesions with scaling, alopecia, and multiple broken-off hairs

significantly added to our knowledge of the pathogenesis of tinea capitis. Observations regarding histopathologic and histochemical studies of tinea capitis were reported from The Skin and Cancer Hospital of Philadelphia in 1960, 1961 and 1964 (BURGOON et al., 1960, 1961; GRAHAM et al.). Studies dealing with dermatophytes causing tinea capitis in Philadelphia have been reported from our institution (SAFERSTEIN et al.; REID et al.). In discussing tinea capitis, reference will frequently be made to basic parasitic patterns, namely endothrix and endo-ectothrix types. Endothrix infections show intrapilary hyphae and arthrospores, and the endo-ectothrix dermatophytes exhibit fungal elements within and surrounding the altered hair shaft. The hair itself is always invaded in both endothrix and endo-ectothrix infections. For purposes of orientation regarding parallel sections through various objective landmarks of the pilosebaceous follicle, see the diagram showing 6 different levels as illustrated in Fig. 1.

2. Microsporum audouinii and Microsporum canis

Introduction: *Microsporum audouinii* is the major pathogen causing tinea capitis in Philadelphia (McCAFFREE et al.) and elsewhere throughout the United

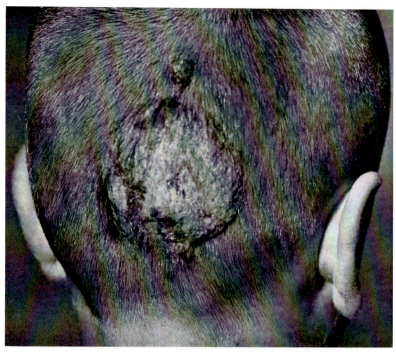

Fig. 3. Tinea capitis of the inflammatory or animal type due to *M.canis* and showing tume-factions, crusting, draining sinuses, and occiptal lymphadenopathy. The changes are characteristic of kerion

States. The latter organism is also the common cause of scalp infections in Canada and Nigeria, whereas, *M. canis* predominates as the common pathogen in Cuba, Puerto Rico, Argentina, Chile, Uruguay, Denmark, Finland, France, Great Britain, Cape Verde Islands, India, Australia and New Zealand (HILDICK-SMITH et al.). *Microsporum canis* is only occasionally isolated as the etiology of tinea capitis in Philadelphia (McCAFFREE et al.), whereas, contrary to most reports, the organism is the most common pathogen causing scalp infections in Montreal, Canada (STRACHAN et al.).

Of the various dermatophytes, more is understood about the pathogenesis of tinea capitis caused by *M. audouinii* and *M. canis* than other pathogens which infect scalp tissue. It is significant that histopathologic studies have played an im-

Fig. 4. Tinea capitis caused by *M.audouinii* showing an essentially normal epidermis except for hypokeratosis and follicular plugging. The corium shows only mild perifollicular and perivascular inflammation, but special stains for demonstration of acid mucosaccharides showed a prominent increase of hyaluronic acid in the extracellular interfibrillar spaces. All of the hair follicles show fungal elements in the form of small ectothrix arthrospores surrounding the altered hair and intrapilary hyphae (PAS, ×55)

Fig. 5. Tinea capitis caused by *M.canis* showing hypokeratosis, spongiosis, exocytosis, intra-epidermal pustule at the left margin, erosion of the stratum Malpighii at the right margin, and moderate irregular acanthosis. A dilated follicular ostium contains an altered hair fragment surrounded and invaded by fungal elements. The papillary corium shows focal inflammation associated with a degenerating pilosebaceous follicle and extruded remnants of keratin. No fungal elements were demonstrated in the perifollicular dermis. The histopathologic changes correlate with patients showing kerion (H & E, ×55)

portant role in our knowledge about the dynamics of the host-parasite relationship
of tinea capitis (KLIGMAN; RIDDELL; BURGOON et al.; GRAHAM et al.). For this

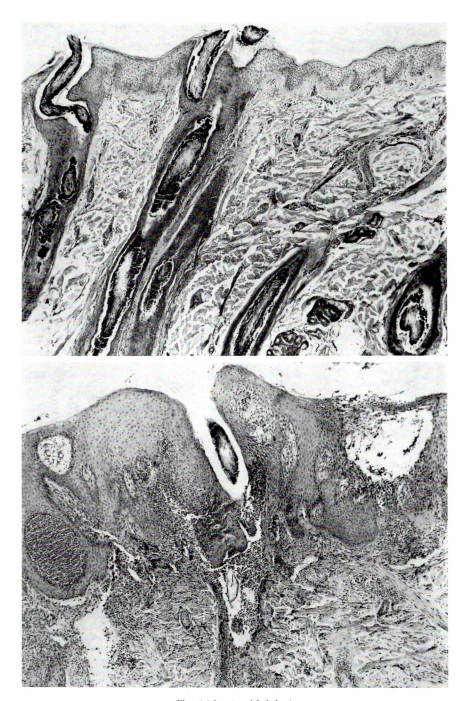

Figs. 4 (above) and 5 (below)

report, biopsy sections were reviewed from 52 children with tinea capitis proven by mycological culture studies to be caused by *M. audouinii* or *M. canis*.

Gross Appearance: Clinically, the majority of patients showed characteristic changes of circinate lesions with broken hairs and scaling, and in some there was erythema (Fig. 2). Some patients showed crusted lesions with posterior cervical and occipital lymphadenopathy, and a few cases exhibited kerion reaction characterized by boggy tumefaction, crusting, and multiple draining sinuses. As a general rule, the disease in patients showing minimal or no gross evidence of inflammation was caused by *M. audouinii*, the human or epidemic form acquired by direct transmission from child to child (Fig. 2). *Microsporum canis*, the cause of animal type tinea capitis, accounted for the disease in most patients showing prominent inflammation or kerion (Fig. 3). Examination under Wood's light usually showed typical, brilliant, greenish-white fluorescence of the involved areas. FORESMAN and BLANK (1967) demonstrated that the fluorescent matter is located only in the cortex and medulla of hairs infected with *Microsporum* species, and that the fungal elements do not fluoresce. The clinical differential diagnosis justifying special studies includes alopecia areata, trichotillomania, secondary syphilis, trichorrhexis nodosa, monilethrix, generalized myxedema with alopecia, seborrheic dermatitis, psoriasis, superficial pyoderma and perifolliculitis capitis abscedens et suffodiens.

Microscopic Observations: Observations were made from parallel and vertical sections stained with H & E for *M. audouinii* and *M. canis* infections and these showed similar changes except there was a greater tendency for inflammation in in tinea capitis caused by *M. canis*. Key illustrations will be utilized in showing significant changes from the follicular ostium to the hair bulb in sections cut vertically to the epidermis. The round trip will be completed by tracing the infection in parallel sections from the hair bulb to the SC. Details about the fungal elements and their relationship to the pilary complex will be discussed under histochemistry and illustrated by the photomicrographs.

In general, the epidermis was not remarkable except for follicular hyperkeratosis, remnants of infected hairs in follicular ostia, spotted parakeratosis, and minimal acanthosis (Fig. 4). Biopsy sections from patients with gross inflammatory changes including kerion showed hypokeratosis, spotted parakeratosis, spongiosis, exocytosis, intraepidermal miliary abscesses, prominent irregular acanthosis, and focal superficial erosion of the stratum Malpighii (Fig. 5). Perifollicular and perivascular inflammation was seen at all levels of the corium and subcutaneous tissue (Figs. 4, 5, 12). The infiltrate generally included lymphocytes, histiocytes, plasma cells, eosinophils and mast cells. In a few instances, multinucleated foreign body giant cells were seen about degenerating follicles at the level of the APM and above in patients with kerion (Fig. 5). In general, the corium showed either diffuse or focal areas in which there were separation and thinning of the connective tissue

---

Fig. 6. Tinea capitis caused by *M. canis* showing the longitudinal plane of an infected hair in the pilosebaceous canal. The level of this vertical field was just above the SG in the follicular infundibulum and beneath the SM-AT. The pilary outer root sheath epithelium shows parakeratosis bordering on the pilosebaceous canal, and a fragment of hair is surrounded and occupied by small arthrospores (microspores). A few intrapilary hyphae can be recognized and inflammatory cells are present in the hair canal and outer root sheath. The patient had gross evidence of kerion (PAS, ×445)

Fig. 7. Tinea capitis caused by *M. audouinii* and showing only intrapilary segmented hyphae. Some hyphae show only a weak staining reaction. The pilary outer root sheath epithelium contains some glycogen. The level of this vertical section is identified by the small sebaceous gland bud present at the lower left margin. The inner root sheath is absent since this component of the pilosebaceous follicle normally disappears at the level of the SG (PAS, ×445)

fibers (Fig. 4). The extracellular interfibrillar spaces showed a basophilic staining substance, and inflammation in these areas was usually minimal or absent (Fig. 4).

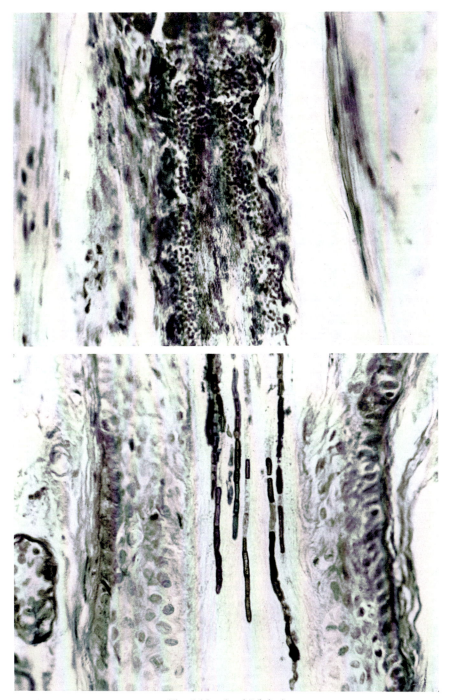

Figs. 6 (above) and 7 (below)

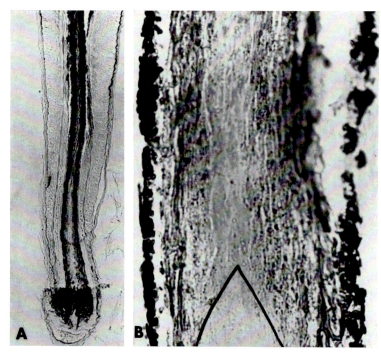

Fig. 8. Tinea capitis caused by *M.audouinii*: A. Section showing an anagen (growing stage) hair follicle in longitudinal plane below the APM and including the hair bulb, KZ, keratinized pigmented hair, inner root sheath and outher root sheath (GMS, ×93). B. High power magnification showing the hair surrounded by ectothrix arthrospores, short segmented hyphae in the hair cortex, and long intrapilary hyphae which appear as clear, white, irregular lines. Adamson's fringe outlined in black ink appears as an inverted V representing the deepest point of fungal penetration in the KZ. The central hair shaft within the inverted V is not completely keratinized, whereas the cortex and altered inner root sheath showed evidence of birefringence when examined polariscopically under polarizer and analyzer lenses (GMS, ×445)

The number of small blood vessels was increased at all levels of the corium, and in most instances there was vascular ectasia. All specimens contained numerous anagen hairs (Fig. 4) although catagen and telogen follicles were identified. The sebaceous glands were small, atrophic, or completely absent (Figs. 7, 16). In most biopsy sections, it was difficult to find more than a rudimentary sebaceous gland bud (Figs. 7, 16C). There were no recognizable alterations of eccrine sweat structures except from inflammation. The connective tissue sheath of anagen follicles was intact, whereas it appeared as a circular, hyalinized structure beneath catagen and telogen follicles. In tissue sections from some cases, fibrosis and granulomatous inflammation occurred about remnants of degenerating pilosebaceous follicles (Fig. 5). Pilary outer root sheath epithelium of anagen follicles appeared vacuolated, and there was evidence of intracellular and intercellular edema (Figs. 11A, 12A, 13A, 15A, 15B). Changes in the outer root sheath epithelium were most pronounced in the regions between the KZ and APM, although some abnormal features were apparent above this level (Figs. 7, 16B, 16D). The inner root sheath was altered in the lower KZ and appeared progressively disorganized until it disappeared at the level of the SG (Figs. 11A, 12A, 13A, 13B, 14, 15A, 15B, 16B). From the level of the APM and above, the outer root sheath of infected follicles showed parakeratosis (Figs. 6, 16B, 16D). Most of the anagen follicles were not infected,

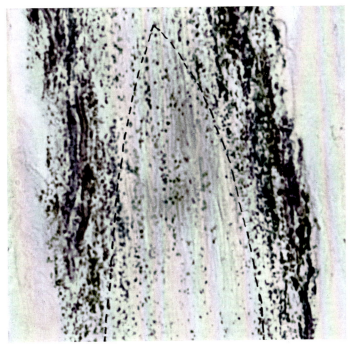

Fig. 9. Tinea capitis caused by *M.audouinii* showing only a few hyphae involving the hair cortex. Hyphae extend down to the critical zone of keratinization at the lateral aspects of Adamson's fringe outlined in the form of an inverted V as a broken line. Numerous melanin granules are present and the longitudinal straight white lines represent spindle-shaped, incompletely keratinized matrix cells of the KZ. No hyphae could be demonstrated in the hair bulb below the level illustrated (GMS, ×655)

although the number involved in a single section varied, particularly in parallel sections and depending on the transverse level from which it came. Extreme examples of this variation were noted at higher levels in which the majority of the follicles were infected, while others showed up to 30 anagen hairs with only 1 involved. It was common to see an infected anagen hair next to an uninvolved one, and in many instances these follicles shared the same APM (Fig. 16A). Sections through the hair bulb showing the dermal papillae and matrix cells did not exhibit significant identifiable pathologic changes (Fig. 10A, 10B, 10C). For purposes of this study, the critical zone of pilar keratinization was established as that level showing birefringence when the sections were examined polariscopically utilizing polarizer and analyzer lenses (Figs. 9, 10C). In general, infected hairs showed fungal elements approximately 25 μ to 30 μ above this critical zone (Fig. 11B). Between the KZ and SM-AT, fungal elements involved the hair shaft and adjacent inner root sheath in a variety of ways best observed in the sections prepared by special techniques.

Histochemistry: Infected and uninvolved anagen hairs showed an abundance of glycogen in the outer root sheath, particularly in the region between the lower KZ and APM (Figs. 4, 7, 11A, 13A, 13B, 14). The fungal elements were PAS-positive and diastase-resistant (Figs. 13A, 13B), however, there was color reaction variability depending on location of the hyphae and small arthrospores (microsporosis, 3 μ) within the infected anagen follicles. The fungal elements were also

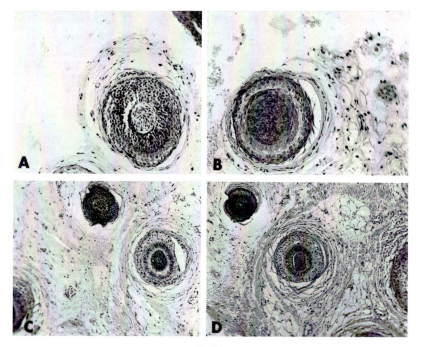

Fig. 10

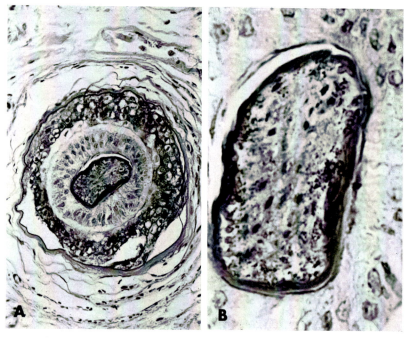

Fig. 11

Fig. 10. Tinea capitis caused by *M. audouinii*: A. Level I, section through the middle region of the hair bulb showing matrix cells surrounding the dermal papilla. Fungal elements are absent (H & E, ×115; AFIP Neg. 59-5894). B. Level I, section through the upper portion of the hair bulb showing a cellular inner root sheath and central suprapapillary matrix cells. No fungal elements could be demonstrated (H & E, ×125; AFIP Neg. 59-5894). C. Level II, section through the critical level of the KZ showing trichohyalin granules in Huxley's layer of the inner root sheath. No spores are present. The perifollicular subcutaneous tissue shows an increase in hyaluronic acid and one other hair follicle (H & E, ×60; AFIP Neg. 59-5894). D. Level II, section through the KZ 25 μ distant from C. A few hyphae are present as illustrated in Fig. 11B (H & E, ×70; AFIP Neg. 59-5894)

Fig. 11. Tinea capitis caused by *M. audouinii*: A. Level II, intermediate magnification of Fig. 10D shows an abundance of glycogen in the outer root sheath and trichohyalin granules are prominent in Huxley's layer of the inner root sheath (PAS, ×195; AFIP Neg. 63-3133). B. Level II, high power magnification shows melanin granules in the hair cortex adjacent to hyphae which appear in transverse plane as clear tube-like structures. Centrally, incompletely keratinized nucleated matrix cells are present. The hair cortex cuticle and cuticle of the inner root sheath appear intact. Polaroscopic examination showed birefringence of the keratinized hair cortex and cuticle of the cortex in the region of the fungal elements (PAS, ×705; AFIP Neg. 63-3183)

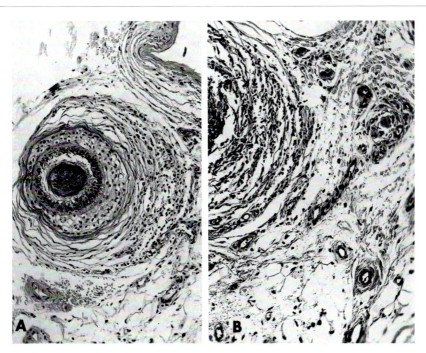

Fig. 12. Tinea capitis caused by *M. audouinii*: A. Level II, section through the low KZ showing perifollicular fibrosis, inflammation, vascular ectasia, and extravasated red blood cells (Movat's pentachrome method, ×125; AFIP Neg. 63-3182). B. Level II, section showing perifollicular inflammation and some capillary-endothelial proliferation through the middle KZ. Special stains demonstrated an increase in stromal hyaluronic acid (Movat's pentachrome method, ×145; AFIP Neg. 63-3182)

demonstrated with Gridley's method, GMS (Figs. 8B, 9), Snook's reticulum stain (Figs. 17B, 17D) and Fontana-Masson silver method. The fungal elements involved infected hairs at all levels from the lower KZ upward in 3 principal ways. The most common pattern was a combination of long, segmented hyphae located in the periphery of the hair shaft surrounded by a sheath of arthrospores, some of

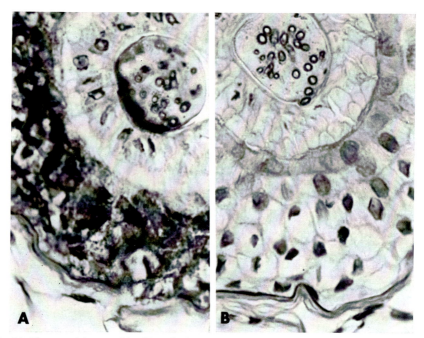

Fig. 13. Tinea capitis caused by *M.audouinii*: A. Transverse section through a level just above the central zone of Adamson's fringe showing intrapilary hyphae. The cuticle of the cortex is intact, and the cell walls of hyphae and glycogen in the outer root sheath are PAS-positive (PAS, ×705; AFIP Neg. 63-3184). B. Transverse section 5 μ above the level of A showing intrapilary hyphae which appear tube-like with central clear area and dark color reaction at the periphery. Glycogen has been removed (PAS with diastase digestion method, ×705; AFIP Neg. 63-3184)

which involve the fringes of the hair cortex (Figs. 8B, 14). Arthrospores were strongly PAS-reactive throughout the entire cell (Figs. 4, 5, 6, 14, 16B, 16D), whereas, segmented hyphae showed a much less intense color reaction outlining the wall in black giving the center a clear appearance (Figs. 11B, 13A, 13B, 14). In parallel and vertical sections, PAS and other special stains for demonstration of fungal elements showed a solid uniform color reaction identifying the arthrospores (Figs. 4, 5, 6, 8B, 14, 16B, 16D, 17B, 17D), and these were easy to distinguish from the clear tube-like segmented hyphae (Figs. 7, 8B, 9, 11B, 13A, 13B, 14, 15A, 15B). The second most common pattern of follicle involvement showed only intrapilary segmented hyphae involving all areas of the hair shaft (Figs. 7, 13A, 13B, 15A, 15B). The hair cortex cuticle was intact between the KZ and SC, and the cell walls generally showed a more prominent PAS-positive color reaction than the cytoplasm giving the hyphae a tube-like appearance (Figs. 7, 13A, 13B, 15A, 15B). The third pattern was a combination of features which included long segmented hyphae and arthrospores involving some or all intrapilary areas, and arthrospores and short segmented hyphae surrounding the altered hairs. Infected hairs appeared more fragmented at levels above the APM and intrapilary arthrospores were commonly seen. The arthrospores and short hyphae routinely showed a strong PAS-positive color reaction when compared with the walls of the long segmented intrapilary hyphae. Combined examination of vertical and parallel sections accurately localized the relationship of fungal elements to the KZ where intrapilary hyphae in their deepest penetration clearly outlined Adamson's (1895) fringe as an inverted

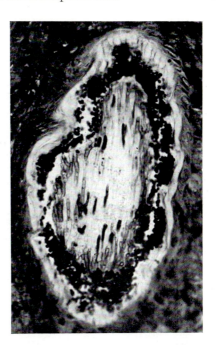

Fig. 14. Tinea capitis caused by *M. audouinii*: Transverse-oblique section of a level between the KZ and APM. Long, intrapilary segmented hyphae and numerous ectothrix arthrospores are prominent at the provisional zone of spore formation. The small arthrospores (3 μ) are located predominantly in the space between the opposing cuticles of the hair cortex and inner root sheath. These structures have been destroyed and arthrospores are present in the periphery of the hair cortex. Trichohyalin granules of Huxley's layer are compressed and disorganized by the larger number of arthrospores. An abundance of glycogen is present in the outer root sheath (PAS, $\times$305; AFIP Neg. 63-3191)

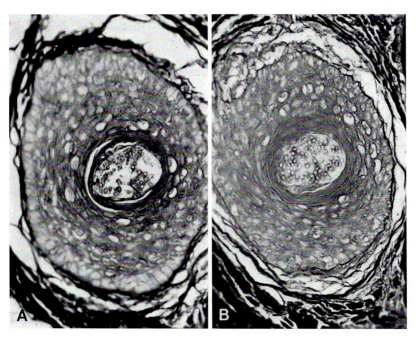

Fig. 15. Tinea capitis caused by *M.audouinii*: Level III. A. The outer root sheath and intrapilary hyphae are colloidal iron-reactive (Colloidal iron stain, $\times$305; AFIP Neg. 63-3189). B. The colloidal iron-reactive material is hyaluronidase-labile and interpreted as hyaluronic acid. After hyaluronidase digestion, the intrapilary hyphae appear in transverse plane as clear tube-like structures (Colloidal iron stain with hyaluronidase digestion method, $\times$305; AFIP Neg. 63-3189)

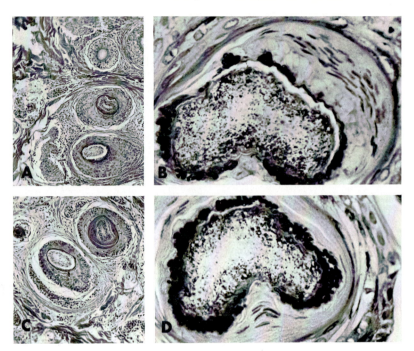

Fig. 16. Tinea capitis caused by *M. audouinii*: Level III and IV. A. Section showing an infected and uninvolved hair sharing the same APM. Mild perifollicular inflammation is present (H & E, ×60; AFIP Neg. 59-5892). B. High power magnification of a section through the APM level showing a few clear tube-like intrapilary hyphae, and arthrospores and short hyphae surrounding the hair. Hyphae, a few arthrospores and melanin granules are present in the peripheral hair cortex. The trichohyalin granules are disorganized and adjacent cells of the outer root sheath show parakeratosis (PAS, ×440; AFIP Neg. 63-3185). C. Section through the SG bud showing an infected hair and noninfected anagen follicle (H & E, ×75; AFIP Neg. 59-5892). D. High power magnification of a section through an infected hair at the SG level. The features are similar to B except the inner root sheath is absent. The arthrospores are adjacent to parakeratotic cells, but do not invade the outer root sheath (PAS, ×440; AFIP Neg. 63-3185)

V (Figs. 8A, 8B, 9, 11B). The terminal intrapilary hyphae were demonstrated laterally in the KZ which showed birefringence because keratinization occurs earlier than in the central part of the hair shaft (Figs. 8B, 9, 11B). Terminal hyphae forming Adamson's fringe did not penetrate nucleated spindle-shaped cells of the KZ, and examination of sections under polarizing lenses failed to exhibit birefringence indicating that the non-keratinized substrate was unacceptable for survival and growth of the fungal elements (Figs. 9, 10A, 10B, 10C, 10D, 11A, 11B). Ectothrix arthrospores were demonstrated in the upper limits of Adamson's fringe and these appeared to form from short terminal extrapilary hyphae by frequent segmentation (Figs. 8A, 8B, 14). When fungal elements surrounded the hair shaft, the cortex cuticle was practically always disrupted. Above the KZ, the cuticle of the inner root sheath was difficult to identify, and Huxley's layer appeared progressively more disorganized as the infected hair was traced upward. Usually between the upper KZ and SG, arthrospores were in direct contact with pyknotic and compressed trichohyalin granules (Figs. 14, 16B). The hyphae and arthrospores did not invade the pilary outer root sheath at any level, and only a few examples showed fungal elements in the SC away from fragments of infected hair in folli-

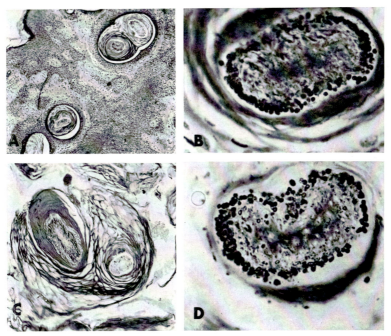

Fig. 17. Tinea capitis caused by *M.audouinii*: Level V and VI. A. Section through the acro-trichium and adjacent SM showing the same anagen hair follicles illustrated in Fig. 16A and C (H & E, ×50; AFIP Neg. 59-5891). B. High power magnification of a section through the acrotrichium showing arthrospores surrounding the altered hair. No fungal elements are present in the keratinized outer root sheath (Snook's reticulum stain, ×440; AFIP Neg. 63-3186). C. Section of SC through the follicular ostia showing the same follicle as illustrated in A (H & E, ×115; AFIP Neg. 59-5891). D. High power magnification through a keratin-plugged follicular ostia showing features similar to B. A few arthrospores are present in the peripheral hair cortex and adjacent SC. Intrapilary hyphae appear as clear-white dots (Snook's reticulum stain, ×440; AFIP Neg. 63-3186)

cular ostia (Figs. 17D, 18A, 18C). Biopsy sections from a few patients showed intense dermal inflammation with granulomatous changes, but in none were fungal elements demonstrated in the eroded stratum Malpighii or subjacent corium.

Colloidal iron reactive material was demonstrated in increased amounts in extracellular interfibrillar spaces and the pilary outer root sheath of infected (Fig. 15A) and uninvolved anagen follicles. Reactive material coated the arthrospores, and to a lesser degree, the segmented hyphae (Fig. 15A). The reactive substance in the corium and outer root sheath, and that associated with the fungal elements was hyaluronidase-labile identifying it as predominantly hyaluronic acid (Figs. 15A, 15B), since chondroitin sulfate B is resistant to hyaluronidase digestion. Undigested colloidal iron positive substance in the pilary outer root sheath prob-ably represents resistant hyaluronic acid, chrondroitin sulfate B, nucleic acids, and possibly sialomucin. Alcian blue pH 2.5 showed identical results for the colloi-dal iron stain except that there was less affinity of alcian blue for the fungal ele-ments. Sites of hyaluronic acid showed a negative reaction with alcian blue pH 0.4. Alcian blue pH 2.5 and 0.4 demonstrated mast cells in slightly increased numbers and these averaged about 5 per high power field. Aldehyde fuchsin pH 1.7 and 0.4

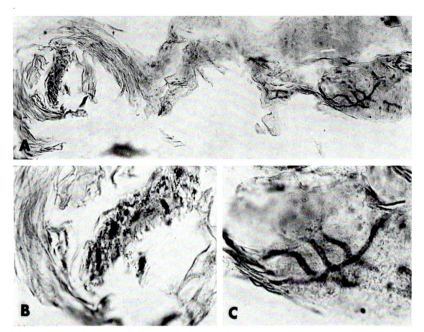

Fig. 18. Tinea capitis caused by *M. audouinii*: A. Level VI, transverse section through the SC showing a few hyphae at the right and intrapilary fungal elements at the left margin (PAS, ×195; AFIP Neg. 63-3193). B. Level VI, high power magnification of A showing a keratin-plugged follicular ostium and remnant of hair containing fungal elements (PAS, ×530; AFIP Neg. 63-3193). C. Level VI, high power magnification of A showing extrafollicular hyphae in the SC (PAS, ×530; AFIP Neg. 63-3193)

demonstrated mast cells and few or no elastic fibers in areas of increased ground substance and where inflammation was dense. Movat's pentachrome method showed general thinning or absence of collagen fibers and elastic fibers in areas of inflammation and increased amounts of hyaluronic acid. Snook's reticulum stain showed a network of reticular fibers in areas of dermal inflammation, but thinning of these fibers where there was an increase in ground substance. The remaining histochemical studies did not show significant changes and will not be described.

Differential Diagnosis: Lewis et al. indicated that *T. ferrugineum* shows considerable clinical resemblance to tinea capitis caused by *M. audouinii* and that infected hairs contain slender entwined filaments packed tightly together, and some may be found near the scalp surface. Direct microscopic examination of infected hairs shows a favus-like invasion of the hair shaft and intrapilary spore formation (Lewis et al.). Infected hairs fluoresce whitish-green and Wood's light examination is an important diagnostic test. *Microsporum distortum*, probably of animal origin, was first reported in New Zealand, where human infection involves small children (Hildick-Smith et al.). Hildick-Smith et al. take the view that infections caused by *M. ferrugineum* and *M. distortum* show small-spore ectothrix hair invasion, and are clinically similar to infections caused by *M. audouinii* and *M. canis*. Ectothrix parasites represented by *M. canis*, *M. audouinii*, *M. ferrugineum* and *M. distortum* show a specialized form of sporulation which occurs on the pilar surface or just beneath the cuticle allowing for dissemination of large quantities of infective material, and the hair usually exhibits a bright green fluoresence (HILDICK-SMITH et al.). *Microsporum audouinii* and *M. canis* are unusual dermatophytes because they parasitize anagen hairs in a variety of ways and involve some by showing an endothrix pattern of segmented intrapilary hyphae at all levels of the follicle.

Comment: Tinea capitis is generally clinically classified as noninflammatory or inflammatory in type. The majority of patients with *M. audouinii* and *M. canis* infections showed only minimal clinical signs of inflammation. The lack of significant gross inflammatory disease contrasts with the histopathologic features of dermal inflammation, and some examples showing intense perifollicular granulomatous changes. The contrast between gross non-inflammatory changes and microscopic features of inflammation strongly suggest that scalp tissue has a unique ability for masking the true nature of the disease process.

The presence of inflammatory changes, and abnormal amounts of hyaluronic acid in extracellular interfibrillar spaces and infected and noninfected hair follicles may be caused by elaboration of enzymes or allergens or both by the fungal elements. These enzymes or allergens injure epithelial and mesenchymal cells stimulating overproduction of hyaluronic acid which may be necessary for survival and propagation of dermatophytes. Cultural requirements of an acidic environment for growth and survival of dermatophytes *in vitro*, indicate that these dermatophytes are in part pH dependent for *in vivo* survival.

The affinity of hyaluronic acid for fungal elements of *M. audouinii* and *M. canis* is a striking histochemical observation. Hyaluronic acid probably diffuses from the outer root sheath of infected anagen follicles and literally coats the fungal elements in meeting their requirements of an acidic environment.

The exact chemical composition of fungal elements demonstrated in *M. audouinii* and *M. canis* is unknown. BLANK (1953) demonstrated that dermatophytes in their parasitic phase use nitrogen-containing keratin for synthesis of chitin, a nitrogen-containing polysaccharide, for skeletal material of their cell walls. Chitin and probably water-soluble polysaccharides in the fungal elements of *M. audouinii* and *M. canis* cause the color reaction with PAS and Gridley's method for demonstrations of fungi. These and the other special histochemical methods represent real progress in our technical ability to demonstrate fungal elements within infected pilosebaceous follicles.

The characteristics of *M. audouinii* and *M. canis* fungal elements to penetrate human hair and fragment hard keratin undoubtedly indicates that these organisms elaborate potent keratinolytic enzymes. DANIELS (1953) demonstrated that *M.canis* was able to digest human hair keratin *in vitro*, and WEARY et al. (1965) demonstrated that 1 strain of *M. canis* was capable of exerting a keratinolytic effect on wool. It is not surprising that evidence of *in vivo* keratinolytic changes should occur in human hair infections from *M. audouinii* and *M. canis*. Keratinases or other enzymes may be responsible for thinning of dermal collagen fibers and elastic tissue changes. Alteration of elastic tissue and collagen in the corium of *M. audouinii* and *M. canis* infections of the scalp may be a result of *in vivo* elastase activity. BLANK, TAPLIN and ZAIAS (1969) reported elastase activity of *T. mentagrophytes* isolates causing human infection in Vietnam, and it is possible that *M. audouinii* and *M. canis* might elaborate similar enzymes, although *in vitro* studies have been negative (RIPPON, 1967; RIPPON and VARADI). RIPPON and LORINCZ reported negative *in vitro* collagenase activity for *M. audouinii* and *M. canis*, but comparing the results of experimental studies with observations on natural disease does not always correlate.

KLIGMAN (1955) published observations on tinea capitis in experimental subjects inoculated with *M. audouinii* and *M. canis*, and microscopic studies showed that during an incubation period of 2—4 days, hyphae were present in the SC and follicular ostia. Hyphae penetrated the follicle growing on the hair surface, and segmented into chains of large cells considered as primary arthrospore formation. Fungal elements proliferated in the SC from the 4th to 12th day, and invaded new follicles in a radial path of growth. Intrafollicular hyphae penetrated the hair shaft on the 6th to 7th day, and descended to the KZ where they formed Adamson's fringe by the 12th day. After Adamson's fringe was formed, ectothrix arthrospores appeared and the origin of primary arthrospores from the external system of segmented hyphae ceased. The provisional zone of spore formation was located just above Adamson's fringe where external branches of segmented intrapilary hyphae can be identified and observed to separate into multiple arthrospores. All patients in our study of tinea capitis from *M. audouinii* and *M. canis* were natural infections of more than 12 days duration, therefore, primary arthrospore formation was not observed.

According to KLIGMAN (1955), terminal intrapilary hyphae have a unique relationship to keratinizing cells of the hair matrix and form Adamson's fringe. ADAMSON (1895) and SABOURAUD observed that terminal tips of intrapilary hyphae stopped "at the neck of the bulb at the point it joins the root stem." Adamson's fringe occurs because an equilibrium is established between the terminal hyphae and hair matrix cells, and fungal elements do not invade deeper than where the keratinized substrate is formed. If hair shaft keratin were formed at a greater rate than the fungal elements, they would gradually be eliminated since the growth rate of hair is about 0.3—0.4 mm per day (MEYERS et al.). During the active period of scalp infection from *M. audouinii* and *M. canis*, proliferation of fungal elements and hair growth rate are equal. Therefore, the host-parasite relationship remains constant forming Adamson's fringe. ADAMSON considered that terminal hyphae bordering on the KZ were external to the hair shaft. Our observations clearly show that intrapilary hyphae extend to the critical zone of keratinization. Their deepest penetration of the KZ occurs in the keratinized peripheral hair cortex, whereas, nucleated spindle-shaped matrix cells in the central hair shaft are free of terminal hyphae.

3. Microsporum Gypseum

Introduction: *Microsporum gypseum* is generally classified as causing an inflammatory type of tinea capitis affecting adults and children. The organism is derived from soil where it grows saprophytically, and occasionally the disease is contracted from animals. AJELLO (1953) believes that animal infection is less important than the saprophytic existence of *M. gypseum* in the soil. This comparatively rare mycosis of the scalp shows a world-wide distribution and has been infrequently observed on all continents and in most countries. Since *M. gypseum* is a comparatively rare cause of tinea capitis, our experience has been limited to examining material from only 1 patient, but we have studied biopsy sections from an additional 3 patients showing smooth skin infections with hair follicle involvement.

Gross Appearance: Only 1 lesion is usually seen, but there may be rarely up to 3 areas of scalp involvement. Clinically, the lesion appears erythematous, edematous, crusted and there is usually evidence of exudation (Fig. 19). The patients may complain of tenderness and experience pain at the involved site. Tinea capitis due to *M. gypseum* shows features similar to the inflammatory or animal type caused by *M. canis* (Fig. 3), and the clinical differential diagnosis includes those diseases confused with infections due to *M. canis* and *M. audouinii*. Wood's light examina-

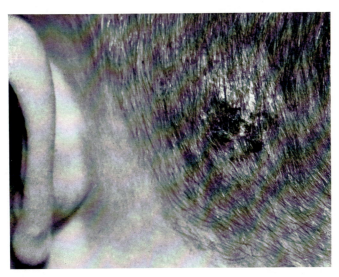

Fig. 19. Tinea capitis caused by *M.gypseum* showing a solitary, erythematous, crusted, boggy lesion involving the left occipital scalp region. The patient, a four-year-old Caucasian boy, complained of a painful and tender scalp lesion for three months. There was a history of frequent exposure to farm animals prior to onset. The gross characteristics are those of an inflammatory or animal type of tinea capitis with striking resemblance to scalp disease caused by *M.canis*

tion may or may not show white-green fluoresence of the stubs of some infected hairs. Kerion lesions with boggy tumefaction usually show absence of fluorescence.

Microscopic Observations: Examination of vertical and parallel serial sections from 2 separate scalp tissue specimens showed similar changes. Significant changes include hypokeratosis, areas of hyperkeratosis, spotted parakeratosis, dilated keratin-plugged follicular ostia containing remnants of altered hairs, spongiosis, exocytosis, and moderate irregular acanthosis. Sections prepared from 1 biopsy specimen showed diffuse dermal inflammation with granulomatous changes. The cellular infiltrate was composed of lymphocytes, histiocytes, plasma cells, and focal miliary abscesses containing neutrophils and eosinophils. Other features of dermal granulomatous inflammation were degenerating pilosebaceous follicles, fragments of hairs, foreign body giant cells, fibrosis, capillary-endothelial proliferation, vascular ectasia, and focal edema-like changes of the stroma. In areas, the epidermis was eroded and filled with fragments of keratin, inflammatory cells, cellular debris, and spicules of hair containing fungal elements. Sections of a second biopsy specimen adjacent to the first one exhibited milder changes (Fig. 20). The epidermis showed slight irregular acanthosis and mild to moderate granulomatous inflammation in the dermis. Multiple anagen hair follicles were present, but none showed fungal elements (Fig. 20). Only rare SG buds could be identified in examining serial sections.

Histochemistry: Special stains for fungal elements demonstrated organisms only in sections from the biopsy specimen showing diffuse granulomatous inflammation. The PAS method demonstrated intrapilary hyphae extending from the KZ to the SC, and at superficial levels these were frequently segmented and showed some large arthrospores (Fig. 21). A few of the arthrospores were small, but the majority surrounding the hair shaft appeared as megaspores, some measuring up

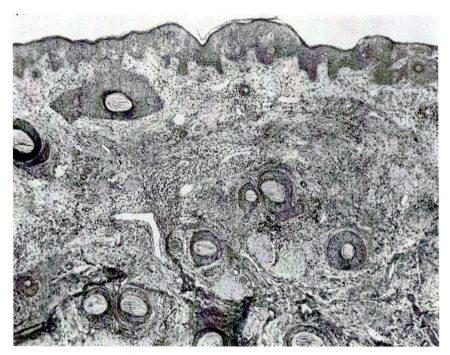

Fig. 20. Tinea capitis caused by *M.gypseum* showing mild irregular acanthosis. Several noninfected anagen hair follicles are seen in transverse plane. The perifollicular stroma shows focal granulomatous inflammation characterized by a mixed cellular infiltrate, foreign body giant cells, fibrosis, interstitial edema, vascular ectasia, and extravasated red blood cells. Sections from an adjacent biopsy specimen showed intense granulomatous inflammation and several infected hairs as illustrated in Fig. 21 (H & E, ×55)

to 10 μ. No fungal elements were identified in the corium even though pilosebaceous follicles showed evidence of degeneration. Special stains for demonstration of connective tissue showed thinning of collagen in areas of granulomatous inflammation, and elastic fibers were almost completely lacking. Mast cells were generally increased, and Snook's reticulum stain showed a reticular fiber hyperplasia in areas of granulomatous inflammation. The remaining histochemical studies did not show significant results.

Differential Diagnosis: Lewis et al. describe *M.gypseum* as showing segmented hyphae which have penetrated the cuticle and some hairs are surrounded by a mosaic of microconida. The microscopic picture simulates that of other *Microspora*, but if the infection has only recently occurred, short filaments in the hair shaft suggest infection with *T. schoenleinii* (Lewis et al.). Emmons et al. compare *M. canis* and *M.gypseum*, because the organisms grow within and outside the hair shaft as small ectothrix arthrospores. Our histopathologic and histochemical observations from 1 patient with tinea capitis due to *M.gypseum* suggest that the hair infection is of the endo-ectothrix type. Large intrapilary arthrospores form from segmented hyphae at all levels above the KZ, and although some surround the hair shaft, large numbers are not seen as is characteristic of microsporosis infections due to *M.audouinii* and *M.canis*.

Comment: The exact chemical composition of *M.gypseum* is unknown, but like other dermatophytes the fungal elements are demonstrated by special histo-

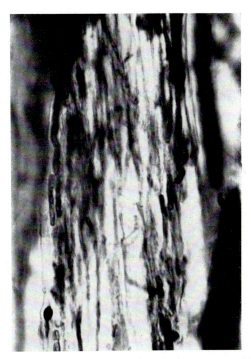

Fig. 21. Tinea capitis caused by *M.gypseum* showing a high power magnification of an infected hair with intrapilary segmented hyphae and a few large arthrospores. Some infected follicles showed arthrospores surrounding the hair shaft and the cuticle of the cortex was disrupted. The parasitic pattern indicates that hair follicle infections from *M.gypseum* are of the endo-ectothrix type with megaspore formation occurring at levels above the KZ by frequent segmentation of intrapilary hyphae as illustrated in Figure 123 (PAS, ×445)

chemical stains because of chitin in their skeletal framework, and probably water-soluble polysaccharides. *Microsporum gypseum* undoubtedly elaborates an enzyme allowing the organism to penetrate hard keratin of human hair, and this is supported by its ability to exert a keratinolytic effect on wood (WEARY et al., 1965). Tinea capitis caused by *M.gypseum* is a rare disease and future histopathologic and histochemical studies on proven cases will be conducted whenever the opportunity arises. Our observations on hair follicle involvement by *M.gypseum* as a megaspore endo-ectothrix parasite seem confirmed by pilar changes seen in biopsy sections from patients with the disease involving other parts of the body.

4. Trichophyton Schoenleinii

Introduction: *Trichophyton schoenleinii* produces a type of tinea capitis historically called favus and the disease often affects other areas of the patient's body. The disease is transmitted from human to human, and more than one member of the same family including several generations may show evidence of favus. Favus is unusual in the United States, but is common in countries bordering the Mediterranean sea, central Europe, South America and India. *Trichophyton schoenleinii* infections are particularly seen in North Africa, Turkey and Iran, and the organism represents one of the most common causes of tinea capitis in these countries. Biopsy sections were reviewed from 10 patients with favus, and this material

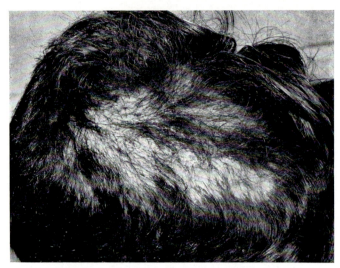

Fig. 22. Favus type of tinea capitis caused by *T.schoenleinii* showing adherent crusts, scaling, atrophy, and scarring alopecia. The patient, a 12-year-old Caucasion boy of Italian ancestory, gave a history of pyoderma followed by poor hair growth for 22 months. The clinical differential diagnosis included post infectious cicatricial alopecia and lupus erythematosus. Identification of fungal elements in the initial biopsy sections and subsequent mycological culture studies proved the disease was caused by *T.schoenleinii*. A 10-year-old brother had similar scalp involvement for eight years

came from Caucasian males of Italian, French-Canadian, middle eastern, and other countries of Mediterranean origin (GRAHAM et al., 1964). The disease occurs in both children and adults. Prior to the advent of griseofulvin, favus was resistant to treatment showing progressive spread from childhood and persisting throughout life causing permanent scarring alopecia.

Gross Appearance: Favus characteristically shows cup-shaped crusts referred to as scutula, and these are composed of dry, crusted material including hair and purulent exudate (Fig. 22). Scarring, atrophy, and permanent alopecia (Fig. 22) are common sequelae of the disease although some patients show only diffuse thinning of the hair with scaling. When scalp hygiene has been neglected, scutula are usually prominent and may elaborate a mousy odor. Removal of *T.schoenleinii* scutula leaves an erythematous moist to oozing base. Wood's light examination shows a dull green fluorescence of relatively long hairs which are not prone to break as in infections due to *M.audouinii* and *M.canis*. The differential diagnosis of favus includes pseudopelade of Brocq, folliculitis decalvans, chronic radiodermatitis, chronic discoid lupus erythematosus, localized scleroderma, tertiary syphilis, lupus vulgaris, burned-out areas of perifolliculitis capitis abscedens et suffodiens, lichen planopilaris, sometimes cutaneous sarcoidosis, and infections caused by other dermatophytes which produce scarring alopecia. Infections showing clinical features of favus are occasionally caused by *T.violaceum* and *M.gypseum*.

Microscopic Observations: Some vertical sections showed epidermal areas of cup-shaped scutula containing dense masses of fungal elements (Figs. 23A, 23B). High power magnification examination of scutula showed prominent intertwining segmented hyphae and small and some large arthrospores at the periphery (Fig. 23B), and principally granular debris and fragmented fungal elements in the central part (Fig. 23A). Fragments of infected hairs were usually present within scutula

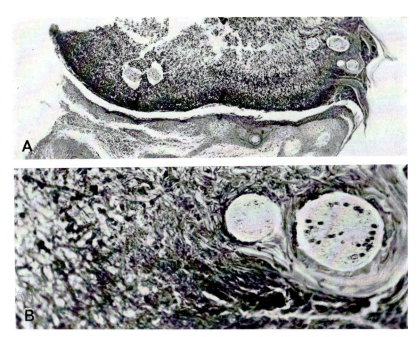

Fig. 23. Tinea capitis showing a scutulum caused by *T.schoenleinii*: A. Scanning view showing a cup-shaped scutulum filled with fungal elements, entrapped hairs, parakeratosis at the right margin, and epidermal atrophy at the base. Inflammatory cells and interstitial edema are present in the upper corium beneath the scutulum (PAS, ×40; AFIP Neg. 63-3204). B. High power magnification of A showing a peripheral zone of intertwined hyphae and small arthrospores. Remnants of two hairs are entrapped in the scutulum, and one shows intrapilary fungal elements (PAS, ×305; AFIP Neg. 63-3204)

(Figs. 23A, 23B). The stratum Malpighii formed the base of scutula and there was no evidence that fungal elements invade deeper layers of the epidermis or subjacent corium (Fig. 23A). The scutula showed either epidermal atrophy or acanthosis at the base, but acanthosis was usually seen at the lateral margins (Fig. 23A).

The epidermis adjacent to scutula showed hyperkeratosis, parakeratosis, superficial crusting, dilated follicular ostia containing remnants of hairs, spongiosis, exocytosis, areas of atrophy, and foci of irregular acanthosis. Granulomatous inflammation with many plasma cells and giant cells was seen in the papillary corium beneath scutula. Inflammation away from scutula was usually associated with degenerating pilosebaceous follicles and fragments of hair at all levels of the corium. Examination of sections under polarized light showed birefringence of remnants of hair, but no fungal elements were identified. Capillary-endothelial proliferation and vascular ectasia were usually present and particularly associated with areas of granulomatous inflammation. Fibrosis was common and in some sections mimicked keloid and folliculitis keloidalis. Ground substance changes and alterations at various levels of the involved hair follicles were similar to *M.audouinii* and *M.canis* infections. Sections of all tissue specimens contained anagen follicles, but these were not as numerous as seen in infections caused by *M.audouinii*, *M.canis* and *M.gypseum*. The number of anagen, catagen, and telogen hair follicles was inversely related to the degree of inflammation and fibrosis. Only a few SG buds were associated with the hair follicles in *T.schoenleinii* infections. Fungal elements were identified in the lower levels of the KZ, and generally more follicles appeared in-

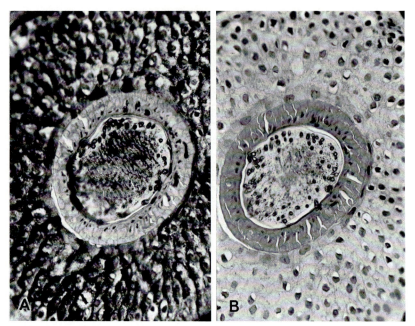

Fig. 24. Tinea capitis caused by *T.schoenleinii*: A. Level II, section showing fungal elements in the peripheral hair cortex, between the cuticles of the cortex and inner root sheath, and in the inner root sheath. Hyphae in Huxley's layer do not cause significant disorganization of the trichohyalin granules. The outer root sheath is rich in glycogen (PAS, ×275; AFIP Neg. 63-3205). B. Level II, section 30 μ distant from A showing similar fungal elements. The fungal elements are diastase-resistant, whereas, glycogen is diastase-labile and removed from the outer root sheath (PAS with diastase digestion method, ×275; AFIP Neg. 63-3205)

fected when compared with *M.audouinii* and *M.canis*. Significant changes will be described under histochemical observations.

Histochemistry: Hyphae and arthrospores were demonstrated by the various histochemical techniques already mentioned for showing fungal elements. Glycogen was present, showed intensity of color reaction, and involved hair follicle sites similar to *M.audouinii* and *M.canis* (Figs. 24A, 24B). Sections cut vertical to the epidermis demonstrated infected hair follicles in longitudinal plane and showed a net-like arrangement of many intercommunicating segmented hyphae which were intrapilary and surrounded the hair shaft at all levels from the KZ to the SC. The intercommunicating network of segmented hyphae within and about the hair shaft was striking and was verified in transverse sections which showed the intrapilary (Fig. 25B) fungal elements and those located between the cortex and inner root sheath cuticles (Figs. 24A—B, 26A—D). Some sections showed short segmented hyphae and arthrospores involving the inner root sheath without significant disorganization of Huxley's layer (Figs. 24A—B). Segmented hyphae showed a tendency to invade the keratinized outer root sheath bordering on the hair canal above the SG level (Figs. 26C—D). The various special techniques for demonstration of fungal elements were particularly striking in showing masses of intercommunicating segmented hyphae and arthrospores within scutula (Figs. 23A—B). Granular amorphous debris and fragmented fungal elements located centrally within scutula were PAS-positive as was glycogen in the spongiotic epidermal base and adjacent stratum Malpighii (Fig. 23A). Special stains did not demonstrate fungal elements

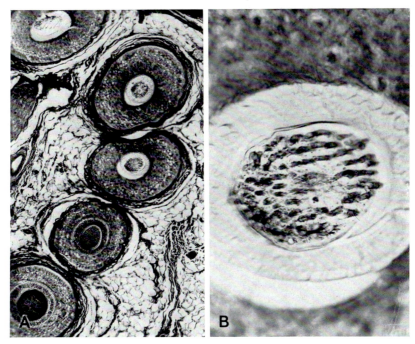

Fig. 25. Tinea capitis caused by *T.schoenleinii*: A. Level II, section showing hyaluronic acid in the perifollicular stroma, and two infected and three uninvolved anagen follicles (Colloidal iron stain, ×60; AFIP Neg. 63-3207). B. Level II, high power magnification of A showing numerous intrapilary segmented hyphae coated with hyaluronic acid (Colloidal iron stain, ×485; AFIP Neg. 63-3207)

in the viable epidermis or corium. The colloidal iron stain showed results identical to those described for *M.audouinii* and *M.canis* infections regarding changes demonstrated in infected and noninfected anagen follicles (Figs. 25A—B). The fungal elements in scutula were coated with colloidal iron reactive material and the majority of this substance was removed with hyaluronidase digestion identifying it as predominantly hyaluronic acid. The alcian blue method showed results similar to the colloidal iron technique, except mast cells were more satisfactorily demonstrated and in numbers up to 20 per field in sections examined under high power magnification. Aldehyde fuchsin and Movat's pentachrome method showed collagen, and elastic fibers were generally thinned or absent in areas of inflammation and where hyaluronic acid was demonstrated in increased amounts. Snook's reticulum stain exhibited a network of reticular fibers in areas of cellular infiltration. In general, hyphae were well demonstrated with special stains, but often the cell wall showed a more prominent color reaction giving a clear appearance to the cytoplasm (Figs. 26A—C). In sections showing the longitudinal plane of infected hairs, and particularly transverse ones, the hyphae appeared as tube-like filaments causing them to mimic bubbles of air or lipid droplets (Figs. 26A—C).

Differential Diagnosis: Scutula in *T.schoenleinii* type of favus, fungal elements invading the keratinized inner and outer root sheaths, and a combination of long, intercommunicating, segmented, intrapilary and external hyphae and arthrospores involving the hair in a net-like fashion are principal differences from endoectothrix follicle infections caused by *M.audouinii*, *M.canis* and *M.gypseum*.

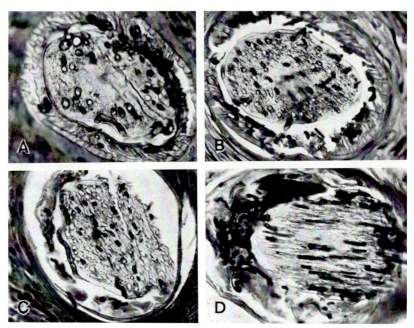

Fig. 26. Tinea capitis caused by *T. schoenleinii* showing transverse sections through various levels of the same infected hair shaft. A. Level III, section through the APM showing segmented hyphae surrounding and within the hair shaft. Hyphae and arthrospores are present in Huxley's layer, but the trichohyalin granules show only minimal disorganization. Large hyphae sectioned transversely appear tube-like and are sometimes called air bubbles. This occurs because the cytoplasm of the hyphae does not stain, whereas, the cell wall is PAS-reactive (PAS, ×305; AFIP Neg. 63-3206). B. Level IV, section through the SG showing a disorganized inner root sheath which blends with the abnormally keratinized inner zone of the outer root sheath. Numerous PAS-positive hyphae and arthrospores involve the hair shaft, disrupted cuticles, and inner root sheath (PAS, ×305; AFIP Neg. 63-3206). C. Level V, section through the SM-AT showing long segmented hyphae surrounding the hair shaft and short hyphae and arthrospores invading the disorganized keratinized layer of the outer root sheath (PAS, ×305; AFIP Neg. 63-3206). D. Level VI, section through the follicular ostium showing many PAS-positive fungal elements which are still intrapilary. Hyphae, and large and small arthrospores also surround the hair shaft and invade the adjacent SC (PAS, ×305; AFIP Neg. 63-3206)

Trichophyton schoenleinii represents an endo-ectothrix hair follicle parasite showing small and some large arthrospores, but not in the quantity and characteristic way demonstrated for microsporosis infections of *M. audouinii* and *M. canis*, or the megaspores of *M. gypseum*. According to Wilson et al., Hildick-Smith et al., Emmons et al., and Lewis et al., *T. schoenleinii* causes an endothrix hair follicle infection but our studies clearly demonstrate that this organism should be classified as an endo-ectothrix parasite. This interpretation is in keeping with the definition of an endo-ectothrix parasitic pattern which shows fungal elements inside and outside of the hair shaft. Blank (1959) included favus as a subdivision of the endo-ectothrix type and mentioned that large arthrospores are seen around and inside the unbroken tunnelled hair. Montgomery indicates that *T. schoenleinii* is strictly an endothrix parasite and that no sheath of spores is formed. Our observations are in agreement with those of Blank (1959) who classifies *T. schoenleinii* as an endo-ectothrix parasite showing intrapilary segmented hyphae, mostly small and some large arthrospores, and an intertwining mass of segmented hyphae and a few arthrospores about the involved hair shaft. Scutula of *T.schoenleinii* are unique in showing masses of segmented hyphae and arthrospores, and within the central granular debris fungal elements can be identified. According to ALLEN (1967) and BLANK et al. (1961), *T.quinckeanum* is a rare etiologic organism which can show manifestations of favus in man.

Comment: Our histopathologic and histochemical studies clearly identify *T.schoenleinii* as causing an endo-ectothrix type of parasitic hair follicle infection. Demonstration of *T.schoenleinii fungal elements*, particularly by the PAS and Gridley's method for fungi can be explained by chitin and polysaccharides in the fungal elements. BISHOP et al. (1965, 1966) identified water-soluble polysaccharides from *T.schoenleinii* fungal elements and characterized these as two galactomannans (I and II) and one glucan. *Trichophyton schoenleinii's* ability to penetrate and alter hair shaft hard keratin undoubtedly indicates keratinolytic activity as described by WEARY and CANBY (1967). Alterations in dermal connective tissue and extra-cellular interfibrillar ground substance may result from elastase (RIPPON; RIPPON and VARADI) and collagenase activity (RIPPON and LORINCZ). *Trichophyton schoen-leinii* produces enzymes capable of lysing the 3 major scleroproteins, keratin, ela-stin, and collagen (RIPPON and VARADI). Brassicasterol (I) and ergosterol peroxide (II and III) have been isolated from *T.schoenleinii* fungal elements (BAUSLAUGH et al.), and it is possible that these sterols may account in part for the so-called air bubbles or lipid-appearing droplets which characterize intrapilary hyphae in tissue sections or those seen by direct microscopic examination of epilated hairs.

5. Trichophyton Mentagrophytes

Introduction: *Trichophyton mentagrophytes* variety *granulosum* is a zoophilic organism isolated from domestic animals and particularly involves populations of wild rodents and other mammals, and is widespread in farming areas throughout the world. This dermatophyte is apparently not well adapted to acting as a parasite for man and proven human infections are rather infrequent in the United States. Transmission from animals to man probably occurs more commonly than realized in rural areas, but the disease is usually not properly diagnosed. Rodents and other animals can harbor the organism without evidence of clinical disease, whereas, human skin manifestations are rather conspicuous and may indicate the first evidence that infected animals are present in the environment. Familial infections occur and individual members may show a variety of manifestations with involve-ment of different areas of the body. *Trichophyton granulosum* is highly infectious representing one of the most common causes of laboratory diseases and epidemics in animal quarters. Because of the rarity of proven cases of tinea capitis caused by *T.mentagrophytes*, the opportunity for obtaining biopsy material has been small. In this report, we shall record our observations of biopsy material from one child with tinea capitis caused by *T.mentagrophytes* variety *granulosum* (Fig. 87) and a second child whose disease was due to *T.mentagrophytes* variety asteroides (Fig. 27). The latter infection originated from a zoophilic species in Vietnam contracted by the patient's father and then transmitted to family members in Philadelphia (Fig. 27). *Trichophyton interdigitale*, another variety of *T.mentagrophytes*, appar-ently does not cause tinea capitis or invade the hair follicle.

Gross Appearance: Tinea capitis caused by *T.mentagrophytes* variety *granu-losum* and variety *asteroides* show prominent inflammation and development of kerion is common (Figs. 27, 87). Scalp lesions usually appear as ill-defined, scaling areas with alopecia. Painful, edematous, and boggy lesions characterize the deve-lopment of kerion (Figs. 27, 87). Superficial small pustules and regional lymphadeno-

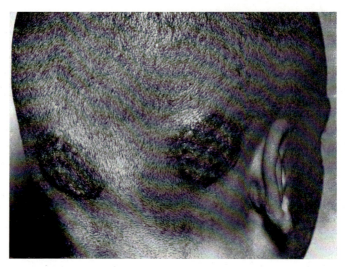

Fig. 27. Nonfluorescent tinea capitis caused by *T.mentagrophytes* variety *asteroides* showing separate 3 cm, erythematous, crusted, oozing, infiltrated, boggy lesions with a few pustules and multiple broken-off hairs on the posterior occipital scalp region. A similar lesion was located on the left temporal scalp region and the patient had bilateral tender cervical and occipital lymphadenopathy. The hairs could be easily epilated and mycological culture studies showed the causative organism was *T.asteroides*. The resemblance to severe pyoderma is striking. The patient, a 10-year-old Negro boy, had two younger sisters with similar disease of the scalp caused by the same organism. The patient's father had been stationed with the Army in Vietnam and developed a cutaneous dermatophytic infection for which he was treated with griseofulvin. On reunion of the family in Philadelphia, the patient's mother contracted fungus disease of the skin, and tinea capitis occurred in his two younger sisters. At the time of biopsy, the scalp lesions had been present for three weeks. The clinical characteristics of the disease are typical for the inflammatory or animal type of tinea capitis and similar to that caused by *T.mentagrophytes* variety *granulosum* as illustrated in Fig. 87

pathy may be seen (Fig. 27). Wood's light examination shows no evidence of fluorescence of the involved hairs. Scalp lesions due to *T.granulosum* and *T.asteroides* are often confused with other inflammatory or animal types of tinea capitis, particularly those caused by *M.canis* and *M.gypseum*. Additional considerations include pyoderma or seborrheic dermatitis which often represents the clinical diagnosis.

Microscopic Observations: Examination of serial sections prepared from 4 biopsy specimens showed hyperkeratosis, parakeratosis, superficial crusting, dilated follicular ostia containing fragments of hair, spongiosis, exocytosis, irregular acanthosis, and focal atrophy (Fig. 28). The corium showed diffuse granulomatous inflammation with many foreign body giant cells, particularly associated with degenerating pilosebaceous follicles (Fig. 28). The granulomatous process included a mixed inflammatory infiltrate, capillary-endothelial proliferation, vascular ectasia, extravasated red blood cells, and fibrosis (Fig. 28). The microscopic features were characteristic of kerion (Fig. 28), and correlated with the clinical disease manifested by two different patients (Figs. 27, 87). Sebaceous glands were not identified, whereas, eccrine sweat structures were present, but appeared altered by the diffuse granulomatous inflammation.

Histochemistry: Special stains for demonstration of fungal elements showed a few infected hairs with intrapilary segmented hyphae and microide (3 μ) arthro-

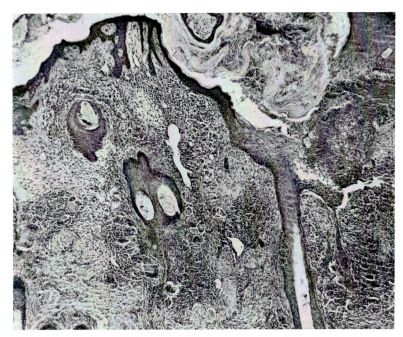

Fig. 28. Tinea capitis caused by *T.mentagrophytes* variety *granulosum* showing hyperkeratosis, parakeratosis, superficial crusting, follicular plugging, mild irregular acanthosis, and areas of atrophy of the outer root sheath at the level of the acrotrichium. Several hair follicles are present and the one showing a large dilated, keratin-filled follicular ostium is eroded at the base. The dermis shows intense granulomatous inflammation characterized by a mixed cellular infiltrate, foreign body giant cells, fibrosis, capillary-endothelial proliferation, vascular ectasia, extravasated red blood cells and interstitial edema. The microscopic features are those of kerion. No fungal elements were observed in the section, but microscopic examination of epilated hairs showed a microide (3 μ) endo-ectothrix parasitic pattern (H & E, ×55)

spores. Several hairs in each biopsy specimen showed only extrapilary hyphae and arthrospores of variable size at different levels from the KZ to the SC. No fungal elements were identified in areas of perifollicular granulomatous inflammation. Significant features demonstrated by histochemical methods showed an abundance of epidermal and hair follicle glycogen, general thinning of collagen, absence of elastic tissue, proliferation of reticular fibers in areas of granulomatous inflammation, foci of extracellular interfibrillar ground substance changes and a prominent increase in mast cells.

Differential Diagnosis: LEWIS et al. classify *T.mentagrophytes* as an ectothrix organism showing extrapilary fungal elements, and the spores tend to form chains and are similar in size to microspora. We agree with EMMONS et al. that *T.mentagrophytes* shows fungal elements inside the hair shaft and also produces a sheath of large and small ectothrix arthrospores on the outside of the hair. KOBLENZER et al. examined epilated scalp hairs from two patients with tinea capitis due to *T.mentagrophytes* variety *granulosum* and demonstrated intrapilary hyphae. Infected hairs pulled from one patient showed endo-ectothrix involvement with extrapilary arthrospores. HILDICK-SMITH et al. refer to a type of hair invasion caused by the ectothrix *Trichophytons* which include zoophilic *T.verrucosum* and *T.mentagrophytes* variety *granulosum*, and anthropophilic *T.megninii*. In these species, chains of relatively large spores when compared to the *Microsporum* infections, are formed outside the hair and no fluorescence occurs (HILDICK-SMITH et al.). The microscopic differential diagnosis of tinea capitis caused by *T. mentagrophytes* variety *granulosum* and variety *asteroides* would logically include other endo-ectothrix parasites and stresses the importance of proving each case by mycological culture studies. *Trichophyton verrucosum* infections involving only the scalp are rare and seen mostly in farming communities among those handling cattle. When *T. verrucosum* is the cause of tinea capitis, the disease is nonfluorescent and usually shows an associated intense inflammatory reaction with kerion. BIRT et al. reported their observations from 13 patients with kerion celsi caused by *T. faviforme* and indicated that the organism was a common cause of suppurative ringworm in North America. *Trichophyton faviforme* infections of the follicle show spores within and surrounding the hair shaft (BIRT et al.). *Trichophyton faviforme (album)* is considered synonymous with *T. verrucosum* variety *album* (AINSWORTH et al.). *Trichophyton megninii* is a rare cause of an inflammatory type of tinea capitis in southwestern Europe and is virtually restricted to Portugal.

Comment: Our experience related to histopathologic and histochemical studies of tinea capitis caused by *T. mentagrophytes* variety *granulosum* and variety *asteroides* is limited, but additional complete studies on one patient with tinea barbae due to *T. granulosum* indicate the organisms infect hair as endo-ectothrix parasites. Some larger arthrospores are formed, but generally they fall into the microide size of not exceeding 3 μ. Kerion formed in about 3 weeks in the two patients from whom biopsy specimens were available and this may account for only a few infected hairs showing intrapilary fungal elements. Kerion is accepted as a host response to the parasite and generally leads to spontaneous cure of the disease and this prevents further development of intrapilary fungal invasion. Enzyme histochemical methods have demonstrated a variety of *in vitro* and *in vivo* enzymatic activities for dermatophytes including some organisms which cause tinea capitis, namely, *T. mentagrophytes*, *T. verrucosum*, *T. schoenleinii*, *T. violaceum*, *M. audouinii*, *M. canis* and *M. gypseum* (MALE et al.). When *T. mentagrophytes* variety *granulosum*, *M. canis*, *M. gypseum*, and other dermatophytes were cultivated on hair keratin, a prominent increase in enzymatic activity occurred (MALE et al.). Leucine aminopeptidase activity was particularly demonstrated *in vivo* for *T. granulosum* hair infections which showed enzymatic reactivity within and adjacent to fungal elements (MALE et al.). Of significance is that leucine aminopeptidase activity in *T. granulosum* and other dermatophytes indicate that peptide splitting enzymes elaborated by these organisms play an important role in keratinolysis of SC soft keratin, and hard keratin of the hair and nail plate. WEARY and CANBY concluded that *T. mentagrophytes* was capable of severely disrupting and fragmenting wool fibers. YU et al. have recently isolated and purified an extracellular keratinase from *T. mentagrophytes* variety *granulosum*. MERCER and VERMA observed changes resembling enzymatic digestion of *T. mentagrophytes* infected hairs by electron microscopic examination. *Trichophyton mentagrophytes* isolated from patients with severe inflammatory infections shows elastase activity (RIPPON; RIPPON and VARADI; BLANK, TAPLIN and ZAIAS). BISHOP et al. (1965, 1966) isolated water-soluble polysaccharides from *T. granulosum* and identified galactomannan I, galactomannan II, and one glucan. Guinea pigs sensitized by cutaneous infections with *T. granulosum* were injected intracutaneously with pure polysaccharides isolated from fungal elements of the dermatophyte and no immediate or delayed reactions were observed, whereas, a delayed response was obtained with commercial trichophytin (SAFERSTEIN et al., 1968). Even though the water-soluble polysaccharides (BISHOP et al., 1965, 1966) are apparently not antigenic in guinea pigs, they along with chitin undoubtedly account for the chemical color reaction of fun-

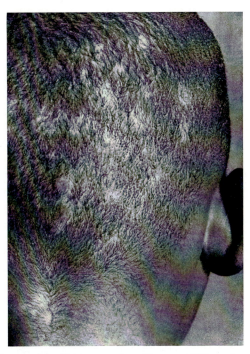

Fig. 29. Tinea capitis caused by *T.tonsurans* in a 10-year-old Negro boy with involvement of the occipital scalp region. Grossly, the disease showed mild scaling and a patchy scarring alopecia characterized by broken-off hairs at the scalp surface. The disease was asymptomatic and initially diagnosed as seborrheic dermatitis

gal elements in tissue with PAS and Gridley's method for fungi. Efforts will be made in the future to obtain more biopsy specimens from proven cases of tinea capitis caused by the various species of *T.mentagrophytes*.

6. Trichophyton Tonsurans and Trichophyton Sulfureum

Introduction: *Trichophyton tonsurans* and *T.sulfureum* infections are transferred from human to human and occur in some geographic areas of the world in epidemic proportions. These two organisms cause tinea capitis predominantly in America, particularly Peru, Mexico, and the southwestern United States. In recent years, there have been numerous reports of tinea capitis caused by these organisms from various geographic areas of the United States and rural eastern Quebec, Canada. Endothrix tinea capitis occurring in Philadelphia has been reported by KLIGMAN and CONSTANT, SAFERSTEIN et al. (1964), REID et al., and McCAFFREE et al. There is a definite tendency for endothrix tinea capitis caused by *T.tonsurans* and *T.sulfureum* to occur in family epidemics and emphasizes the need for investigation of each patient's family and household contacts. In Philadelphia, endothrix tinea capitis from *T.tonsurans* and *T.sulfureum* occurs predominantly in children under 10 years old and has been seen only in Negroes, although the disease has been reported in Caucasians by many investigators. Several investigators have correlated the spread of endothrix tine capitis due to the movement of migratory farm workers from Texas and southern California, but this does not seem valid with regard to patients seen with the disease in Philadelphia. This is also supported by

16*

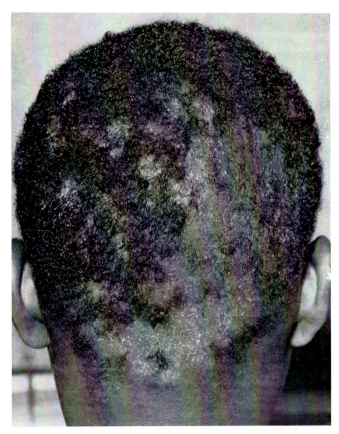

Fig. 30. Tinea capitis caused by *T. sulfureum* in a 10-year-old Negro boy who had siblings with similar disease. Grossly, the disease appeared as erythematous, circinate, scaling, crusted lesions with prominent alopecia on the posterior parietal and occipital scalp regions. Small pustules were present and the hairs were broken off at the scalp surface. Mycological culture studies of epilated hairs from the patient and other members of the family identified the causative organism as *T. sulfureum*

70 patients reported with endothrix tinea capitis from rural eastern Quebec, Canada, where there have been no migratory farm workers moving into the area and no immigrants for over 100 years (Blank, 1958; Blank and Strachan). For this report, we reviewed biopsy sections from 15 children with endothrix tinea capitis proven by mycological culture studies to be caused by *T. tonsurans* or *T. sulfureum*.

Gross Appearance: Endothrix tinea capitis caused by *T. tonsurans* and *T. sulfureum* shows a wide variety of clinical manifestations including smooth skin involvement. The scalp lesions are characterized by various degrees of erythema, scaling, broken-off hairs, weeping, serous or purulent crusts, pustules, papules or combinations of these (Figs. 29, 30). The involved areas are often poorly circumscribed and vary in shape from round to irregular patches (Fig. 29).

The disease may be highly inflammatory (Fig. 30) with kerion and easily mistaken for pyoderma or it can appear nonimflammatory and cause confusion with seborrheic dermatitis (Fig. 29). Scalp disease from these two organisms may lack distinction (Fig. 29) and typical, round, circumscribed, scaling patches with broken

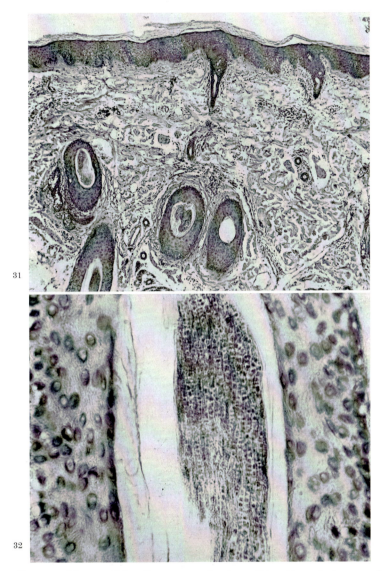

Fig. 31. Tinea capitis caused by *T.tonsurans* showing mild epidermal changes of minimal acanthosis. Infected anagen hair follicles are present, and the dermis shows mild perifollicular inflammation and extracellular interfibrillar ground substance changes. Eccrine sweat structures appear uninvolved and one anagen follicle shows an associated SG bud (H & E, ×55)

Fig. 32. Vertical section of tinea capitis due to *T.tonsurans* showing the longitudinal plane of an infected hair with intrapilary arthrospores in linear arrangement. The cuticle of the hair cortex is intact and the inner root sheath appears uninvolved except for some compression. The pilary outer root sheath epithelium appears normal except for vacuolization of cells adjacent to the basement membrane (H & E, ×445)

off hairs are the exception rather than the rule. Hairs infected with *T.tonsurans* and *T.sulfureum* do not fluoresce under Wood's light. *Trichophyton tonsurans* is frequently mentioned as producing typical "black-dot" tinea capitis showing disse-

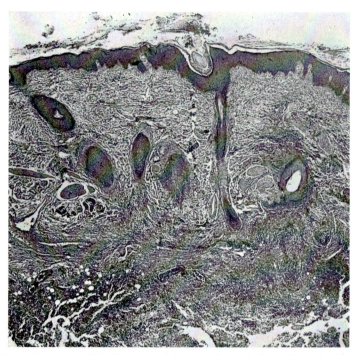

Fig. 33. Tinea capitis caused by *T. tonsurans* showing histopathologic characteristics of kerion. The reticular dermis and subcutaneous tissue shows diffuse granulomatous inflammation, miliary abscesses and disruption of hair follicles (H & E, ×20)

minated, patchy hair loss and must be distinguished from alopecia areata, trichotillomania, secondary syphilis, generalized myxedema with alopecia, and scalp disease caused by *T. violaceum* and *T. ferrugineum*. In some patients, *T. tonsurans* and *T. sulfureum* cause permanent scarring alopecia, and the clinical differential diagnosis includes lupus erythematosus, chronic radiodermatitis, pseudopelade of Brocq, folliculitis decalvans, coup de sabre scleroderma, benign late syphilis and lupus vulgaris.

Microscopic Observations: The histopathologic tissue changes caused by *T. tonsurans* and *T. sulfureum* were similar. Sections cut vertically to the epidermis showed slight hyperkeratosis, spotted parakeratosis, dilated keratin-plugged follicular ostia containing infected remnants of hair, and mild irregular acanthosis (Figs. 31, 33). The pilary outer root sheath cells often appeared vacuolated, particularly those showing intrapilary arthrospores (Fig. 32). Biopsy sections from patients showing gross evidence of inflammation exhibited epidermal changes of spongiosis, exocytosis, and a greater degree of irregular acanthosis (Fig. 33). All biopsy sections showed varying degrees of perifollicular inflammation comprised of a mixed cellular infiltrate (Figs. 31, 33). At least seven patients had biopsy sections showing perifollicular granulomatous inflammation with plasma cells, foreign body giant cells, miliary abscesses, fibrosis, capillary-endothelial proliferation, vascular ectasia and interstitial edema (Figs. 33, 34A—B, 35). In some sections there was degeneration of pilosebaceous follicles at all levels of the corium with extension of granulomatous inflammation into the subcutaneous tissue (Fig. 33). Foreign body giant cells were numerous and formed about melanin granules and

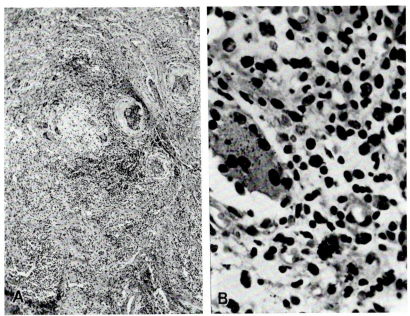

Fig. 34. Tinea capitis due to *T.sulfureum*: A. Level I, transverse section showing the corium and subcutaneous tissue replaced by granulomatous inflammation at the hair bulb level. The features show foreign body giant cells, fibrosis, and remnants of hair follicle epithelium (H & E, ×50; AFIP Neg. 63-3198). B. Level I, high power magnification showing granulomatous inflammation including a foreign body giant cell containing phagocytized melanin granules from disrupted hair matrix melanocytes (H & E, ×485; AFIP Neg. 63-3198)

spicules of hair (Figs. 34A—B, 35). Extracellular interfibrillar ground substance changes (Fig. 31) and the number of infected anagen follicles were similar, but usually less (Fig. 31) than observed in infections due to *M.audouinii* and *M.canis*. Transverse sections through various hair follicle levels showed intrapilary fungal elements from the middle of the KZ to the SC (Figs. 36, 37A—D, 38A—B). Only small SG buds were associated with the anagen hair follicles (Fig. 31). Eccrine sweat structures were present and not significantly altered except in sections showing granulomatous inflammation (Fig. 33).

Histochemistry: The fungal elements were demonstrated by various histochemical methods described and illustrated under discussion of other dermatophytes causing tinea capitis. The PAS method showed an accumulation of glycogen in the pilary outer root sheath and PAS tinctorial reactions for fungal elements were similar to microsporosis infections caused by *M.audouinii* and *M.canis* (Figs. 35, 36, 37A—D, 38A—B). Intrapilary arthrospores were positive with the various methods used for demonstrating them and they showed a prominent uniform color reaction (Figs. 35, 36, 37A—D, 38A—B). Arthrospores were observed from the middle KZ (Fig. 36) and at all levels above they appeared confined by an intact hair cortex cuticle (Figs. 36, 37A—B, 37C—D, 38A—B). Vertical sections showing the longitudinal plane of infected follicles demonstrated the linear arrangement of intrapilary arthrospores (Fig. 32). This feature was also seen when parallel sections showed a transverse, slightly oblique plane of the hair shaft (Fig. 38A). No arthrospores were demonstrated between the hair cortex and inner root sheath cuticles or any part of the viable epidermis. Serial sections showed remnants of

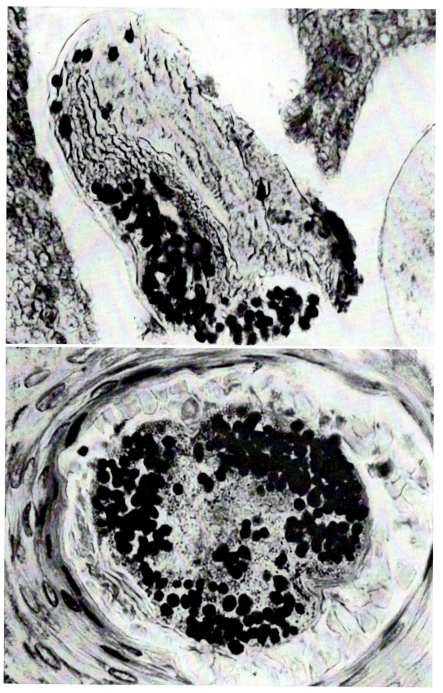

Figs. 35 (above) and 36 (below)

Fig. 35. Tinea capitis caused by *T.tonsurans* showing a spicule of hair in transverse section at a level between the KZ and APM. The hair fragment is located in a perifollicular miliary abscess with adjacent granulomatous inflammation and contains intrapilary endothrix arthrospores. No arthrospores could be identified singly or in groups away from the infected hair (PAS with diastase digestion method, ×655)

Fig. 36. Tinea capitis caused by *T.tonsurans* showing a transverse section at Level II through an infected hair with endothrix arthrospores in the upper KZ. The arthrospores show a uniform color reaction with the PAS method and are localized to the peripheral hair cortex, but confined by an intact cuticle (PAS, ×655)

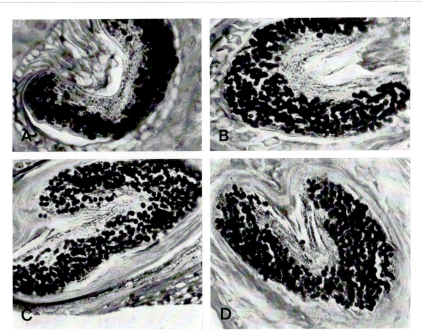

Fig. 37. Endothrix tinea capitis caused by *T.tonsurans* showing transverse sections through various levels of the same infected hair: A. Level II, section through the upper KZ showing intrapilary arthrospores. The cuticle of the cortex is intact (PAS, ×400; AFIP Neg. 63-3195). B. Level III, section through the APM level showing intrapilary endothrix arthrospores (PAS with diastase digestion method, ×350; AFIP Neg. 63-3195). C. Level IV, section through the SG showing arthrospores in a mosaic arrangement (PAS, ×300; AFIP Neg. 63-3195). D. Level V, section through the SM-AT showing an intact hair cortex cuticle and no evidence of invasion of the keratinized pilary outer root sheath by arthrospores (PAS, ×350; AFIP Neg. 63-3195)

hair located in miliary abscesses at sites of perifollicular granulomatous inflammation and some still contained intrapilary arthrospores (Fig. 35), but no fungal elements were demonstrated either singly or in groups away from the involved hairs. The colloidal iron stain showed an increase in extracellular interfibrillar hyaluronic acid, but there was no affinity of this substance for coating intrapilary arthrospores characteristic of infections caused by *M.audouinii*, *M.canis* and *T.schoenleinii*. The alcian blue and aldehyde fuchsin methods showed changes similar to other dermatophytes, and in general, mast cells were present as high as 20 per high power magnification field. Connective tissue stains showed general thinning of collagen and elastic fibers, particularly in areas of granulomatous inflammation and extracellular interfibrillar ground substance changes. Snook's reticulum stain

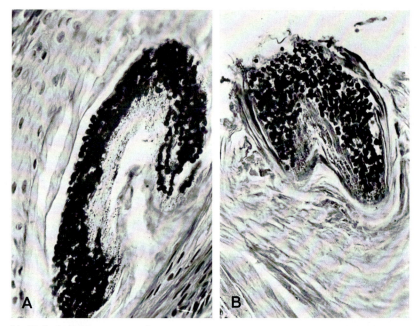

Fig. 38. Endothrix tinea capitis due to *T.tonsurans*: A. Level III, transverse-oblique section above the APM showing intrapilary arthrospores in linear arrangement. Remnants of the inner root sheath are seen and the outer root sheath shows some parakeratosis (PAS with diastase digestion method, ×350; AFIP Neg. 63-3196). B. Level VI, transverse section through the SC showing endothrix arthrospores still confined by an intact hair cortex cuticle. No fungal elements are present in the dilated keratin-plugged follicular ostium (PAS with diastase digestion method, ×300; AFIP Neg. 63-3196)

demonstrated the intrapilary fungal elements and showed a proliferation of reticular fibers in areas of inflammation. Fontana-Masson silver method demonstrated the arthrospores and was particularly good for showing melanin granules free and within giant cells and melanophages in areas of perifollicular granulomatous inflammation. The Ziehl-Neelsen method for acid-fast bacteria stains hair an intense red color and was excellent for identifying pilar fragments in areas of granulomatous inflammation.

Differential Diagnosis: The histopathologic and histochemical differential diagnosis of tinea capitis caused by *T.tonsurans* and *T.sulfureum* includes black-dot endothrix tinea capitis caused by *T.violaceum*. Black-dot variety of tinea capitis seems to be an exception in our case material, but when seen shows dilated follicular ostia containing colored debris, hair fragments and fungal elements. Other dermatophytes causing endothrix tinea capitis have been reported and these include *T. Yaoundei* (GEORG et al.), *T.soudanense* (JOHNSON and ROSENTHAL) and *M.nanum* (BROCK). *Trichophyton simii* (RIPPON, ENG and MALKINSON), isolated from a patient with tinea corporis produced an endothrix infection in guinea pigs with brilliant light green fluorescence under Wood's light, but human cases of tinea capitis caused by this organism have not been reported. *Trichophyton rubrum* in more tropical regions can rarely cause tinea capitis. HILDICK-SMITH et al. in their classification of fungi based on the pattern of pilar invasion listed *T.rubrum* as involving the hair shaft producing an endothrix infection. MACKENNA et al. examined hairs from *T.rubrum* infection on the leg and demonstrated a large-spored endothrix pattern of involvement. Contrary to this, WEBER and ULRICH obtained study material from a patient showing kerion caused by *T.rubrum* and indicated that the hair shafts were covered by spores. BLANK and TELNER (1956) studied multiple *T.rubrum* infected hairs from a man with pustular folliculitis of the beard and demonstrated three different parasitic patterns, namely, extrapilary segmented hyphae, intrapilary segmented hyphae, and extrapilary segmented hyphae associated with invasion of the cortex cuticle by large arthrospores. BLANK and TELNER concluded the endo-ectothrix pattern in *T.rubrum* hair infections constitute a transitory form of the ultimate endothrix parasitic growth phase. We have not had the opportunity to study biopsy material from patients with tinea capitis caused by *T.rubrum*, but our observations of chronic disease involving smooth skin hair follicles indicates that this dermatophyte parasitizes hair showing an endo-ectothrix pattern with intrapilary hyphae and a surrounding combination of segmented hyphae and large arthrospores (megaspores).

Comment: Our observations confirm that *T.tonsurans* and *T.sulfureum* represent true endothrix parasites. Kerion produced by these organisms can show spicules of hair with intrapilary arthrospores in foci of perifollicular granulomatous inflammation, but apparently the keratinophilic fungal elements do not survive and propagate in a mesenchymal substrate. In classifying dermatophytes, most observers consider *T.sulfureum* as a variety of *T.tonsurans* (WILSON et al.; HILDICK-SMITH et al.; EMMONS et al.; LEWIS et al.). GEORG (1956) concluded that species such as *T.sulfureum*, *T.sabouraudii* and *T.epilans* can be regarded as unusual variants of a single species, namely, *T.tonsurans*. BLANK (1959) reported there was not enough evidence to lump *T.tonsurans*, *T.sulfureum* and *T.sabouraudii* in one species, and it was recommended by the Medical Mycology Committee of the British Medical Research Council to keep these species distinct. BLANK (1959) cited his experience with endothrix tinea capitis in villages of eastern Quebec, Canada, and always isolated only either *T.tonsurans* or *T.sulfureum* from patients in each village. The primary isolates were always typical individual species from each village, and repeated follow-up cultures over a 3-year-period showed the same colony characteristics for either *T.tonsurans*, *T.sabouraudii* or *T.sulfureum* (BLANK, 1959). Because no international agreement exists with regard to grouping these organisms, BLANK (1959) prefers to consider *T.tonsurans*, *T.sulfureum*, and *T.sabouraudii* as distinct since lumping them may conceal interesting epidemiological and clinical data. BLANK (1959) advises that alterations in the taxonomy of dermatophytes should be undertaken with caution and only after complete careful consideration of all viewpoints. Only a close cooperation of all specialties dealing with dermatophytes can provide a firm basis for better taxonomy of these organisms (BLANK, 1959).

Results of histochemical studies in demonstrating the fungal elements of *T.tonsurans* can be explained by chitin in the skeletal framework and isolation of nitrogen free water-soluble neutral polysaccharides which have been identified as galactomannan I, galactomannan II, and a glucan (GRAPPEL et al.). GRAPPEL et al. have also isolated variable amounts of these water-soluble neutral polysaccharides from *M.praecox*, *T.ferrugineum* and *T.sabouraudii*. *Trichophyton tonsurans* exhibits *in vitro* elastase activity (RIPPON; RIPPON and VARADI) and may account for thinning to absence of dermal elastic tissue in biopsy sections from patients with tinea capitis caused by this endothrix parasite. Future studies will undoubtedly isolate a potent keratinolytic enzyme from *T.tonsurans* and *T.sulfureum*, since the endothrix pattern seen by light microscopy indicates prominent damage to the hair shaft hard keratin.

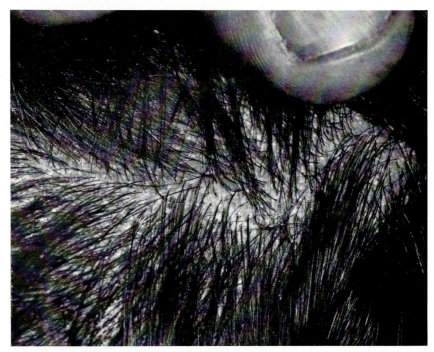

Fig. 39. Endothrix tinea capitis caused by *T. violaceum* in a 6-year-old Caucasian girl of Italian ancestory. The disease was asymptomatic and showed only mild erythema, scaling, follicular plugging and a few broken-off hairs with alopecia in the mid-parietal scalp region. The patient's mother had skin lesions on the extremities. Mycological culture studies showed the disease in both individuals was due to *T. violaceum*

7. Trichophyton Violaceum

Introduction: *Trichophyton violaceum* causes endothrix scalp disease usually referred to as black-dot tinea capitis. The disease is widely distributed throughout the world and is particularly seen in Russia, Poland, Italy, Spain, Portugal, Yugoslavia, South America, India, North Africa, Israel and Australia. Infections in the United States occur chiefly in immigrants or their siblings, but some cases have been reported in native stock. Most initial infections occur in children, and the disease may persist into adulthood. The infection is transmitted from human to human and probably by indirect contact through hats, combs, and hair bands. Our histopathologic and histochemical observations were made from review of biopsy sections from two children and one adult with endothrix tinea capitis proven by mycological culture studies to be caused by *T. violaceum*.

Gross Appearance: Clinically, there is usually only mild inflammation localized to perifollicular scalp tissue (Fig. 39), and small pustules and follicular crusts tend to form, followed by permanent scarring. Kerion rarely develops, and the usual features are "black dots" caused by hairs breaking off near the scalp surface with superficial scaling (Fig. 39). Sequelae of longstanding disease includes atrophy, scarring, and permanent alopecia. The clinical differential diagnosis includes other dermatophytes causing endothrix tinea capitis, and diseases listed in the consideration of infections due to *T. tonsurans* and *T. sulfureum*. Because the disease is manifested in some patients only in the form of minimal scaling (Fig. 39), the resem-

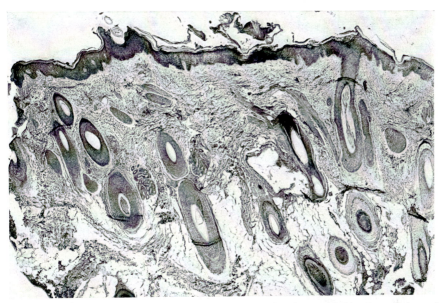

Fig. 40. Endothrix tinea capitis caused by *T.violaceum* showing multiple anagen hairs, only two of which are infected. The epidermis shows focal hyperkeratosis and minimal acanthosis. Perifollicular inflammation is slight, but high power magnification showed some extracellular, interfibrillar ground substance changes (H & E, ×20)

blance to seborrheic dermatitis is often striking. Examination of the infected patient under Wood's lamp is negative, and according to MACKENZIE, clinical diagnosis of nonfluorescent scalp ringworm is not reliable. MACKENZIE discarded clinical examinations in favor of the hair-brush diagnosis of nonfluorescent tinea capitis by repeated recovery of the causative organism from sterilized hairbrushes.

Microscopic Observations: The microscopic changes were similar to *T.tonsurans* and *T.sulfureum*, except there was less perifollicular inflammation (Fig. 40). Examination of serial sections showed spotted parakeratosis, follicular plugging with entrapped remnants of infected hairs, and mild irregular acanthosis (Fig. 40). Multiple anagen follicles were identified and only a few contained infected hairs (Fig. 40). The infected hairs were altered and sometimes showed a serpentine appearance in the hair canal (Fig. 40). Transverse sections of infected hairs showed only intrapilary fungal elements from the upper KZ to the follicular ostia SC (Figs. 42A—D). The dermis showed only a mild perifollicular mixed cellular infiltration (Fig. 40) and no changes of kerion were observed. Extracellular interfibrillar ground substance changes, connective tissue alterations, and rarity of sebaceous glands were similar to *M.audouinii* and *M.canis* infections.

Histochemistry: Intrapilary arthrospores were strongly PAS-reactive (Figs. 41, 42A—D, 43A) and positive with the other methods for demonstrating fungal elements. Transverse sections through infected follicles showed arthrospores confined to the hair shaft by an intact cuticle of the cortex, and fungal elements were observed no deeper than the upper regions of the KZ (Fig. 42A). Linear arrangement of the arthrospores (Figs. 43A—B) in vertical sections showing the longitudinal plane of infected hairs was even more prominent than described for *T.tonsurans* and *T.sulfureum*. Special histochemical methods demonstrated the relationship of intrapilary arthrospores to altered hairs which sometimes showed a serpentine

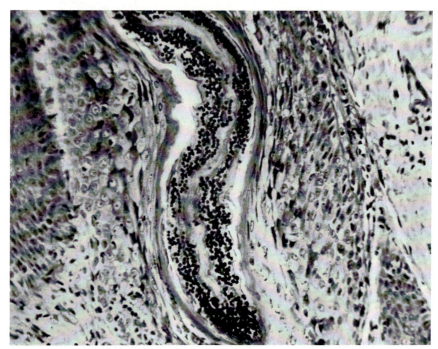

Fig. 41. Endothrix tinea capitis due to *T. violaceum* showing a section vertical to the epidermis with an involved hair follicle in longitudinal plane. The section represents a high power magnification of the follicular infundibulum above the SG level, and shows a serpentine configuration of the hair canal and remnants of a hair shaft infected with intrapilary arthrospores. The arthrospores show a definite predilection for the peripheral hair cortex, but are contained by an intact cuticle with no involvement of the adjacent keratinized and parakeratotic outer root sheath (PAS, ×190)

appearance (Fig. 41) and the hair canal contour was similar. The colloidal iron stain demonstrated an increase of hyaluronic acid in extracellular interfibrillar spaces, lesser amounts in the outer root sheath and none associated with intrapilary arthrospores. Mast cells were present in increased numbers in the dermis, and collagen and elastic fibers were generally thinned or absent in areas of increased ground substance. Areas of perifollicular inflammation showed a network of reticular fibers

Fig. 42. Endothrix tinea capitis caused by *T. violaceum* showing transverse sections through various levels of the same infected hair: A. Level II, section through the upper KZ showing endothrix arthrospores. The cuticle of the cortex is intact (PAS, ×440; AFIP Neg. 63-3199). B. Level III, section through the APM showing intrapilary arthrospores and no fungal elements involving the inner root sheath which appears well organized (PAS, ×440; AFIP Neg. 63-3199). C. Level IV, section through the SG showing endothrix arthrospores with an intense PAS color reaction. No fungal elements are seen in the keratinized outer root sheath bordering on the hair canal (PAS, ×305; AFIP Neg. 63-3199). D. Level V, section through the SM-AT showing an infected and uninvolved hair sharing the same keratin-plugged follicular ostium. No fungal elements are seen in the adjacent SC (PAS, ×305; AFIP Neg. 63-3199)

Fig. 43. Endothrix tinea capitis caused by *T. violaceum* showing vertical longitudinal sections of infected hairs: A. Section at APM level showing linear arrangement of intrapilary arthrospores. Glycogen has been removed from the outer root sheath (PAS with diastase digestion method, ×305; AFIP Neg. 63-3201). B. Section at APM level showing endothrix arthrospores in linear arrangement and confined by an intact cuticle of the cortex. The argyrophilic granules in the inner root sheath and outer root sheath represent melanin pigment (Snook's reticulum stain, ×305; AFIP Neg. 63-3201)

with Snook's reticulum stain. No fungal elements were demonstrated in the corium
or living epidermis. The intrapilary arthrospores were still in fragments of hair
even within dilated, keratin-plugged, follicular ostia. The pilary outer root sheath
showed a prominent increase in glycogen similar to that described for *M.audouinii*

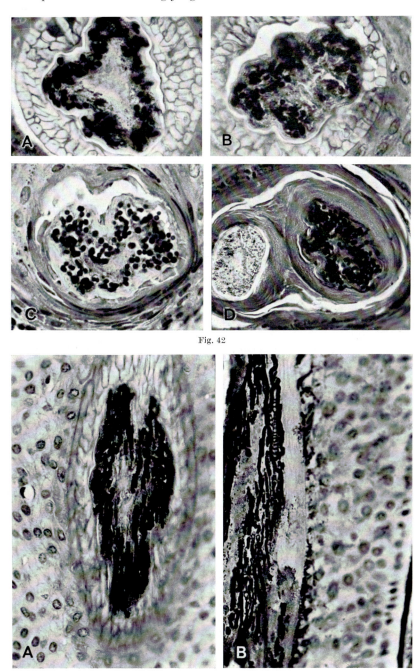

Fig. 42

Fig. 43

and *M. canis*. The remaining histochemical studies did not show significant results and were similar to observations described for other dermatophytes causing tinea capitis.

Differential Diagnosis: The histopathologic and histochemical differential diagnosis of endothrix tinea capitis caused by *T. violaceum* is similar to *T. tonsurans* and *T. sulfureum*.

Comment: Our studies confirm observations made by others that endothrix tinea capitis caused by *T. violaceum* shows only intrapilary arthrospores and these occur from the upper KZ to the SC. *In vitro* elastase activity to *T. violaceum* shows negative activity at 1 week (Rippon and Varadi), yet our histochemical studies indicate dermal elastic tissue thinning without prominent inflammatory changes. Morphologic alterations of the hair shaft in *T. violaceum* infections indicate an intense keratinolytic enzyme activity similar to that described for *T. mentagrophytes* (Yu et al.), *M. canis* (Daniels), *T. schoenleinii* and *T. rubrum* (Weary et al., 1967).

Two patients in our group of 3 with tinea capitis from *T. violaceum* were of European ancestry, but 1 child was from native stock born in Philadelphia and no history of travel outside the United States. The 2 children in our study had other members of the family with similar disease including involvement of glabrous skin. The sterilized hairbrush diagnosis technique (Mackenzie) was of value in isolating *T. violaceum* from the scalp of siblings without obvious evidence of clinical disease.

8. Summary and Conclusions

Histopathologic and histochemical evaluation of biopsy sections from patients with tinea capitis due to *M. audouinii*, *M. canis*, *M. gypseum*, *T. schoenleinii*, *T. mentagrophytes*, *T. tonsurans*, *T. sulfureum* and *T. violaceum* shows fungal elements rich in polysaccharides and defines the hair follicle parasitic pattern of these pathogenic dermatophytes. Abnormal amounts of hyaluronic acid are present in the dermal stroma, outer root sheath of anagen hair follicles, and this substance shows an affinity for fungal elements in *M. audouinii*, *M. canis* and *T. schoenleinii* infections. It is clearly demonstrated that *M. audouinii*, *M. canis*, *M. gypseum*, *T. schoenleinii*, *T. asteroides*, and *T. granulosum* cause endo-ectothrix scalp infections, and that the other dermatophytes studied represent true endothrix parasites. Observations suggest that survival and propagation of dermatophytes is pH dependent, and may be related to increased amounts of hyaluronic acid in the extracellular interfibrillar spaces and pilary outer root sheath. The noninflammatory clinical appearance of many infections due to *M. audouinii*, *T. tonsurans*, *T. sulfureum* and *T. violaceum* contrasts sharply with the intense histopathologic changes and indicates that scalp tissue has a unique ability for masking the true nature of disease processes. In general, the diagnosis of tinea capitis is easily made by thorough clinical and mycological study of the patient. The value and justification for doing biopsies on patients with tinea capitis is apparent since considerable information can be gained and knowledge increased regarding pathogenesis. Histopathologic and histochemical observations often suggest new problems for investigation by a variety of sophisticated approaches.

Blank opened the discussion on "Tinea Capitis", read by Graham et al., before the Section on Dermatology at the 112th Annual Meeting of the American Medical Association, Atlantic City, New Jersey, June 17, 1963, and his remarks seem appropriate to be included here as follows: Microscopic observations of hairs removed from patients with tinea capitis were made by Remak (cited by Sabouraud) and Gruby more than a century ago. These studies established the mycotic etiology of tinea capitis and suggested that more than one organism could cause the disease. If dermatologists at the turn of the century had paid more attention to GRUBY's published observations, SABOURAUD would not have encountered so much opposition from his doctrinaire colleagues who refused to alter their opinions and recognize that different organisms could cause tinea capitis.

Two main parasitic patterns of hair involvement exist; endothrix and endo-ectothrix types. In both types, the hair is invaded, however, endothrix infections show intrapilary fungal elements consisting of arthrospores, i.e., broken-up hyphae. In endo-ectothrix infections, hyphae are found inside the hair and arthrospores and/or hyphae surround the invaded hair. In the endo-ectothrix pattern, fungal elements are not always recognizable on direct microscopic examination, although cross sections of an infected hair will reveal intrapilary hyphae. It is unfortunate that this type of parasitic pattern is often referred to as an ectothrix infection. This has made many forget that each parasitized hair regardless of the dermatophytic infection always shows fungal elements inside the hair shaft.

Invasion of keratinized hair by dermatophytes has been clearly demonstrated. Electron microscopic investigations by MERCER and VERMER leave little doubt that dermatophytes are keratinolytic and feed on keratin of the invaded hair. Our own studies demonstrate keratinolytic enzymes in dermatophytes and this has to be regarded as one of their most pathogenic traits (these observations have recently been corroborated by YU et al., by isolation of a keratinolytic enzyme from *T. mentagrophytes* variety *granulosum* which digests hair *in vitro*). A difference in keratinolytic enzymes of various dermatophytes could conceivably account for the variation in parasitic patterns seen.

Application of histochemical methods to the study of tinea capitis has opened new avenues which may aid in better understanding the disease process. The variable, but regularly observed microscopic inflammatory response in infections due to *M. audouinii*, *T. tonsurans*, *T. sulfureum*, *T. violaceum* and *T. schoenleinii* may be a surprise to the clinician. It indicates that there are only quantitative differences in the host tissue response and that clinical distinction between inflammatory and noninflammatory types of tinea capitis is meaningless. Chemical investigations have shown that the water-soluble polysaccharides of each dermatophyte consist of a glucan and two different galactomannans. The glucans and galactomannans differ from species to species. It might therefore be expected that different immunological reactions of the host tissue are due to different allergens, probably glycopeptides or polysaccharide-protein complexes, varying from species to species. Further investigations of keratinolytic enzymes and allergens isolated from different species together with an extension of histochemical studies of parasitized host tissues will provide a better understanding of the host-parasite relationship of dermatophytic scalp infections in the same way as earlier microscopic observations aided in recognition of fungi as the cause of tinea capitis.

Tinea Barbae, Tinea Faciei, Tinea Corporis, Tinea Manuum, Tinea Cruris, Tinea Pedis, and Tinea Unguium

1. Introduction

As with tinea capitis, dermatophytic infections involving other cutaneous sites including nails will be considered from an etiological viewpoint. Certain species show a predilection for particular anatomical locations, and for this reason, prototypes will be selected to point out significant tissue changes. When certain data have already been mentioned for a species causing tinea capitis, repeat information will not be given.

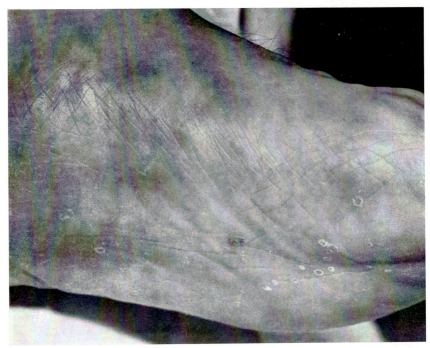

Fig. 44. Tinea pedis caused by *T. rubrum* showing erythematous scaling of the plantar surface of a foot. One lesion shows crusting and close inspection revealed minute vesicles. The patient also had vesicular lesions on the fingers and *T. rubrum* infection on other parts of the body

2. Trichophyton Rubrum

Introduction: One of the most common dermatophytes with a worldwide distribution and causing cutaneous human fungal disease is *T. rubrum*. This organism produces a wide range of clinical and histopathologic changes that frequently lead to mis-diagnosis. In comparison with other dermatophytes, *T. rubrum* is responsible for cutaneous infections in varying ratios in different countries, and disease from this organism has been increasing during the past decade. There has been a great increase in the incidence of *T. rubrum* infections since World War II, and this organism is thought to be one of the most recently introduced pathogens into western countries. *Trichophyton rubrum* is the second most common pathogen causing superficial cutaneous fungal infections isolated from the case material studied at The Skin and Cancer Hospital of Philadelphia (McCaffree et al.), and particularly from patients with tinea pedis (Figs. 44, 74, 82), onychomycosis (Figs. 74, 82), tinea cruris (Fig. 58), tinea corporis (Figs. 50, 54, 56, 61, 67, 74) and tinea manuum (Fig. 47). Except for tinea capitis, our experience with *T. rubrum* infections indicates that the organism involves the glaborous skin (Figs. 50, 54, 56, 61, 67, 74), hands (Fig. 47), feet (Figs. 44, 74, 82), groin (Fig. 58), and nails (Figs. 74, 82). The host tissue response elicited by *T. rubrum* varies from a relatively mild inflammatory one to that which is quite intense producing a spectrum of clinicopathologic reactions showing a striking resemblance to other dermatoses. Each of the important reaction patterns produced by *T. rubrum* and the significant results of histochemical studies will be discussed. This report is based on observations of one or more biopsies from 75 patients with *T. rubrum* infections, and all but a few of the individuals were adults.

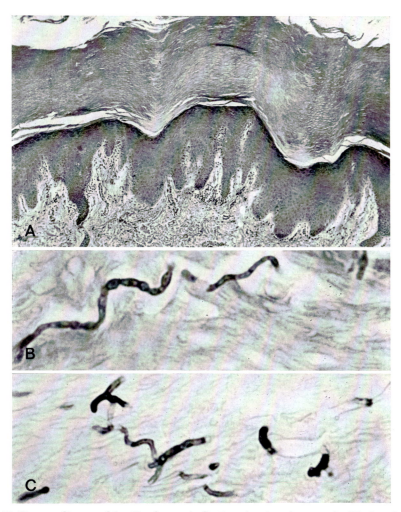

Fig. 45. Tinea pedis caused by *T.rubrum*: A. Section showing changes of mild chronic dermatitis characterized by hyperkeratosis, spotted parakeratosis, irregular acanthosis, and a minimal perivascular infiltrate of lymphocytes and histiocytes (H & E, ×55). B. High power magnification of the SC showing frequently segmented hyphae (PAS, ×655). C. High power magnification of the SC in A showing multiple hyphae, some of which are branched (GMS, ×655)

Gross Appearance: Anatomically, biopsy material was studied from *T.rubrum* infections involving the face (Figs. 50, 61), neck (Figs. 56, 61), arms (Fig. 54), hands (Fig. 47), back, abdomen, flank, buttocks, groin (Fig. 58), legs (Figs. 67, 74), ankles (Fig. 74), feet (Figs. 44, 74, 82) and nails (Figs. 74, 82). Over 80% of the patients showed disease in more than one anatomical location. Grossly, *T.rubrum* infections showed erythema, purpura, scaling, urticarial changes, annular infiltrated plaques, papules, nodules, vesicles, bullae, pustules, follicular pustules, excoriations, papulonecrotic lesions and deep seated follicular nodules and plaques, some of which were tender and painful (Figs. 44, 47, 50, 54, 56, 58, 61, 67, 74, 82). Onychomycosis from *T.rubrum* showed dull gray, opaque, thickened, elevated, distorted nails with irregular margins and distal subungual powdery hyperkeratosis (Figs. 74, 82). Some

17*

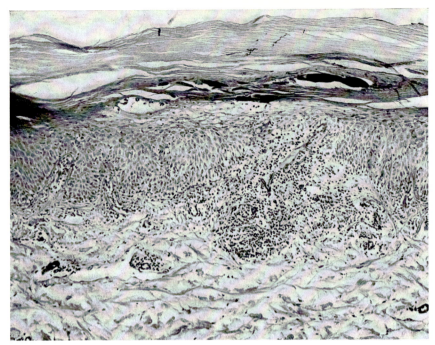

Fig. 46. Tinea pedis caused by *T.rubrum* showing changes of subacute dermatitis characterized by spongiosis, intracellular edema, exocytosis, angiitis, and a perivascular infiltrate of lymphocytes, histiocytes, neutrophils and eosinophils. Hyphae are demonstrated in the SC which shows accumulations of lymph fluid (PAS, ×93)

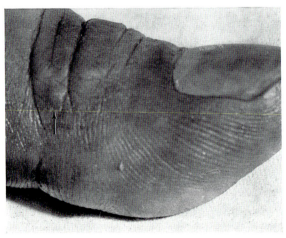

Fig. 47. Tinea manuum caused by *T.rubrum* occurring in the same patient illustrated by Fig. 44. A close-up view (arrow) shows an isolated vesicular lesion on the thumb

Fig. 48. Tinea manuum due to *T.rubrum* showing an acute vesicular dermatitis mimicking contact dermatitis. The section shows hyperkeratosis, parakeratosis, accumulations of lymph fluid in the SC, intraepidermal vesicles, spongiosis, exocytosis, and moderate irregular acanthosis. A mild inflammatory infiltrate is present in the upper corium (H & E, ×32)

Fig. 49. Tinea manuum caused by *T.rubrum*: A. High power magnification of Fig. 48 showing intraepidermal multilocular vesicles containing lymph fluid and mononuclear cells similar to allergic contact dermatitis (H & E, ×155). B. High power magnification of A demonstrating segmented hyphae in the SC and adjacent to the intraepidermal vesicles (PAS, ×655)

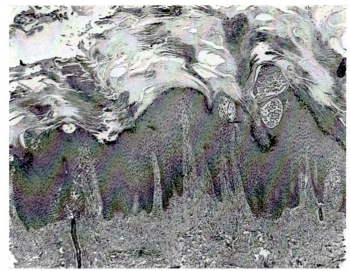

Fig. 48

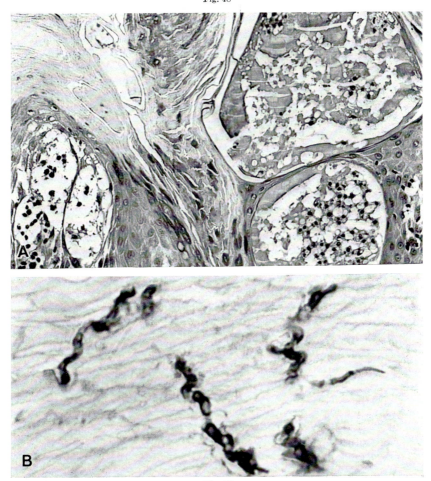

Fig. 49

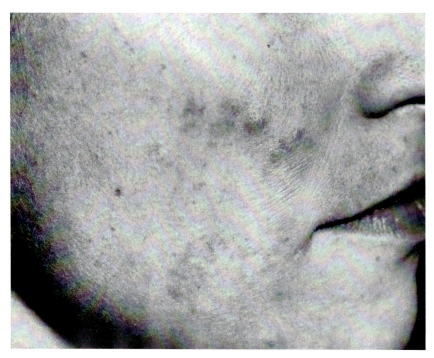

Fig. 50. Tinea corporis (tinea faciei) caused by *T. rubrum* showing erythematous, macular, papular, and vesicular lesions on the right cheek. The clinical differential diagnosis included nummular eczema, contact dermatitis, lupus erythematosus, and polymorphous light eruption

of the patients with *T. rubrum* infections showed a variety of cutaneous id eruptions. In addition to dermatophytosis, a variety of diseases was considered in the clinical differential diagnosis, and in order of frequency, these included: silica granuloma, granuloma annulare (Figs. 54, 56, 61), nummular eczema (Fig. 50), lupus erythematosus (Figs. 50, 61), polymorphous light eruption (Figs. 50, 61), erythema perstans (Figs. 54, 56, 61), parapsoriasis en plaque, chronic vesicular eruption (Figs. 44, 47), dermatitis herpetiformis, allergic angiitis, necrobiosis lipoidica diabeticorum (Fig. 67), cutaneous sarcoidosis, benign lymphocytic infiltration of Jessner-Kanof (Figs. 50, 61), folliculitis (Figs. 67, 74), pyoderma, erythema annulare centrifugum (Figs. 54, 56, 61), familial benign chronic pemphigus, tinea versicolor, sporotrichosis, lichen simplex chronicus (Fig. 67), papulosquamous drug eruption, contact dermatitis (Fig. 50) and cellulitis (Figs. 67, 74).

Microscopic Observations: A previous report (GRAHAM, BLANK, JOHNSON and GRAY) from The Skin and Cancer Hospital of Philadelphia recorded *T. rubrum* infections causing a variety of histopathologic reactions showing remarkable resemblance to other inflammatory skin diseases. From our additional experience and for purposes of this report, cutaneous reactions caused by *T. rubrum* have been classified into the following clinicopathologic types: chronic dermatitis (Figs. 44, 45A), subacute dermatitis (Figs. 44, 46), acute vesicular dermatitis of the contact type and mimicking nummular eczema (Figs. 47, 48, 50, 51), erythema multiforme type (Figs. 54, 55A), erythema perstans (Figs. 56, 57A—B), purpuric dermatitis (Figs. 58, 59), granuloma faciale (Figs. 61, 62), granuloma annulare (Figs. 61, 64, 65), pustular dermatitis (Figs. 67, 68), papulonecrotic dermatitis with allergic

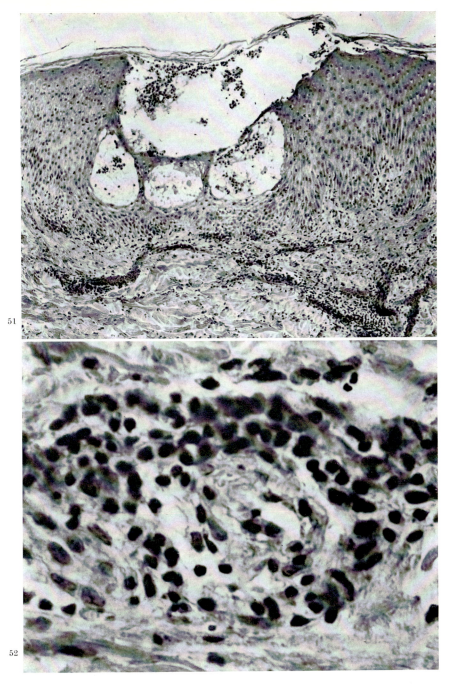

Fig. 51. Tinea faciei due to *T. rubrum* showing multilocular intraepidermal vesicles containing mononuclear cells, spongiosis, exocytosis, and acanthosis. In the papillary corium there are moderately intense angiitis and perivascular inflammation. The features are strikingly similar to nummular eczema, contact dermatitis and vesicular id eruption (H & E, ×93)

Fig. 52. High power magnification of tinea faciei caused by *T. rubrum* showing a small blood vessel with thickening, endothelial swelling and inflammatory infiltration of its wall. The vascular changes are those suggesting allergic angiitis (H & E, ×655)

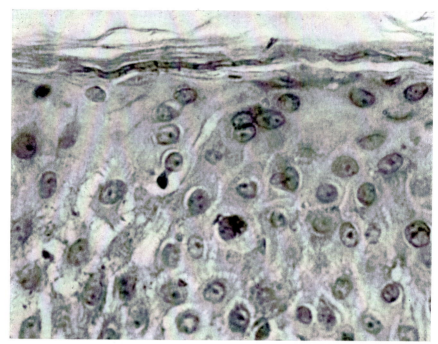

Fig. 53. Tinea faciei caused by *T. rubrum* showing long segmented hyphae in the SC. The stratum Malpighii is altered in the form of spongiosis, intracellular edema, and the presence of multinucleated epithelial cells (PAS, ×655)

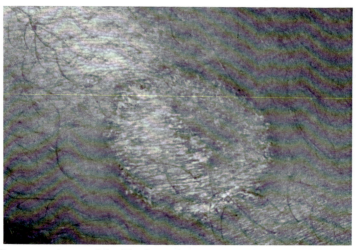

Fig. 54. Tinea corporis caused by *T. rubrum* showing an erythematous, annular, target-type lesion on the arm and mimicking erythema multiforme. The periphery and central part of the lesion showed gross evidence of vesiculation

angiitis (Figs. 67, 70A—B), folliculitis and perifolliculitis (Figs. 67, 71), nodular granulomatous perifolliculitis (Figs. 74, 75) showing features of allergic granulomatosis and reactive lymphoid hyperplasia, and onychomycosis (Figs. 74, 82, 83). Each host-parasite tissue reaction pattern including significant nail changes will

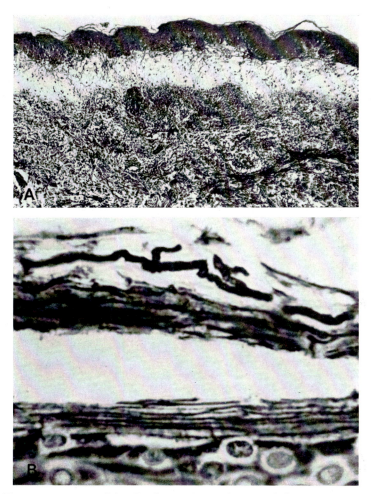

Fig. 55. Tinea corporis caused by *T.rubrum*: A. Erythema multiforme reaction showing a subepidermal multilocular bulla and angiitis of the small papillary dermal blood vessels (Movat's pentachrome method, ×66). B. High power magnification of the SC in A showing silver-positive hyphae (Snook's reticulum stain, ×655)

be described because of confusion with other inflammatory, allergic, granuloma-tous and reactive dermatoses.

Depending on the anatomical location, stage, and duration of the lesion, all clinicopathologic types of *T. rubrum* infection can show changes of mild to moderate chronic dermatitis (Fig. 45A). The usual features included combinations of hyper-keratosis, hypokeratosis, spotted parakeratosis, hypergranulosis, hypogranulosis, spongiosis, intracellular edema, exocytosis of mononuclear cells and mild to mod-erate irregular acanthosis (Fig. 45A). The upper corium showed mild to moderate perivascular inflammation composed of lymphocytes and histiocytes (Fig. 45A). Plasma cells and eosinophils were sometimes seen in the cellular infiltration along with vascular ectasia and edematous stromal changes. Because of nonspecific features, fungal elements in the SC were often overlooked and the changes con-fused with dermatitis-eczema dermatoses and various papulosquamous diseases.

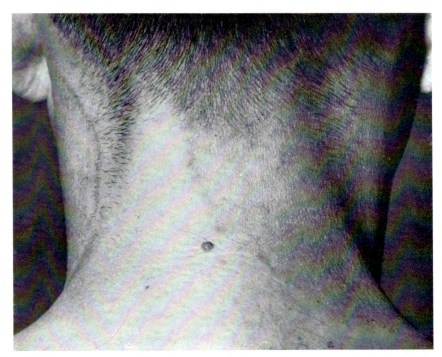

Fig. 56. Tinea corporis caused by *T. rubrum* showing erythematous, scaling lesions with an elevated infiltrated peripheral border located on the neck, and mimicking erythema perstans. The disease extended into the occipital scalp region but there was no evidence of fungal elements invading pilosebaceous follicles to cause tinea capitis

Subacute dermatitis (Fig. 46) showed changes similar to chronic dermatitis (Fig. 45A), but additional features were superficial crusting, lymph fluid in the SC, prominent spongiosis, intracellular edema, moderate exocytosis and intraepidermal microabscesses containing mononuclear cells (Fig. 46). The upper corium usually showed edematous stromal changes, a mixed inflammatory infiltrate, and an angiitis of the small blood vessels characterized by endothelial swelling, thickening and infiltration of their walls by inflammatory cells (Fig. 46). Acute vesicular dermatitis (Figs. 48, 49A, 51) of the contact type or mimicking nummular eczema showed some features already mentioned for subacute and chronic dermatitis, but particularly spongiosis, exocytosis of mononuclear cells, reticular degeneration, and intraepidermal unilocular and multilocular vesicles (Figs. 48, 49A, 51). Some examples of acute vesicular dermatitis caused by *T. rubrum* showed vascular changes of allergic angiitis (Fig. 52).

Erythema multiforme type reactions (Fig. 55A) caused by *T. rubrum* were characterized by prominent subepidermal multilocular bullae containing acute inflammatory cells, lymph fluid, red blood cells and fibrin (Fig. 55A). Stretched and thinned collagen fibers traversed the subepidermal bullae and inserted into the overlying dermoepidermal junction (Fig. 55A). The epidermal bulla roof was generally not significantly altered and the dermoepidermal basement membrane appeared intact (Fig. 55A). Small blood vessels in the upper corium and middle corium showed changes of allergic angiitis. The perivascular stroma showed interstitial edema, extravasated red blood cells, and an infiltrate of lymphocytes, histiocytes, neutrophils and eosinophils (Fig. 55A).

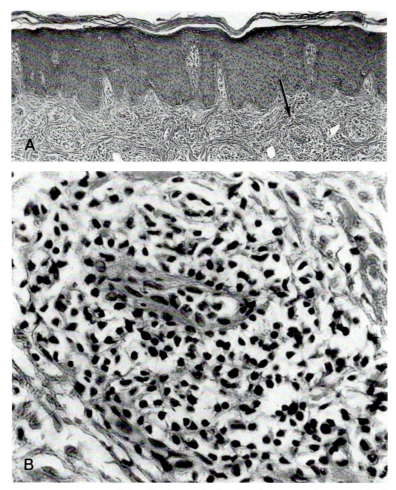

Fig. 57. Tinea corporis caused by *T.rubrum*: A. Section showing uniform acanthosis of the epidermis and special stains demonstrated fungal elements in the SC. The papillary corium shows an angiitis of small blood vessels, vascular ectasia and mild interstitial edema (H & E, ×55). B. High power magnification of A showing a small blood vessel (arrow) surrounded by lymphocytes and histiocytes. The cuffing of inflammatory cells about small blood vessels showing endothelial swelling, thickening, and infiltration of their walls is characteristic of erythema perstans and other persistent erythemas. The tissue changes suggest a hyper-sensitivity vasculitis (H & E, ×445)

Erythema perstans type reactions (Figs. 57A—B) generally showed minimal epidermal changes, but some examples exhibited hyperkeratosis, spotted para-keratosis, intraepidermal microabscesses containing mononuclear cells, acanthosis, and focal liquefaction degeneration. The most consistent change was vascular in-volvement characterized by an angiitis of small blood vessels (Figs. 57A—B) at various levels of the corium. The typical features were a broad mantle of lympho-cytes and histiocytes about small thickened blood vessels showing endothelial swel-ling and infiltration of their walls (Figs. 57A—B). Red blood cells, eosinophils and neutrophils were sometimes seen in the perivascular cellular infiltrate and the stroma showed variable degrees of extracellular interfibrillar ground substance changes.

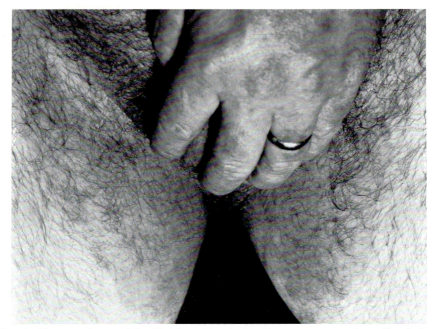

Fig. 58. Tinea cruris caused by *T.rubrum* showing erythematous, purpuric, scaling lesions, with an active peripheral border involving the medial aspects of the upper thigh and adjacent inguinal regions. The patient also had tinea pedis, onychomycosis, folliculitis, and deep seated nodular lesions on the extremities showing clinicopathologic and histochemical features of nodular granulomatous perifolliculitis

Purpuric dermatitis reactions (Fig. 59) were characterized by focal changes of hypokeratosis, parakeratosis, exocytosis, liquefaction degeneration, and red blood cells in areas of spongiosis (Figs. 59, 60). The subjacent papillary corium showed perivascular inflammation, extravasated red blood cells, angiitis, and edematous stromal changes (Fig. 59).

Granuloma faciale type reactions (Fig. 62) showed an essentially normal epidermis except for effacement of the rete ridges (Fig. 62). A grenz zone of relatively uninvolved connective tissue always separated the epidermis and pilosebaceous follicles from an adjacent cellular infiltration of neutrophils, eosinophils, lymphocytes, histiocytes, and plasma cells (Fig. 62). Hemosiderin and red blood cells were sometimes intermingled with the inflammatory cells, and edematous stromal changes showed an increase in ground substance with special stains (Fig. 62). Striking was the relationship of inflammatory cells to small dilated blood vessels (Fig. 62).

Changes mimicking granuloma annulare (Fig. 64) showed focal stromal alterations consisting of an increase in extracellular interfibrillar ground substance,

Fig. 59. Tinea cruris caused by *T.rubrum* showing changes of purpuric dermatitis. The section shows hypokeratosis, spongiosis, mild exocytosis, focal liquefaction degeneration, and migration of red blood cells into the epidermis in the region of the disrupted dermoepidermal junction. The upper corium shows mild inflammation, extravasated red blood cells, vascular ectasia and interstitial edema. The microscopic features mimic those seen in purpuric drug eruption and pityriasis rosea (H & E, ×155)

Fig. 60. Tinea cruris caused by *T.rubrum* showing a few short hyphae in the SC and red blood cells in the epidermis adjacent to the dermoepidermal junction (GMS, ×445)

minimal inflammation, and a tendency for palisaded arrangement of fibrocytes and histiocytes about necrobiotic centers (Figs. 64, 65). The corium adjacent to areas of necrobiosis usually showed a mixed inflammatory infiltrate (Fig. 64) and

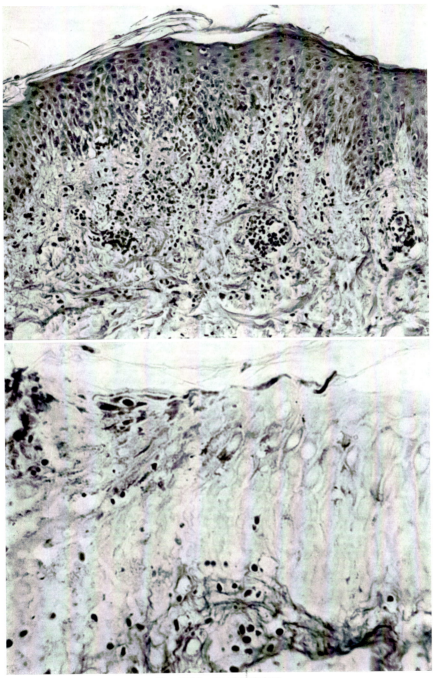

Figs. 59 (above) and 60 (below)

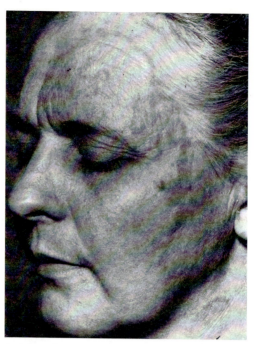

Fig. 61. Tinea corporis (tinea faciei) caused by *T. rubrum* showing erythematous scaling, annular, infiltrated plaques with elevated borders on the face and neck. The clinical differential diagnosis included granuloma annulare, granuloma faciale, erythema perstans, lupus erythematosus, and polymorphous light eruption

vascular changes of allergic angiitis. The combination of granulomatous features and vascular and extravascular changes suggested a tissue reaction pattern of allergic granulomatosis (Figs. 64, 65).

Examples of pustular dermatitis (Fig. 68) showed extrafollicular subcorneal to intraepidermal abscesses containing neutrophils with adjacent spongiosis, exocytosis, intracellular edema and acanthosis (Figs. 68, 69A). The upper corium exhibited a mixed inflammatory infiltrate including many neutrophils, vascular ectasia and edema-like stromal changes (Fig. 68).

Papulonecrotic dermatitis (Fig. 70) showing vascular changes of allergic angiitis was characterized by focal, segmental, V-shaped, necrotic, epidermal ulcerations with marginal hyperkeratosis, parakeratosis, superficial crusting, spongiosis, exocytosis and acanthosis (Fig. 70A). Ulcer defects usually contained inflamma-

---

Fig. 62. Tinea faciei caused by *T. rubrum* showing tissue changes seen in granuloma faciale. The epidermis is normal except for follicular plugging and effacement of the rete ridges. Striking is the presence of a grenz zone of relatively uninvolved connective tissue separating the epidermis from an underlying infiltration of lymphocytes, histiocytes, plasma cells, neutrophils, and eosinophils localized about small dilated blood vessels. High power magnification of the dermal cellular infiltration showed extravasated red blood cells and hemosiderin deposits. Special stains showed an increase of hyaluronic acid in the extracellular interfibrillar spaces, and thinning of collagen and elastic fibers. Reticular fibers were increased in areas of perivascular inflammation (H & E, ×83)

Fig. 63. Tinea faciei caused by *T. rubrum* showing segmented hyphae in the dilated, keratin-plugged follicle illustrated in Fig. 62 (PAS, ×445)

tory cells, cellular debris, red blood cells and fibrin (Fig. 70A). Angiitis of small blood vessels showed fibrinoid degeneration, and vascular occlusion was seen in the papillary corium subjacent to segmental infarcts (Figs. 70A—B). The extravascular stroma showed edema, fibrinoid degeneration, extravasated red blood cells, and a

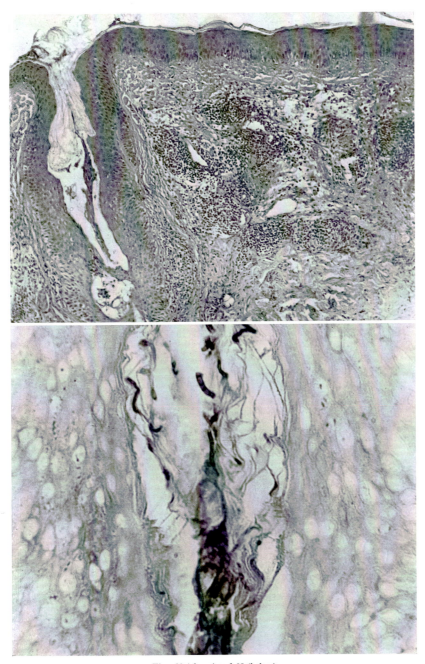

Figs. 62 (above) and 63 (below)

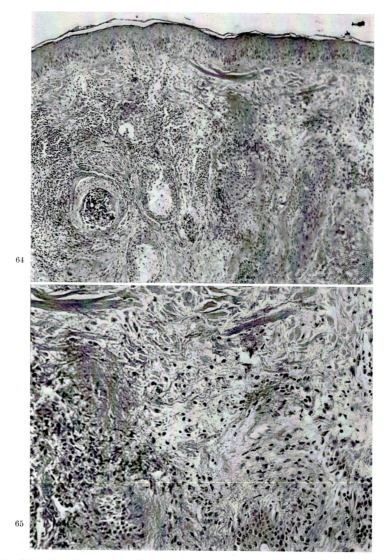

Fig. 64. Tinea faciei caused by *T. rubrum* showing a deep follicular abscess with adjacent stromal changes simulating granuloma annulare. The perifollicular stroma is infiltrated with inflammatory cells, whereas, special stains demonstrated an increase in hyaluronic acid and thinning of collagen and elastic tissue in the area mimicking granuloma annulare (H & E, ×75)

Fig. 65. Tinea faciei caused by *T. rubrum* showing a high power magnification of granuloma annulare changes seen in Fig. 64. The connective tissue exhibits necrobiosis, minimal cellular infiltration, and special stains demonstrated acid mucosaccharides in the form of extracellular interfibrillar hyaluronic acid (H & E, ×155)

mixed inflammatory infiltrate which also invaded the altered blood vessels (Figs. 70A—B).

The reaction pattern showing folliculitis and perifolliculitis (Fig. 71) was considered to represent a precursor stage for development of nodular granulomatous perifolliculitis (Fig. 75). The features of folliculitis were characterized by sub-

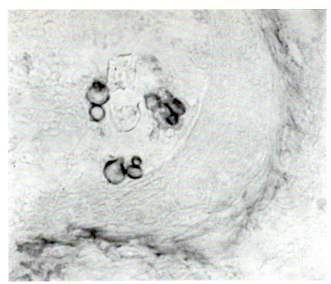

Fig. 66. Tinea faciei caused by *T.rubrum* showing a high power magnification of the follicular abscess illustrated in Fig. 64. Large arthrospores (megaspores) are demonstrated, and some show single budding type of sporulation. The walls of the arthrospores are reactive with aldehyde fuchsin pH 1.7, but negative at pH 0.4. These results indicate the presence of a nonsulfated mucosubstance (Aldehyde fuchsin pH 1.7, ×655)

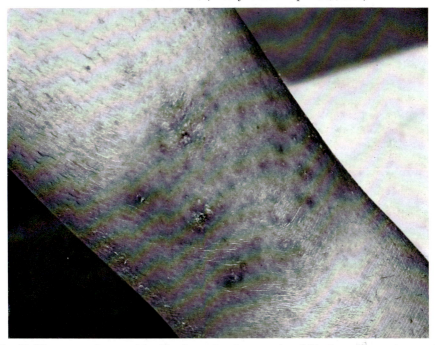

Fig. 67. Tinea corporis caused by *T.rubrum* showing pustular, follicular, and papulonecrotic lesions within an erythematous, scaling, atrophic, scarred area on the dorsum of the shin. The initial clinical diagnosis was foreign body granuloma or chronic bacterial cellulitis, but the latter interpretation was ruled out by repeated sterile cultures. The disease persisted for ten months with episodes of acute cellulitis, and subsequent diagnoses included necrobiosis lipoidica, necrobiosis lipoidica diabeticorum, stasis dermatitis, and atrophie blanche of Milian. Biopsy sections from different areas showed a variety of tissue changes, and mycological culture studies isolated *T.rubrum* as the causative organism

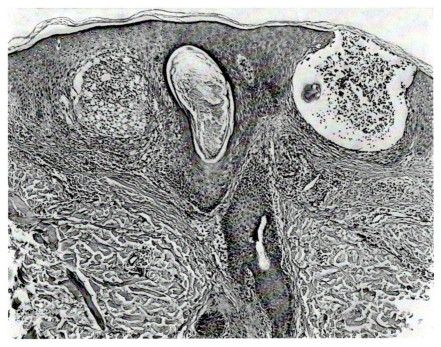

Fig. 68. Tinea corporis caused by *T.rubrum* and showing intraepidermal pustules adjacent to an uninvolved hair follicle. The upper corium exhibits inflammation and interstitial edema (H & E, ×66)

corneal pustules involving follicular ostia and adjacent stratum Malpighii with spongiosis and exocytosis of the pilary outer root sheath. Remnants of hair showing fungal elements were usually seen in the follicle canal in examining serial sections (Figs. 71, 72). Intact intrafollicular pustules were covered with thickened horny material showing parakeratosis. Changes of perifolliculitis were characterized by follicular involvement associated with adjacent stromal inflammation, fibrosis, capillary-endothelial proliferation, vascular ectasia, edema-like alteration of the stroma and extravasated red blood cells (Fig. 71). Some examples showed perifollicular granulomatous inflammation with dermal abscesses, areas of necrosis, foreign body giant cells, fragments of keratin, spicules of hair, and an angiitis of small blood vessels. Deep intrafollicular abscesses were sometimes seen, particularly in tinea barbae. Examination of sections under polarized light showed birefringence of keratinized particles in the perifollicular stroma and this endogenous foreign material served to elicit a host reaction pattern in the form of granulomatous inflammation mimicking foreign body granuloma and sometimes allergic granulomatosis.

Examples of folliculitis and perifolliculitis with granulomatous inflammation and fungal elements in the corium were classified as nodular granulomatous perifolliculitis (Fig. 75). The subcorneal intrafollicular pustule often showed 1 or 2 hairs piercing it with partial to complete degeneration of the acrotrichium, follicle infundibulum and deeper structures of the pilary complex (Fig. 75). All cases showed prominent perifollicular granulomatous changes (Figs. 75, 76), and some examples exhibited prominent connective tissue necrosis, epithelioid cells and tubercles. Remnants of the pilary outer root sheath were usually identified (Figs. 75, 76) in

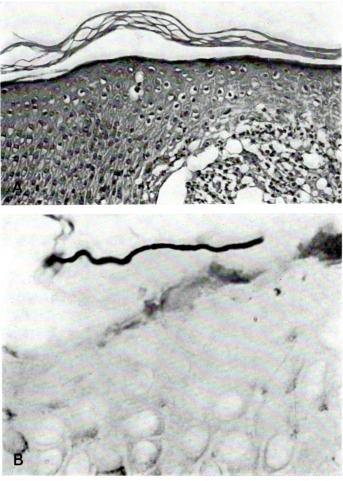

Fig. 69. Tinea corporis caused by *T. rubrum*: A. High power magnification of an intraepidermal pustule showing many neutrophils (H & E, ×155). B. High power magnification of the SC in A and showing a long hypha (GMS, ×655)

areas showing a foreign body giant cell reaction (Fig. 76), and serial sections often revealed fragments of hair (Fig. 78) and fungal elements in miliary abscesses (Figs. 78, 79B, 80, 81A—D). Blood vessel changes suggested a hypersensitivity reaction, and the combination of vascular and extravascular connective tissue damage resembled allergic granulomatosis. Some examples of nodular granulomatous perifolliculitis showed changes of reactive lymphoid hyperplasia with follicular pattern and germinal centers. The cellular infiltrate was always polymorphous and examination of serial sections usually showed foci of granulomatous inflammation, blood vessel changes of allergic angiitis, remnants of pilosebaceous follicles, and epidermal features of hyperkeratosis, spotted parakeratosis and irregular acanthosis. Biopsies from patients showing lesions of nodular granulomatous perifolliculitis were anatomically located on the legs, forearms, trunk, and face.

Onychomycosis (Figs. 74, 82) caused by *T. rubrum* showed subungual hyperkeratosis and loss of normal architecture of thickened nail plate substance at all

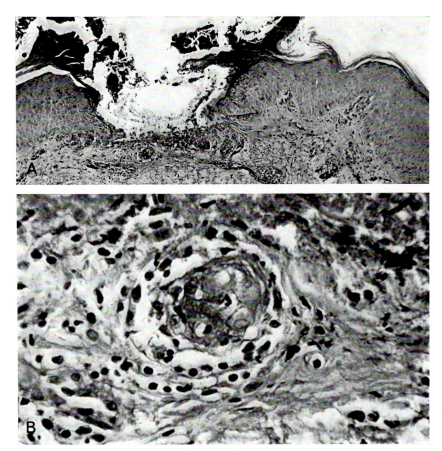

Fig. 70. Tinea corporis caused by *T. rubrum*: A. Section showing a papulonecrotic lesion with marginal hyperkeratosis, parakeratosis, and acanthosis. There is segmental epidermal necrosis showing an ulcer filled with inflammatory cells, red blood cells, fibrin, and cellular debris. High power magnification revealed a few short hyphae in the thickened SC at the ulcer margin. The base of the ulcer shows fibrinoid degeneration and there is perivascular inflammation in the upper corium (PAS, ×66). B. High power magnification of A showing an occluded small blood vessel at the base of the V-shaped area of epidermal necrosis. The involved blood vessel shows changes of allergic angiitis characterized by perivascular inflammation, infiltration of its wall and fibrinoid degeneration (PAS, ×445)

levels (Figs. 83, 84, 85). The altered nail plate keratin exhibited numerous cleavages with parakeratosis, microabscesses containing mononuclear cells and neutrophils, and aggregates of lymph fluid (Figs. 83, 84, 85). The nail bed epithelium showed abnormal keratinization in the form of hyperkeratosis and parakeratosis, and additional changes included combinations of hypogranulosis or hypergranulosis, vacuolated cells, spongiosis, exocytosis, acanthosis, elongated rete ridges and an undulating pattern caused by stromal papillomatosis (Figs. 83, 84). The altered nail bed epithelium was apparently producing soft keratin in abnormal amounts, and accounted for elevation of the abnormal nail plate. The papillary stroma showed fibrosis, inflammation, edema and vascular ectasia.

Histochemistry: In all clinicopathologic tissue reaction patterns, segmented hyphae were demonstrated in the SC, keratin-plugged follicles or altered nails by

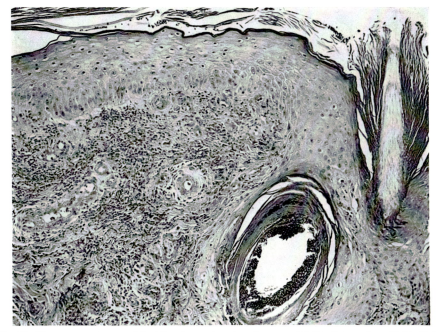

Fig. 71. Tinea corporis caused by *T. rubrum* showing changes of folliculitis and perifolliculitis. The follicular ostium contains an intact hair, whereas, the adjacent keratin-plugged follicular infundibulum shows arthrospores outlining the space where a hair was located. The perifollicular stroma shows inflammation, fibrosis and capillary-endothelial proliferation (H & E, ×93)

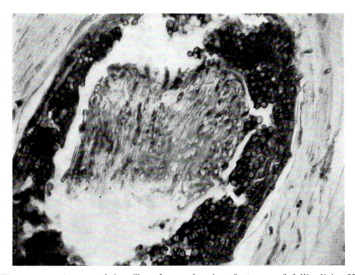

Fig. 72. Tinea corporis caused by *T. rubrum* showing features of folliculitis. High power magnification of a section 5 μ from Fig. 71 shows an intrafollicular remnant of hair with intrapilary segmented hyphae and a sheath of large arthrospores, some measuring up to 15 μ. The keratinized outer root sheath adjacent to many megaspores shows segmented hyphae and parakeratosis. Follicle invasion by *T. rubrum* clearly indicates the organism parasitizes the hair showing an endo-ectothrix pattern with formation of large arthrospores from intrapilary hyphae at all levels above the KZ (PAS, ×445)

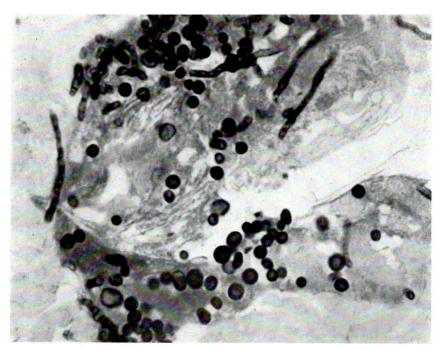

Fig. 73. Tinea corporis caused by *T. rubrum* and showing clinicopathologic features of folliculitis. High power magnification of a dilated, keratin-plugged hair follicle shows segmented hyphae and arthrospores of variable size. Water-soluble neutral polysaccharides in the fungal elements are PAS-positive and diastase-resistant (PAS with diatase digestion method, ×665)

the various histochemical methods for fungal elements (Figs. 45B—C, 46, 49B, 53, 55B, 60, 63, 66, 69B, 72, 73, 77, 79A, 84, 85). As a general rule, hyphae and arthrospores were more concentrated in newly formed epidermal and altered nail bed soft keratin just above the stratum granulosum (Figs. 49B, 53, 55B, 60, 69B, 77, 79A, 84, 85) with fewer numbers in the middle horny layer (Figs. 45B—C, 46) and rare forms in the superficial layers of the SC or abnormal nail plate keratin. In reaction patterns such as granuloma faciale, granuloma annulare (Fig. 66), pustular dermatitis, folliculitis and perifolliculitis (Figs. 71, 72, 73), nodular granulomatous perifolliculitis (Figs. 77, 78, 79A, 80) and onychomycosis (Fig. 85), some of the hyphae were frequently segmented forming rectangular ovoid 10 μ arthrospores, but occasionally measuring up to 40 μ (megaspores). Focally, older, broad segmented hyphae showed large, deep staining, thick-walled ovoid to triangular and rectangular enlargements (Figs. 73, 77, 79A), and small spores along the surface and terminal ends of branching filaments (Figs. 73, 77, 79A). Short and long hyphae immediately

Fig. 74. Tinea corporis caused by *T. rubrum* showing a deep seated, erythematous, follicular, pustular, indurated lesion with gross characteristics of nodular granulomatous perifolliculitis, and located on the dorsum of the right shin. The patient had tinea pedis, onychomycosis, and evidence of *T. rubrum* infection on other parts of the body

Fig. 75. Tinea corporis caused by *T. rubrum* showing clinicopathologic features of nodular granulomatous perifolliculitis. The section shows hair piercing a follicular and perifollicular intraepidermal pustule with necrosis of the pilary outer root sheath. A small island of outer root sheath epithelium with adjacent inflammation is present in one area of the upper corium
(H & E, ×55)

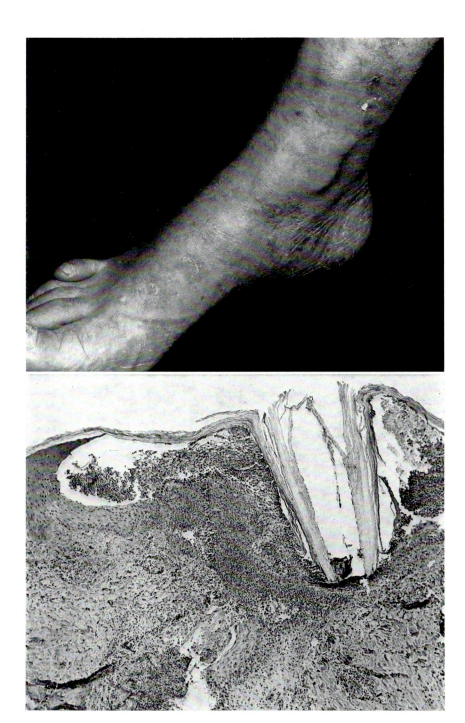

Figs. 74 (above) and 75 (below)

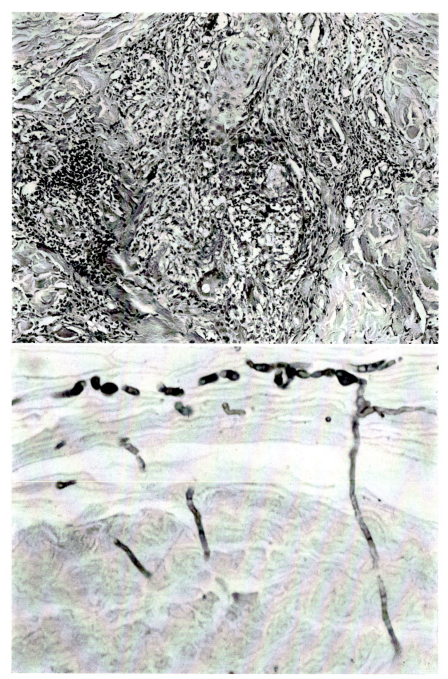

Figs. 76 (above) and 77 (below)

adjacent to the stratum Malpighii showed ill-defined septae and reacted lightly with PAS and Gridley's method, although deeper staining was observed with the various silver techniques (Figs. 53, 55B, 60, 69B). Large, broad hyphae at higher

Fig. 76. Tinea corporis caused by *T. rubrum* showing changes of perifollicular granulomatous inflammation characteristic of nodular granulomatous perifolliculitis. In the upper part of the section there is an island of pilary outer root sheath epithelium, and the adjacent stroma shows fibrosis, capillary-endothelial proliferation and inflammation including lymphocytes, histiocytes, plasma cells, neutrophils, eosinophils and multinucleated giant cells (PAS, ×107)

Fig. 77. Tinea corporis caused by *T. rubrum* with clinicopathologic features of nodular granulomatous perifolliculitis. The SC forms the roof of an intrafollicular abscess and shows hyphae which are frequently segmented. Striking is the presence of a long segmented hypha which shows its origin in the SC and penetrates the abscess (Gridley's method for fungi, ×655)

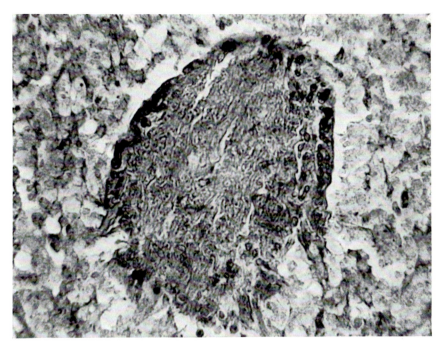

Fig. 78. Tinea corporis caused by *T. rubrum* showing clinicopathologic and histochemical features of nodular granulomatous perifolliculitis. High power magnification exhibits a fragment of hair in a deep dermal miliary abscess with intrapilary hyphae, and short segmented hyphae and arthrospores in the peripheral cortex. The fungal elements still show preference for a keratin substrate (PAS, ×445)

levels of the SC exhibited prominent segmentation and focally they were deeply colored by all methods for demonstration of fungal elements (Figs. 45B—C, 46, 77, 79A). Arthrospores were seen in the SC (Figs. 77, 79A), within follicular pustules (Fig. 73), inside and external to the hair shaft (Figs. 71, 72), involving spicules of hair in perifollicular dermal abscesses (Fig. 78), and singly (Figs. 81B—C) or in groups (Figs. 79B, 81A, 81D) scattered throughout foci of dermal granulomatous inflammation. Groups of arthrospores in dermal abscesses sometimes showed radiate formation with a peripheral zone of acidophilic material simulating a radiating granule (Fig. 79B).

Examination of vertical and parallel serial sections from patients with tissue reaction patterns classified as folliculitis, perifolliculitis, and nodular granulomatous perifolliculitis clearly indicates *T. rubrum* invades body hair most often as an endo-ectothrix parasite (Figs. 72, 78). Some hairs showed an endothrix pattern of

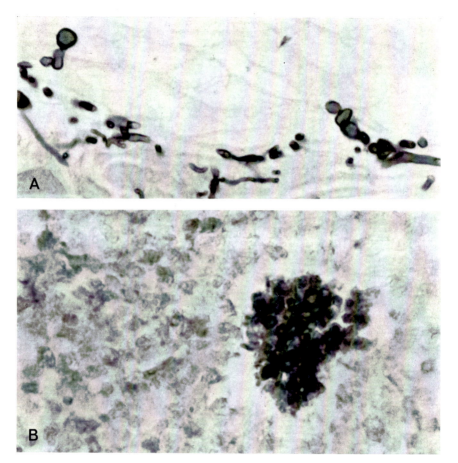

Fig. 79. Tinea corporis caused by *T. rubrum* showing clinicopathologic characteristics of nodular granulomatous perifolliculitis: A. High power magnification of the SC forming the roof of an intrafollicular abscess showing segmented hyphae forming large arthrospores (Gridley's method for fungi, ×655). B. High power magnification showing radiate formation of large arthrospores in a deep perifollicular dermal abscess. No remnants of hair could be identified indicating the ability of the fungal arthrospores to adapt to a mesenchymal substrate. *Trichophyton rubrum* is generally considered a keratinophilic dermatophyte, but shows a definite tendency in certain patients to invade nonkeratinizing tissues (PAS with diastase digestion method, ×655)

only intrapilary segmented hyphae and arthrospores from the KZ to the SC, but most follicles exhibited intrapilary fungal elements with arthrospores and segmented hyphae surrounding parasitized hairs (Figs. 71, 72, 73, 78). Some endo-ectothrix examples even showed fungal elements invading the adjacent keratinized pilary outer root sheath above the SG level (Fig. 72). Rarely infected follicles showed only fungal elements about the hair shaft.

In onychomycosis, fungal elements demonstrated by the various histochemical methods were located predominantly in soft keratin adjacent to the stratum Malpighii and in deep levels of the altered nail plate (Figs. 84, 85). Some fungi were in the middle layers of the nail substance (Fig. 84), and in the superficial part. Serial sections of transverse and longitudinal nail wedges from *T. rubrum* onycho-

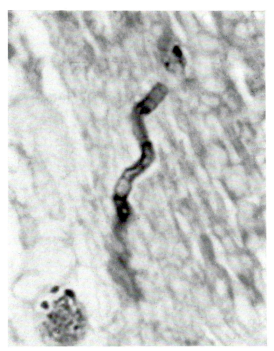

Fig. 80. *Trichophyton rubrum* infection of the lower leg with clinicopathologic and histochemical features of trichophytic granulomatous disease. Patients with lesions of this type have been diagnosed as having nodular vasculitis, migratory thrombophlebitis or a type of panniculitis. Biopsy sections from this patient showed many short and long segmented hyphae in the SC, and a lesser number in areas of perifollicular granulomatous inflammation at the level of the middle corium (From Telner, Blank & Schopflocher. By permission of F. BLANK. PAS, ×790)

mycosis showed long and short hyphae, some of which segmented frequently to form large arthrospores in linear arrangement (Fig. 85). The fungal elements showed no tendency for invading the nail bed epithelium or subjacent stroma.

Arthrospores located in perifollicular dermal granulomas showing single budding sporulation were PAS-positive (Fig. 81A), diastase-resistant (Fig. 81B), demonstrated with the various silver stains, positive with colloidal iron (Fig. 81C), resistant to hyaluronidase digestion (Fig. 81C), reactive with alcian blue pH 2.5, negative with alcian blue pH 0.4, aldehyde fuchsin pH 1.7 reactive (Fig. 81D), and negative with aldehyde fuchsin pH 0.4. These results indicated the presence of neutral polysaccharides and nonsulfated acid mucosaccharides other than hyaluronic acid. The colloidal iron, alcian blue and aldehyde fuchsin color reactions could result from one or a combination of fatty acids, nucleic acids, or sialomucins. The pattern of positive color reaction of *T. rubrum* megaspores with colloidal iron and alcian blue pH 2.5 showed a striking resemblance to that demonstrated by tissue yeast spores of *Cryptococcus neoformans*. Our studies demonstrated that the capsule material of *Cryptococcus neoformans* was colloidal iron positive, resistant to hyaluronidase digestion, alcian blue reactive at pH 2.5, and alcian blue negative at pH 0.4. These results indicate that the capsule acidic substance of the spherical organisms of *Cryptococcus neoformans* probably represents a nonsulfated acid mucosaccharide consistent with sialomucin. The positive staining reaction of *T. rubrum* arthrospores with aldehyde fuchsin pH 1.7 (Fig. 81D) and the negative results at pH 0.4 indicate

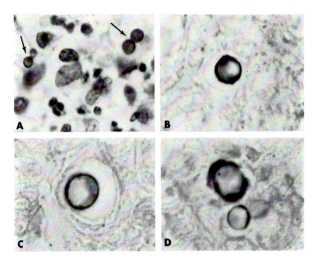

Fig. 81. Tinea corporis caused by *T. rubrum* with clinicopathologic and histochemical features of nodular granulomatous perifolliculitis: A. Arthrospores in the deep corium multiplying by single budding sporulation (arrows) and independent of keratin as a substrate (PAS, × 1400). B. Single arthrospore in a deep dermal abscess and all but the central part is intensely PAS-reactive due to water-soluble neutral polysaccharides in the skeletal wall (PAS with diastase digestion method, × 1400). C. Large arthrospore located in a deep perifollicular dermal abscess showing reactivity of the cell wall with modification of Mowry's 1958 colloidal iron stain for acid mucosaccharides. The cytoplasm of the megaspore is essentially nonreactive and the cell wall color intensity is not altered by hyaluronidase digestion. The results indicate the presence of an unidentified acid mucosaccharide in the peripheral skeletal structure of the organism (Colloidal iron stain with hyaluronidase digestion method, × 1400). D. Two arthrospores in a deep dermal abscess showing aldehyde fuchsin pH 1.7 reactivity of the peripheral cell wall with a clear appearance to the central cytoplasm. The cell wall of megaspores is nonreactive with aldehyde fuchsin pH 0.4 and this rules out the presence of sulfated mucosubstances (Aldehyde fuchsin pH 1.7, × 1400)

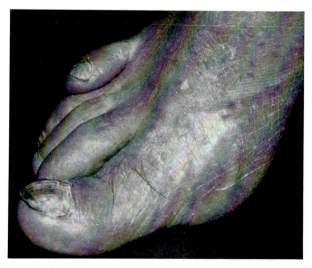

Fig. 82. Close-up view of a patient with onychomycosis who showed evidence of other skin disease caused by *T. rubrum* as illustrated in Fig. 74

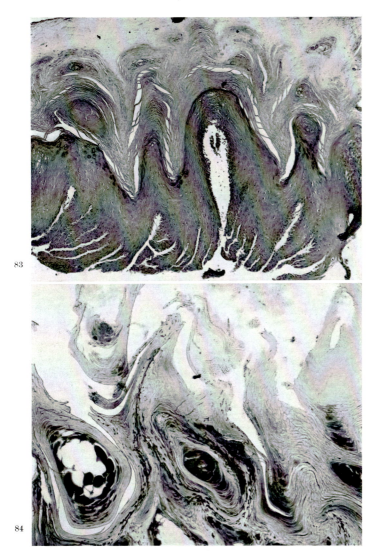

Fig. 83. Onychomycosis due to *T. rubrum* showing an abnormal thickened nail plate with parakeratosis. The nailbed epithelium exhibits focal hypergranulosis, acanthosis, and elongated rete ridges. The nailbed stroma is absent, but the combination of dermal papillae outlined as empty spaces and the nailbed epithelium configuration indicates papillomatosis (H & E, ×66)

Fig. 84. Onychomycosis caused by *T. rubrum* showing hyperkeratosis, parakeratosis, fungal elements, and accumulations of lymph fluid in the altered nail plate (PAS, ×93)

that at least some of the acidic material represents a nonsulfated mucosubstance, probably sialomucin.

Significant results of histochemical studies, other than the demonstration of fungal elements, showed hyaluronic acid in the interstices of epidermal cells, pilary outer root sheath, and in dermal extracellular interfibrillar spaces. As suggested for tinea capitis, dermatophytes involving smooth skin may require an acidic environment for growth and survival. Connective tissue stains showed that elastic

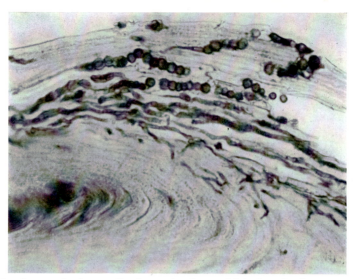

Fig. 85. Onychomycosis due to *T. rubrum* showing multiple long hyphae, some of which segment frequently forming large arthrospores. The fungal elements are located in the thickened altered keratin of the nail plate (PAS, ×655)

and collagen fibers were thinned in areas of dermal inflammation, whereas there was usually a proliferation of argyrophilic reticular fibers. Glycogen was diastase-labile and was demonstrated in variable amounts in the epidermis, pilosebaceous follicles, eccrine sweat glands, and areas of perifollicular granulomatous inflammation. In general, the more intense inflammatory reaction patterns showed greater accumulations of glycogen at the various sites mentioned. Reaction patterns showing vascular changes of allergic angiitis and allergic granulomatosis sometimes exhibited fibrinoid degeneration of blood vessels and extravascular stroma, and this alteration was PAS-positive, diastase-resistant, and demonstrated with PTAH and Movat's pentachrome method.

Differential Diagnosis: Observations indicate that *T. rubrum* is a versatile organism capable of adapting to different tissues and the arthrospores are independent of keratin for survival. The wide spectrum of gross and histopathologic reactions can cause confusion with a variety of dermatoses and often leads to an erroneous clinical and microscopic diagnosis. The microscopic differential diagnosis of acute vesicular dermatitis, subacute dermatitis, and chronic dermatitis caused by *T. rubrum* includes certain stages of contact dermatitis, nummular eczema, atopic dermatitis, allergic id eruption, incontinentia pigmenti, lichen simplex chronicus, prurigo nodularis, pompholyx, lichen striatus, seborrheic dermatitis, exfoliative dermatitis, parapsoriasis en plaques, parapsoriasis guttata, psoriasis, pityriasis rosea, keratoderma palmaris et plantaris, polymorphous light eruption, persistent light reaction, papular urticaria, pityriasis alba, asteatosis and acrodermatitis enteropathica. Erythema multiforme type reaction mimics diseases which show subepidermal multilocular bullae such as erythema multiforme, polymorphous light eruption, allergic dermal type of contact dermatitis, papular urticaria, bullous urticaria pigmentosa, and porphyria cutanea tarda. Erythema perstans type of reaction shows a striking resemblance to erythema perstans, erythema annulare centrifugum, erythema marginatum and other persistent erythemas, and certain stages of urticaria, papular urticaria, polymorphous light eruption, erythema multiforme, pityriasis lichenoides et varioliformis acuta, and secondary syphilis. Purpuric dermatitis caused by *T.rubrum* can mimic certain stages of purpuric drug eruption, pityriasis rosea, pityriasis lichenoides et varioliformis acuta and purpura pigmentosa progressiva. Erythematous, infiltrated, annular, cutaneous plaques caused by *T.rubrum* can show histopathologic changes strikingly similar to granuloma faciale, granuloma annulare, necrobiosis lipoidica diabeticorum, and reactive lymphoid hyperplasia such as are seen in insect or arthropod bite reactions. The features of pustular dermatitis can be confused with impetigo contagiosa, subcorneal pustular dermatosis, pustular psoriasis, pustular bacterid, miliaria pustulosa, pustulosis palmeris et plantaris, acrodermatitis continua of Hallopeau, Reiter's disease, keratoderma blenorrhagica, pyoderma gangrenosum, cutaneous candidiasis, primary irritant contact dermatitis, erythema toxicum, scabies, creeping eruption, and pustular forms of papular urticaria. Papulonecrotic reaction pattern with allergic angiitis and segmental, V-shaped, epidermal infarcts, resembles atrophie blanche of Milian, varioliform stage of pityriasis lichenoides et varioliformis acuta, papulonecrotic tuberculid, insect bite reaction, and drug reactions showing papulonecrotic purpuric lesions. *Trichophyton rubrum* folliculitis and perifolliculitis can be confused with superficial folliculitis, impetigo of BOCKHART, sycosis vulgaris, pustular acne, pustular rosacea, *Pityrosporum* folliculitis and perforating folliculitis. Nodular granulomatous perifolliculitis shows a tissue reaction pattern similar to that seen in cystic acne, perifolliculitis capitis abscedens et suffodiens, hidradenitis suppurativa, folliculitis keloidalis, folliculitis decalvans, foreign body granuloma, allergic granulomatosis, insect bite granuloma, tick bite granuloma, bromide granuloma, deep mycoses, atypical *Mycobacterium* infection, *Staphylococcus* actinophytosis, *Candida* granuloma, and reactive lymphoid hyperplasia causing confusion with some malignant lymphomas.

Trichophyton rubrum is the most common cause of onychomycosis, although other dermatophytes invade the nail plate such as *T.mentagrophytes*, *T.schoenleinii*, *T.violaceum*, *T.sulfureum* and *E.floccosum* (HILDICK-SMITH et al.). The clinical differential diagnoses of onychomycosis with overlapping histopathologic changes include monilial paronychia, psoriasis, bacterial onychitis, contact onychitis, atopic dermatitis, acrodermatitis perstans, lichen planus, various dystrophic nail diseases, and onychogryphosis (HILDICK-SMITH et al.). The histopathology of onychomycosis and psoriatic nails are strikingly similar except for hyphae and spores in the nail plate or subungual keratin (WHITE et al.).

Comment: As is evident in the illustrations of cutaneous tissue reaction patterns caused by other dermatophytes, *T.rubrum* can mimic them and produce a variety of additional clinicopathologic changes similar to a spectrum of dermatoses. BAKER (1947) reported his observations on a large series of patients with mycotic infections including some involving the skin, and indicated there was considerable variation and many differences in the tissue changes produced by pathogenic fungi.

Erythematous skin manifestations of *T.rubrum* simulate eruptions described as chronic and atypical varieties of erythema multiforme (WAISMAN). Erythema simplex gyratum, erythema figuratum perstans, erythema annulare centrifugum and erythema chronicum migrans show transitional forms and have been unified under the term of erythema perstans (WAISMAN). This type of chronic isolated, erythematous, multiform, urticarial, and ringed to serpiginous eruption can be caused by *T.rubrum* (WAISMAN). Case 4 reported by WAISMAN (1954) was diagnosed as granuloma annulare, but biopsy sections showed typical changes of erythema perstans and *T.rubrum* fungal elements were demonstrated in the horny layer. Patients with erythema perstans type lesions caused by *T.rubrum* generally show only a few segmented hyphae in the SC and this may result from host-parasite relationship immunologic mechanisms indicated by vascular changes of allergic angiitis. Localized urticarial reactions associated with *T. rubrum* infections of the skin have been confused with contact dermatitis, urticaria, angioedema, insect bite reaction, and erythema perstans (WEINER et al.).

TOLMACH and SCHWEIG reported a patient with extensive cutaneous *T. rubrum* infection mimicking dermatitis herpetiformis, but histopathologic changes showed only a simple inflammatory process involving the epidermis and upper cutis. At times, the diagnosis of *T. rubrum* infections are made with certainty only from culture studies, and the various clinical manifestations simulate psoriasis, seborrheic dermatitis, arsenical keratosis, neurodermatitis, atopic dermatitis, eczema, callus, sycosis vulgaris, impetigo contagiosa, pyoderma, folliculitis, and erythema annulare centrifugum (LEWIS, MONTGOMERY and HOPPER; LEWIS et al.). Tinea faciei caused by *T. rubrum* and simulating chronic discoid lupus erythematosus was reported in 1960 by SHANON and RAUBITSCHEK.

Trichophyton rubrum can mimic other superficial fungus diseases and this is indicated by PARTRIDGE who reported multiple fungus infections occurring in the same patient and isolated *T. rubrum* as one of the causative organisms in 25 of 29 cases. The associated dermatophyte was rarely suspected until isolated by mycological culture studies (PARTRIDGE).

LEWIS, HOPPER and SCOTT observed three patients with widespread cutaneous *T. rubrum* infections who had coexistent lymphatic leukemia, lymphosarcoma and monocytic leukemia, respectively. ROTHMAN (1953) reported systemic abnormalities of carbohydrate metabolism in recalcitrant *T. rubrum* infections. Cushing's syndrome may be associated with widespread *T. rubrum* infection and this dermatophytic disease can also occur in patients with acute disseminated lupus erythematosus and diabetes mellitus (NELSON et al.; CANIZARES et al.). Cutaneous ichthyotic nevoid anomalies associated with extensive *T. rubrum* infections have been reported (LANE; SWARTZ et al.; BAER et al.). WILSON in discussing the paper by WILLIAMS (1960) on griseofulvin and *Trichophyton rubrum* infections indicated that individuals with the disease possess immunologic defects not corrected by treatment, although patients do well on the drug who also have concomitant diabetes, nephritis, lupus erythematosus, Cushing's syndrome from pituitary tumor and steroid administration, arthritis, sarcoidosis, scleroderma, tuberculosis, polycythemia vera and pernicious anemia. CALLAWAY reported widespread *T. rubrum* infection in a child with lymphatic leukemia and concluded the dermatophyte should be considered as "opportunistic." BLANK and SMITH reported a young adult man with multiple nodular granulomatous lesions caused by *T. rubrum* and he also had rheumatoid arthritis for which continuous corticosteroids were used for 6 years. In our experience, widespread *T. rubrum* infections have been studied in patients with pemphigus erythematosus, lupus erythematosus and mycosis fungoides, and all were receiving systemic steroids or antimetabolites.

Growth of dermatophytes in the dermis is unusual since these organisms usually parasitize only keratinized epidermal structures and its appendages such as the SC, hair and nails. Since MAJOCCHI's (1883) original report on *Trichophyton* granuloma, there has been an increasing awareness of *T. rubrum* showing invasion of deep non-keratinized structures of the smooth skin (HARRIS et al.; WILSON; CREMER; WILSON et al.; TELNER et al.; LEWIS et al.; BLANK and SMITH; HILDICK-SMITH et al.; COOPER et al.; SCHREIBER et al.). Diseases to be considered in the clinicopathologic differential diagnosis of cutaneous granulomatous infiltrations caused by *T. rubrum* include Darier-Roussy sarcoid, multiple inflammatory nodules of the hypoderm, erythrocyanosis, erythema induratum, pyoderma, pernio, erythema nodosum, periphlebitis nodularis necrotisans, ulcerating white atrophy, primary recurrent idiopathic thrombophlebitis, drug eruptions particularly from halogens, periarteritis nodosa, recurrent erysipelas, lymphedema, thrombophlebitis and panniculitis (WILSON et al.; LEWIS et al.; TELNER et al.). WILSON et al. (1954) indicated that nodular vasculitis was the most difficult disease to differentiate from nodular granulomatous perifolliculitis by clinical means alone. LEWIS et al. referred to the work of THOMPSON (1941, 1942) who implicated *Trichophyton* species and *T. rubrum* infections with thromboangiitis obliterans and other peripheral vascular disorders, but definite confirmation of a relationship was lacking. LEWIS and CORMIA reported a patient with *T. rubrum* infection of the feet and generalized cutaneous eosinophilic granulomas and speculated about the relationship of the two diseases, but definite proof for this was lacking.

Confinement of *T. rubrum* fungal elements to keratinized tissue in most cutaneous infections seemed related to a human host serum factor which prevents dermal invasion since controlled *in vitro* organ cultures studies without fungistatic serum activities showed invasion of living epithelium by hyphae (BLANK, SAGAMI, BOYD and ROTH; BLANK and ROTH). Isolation of *T. rubrum* as a rare cause of natural infections in animals has been recorded by CHAKRABORTY et al., and successful inoculations of experimental animals with this organism have been reported (REISS; CHAKRABORTY et al.). STERNBERG et al. injected mycelial suspension of *T. rubrum* intraperitoneally into mice with the development of chronic granulomatous lesions involving the omentum, liver, spleen and muscles. Viable organisms were subsequently isolated on culture media and the Hotchkiss-McManus PAS method demonstrated fungal elements in tissue sections (STERNBERG et al.). NEWCOMER et al. demonstrated viability of *T. rubrum* in subcutaneous tissue granuloma pouches in rats. These experimental studies demonstrate the ability of dermatophytes to adapt to a living mesodermal substrate and support the occurrence of human dermal invasion by *T. rubrum*.

Histologic studies on *T. rubrum* onychomycosis have been reported by SAGHER (1948) and HANUSOVA (1967). Significant information related to pathogenesis of onychomycosis has been reviewed by HILDICK-SMITH, BLANK and SARKANY (1964). We are in agreement with SAGHER that *T. rubrum* fungal elements occur in the deep layers and middle part of the altered nail plate, but our studies show that most of the organisms involve a zone of subungual hyperkeratosis representing newly formed soft keratin adjacent to the stratum Malpighii. Similar to our description of *T. rubrum* arthrosrores in linear arrangement involving the disturbed nail plate and zone of subungual hyperkeratosis, SAGHER observed chains of spores only with certainty in the subungual horny substance. *Trichophyton rubrum* onychomycosis shows fungal elements more often at the nail root than in the distal or lateral parts of infected nails and appear to grow longitudinally in the abnormal plate (SAGHER). *Trichophyton rubrum* apparently does not enter the superficial nail plate layers as does *T. violaceum*, but invades from the distal hyponychium, lunula region or lateral nail fold (SAGHER). HANUSOVA noted irregular rows of *T. rubrum* spores and filaments predominantly in hyponychial and eponychial cornified desquamating tissue and rarely in the nail plate. The observations of SAGHER and HANUSOVA suggest that fungal elements of *T. rubrum* invade the nail plate predominantly through the hyponychium and lateral nail folds.

SAGHER observed that when *T. rubrum* penetrated the hyponychium, organisms proliferated opposite to that of nail growth, whereas, when the infection entered via the lunula, fungal elements followed the growing nail. Our histopathologic studies are incomplete when compared with observations on tinea capitis, but it is likely that *T. rubrum* fungal elements establish a relationship to nail matrix cells and subungual soft keratin similar to hair follicle parasites forming Adamson's fringe at the KZ and not penetrating the nonkeratinized substrate. It appears that a similar equilibrium is established between fungal elements and the epidermis and nail bed epithelium since the organisms usually invade no deeper than fully keratinized cells adjacent to the stratum granulosum.

Penetration of human soft and hard keratin by *T. rubrum* fungal elements must result from elaboration of potent substances similar to wool substrate keratinolytic activity (WEARY and CANBY) and intense histochemical enzymatic reactions demonstrated in nail infections caused by *T. rubrum* and *T. interdigitale* (MALE et al.). It seems reasonable that fungal enzymes capable of altering soft and hard keratin in *T. rubrum* infections could account for some of the dermal features we have described including inflammation, connective tissue alterations and ground substance changes.

HANUSOVA described branching filaments from *T. rubrum* onychomycosis as having a length of 15—17 μ and a width of 1—4 μ showing small surface protrusions and inner structures. *Trichophyton rubrum* spores and filaments show an outer membrane with strong light refraction characteristics and chlamydospores are seen only in mycelia close to the altered nail plate surface (HANUSOVA). HANUSOVA described Sudan black B staining of *T. rubrum* filaments and spores, and observed lipidized cells with intracellular lipoid granules in the cornified sealing barrier of the disrupted eponychium and hyponychium. BLANK, TAPLIN and ROTH (1960) demonstrated homogenous irregularly shaped inclusions by electron microscopy in *T. rubrum* fungal elements, and considered them as lipid storage granules. TAPLIN and BLANK (1961) interpreted refractile lipid droplets in *T. rubrum* fungal elements as a sign associated with cell death and observed that hyphae which contain an abundance of lipid material do not regenerate when placed in a fresh culture medium. Griseofulvin treated *T. rubrum* fungal elements show extremely large lobulated lipid granules as a sign of approaching death (BLANK, TAPLIN and ROTH). Sudanophilic lipids in *T. rubrum* fungal elements can be explained in part by brassicasterol (WIRTH, BEESLEY and MILLER) since this sterol and ergosterol occur among the *Trichophyton* species (BLANK, SHORTLAND and JUST). WIRTH et al. isolated ergosterol from a strain of *T. rubrum* and subsequently WIRTH and ANAND identified fatty acids in *T. rubrum* fungal elements. Except for behenic acid (WIRTH and ANAND), the spectrum of fatty acids in *T. rubrum* is similar to *T. mentagrophytes* (AUDETTE et al.). A combination of fatty acids and sialomucin in *T. rubrum* fungal elements may explain our histochemical demonstration of acidic material in large arthrospores of nodular granulomatous perifolliculitis. Water-soluble polysaccharides in the form of one mannan (BISHOP et al., 1965), one galactomannan (BISHOP and PERRY), and one glucan (BISHOP et al., 1966) have been identified from the fungal elements of *T. rubrum* (GRAHAM et al., 1965). These neutral polysaccharides and chitin (BLANK, 1953) undoubtedly account for the positive reaction of *T. rubrum* fungal elements with the PAS and Girdley's method for fungi.

Morphologic studies on *T. rubrum* fungal elements by GÖTZ (1960) showed the following significant observations: 1. The diameters of hyphae measure 1.5—2.5 μ from the 600 μ thick SC of the palms and soles, and 3—4.5 μ from the inguinal region SC which only shows a thickness of 30 μ. 2. Arthrospores from the inguinal region showed highly refractile intracellular bodies. 3. Arthrospores form from filaments by division into rectangular to oval cells or by localized swelling of hyphae due to retraction of the adjacent protoplasm. 4. Bizarre branching hyphae occur. 5. Small round 1.5—2.5 μ bodies were located on the surface of short hyphae. 6. Young hyphae stained a faint rose-color and were nonseptate or had only thin septa, whereas the more mature filaments showed prominent thick segmentation and stained deeply. 7. Hyphae were identified in localized areas of only the lower third of the SC. 8. The inguinal region and dorsum of the hands showed hyphae in a thin horny layer extending only to the stratum spinosum. 9. Inguinal region infections showed fungal filaments extending deep into the hair follicle. 10. Fungus spores appeared to be disseminated from the superficial horny layers. Our observations of small spores developing from *T. rubrum* hyphae are similar to protrusions extending from the surface of filaments from nail infections described by HANUSOVA and 1.5—2.5 μ bodies located on short hyphae from skin infections (GÖTZ, 1960). Intracellular refractile bodies in arthrospores described by GÖTZ (1960) may represent lipid vacuoles that stain sudanophilic (HANUSOVA). Localized hyphal swellings (GÖTZ, 1960) could compare to chlamydospores observed in *T. rubrum* onychomycosis (HANUSOVA), and what we described as large, thick-walled deep staining enlargments of varying configuration seen focally along segmented hyphae. Our observations of large arthrospores in *T. rubrum* infections, particularly nodular granulomatous perifolliculitis, correspond to those of others (WILSON; WILSON et al., 1954; COOPER et al.; SCHREIBER et al.). Segmented hyphae within fragments of hair in perifollicular dermal abscesses observed in serial biopsy sections from our patients with *T. rubrum* nodular granulomatous perifolliculitis were similar to those made by COOPER and MIKHAIL. In our experience, *T. rubrum* segmented hyphae away from hair spicules in nodular perifollicular dermal granulomas are unusual, but we have rarely observed filaments similar to those described by CREMER, TELNER et al., and BLANK and SMITH. The same patient reported in publications by BLANK and SMITH, BLANK and ROTH, and HILDICK-SMITH et al. showed numerous *T. rubrum* segmented hyphae and spores in areas of dermal granulomatous inflammation with epithelioid tubercles. That *T. rubrum* fungal elements elicit a dermal sarcoid type of granuloma is not surprising and is additional evidence of another clinicopathologic reaction pattern which the host-parasite relationship can produce. In general, our experience and that of others regarding *T. rubrum* infections with dermal granulomatous inflammation indicate that arthrospores are the predominant fungal element. DESAI and BHAT observed that whenever the circumstances are not favorable for mycelial growth, spores are formed. This observation would apply to our cases of *T. rubrum* nodular granulomatous perifolliculitis which showed varying sized arthrospores in mesenchymal tissue away from any vestige of a keratin substrate. *Trichophyton rubrum* fungal elements are capable of survival and propagation in a mesenchymal environment, but this must occur only in the proper host with absence or diminished levels of fungistatic inhibitory serum factor. Adverse conditions of the dermal mesoderm may alter the function, metabolism and chemistry of *T. rubrum* arthrospores and may account for histochemical characteristics suggesting acid mucosaccharides in their skeletal framework and cytoplasm. *Trichophyton rubrum* fungal elements contain a variety of lipid substances and it is probable that *T. rubrum* arthrospores surviving under adverse conditions away from keratin show an increase in acidic substances such as fatty acids and account in part for the histochemical results we obtained. Radiate formation of pathogenic fungi in human tissue has been reported by MOORE (1946), and recently this observation was recorded in *T. rubrum* perifolliculitis (COOPER et al., 1966). Our own observations identified groups of *T. rubrum* arthrospores in perifollicular dermal granulomas showing radiate formation of peripheral acidophilic material. The significance of radiate formation from aggregates of thick-walled *T. rubrum* arthrospores is not definite, but probably represents a manifestation of host-parasite relationship dealing with fungal elements in a non-keratinized substrate. It may be that this phenomenon occurs in patients with partial fungistatic serum factor activity or indicates localization of arthrospores

19*

by specific immunological mechanisms. That hypersensitivity plays a role in *T. rubrum* infections is well established and supported by our observations of allergic angiitis as an important basic pathologic change accounting for some of the various clinicopathologic tissue reaction patterns.

The parasitic pattern of hair follicle invasion exhibited by *T. rubrum* is a controversial matter. Some investigators consider *T. rubrum* as causing an endothrix infection (HILDICK-SMITH et al.; MacKENNA et al.; CREMER; BLANK and TELNER), others show evidence supporting an endo-ectothrix pattern of hair shaft involvement (CREMER; WILSON et al., 1954; COOPER et al.; BLANK and TELNER), and there are reports of this pathogen producing strictly an ectothrix type of pilar disease (HARRIS et al.; MOORE et al.; WILSON, 1952; CREMER; WEBER et al.; WILSON et al., 1954; MOORE et al.; LEWIS et al.; BLANK and TELNER). It would appear that these observations are all valid regarding various patterns of hair follicle invasion by *T. rubrum* and indicate the versatility of this organism. Our experience of examining vertical and transverse serial sections of *T. rubrum* follicle infections supports observations that this dermatophyte can cause three different types of hair invasion, but shows predominantly an endo-ectothrix parasitic pattern.

In summary, the spectrum of clinicopathologic reactions caused by *T. rubrum* is striking, and other than fungal elements in tissue sections, the changes are similar to a wide variety of dermatoses. The tissue reaction patterns varied from mild chronic dermatitis to subacute dermatitis, contact or nummular eczema type of acute vesicular intraepidermal multilocular dermatitis, erythema multiforme type of bullous subepidermal multilocular dermatitis, erythema perstans with angiitis, purpuric dermatitis with angiitis, granuloma faciale type changes, allergic granulomatosis mimicking granuloma annulare, allergic angiitis with papulonecrotic features, pustular dermatitis, superficial folliculitis, perifolliculitis with dermal abscess formation, granulomatous perifolliculitis, reactive lymphoid hyperplasia, sarcoid type of granulomatous inflammation, and destructive nail involvement. It is hoped that our observations and experience will alert pathologists and other physicians to establish a high index of suspicion for the disease spectrum which *T. rubrum* can cause in the human host. *Trichophyton rubrum* should rightfully take its place along with *Treponema pallidum* and drugs as being a mimicker of many cutaneous diseases including those caused by other superficial fungal parasites.

3. Trichophyton Mentagrophytes

Introduction: Isolations made from patients seen at The Skin and Cancer Hospital of Philadelphia during a four and a half year period showed that *T. mentagrophytes* variety *interdigitale* accounted for the third largest number of dermatophytic infections involving the smooth skin (McCAFFREE et al.). *Trichophyton interdigitale* which is not transmitted by animals was second only to *T. rubrum* as the cause of infections involving the feet and toenails (McCAFFREE et al.). HILDICK-SMITH et al. indicate that infections from *T. mentagrophytes* occur in all countries of the world as a parasite of man and lower animals; the downy form (T. *interdigitale*) being associated with chronic human infections, and *T. granulosum* causing predominantly animal ringworm and acute dermatophytosis in man. A recent study by BLANK, TAPLIN and ZAIAS reported that the most common cause of skin disease in Vietnam was a granular form of *T. mentagrophytes* which produces a highly inflammatory type of dermatophytosis. Recent reports (KOBLENZER et al.; SAFERSTEIN and BLANK) have recorded the occurrence of zoophilic *T. granulosum* infections in Philadelphia causing tinea faciei, tinea barbae, tinea corporis and tinea manuum. BLANK (1955) reviewed information about dermatophytes of animal

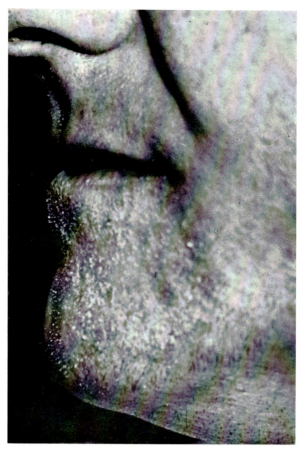

Fig. 86. Tinea barbae due to *T.mentagrophytes* variety *granulosum* showing an erythematous, scaling area with fairly sharply demarcated margins involving the bearded area of the chin. Subsequently, the patient developed gross and microscopic evidence of hair follicle involvement. His son had tinea capitis caused by the same organism and the gross disease is illustrated in Fig. 87

origin transmissible to man and among these were the granular forms of *T.mentagrophytes*.

Since the report of McCaffree et al., *T.rubrum* continues as the predominant cause of smooth skin and nail infections in our case material, but this may be due to chronicity of the disease causing the affected individual to seek medical attention. It is probable that many *T.mentagrophytes* infections are of short duration and show favorable response to patient self-treatment or remedies received from general practitioners, and these people never seek attention from a dermatologist who might be maintaining epidemiological records. For this report, we shall record our experience and observations of biopsies from 35 patients with infections caused by *T.mentagrophytes* variety *interdigitale*, variety *niveum* (*radians*, Sabouraud), variety *granulosum* and variety *asteroides*.

Gross Appearance: Biopsy specimens available for study came from the face (Fig. 86), arms (Fig. 89), hands (Fig. 91), trunk, legs and feet (Fig. 94). Grossly, the infections showed some variation in appearance depending on anatomical loca-

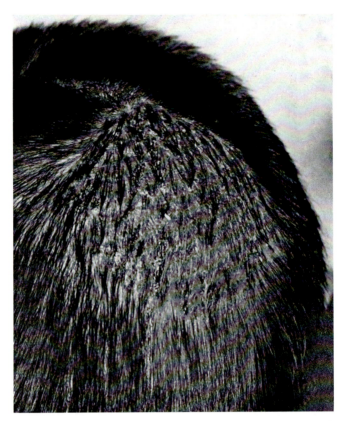

Fig. 87. Non-fluorescent tinea capitis caused by *T.mentagrophytes* variety *granulosum* showing an 8 × 7 cm erythematous, crusted, exudative, infiltrated, boggy area of partial alopecia on the posterior parietal scalp region. Hairs could be easily epilated and mycological culture studies isolated *T.granulosum* as the causative organism. Initially, severe pyoderma was the clinical diagnosis. The patient, a 12-year-old Caucasian boy, had been in contact with farm animals and also had a dog and cat at home. Subsequently, the patient's father was proven to have tinea barbae caused by *T.granulosum* as illustrated in Fig. 86

tion and variety of organism causing the disease. Clinically, tinea barbae caused by *T.granulosum* can show erythematous annular lesions with scaling, central clearing, and spreading peripheral margins (Fig. 86). Papules, vesicles, pustules and follicular lesions may occur, but purulent exudation is usually not prominent. A more tender, inflammatory form of the disease shows erythematous, nodular, boggy lesions with pustules, crusting, sinus formation, purulent drainage and regional lymphadenopathy. The clinical features of this type of infection of the face and neck with deep hair follicle involvement is essentially identical to tinea capitis with kerion (Figs. 27, 87). Similar hair follicle involvement may occur on other areas of the body, particularly the extremities.

Dermatophytosis from *T.granulosum*, *T.asteroides* and *T.niveum* (variety *radians*, Sabouraud) (Fig. 89) involving smooth skin of the trunk and extremities initially shows prominent inflammation characterized by erythematous, papular, follicular and sometimes circinate lesions. The eruption may be generalized or localized (Fig. 89) and occur as circular to irregular, erythematous, papular, vesicular, pustular, excoriated, scaly, edematous patches with sharply defined borders

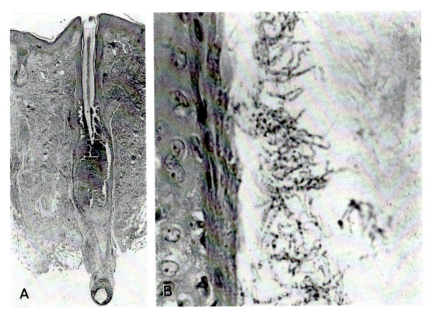

Fig. 88. Tinea barbae caused by *T. mentagrophytes* variety *granulosum*: A. Vertical section showing the longitudinal plane of an infected hair with a deep intrafollicular abscess, necrosis of the outer root sheath, and inflammation in the adjacent stroma. The involved hair is in the anagen growth phase indicating a predilection of *T. granulosum* for this type of mature keratin substrate similar to patients with tinea capitis caused by the same organism (H & E, × 10). B. High power magnification of an area at the SG level showing the outer root sheath, para-keratosis bordering on the hair canal, numerous segmented hyphae, a few arthrospores, and the adjacent hair shaft. Examination of vertical and parallel oriented serial sections with the technical aid of special histochemical stains demonstrated segmented hyphae and small arthrospores of microide (3 μ) size which were intrapilary and external to the hair shaft. Similar fungal elements were located in perifollicular dermal abscesses surrounded by granu-lomatous inflammation, and the microscopic features resembled kerion and nodular granulo-matous perifolliculitis (H & E, × 445)

and no evidence of central clearing (Fig. 91, right). More chronic lesions appear as scaling to psoriasiform patches (Fig. 91, left). *Trichophyton interdigitale* infections of the smooth skin other than the hands and feet may initially show vesicles, but usually appear as scaling, ill-defined areas of involvement.

Trichophyton interdigitale spares the hair follicle and commonly causes tinea pedis (Fig. 94), rarely superficial onychomycosis of the toenails, and sometimes tinea manuum. Tinea pedis initially appears as an acute inflammatory disease often assoc-iated with vesicles and bullae involving multiple areas of the volar surface (Fig. 94). Localized, discrete vesicles sometimes show an erythematous base. Pustules, scaling, fissuring and maceration, particularly the latter two changes between the toes, are seen in subacute to chronic stages of the disease (Fig. 94). Toenail involvement from *T. interdigitale* may show only superficial leukonychia on the surface or within the nail substance. More advanced destructive lesions occur with distal or marginal separation of the nail plate from its base giving a dull yellow, opaque appearance and finally friable debris. Subungual hyperkeratosis and dystrophic changes are frequent. A variety of localized and disseminated morphologic types of cutaneous id eruptions occur from *T. mentagrophytes* infections and these are discussed in detail by Peck (1930), and Lewis et al. (1958).

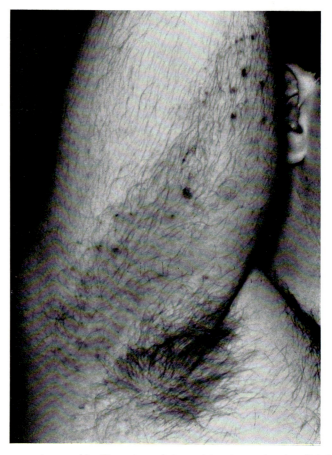

Fig. 89. Tinea corporis caused by *T.mentagrophytes* variety *niveum* showing slightly erythematous, papular, scaling, and excoriated lesions adjacent to the axilla and extending down the inner aspect of the right arm. The patient showed good response to treatment with complete clearing and an interesting feature was that one year later he developed erythrasma of the axillae and groin

The clinical differential diagnosis of dermatophytosis caused by *T.mentagrophytes* includes many diseases listed for *T.rubrum* infections. In particular, inflammatory lesions may mimic miliaria rubra, folliculitis, contact dermatitis, nummular eczema and psoriasis. *Trichophyton interdigitale* infections of the feet and hands can be confused with cutaneous candidiasis, pyoderma, contact dermatitis, vesicular id eruption, pompholyx, nummular eczema, pustular psoriasis, pustulosis palmaris et plantaris, pustular bacterid and dermatitis repens. Intertriginous disease of the feet caused by *T.interdigitale* and *T.rubrum* usually appear identical. According to LEWIS et al., secondary syphilis may produce lesions difficult to distinguish from tinea pedis. Soft corns of the feet may show superimposed dermatophytic disease and when present at the base of interdigital webs may on superficial examination suggest the diagnosis of tinea pedis (LEWIS et al.). Tinea barbae is most often caused by *T.granulosum*, but similar features occur from *T.verrucosum*, *T.rubrum*, *T.violaceum*, *M.canis*, sycosis vulgaris, cystic acne, rosacea, and drug eruptions such as iododerma and bromoderma. The differential diagnosis of

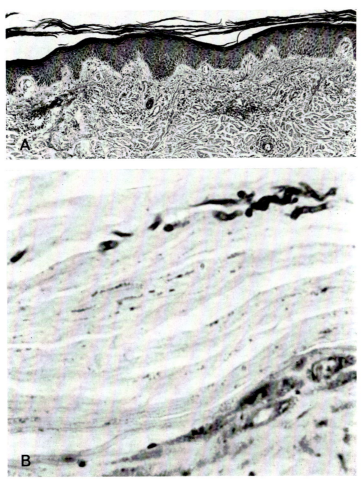

Fig. 90. Tinea corporis caused by *T.mentagrophytes* variety *niveum*: A. Scanning view of a section showing slight hyperkeratosis, spotted parakeratosis, minimal spongiosis, mild irregular acanthosis, and a few inflammatory cells about small blood vessels in the papillary corium (H & E, ×55). B. High power magnification of A showing segmented hyphae in the SC. The fungal elements show no tendency to invade the living epidermis or corium (PAS with diastase digestion method, ×445)

toenail infections due to *T.interdigitale* is similar to that for onychomycosis from *T.rubrum*.

Microscopic Observations: Superfical forms of tinea barbae caused by *T.granulosum* showed changes seen in *T.rubrum* infections including chronic dermatitis (Fig. 90A), subacute dermatitis (Figs. 92, 93), acute vesicular dermatitis (Fig. 51), pustular dermatitis (Fig. 68) and folliculitis (Fig. 71). Deep inflammatory follicular tinea barbae from *T.granulosum* (Figs. 88A, 88B) showed changes of folliculitis and perifolliculitis (Fig. 71), and nodular granulomatous perifolliculitis (Figs. 75, 76) from *T.rubrum*. Inflammatory lesions of the trunk and extremities caused by zoophilic organisms including *T.granulosum*, *T.asteroides* and *T.niveum* (variety radians, Sabouraud) showed changes similar to the superficial scaling form of tinea barbae and *T.rubrum* infections. Acute and subacute stages usually showed pro-

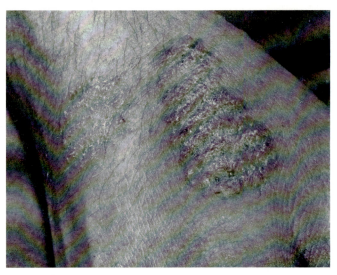

Fig. 91. Tinea manuum caused by *T. mentagrophytes* variety *granulosum* showing erythematous, circinate, scaling, crusted, pustular and coalescing lesions on the dorsum of the right hand. One week before onset, the patient acquired a stray white rat as a pet. The animal was captured by a friend, and had been handled freely by both of them and the patient's girl friend. The granular strain of *T. mentagrophytes* was isolated from the patient and his girl friend. The friend who captured the rat had lesions on his thighs, but he was not available for study. *Trichophyton granulosum* was isolated from the pet rat by the sterile brush technique

minent small blood vessel changes suggesting allergic angiitis. There was a predilection for the three organisms of animal origin to involve follicular ostia showing changes of folliculitis, whereas, *T. interdigitale* spared pilar structures. *Trichophyton interdigitale* infections of the glabrous skin other than the hands and feet usually showed changes of chronic dermatitis, but early lesions exhibited features of acute vesicular dermatitis, subacute dermatitis, and pustular dermatitis. Acute *T. interdigitale* infections of the soles and palms commonly showed vesicular dermatitis of the contact or nummular eczema type (Fig. 95A). Older and resolving lesions showed features of pustular dermatitis, subacute dermatitis (Fig. 46) and chronic dermatitis (Fig. 45A) similar to biopsy sections from patients with tinea pedis caused by *T. rubrum*.

Histochemistry: As with *T. rubrum* infections, *T. mentagrophytes* fungal elements were demonstrated by the various histochemical methods. Vertical and parallel serial sections of *T. granulosum* tinea barbae showed fungal elements

Fig. 92. Tinea manuum caused by *T. mentagrophytes* variety *granulosum* showing slight hyperkeratosis, spotted parakeratosis, one foci of superficial crusting, spongiosis, exocytosis, moderate acanthosis, and an intraepidermal microabscess containing neutrophils. The upper corium shows perivascular inflammation, angiitis of the small blood vessels, extravasated red blood cells and interstitial edema. A few short hyphae are present in the corneal layer (PAS with diastase digestion method, ×55)

Fig. 93. Tinea manuum caused by *T. mentagrophytes* variety *granulosum* showing a high power magnification of an area from Fig. 92. The field shows basket-weave hyperkeratosis, segmented hyphae adjacent to cells of the stratum Malpighii, absence of the granular layer, spongiosis, and an intraepidermal microabscess containing neutrophils. The section was digested with diastase for removal of glycogen, but because of the large amount present, not all of it was removed (PAS with diastase digestion method, ×445)

involving the follicles from the KZ upward in two principal ways: 1. Some hairs
showed a network of extrapilary segmented hyphae and predominantly microide
(3 μ) arthrospores, but a few larger arthrospores were observed and measured up

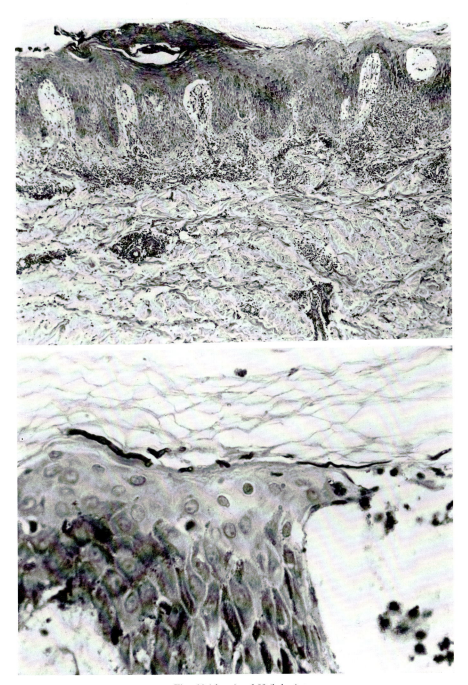

Figs. 92 (above) and 93 (below)

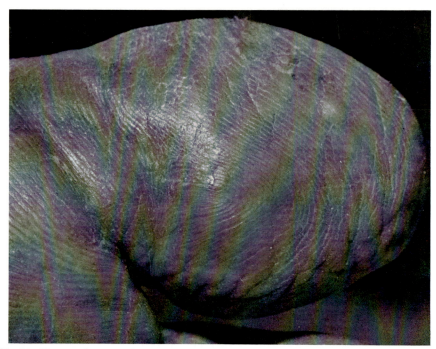

Fig. 94. Tinea pedis caused by *T.mentagrophytes* variety *interdigitale* showing erythema, scaling, minute vesicles, and pustular lesions on the volar surface of the right large toe

to 10 μ. 2. A few hairs exhibited similar fungal elements about the hair shaft, and intrapilary segmented hyphae and some small arthrospores. Branching segmented hyphae penetrated the hair follicle to deep levels of the KZ and formed Adamson's fringe as an inveted V similar to that described for *M.audouinii* and *M.canis* infections. Serial sections of tissue from the patient with tinea barbae illustrated by photomicrographs in Figure 88 showed intrapilary and extrapilary fungal elements, and special stains demonstrated bizarre branching segmented hyphae and arthrospores in areas of perifollicular granulomatous inflammation. The fungal elements showed only a light color reaction with the PAS and Gridley's method, whereas, they stained deeply with silver, particularly GMS. Special stains performed on biopsy sections of tinea corporis (Fig. 90B), tinea manuum (Figs. 92, 93) and tinea pedis (Fig. 95B) demonstrated predominantly segmented hyphae and a few small arthrospores adjacent to the stratum Malpighii (Figs. 92, 93), but fungal elements were also demonstrated in more superficial layers of the SC (Figs. 90B, 95B). Other than in one patient with tinea barbae from *T.granulosum*, fungal elements were confined to involving the epidermal SC, and within and external to the hair shaft as an endo-ectothrix parasite. Histochemical alterations of the epidermis, hair follicle, sweat glands, mast cells, connective tissue and ground substance were similar to descriptions given for *T.rubrum* infections.

Differential Diagnosis: The histopathologic and histochemical differential diagnosis of *T.mentagrophytes* infections is similar to that given for *T.rubrum*, but with a more limited spectrum of tissue reaction patterns. The differential considerations relate mainly to diseases showing features of folliculitis, perifolliculitis, nodular granulomatous perifolliculitis, chronic dermatitis, subacute dermatitis, acute vesicular dermatitis and pustular dermatitis.

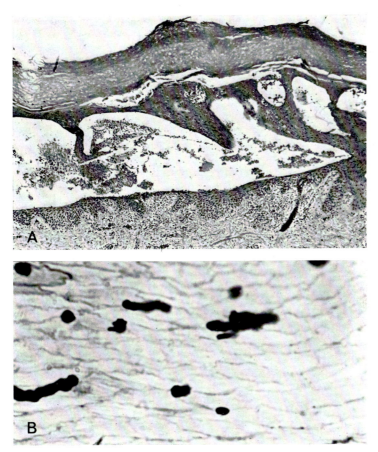

Fig. 95. Tinea pedis caused by *T.mentagrophytes* variety *interdigitale*: A. Low power magnification showing hyperkeratosis, spotted parakeratosis, hypogranulosis, intraepidermal microabscesses containing mononuclear cells, spongiosis, intracellular edema, exocytosis, intraepidermal multilocular bullae, and acanthosis. The bullae contain red blood cells, fibrin and inflammatory cells. The upper corium shows perivascular inflammation and an angiitis of the papillary capillaries (H & E, ×55). B. High power magnification of the SC in A showing short segmented hyphae (GMS, ×655)

Comment: Comments made regarding tinea capitis infections from *T.granulosum* and *T.asteroides* apply similarly to *T.niveum* (*T.radians*, Sabouraud). Consideration of these three zoophilic dermatophytes together is realistic since they cause inflammatory cutaneous disease with predilection for involving the hair follicle. *Trichophyton interdigitale* consistently spares the hair follicle and shows its greatest predilection for causing acute vesicular dermatitis of the feet, an anatomical site not affected in our case material by the granular forms of *T.mentagrophytes*. Based on clinicopathologic, anatomic and mycological characteristics, it would seem logical to separate *T.interdigitale* from the granular forms of *T.mentagrophytes* and consider the organism as a distinct dermatophytic pathogen. The predilection of *T.mentagrophytes* (granular forms) to involve the hair follicle has been discussed under tinea barbae by HILDICK-SMITH et al., and recently, BLANK, TAPLIN and ZAIAS observed follicular changes in dermatophytic infections caused by this organism in Vietnam. Isolation of *T.asteroides* from several members of a Philadelphia family strongly suggested that the organism was transmitted by the male head of the household who had acute inflammatory dermatophytosis in Vietnam while stationed there with the Army. It is possible that some of the zoophilic granular forms of *T.mentagrophytes* which accounted for cutaneous infections in Vietnam as reported by Blank, Taplin and Zaias could have resulted from *T.asteroides*. Figure 5 in the paper by Blank, Taplin and Zaias illustrates microide ectothrix arthrospores about an altered hair, and although not definite, suggests intrapilary fungal elements similar to our observations of hair follicle infections due to *T.granulosum* and *T.asteroides*. Blank, Taplin and Zaias referred to the hair follicle changes in Fig. 5 of their publication as similar to Majocchi's granuloma, but made no definite statement about fungal elements in the perifollicular stroma. One patient we studied with tinea barbae caused by *T.granulosum* is unique in our experience and showed fungal elements in areas of perifollicular granulomatous inflammation similar to nodular granulomatous perifolliculitis caused by *T.rubrum*, *T.epilans*, and *M.gypseum*. The ability of *T.granulosum* to invade the human dermis and survive in a mesodermal substrate seems supported by Newcomer et al. who demonstrated viable *T.mentagrophytes* fungal elements in granuloma pouches of rats for as long as 40 days post-inoculation, and some even showed dissemination to the liver and spleen.

Regarding morphology of the fungal elements in *T.mentagrophytes* infections, Götz reported the following significant observations: 1. Numerous filaments are present in the horny layer and there is little tendency to branching. 2. In the superficial SC most of the filaments are septate and more prominent than for *T.rubrum* hyphae. 3. As with *T.rubrum*, 1.5—2.5 μ spore-like round balls were located on top of short hyphae. 4. The youngest hyphae grow in the deep SC and many are nonseptate and show a faint rose-colored tint.

Trichophyton granulosum was the first organism from which a water-soluble polysaccharide, galactomannan containing D-galactose (16%) and D-mannose (84%) was isolated (Bishop et al., 1962). Subsequent complete studies (Bishop et al., 1965, 1966) verified the presence of water-soluble polysaccharides in *T.granulosum*. The combination of a water-insoluble polysaccharide identified as chitin (Blank, 1953) and three water-soluble polysaccharides in the cell wall of *T.granulosum* fungal elements accounts for histochemical demonstration of the organism in tissue sections from cutaneous disease caused by this dermatophyte. In *T.mentagrophytes* infections, the polysaccharides are of antigenic immuno-

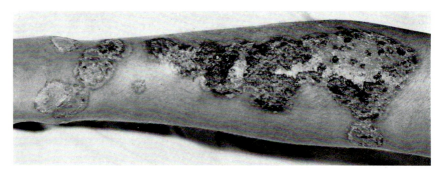

Fig. 96. Tinea corporis caused by *T.verrucosum* variety *discoides* showing circinate to coalescing, scaling, and crusted lesions on the dorsum of the right leg and ankle. The patient, a 14-year-old German refugee, lived on a farm and had frequent contact with domestic animals. The initial clinical diagnosis was pyoderma, but the disease failed to respond to topical and systemic antibacterial therapy

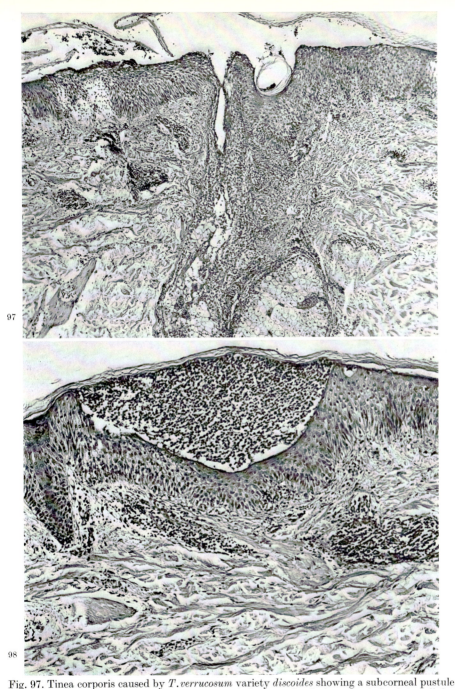

97

98

Fig. 97. Tinea corporis caused by *T. verrucosum* variety *discoides* showing a subcorneal pustule containing neutrophils. The epidermal base of the pustule shows spongiosis, intracellular edema, exocytosis, and acanthosis. Remnants of one pilosebaceous follicle are also included in the area of the subcorneal pustule and this shows changes of folliculitis. In the upper corium and perifollicular stroma there are inflammatory cells and interstitial edema (H & E, ×55)

Fig. 98. Tinea corporis due to *T. verrucosum* variety discoides showing a subcorneal abscess mimicking the changes seen in impetigo contagiosa, pustular psoriasis, pustular bacterid, and subcorneal pustular dermatosis. The epidermal base of the pustule is compressed, and shows spongiosis, intracellular edema, exocytosis and mild acanthosis. The upper corium exhibits a perivascular inflammatory infiltrate and interstitial edema (H & E, ×93)

chemical importance and histochemical characteristics allow for localization of fungal elements in the skin tissue sections.

It is our opinion that correct recognition and improved isolation techniques for identifying the different varieties of *T.mentagrophytes* as a cause of cutaneous disease may prove in the future that this group of organisms represents the predominant pathogen producing human dermatophytic infections. With continued advancing means for rapid transportation and movement of United States civilian and military personnel in and out of multiple geographic areas of the world, there may well evolve continued changes in dermatophytic flora such as the prominent increase in *T.rubrum* infections which occurred in western countries following World War II.

4. Trichophyton Verrucosum

Introduction: *Trichophyton verrucosum* is a zoophilic organism isolated from domestic animals, and the origin of human disease is often from infected cattle and horses. Instances of laboratory workers contacting *T.verrucosum* infections from rabbits and white mice have been reported (LEWIS et al.). Several members of the same family may be affected and children are particularly susceptible. The disease is encountered most often in rural areas, and human infections from *T.verrucosum* have been reported from the United States, Canada, England and Portugal. A total of nine isolations of *T.verrucosum* variety *discoides* from four patients has been reported from The Skin and Cancer Hospital of Philadelphia by McCAFFREE et al. For this report, we shall review our observations of biopsy sections from five patients with tinea corporis caused by *T.verrucosum*.

Gross Appearance: Biopsy specimens were from the face, trunk and legs (Fig. 96). Once the infection occurs, the clinical disease develops rapidly showing erythema, edema, papules and vesicles. Subsequently, coalescing, circinate plaques develop and these show little tendency for central clearing because of crusting, scaling, exudation and pustules (Fig. 96). Gross changes of folliculitis occur and lesions of the bearded area show prominent inflammation with tender, deep seated, boggy nodules, broken off hairs, crusting, and drainage of purulent exudate from sinuses. These latter changes are those of kerion similar to inflammatory tinea capitis caused by *T.verrucosum* and other zoophilic dermatophytes. *Trichophyton verrucosum* infected hairs can be easily epilated and are nonfluorescent when examined under Wood's light. JILLSON and BUCKLEY indicated that *T.faviforme* (*T.verrucosum* is a synonym, AINSWORTH et al.) causes four clinical forms of infection: ringworm-like patches; folliculitis showing grouped follicular pustules; kerion with boggy, crusted masses; and granulomatous changes of the Majocchi type.

Fig. 99. Tinea corporis caused by *T.verrucosum* variety *discoides* showing an intermediate power magnification of a few short hyphae in the stratum corneum, hypogranulosis, spongiosis, intracellular edema, exocytosis, and intraepidermal microvesicles containing mononuclear cells. Clinically, the eruption appeared papulovesicular suggesting an allergic id, and this may account for mononuclear cells in the intraepidermal microvesicles (PAS, ×190)

Fig. 100. Tinea corporis caused by *T.verrucosum* variety *discoides* showing a subepidermal, multilocular bulla with striking resemblance to erythema multiforme. The epidermal bulla roof shows spongiosis, intracellular edema and exocytosis, but the dermoepidermal basement membrane appears intact as is characteristics of erythema multiforme. The papillary corium at the base of the bulla shows perivascular inflammation and interstitial edema. A few short fragmented hyphae are present in the altered corneal layer which shows hypokeratosis and parakeratosis. Glycogen has been removed from the epidermis (PAS with diastase digestion method, ×190)

The clinical differential diagnosis of *T.verrucosum* infections of the glabrous skin includes several diseases given for dermatophytosis caused by *T.rubrum*, but with a more limited spectrum similar to lesions caused by granular forms of *T.mentagrophytes*.

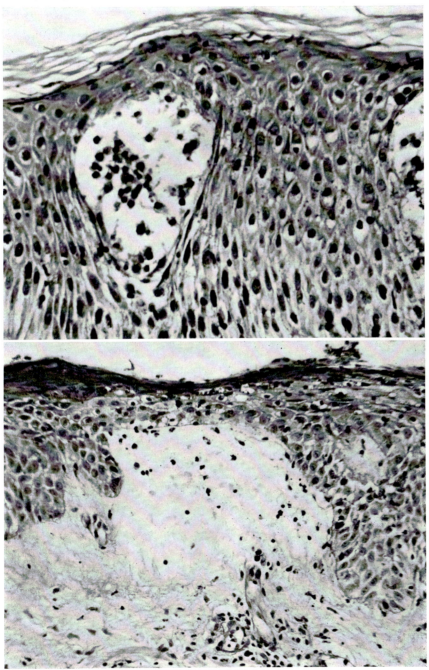

Figs. 99 (above) and 100 (below)

20

Trichophyton verrucosum infections are frequently diagnosed clinically as pyoderma (Fig. 96), or bacterial folliculitis and antibiotic treatment is instituted but without response. Disseminated papular and follicular id eruptions can occur as an allergic manifestation of fungal element cell wall polysaccharides and other antigenic substances elaborated by the organism.

Microscopic Observations: Early lesions showed changes of an angiitis with acute vesicular dermatitis (Fig. 99), and focally there were small subepidermal, multilocular bullae resembling erythema multiforme (Fig. 100). Subacute lesions were usually pustular (Figs. 97, 98) and serial sections showed hair follicle involvement with changes of folliculitis (Fig. 97) and perifolliculitis (Fig. 97). Older lesions showed features of chronic dermatitis and some exhibited perifollicular granulomatous inflammation.

Histochemistry: *Trichophyton verrucosum* fungal elements were demonstrated by the various histochemical techniques and the organisms appeared limited to the SC (Figs. 99, 100, 101), hair shaft and extrapilary in the follicle canal (Fig. 102). Frequently segmented hyphae and a few small arthrospores were located predominantly adjacent to the stratum Malpighii (Fig. 101), although a few fungal elements were demonstrated at higher levels of the SC. A few short segmented hyphae and arthrospores of variable size were present within intraepidermal and follicular pustules. Serial sections of *T. verrucosum* infected hairs showed fungal elements involving the follicles from the KZ and above as follows: the majority of hairs were surrounded by frequently segmented hyphae (Fig. 102) and small and large arthrospores, but some also contained intrapilary fungal elements. No fungal elements were demonstrated in the perifollicular stroma. Histochemical alterations of other structures and substances were similar to those observed in infections caused by *T. rubrum* and *T. mentagrophytes*.

Differential Diagnosis: The histopathologic and histochemical differential diagnosis of *T. verrucosum* infections is similar to those given for *T. mentagrophytes*, but also with some tissue reaction patterns discussed under *T. rubrum*.

Comment: Our observations agree with Birt et al. that *T. verrucosum* fungal elements can occur within and surround the hair shaft as an endo-ectothrix parasite. The hyphae segment frequently to form arthrospores, some of which are large, of the megasporosis type. Jillson and Buckley studied 16 cases of "barn itch" and isolated *T. faviforme* as the causative organism which they classified as a large-spore ectothrix parasite of the hair follicle. Lewis et al. also classified *T. verrucosum* as an ectothrix *Trichophyton*, but in their textbook illustrated an infected hair showing chains of intrapilary arthrospores. Dermal granulomatous inflammation has been reported in *T. verrucosum* infections (Jillson et al.; Birt et al.), but no fungal elements have been demonstrated in the perifollicular stroma. It is likely that some patients with deep follicular nodular lesions do extrude fungal elements into the corium, but immune mechanisms of the human host prevent propagation of the organism.

Fig. 101. Tinea corporis caused by *T. verrucosum* variety discoides showing hyphae limited to the horny layer. The epidermis contains numerous melanin granules and reticular fibers are demonstrated in the papillary corium (GMS, ×190)

Fig. 102. Tinea corporis due to *T. verrucosum* variety *discoides* showing clinicopathologic features of folliculitis. A high power magnification shows the follicular infundibulum above the SG and the follicle canal contains a remnant of hair surrounded by segmented hyphae. Serial sections showed some hairs with intrapilary segmented hyphae and small arthrospores. Diastase digestion removed glycogen from the outer root sheath, whereas, the water-soluble polysaccharides in the fungal elements were diastase-resistant (PAS with diastase digestion method, ×445)

Histochemical methods for the demonstration of *in vitro* enzyme activity performed by MALE and HOLUBAR on *T. verrucosum* fungal elements gave positive results similar to granular forms of *T. mentagrophytes* and support *in vivo* keratino-

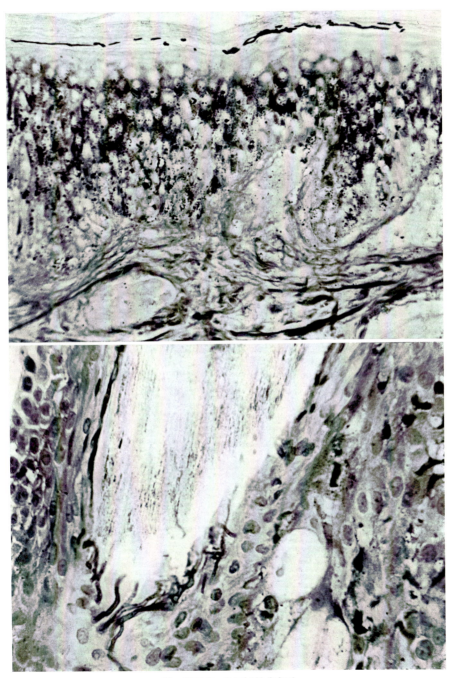

Figs. 101 (above) and 102 (below)

20*

lysis of soft and hard keratin by these organisms. RIPPON (1967), and RIPPON and VARADI (1968) demonstrated *in vitro* elastase activity of some isolates of *T. verrucosum* and this supports the ability of enzymes elaborated by the organism to play an *in vivo* role in scleroproteolysis. The complete chemical composition of *T. verrucosum* is not known, although BLANK (1953) has identified chitin in the cell wall skeletal material of *T. discoides* (now classified as a variety of *T. verrucosum*). Chitin and other polysaccharide substances undoubtedly account for the histochemical properties of *T. verrucosum* which are so important for locating fungal elements in tissue sections. Of the *Trichophyton* species, *T. discoides* and *T. violaceum* are interesting because their fungal elements contain brassicasterol (BLANK, SHORTLAND and JUST, 1962). *Trichophyton megninii* also elaborates brassicasterol, although traces of ergosterol have been identified (BLANK et al., 1962).

Our limited source of case material from patients infected with *T. verrucosum* suggests that the disease is rare, but we tend to agree with BIRT et al. that the organism is a common cause of highly inflammatory dermatophytosis in rural areas of North America. Transmission of *T. verrucosum* infections from farm animals to man probably occurs much more frequently than epidemiological records indicate, but the disease is usually not diagnosed properly because of confusion with pyoderma or folliculitis, and spontaneous healing often results before the patient consults a physician.

5. Trichophyton Violaceum

Introduction: Some of the comments made regarding *T. violaceum* as a cause of tinea capitis apply here and will not be repeated. The organism can cause chronic forms of tinea barbae, onychomycosis and dermatophytosis of the glabrous skin. Several members of the same family may be affected. Our histopathologic and histochemical observations of tissue changes from *T. violaceum* infections are limited. Observations were made by reviewing biopsy sections from two patients with lesions of the trunk and extremities. One patient also had tinea capitis.

Gross Appearance: Lesions showing only mild inflammation may occur on the bearded area of men and appear similar to tinea capitis caused by *T. violaceum*. Some examples of *T. violaceum* beard infections cause chronic follicular lesions mimicking sycosis vulgaris of bacterial origin. Nails infected with *T. violaceum* appear yellow, opaque, and are crumbly (LEWIS et al.). Smooth skin disease shows superficial, erythematous, sharply defined, circinate plaques and scattered papules, follicular lesions and crusted nodules (Fig. 103).

The clinical differential diagnosis includes consideration of other dermatophytic infections of the beard, nails and glabrous skin, particularly those caused by *T. rubrum*. Other inflammatory diseases can be mimicked by *T. violaceum* similar to some listed in the differential diagnosis for *T. rubrum*.

Microscopic Observations: Limited biopsy material from *T. violaceum* infections indicate tissue reaction patterns of chronic dermatitis, subacute dermatitis (Fig. 104), purpuric dermatitis and erythema perstans. Onychomycosis caused by *T. violaceum* shows long, segmented hyphae in the superficial parts of the nail plate without causing any reaction in the surrounding nail substance (SAGHER).

Histochemistry: Histochemical methods for demonstration of fungal elements showed hyphae which were frequently segmented, forming arthrospores adjacent to the stratum granulosum. Fungal elements were not observed in the deep epidermal layers or corium. Other histochemical changes were similar to those described for *T. rubrum*.

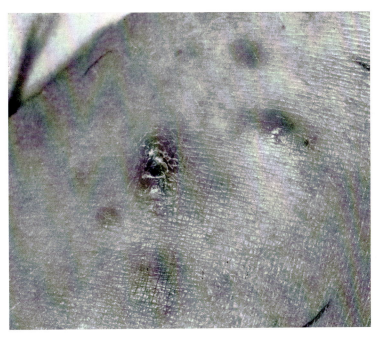

Fig. 103. Tinea corporis caused by *T.violaceum* showing erythematous, papular, crusted and deep nodular lesions on the right arm. The patient had similar lesions on the legs and trunk, and her daughter had tinea capitis caused by *T.violaceum* illustrated in Fig. 39

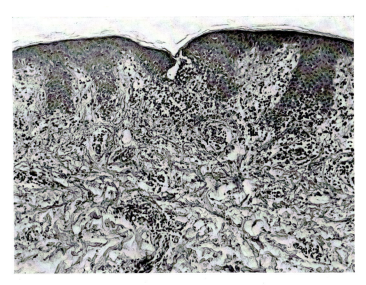

Fig. 104. Tinea corporis caused by *T.violaceum* showing mild spongiosis, exocytosis, and irregular acanthosis. Centrally, there is a small microabscess containing mononuclear cells. The upper corium exhibits interstitial edema, and a perivascular inflammatory infiltrate of lymphocytes and histiocytes. Special stains for demonstration of fungal elements showed a few short segmented hyphae in the SC (H & E, ×107)

Differential Diagnosis: The histopathologic and histochemical differential considerations include some diseases listed for the various tissue reaction patterns caused by *T.rubrum*.

Comment: *In vitro* enzymatic activity of fungal elements as reported by Male and Holubar probably indicates that some of the cutaneous tissue changes, particularly those of keratin and connective tissue, result from keratinases elaborated by *T.violaceum*. Some of the fungal keratinases show *in vitro* ability to digest hair, nails, soft keratin, and probably other scleroproteins such as collagen and elastin. Blank (1953) identified chitin as a component of the skeletal cell wall of *T.violaceum* fungal elements and indicated there was no evidence of cellulose or other high polymeric substances in the membranes. Blank, Ng and Just (1966), in a continuing program of investigating chemical constituents of dermatophytes, have identified vioxanthin and viopurpurin from *T.violaceum* fungal elements, and indicated that xanthomegnin was found to be the major component of the pigment mixture.

The spectrum of glabrous skin tissue changes caused by *T.violaceum* is probably similar to those of *T.rubrum*, but definite proof is lacking in our limited material which showed only a few reaction patterns. Gross features of infiltrated papules, deep nodules, and crusted lesions suggest papulonecrotic changes, angiitis of small blood vessels, allergic granulomatosis, folliculitis, perifolliculitis and even nodular granulomatous perifolliculitis. As the opportunity arises, additional histopathologic and histochemical studies will be performed on proven smooth skin infections caused by *T.violaceum*.

6. Trichophyton Concentricum

Introduction: Tinea imbricata (tokelau), a fungus infection of the tropics caused by *T.concentricum*, has been identified from patients with a chronic itching cutaneous disease who live in the Pacific islands, Malaya, China, Ceylon, Southern India, Burma, South America, Central America and South Africa. The disease affects males and females and there is no age predilection. The organism is transmitted from human to human and multiple infections in the same family may indicate an hereditary susceptibility to the disease (Wilson et al., 1965). The disease affects individuals native to the geographic area, but tends to spare Caucasian immigrants. Histopathologic and histochemical observations were made from the study of a surgical biopsy specimen removed from one patient with typical tinea imbricata.

Gross Appearance: Initially, the disease shows single or multiple small brown pigmented scales which slowly enlarge to form concentric overlapping lesions because of the continous development of new lesions in the center of older ones. Erythema is usually minimal or absent. Typically, the scales are attached at the periphery with central clearing because of fissuring and separation of the horny layer, development of rolled up flaky margins and eventual exfoliation (Fig. 105). The disease may involve most of the cutaneous surface with serpiginous and polycyclic lesions, although the scalp, axillae, palms and soles are usually spared. Severe examples of tinea imbricata show coalescence of concentric rings with diffuse scaling, lichenification, and loss of the usual pattern. Nail involvement has been reported, but others dispute this (Lewis et al.). No characteristics fluorescence is seen when the smooth skin lesions are examined under Wood's light. Resolving lesions can leave residual brownish pigmentation (Allen, 1967).

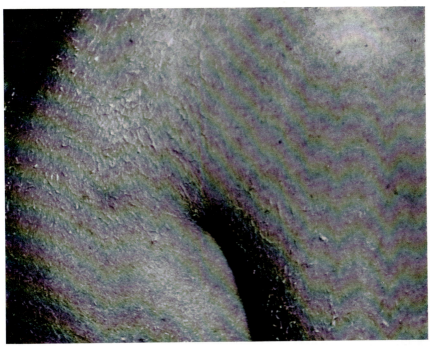

Fig. 105. Tinea imbricata caused by *T.concentricum* showing involvement of the upper back region and adjacent left arm. The hyperkeratotic lesions show a tendency for lamellar configuration with rolled-up scaly margins and exfoliation. The patient was an adult man native to Okinawa

The clinical differential diagnosis includes ichthyosis vulgaris, ichthyosis congenita, exfoliative dermatitis, and dermatophytosis caused by pathogens which sometimes form concentric lesions.

Microscopic Observations: Examination of multiple sections showed changes of mild chronic dermatitis characterized by basket-weave hyperkeratosis, focal parakeratosis, areas of hypergranulosis, regular psoriasiform acanthosis, papillomatosis, epidermal hypopigmentation, and thinning of some suprapapillary plates (Fig. 106A). The papillary corium showed mild capillary-endothelial proliferation, vascular ectasia, perivascular round cell inflammation, and incontinence of melanin pigment free and within melanophages (Fig. 106A). Pilosebaceous follicles showed follicular hyperkeratosis and some parakeratosis, but otherwise these structures did not appear significantly altered.

Histochemistry: Long and short frequently segmented hyphae and small arthrospores were demonstrated by special histochemical methods for fungi. The organisms were limited to the thickened horny layer (Fig. 106B). The PAS method identified many fungal elements in the SC adjacent to the stratum granulosum. Fungal elements in superficial levels of the SC were only faintly colored with PAS, whereas they were demonstrated quite satisfactorily with the silver stains (Fig. 106B). Keratin-plugged follicular ostia showed some fungal elements, but the hairs were not involved. Melanin was demonstrated in the upper corium and was localized predominantly about small blood vessels. The remaining histochemical studies did not show significant results and changes were similar to those described for chronic dermatitis caused by other dermatophytes.

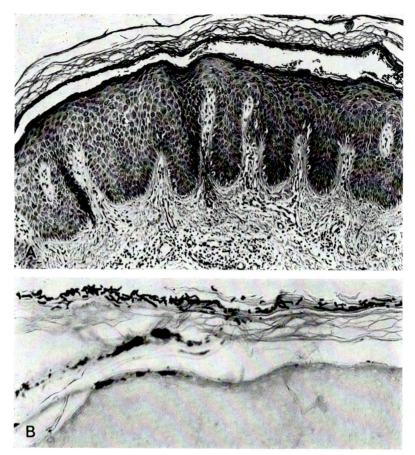

Fig. 106. Tinea imbricata caused by *T.concentricum*. A. Section showing changes of mild chronic dermatitis characterized by hyperkeratosis, granular layer intact, uniform acanthosis, and a mild cellular infiltrate about the small blood vessels in the upper corium (H &E, ×93). B. Numerous segmented hyphae are present in the thickened horny layer. There is no evidence of invasion of the living epidermis or corium by the fungal elements (GMS, ×155)

Differential Diagnosis: The histopathologic and histochemical differential diagnosis includes dermatophytic infections with mild chronic dermatitis, psoriasis, psoriasiform inflammatory dermatoses and fixed drug eruption.

Comments: Patients with tinea imbricata fail to develop local tissue immunity and this accounts for the continued growth of fungal elements at the center of overlapping lesions with the development of chronic widespread disease (EMMONS et al.). Epidermal hypopigmentation resulting from incontinence of melanin accounts for papillary dermal melanosis similar to fixed drug eruption. The brown pigmented color of the scaling macules seen grossly results from dermal melanosis. Apparently, melanin can remain fixed in the upper corium even after the active disease resolves. It is possible that melanin granules released from the melanocytes of the dermo-epidermal junction are phagocytized by Schwann cells and other cutaneous neural structures in the papillary corium, rather than by melanophages of histiocytic origin (BUTTERWORTH and GRAHAM). Even after the fungal elements disappear, the melanin pigment may remain fixed in the dermal neural structures and cause

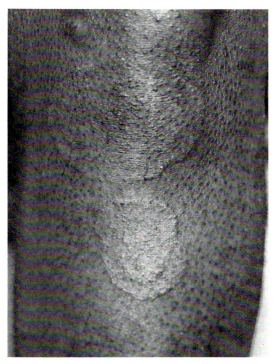

Fig. 107. Tinea corporis caused by *T.sulfureum* showing erythematous, scaling lesions with a definite circinate ringed pattern located on the dorsum of the leg below the knee. The patient had lesions on other parts of the body. Similar cutaneous disease is seen in patients with tinea corporis due to *T.tonsurans*

pigmented lesions similar to a tattoo. Very little investigative work has been done on human cutaneous disease caused by *T.concentricum* and additional tissue studies should be performed. The information gained might open new avenues for research and lead to a better understanding of tinea imbricata.

7. Trichophyton Tonsurans and Trichophyton Sulfureum

Introduction: Remarks made about *T.tonsurans* and *T.sulfureum* under tinea capitis apply here and will not be repeated. McCaffree et al. in a report dealing with the dermatophytic flora of Philadelphia isolated *T.sulfureum* or *T.tonsurans* on 55 occasions from 53 patients with glabrous skin infections. Fifteen of 53 (30%) patients with smooth skin lesions also had tinea capitis (McCaffree et al.). Pipkin (1952) reported that 59% of adults with tinea capitis from *Trichophyton* organisms also had glabrous skin lesions. For this report, we reviewed biopsy sections from five patients with *T.sulfureum* or *T.tonsurans* infections involving the face, neck, trunk and extremities.

Gross Appearance: Glabrous skin lesions caused by *T.tonsurans* or *T.sulfureum* show well demarcated, erythematous, circinate, scaling areas with little tendency for central clearing (Fig. 107). Some lesions show a definite ringed pattern of papular, pustular and follicular lesions (Fig. 107). Occasionally, ill-defined, erythematous, scaling lesions occur. The fingernails may be involved and the disease resembles onychomycosis caused by *T.rubrum* (Lewis et al.). Pipkin

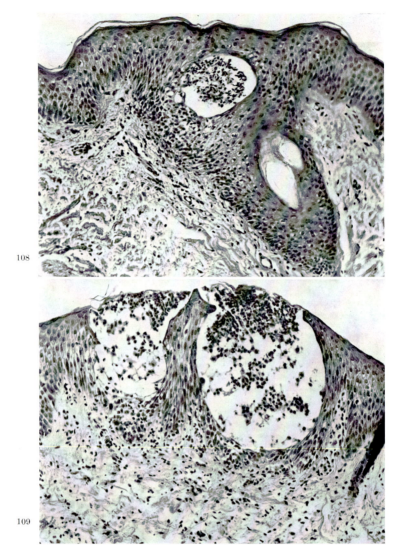

Fig. 108. Tinea corporis caused by *T. sulfureum* showing microscopic features of folliculitis. The section exhibits an intrafollicular pustule containing neutrophils and spongiosis of the pilary outer root sheath. The perifollicular stroma shows interstitial edema (H & E, ×155)

Fig. 109. Tinea corporis caused by *T. sulfureum* showing clinicopathologic changes of a pustular dermatitis characterized by intraepidermal abscesses filled with neutrophils. The adjacent stratum Malpighii shows spongiosis, exocytosis and mild acanthosis. Minimal inflammation and interstitial edema is present in the subjacent dermis (H & E, ×155)

(1952) reported nail involvement in 25% of adult patients and in 18% of children who had *Trichophyton* scalp infections. Papular, pustular and follicular id eruptions can occur in patients infected with *T. sulfureum* or *T. tonsurans*.

The clinical differential diagnosis is similar to that of *T. rubrum* and other organisms causing dermatophytosis except for the absence of volar and palmar skin lesions in patients with infections caused by *T. tonsurans* or *T. sulfureum*.

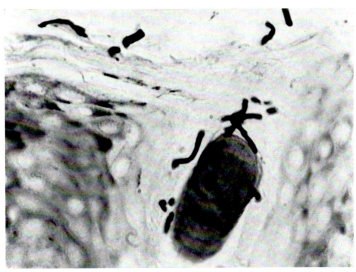

Fig. 110. Tinea corporis caused by *T.sulfureum* showing clinicopathologic and histochemical features of folliculitis. Fungal elements are in the SC and follicular ostium and surround a fragment of hair at this latter site. No fungal elements were demonstrated in the stratum Malpighii or corium (GMS, ×655)

Microscopic Observations: The spectrum of smooth skin tissue reaction patterns caused by *T.sulfureum* or *T.tonsurans* is limited when compared with *T.rubrum*. The microscopic changes were classified as chronic dermatitis, subacute dermatitis, folliculitis (Figs. 108, 110), perifollicultitis and pustular dermatitis (Fig. 109).

Histochemistry: The fungal elements were demonstrated histochemically as described for *T.tonsurans* and *T.sulfureum* under tinea capitis. Segmented hyphae and a few arthrospores were observed in the SC, within pustules and in keratin-plugged follicular ostia (Fig. 110). Fungal elements were located predominantly in the SC adjacent to the stratum Malpighii, although some were identified at more superficial levels. No organisms penetrated the stratum Malpighii or dermis. The results of other histochemical studies were similar to those reported for *T.rubrum*.

Differential Diagnosis: The histopathologic and histochemical differential diagnosis includes some of the diseases listed for *T.rubrum*, and smooth skin lesions caused by *T.verrucosum* and granular forms of *T.mentagrophytes*.

Comment: Much of the discussion for *T.tonsurans* and *T.sulfureum* under comments dealing with tinea capitis can apply to the consideration of glabrous skin disease and will not be repeated. Clinicians and pathologists should be alert to the apparent increase of dermatophytosis caused by these organisms. When glabrous skin lesions are identified as being caused by *T.tonsurans* or *T.sulfureum*, the patient and other family members should be examined thoroughly to check for additional smooth skin, scalp and nail disease.

8. Trichophyton Epilans

Introduction: *Trichophyton epilans* causing dermatophytosis has been reported from Canada by BLANK et al. (1957). Through the courtesy of Dr. F. BLANK, we were able to study biopsy sections and perform histochemical studies on material from 2 adult sisters with *T.epilans* dermatophytosis. GEORG (1956) considers

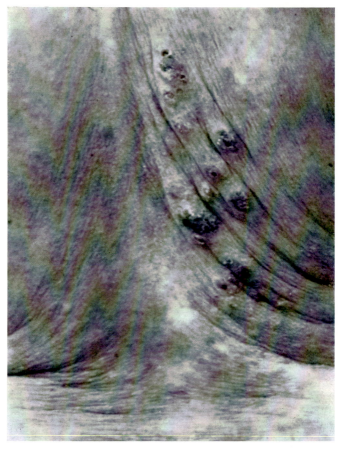

Fig. 111. Tinea corporis caused by *T. epilans* showing nodular, eroded, granulomatous lesions on the right back region below the scapula. Several areas manifest residual scarring with hypopigmentation. The patient had multiple lesions involving the scalp, face, neck, arms, thighs, nails, and there was almost complete alopecia with scarring and atrophy. The patient, a 65-year-old French-Canadian woman had the disease since she was age eight and her younger sister had a similar infection (From Blank, Schopflocher, Poirier and Riopelle, and by permission of F. Blank)

T. epilans as a variant of *T. tonsurans*, whereas Blank (1959) feels these conclusions should be corroborated prior to general acceptance. *Trichophyton epilans* as a cause of human granulomatous skin disease in Europe has been reported by Sabouraud (1910), Sequeira (1912) and Majocchi (1920). Blank (1955) reviewed the dermatophytes of animal origin transmissible to man. The summarized observations indicate that *T. epilans* is a zoophilic organism because it is isolated from cats and horses, it is frequent among patients from rural areas, and is a common cause of sycosis barbae. *Trichophyton epilans* causing dermatophytosis has been reported from Argentina, Germany, Denmark, Italy and Hungary.

Gross Appearance: Anatomically, biopsy material was studied from *T. epilans* infection involving the neck, anterior chest and back (Fig. 111). The 2 patients from whom biopsies were obtained had multiple lesions involving the scalp, face, neck, trunk, extremities, and fingernails. The youngest sister showed a mild

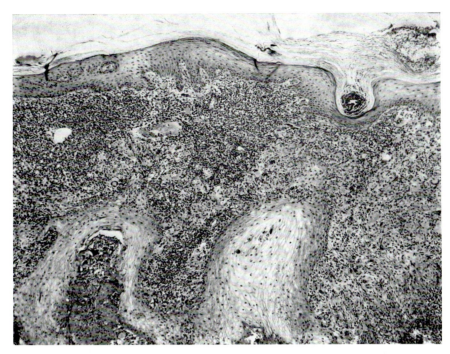

Fig. 112. Tinea corporis showing extensive *Trichophyton* infection of about 50 years duration caused by *T. epilans* and from the patient illustrated in Fig. 111. The section shows changes of a trichophytic granuloma similar to that first described by Majocchi. The features are those of hyperkeratosis, parakeratosis, follicular plugging, irregular acanthosis, deep intrafollicular abscesses and a diffuse granulomatous inflammation in the corium. High power magnification showed necrosis and disruption of the pilary outer root sheath at the depth of the intrafollicular abscesses. The granulomatous inflammation was characterized by a mixed cellular infiltration of lymphocytes, histiocytes, plasma cells, neutrophils, eosinophils, epithelioid cells, epithelioid tubercles, and giant cells of the Langhans' and foreign body type (H & E, ×55)

cutaneous infection characterized by erythema, papules, vesicles, pustules, scaling, lichenification, thickening, excoriations and white residual scars. There was almost complete scalp alopecia and some of the fingernails appeared grey, thickened and brittle. The older patient had lesions similar to her younger sister, but she also showed ill-defined, scaly, eczematous patches and multiple single or grouped nodular lesions (Fig. 111). The nodules were bluish-red, dome-shaped, hard, freely moveable and some lesions showed a peripheral rim of vesicles. A few nodules were soft, crusted and showed drainage of sanguinous fluid. All the fingernails were thickened, and there was almost total alopecia and atrophy of the scalp. Multiple residual white scarred lesions were scattered over areas showing active disease. *Trichophyton epilans* apparently causes tinea barbae since the organism was isolated as the pathogen responsible for epidemics of sycosis barbae in Germany (BLANK, 1955).

The clinical differential diagnoses for *T. epilans* infection include many of those confused with dermatophytosis from *T. rubrum*, particularly lesions classified as nodular granulomatous perifolliculitis. Mycosis fungoides, other malignant lymphomas, periarteritis nodosa, allergic granulomatosis, deep mycoses, and other infectious granulomas have to be considered because of the gross morphology of the nodular lesions.

Microscopic Observations: Multiple biopsy sections stained with H & E were examined from the youngest patient with *T.epilans* dermatophytosis, and the changes were classified as chronic dermatitis and subacute dermatitis. The microscopic features of the nodular lesions from the older patient were those of diffuse granulomatous inflammation (Figs. 112, 113, 114). The changes were like those seen in nodular granulomatous perifolliculitis, but plasma cells, epithelioid cells, tubercles, giant cells and necrosis were more prominent (Figs. 112, 113, 114). Remnants of acanthotic pilary outer root sheath epithelium and deep intrafollicular abscesses were observed in examining multiple sections (Fig. 112). No spicules of hair were identified in the material available for study.

Histochemistry: Fungal elements were demonstrated by special histochemical methods as described for other dermatophytes. Tissue reaction patterns of chronic dermatitis and subacute dermatitis showed a few short segmented hyphae limited to the horny layer which exhibited areas of hyperkeratosis and superficial crusting. Nodular lesions characterized by diffuse granulomatous inflammation contained numerous fungal elements associated predominantly with epithelioid tubercles and giant cells (Figs. 114, 115A—B), although a few organisms were observed in areas of necrosis. The fungal elements were present in the form of long and short segmented hyphae (Figs. 114, 115A—B), and a few large and small arthrospores (Fig. 115A). The arthrospores appeared to originate as terminal single budding organisms or as single to multiple intercalary cells along the course of filaments (Fig. 115A). No fungal elements were observed in the SC or associated with remnants of pilosebaceous follicles. Some of the segmented hyphae showed branching and were bizarre in appearance (Figs. 115A—B). A striking feature was an increase in hyaluronic acid in areas of granulomatous inflammation, and hyaluronidase resistant acid mucosaccharides associated with the fungal elements. Collagen showed prominent thinning in areas of granulomatous inflammation and elastic tissue was almost completely absent, whereas reticular fiber proliferation was striking (Fig. 115B). Mast cells were generally increased in association with the epithelioid tubercles and throughout other areas of granulomatous inflammation.

Differential Diagnosis: The histopathologic and histochemical differential diagnosis of tissue reaction patterns caused by *T.epilans* and showing features of chronic dermatitis, subacute dermatitis and nodular granulomatous perifollicultis is similar to that given for *T.rubrum*. Because of the diffuse dermal granulomatous inflammation with prominent epithelioid cells other diagnoses might be beryllium granuloma, zirconium granuloma, necrobiosis lipoidica diabeticorum, tertiary syphilis, lupus vulgaris and tuberculosis verrucosa cutis.

Comment: The multiple nodular granulomatous lesions, caused by *T.epilans*, from the older patient, presented a tissue reaction pattern like that of *T.rubrum* in the case reported by Blank and Smith (1960). The authors (Blank and Smith) described their patient as having the lowest level of serum antifungal activity of any subject they tested. It is likely that the immune response and serum antifungal activity, of the patient from whom we studied material, was abnormal because her sister also had chronic widespread *T.epilans* infection, but tissue sections showed no granulomatous reaction pattern nor could fungal elements be demonstrated in the dermis. We would classify the patient with *T.epilans* granulomatous dermatitis referred to in this report and the case reported by Blank and Smith (1960) as representing typical examples of Majocchi's trichophytic granuloma. Overlapping features are seen in tissue reaction patterns of the nodular granulomatous perifolliculitis type caused by *T.rubrum*, *T.mentagrophytes* variety *granulosum* and *M.gypseum*, but certain differences are apparent. The granu-

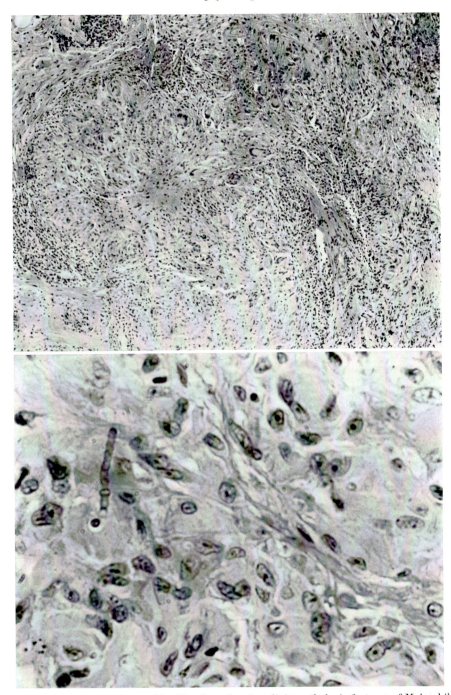

Fig. 113. Tinea corporis caused by *T.epilans* showing clinicopathologic features of Majocchi's trichophytic granuloma. The section shows granulomatous inflammation with epithelioid tubercles, numerous giant cells, and focal necrosis at the upper right margin (H&E, ×93)

Fig. 114. High power magnification of Majocchi's trichophytic granuloma caused by *T.epilans* showing an epithelioid tubercle with giant cells and a segmented hypha (PAS, ×655)

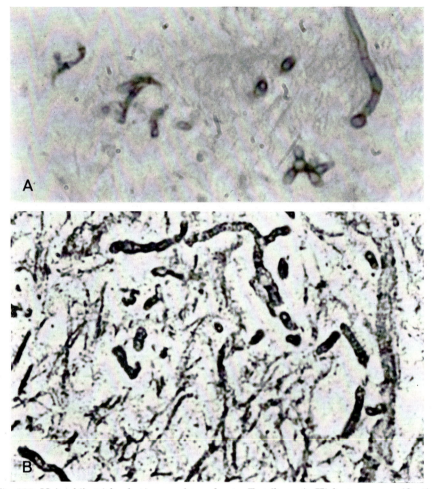

Fig. 115. Majocchi's trichophytic granuloma due to *T.epilans*: A. High power magnification showing segmented hyphae and some large budding arthrospores located in an area of dermal granulomatous inflammation (Gridley's method for fungi, ×655). B. High power magnification showing multiple hyphae located in an area of deep dermal granulomatous inflammation. Snook's silver stain shows a prominent reticular fiber hyperplasia associated with the granulomatous inflammation (Snook's reticulum stain, ×655)

lomatous tissue reaction elicited by *T.epilans* and *T.rubrum* in certain patients with an altered host-parasite relationship shows a much more diffuse reaction with many plasma cells, epithelioid cells, tubercles, and prominent necrosis. Evidence of altered pilosebaceous follicles in the sections we studied favors the penetration of the fungal elements into the corium via the pilary complex. Involved hairs were not identified in the sections we studied, but Sabouraud who first isolated *T.epilans* classified the organism as an endo-ectothrix parasite and separated it from endothrix infections caused by *T.tonsurans*. *Trichophyton tonsurans* infections are transferred from human to human, whereas *T.epilans* is of animal origin (Blank, 1955). Significant clinical differences exist in the nature of infections caused by *T.epilans* and *T.tonsurans*, and Sabouraud pointed out the frequency with which zoophilic dermatophytes cause granulomatous skin disease.

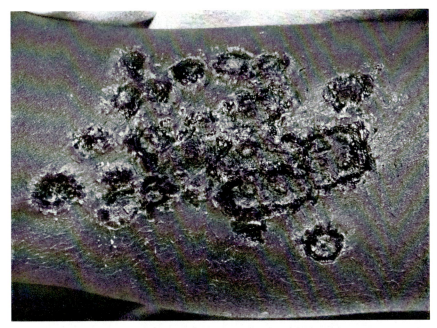

Fig. 116. Tinea corporis caused by *M.audouinii* showing highly inflammatory, circinate, crusting lesions on the right arm. The patient was an 8-year-old Negro girl

The presence of acid mucosaccharides in the cell wall of *T.epilans* fungal elements is interesting and similar to those described for *T.rubrum*. The exact chemical nature of *T.epilans* fungal elements is unknown, although based on our histochemical results future investigations will probably identify chitin, water-soluble polysaccharides and other substances. When recognized and isolated from unusual cases such as the patients reported by BLANK et al. (1957), *T.epilans* should be studied in greater detail by modern sophisticated techniques. The organism at one time in Europe apparently caused human skin disease in epidemic proportions, and sometime in the future, when the conditions are right, *T.epilans* will undoubtedly reappear as a more common cause of dermatophytosis.

9. Microsporum Audouinii and Microsporum Canis

Introduction: Comments made about *M.audouinii* and *M.canis*, in consideration of these organisms as causes of tinea capitis, can apply here and will not be repeated. As a cause of glabrous skin disease in Philadelphia, these two organisms were isolated 164 times during a four and a half year period (McCAFFREE et al.). Most of these cases were associated with scalp infections. For this report, biopsy sections were reviewed from ten patients with glabrous skin dermatophytosis caused by *M.audouinii* or *M.canis*.

Gross Appearance: Biopsy material from *M.audouinii* or *M.canis* infections were studied from the face, neck, trunk and extremities. Dermatophytosis from *M.audouinii* usually shows evidence of only mild inflammation characterized by slightly erythematous, annular, scaling lesions with central clearing. Sometimes, lesions caused by *M.audouinii* are highly inflamed and show vesicles, pustules, crusting, exudation and little or no tendency for central clearing (Fig. 116).

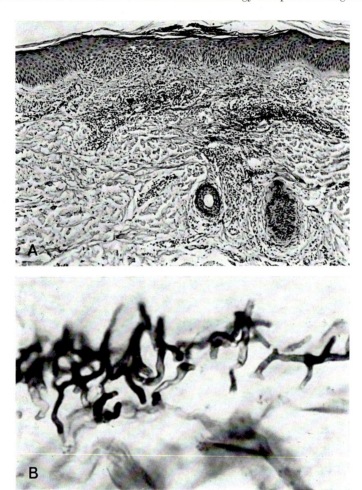

Fig. 117. Tinea corporis caused by *M.audouinii*: A. Low power magnification showing hypo-keratosis, focal parakeratosis, spongiosis, exocytosis, and mild acanthosis. In the upper corium there is perivascular inflammation involving small blood vessels showing changes of angiitis characterized by endothelial swelling, thickening, and infiltration of their walls (H & E, ×66).
B. High power of the SC showing multiple branching, segmented hyphae (PAS, ×655)

Lesions of *M.audouinii* show peripheral enlargenemt, but usually stop spreading after attaining the size of several centimeters. Dermatophytosis caused by *M.canis* can show lesions similar to those described for *M.audouinii* with mild, moderate or severe inflammatory changes (Fig. 118). Sometimes, *M.canis* infections occur as multiple overlapping ringed lesions and vesicles which are occasionally observed in the spreading peripheral margins (Fig. 118). Nail involvement rarely occurs with *M.audouinii* and *M.canis* infections and has not been a feature of case material studied at The Skin and Cancer Hospital of Philadelphia. When the nails are involved, they appear yellow, opaque and lusterless. *Microsporum canis* can rarely cause tinea barbae, although we have not observed such an infection in our case material. Allergic dermatophytid eruptions sometimes occur in the form of papular, lichenoid, follicular and erythema perstans type lesions, and these are more often seen in zoophilic *M.canis* infections with kerion.

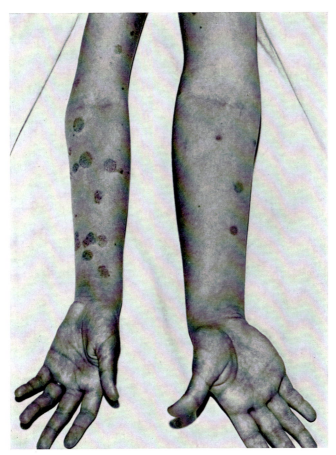

Fig. 118. Tinea corporis caused by *M.canis* showing the disease in 11-year-old Caucasian twin girls. The lesions appear erythematous, circinate, scaly and crusted, and are located on the flexor surface of their upper extremities

The clinical differentiation of *M.audouinii* and *M.canis* infections is often difficult and usually requires the results of mycological culture studies to identify the causative organism. The clinical differential diagnosis is similar to that given for other dermatophytes causing glabrous skin infections. Distinction from papulosquamous inflammatory dermatoses and bacterial disease such as impetigo contagiosa is sometimes difficult.

Microscopic Observations: Tissue reaction patterns were classified as chronic dermatitis, subacute dermatitis, purpuric dermatitis, erythema perstans (Fig. 117A), pustular dermatitis (Fig. 119A), folliculitis (Fig. 120) and perifolliculitis. An angiitis of the small papillary blood vessels was frequently observed in the various tissue reaction patterns (Figs. 117A, 119A).

Histochemistry: Fungal elements were demonstrated in the SC (Figs. 117B, 119B) and serial sections showed organisms involving some hair follicles (Fig. 120). Segmented hyphae and a few small arthrospores were located predominantly adjacent to the stratum Malpighii (Fig. 119B), but some fungal elements were identified at more superficial levels of the horny layer (Fig. 117B). Sometimes, the

21*

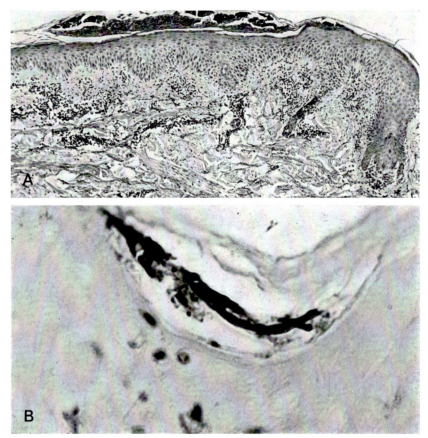

Fig. 119. Tinea corporis caused by *M.canis*: A. Scanning view showing superficial crusting, parakeratosis, spongiosis and mild acanthosis. In the upper corium there is perivascular inflammation composed of lymphocytes, histiocytes and neutrophils. The stroma shows interstitial edema (H & E, ×71). B. High power magnification of an area from A showing hyphae located in a follicular ostium (GMS, ×655)

hyphae occurred as multiple bizarre branching forms (Fig. 117B). The frequent branching of segmented hyphae in the SC was a feature noted in tinea capitis, and particularly when the infection was caused by *M.audouinii* (Fig. 18C). Fungal elements of *M.audouinii* and *M.canis* involved the glabrous skin hair as endo-ectothrix parasites, atlhough some follicles showed only intrapilary segmented hyphae (Fig. 120) similar to that observed in tinea capitis (Figs. 7, 13A—B, 15A—B). No fungal elements were demonstrated in the stratum Malpighii or dermis.

Differential Diagnosis: The histopathologic and histochemical differential diagnosis for tissue reaction patterns elicited by *M.audouinii* and *M.canis* is similar to diseases considered for those caused by *T.rubrum*. Multiple branching hyphae occur in the SC of some *M.audouinii* infections, but generally fungal element morphology in tissue sections is not specific and makes it difficult to distinguish a particular dermatophyte as the cause of a given superficial fungus disease.

Comment: Many of the remarks made about *M.audouinii* and *M.canis* infections under the section related to these organisms causing tinea capitis apply

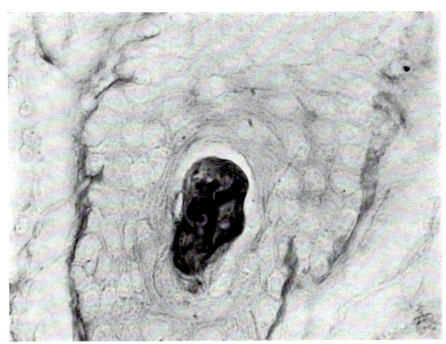

Fig. 120. Tinea corporis caused by *M.canis* showing high power magnification of intrapilary hyphae confined by an intact cuticle of the cortex. A similar parasitic pattern occurs in infected scalp hairs from *M.canis* and no sheath of ectothrix arthrospores is seen (PAS, ×655)

here and need not be repeated. Patients with tinea capitis caused by *M.audouinii* and *M.canis* should always be inspected closely to check for glabrous skin disease caused by these dermatophytes.

10. Microsporum Gypseum

Introduction: In this section, we shall report our histopathologic and histochemical observations from three patients with *M.gypseum* glabrous skin infections involving the left thigh, left knee, and left leg below the knee (Fig. 121). Microsporum gypseum is an interesting organism which causes an inflammatory type of tinea capitis (Fig. 19) and even in tinea corporis this dermatophyte shows a predilection for involving the hair follicle. Hair involvement and even dermal invasion occurred in one patient we studied, and this case represents the same individual reported by Luscombe and Bingul as nodular granulomatous perifolliculitis caused by *M.gypseum*. Ajello (1953) considers *M.gypseum* as mainly a soil saprophyte from which human infections are contracted. Gordon reviewed the occurrence of *M.gypseum* infections in horses, dogs and cats, and considered the possibility that they perhaps acted as animal vectors of human disease from this primary soil saprophyte. Nine patients with glabrous skin dermatophytosis showed isolates of *M.gypseum* identified by the Section of Medical Mycology, The Skin and Cancer Hospital of Philadelphia (McCaffree et al.).

Gross Appearance: *Microsporum gypseum* infections usually appear as single, discrete, erythematous, annular, scaling lesions with some tendency for central clearing (Fig. 121). Papules, vesicles, pustules, follicular lesions and nodules may occur (Fig. 121), and when inflammation is prominent, exudation and crusting

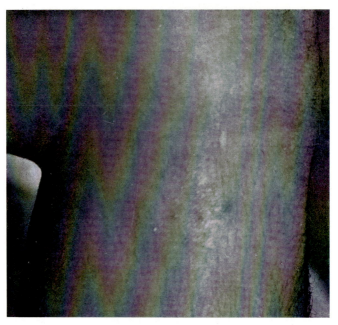

Fig. 121. Tinea corporis caused by *M.gypseum* showing ill-defined, erythematous, circinate, papular nodular lesions on the medial aspect of the left leg below the knee. The lesion was single with no other similar ones on other areas of the body

result. In follicular-pustular lesions, hair can be easily epilated and may show white to greenish fluorescence under Wood's light.

The clinical differential diagnosis includes dermatophytosis caused by zoophilic organisms, particularly *M.canis* and *T.verrucosum*. Distinguishing inflammatory superficial fungus infections from pyoderma, bacterial folliculitis, eczematous dermatoses and papulosquamous diseases is difficult and requires a high index of suspicion for cutaneous reactions caused by the various dermatophytes. The patient reported by Luscombe and Bingul (1964) was initially thought to have Bowen's disease or psoriasis, but results of biopsy and mycological culture studies subsequently revealed the true nature of the process caused by *M.gypseum*.

Microscopic Observations: The tissue reaction patterns caused by *M.gypseum* in the sections we studied include chronic dermatitis, subacute dermatitis, pustular dermatitis, folliculitis (Figs. 122, 123), perifolliculitis (Fig. 122) and nodular granulomatous perifolliculitis (Figs. 124, 125, 126, 127, 128A—B).

Fig. 122. Tinea corporis caused by *M.gypseum* showing a subcorneal intrafollicular pustule filled with neutrophils. A remnant of hair contains fungal elements. The pustule roof is made up of a thickened SC with parakeratosis and entrapped inflammatory cells. The lateral epidermal margins show acanthosis, and glycogen is demonstrated with the PAS method. The pilary outer root sheath at the base of the pustule shows partial erosion and there is inflammation in the adjacent corium (PAS, ×66)

Fig. 123. Tinea corporis caused by *M.gypseum* shows intrapilary and external hyphae which frequently segment to form large arthrospores (megaspores) involving the remnant of hair illustrated in Fig. 122. The pattern of hair involvement by the fungal elements indicates that *M.gypseum* should be classified as an endo-ectothrix parasite and the organism falls into the megasporosis group of dermatophytes (PAS with diastase digestion method, ×445)

Histochemistry: Fungal elements were demonstrated by the techniques described for other dermatophytes. Segmented hyphae and arthrospores were observed in the SC adjacent to the stratum granulosum. Some fungal elements

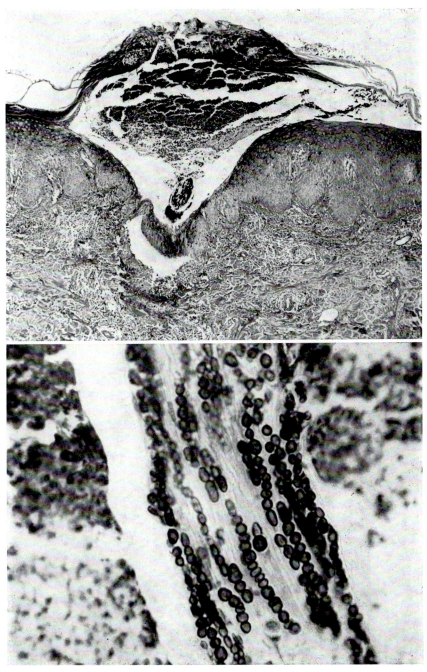

Figs. 122 (above) and 123 (below)

were present at more superficial levels of the horny layer, particularly in areas of superficial crusting related to intraepidermal and follicular pustules. Short segmented hyphae and large arthrospores were identified within these pustules and related to spicules of hair in altered follicular ostia (Figs. 122, 123). Examination of serial sections showed two predominant parasitic patterns of hair involvement:
1. Intrapilary segmented hyphae extending from the KZ to the SC (Fig. 124).
2. Intrapilary segmented hyphae and arthrospores and a sheath of similar fungal elements surrounding the involved hairs (Figs. 122, 123, 127). The arthrospores were predominantly of the megasporosis type, some measuring up to 20 μ (Fig. 123). Biopsy sections from one patient showed histopathologic features of nodular granulomatous perifolliculitis with fungal elements in perifollicular dermal abscesses (Fig. 125, 126, 127, 128A—B). Spicules of hair which were apparently extruded into the corium from degenerated pilosebaceous follicles showed intrapilary segmented hyphae and arthrospores (Fig. 127). Arthrospores were scattered singly (Fig. 128A) and in groups (Fig. 128B) throughout areas of dermal abscess formation. Some of the fungal elements in the corium were formed by single budding sporulation (Fig. 128B) and special techniques for the demonstration of acid mucosaccharides showed that the positive organisms (Fig. 128B) were identical to those described for nodular granulomatous perifolliculitis caused by $T.rubrum$. The results of other histochemical studies were similar to those described for $T.rubrum$.

Differential Diagnosis: The histopathologic and histochemical differential diagnosis is identical to that given for $T.rubrum$ tissue reaction patterns of chronic dermatitis, subacute dermatitis, pustular dermatitis, folliculitis, perifolliculitis and nodular granulomatous perifolliculitis. Vesicles are sometimes seen grossly in smooth skin infections caused by $M.gypseum$, but multiple sections prepared from three biopsy specimens did not show this reaction pattern in our case material.

Comment: Our observations of glabrous skin lesions with hair follicle involvement caused by $M.gypseum$ support the classification of the organism as an endoectothrix megasporosis parasite as was done in tissue studies on tinea capitis. Glabrous skin hair follicle involvement by $M.gypseum$ is supported by Gordon (1953) who inoculated fungal elements into an adult subject, and subsequently there developed an impetiginous reaction. After 21, 28 and 37 days, epilated hairs showed large ectothrix spores (Gordon, 1953). Intrapilary fungal elements could have been missed in hairs examined by Gordon. It is possible that host-parasite relationship factors prevented the organism from penetrating the hair shaft and explains spontaneous healing of the lesion after eight weeks. Penetration of the

Fig. 124. Tinea corporis caused by $M.gypseum$ showing clinicopathologic and histochemical features of nodular granulomatous perifolliculitis. High power magnification shows only intrapilary segmented hyphae at the SG level. Serial sections showed some infected hairs containing intrapilary segmented hyphae and arthrospores, and a surrounding sheath of megaspores similar to that seen in tinea capitis due to $M.gypseum$ (Snook's reticulum stain, ×445)

Fig. 125. Tinea corporis caused by $M.gypseum$ showing clinicopathologic features of nodular granulomatous perifolliculitis. The section shows a remnant of outer root sheath epithelium with necrosis at the base and perifollicular granulomatous inflammation. The granulomatous process is characterized by a mixed cellular infiltrate, multinucleated giant cells, necrosis, fibrosis, capillary-endothelial proliferation, vascular ectasia, extravasated red blood cells, and interstitial edema (H & E, ×93)

dermis by *M.gypseum* arthrospores is not surprising since geophilic dermatophytes seem to show a potential for adapting to a mesenchymal substrate in the
proper host.

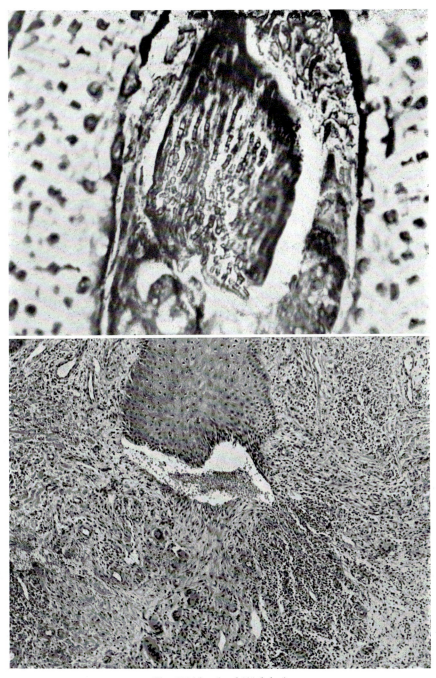

Figs. 124 (above) and 125 (below)

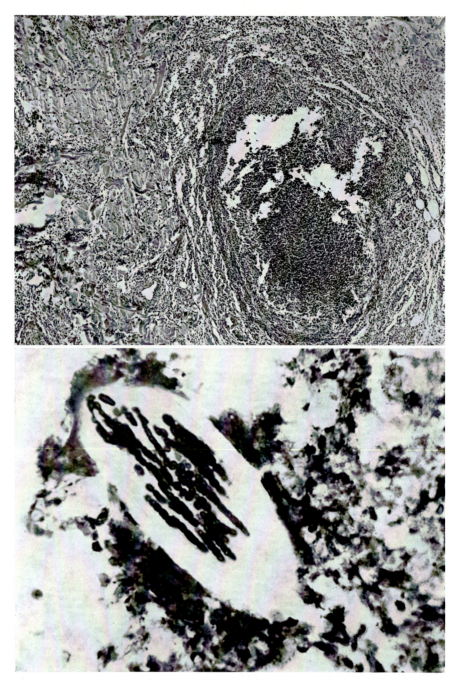

Figs. 126 (above) and 127 (below)

The large *M. gypseum* arthrospores located in deep dermal perifollicular abscesses contain substances with histochemical properties of acid mucosaccharides. Similar acid mucosaccharides were demonstrated in *T. rubrum* arthro-

Fig. 126. Tinea corporis caused by *M.gypseum* showing clinicopathologic changes of nodular granulomatous perifolliculitis. The section shows a deep perifollicular miliary abscess located at the level of the corium and subcutaneous tissue. The abscess contains neutrophils centrally and a peripheral margin of lymphocytes, histiocytes, plasma cells, eosinophils, and some foreign body giant cells. Special stains for demonstration of fungal elements showed megaspores scattered throughout the abscess (H & E, ×66)

Fig. 127. Tinea corporis caused by *M.gypseum* showing clinicopathologic and histochemical changes of nodular granulomatous perifolliculitis. High power magnification of a deep perifollicular dermal abscess showing a fragment of hair with intrapilary segmented hyphae and arthrospores (PAS, ×445)

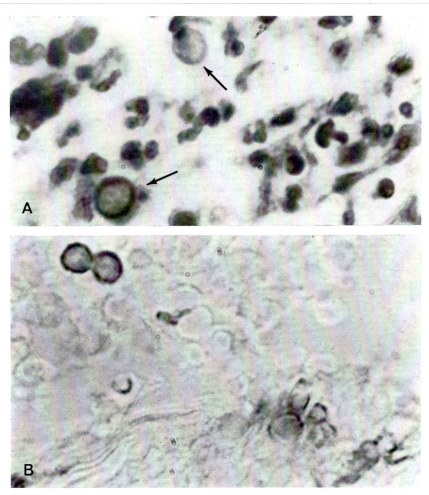

Fig. 128. Tinea corporis caused by *M.gypseum* showing clinicopathologic and histochemical features of nodular granulomatous perifolliculitis. A. Oil immersion magnification showing megaspores (arrow) in a deep perifollicular dermal abscess with a striking resemblance to those seen in nodular granulomatous perifolliculitis caused by *T.rubrum*. Some individual megaspores measure up to 20 μ (PAS, ×1400). B. Oil immersion magnification of arthrospores in a deep perifollicular dermal abscess showing division by single budding sporulation. The cell walls are colloidal iron positive and hyaluronidase resistant indicating the presence of acid mucosaccharides other than hyaluronic acid. A group of the arthrospores show some staining reaction of their walls at the lower right margin (Colloidal iron stain with hyaluronidase digestion method, ×1400)

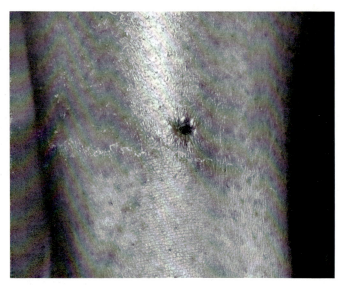

Fig. 129. Tinea corporis caused by *E. floccosum* showing mild erythematous, scaling lesion on the dorsum of the skin. The biopsy site is seen in the central part of the photograph. The patient was treated with oral griseofulvin and subsequently developed an annular lesion on the posterior neck region diagnosed as fixed drug eruption resulting from the antifungal therapy

spores and associated with the fungal elements in *T. epilans* infection showing dermal granulomatous inflammation. Acidic material in *M. gypseum* arthrospores probably represents a combination of fatty acids, nuclei acids and sialomucin.

Clinicians and pathologists should know that *M. gypseum*, as a cause of glabrous skin dermatophytosis, mimics other diseases, and that the organism can penetrate the dermis with clinicopathologic features of nodular granulomatous perifolliculitis.

11. Epidermophyton Floccosum

Introduction: Dermatophytosis from *E. floccosum* occurs as a world-wide disease causing infections predominantly of the groin and feet. A total of 62 isolations of *E. floccosum* were made from 52 patients reported by McCaffree et al., and anatomically, in order of frequency, the lesions involved the feet, groin, trunk, extremities, hands and nails. Blank and Prichard (1962) reported epidemic ringworm of the groin caused by *E. floccosum* from Montreal, Canada, and mentioned its familial and conjugal transmission. The exact method of spread of *E. floccosum* human disease is not definite, but probably it is through infected athletic equipment and clothing. Blank and Pritchard believed that their cases of eczema marginatum caused by *E. floccosum* developed from infected climbing ropes in a boys high school gym, and macerated cutaneous material provided the source of inoculum. For this report, we shall record our observations of biopsy sections from five patients with *E. floccosum* infections proven by mycological culture studies. The tissue specimens came from the feet, legs (Fig. 129) and inner aspect of the thigh.

Gross Appearance: Lesions of the feet appear dry and scaly with evidence of interdigital maceration particularly between the 4th and 5th toes. The groin and inner aspects of the thighs usually show erythematous, scaly, annular lesions which

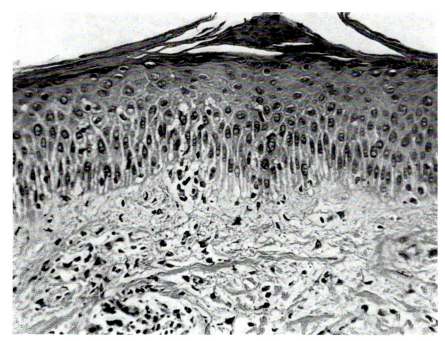

Fig. 130. Tinea corporis caused by *E. floccosum* showing hypokeratosis, parakeratosis, hypogranulosis, spongiosis, mild acanthosis and a central area of liquefaction degeneration. The upper corium shows interstitial edema and a mild perivascular inflammatory infiltrate. Special stains for fungal elements demonstrated segmented hyphae in the altered horny layer. There was no evidence of epidermal or dermal invasion by the fungal elements (H & E, ×190)

are sharply marginated with little or no tendency for central clearing. The peripheral margins of *E. floccosum* lesions may be raised and show minute vesicles and pustules. The groin lesions are usually bilateral and symmetrical. Sometimes, dermatophytosis from *E. floccosum* involving sites other than the groin appear as asymptomatic, ill-defined, slightly erythematous, scaling lesions which are easily missed (Fig. 129). Initially, infected nails appear white, opaque and lusterless, but eventually show changes similar to *T. rubrum* onychomycosis. Widespread verrucous epidermophytosis has been reported (FISHER et al.) and patients of this type may have serious immunological abnormalities (COISCOU et al.).

The clinical differential diagnosis includes dermatophytosis of the groin and feet caused by *T. rubrum*. Confusion with erythrasma and cutaneous candidiasis can also occur. Sometimes distinction from papulosquamous diseases, particularly seborrheic dermatitis and psoriasis is difficult and may lead to an erroneous clinical diagnosis. Patients with lesions of verrucous epidermophytosis may be confused with having bromide granuloma, lupus vulgaris, tuberculosis verrucosa cutis or one of the deep cutaneous mycotic infections.

Microscopic Observations: The microscopic changes of *E. floccosum* infections showed tissue reaction patterns of chronic dermatitis (Figs. 130, 131A), subacute dermatitis and pustular dermatitis. The follicle was spared with no evidence of hair invasion by *E. floccosum* fungal elements.

Histochemistry: Segmented hyphae and a few arthrospores were demonstrated in the SC by the various histochemical methods utilized for fungal elements (Fig. 131B). A few of the fungal elements extended to the stratum granulosum,

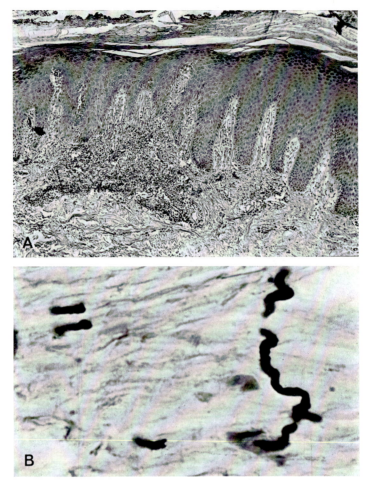

Fig. 131. Tinea pedis caused by *E. floccosum*: A. Scanning magnification showing prominent parakeratosis, granular layer intact and a moderate irregular acanthosis. Focally, the upper corium shows a dense cellular inflammatory infiltrate (H & E, ×55). B. High power magnification of A and showing multiple hyphae in the SC. No fungal elements were demonstrated in the living epidermis or dermis (GMS, ×655)

but the majority were located at more superficial levels of the horny layer and this was particularly well demonstrated in examples of tinea pedis (Fig. 131B). No fungal elements were identified in the stratum Malpighii or corium. Histochemical alterations of the epidermis, sweat glands, mast cells, connective tissue and ground substance were similar to descriptions given for *T. rubrum* infections.

Differential Diagnosis: The histopathologic and histochemical differential diagnosis of *E. floccosum* infections is similar to that for *T. rubrum* dermatophytosis showing tissue reaction patterns of chronic dermatitis, subacute dermatitis and pustular dermatitis. The superficial location in the SC of most *E. floccosum* fungal elements appears to be different from other dermatophytes which show segmented hyphae and arthrospores predominantly adjacent to the stratum granulosum or stratum Malpighii. This is worth considering as a differential feature favoring *E. floccosum* as the causative dermatophyte when examining tissue sections which show fungal elements in biopsy specimens from the feet, legs, thighs and groin. Absence of follicular involvement by fungal elements in *E.floccosum* dermatophytosis is similar to that occurring in glabrous skin infections caused by *T.interdigitale* and *T.concentricum*. Tissue changes of folliculitis with hair involvement should represent an aid in eliminating *E.floccosum*, *T.interdigitale* and *T.concentricum* as a cause of the patient's disease.

Comments: The feature of *E.floccosum* fungal elements being localized more to the superficial layers of the SC probably represents an indication of host-parasite relationship and from fungistatic serum activity which prevents deeper penetration of the horny layer by the organism. Unusual examples of *E.floccosum* infections like those in the patient with verrucous epidermophytosis reported by FISHER et al. showed numerous fungal elements penetrating to the deep layers of the SC adjacent to the stratum granulosum. Patients with this form of host response to *E.floccosum* who show resistance to griseofulvin therapy (COISCOU et al.; FISHER et al.) undoubtedly have serious immunological abnormalities and/or a lowered antifungal serum factor. FRANKS and FRANK (1951) reported a patient with extensive verrucous dermatitis associated with dermatophytosis and onychomycosis due to *T.gypseum* and the resemblance is striking to the cases reported by FISHER et al. and COISCOU et al.

Tinea cruris caused by *E.floccosum* is still referred to by some as eczema marginatum which was the term first used by HEBRA in 1860, and in India the disease is known as dhobie itch (LEWIS et al.). It is likely that *E.floccosum* infections are more common than records indicate because the usual form of the disease responds well to topical treatment and makes it difficult to conduct accurate epidemiological studies on this cosmopolitan species as a cause of dermatophytosis.

Cutaneous Candidiasis

Introduction: Candidiasis will be discussed in detail elsewhere in this textbook (WINNER, Chapter XIX) and in depth consideration other than skin and mucocutaneous involvement will not be attempted here. *Candida albicans* is the most frequent cause of cutaneous candidiasis although *C.parapsilosis*, *C.guilliermondii*, *C.tropicalis*, *C.pseudotropicalis*, *C.krusei* and *C.stellatoidea* have all been isolated from pathologic lesions. In general, *Candida* species are present in saprophytic yeast form in many organs of the body, but under certain conditions the host-parasite relationship becomes disturbed and a mycelial phase develops. Hyphae and spores represent the morphology of *Candida* organisms encountered in diseased tissue. Intertriginous candidiasis is encountered in patients with obesity, diabetes mellitus, alcoholics with malnutrition, housewives, fruit canners, infants and children. Cutaneous and mucocutaneous candidiasis of the generalized type seems more prone to develop in patients with systemic diseases such as carcinomatosis, diabetes, hypoparathyroidism, hypofunction of the adrenals, acrodermatitis enteropathica, celiac syndrome, hypothyroidism and congenital ectodermal defects. Relapses after treatment with nystatin among 94 patients with *C.albicans* infections of the skin and mucosa were encountered in cases of pemphigus vulgaris, systemic lupus erythematosus, leukemia, diabetes and other severe systemic diseases (GRAHAM et al., 1955). Candidiasis of the nails is common in Great Britain and seen among barmaids, pastry cooks, chefs and fishmongers (HILDICK-SMITH et al.). For this report, we shall record our observations of biopsy sections from 30 patients with skin, mucocutaneous and nail infections caused predominantly by *C.albicans*.

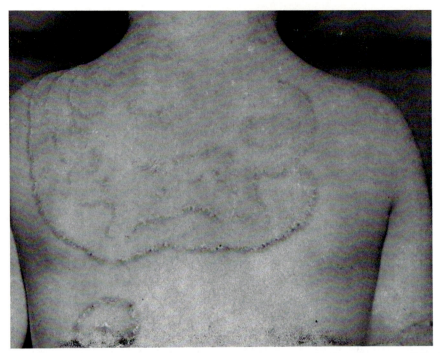

Fig. 132. The patient, a 4-year-old Caucasian boy, showed generalized cutaneous candidiasis caused by *C.albicans*. The back shows annular to serpiginous, erythematous, scaling lesions, and the peripheral borders are elevated and studded with pustules. An associated systemic disease was suspected but thorough investigative studies revealed nothing of significance

Gross Appearance: Biopsy specimens were studied from the lips, fingers, fingernails, arms, anogenital region, abdomen, back (Fig. 132), thigh, legs and feet. Clinically, intertriginous candidiasis shows erythematous, eczematous, scaling, eroded areas with scattered papules, vesicles, pustules and follicular lesions. There is usually an accentuated peripheral margin of papules and pustules. Satellite pustules and follicular pustules are common adjacent to eroded areas and/or the peripheral margin of *Candida* lesions. There is little or no tendency for central clearing, and secondary changes of exudation, crusting, maceration, fissuring and edema can occur. Localized forms of intertriginous candidiasis have been referred to as intertrigo, erosio interdigitalis blastomycetica (intertrigo affecting the interdigital webs), perleche, perianal candidiasis, candidal vulvovaginitis and candidal balanoposthitis. Mucocutaneous lesions appear as erythematous to white, crusted, thickened plaques which may show pustules, exudation and eroded areas. Nail infections are usually painful and characterized by nonpurulent erythema and edema of the paronychia and adjacent skin. The nails may show depressions, striations, hypertrophic areas and appear yellow to brown or greenish-brown in color. Separation of the nail plate from the nail bed epithelium usually occurs along the lateral margins. Tabulation of data from the Section of Medial Mycology, The Skin and Cancer Hospital of Philadelphia, during the period from July 1, 1962 through December 31, 1968, revealed a total of 186 isolations of *Candida* species from fingernail infections. Identification of the species showed that 121 of the isolations were *C.albicans* and the remaining 65 had characteristics of *C.parapsilosis*.

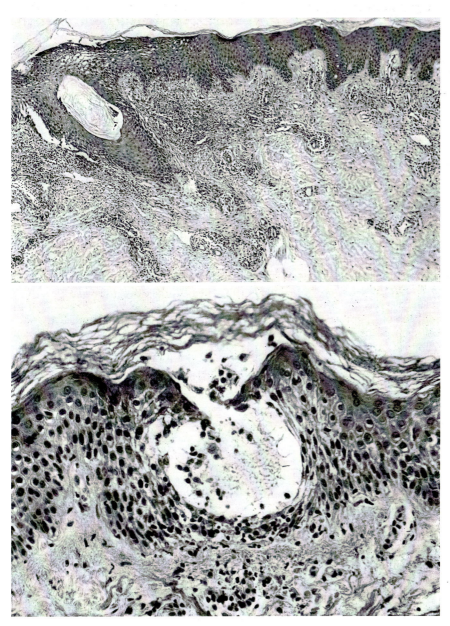

Fig. 133. Cutaneous candidiasis showing microscopic changes of subacute dermatitis. Spongiosis, intracellular edema, exocytosis, and mild irregular acanthosis is seen in relationship to a keratin-plugged follicular ostium. The upper corium shows a perifollicular inflammatory infiltrate, and there is some capillary-endothelial proliferation. Special stains demonstrated filamentous hyphae and spores in the SC (H & E, ×66)

Fig. 134. Cutaneous candidiasis caused by *C. albicans* showing an intraepidermal microvesicle with mononuclear cells similar to nummular eczema or allergic contact dermatitis. A mild cellular infiltrate of lymphocytes and histiocytes is seen in the upper corium. Special stains demonstrated pseudohyphae and spores in the corneal layer (H & E, ×190)

Generalized cutaneous candidiasis can show nail changes, intertriginous involvement, and erythematous, annular to serpiginous scaling lesions with sharply demarcated elevated margins comprised of papules, vesicles, pustules and follicular pustules (Fig. 132). An unusual form of extensive cutaneous candidiasis is *Candida* granuloma as reported by Hauser and Rothman. More recently, reports and reviews of *Candida* granuloma have been documented (Rothman; Kugelman et al.; Montgomery; and Imperato et al.). Individual skin lesions of *Candida* granuloma differ from the common forms of cutaneous candidiasis and show hyperkeratotic granulomatous lesions involving the face, scalp, trunk, intertriginous areas, extremities, feet, hands and fingernails. The clinical lesions vary from primary vascularized papules covered with thick, adherent, yellow-brown crusts surrounded by edema and erythema, to hornlike structures which can be stripped off leaving a bleeding granulomatous base (Hildick-Smith et al.). Candidids or monolids may develop with any cutaneous form of candidiasis. The lesions occur as localized or disseminated erythematous, papular, vesicular lesions, and resemble dermatophytids caused by *Trichophyton* species.

The clinical differential diagnosis includes a number of inflammatory dermatoses, particularly pyoderma, folliculitis, miliaria, seborrheic dermatitis and atopic dermatitis. Confusion can occur between cutaneous candidiasis and dermatophytic infections because most of the pathogens elicit a pustular tissue reaction pattern. *Candida* granuloma may be difficult to distinguish from dermatophytes showing unusual verrucous lesions such as those caused by *E. floccosum* and *T. gypseum*. Confusion of *Candida* granuloma with favus from *T. schoenleinii* and *M. quinckeanum* can occur, and additional considerations include bromide granuloma, dermatitis vegetans, tuberculosis cutis with vegetating lesions and deep cutaneous mycotic diseases.

Microscopic Observations: The various tissue reaction patterns caused by *C. albicans* and *C. parapsilosis* were essentially similar to those described for *T. rubrum* and classified as chronic dermatitis, subacute dermatitis (Fig. 133), acute vesicular dermatitis (Fig. 134), purpuric dermatitis, pustular dermatitis, folliculitis (Figs. 133, 136, 137) and perifolliculitis (Figs. 133, 136). *Candida* granuloma showed features of pseudoepitheliomatous hyperplasia with granulomatous inflammation. Fingernail infections or paronychia caused by *C. albicans* and *C. parapsilosis* showed histopathologic changes of inflammation with reaction patterns similar to chronic dermatitis, subacute dermatitis, and pustular dermatitis. The cellular inflammatory infiltrate and angiitis of small blood vessels was usually a fairly prominent change in the various reactions caused by *C. albicans* and *C. parapsilosis*. *Candida* granuloma showed tissue changes overlapping with those described for nodular granulomatous perifolliculitis. Additional features were pseudoepitheliomatous hyperplasia, superficial crusting, spongiosis, exocytosis, microabscesses containing neutrophils, and miliary abscesses in the corium and areas of squamous cell hyperplasia. There were deep keratin-filled

Fig. 135. Cutaneous candidiasis caused by *C. albicans* showing a thickened stratum corneum with numerous hyphae (pseudohyphae) and spores. The stratum Malpighii contains melanin and a reticular fiber hyperplasia is seen in the papillary corium. There is no evidence of invasion of these structures by the fungal elements (GMS, ×190)

Fig. 136. Cutaneous candidiasis caused by *C. albicans* showing follicular involvement in a patient with vulvar disease. The section shows parakeratosis, follicular plugging, spongiosis, exocytosis, and irregular acanthosis. Numerous fungal elements are demonstrated in the keratin-plugged follicular ostia. The upper corium shows inflammation, vascular ectasia and interstitial edema (PAS, ×66)

follicular crypts with parakeratosis and some sections showed remnants of hair. Plasma cells, eosinophils and neutrophils were prominent in the dermal cellular infiltrate.

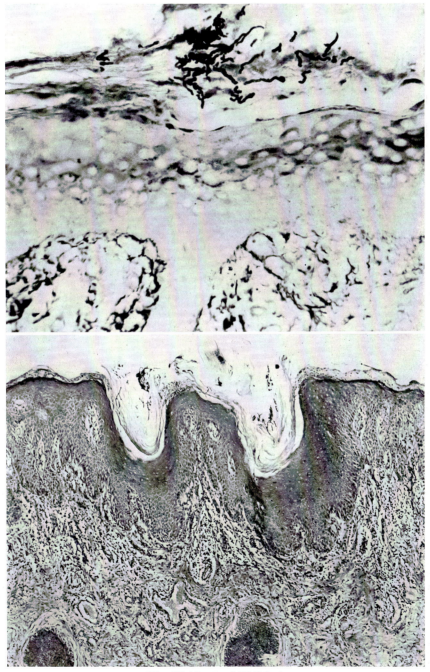

Figs. 135 (above) and 136 (below)

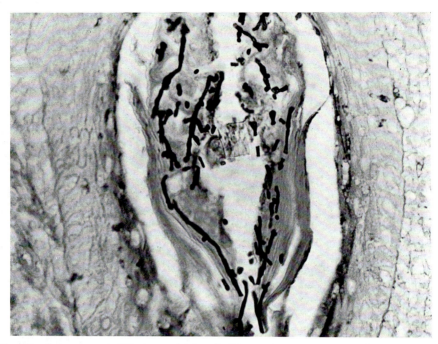

Fig. 137. Cutaneous candidiasis caused by *C.albicans* showing a keratin-plugged follicular ostium with numerous short and long branched segmented hyphae and spores. In general, the germ tubes (pseudohyphae) of *C.albicans* in tissue show less tendency for cross segmentation than do the dermatophytes (PAS, ×265)

Histochemistry: Hyphae and spores characteristic of the pathogenic tissue phase of *C.albicans* and *C.parapsilosis* were demonstrated by special histochemical techniques utilized for fungal elements in dermatophytic infections (Figs. 135, 136, 137). *Candida* hyphae or pseudohyphae were not as frequently segmented as those observed in the various dermatophytes causing human disease (Fig. 135). The germ tubes of *Candida* species appeared quite long with infrequent septae, but some examples showed greater segmentation and multiple branching hyphae (Figs. 136, 137). Spores approximately 4 μ in size or larger were observed singly and in groups, and appeared to form as terminal, intercalary, or small nodular cells along the surface of hyphae (Figs. 135, 137). *Candida* fungal elements were identified in the SC (Fig. 135), keratin-plugged follicular ostia (Figs. 136, 137), and within intraepidermal pustules and miliary abscesses. In general, *Candida* organisms were concentrated in the superficial levels of the horny layer (Fig. 135). Multiple sections showed branching hyphae and spores surrounding hairs, but with no evidence of intrapilary invasion by the fungal elements. No hyphae or spores were identified in the corium. In *Candida* granuloma, hyphae and spores extended to the stratum Malpighii, into deep keratin-filled follicular crypts, and were even seen in intraepidermal intercellular spaces adjacent to miliary abscesses. Histochemically, some *Candida* spores in the SC reacted positive for acidic substances similar to results obtained for *T.rubrum*, *T.epilans* and *M.gypseum*. Histochemical alterations of the epidermis, hair follicle, sweat glands, mast cells, connective tissue and ground substance were similar to descriptions given for the various dermatophytes. Granulomatous inflammation in *Candida* granuloma showed 20—30 mast cells per high power magnification field.

Differential Diagnosis: The histopathologic and histochemical considerations for cutaneous, mucocutaneous and nail reaction patterns caused by *C.albicans* and *C.parapsilosis* are similar to those given for *T.rubrum*. Confusion of cutaneous reaction patterns caused by *Candida* species and zoophilic dermatophytes occur, but the superficial location of organisms in the SC and numerous spores aid in distinguishing yeast infections. Dermatophytes such as *E.floccosum*, *T.mentagrophytes* (*gypseum*), *T.rubrum*, *T.schoenleinii* and *M.quinckeanum* can rarely cause verrucous lesions that histologically resemble *Candida* granuloma. Granulomatous inflammation caused by *C.albicans* can produce skin tissue changes mimicking squamous cell carcinoma, irritated verruca, bromide granuloma, condyloma lata, granuloma inguinale, tuberculosis verrucosa cutis, botryomycosis, actinomycosis, nocardiosis, maduromycosis, deep mycotic diseases and other infectious granulomas.

Comments: In general, reported microscopic observations of cutaneous candidiasis indicate that the fungal elements are limited to the SC. In examining multiple tissue sections from each biopsy specimen, we observed hyphae and spores in follicular ostia and surrounding remnants of hair, but no definite evidence of invasion of pilar structures. Follicular involvement and hair invasion by *Candida* organisms probably occur more often than published reports indicate. HELLIER et al. (1963) described a patient with *Candida* granuloma who showed extrapilary fungal elements and hair invasion by mycelium. Additional support for *in vivo* SC, hair and nail keratinolytic activity of *C.albicans* and *C.parapsilosis* is the ability of these organisms to digest keratin *in vitro* (KAPICA and BLANK, 1957, 1958).

Invasion of the mesodermal stroma by fungal elements was not seen in tissue sections of our case material of cutaneous and mucocutaneous candidiasis. KUGELMAN et al. (1963) reviewed the subject of *Candida* granuloma and reported a patient with severe generalized mucocutaneous candidiasis who had an ankle lesion from which biopsy sections showed many mycelia in the SC and dermis. KUGELMAN et al. referred to reported cases of *Candida* granuloma and referred to several investigators who had studied tissue from patients that showed large numbers of hyphae and spores in the SC and occasionally in the dermis. EMMONS et al. illustrated a granulomatous lesion of the lip from a patient thought to have tuberculosis, but special stains showed granulomatous inflammation with numerous *C.albicans* spores and hyphae, some located in giant cells. In patients with *Candida* granuloma, fungal elements probably invade the dermis via the pilosebaceous follicle similar to *T.rubrum*, *T.mentagrophytes* variety *granulosum* and *M.gypseum*, all of which can cause a reaction pattern of granulomatous inflammation. *Candida* hyphae and spores may also penetrate the underlying stroma through the inflamed epidermis or mucosa via spongiotic intercellular spaces, miliary abscesses and foci of epithelial ulceration. It can generally be assumed that patients showing *Candida* organisms in mesenchymal tissues of cutaneous and mucocutaneous infections have an altered host-parasite relationship. It would appear that in all cases of *Candida* granuloma, the host is abnormal in some way (IMPERATO et al.).

Histochemical methods demonstrating *Candida* hyphae and spores in tissue sections gave results similar to those observed for dermatophytes, and can be explained on the basis of chitin, a glucan and a mannan in the cell wall polysaccharides of *C.albicans* (BISHOP et al., 1960). The explanation of why *Candida* spores show histochemical evidence of containing acidic substances is not certain, but the reactive material probably represents a combination of fatty acids, nucleic acids and sialomucin. *Candida albicans* spores and hyphae show selective staining and exhibit a yellow-green color when prepared by a fluorescent method for mucin

(Pickett et al., 1960). The results of Pickett et al. tend to support our interpretation that *Candida* spores contain sialomucin similar to *Cryptococcus neoformans*, *T.rubrum*, *T.epilans* and *M.gypseum*.

Recent studies have shown that extracts of *C.parapsilosis*, and probably those from several other fungi contain compounds with carcinogenic activity for mice (Blank et al., 1968). Carcinogenic activity in white mice was suggested with fungal element lipid extracts of *Microsporum*, *Trichophyton*, *Epidermophyton* and *Scopulariopsis* by the appearance of subcutaneous sarcomas, leukemia and pulmonary tumors (Blank et al., 1968). Candidiasis and concurrent dermatophytic infections in man occur, and have particularly been reported in patients with *Candida* granuloma (Kugelman et al.). *Candida parapsilosis* and *C.albicans* are often found associated with cutaneous and mucocutaneous disorders of man, and are known to cause generalized candidiasis in patients with debilitating diseases such as leukemia, malignant lymphoma and other types of systemic cancer (Hutter et al., 1962). The carcinogenic role of *Candida* species is unknown in man, but experimental and human tissue studies stress the importance of accurate epidemiologic surveys dealing with pathogens causing superficial fungus diseases.

Tinea Versicolor

Introduction: Tinea versicolor is commonly referred to under the synonym of pityriasis versicolor caused by *Malassezia furfur*. The fungal elements of *M.furfur* are easily demonstrated by direct microscopic examination of superficial scrapings from the SC, but the organism is extremely difficult to culture with any regularity and uniformity of results. Considerable evidence indicates a relationship between *Pityrosporum orbiculare* and *M.furfur*, and some investigators conclude that the two organisms are identical (Keddie et al.; Emmons et al.; Hildick-Smith et al.). Tinea versicolor has a worldwide disrtibution including temperate zones, but occurs more often in tropical and humid climates. In certain coastal regions of Mexico and Western Samoa, the disease involves 50% of the people living in these geographic areas (Keddie et al.; Wilson et al.). Tinea versicolor shows no significant sex or racial predilection, but does seem more apparent among dark-skinned people who predominantly inhabit geographical areas with tropical and humid climates. Tinea versicolor affects all ages including infants (Michalowski et al.), but young adults seem more commonly involved with the disease. *Malassezia furfur* has not been isolated from domestic, wild or laboratory animals and the disease is probably spread from person to person, or *in vivo* alterations occur in the individual human host which allow a cutaneous lipophilic saprophyte such as *P.orbiculare* to become pathogenic. For this report, we reviewed histologic material from 22 patients with tinea versicolor, and 10 of the cases were biopsied because the exact clinical diagnosis was in doubt.

Gross Appearance: Biopsy specimens came from the upper arm, neck, anterior chest, shoulder, subscapular area and abdomen. Multiple areas of the trunk were often involved, and some patients showed lesions of the face, axillae and lower extremities. Lewis et al. indicate that tinea versicolor may involve any area of the skin including the scalp, inguinal regions, palms and soles. Mucous membranes, hair, or nails are never involved (Wilson et al., 1965). Clinically, the disease shows discrete to confluent, yellowish-brown or erythematous, macular, papular, follicular, scaling lesions of varying size (Fig. 138). In some patients the involved areas appear hyperpigmented and/or hypopigmented and a combination of light and dark lesions gives a mottled pattern. Initially, the disease starts with single or multiple foci of small lesions which enlarge to form annular and gyrate plaques.

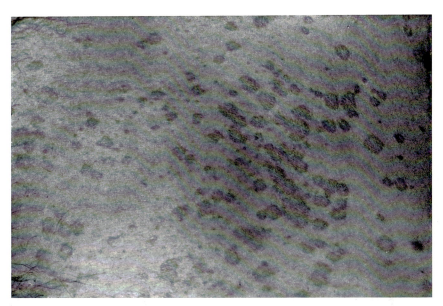

Fig. 138. Tinea versicolor caused by *M. furfur* showing slightly erythematous to brown, superficial, circinate, scaling lesions on the trunk

There is a tendency for tinea versicolor to fade in color during the cooler months of the year and then become darker in the summer. In general, the disease is asymptomatic, but some patients experience itching, particularly when they are hot and sweaty. Lewis et al. reported that tinea versicolor fluoresces when affected areas are examined under filtered ultraviolet rays (Wood's light), and depending on the amount of pigment in the lesions, the color varies from golden yellow to light brown. Newcomer in a recent report on superficial fungus infections described tinea versicolor lesions as sometimes showing a gold to orange fluorescence when examined under Wood's light. Tinea versicolor in children is misleading and difficult to diagnose since patches of disease often appear invisible by daylight, but fluoresce a yellow-green under Wood's light (Michalowski et al.). Fluorescent characteristics of tinea versicolor is important in diagnosis and an aid in determining the extent of the lesions.

Lewis et al. indicate that tinea versicolor is rarely confused clinically with other diseases, but depending on the amount of pigmentation can resemble chloasma, erythrasma, vitiligo, pinta, syphilitic leukoderma, and postinflammatory depigmentation occurring after a variety of dermatoses. In our group of 22 patients, tinea versicolor was the established clinical diagnosis for 12 cases. The remaining ten patients were initially considered as having a variety of dermatoses such as guttate psoriasis, guttate parapsoriasis, pityriasis rosea, lichen planus, papulosquamous drug eruption, lichen sclerosus et atrophicus, erythema multiforme, urticaria, erythema perstans, polymorphous light eruption, actinic dermatitis, lupus erythematosus, nummular eczema and cutaneous sarcoidosis. Pityriasis alba and seborrheic dermatitis also represent diseases which are sometimes clinically confused with tinea versicolor.

Microscopic Observations: Typically, the sections showed mild chronic dermatitis with basket-weave hyperkeratosis, follicular plugging, vacuolated cells in areas of hypergranulosis and mild acanthosis (Figs. 139, 140). The hypergranulosis

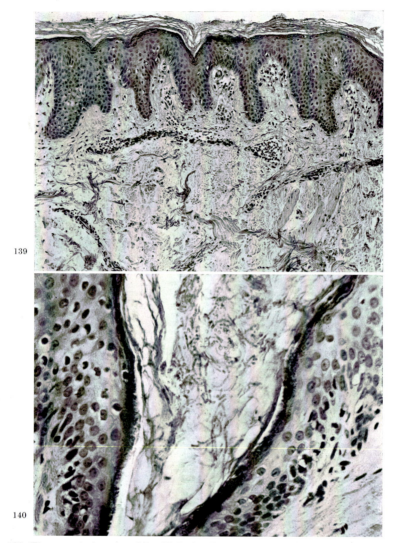

Fig. 139. Tinea versicolor caused by *M. furfur* showing slight hyperkeratosis, hypergranulosis and mild acanthosis. Higher magnification reveals numerous short hyphae and spores limited to the SC. The upper corium shows a mild, perivascular cellular infiltrate of lymphocytes and histiocytes (H & E, × 107)

Fig. 140. Tinea versicolor caused by *M. furfur* showing numerous short and some long segmented hyphae in a keratin-plugged follicular ostium. Spores in the form of spherical cells are intermingled with the hyphae. There is no evidence of invasion of the pilary outer root sheath or adjacent corium (H & E, × 265)

and vacuolated cells were apparent in some pilosebaceous follicles showing follicular plugging (Fig. 140). Hypopigmentation of the epidermal basal layer was sometimes observed when biopsies came from hypopigmented lesions. Brown lesions usually showed prominent epidermal pigmentation with incontinence of melanin, and granules were free and within melanophages in the upper corium. Some sections showed mild perifollicular inflammation adjacent to the hair follicle

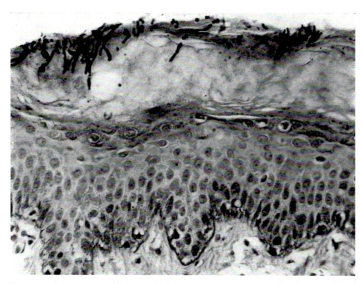

Fig. 141. Tinea versicolor caused by *M. furfur* showing numerous short hyphal filaments and spores limited to the upper SC where a few spherical cells show single budding type of sporulation. The epidermis exhibits hypergranulosis and an intact basement membrane at the dermo-epidermal junction (PAS with diastase digestion method, ×265)

infundibulum and sebaceous glands. In some examples, perivascular inflammation was more pronounced in the upper corium and the small blood vessels showed changes of an angiitis. The clinical features were usually atypical and erroneously diagnosed as urticaria, erythema multiforme, erythema perstans, papulosquamous drug eruption or some other erythematous inflammatory dermatoses. Even in biopsy sections stained with H & E, the fungal elements of *M. furfur* were easily identified in the SC and keratin-plugged follicular ostia (Fig. 140).

Histochemistry: *Malassezia furfur* fungal elements were demonstrated in tissue sections by the histochemical methods used for showing dermatophytic hyphae and arthrospores, and *Candida* organisms. Hyphae and yeast-like spores observed in sections of tinea versicolor were limited to superficial layers of the SC and keratin-plugged follicular ostia (Figs. 140, 141). Examination of multiple sections showed that organisms were sometimes located about glabrous skin hair in the acrotrichium canals, but there was no evidence of pilar invasion by the fungal elements. No organisms were identified in the stratum Malpighii or corium. The fungal elements were present in the form of wavy or serpentine hyphae and multiple spores. The spores varied in size from 2—8 μ and had double-contoured walls. Occasionally, long segmented filaments were seen, but the usual morphology was that of short hyphal conidiophores showing formation of terminal conidia (phialospores). Some individual conidia showed germinating conidium with evident collarette appearance at the point of separation of the budding spore and parent cell. The hyphae and spores of *M. furfur* stained blue and were considered Gram positive with the BROWN and BRENN method for Gram positive and Gram negative bacteria. Movat's pentachrome method stained the fungal elements red, but they were difficult to identify because the horny layer stains similarly. Mallory's PTAH method stained the spores and hyphae a blue to purple color and nicely outlined the double-contoured walls of the conidia. The remaining histochemical studies were not significant, but did show some mild changes similar to those described for *T. rubrum*.

Differential Diagnosis: The histopathologic and histochemical differential diagnosis of tinea versicolor includes some diseases considered under *T. rubrum* showing a reaction pattern of chronic dermatitis. Examples of *M. furfur* infection which showed an angiitis suggesting an urticarial tissue reaction pattern coincided with atypical cases of the disease and probably accounted for some of the erroneous diagnoses made clinically. When hyperpigmentation was prominent, incontinence of melanin produced changes similar to fixed drug eruption, pigmented stage of incontinentia pigmenti, chloasma and postinflammatory pigmentation. Biopsies from hypopigmented areas of tinea versicolor with minimal inflammation showed changes suggesting vitiligo, postinflammatory leukoderma and pityriasis alba. It is usually easy to distinguish *M. furfur* organisms in tissue section from dermatophytic fungal elements, but confusion can sometimes occur with cutaneous candidiasis. Atypical cases of tinea versicolor with angiitis and prominent inflammation can suggest *Candida* infection, but distinguishing morphological features of *M. furfur* include the method of spore formation and double contour of the cell walls. The morphology of *M. furfur* phialospores and germinating conidium appears essentially identical in skin tissue sections to organisms we have observed in *Pityrosporum* folliculitis.

Comment: Most publications regarding the clinical features and microscopic pathology of tinea versicolor refer to the disease as a noninflammatory process. Approximately 46% of the patients from whom we studied biopsy sections were erroneously diagnosed clinically, and this indicates that *M. furfur* can elicit an inflammatory cutaneous response in the human host. The term versicolor indicates a variable color of the lesions and perhaps multiform should also be used because some erythematous, macular, papular and follicular lesions show morphological characteristics which may account for clinical diagnoses such as urticaria, erythema multiforme, erythema perstans, polymorphous light eruption, lichen planus, lupus erythematosus, pityriasis rosea, papulosquamous drug eruption, psoriasis and guttate parapsoriasis.

The histochemical features of *M. furfur* fungal elements are similar to dermatophytes and although identification studies of the chemical composition of the spore walls have not been done, chitin and other polysaccharides are undoubtedly present. Our histochemical observations on the morphology of *M. furfur* fungal elements in tissue sections are in agreement with those of KEDDIE and SHADOMY (1963). Detailed descriptions of *M. furfur* hyphae and spores were made in 1962 by HANUSOVA. The hyphae and spores of *M. furfur* are Gram positive and this is a distinct histochemical difference from dermatophytic fungal elements. The Gram positive nature and morphology of *M. furfur* yeast-like spores is strikingly similar to *P. orbiculare* and has common histochemical characteristics of staining blue to purple in tissue sections similar to the Gram positive filaments of *Nocardia* and *Actinomyces*. The similar histochemical and morphological characteristics of *M. furfur* and *P. orbiculare* supports the taxonomic relationship of these organisms and additional studies will probably group them together under the same genus as a single lipophilic yeast, belonging to the Cryptococcaceae family. MARPLES in discussing the relationship of *P. orbiculare* to *M. furfur* concludes that the two organisms are essentially identical and made comparisons with the dimorphism of the saprophytic yeast phase and pathogenic mycelial form of *C. albicans*.

Clinicians are advised to be alert to the variability of lesions sometimes manifested by patients with tinea versicolor. All diagnostic aids should be utilized in

Fig. 142. Pityrosporum folliculitis thought to be caused by *P.ovale* showing papular, pustular, and follicular lesions on the upper back. The patient had similar lesions scattered over the upper part of the trunk

suspected cases including skin strippings, skin scrapings, examination under Wood's light, cultures and cutaneous biopsies for histopathologic and histochemical studies. The pathologist should be aware of *M.furfur* and its morphological tissue characteristics in typical cases of tinea versicolor so that proper recognition can be made in unusual examples of the disease. *Pityrosporum* species are present on the skin surface as saprophytic lipophilic fungi and the pathologist should also be aware of these organisms occurring routinely in biopsy tissue sections from seborrheic areas of the body. Only experience and being aware of saprophytic fungi occurring on the skin can allow for their proper recognition in tissue sections. This is extremely important in arriving at the final decision regarding the role of fungal elements observed in biopsy sections and whether they contribute or cause the tissue changes seen.

Pityrosporum Folliculitis

Introduction: For at least 6 years, we have coded skin biopsies showing yeast-like organisms associated with pilosebaceous inflammation under the diagnosis of *Pityrosporum* folliculitis. The involved patients varied in age from 14—58 years and there was an equal sexual distribution. No racial predilection or seasonal variation was apparent and the stated duration of the disease varied from 1 week to 12 years. Some patients experienced periodic itching of their lesions, but most of them stated that the disease was asymptomatic. For this report, we shall record our experience and observations of biopsy sections from twelve patients who were coded in the files of The Skin and Cancer Hospital of Philadelphia under the tissue diagnosis of *Pityrosporum* folliculitis.

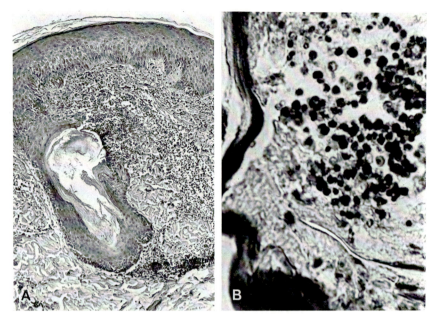

Fig. 143. Pityrosporum folliculitis presumably caused by *P.ovale* or possibly *P.orbiculare*: A. Scanning view showing a dilated keratin-plugged follicle with obvious disruption of the pilary outer root sheath in one area and perifollicular inflammation. The overlying epidermis appears essentially normal except for mild spongiosis (H & E, ×66). B. High power magnification showing numerous spherical cells present in the dilated keratin-plugged follicular ostium illustrated by A. Similar spores were demonstrated in areas of perifollicular inflammation (Brown and Brenn method, ×655)

Gross Appearance: The skin tissue sections we studied represented biopsy specimens from the shoulders, scapular areas and proximal portion of the arms. Anatomically, multiple lesions were common and predominantly involved the upper back, shoulders, and anterior chest. Some of the patients also showed lesions on the face, posterior neck region, axillae, abdomen, and thighs. Grossly, the disease showed primary lesions which appeared as 2—4 mm discrete, erythematous to brown, papular, follicular lesions (Fig. 142). Some lesions in all patients appeared as acneiform, follicular vesiculopustules (Fig. 142). The lesions were usually firm with some tendency for grouping. Scaling was apparent at sites of older lesions and small residual pitted scars were noticeable in some patients. With scratching or manual pressure, a clear to purulent exudate oozed from the follicular vesiculopustular lesions.

Clinically, the disease was most often diagnosed as folliculitis or acne vulgaris, but the differential diagnosis included allergic id eruption, papular urticaria, urticaria pigmentosa, allergic drug eruption, dermatitis herpetiformis, familial benign chronic pemphigus and cutaneous candidiasis.

Microscopic Observations: Examination of multiple sections from each biopsy specimen always showed features of folliculitis and perifolliculitis with granulomatous inflammation and dermal abscess formation (Figs. 143A—B, 144, 145A—B). The involved pilosebaceous follicle appeared dilated and was filled with keratin and inflammatory cells. Remnants of hair could sometimes be identified in the follicular canal. The pilary outer root sheath was always focally disrupted with necrosis of the epithelium. Fragments of keratin in the dilated follicular ostia

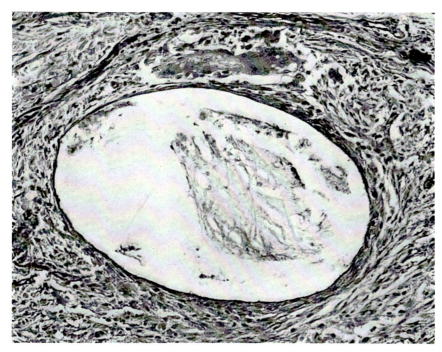

Fig. 144. Pityrosporum folliculitis caused by *P.ovale* showing remnants of a dilated keratin-plugged atrophic pilosebaceous follicle with surrounding granulomatous inflammation characterized by a mixed cellular infiltrate including foreign body giant cells, fibrosis, and capillary-endothelial proliferation. High power magnification revealed a few spores morphologically resembling *P.ovale* in the keratinous cyst and adjacent granulomatous inflammation (PAS, ×155)

showed direct continuity and evidence of extrusion into areas of inflammation (Figs. 143A, 144). The perifollicular inflammation generally showed central abscess formation with neutrophils and a surrounding cellular infiltrate of lymphocytes, histiocytes, eosinophils, plasma cells and variable numbers of multinucleated foreign body giant cells (Figs. 143A, 144, 145A). Sections of older lesions or those through the periphery of involved pilosebaceous follicles with atrophy sometimes appeared as dilated miniature inclusion cysts containing remnants of keratin (Fig. 144). Fragments of keratin and even spicules of hair were sometimes seen in the perifollicular granulomatous inflammation (Fig. 144). The epidermis adjacent to the involved hair follicle usually showed mild acanthosis, spongiosis and exocytosis. Small blood vessels in the perifollicular edematous stroma and adjacent to dermal abscesses were thickened, sometimes dilated and surrounded by inflammation. Some sections showed extravasated red blood cells and incontinence of pigment, and melanin granules were free and within melanophages in the upper corium. Sebaceous glands were identified in some sections from all biopsies and only those associated with the involved hair follicle appeared altered by inflammation. The eccrine sweat structures were spared. Small yeast-like organisms could be easily identified in sections stained with H & E, but were best demonstrated with special stains.

Histochemistry: Yeast-like spores observed in skin biopsies diagnosed as *Pityrosporum* folliculitis were demonstrated by special stains for fungi similar to

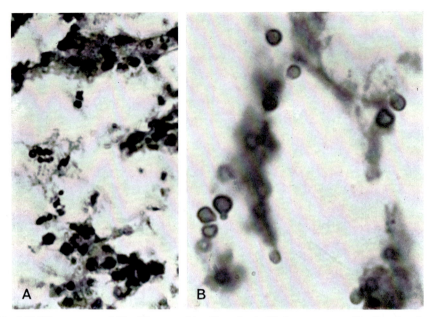

Fig. 145. Pityrosporum folliculitis caused by *P. ovale*: A. High power magnification showing a perifollicular dermal abscess containing small spherical cells singly and in clusters (PAS, ×655). B. Oil immersion magnification showing numerous spherical cells within a perifollicular dermal abscess. The yeast-like organisms show single budding sporulation strikingly similar to that demonstrated for *M. furfur*. The spherical spores are morphologically identical with *P. ovale*, but could represent *P. orbiculare* (PAS, ×1400)

M. furfur organisms in tissue sections (Figs. 143B, 145A—B). The spores were best demonstrated with the BROWN and BRENN, and PAS methods and appeared as small spherical cells (Fig. 143B). Most of the spores were 2—4 μ, but some measured up to 10 μ (Figs. 143B, 145A—B). The cell walls were stained best by the various histochemical methods and sometimes the cytoplasm showed only a pale color. The yeast-like organisms exhibited a single budding type of sporulation with development of a daughter cell from one pole of the parent spore (Fig. 145B). Separation occurred after formation of a septum between the polar bud and parent spore (Fig. 145B). No multiple budding cells or mycelial forms were observed in the biopsy sections studied from our case material. Generally, the spores were aggregated together, but sometimes they occurred singly. Spores were routinely identified in the SC overlying involved pilosebaceous follicles, within dilated keratin-plugged follicular ostia (Fig. 143B), and intermingled with inflammatory cells in areas of dermal abscess formation. Some spores had apparently been phagocytized and were located in the cytoplasm of foreign body giant cells. Spores were sometimes observed surrounding remnants of hair in the dilated, keratin-plugged follicular canal, but there was no evidence of intrapilary penetration by the yeast-like organisms. Collagen and elastic fibers were thinned to absent in areas of perifollicular inflammation with granulomatous changes and dermal abscess formation. Mast cells were generally increased in the same areas. Some sections showed a few Gram positive bacteria in keratin-plugged follicular ostia, but none were observed in areas of perifollicular inflammation.

Differential Diagnosis: The common histopathologic classification we use for *Pityrosporum* folliculitis prior to 1963 was simply folliculitis and perifolliculitis with granulomatous inflammation. This latter nomenclature characterized the tissue reaction pattern and involvement of the pilosebaceous follicle, but the etiology was unknown. Diseases showing changes of folliculitis that can be confused with *Pityrosporum* follicultits include impetigo of Bockhart, sycosis vulgaris, acne vulgaris, rosacea, perforating folliculitis (MEHREGAN and COSKEY), dermatophytosis, candidiasis and certain drug eruptions with follicular involvement such as iododerma. *Cryptococcosis neoformans* can cause erythematous, acneiform, papular, cutaneous lesions and the organism in areas of dermal granulomatous inflammation mimic the spores seen in *Pityrosporum* folliculitis. The similarity is even more striking because of single budding characteristics of the spherical spores seen in the two diseases. Differentiation is important and can be made on the basis of special staining methods since the yeast organisms of *Cryptococcosis neoformans* show reactive mucinous material in their capsules with histochemical characteristics of sialomucin. If the plane of the biopsy section is off center in tissue specimens of *Pityrosporum* folliculitis, the follicular involvement may not be appreciated and confusion can occur with reactive perforating collagenosis (MEHREGAN et al.), hyperkeratosis follicularis et parafollicularis in cutem penetrans (Kyrle's disease) and elastosis perforans serpiginosa. Likewise, if the plane of the tissue section from Staphylococcic actinophytosis does not include a bacterial granule in areas of dermal abscess formation, the changes are similar to *Pityrosporum* folliculitis.

The essential criteria we require before coding a skin tissue specimen as *Pityrosporum* folliculitis include compatible clinical features, follicular involvement, yeast-like spores in dilated keratin-plugged follicular ostia showing inflammation, and single budding organisms in perifollicular dermal abscesses with surrounding granulomatous inflammation.

Comment: We cannot be completely sure about the identity of organisms routinely demonstrated in *Pityrosporum* folliculitis, but favor the view that they represent spores of *P. ovale* or other *Pityrosporum species* which normally inhabit human skin as saprophytic lipophilic fungi. MARPLES describes *P. ovale* as a small yeast-like organism, the cells of which are oval and show considerable variation in size, occurring singly or in pairs, and reproduce by a rather unusual form of budding. A single polar bud is formed on a wide base, and separation results from the formation of a septum (MARPLES, 1965). MARPLES description of *P. ovale* organisms is identical to characteristics of spores we have observed in *Pityrosporum* folliculitis. The morphology of yeast-like spores in *Pityrosporum* folliculitis shows a striking resemblance to the individual conidia of *M. furfur* and *P. orbiculare*. The absence of short hyphal conidiophores in all of our cases of *Pityrosporum* folliculitis tends to rule against *M. furfur* or *P. orbiculare* being of etiological significance in the disease. The histochemical characteristics of yeast-like spores assumed to represent *P. ovale* in *Pityrosporum* folliculitis stain identical to results we obtained for *M. furfur* and *P. orbiculare* and lends support to the close relationship of these organisms. The cell walls of *P. ovale* spores undoubtedly contain chitin and other polysaccharides to account for their histochemical staining characteristics. The BROWN and BRENN method stains *P. ovale* organisms and the yeast-like spores in *Pityrosporum* folliculitis Gram positive and similar results were obtained for *M. furfur* fungal elements. In general, dermatophytic fungal elements are not demonstrated with the BROWN and BRENN method, although sometimes *Microsporum* microspores and microide arthrospores in granular forms of *T. mentagrophytes* exhibit Gram positive staining characteristics.

In signing out the daily surgicals, we routinely observe yeast-like organisms in tissue sections prepared from biopsy and surgical specimens located on seborrheic areas of the body. Organisms of the genus *Pityrosporum* belong to the family Cryptococcaceae and commonly occur in the hyperkeratotic horny layer of lesions such as seborrheic keratosis, lichenoid benign keratosis, solar keratosis, Bowen's disease, epithelial nevi and some inflammatory dermatoses. We consider these yeast-like organisms as predominantly lipophilic saprophytes of *P. ovale* even when they are present in large numbers. In a few keratoses, we have observed yeast-like spores associated with hyphal elements and considered these fungal elements as representing those of *P. orbiculare*.

The causal relationship of *P. ovale* in seborrhea and seborrheic dermatitis has been reviewed by MARPLES, and there seems to be ample evidence that the yeast-like cells are much more numerous in scrapings taken from these dieseases, but controlled studies do not suggest a definite pathogenic role. The increased population of *P. ovale* is probably secondary and related to an abnormal quantity of sebaceous material in chronic seborrheic conditions, rather than being of etiological significance (MARPLES). Scientific evidence that *P. ovale* is definitely acting as a pathogen in *Pityrosporum* folliculitis is lacking, but yeast-like spores in areas of perifollicular granulomatous inflammation strongly suggests a causal relationship. One of us (GRAHAM) in discussing Weary's (1968) paper on *Pityrosporum ovale* dealing with observations on some aspects of host-parasite interrelationship, mentioned our experience with patients who had *Pityrosporum* folliculitis. Weary's response lends some scientific credibility to our observations of *P. ovale* as a cause of *Pityrosporum* folliculitis since he referred to a lady who developed an acneiform eruption regularly after receiving broad spectrum antibiotics and *Pityrosporum* organisms were repeatedly cultured from pustular lesions.

Clinicians and pathologists are encouraged to question the nature of unexplained cases showing clinicopathologic features of folliculitis. Tissue sections should be carefully screened for yeast-like organisms located in dilated keratin-plugged follicular ostia and perifollicular dermal abscesses. Mycological studies from intact pustules utilizing the culture media reported by Weary is recommended. Only future studies will definitely determine whether *P. ovale* plays a significant role in causing otherwise unexplained cases of folliculitis similar to what we have reported. Our opinion is that some examples of follicular disease currently being reported as perforating folliculitis may represent examples of *Pityrosporum* folliculitis.

Tinea Nigra

Introduction: The clinical disease of tinea nigra in the Western Hemisphere is caused by *C. werneckii*. *Cladosporium mansoni* is isolated from the Oriental variant of the infection. The genus *Cladosporium* occurs in soil usually where there is an abundance of plant residue and it has been shown that the spores are present in the air in large numbers (MARPLES). It seems likely that *C. werneckii* probably occurs in the soil, sewage, and on the surface of dead and living plants. It is not definite as to how human disease is contracted, but organisms may be introduced onto the skin surface from trauma. SMITH et al. (1958) made attempts at experimental reproduction of tinea nigra by inoculation of *C. werneckii* infected scales and culture material into the epidermis of human volunteers, but were unsuccessful. According to EMMONS et al. (1963), a superficial type of cutaneous infection can be produced experimentally in man and guinea pigs. LEEMING (1963) cites Castellani who easily reproduced tinea nigra by scarifying the horny layer and applying a pure culture of organisms; the incubation period was 10—15 days. RITCHIE and TAYLOR (1964) experimentally produced tinea nigra palmaris in a human host and an eruption clinically identical to the naturally acquired disease appeared 7 weeks after inoculation. MERWIN (1965) reviewed the literature regarding tinea nigra palmaris and referred to the work of others who have experimentally reproduced tinea nigra in man and animals. The occurrence of spontaneous disease in animals is unknown (MARPLES). There is no definite evidence of human to human transmission of the disease, although the familial occurrence of tinea nigra has been reported. The limited number of familial cases indicates *C.werneckii* has a low degree of contagion (VAN VELSOR et al.). Natural or acquired immunity apparently does not occur (LEEMING). Tinea nigra shows a predilection for affecting females, and although the disease occurs in all age groups, there is a definite tendency to involve younger individuals below 20 (MERWIN). Tinea nigra has not been reported in Negroes (LEEMING; VAN VELSOR et al.; WILSON et al. 1965; MERWIN). Human infections from *C.werneckii* have been recorded in Brazil, Colombia, Venezuela, Panama, other parts of South America and Central America, Cuba, Puerto Rico, United States, South Africa and Australia. Tinea nigra also occurs in Ceylon, India, Burma, South China, Java, Sumatra, Borneo and other tropical countries of the Far East, but most of the cases reported are caused by *C.mansoni*. Tinea nigra in the United States has been diagnosed with increasing frequnecy and this subject was reviewed in 1964 by VAN VELSOR and SINGLETARY, and more recently by MERWIN (1965). It is striking that tinea nigra in the United States is reported predominantly from coastal states. For this report, we shall record our histopathologic and histochemical observations of skin biopsy sections from two patients with typical tinea nigra palmaris who lived in Venezuela, South America.

Gross Appearance: Clinically, tinea nigra caused by *C.werneckii* shows pigmented, macular, slightly scaly plaques or patches with sharply demarcated borders (Fig. 146). The color varies and may appear dark green, black, brown (Fig. 146), or show shades of bluish-gray. The pigmented plaques can appear mottled and are usually round and discrete. However, the peripheral margins may be irregular and show a serpiginous, polycyclic, arcuate, or festooning pattern. Multiple lesions sometimes occur and show confluence with considerable variation in size and shape. Tinea nigra from *C.werneckii* begins insidiously as a small, asymptomatic, pigmented, macular lesion, and shows gradual peripheral extension over a period of weeks to months and varies in size from several millimeters to 8 cm, or larger (MERWIN). The lesions may persist for years before the patient seeks medical attention because of the innocuous nature of the disease (MERWIN). Subjective symptoms are usually lacking, although slight pruritus is experienced by some individuals. Most patients with tinea nigra caused by *C.werneckii* show lesions of the palms, but the disease can involve the finger webs, palmar aspect of the fingers, sides of the fingers, dorsum of the hands, wrists, ulnar aspect of the forearm, thorax and neck. A patient with tinea nigra from Lancaster, Pennsylvania, probably contracted the disease while vacationing in Florida and is illustrated in Fig. 146 with a discrete, brown, superficial lesion involving the arch of the left foot. The initial diagnosis was pigmented junction nevus or malignant melanoma, but skin scrapings for direct microscopic examination and mycological culture studies revealed the true nature of the disease as tinea nigra plantaris caused by *C.werneckii*. Our review of the literature indicates that tinea nigra plantaris must be rare or misdiagnosed since only a few cases have been reported showing this anatomical site of involvement (YAFFEE et al.; MILES et al.). MARPLES (1965) reported that tinea nigra showing lesions of the soles had never been recorded. RITCHIE and TAYLOR (1964) recorded a predilection of tinea nigra for involving the left palm, but did refer to cases published by REYNOLDS who observed the infection about equally divided between the right and left palm.

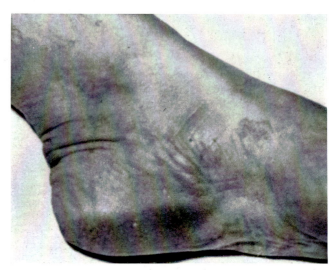

Fig. 146. Tinea nigra caused by *C.werneckii* showing a discrete brown, superficial lesion involving the arch of the left foot. The diagnosis was confirmed by direct microscopic demonstration of fungal elements and isolation of *C.werneckii* by mycological culture studies. The patient apparently acquired the infection while vacationing in Florida (courtesy of Dr. C. Walter Hassel, Jr.)

Merwin in his review reported there is little difference between the two hands, and referred to three instances of bilateral palmar involvement from tinea nigra.

Tinea nigra caused by *C.mansoni* shows a predilection for involving the face, neck and chest, although rare lesions on the hands have been reported. Some observers consider tinea nigra caused by *C.mansoni* and *C.werneckii* are not the same disease. In spite of anatomical differences, the two forms of tinea nigra appear to be fundamentally related and this view is generally accepted (Leeming).

The important clinical differential diagnosis of tinea nigra caused by *C.werneckii* is pigmented junction nevus and malignant melanoma, and sometimes unnecessary surgery is performed. Other clinical considerations include ephelide, lentigo, additional forms of nevus cell nevi, melanocytic nevi such as café au lait spots, Addison's disease, fixed drug eruption, postinflammatory dermal melanosis, chromhidrosis, hematoma showing extravasation of blood into the horny layer, traumatic tattoo, chemical stains such as from silver nitrate, contact dermatitis from compounds showing a tendency for causing pigmentation, tinea versicolor, dermatophytosis, pinta and secondary syphilis. In general, dermatophytes causing tinea manuum and tinea pedis show gross features of inflammation and should be easily distinguished from tinea nigra. Tinea nigra caused by *C.mansoni* showing lesions on the trunk is difficult to distinguish from tinea versicolor and some authors still confuse the two diseases (Leeming).

Microscopic Observations: Examination of sections stained with H & E from two examples of tinea nigra palmaris showed epidermal features of hyperkeratosis, normal granular layer and mild irregular acanthosis. Numerous cleavages were present in the thickened horny layer and these cleft-like spaces usually showed relationship to fungal elements (Figs. 147A, 148A—B, 149A—B). Splitting of the SC occurred predominantly beneath the fungal elements which were localized to the superficial levels of the horny layer (Figs. 147A, 148A—B, 149A). Sometimes, separated layers of the SC were apparent above fungal elements located at deeper

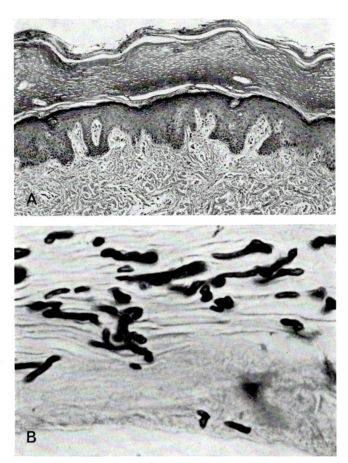

Fig. 147. Tinea nigra caused by *C.werneckii*: A. Scanning magnification showing hyper-keratosis, normal granular layer and mild acanthosis. Inflammation is absent in the corium. Light-brown fungal elements are present in the superficial SC (H & E ×66). B. High power magnification of the SC in A showing numerous hyphae and spores (Gridley's method for fungi, ×655)

levels of the thickened horny layer (Fig. 149B). The epidermis was generally hypopigmented, although focally a few cells containing melanin granules were recognized in the basal layer. Inflammation was essentially absent (Fig. 147A), although some sections showed a few lymphocytes and histiocytes localized about small blood vessels in the papillary corium. The small blood vessels in the dermis showed some slight thickening of their walls. The connective tissue, nerves, neural end organs, and eccrine sweat structures appeared essentially normal for palmar skin. Although we have not studied sections of tinea nigra from hairy areas of the body, there is apparently no gross evidence of pilosebaceous follicle involvement. *Cladosporium werneckii* organisms were easily identified in the thickened palmar SC of H & E stained sections because the yellow to brown melanoid pigment associated with hyphae and spores represents an excellent *in vivo* color for demonstrating the fungal elements.

Histochemistry: Hyphae and spores of *C.werneckii* were satisfactorily demonstrated by the various histochemical methods utilized for showing organisms in

23*

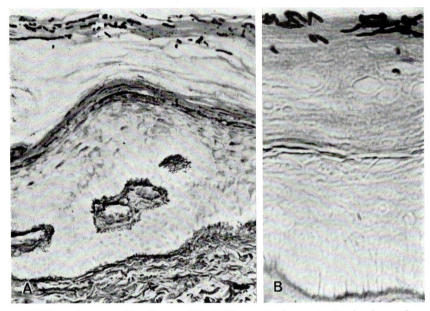

Fig. 148. Tinea nigra caused by *C.werneckii*: A. Silver stain demonstrating hyphae and spores localized to the superficial SC. No fungal elements are seen in the living epidermis or corium (Snook's reticulum stain, ×190). B. The polysaccharide in the fungal elements is PAS-positive and diastase-resistant localizing the hyphae and spores to the upper levels of the SC with no evidence of invasion of the living epidermis (PAS with diastase digestion method, ×265)

other superficial fungus diseases. Some of the histochemical results were unusual and these will be described. Multiple hyphae which showed frequent segmentation and spores (blastospores) were located predominantly in the superficial layers of the SC, although a few fungal elements extended to deeper levels in the thickened horny layer (Figs. 147B, 148A—B, 149A—B). The stratum lucidum was easily identified in sections stained by Gridley's (Fig. 147B) and PAS (148B) methods for fungi, and no fungal elements were observed beneath this layer of the epidermis. In general, horny material overlying the acrosyringium was free of fungal elements (Fig. 147A). The various silver stains such as Snook's reticulum (Fig. 148A), GMS and Fontana-Masson demonstrated the fungal elements extremely well. Segmented hyphae of *C.werneckii* were of variable width (1—6 μ), length and shape (curved and serpentine), and some showed single to multiple branching filaments (Figs. 147B, 148B, 149B). Hyphal septae and skeletal walls appeared thick and were well demonstrated by the various histochemical methods, particularly the Fontana-Masson silver stain. The cytoplasm of fungal elements often stained a pale color. Multiple yeast-like spores (Figs. 147B, 148A—B) 3—5 μ in size were present in the SC and a few larger ones measured up to 10 μ. The spores occurred singly and in groups and most of them appeared to form as terminal conidia from broad hyphae (Figs. 147B, 148A, 149A—B). In some instances, yeast-like arthrospores appeared to develop by multiple segmentation of short broad hyphae. Small conidia occurred from short conidiophores along the surface of longer filaments, many of which were branched (Figs. 147B, 149B). The fungal elements of *C.werneckii* showed the following additional histochemical characteristics: colloidal iron positive and hyaluronidase resistant; reactive with alcian blue pH 2.5 and negative at pH 0.4; aldehyde-fuchsin pH 1.7 positive (Fig. 149A) and

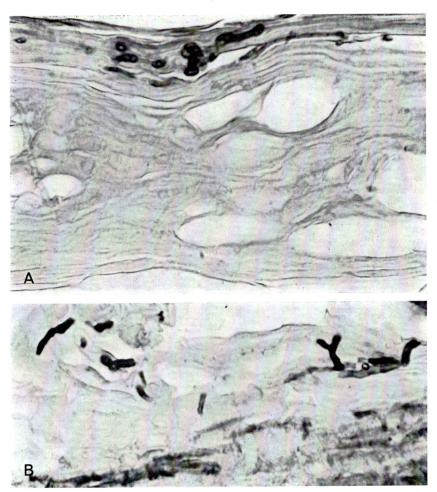

Fig. 149. Tinea nigra caused by *C.werneckii*: A. The fungal elements are aldehyde fuchsin pH 1.7 reactive, but show negative results with aldehyde fuchsin pH 0.4. The results indicate nonsulfated acid mucosubstances are present in the skeletal wall of the fungal elements. Numerous cleavages in the horny layer are seen beneath the fungal elements (Aldehyde fuchsin pH 1.7, ×655). B. The fungal elements of *C.werneckii* in tinea nigra are strongly reactive with basic fuchsin, and the positive results favor the presence of mucosubstances (BROWN and BRENN method, ×655)

negative at pH 0.4; and demonstrated by the BROWN and BRENN method (Fig. 149B). The spores were well outlined by a blue to green color with the colloidal iron and alcian blue pH 2.5 methods for acid mucosaccharides. The BROWN and BRENN method stained *C.werneckii* hyphae and spores Gram positive (Fig. 149B). The Fontana-Masson silver method for melanin demonstrated only a small amount of pigment in focal areas at the dermoepidermal junction, whereas, melanoid granules associated with fungal elements were stained. Special stains for iron pigment were negative. Histochemical methods for demonstration of collagen, elastic fibers, and extracellular interfibrillar ground substance showed essentially normal results. Mast cells were increased in the upper corium and numbered up to ten per field under high power magnification.

Differential Diagnosis: The histopathologic and histochemical differential diagnosis of tinea nigra caused by *C.werneckii* realistically only includes superficial fungus diseases showing hyphae and spores in the horny layer. Yellow to brown pigment associated with fungal elements and cleavages in the SC represent differential features in tissue sections of tinea nigra not seen in other superficial fungus infections. We have not had the opportunity to study material from tinea nigra occurring in the Orient nor can we find a description of the pathology to indicate that *C.mansoni* produces changes differing from those minimal tissue alterations caused by *C.werneckii*. Histochemical characteristics of fungal elements in tinea nigra palmaris overlap with those of other superficial fungus infections. This undoubtedly indicates that chitin and other polysaccharides are present in the skeletal framework of *C.werneckii* fungal elements, although definite chemical isolation studies have not been done. It is our opinion that *C.werneckii* fungal elements showing positive histochemical reactions for nonsulfated acidic mucosubstances probably result from one or a combination of sialomucins, nuclei acids or fatty acids similar to reactive material in organisms of *T.rubrum*, *T.epilans*, *M.gypseum* and *C.albicans*. The principal histochemical difference of *C.werneckii* hyphae and spores from these latter organisms is the Gram positive staining of tinea nigra fungal elements. Gram positive fungal elements are seen in tinea versicolor and *Pityrosporum* folliculitis, and this appears to single out *M.furfur*, *P.ovale* and *C.werneckii* as being histochemically similar probably because of their yeast-like characteristics.

Comments: From our review of the literature, it would appear that the first histopathologic description for tinea nigra caused by *C.werneckii* was published by NEVES and COSTA (1947, 1953). Since this original report (NEVES et al., 1947) which documented the essential pathology of tinea nigra, only a few other cases with histologic tissue studies have been recorded (SLEPYAN et al.; SMITH et al.; HITCH). Most other publications giving histopathologic information about tinea nigra (CONANT et al.; LEWIS et al.; EMMONS et al.; GÖTZ; HILDICK-SMITH et al.; MARPLES; WILSON et al.) appear to mention either NEVES et al. (1947, 1953), SLEPYAN et al., SMITH et al., or HITCH as the source of their descriptions. HITCH stressed the value of biopsy as an aid in establishing the nature of tinea nigra palmaris. Five of nine patients with tinea nigra reported in the United States before 1961 were initially erroneously diagnosed, and in some instances, received unnecessary surgical removal of the lesion because it was considered to represent a pigmented nevus (HITCH).

The epidermis beneath *C.werneckii* fungal elements is generally hypopigmented and special stains for melanin show only focal areas with argentaffin granules in the basal layer. This histochemical observation indicates the gross color of tinea nigra lesions is caused by the yellow to brown pigment associated with *C.werneckii* hyphae and spores. The mottled appearance of some tinea nigra lesions may result from areas showing only a small population of pigmented fungal elements such as the small number overlying sweat pores. Melanin occurring only focally at the dermoepidermal junction may also represent a contributing factor to account for a mottled pattern of pigmentation. The chemical nature of the pigment in tinea nigra is unknown, although affinity of silver stains for *C.werneckii* fungal elements suggests melanin-like characteristics.

The increasing number of patients being reported with tinea nigra from temperate climates of the United States seems to indicate that the disease is much more prevalent than generally realized, and the report of VAN VELSOR et al. from coastal North Carolina strongly suggests endemic foci of *C.werneckii* outside of tropical areas. An increased awareness of tinea nigra should be established by clinicians since the correct diagnosis may save the patient from receiving unnecessary treatment for confusing pigmented diseases. Tinea nigra plantaris is probably more common than reported in the literature and the disease should be considered in the clinical differential diagnosis of pigmented macular lesions affecting the feet. Clinicians should use every aid at their command to establish the correct diagnosis of tinea nigra. The important procedures include cutaneous scrapings for direct microscopic examination, scotch tape skin strippings, cultures, and biopsy studies.

Piedra

Introduction: Piedra is an infection limited to hair caused by 2 different organisms, and synonyms for the disease include trichosporosis, tinea nodosa, piedra nostros, trichomycosis nodularis, trichomycosis nodosa, chignon disease, Beigel's disease, black piedra and white piedra.

Black piedra is due to *Piedraia (P.) hortai*, an ascomycete, and the disease occurs in humid, wet, tropical areas of the world such as South America (Brazil, Paraguay, Ecuador, Argentina, Uruguay, Colombia, Venezuela, Guiana), Central America, West Indies, East Indies, Vietnam and Thailand. The occurrence of black piedra in the United States has been reported (BURDICK; HITCH, 1959), but definite identification of the causative organism was not made. The natural habitat of *P. hortai* other than mammalian hair is not known, although the organism may be located on the surface of plants (MARPLES). The small black nodule on the hair shaft of black piedra is the ascostioma of *P. hortai* belonging to the Asterinae, a family of fungi parasitic on the leaves of trees in very humid climates (MANSON-BAHR; HILDICK-SMITH et al.). Relationship of *P. hortai* to stagnant water in certain geographic areas is suggested because of the disease being common in individuals who wash their hair or are regular swimmers in the local rivers (LEWIS et al.; WILSON et al., 1965). However, it is possible that frequent wetting of hair may merely reduce resistance to infection (KAPLAN, 1959). In Colombia and Paraguay, black piedra has been commonly attributed to hair-oils used by women (SIMONS). An unusual feature in Argentina, Colombia and Guiana is that black piedra has been observed fairly often in students and medical men (SIMONS). The disease has been reported in almost epidemic proportions in Jakarta, Indonesia (SIMONS). Black piedra occurs commonly on the pelts of lower primates such as monkeys and chimpanzees, but no definite knowledge is known about the way in which human infections occur (KAPLAN; MARPLES; WILSON et al., 1965). Black piedra affecting pelts from primates indigenous to Africa, Asia and the New World suggests a widespread reservoir of infection in the forests of these continental land masses (KAPLAN, 1959). A direct mode of piedra infection was suggested in school children who were in the habit of wearing each others hats (SIMONS). Attempts to experimentally infect man and animals have been unsuccessful (MARPLES). Smearing pure cultures of piedra into guinea pigs and human subjects gave negative results, although successful experimental infections in rats have been reported (SIMONS). In most areas of the world where black piedra occurs, the disease is more common in males than in females, but in Colombia and Paraguay, women are commonly affected (MARPLES). Black piedra in Brazil shows an equal sex distribution, although some Brazilian authors report the disease is more common in men (FISCHMAN, 1965). Black piedra occurs in all ages, but in Brazil the disease more frequently involves patients from 10—49 years old (FISCHMAN). Human cases of black piedra have not been reported from Africa, and it has been suggested that Negro hair is unsusceptible to infection (KAPLAN; MARPLES). SIMONS (1953) referred to the particular susceptibility of persons with straight hair for developing piedra and mentioned that the disease had not been observed in a Negro. FISCHMAN recorded black piedra in Brazil as occurring in 47 white people and 84 were from colored individuals. WILSON et al. (1965) indicate that black piedra shows no predilection based on age, sex or skin color.

White piedra is caused by the imperfect yeast-like fungus, *Trichosporon (T.) beigelii*, but the organism has been called a variety of names and is currently referred to by most observers as *T.cutaneum (cutanum)*. SCOTT (1951) reported the first case of white piedra from the United States under the name of *Trichosporum beigelii* and listed multiple synonyms. *Trichosporon beigelii* is related to common fungi known as *Geotrichum, Oidium* or *Mycoderma*, and white nodules on the hair are formed of masses of mycelium (MANSON-BAHR; HILDICK-SMITH et al.). White piedra shows a geographical distribution to tropical and temperate climates, and occurs in South America (Colombia, Venezuela, Brazil, Argentina, Paraguay and Uruguay), Southern Asia, Japan, England, Central Europe and Western Europe. White piedra occurs occasionally in the United States (SCOTT; DALY; PATTERSON et al.), but only the case reported by PATTERSON et al. was proven by culture studies to be caused by *T.beigelii*. There is evidence that the natural habitat of *T.beigelii* is primarily in soil and plant residues since the organism has been isolated from those sources (MARPLES). *Trichosporon cutaneum* has been isolated from a variety of natural substrates including wood pulp in Sweden and Italy, dairy plant sewage in England, and from soil and decaying plant material in Israel (KAPLAN, 1959). White piedra organisms have been isolated from the spider monkey and is common in horses, but definite knowledge about transmission of the infection to man is lacking (KAPLAN, 1959). KAPLAN (1959) reported the first simian infection of white piedra in a pet black spider monkey, but found no evidence of transmission to the human owner or members of his family. There is very little evidence to suggest that white piedra is transferred directly from infected horses and monkeys to human hair (WILSON and PLUNKETT). According to MARPLES, white piedra in man is rare and sporadic, and the incidence appears to be lower than the disease caused by *P.hortai*. In Brazil, black piedra is much more frequent than white piedra and only three cases of the latter disease were found (FISCHMAN, 1965). White piedra affects all age groups, and both sexes are involved (SCOTT; LEWIS et al.). WILSON and PLUNKETT (1965) indicate that white piedra shows no predilection for involving the hair of individuals of a particular skin color.

For this report, we shall record our gross, histopathologic, histochemical and polariscopic observations on infected hair from two patients each with piedra caused by *P.hortai* and *T.beigelii*. The four patients were all from South America; one with each type of piedra came from Venezuela, and Brazil, respectively.

Gross Appearance: Black piedra is essentially limited to scalp hair characterized by asymptomatic dark brown to black, fusiform concretions firmly attached to the shaft and usually involving the distal one-third (Fig. 150A). Each affected hair can show one or several stony hard accretions measuring about 1 mm and fully developed irregular nodules encircle the hair shaft to form ring-like structures (Fig. 150A). Individual lesions vary from minute black dots to larger ones which only partially surround the hair. Pigmented nodules vary in size and shape, but usually the circumference is greater at one pole with tapering at the opposite end (Fig. 150A). Some nodules are largest in their central part and taper distally and proximally. Figure 9 in the publication by LANGERON (1936) illustrates a wide morphological spectrum of how black piedra nodules involve the hair shaft. There is no evidence of pilosebaceous follicle disease below the skin surface and lesions are thought to initially start on the hair just about the scalp level. The scalp and hair generally appear normal in patients with black piedra, but palpation or drawing affected hairs through the fingertips gives a rough, gritty, sandy or granular sensation. The hair is said to crepitate when combed (SIMONS), or a sharp metallic sound is produced (CONANT et al.).

In contrast to black piedra, white piedra affects chiefly coarse hairs of the body (MANSON-BAHR; HILDICK-SMITH et al.). *Trichosporon beigelii* usually involves hairs of the beard or moustache (CONANT et al.; EMMONS et al.; MARPLES). Infection of scalp hairs, eyebrows and eyelashes were referred to by SCOTT (1951), and PATTERSON et al. reported a patient with involvement of the pubic hair. SIMONS referred to white piedra involving human pubic hairs and indicated that rare cases affecting axillary hair were observed in South America. White piedra is characterized by asymptomatic, pale to light brown nodules on the affected hairs (Figs. 153A—B). Fully developed nodules surround the entire hair shaft and some show coalescence to cover several millimeters length of hair surface (Fig. 153A). The nodes are usually thickest in their central parts, but may show considerable irregularity with variation in size and shape (Figs. 153A—B). Generally, white piedra nodules are not quite as large as those caused by *P.hortai* (Figs. 150A, 153A). *Trichosporon beigelii* produces soft to firm, but not stony hard nodules, and the fungal masses can easily be stripped from the affected hairs (WILSON and PLUNKETT, 1965). White piedra nodules form as hairs emerge from the follicles (SCOTT; WILSON and Plunkett), harden with pilar growth, and fungal elements disrupt the shaft causing structural weakening (WILSON and PLUNKETT, 1965). Often, the distal end of affected hairs appear enlarged because the fractured nodules separate (EMMONS et al.). According to SCOTT's (1951) observations, white piedra nodules are usually located on the distal portion of long scalp hairs and these do not break easily.

Examination of patients with black piedra and white piedra under Wood's light gives negative results and this is a valuable differential aid in distinguishing trichomycosis nodosa of the yellow variety which shows prominent fluorescence. Trichomycosis nodosa involves hair of the axillae and pubis, and these anatomical sites are sometimes affected by white piedra. *Nocardia tenuis* has long been regarded as the cause of trichomycosis nodosa (trichomycosis axillaris or leptothrix) which shows yellow, black or red concretions. Recent studies suggest that the organism causing trichomycosis axillaris has cultural characteristics of Cornyebacterium for which the name of *Cornyebacterium tenuis* has been proposed (HILDICK-SMITH et al.). Additional diseases to be considered in the clinical differential diagnosis of piedra include pediculosis nits, monilethrix, trichorrhexis nodosa, trichonodosis, and abnormalities of hair due to artefacts. The essential distinguishing feature of piedra from other diseases showing nodular lesions of the hair is by direct microscopic examination for demonstration of *P.hortai* or *T.beigelii* fungal elements. Confirmatory mycological culture studies on each case of piedra is important to identify the exact organism causing the patient's disease.

Microscopic Observations: Direct microscopic examination of infected unstained hairs showed that older black piedra lesions were composed of hyphae in linear arrangement best observed at the periphery of pigmented nodules. The hyphae were frequently segmented to form multiple thick-walled cells or arthrospores (Fig. 150B). The main mass of older black piedra nodules showed so much pigment that fungal element details and the underlying hair shaft were indistinct (Figs. 150A—B). Multiple black specks were associated with segmented hyphae and arthrospores at the periphery of older nodules (Fig. 150A), and throughout the entire lesion of small brown-colored ones. Fungal cell details were much better observed in small lesions which only partially surrounded the hair shaft. The keratinized hair cortex cuticle was clearly elevated over *P.hortai* fungal elements

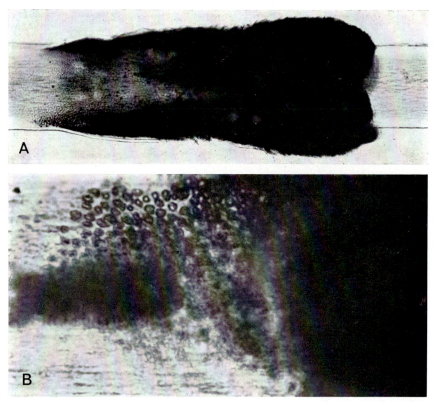

Fig. 150. Black piedra caused by *P. hortai*: A. Gross scalp hairs showing dark concretion attached to the hair shaft. The irregular nodules are extremely hard, and some encircle the hair shaft to form ring-like structures. The nodule is larger at one end, but some show this feature in the central part with a tendency for tapering distally and proximally. Examination of several concretions will usually show a variation in their size and shape. (Gross hair, × 130). B. High power magnification showing a black concretion at one pole comprised of hyphae which frequently segment into arthrospores (Gross hair, × 655)

in small brown pigmented lesions and at the tapering peripheral end of older black nodules (Fig. 150A). Examination of infected gross hairs under polarized light showed white birefringence of the fragmented cortex cuticle elevated over large nodules of *P. hortai* organisms. The main elevated mass of pigmented fungal elements making up large black piedra nodules surrounding the hair shaft showed dull yellow birefringence under polarized light. Small brown lesions showed more prominent yellow to orange polariscopic color characteristics. The hair shaft subjacent to tapering ends of large black nodules and beneath most of the small brown lesions showed some weak yellow-orange birefringence. This contrasted with striking polychroism (multiple colors) exhibited by uninvolved hair between nodules. Direct microscopic examination of crushed nodules of black piedra showed numerous asci containing 2—8 single-celled, fusiform, slightly curved ascospores with a single polar filament at each end. Short segments of several infected hairs surrounded by nodules of Brazilian black piedra were blocked together on end in paraffin and serial sectioned for transverse views of the involved shaft. Sections through thick black nodules stained with H & E showed hyphae in linear radial rosette arrangement extending from the hair shaft cortex

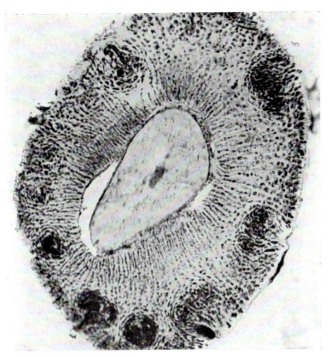

Fig. 151. Black piedra caused by *P. hortai* showing a transverse section of the hair shaft surrounded by a concretion of fungal elements. An intermediate magnification exhibits numerous segmented hyphae in linear radial arrangement forming arthrospores. Peripherally, the concretion shows asci containing ascospores. The hair shaft cortex and medulla are free of fungal elements (Mallory's PTAH stain, ×194)

outward (Fig. 151). The hyphae were frequently segmented to form rectangular nucleated cells or arthrospores which varied from 4—8 μ in size (Figs. 151, 152). An abundance of brown melanoid pigment was associated with the hyphae and arthrospores, and many granules appeared entrapped in a dark colored, cement-like substance occupying prominent intercellular spaces. The melanoid granules did not involve the cortex or medulla, but showed dense accumulations of pigment adjacent to the hair shaft. Asci appearing as pale staining, nonpigmented, circumscribed areas were observed at the periphery of nodules, and these usually contained up to eight single-celled fusiform and spirally curved ascospores lying in close proximity (Figs. 151, 152). Asci, sometimes referred to as bright spots or Horta's cysts, showed exit points to the surface of black piedra nodules, and these were interpreted as representing focal escape points for ascospores (Fig. 151). Remnants of hair shaft cuticle were identified surrounding fungal elements, but there was no evidence of invasion of the cortex or medulla by *P. hortai* hyphae and arthrospores (Fig. 151). Examination of transverse sections stained with H & E, under polarized light, showed white birefringence of the hair shaft and the adjacent region of large piedra nodules exhibited similar doubly refractile material separating and surrounding the fungal elements. The birefringent substance corresponded in location to cement-like material between fungal elements and extended from the hair shaft outward in a radial pattern. At the periphery of black piedra nodules, birefringent strands surrounded circumscribed, cyst-like asci in a concentric or lamellar fashion. Cross sections through small nodules or the tapering

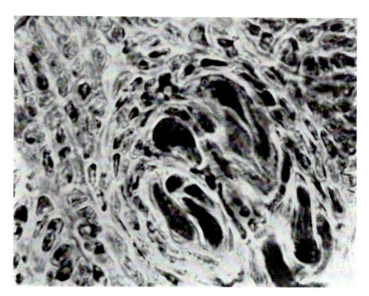

Fig. 152. Black piedra caused by *P.hortai* showing oil immersion magnification of an ascus containing approximately eight single-celled fusiform and spirally curved ascospores lying closely together. The adjacenr pseudoparenchyma is comprised of numerous arthrospores in linear arrangement (Mallory's PTAH stain, ×1400)

ends of large black piedra lesions showed single to a few layers of *P.hortai* arthrospores separating the hair shaft cuticle away from the cortex. This contrasted with cross sections of hair which showed no organisms and the cuticle appeared firmly attached to the cortex. Focally, small black piedra nodules showed disruption of the slightly elevated cuticle suggesting that these sites represented areas of initial penetration by *P.hortai* fungal elements. Some intermediate sized and large black piedra nodules showed a surrounding hair cortex cuticle, but it was disrupted in multiple areas caused by pressure from expanding fungal elements.

Direct microscopic examination of unstained infected hairs without the use of keratinolytic agents showed that nodules of white piedra were composed of light colored, homogeneous to granular substance and segmented hyphae surrounding the hair shaft (Figs. 153A—B). Direct examination of crushed specimens showed only arthrospores and blastospores with no evidence of asci or ascospores. The hair shaft traversing white piedra nodules was easily observed and showed the cortex cuticle focally elevated over fungal elements (Figs. 153 A—B). Some white piedra nodules showed definite evidence of the hair cortex cuticle beneath the fungal elements. In some nodules it even appeared that intracuticular cleavage from fungal elements occurred with parts remaining adherent to the hair cortex and remnants elevated over the white piedra organisms. Direct microscopic examination of white piedra nodules under polarized light showed dichroism to polychroism of the underlying hair shaft. This was characterized by greenish-blue to multicolored birefringence of the medulla and most of the cortex. The peripheral parts of the hair cortex and cuticle showed a bright yellow-orange birefringence. Most of the hair cortex cuticle appeared intact, although some doubly refractile fragments of this structure were identified over the fungal elements. Most areas of individual *T.beigelii* nodules showed dull gray to white birefringence of the fungal masses. The pilar shaft intervening between white

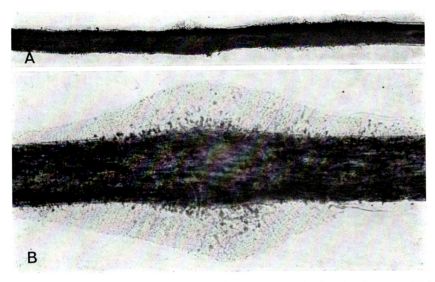

Fig. 153. White piedra caused by *T. beigelii*: A. Scanning magnification showing several light-colored, irregular nodules on the hair shaft which are firm to palpation. Some of the nodules coalesce and surround the entire hair shaft (Gross hair, ×55). B. Intermediate power magnification showing an individual white nodule adhering to the hair shaft with tapering distally and proximally (Gross hair, ×190)

piedra nodules showed multicolored birefringence similar to that described for noninvolved areas of hairs from patients with black piedra. Striking was altered pilar birefringence underlying some white piedra nodules which showed absence of polychroism, and the hair shaft appeared white to yellow with gross physical abnormalities. Dark granularity of white piedra nodules overlying altered hairs was prominent. Some hairs showed transverse fracture lines of the underlying shaft and this feature suggested sites of separation. Parts of nodules were located at broken ends of some gross hairs which verified that separation did occur in the region of abnormal white piedra lesions. The fungal elements showed no definite evidence of invading the hair cortex or medulla. Multiple short segments of hair showing Brazilian white piedra lesions were blocked together on end in paraffin and serially sectioned to demonstrate cross sections of the shaft traversing *T. beigelii* nodules. Paraffin sections stained with H & E showed segmented hyphae with a tendency toward linear radial rosette arrangement extending from the hair shaft outward (Fig. 154). Segmentation of hyphae occurred frequently to form groups of 2—4 thick-walled yeast-like arthrospores and budding terminal blastospores (Fig. 154). The arthrospores and blastospores were oval to rectangularly shaped cells and varied from 4—10 μ in size (Fig. 154). An homogeneous cement-like substance separated the fungal elements and served to bind hyphae, arthrospores and blastospores together as a cohesive mass surrounding and adherent to the hair shaft. Transverse sections of white piedra nodules stained with H & E showed hair shaft birefringence. The cortex cuticle appeared essentially intact beneath the fungal elements and was doubly refractile. There was weak birefringence in areas corresponding to the location of intercellular cement-like substance, but this was not prominent when compared with polarization characteristics exhibited by black piedra. The cortex cuticle was focally disrupted, but no fungal elements invaded the hair shaft below this level. No melanoid pigment, asci or

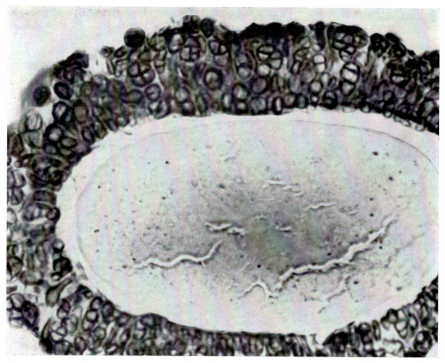

Fig. 154. White piedra caused by *T.beigelii* showing a transverse section of the hair shaft surrounded by multiple yeast-like arthrospores with tendency for linear arrangement. No asci are demonstrated and there is no evidence of invasion of the hair shaft (PAS, ×655)

ascospores were observed. Some of the white piedra nodules in cross section showed fracture lines of the adjacent pilar cortex and medulla and indicated sites of hair weakening beneath the fungal masses.

Histochemistry: The usual histochemical methods for demonstration of fungal elements showed *P.hortai* hyphae and arthrospores, but there was a tendency for the organisms to stain deeply with PAS and Gridley's methods for fungi. Asci were identified as lighter staining areas within nodules, although ascospore details were difficult to see. Mallory's PTAH method demonstrated asci best as purple colored circumscribed areas of ascospores contrasting with adjacent pigmented hyphae and arthrospores containing blue staining nuclei (Figs. 151, 152). Birefringent characteristics of sections stained with PTAH were similar to those described for H & E. The various silver techniques stained *P.hortai* fungal elements so intensely that details of the organisms could not be made out. The deep homogeneous black color of fungal masses produced by silver resulted from the brown melanoid pigment observed in sections stained with H & E. Histochemical methods for demonstration of fungal elements were particularly valuable in small lesions for showing organisms beneath the cuticle with separation of this structure from the hair cortex. Larger nodules showed fragments of the hair cortex cuticle at the periphery of black piedra masses. The ZIEHL-NEELSON method colored hair shaft keratin bright red and showed the cortex cuticle elevated over nonstaining black piedra fungal elements. *Piedraia hortai* arthrospores and hyphae showed some deep blue Gram positive staining with the BROWN and BRENN method. The fungal elements were nonreactive with various methods for demonstration of acidic mucosaccharides and other acid substances. No fungal elements involved the hair cortex or medulla in the material studied (Fig. 151).

White piedra hyphae, arthrospores and blastospores of *T.beigelii* were demonstrated by histochemical techniques for fungal elements (Fig. 154); but certain differences from *P.hortai* were observed. The fungal elements of *T.beigelii* were demonstrated with silver techniques, but the cell walls were predominantly stained and only a light black because of absence of pigment. The Brown and Brenn method stained the yeast-like fungal elements of *T.beigelii* Gram negative. Methods for demonstration of nonsulfated acidic substances, particularly the colloidal iron stain showed arthrospores, blastospores and cement-like substance to be reactive giving a blue color. Sections stained with PTAH showed a blue color reaction for fungal element nuclei, but no asci or ascospores were observed. Some sections stained by the various histochemical methods showed weak birefringence of areas corresponding to the intercellular cement-like substance. The hair shaft was doubly refractile with bright white to yellow birefringence of the cuticle best seen in sections stained with GMS and this structure appeared essentially intact beneath the yeast-like organisms. None of the serial cross sections stained by various histochemical techniques showed organisms invading the hair cortex or medulla, and in most nodules even the cuticle appeared intact (Fig. 154).

Differential Diagnosis: The histopathologic and histochemical differential diagnosis of piedra realistically includes only those differences between the black and white varieties. Gross irregular fusiform concretions of trichomycosis nodosa on the hair shaft may cause confusion with piedra, but the microscopic presence of diphtheroids, micrococci and short rounded bacilli distinguish the disease. Piedra nodules are easily differentiated from the eggs of pediculosis by microscopic identification of hyphae, arthrospores and other fungal elements. Significant distinguishing features of black piedra from white piedra include: 1. Melanoid pigment. 2. Invasion beneath the hair cortex cuticle with elevation of this structure over fungal masses. 3. Asci and ascospores. 4. Gram positive staining of fungal elements. 5. Negative staining of fungal elements for acid mucosaccharides.

White piedra nodules show important differences from *P.hortai* lesions as follows: 1. Absence of pigment. 2. Minimal disruption of the hair cortex cuticle. 3. Groups of 2—4 yeast-like organisms with blastospores. 4. Gram negative staining of fungal elements. 5. Positive histochemical staining of fungal elements for nonsulfated acid mucosaccharides. Polariscopic characteristics of black piedra and white piedra are similar. However, there are quantitative and qualitative differences. For example, gross pilar specimens affected with black piedra nodules showed only weak birefringence of fungal masses because of dense pigmentation, whereas, paraffin cross sections of lesions showed fairly prominent bright white doubly refractile material separating and even surrounding the fungal elements.

Comment: The etiologic agent of black piedra, the fungus *P.hortai*, is considered by some to be the sole authentic causative agent of all types of piedra (Hildick-Smith et al.). Simons (1953) in his review of the literature discussed the characteristics of black piedra and white piedra regarding their representing variants of the same disease. It would appear from our gross, histopathologic, histochemical and polaroscopic observations that piedra affecting human hair is caused by two distinct organisms. There are a sufficient number of differences in the way *P.hortai* and *T.beigelii* parasitize hair to clearly separate piedra into black and white varieties. In paraffin cross sections of hair nodules, birefringence was striking for black piedra and quantitatively greater when compared with white piedra. Polarization characteristics of fungal masses in both types of piedra probably results from a high concentration of chitin in the skeletal walls and intercellular cement-like substance. Some of the birefringence could result from strands of keratin being carried out from the hair cortex cuticle by proliferating fungal elements, and this possibility cannot be ruled out. The doubly refractile material separating and even surrounding piedra fungal elements represents chitin in part, since this water-insoluble polysaccharide is known to be present in many fungal species (Blank, 1953). Polariscopic studies which we conducted on chitin from *T. interdigitale* extracted and oxidized from mycelia by Blank (1953) support our opinion that the birefringent material in piedra sections results predominantly from a water-insoluble polysaccharide. We placed *T. interdigitale* chitin on a clean glass slide in synthetic mounting resin and cover-slipped the fragments, and allowed the preparation to dry overnight. Examination of chitin fragments under polarized light showed gray to white birefringence similar to that observed in transverse paraffin sections of human hair piedra nodules. Additional explanation for piedra lesions showing birefringence of chitin in gross and cross sectioned specimens is probably based on quantitative factors resulting from the large number of fungal elements concentrated together forming a pseudoparenchyma without tissue components other than the underlying hair shaft. We routinely examined paraffin sections of other superficial fungus infections under polarized light, but no birefringence of fungal elements was detected. Even large concentrations of fungal elements in tissue such as *T. schoenleinii* scutula fail to show definite birefringence when sections are examined under polarized light.

No studies have been made to identify chemically the polysaccharides of *P. hortai* and *T. beigelii*, but a high concentration of doubly refractile chitin could account in part for the positive histochemical staining reactions such as with PAS and Gridley's methods for fungal elements. Chitin is widely distributed in nature and is thought to be present in bacterial cell walls (Salton, 1964). The analysis of bacterial cell walls after acid hydrolysis revelaed glucosamine, muramic acid, and several other amino acids (Davis et al.). Salton in an extensive review reported that the two amino sugars N-acetylglucosamine and N-acetylmuramic acid occur in the cell walls of most bacterial species so far examined. Muramic acid is an amino sugar and it is possible that this important component of bacterial cell walls may also be present in the skeletal framework of certain fungal species. If present in fungi, muramic acid could in part account for our histochemical demonstration of acidic substances in the skeletal cell walls of *T. beigelii*, although the yeast-like fungal elements may contain combinations of other acid mucosaccharides, sialomucin and fatty acids. Similar to *T. beigelii* arthrospores and blastospores, acidic substances have been histochemically demonstrated in the fungal elements of *T. rubrum*, *T. epilans*, *M. gypseum*, *C. albicans* and *C. werneckii*, and it is possible that these superficial fungi may also contain varying amounts of muramic acid in their skeletal framework. It is likely that future studies will identify the exact chemical composition of *P. hortai* and *T. beigelii* cell wall substance, and that not only will chitin be identified but variable amounts of water-soluble polysaccharides.

Morphologic evidence for keratinase acitivity of *P. hortai* seems supported on the basis of microscopic evidence which shows fungal elements invading beneath the cortex cuticle with separation and elevation of this structure over black piedra fungal elements. We observed less tendency for microscopic disruption of the cortex cuticle in white piedra. It is possible that keratinases elaborated by *T. beigelii* fungal elements penetrate hard keratin and account for fracture lines and eventual separation of the hair shaft beneath white piedra nodules.

Invasion of the hair cortex and medulla by piedra organisms was not observed in our study, but review of the literature indicates that this represents a controversial point not agreed on by various investigators. MARPLES reported that *P.hortai* organisms probably initially invade susceptible hair at the scalp level by penetrating the cortex cuticle with proliferation of fungal elements beneath this structure and gradual breaking through to surround the shaft. CONANT et al. report that *P.hortai* invades beneath the cuticle, then expands and ruptures this structure to spread around the hair shaft, forming dark brown to black nodules held together by a cement-like secretion material. SIMONS in his review indicated that early descriptions of piedra referred to the disease as an ectothrix infection, but subsequent investigators described it as partly or entirely endothrix because of fungal elements penetrating the hair cuticle. SIMONS favored black piedra as an ectothrix disease and used this terminology in Fig. 809 of his publication in 1953. Some investigators have referred to piedra as an endo-ectothrix parasitic disease based on fungal elements surrounding the hair in the central part of nodules and invasion of the shaft at the periphery (SIMONS). LANGERON's (1936) detailed publication clearly shows in a series of illustrations the pathogenesis of hair cortex cuticle invasion by *P.hortai* organisms with subsequent proliferation of fungal elements to disrupt and elevate this structure over the black piedra nodule. EMMONS et al. in their discussion of black piedra indicated that fungal elements occur within the pilar shaft as well as on the surface and may so weaken affected hair that it breaks easily. KAPLAN in his report on piedra in lower animals referred to observations that five chimpanzee museum pelts showed black piedra fungal elements affecting the hair cortex and medulla, resulting in destruction of the involved shaft. KAPLAN subsequently reported on the occurrence of black piedra in primate pelts and observed distinct patterns of hair involvements: 1. Fungal elements penetrated beneath the cuticle, proliferated, and eventually broke out to form a nodule surrounding the hait shaft identical to human black piedra. 2. Organisms invaded the cortex and medulla causing prominent pilar damage, and in some cases the fungal masses were surrounded by the cuticle. 3. Enlargements were composed of fungal elements with severe pilar involvement of the cuticle, cortex and medulla, and the hairs were frequently broken at sites of nodule formation. It would appear from our limited observations of human black piedra affecting two individuals that *P.hortai* should be classified as a modified type of endo-ectothrix parasite. Fungal elements penetrate only beneath the cuticle with no evidence of hair cortex or medulla invasion in cross sections of black piedra nodules.

CONANT et al. indicated that *T.beigelii* infection occurs only in previously damaged hair. The infected hair may show only a raised cuticle, but more often it is altered severely with trichorrhexis (CONANT et al.). EMMONS et al. reported that white piedra may extend as a sheath around the shaft, but subcuticular or intrapilar changes are prominent producing nodular swellings which vary in size from a microscopic increase to twice the diameter of a hair, and fractures occur at the nodule sites. MARPLES stated that the fungal elements of white piedra are not confined to the pilar surface, but may invade the cortex and break or split the hair. SCOTT reported that initially the minute fungal concretions only partially surround the hair shaft, but eventually the entire circumference is encircled. The scalp, hair follicle and follicular portions of the shaft are not affected (SCOTT). SCOTT believed that the hairs were initially infected near the scalp and that individual nodules enlarged so slowly as to become visible only after the hair lengthened several millimeters. KAPLAN stated that the fungal elements of human white piedra frequently invade the hair shaft causing prominent pilar damage. White piedra of horses and black spider monkeys shows fungal elements invading the cortex and medulla with eventual destruction of the involved hair shaft (Kaplan). Kaplan in reporting his observations of white piedra in a monkey observed proliferation of fungal elements under the cuticle or interior hair shaft with complete pilar destruction, and some hairs were broken at the nodule sites. Daly reported white piedra in a 7-year-old Caucasian boy and noted that the hair shaft was not invaded, but simply overlaid with fungal elements. Our study of infected hairs from two patients with white piedra showed some nodules with underlying abnormalities of the hair shaft, but no intrapilary fungal elements were observed. Transverse paraffin-sections of white piedra lesions showed no invasion of the hair cortex or medulla and only minimal disruption of the cuticle. Based on our observations of two white piedra cases, it appears that *T. beigelii* affects the hair predominantly as an ectothrix infection. There is some tendency for involvement of the cortex cuticle requiring that white piedra also be classified as a partial or modified endo-ectothrix infection.

Our gross, histopathologic, histochemical and polaroscopic observations of piedra in four patients should be corroborated or modified by other investigators, and we urge that this be done by those having the opportunity of easily obtaining infected human hair specimens. It is our recommendation that the most valid information can be derived from studying serial cross sections through multiple piedra nodules similar to those prepared in our laboratory and described under materials and methods. A recent report (Shelley et al.) describes a new technique for cross sectioning hair specimens, and this method should also be a satisfactory one for studying piedra nodules.

Erythrasma

Introduction: Historically, for over a century, erythrasma has been grouped with superficial fungus diseases, but it is now known to represent an unusual type of cutaneous bacterial infection. Investigations have established that erythrasma in all its forms is caused by a diphtheroid, *Corynebacterium minutissimum* (Hildick-Smith et al.) Erythrasma occurs as a worldwide disease and was long considered to represent a superficial fungus infection caused by an actinomycete, *Nocardia minutissima* (Manson-Bahr, 1960) until the organism was given the name of *Corynebacterium minutissimum* by Sarkany, Taplin and Blank (1962, 1963). Human inoculation experiments with pure cultures of *Corynebacterium minutissimum* produced scaly lesions with typical fluorescence (Sarkany et al., 1961, 1962, 1963; Hildick-Smith et al., 1964). Experimental inoculations into human subjects were of relatively short duration and failed to persist as clinical erythrasma, but cultures from scales yielded fluorescent colonies containing Gram positive bacilli with subterminal granules (Sarkany et al., 1961). No detailed animal experiments have been conducted and it is not known if species other than humans are susceptible to the organism causing erythrasma (Hildick-Smith et al.). Based on studies that have been conducted and response to antibiotic treatment, most investigators conclude that *Corynebacterium minutissimum* represents the causative organism of erythrasma (Sarkany et al., 1961, 1962, 1963; Munro-Ashman et al.; Hildick-Smith et al.; Marples). The disease occurs in temperate geographic zones, but is more common in wet, humid and hot tropical climates. Erythrasma affects both sexes, all social groups, and the disease has been observed involving old and young individuals. Sarkany et al. (1961, 1962, 1963) documented erythrasma in a one-year-old child with toeweb lesions and reported the disease affecting a 73-year-old man who exhibited an infection of the axillae and groin. MUNRO-ASHMAN (1963) reported on erythrasma in adolescence, and *Corynebacterium minutissimum* was cultured from 58 (14%) of 410 boys. In 1951, the incidence of erythrasma was quoted as 4.5% of a group of dermatomycoses cases referred to by SARKANY et al. (1962) and HILDICK-SMITH et al. (1964). Mild infections and subclinical examples of *Corynebacterium minutissimum* skin disease are being recognized, and the incidence in the general population may be as high as 23—25% (SARKANY et al., 1961, 1962; MUNRO-ASHMAN et al.). TEMPLE and BOARDMAN (1962) in reporting on erythrasma of the toewebs found a frequency of 14.3%, but noted a significant variation in sex incidence (approximately 17.5% males and 6.5% females). Recent studies on tinea pedis and erythrasma at a chiropody clinic in England revealed that 37% of 200 new patients examined under Wood's light showed fluorescence characteristics of erythrasma (ENGLISH et al., 1968).

In this report, we shall record our histopathologic, fluorescent microscopic, and histochemical observations of biopsy sections from two adult men with typical erythrasma of the axillae and groin.

Gross Appearance: Three clinical types of erythrasma have been recognized and it is generally agreed that all forms are caused by *Corynebacterium minutissimum*. It appears that a mild variety is the most common form of erythrasma characterized by maceration, scaling and fissures between the toes. The disease involves all age groups and the interdigital tissues of the lateral two toewebs of each foot are usually affected (HILDICK-SMITH et al.; TEMPLE et al.). The interdigital toeweb form of erythrasma is probably more common in younger age group males and may account for unexplained cases of scaling and fissuring of the clefts which are not due to fungus (TEMPLE et al.; MUNRO-ASHMAN; HILDICK-SMITH et al.). The classical subacute form of erythrasma affects predominantly adult men (Fig. 155) and involves the upper inner thighs (Fig. 155), crural folds (Fig. 155), perineum, scrotum, pubis and axillae. Genitocrural involvement in men is generally more prominent on the left side because of contact with the scrotum, which is usually affected by the disease process (SARKANY et al., 1961). The subacute form of erythrasma in women affects the axillae and genitocrural regions, but in addition, inframammary, periumbilical and intergluteal cleft regions may be involved. AYRES and MIHAN (1968) observed one patient with erythrasma of the ear canals and vestibules, and referred to the disease in patients with intractable pruritus ani. Clinically, the typical subacute disease appears as dry, irregularly shaped, brown, superficial scaling lesions and the periphery may be accentuated showing a slightly erythematous margination (Fig. 155). Erythrasma may appear orange, yellow, brown, or red, and a combination of color shades can occur. Initially, erythrasma begins as small scaling macules which gradually enlarge to form larger lesions varying in size. Gross evidence of papules, vesicles and follicular lesions are not seen (LEWIS et al., 1958). The disease is almost invariably asymptomatic (WILSON and PLUNKETT, 1965), although mild itching is sometimes experienced and this increases in intensity with activity (HILDICK-SMITH et al.). A widespread chronic itching type of erythrasma is most commonly seen in middle-aged Negro women living in tropical or subtropical climates, and the lesions appear as well-defined, scally, lamellated plaques on the trunk and proximal parts of the extremities (HILDICK-SMITH et al.).

Wood's light examination of erythrasma shows typical coral-red fluorescence of the affected areas, although varying shades of color may occur in different foci of the irregularly shaped patches. PARTRIDGE and JACKSON (1962) reviewed the historical aspects of Wood's light characteristics of erythrasma and reported

24*

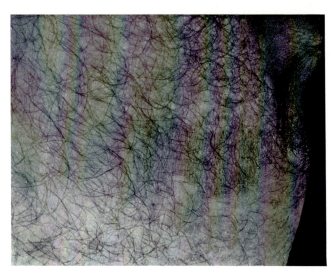

Fig. 155. Erythrasma caused by *Corynebacterium minutissimum* showing slightly erythematous to brown, superficial, scaling lesions on the inner aspect of the thigh. The patient had symmetrical involvement of the groin and axillae

fluorescence was not seen in all lesions, but when present, it appeared only within limits of scaling either covering the entire area, as focal patches, or at the border. Partridge and Jackson (1962) observed that Gram positive bacilli belonging to the genus *Bacillus* grow excessively on susceptible subjects and it was their opinion that these organisms contributed to the fluorescence of erythrasma and some other skin conditions. Munro-Ashman in reporting on erythrasma in adolescence stressed Wood's light examination as very helpful in diagnosis because toe cleft lesions show various shades of red fluorescence. Wood's light examination is valuable when erythrasma is considered clinically since the pink or red fluorescence of lesions can serve as a rapid aid for diagnosis because *Corynebacterium minutissimum* requires special tissue culture media to grow (Halprin, 1967). Hildick-Smith et al. indicate Wood's light examination is invaluable, particularly in confirming the diagnosis of toe cleft erythrasma and in identyfying fluorescent colonies of *Corynebacterium minutissimum* in cultures. The substances responsible for red fluorescence in erythrasma appears to be from porphyrins (Sarkany et al., 1962, 1963; Hildick-Smith et al.; Ayres et al.).

The clinical differential diagnosis of erythrasma, particularly when the disease is irritated, includes tinea pedis, tinea versicolor, tinea cruris, intertrigo, lichen simplex chronicus, and other forms of dermatitis eczema such as pruritus ani. The more generalized form of erythrasma may be particularly confused with tinea versicolor and psoriasis (Hildick-Smith et al.). Tinea versicolor shows less tendency for involving intertriginous areas and an erythematous margin of the lesions is uncommon (Lewis et al.). The long duration, lack of inflammation, and absence of satellite lesions tend to rule against tinea cruris (Lewis et al.). Wood's light characteristics showing coral-red fluorescence of erythrasma lesions is a significant differential feature from other diseases, although tinea versicolor can exhibit varying shades of color when examined under filtered ultraviolet rays. Partridge and Jackson (1962) studied a patient with tinea versicolor who showed red fluorescence of follicular plugs in areas of disease located on the lower back from which they recovered Gram positive bacilli resembling *Bacillus licheni-formis*. Tinea pedis is the disease most difficult to distinguish from toeweb erythrasma. TEMPLE and BOARDMAN reported that 16 (30%) of 53 individuals who showed evidence of superficial fungus infections of the toewebs by direct microscopic examination and/or results of mycological culture studies also exhibited fluorescence characteristics of erythrasma. ENGLISH et al. demonstrated coral-red fluorescence of toeweb lesions in 37% of 200 patients examined and from 5.5% of the cases they isolated a dermatophyte. ENGLISH and TURVEY (1968) failed to isolate *Corynebacterium minutissimum* on culture media from their patients and even observed fluorescence in a lesion-free patient. PARTRIDGE et al. (1962) reported pink pigment production and coral-red fluorescence of genus *Bacillus* organisms grown on enriched and most routine laboratory media, and concluded that these aerobic, spore-forming bacilli, commonly found on skin, play some part in changes associated with erythrasma. Genus *Bacillus* organisms do not normally colonize the skin, but alterations brought about by other cutaneous diseases such as erythrasma allow them to multiply and contribute to scaling and fluorescence (PARTRIDGE et al., 1962). Further investigations into the cause or causes of coral-red fluorescence should be performed (ENGLISH et al.).

Microscopic Observations: Skin tissue sections stained with H & E showed hyperkeratosis, hypergranulosis, numerous vacuolated cells in the granular layer and upper part of the stratum granulosum, mild acanthosis, focal atrophy, and a few elongated rete ridges (Fig. 156A). The thickened corneal layer was focally compact with intervening basket-weave hyperkeratosis. Vacuolated cells were striking (Fig. 156A) and in some sections they extended from beneath the horny layer to a level just above the stratum basale. Examination of serial sections showed focal spongiosis, exocytosis of mononuclear cells, and overlying changes of minimal parakeratosis. The sides and tips of some elongated and broadened dermal papillae showed an increase in melanin in the basal layer. The papillary corium showed mild to moderate inflammation, interstitial edema, minimal capillary-endothelial proliferation, and some vascular ectasia (Fig. 156A). A cellular infiltrate of lymphocytes and histiocytes was predominantly perivascular in location, although some cells involved the intervening stroma. A few small dilated blood vessels were engorged with red blood cells. Extravasated red blood cells were intermingled with the cellular infiltrate in an occasional dermal papillae and some disruption of the dermoepidermal junction was present. Incontinence of pigment was present and melanin granules were free and within melanophages in the upper corium. Pilosebaceous follicles and sweat glands appeared essentially normal. Sections stained with H & E colored the organisms blue and they appeared more concentrated in areas showing a compact type of hyperkeratosis.

Histochemistry: The same series of special stains performed on superficial fungus diseases were done on tissue sections of erythrasma. In addition, unstained sections of erythrasma were examined for autofluorescence with a Leitz Ortholux microscope equipped with an Osram HBO 200 W light source, a UGI excitor, and an ultraviolet absorbing barrier filter.

Rodlike organisms, filaments and coccoid forms of *Corynebacterium minutissi-mum* were demonstrated similarly by histochemical techniques that routinely stained fungal elements of superficial fungus infections. The B & B method best demonstrated blue staining Gram positive organisms confined to superficial layers of the SC (Fig. 156B). The organisms were focally concentrated together forming colonies in the stratum disjunctum (Fig. 156B) with intervening areas showing absence of bacteria. In most colonies, rodlike organisms and coccoid forms

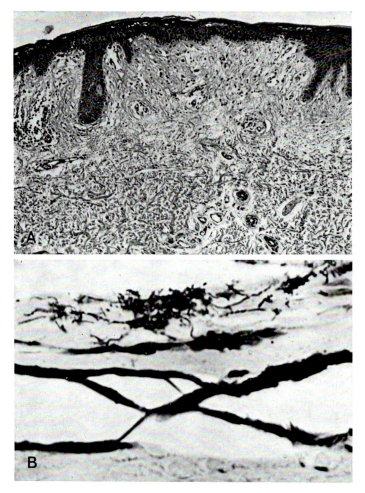

Fig. 156. Erythrasma caused by *Corynebacterium minutissimum*: A. Scanning magnification showing hypergranulosis, numerous vacuolated cells in the stratum granulosum, atrophy, and a few elongate acanthotic rete ridges. The upper corium shows mild inflammation and interstitial edema (H & E, ×93). B. High power magnification showing multiple organisms of *Corynebacterium minutissimum* in the superficial SC. Filamentous forms predominate, but short rods are present and demonstrated as Gram positive bacilli. The organisms do not invade the epidermis or corium (Brown and Brenn method, ×655)

predominated, but definite non-branching segmented filaments of variable length were seen (Fig. 156B). In general, filaments were more prominent at the periphery of bacterial colonies (Fig. 156B). Some rodlike organisms and filaments showed terminal deep staining spores, and after separation these forms appeared as coccoid bodies. Some of the coccoid bodies were paired and appeared as diplococci. Erythrasma diphtheroid organisms were PAS-positive and diastase resistant and demonstrated with the Gridley's method. *Corynebacterium minutissimum* organisms were acid-fast negative with the Ziehl-Neelson method which stained the organisms a light blue color. Wolbach's Giemsa method and PTAH stained the organisms a deep blue to purple color. The morphological forms of *Corynebacterium minutissimum* in tissue sections were demonstrated with silver, but Grocott's method was the most satisfactory technique. The diphtheroid organisms did not involve the intracorneal eccrine sweat pores or keratin within follicular ostia. None of the special stains demonstrated bacterial forms of *Corynebacterium minutissimum* invading the living epidermis or corium. The FONTANA-MASSON silver method showed a prominent increase of melanin in all epidermal layers including the vacuolated cells and horny layer. Argyrophilic melanin granules were also demonstrated in the upper corium. Gomori's method for iron pigment was negative. Some of the special techniques, particularly Movat's pentachrome method, PTAH, and Giemsa stain showed numerous vacuolated cells in striking contrast to normal appearing epidermal cells of the granular layer and stratum Malpighii. Keratohyalin material was prominent in the stratum granulosum and some vacuolated cells contained round to irregular and angulated granules similar to inclusion bodies. Some of the vacuolated cells showed pyknotic nuclei compressed to the periphery or they were completely absent. Methods for demonstration of acid mucosaccharides and other acidic substances did not show significant results exoept that mast cells were generally increased up to 20 per high power field in the papillary corium. Connective tissue stains demonstrated some thinning of collagen, reticulum and elastic fibers in the edematous upper corium, otherwise, these structures appeared essentially normal. Small thickened blood vessels in the papillary corium showed some increase in PAS-positive and diastase resistant material in their walls.

Deparaffinized unstained tissue sections of erythrasma were mounted in buffered glycerol medium, cover slipped and examined under ultraviolet light. The stratum disjunctum corresponding in location to numerous diphtheroid organisms showed a striking ice blue autofluorescence and contrasted with the dull gray color of the subjacent horny material and epidermis. Using different filters caused the fluorescent zone to appear yellow, but in no instance was a definite coral-red color visualized. Dermal elastic tissue in the reticular corium showed bright white autofluorescence characteristic for normal fibers. Control sections of normal skin showed autofluorescence of elastic tissue, whereas, all levels of the SC exhibited a dull gray color.

Differential Diagnosis: The histopathologic and histochemical differential diagnosis of erythrasma rarely presents any real confusion with superficial fungus diseases. The size and morphology of *Corynebacterium minutissimum* organisms located in the stratum disjunctum should in no way be confused with the fungal elements of dermatophytic infections, cutaneous candidiasis, tinea versicolor, *Pityrosporum* folliculitis or tinea nigra. Because the diphtheroid organisms of erythrasma are small, they could be missed in tissue sections and lead to a tissue diagnosis of chronic dermatitis. The vacuolated cells in the epidermis of erythrasma resemble those seen in verruca plana, some epithelial nevi, familial forms of keratoderma palmaris et plantaris, congenital ichthyosiform erythroderma (epidermolytic hyperkeratosis), and bullous lesions of pachyonychia congenita. Elongated, finger-like rete ridges showing an increase in melanin along their sides and tips resemble lentigo or melanocytic epithelial nevi.

Comment: Only brief histopathologic descriptions of tissue changes in erythrasma have been recorded (GÖTZ, 1963; HILDICK-SMITH et al., 1964; MARPLES, 1965; MONTES et al., 1969). HILDICK-SMITH et al. refer to the histopathologic changes in erythrasma as showing hypergranulosis, vascular dilatation, and a mild perivascular lymphocytic infiltrate. Most of the descriptions about erythrasma organisms deal with observations made from scales from gross lesions which were removed for direct microscopic examination, and methylene blue, Gram, Giemsa or PAS show rodlike organisms, filaments and coccoid forms (Hildick-Smith et al.). The filaments are tortuous, divided into segments, and measure 5—25 μ in length and 1 μ in diameter (Hildick-Smith et al.). The average length of individual filament segments is 4—7 μ, but shorter and longer forms are frequently seen (Sarkany et al., 1961; Hildick-Smith et al.). Dark staining granules are often seen within filaments and short bacilli, and this later form of *Corynebacterium minutissimum* measures 1—3 μ in length and 0.5 μ in diameter (Sarkany et al., 1961, 1962, 1963; Hildick-Smith et al.).

The exact nature of vacuolated cells observed in the epidermis of erythrasma cannot definitely be determined on the basis of histopathologic, histochemical and fluorescent studies we performed. Epidermal hyperpigmentation and melanin granules in the cytoplasm of vacuolated cells suggest that they could represent effete or worn out melanocytes being exfoliated with neighboring keratinocytes. The vacuolated cells could also represent epidermal kerationocytes altered by bacterial enzymes, and an abnormal proliferation of Langerhans cells would have to be considered. It is obvious that additional studies need to be done to explain the origin and significance of vacuolated cells in tissue sections of erythrasma. Electron microscopic studies on *Corynebacterium minutissimum* in gross lesion scales and tissue sections of erythrasma have been done, but only descriptions of organisms lying within and between horny layer cells were recorded (Sarkany et al., 1961, 1962, 1963; Hildick-Smith et al.; Montes, 1967; Montes et al., 1969).

Our histopathologic and histochemical observations of epidermal and dermal hypermelanosis help explain the pigmented color of gross erythrasma lesions involving the genitocrural and axillary regions. The pigmented appearance could result indirectly from porphyrins elaborated by *Corynebacterium minutissimum* organisms which stimulate epidermal melanocytes to synthesize increased amounts of melanin. Vascular dilation of small dermal blood vessels engorged with red blood cells may also play a role in accounting for the color changes of classical erythrasma.

Histochemical studies on erythrasma organisms in tissue sections showed results similar to superficial fungus infections, and probably indicate water-soluble polysaccharides and chitin in the bacterial cell walls of *Corynebacterium minutissimum*. Our ultraviolet microscopy observations of autofluorescence limited to the stratum disjunctum in sections of erythrasma is a feature different from superficial fungus infections. The substance causing ice blue autofluorescence may result from porphyrins considered responsible for the coral-red color of gross erythrasma lesions. It is probable that other unknown substances elaborated by diphtheroid organisms play a role in the ultraviolet microscopy autofluorescent characteristics of erythrasma.

It is now generally accepted that erythrasma represents an usual form of cutaneous bacterial disease, but no great criticism can be leveled at earlier investigators who classified the organism as causing a type of superficial fungal disease. The association of erythrasma with superficial fungus infections is well recorded in the literature. The occurrence of erythrasma and tinea versicolor together has been reported (Franks et al.; Sarkany et al., 1962; Montes et al.), and sometimes these two diseases can be confused clinically. Recognition in recent years of toeweb erythrasma has caused an appreciation of the clinical confusion which can occur with tinea pedis and of how frequently the two diseases occur together in the same patient (Temple and Boardman, 1962). Combinations of erythrasma and dermatophytosis have been reported and some of the pathogens identified by mycological culture studies include *T. mentagrophytes* variety *interdigitale, E. floccosum* and *T. rubrum* (SARKANY et al., 1961, 1962, 1963; MUNRO-ASHMAN; MARPLES; TEMPLE et al.; ENGLISH et al.; MONTES et al.). Figure 89 of this manuscript illustrates a patient with tinea corporis caused by *T. mentagrophytes* variety *niveum* who also developed erythrasma of the axillae and groin. Erythrasma associated with diabetes mellitus has been reported (SARKANY et al., 1961), and some patients show superimposed *T. rubrum* infection in areas of typical coral-red fluorescence (MONTES et al., 1969). Erythrasma occurring in patients with diabetes mellitus probably represents another example of how debilitating diseases predispose to the development of bacterial and fungal infections from opportunistic organisms.

AYRES and MIHAN observed that patients with erythrasma responded to a topically applied fungicide as well as from antibacterial antibiotics, and for this reason, suggested that the etiology of the disease merits further study. Studies on erythrasma by PARTRIDGE and JACKSON (1963) raised some doubts in the minds of these investigators regarding the role of a single fluorescent organism as a cause for the disease. ENGLISH and TURVEY (1968) demonstrated toeweb fluorescence characteristics of erythrasma in 37% of 200 patients, but were unable to culture *Corynebacterium minutissimum* from the involved areas. ENGLISH and TURVEY agree with those who contend that further investigations into the cause or causes of coral-red fluorescence in erythrasma should be done, and indicated the results of such studies could be rewarding.

We are in general agreement with those who interpret erythrasma as a bacterial disease based on recent investigations. Our histopathologic, histochemical and fluorescent microscopy observations support *Corynebacterium minutissimum* as the causative organism of classical erythrasma. Erythrasma shows some clinico-pathologic, histochemical and fluorescent characteristics which overlap with those seen in superficial fungus infections. Even though erythrasma is bacterial in origin, consideration with pathogens causing superficial fungus diseases is in order. It is recommended that a high index of suspicion be maintained for erythrasma when the clinical differential diagnosis includes superficial fungus diseases such as tinea pedis, tinea cruris and tinea versicolor. Indeed, investigators are encouraged to conduct additional studies to broaden our knowledge about erythrasma which until 1961 was considered of fungal nature caused by *Nocardia minutissima*.

Acknowledgement: We wish to acknowledge with appreciation the contributions of F. BLANK, Dr. Sc. Nat., Dr. Sc. Techn., Professor in Dermatology (Medical Mycology), Temple University School of Medicine, and Director, Section of Medical Mycology, The Skin and Cancer Hospital of Philadelphia; and Mr. GERALD PEARLMAN, Staff Photographer, The Skin and Cancer Hospital of Philadelphia.

References

ADAMSON, H. G.: Observations on the parasites of ringworm. Brit. J. Derm. **7**, 201 (1895). — AINSWORTH, G. C., GEORG, L. K.: Nomenclature of the faviforme *Trichophytons*. Mycologia **46**, 9 (1954). — AJELLO, L.: Dermatophyte *Microsporum gypseum* as saprophyte and parasite. J. invest. Derm. **21**, 157 (1953). — ALLEN, A. C.: The skin: A clinicopathological treatise (ed. 2). New York: Grune & Stratton, Inc. 1967. — AUDETTE, R. C. S., BAXTER, R. M., WALKER, G. C. A.: A study of the lipid content of *Trichophyton mentagrophytes*. Canad. J. Microbiol. **7**, 282 (1961). — AYRES, S., JR., MIHAN, R.: Erythrasma — response to tolnaftate, an antifungal medication. Arch. Derm. **97**, 173 (1968). — BAER, R. L., MUSKABILT, E.: Extensive *Tricho-phyton purpureum* infection with nevoid anomaly of the skin. Report of a case, together with mycologic and physiologic studies. Arch. Derm. **56**, 834 (1947). — BAKER, R. D.: Tissue chan-ges in fungous disease. Arch. Path. **44**, 459 (1947). — BAUSLAUGH, G., JUST, G., BLANK, F.: Isolation of ergosterol peroxide from *Trichophyton schoenleinii*. Nature (Lond.) **202**, 1218 (1964). — BIRT, A. R., WILT, J. C.: Mycology, bacteriology, and histopathology of suppurative ringworm. Arch. Derm. **69**, 441 (1954). — BISHOP, C. T., BLANK, F., HRANISAVLJEVIC-JAKOVL-JEVIC, M.: The water-soluble polysaccharides of dermatophytes. 1. A galactomannan from

Trichophyton granulosum. Canad. J. Chem. **40**, 1816 (1962). — BISHOP, C.T., BLANK, F., GARDNER, P. E.: The cell wall polysaccharides of *Candida albicans*: Glucan, mannan, and chitin. Canad. J. Chem. **38**, 869 (1960). — BISHOP, C.T., PERRY, M.B.: The water-soluble polysaccharides of dermatophytes. V.Galactomannans II from *Trichophyton granulosum, Trichophyton interdigitale, Microsporum quinckeanum, Trichophyton rubrum* and *Trichophyton schoenleinii*. Canad. J. Chem. **44**, 2291 (1966). — BISHOP, C.T., PERRY, M.B., HULYALKAR, R.K.: The water-soluble polysaccharides of dermatophytes. VI. Glucans from *Trichophyton granulosum, Trichophyton interdigitale, Microsporum quinckeanum, Trichophyton rubrum*, and *Trichophyton schoenleinii*. Canad. J. Chem. **44**, 2299 (1966). — BISHOP, C.T., PERRY, M.B., BLANK, F., COOPER, F.P.: The water-soluble polysaccharides of dermatophytes. IV. Galactomannans I from *Trichophyton granulosum, Trichophyton interdigitale, Microsporum quinckeanum, Trichophyton rubrum*, and *Trichophyton schoenleinii*. Canad. J. Chem. **43**, 30 (1965). — BLANK, F.: On the isolation and classification of dermatophytes. In: Current problems in dermatology, Vol. I, Schuppli. Basel: S. Karger 1959. ~ The chemical composition of the cell walls of dermatophytes. Biochim. Biophys. Acta **10**, 110 (1953). ~ Dermatophytes of animal origin transmissible to man. Amer. J. med. Sci. **229**, 302 (1955). ~ Endothrix ringworm endemic in rural eastern Quebec. Canad. J. Publ. Hlth. **49**, 157 (1958). ~ *Tinea capitis*. A histopathological and histochemical study by J.H. GRAHAM, W.C. JOHNSON, C.F. BURGOON, JR., and E.B. HELWIG. Unpublished opening discussor remarks of paper read before the Section on Dermatology, 112th Annual Meeting, American Medical Association, Atlantic City, New Jersey, June 17, 1963. — BLANK, F., CHIN, O., JUST, G., MERANZE, D.R., SHIMKIN, M.B., WIEDER, R.: Carcinogens from fungi pathogenic for man. Cancer Res. **28**, 2276 (1968). — BLANK, F., LECLERC, G., TELNER, P.: Clinical manifestations of mouse favus in man. Arch. Derm. **83**, 587 (1961). — BLANK, F., NG, A.S., JUST, G.: Metabolites of pathogenic fungi. V. Isolation and tentative structures of vioxanthin and viopurpurin, two colored metabolites of *Trichophyton violaceum*. Canad. J. Chem. **44**, 2873 (1966). — BLANK, F., PRICHARD, H.: Epidemic ringworm of the groin. Arch. Derm. **85**, 410 (1962). — BLANK, F., SCHOPFLOCHER, P., POIRIER, P., RIOPELLE, J.L.: Extensive *Trichophyton* infection of about fifty years' duration in two sisters. Dermatologica (Basel) **115**, 40 (1957). — BLANK, F., SHORTLAND, F.E., JUST, G.: The free sterols of dermatophytes. J. invest. Derm. **39**, 91 (1962). — BLANK, F., STRACHAN, A.A.: Infections due to *Trichophyton tonsurans* and *Trichophyton sulfureum* in rural eastern Quebec. Mycopathologia (Den Haag) **18**, 207 (1962). — BLANK, F., TELNER, P.: Note on the parasitic growth-phase of *Trichophyton rubrum* in hairs. Canad. J. Microbiol. **2**, 402 (1956). — BLANK, H., ROTH, F.J., JR.: Systemic control of cutaneous fungous infections. Amer. J. med. Sci. **240**, 466 (1960). — BLANK, H., SAGAMI, S., BOYD, C., ROTH, F.J., JR.: The pathogenesis of superficial fungous infections in cultured human skin. Arch. Derm. **79**, 524 (1959). — BLANK, H., SMITH, J.G., JR.: Widespread *Trichophyton rubrum* granulomas treated with griseofulvin. Arch. Derm. **81**, 779 (1960). — BLANK, H., TAPLIN, D., ROTH, F.J., JR.: Electron microscopic observations of the effects of griseofulvin on dermatophytes. Arch. Derm. **81**, 667 (1960). — BLANK, H., TAPLIN, D., ZAIAS, N.: Cutaneous *Trichophyton mentagrophytes* infections in Vietnam. Arch. Derm. **99**, 135 (1969). — BROCK, J.M.: *Microsporum nanum*, a cause of tinea capitis. Arch. Derm. **84**, 504 (1961). — BURDICK, K.H.: Piedra in mother and daughter. Arch. Derm. **73**, 386 (1956). — BURGOON, C.F., JR., GRAHAM, J.H., KEIPER, R.J., URBACH, F., BURGOON, J.S., HELWIG, E.B.: Histopathologic evaluation of griseofulvin in *Microsporum audouini* infections. Arch. Derm. **81**, 724 (1960). ~ Griseofulvin in tinea capitis. A clinical and histopathologic evaluation. Kansas City: American Academy of General Practice 1961. — BUTTERWORTH, T., GRAHAM,J. H.:Linear papular ectodermal-mesodermal hamartoma.Arch.Derm.**101**,191(1970).— CALLAWAY, J.L.: Dermatophytes as opportunistic organisms. Lab. Invest. **11** (part 2), 1132 (1962). — CANIZARES, O., SHATIN, H., KELLERT, A. J.: Cushing's syndrome and dermatomycosis. Arch. Derm. **80**, 705 (1959). — CHAKRABORTY, A.N., GHOSH, S., BLANK, F.: Isolation of *Trichophyton rubrum* (Castellani) Sabouraud, 1911, from animals. Canad. J. comp. Med. **18**, 436 (1954). — COISCOU, A.G., KOURIE, M.: Epidermofitosis verrucosa. Reporte de un caso. Rev. Dom. Dermat. **2**, 112 (1968). — CONANT, N.F., SMITH, D.T., BAKER, R.D., CALLAWAY, J.S., MARTIN, D.S.: Manual of clinical mycology (ed. 2). Philadelphia: W.B. Saunders Co. 1954. — COOPER, J.L., MIKHAIL, G.R.: *Trichophyton rubrum*. Perifolliculitis on amputation stump. Arch. Derm. **94**, 56 (1966). — CREMER, G.: A special granulomatous form of mycosis of the lower legs caused by *Trichophyton rubrum* Castellani. Dermatologica (Basel) **107**, 28 (1953). — DALY, J.F.: Piedra in Vermont. Arch. Derm. **75**, 584 (1957). — DANIELS, G.: The digestion of human hair keratin by *Microsporum canis* Bodin. J. gen. Microbiol. **8**, 289 (1953). — DAVIS, B.D., DULBECCO, R., EISEN, H.N., GINSBERG, H.S., WOOD, W.B., JR.: Microbiology. New York: Harper & Row 1967.— DESAI, S.C., BHAT. M.L.A.: Effect of griseofulvin on *T.rubrum* and *T.violaceum* infections. Arch. Derm. **81**, 849 (1960). ~ Studies on experimental infections with *T. rubrum* in humans and the mechanism of griseofulvin effect. J. invest. Derm. **35**, 297 (1960). — EMMONS, C.W., BINFORD, C.H., UTZ, J.P.: Medical mycology. Philadelphia: Lea & Febiger 1963. — ENGLISH, M.P., TURVEY, J.: Studies in the epidemiology of tinea pedis.

IX. Tinea pedis and erythrasma in new patients at a chiropody clinic. Brit. med. J. **4**, 228 (1968). — FISCHMAN, O.: Black piedra in Brazil. A contribution to its study in Manaus (State of Amazonas). Mycopathologia (Den Haag) **25**, 201 (1965). — FISHER, B.K., SMITH, J.G., JR., CROUNSE, R.G., ROTH, F.J., JR., BLANK, H.: Verrucous epidermophytosis. Its response and resistance to griseofulvin. Arch. Derm. **84**, 65 (1961). — FORESMAN, A.H., BLANK, F.: The location of the fluorescent matter in *Microsporon* infected hair. Mycopathologia (Den Haag) **31**, 314 (1967). — FRANKS, A.G., FRANK, S.B.: Extensive verrucous dermatitis associated with dermatophytosis and onychomycosis due to *Trichophyton gypseum*. Arch. Derm. **63**, 489 (1951). — FRANKS, A.G., GOLDFARB, N.: Erythrasma and tinea versicolor. Arch. Derm. **71**, 405 (1955). — GANS, O., STEIGLEDER, G.K.: Histologie der Hautkrankheiten (ed. 2). Berlin-Göttingen-Heidelberg: Springer 1957. — GEORG, L.K.: Studies on *Trichophyton tonsurans*. I. The taxonomy of *T.tonsurans*. Mycologia **48**, 65 (1956). — GEORG, L.K., DOUPAGNE, P., PATTYN, S.R., NEVES, H.: *Trichophyton yaoundei*. A dermatophyte indigenous to Africa. J. invest. Derm. **41**, 19 (1963). — GORDON, M.A.: The occurrence of dermatophyte, *Microsporum gypseum*, as a saprophyte in soil. J. invest. Derm. **20**, 201 (1953). — GÖTZ, H.: Zur Morphologie der Pilzelemente im Stratum corneum bei Tinea (Epidermophytia) pedis, Manus et inguinalis. Mycopathologia (Den Haag) **12**, 124 (1960). ~ Die Pilzkrankheiten der Haut durch Dermatophyten. In: JADASSOHN, Handbuch der Haut- und Geschlechtskrankheiten, Ergänzungswerk Vol. IV/3, MARCHIONINI and GÖTZ. Berlin-Göttingen-Heidelberg: Springer 1962. ~ Die Pilzkrankheiten der Haut durch Hefen, Schimmel, Actinomycetin und verwandte Erreger. In: JADASSOHN, Handbuch der Haut- und Geschlechtskrankheiten, Ergänzungswerk Vol. IV/4, MARCHIONINI and GÖTZ. Berlin-Göttingen-Heidelberg: Springer 1962. — GRAHAM, J.H., JOHNSON, W.C., BURGOON, C.F., JR., HELWIG, E.B.: Tinea capitis. Arch. Derm. **89**, 528 (1964). — GRAHAM, J.H., BLANK, F., JOHNSON, W.C., GRAY, H.R.: *Trichophyton rubrum* infections. A histopathological, histochemical and chemical study. Amer. J. Path. **46**, 34a (1965). — GRAHAM, J.H., WRIGHT, E.T., NEWCOMER, V.D., STERNBERG, T.H.: The use of nystatin as a topical antifungal agent. In: Therapy of fungus diseases. Ed. by STERNBERG and NEWCOMER. Boston: Little, Brown & Co. 1955. — GRAPPEL, S.F., BLANK, F., BISHOP, C.T.: Immunological studies on dermatophytes. IV. Chemical structures and serological reactivities of polysaccharides from *Microsporum praecox*, *Trichophyton ferrugineum*, *Trichophyton sabouraudii* and *Trichophyton tonsurans*. J. Bact. **97**, 23 (1969). — GRIDLEY, M.F.: A stain for fungi in tissue sections. Amer. J. clin. Path. **23**, 303 (1953). — GROCOTT, R.G.: A stain for fungi in tissue sections and smears using Gomori's methenamine silver nitrate technic. Amer. J. clin. Path. **25**, 975 (1955). — GRUBY, D.: Quoted from S.J. ZAKON and T. BENEDEK: "David Gruby and The Centenary of Medical Mycology, 1841—1941." Bull. Hist. Med. **16**, 155 (1944). — HALPRIN, K.M.: Diagnosis with Wood's light: Tinea capitis and erythrasma. J. Amer. med. Ass. **99**, 841 (1967). — HANUSOVA, S.: Pityriasis versicolor im Flächenbild. Arch. klin. exp. Derm. **215**, 33 (1962). ~ Onychomycosis im morphologischen Bild. I. Das Verhalten der Pilze im Nagelapparat. Arch. klin. exp. Derm. **227**, 1014 (1967). ~ Onychomycosis im morphologischen Bild. II. Reaktion des Nagelapparates auf die Anwesenheit von Pilzen. Arch. klin. exp. Derm. **227**, 1026 (1967). — HARRIS, J.H., LEWIS, G.M.: *Trichophyton purpureum* (Bang) as a deep invader of the skin. Report of a case. Arch. Derm. **22**, 1 (1930). — HAUSER, F.V., ROTHMAN, S.: Monilial granuloma. Report of a case and review of the literature. Arch. Derm. **61**, 297 (1950). — HELLIER, F.F., LATOUCHE, C.G., ROWELL, N.R.: Monilial granuloma treated by amphotericin B in a achondroplastic with bronchiectasis. Brit. J. Derm. **75**, 375 (1963). — HILDICK-SMITH, G., BLANK, H., SARKANY, I.: Fungus diseases and their treatment. Boston: Little, Brown & Co. 1964. — HITCH, J.M.: Piedra. Report of a fifth case originating in the U.S.A. Arch. Derm. **79**, 99 (1959). ~ Tinea nigra palmaris. Report of a case originating in North Carolina. Arch. Derm. **84**, 318 (1961). — HUTTER, R.V.P., COLLINS, H.S.: The occurrence of opportunistic fungus infections in a cancer hospital. Lab. Invest. **11** (part 2), 1035 (1962). — IMPERATO, P.J., BUCKLEY, C.E., III, CALLAWAY, J.L.: *Candida* granuloma. A clinical and immunologic study. Arch. Derm. **97**, 139 (1968). — JILLSON, O.F., BUCKLEY, W.R.: Fungous diseases in man acquired from cattle and horses (due to *Trichophyton faviforme*). New Engl. J. Med. **246**, 996 (1952). — JOHNSON, J.A., ROSENTHAL, S.A.: Superficial cutaneous infection with *Trichophyton soudanese*. Arch. Derm. **97**, 428 (1968). — JOHNSON, W.C.: Histochemistry of cutaneous ground substance. In: Methods and achievements in experimental pathology, Vol. I, ed. by BAJUSZ and JASMIN. Basel: S. Karger 1966. — KAPICA, L., BLANK, F.: Growth of *Candida albicans* on keratin as sole source of nitrogen. Dermatologica (Basel) **115**, 81 (1957). ~ Growth of *Candida parapsilosis* with keratin as sole source of nitrogen. Dermatologica (Basel) **117**, 433 (1958). — KAPLAN, W.: Piedra in lower animals. A case report of white piedra in a monkey and a review of the literature. J. Amer. vet. med. Ass. **134**, 113 (1959). ~ The occurrence of black piedra in primate pelts. Trop. geogr. Med. **11**, 115 (1959). — KEDDIE, F., SHADOMY, S.: Etiological significance of *Pityrosporum orbiculare* in tinea versicolor. Sabouraudia **3**, 21 (1963). — KLIGMAN, A.M.: The pathogenesis of tinea capitis due to *Microsporum audouini* and *Microsporum canis*. I. Gross observations following the inoculation of humans. J. invest. Derm. **18**,

231 (1952). ∼ Tinea capitis due to *M. audouini* and *M. canis*. II. Dynamics of host-parasite relationship. Arch. Derm. **71**, 313 (1955). — KLIGMAN, A. M., CONSTANT, E. R.: Family epidemic of tinea capitis due to *Trichophyton tonsurans* (variety *sulfureum*). Arch. Derm. **63**, 493 (1951). — KLIGMAN, A. M., MESCON, H., DELAMATER, E. D.: The Hotchkiss-McManus stain for the histopathologic diagnosis of fungus diseases. Amer. J. clin. Path. **21**, 86 (1951). — KOBLENZER, P. J., LOPRESTI, P. S., BLANK, F.: Non-fluorescent ringworm of the scalp due to *Trichophyton mentagrophytes* var. *granulosum*. Clin. Pediat. **6**, 217 (1967). — KUGELMAN, T. P., CRIPPS, D. J., HARRELL, E. R., JR.: *Candida* granuloma with epidermophytosis. Report of a case and review of the literature. Arch. Derm. **88**, 150 (1963). — LANE, C. G.: Tinea corporis (*Trichophyton purpureum*). Moniliasis of feet; ichthyosis. Arch. Derm. **40**, 119 (1939). — LANGERON, M.: Piedra. In: Nouvelle pratique dermatologique, Vol. II. Ed. by DARIER, SABOURAUD, GOUGEROT, MILIAN, PAUTRIER, RAVAUT, SEZARY and SIMON. Paris: Masson et Cie 1936. — LEEMING, J. A. L.: Tinea nigra. Brit. J. Derm. **75**, 392 (1963). — LEVER, W. F.: Histopathology of the skin (ed. 4). Philadelphia: J. B. Lippincott Co. 1967. — LEWIS, G. M., CORMIA, F. E.: Eosinophilic granuloma. Theoretic and practical considerations based on the study of a case. Arch. Derm. **55**, 176 (1947). — LEWIS, G. M., HOPPER, M. E., SCOTT, M. J.: Generalized *Trichophyton rubrum* infection associated with systemic lymphoblastoma. Report of three cases. Arch. Derm. **67**, 247 (1953). — LEWIS, G. M., HOPPER, M. E., WILSON, J. W., PLUNKETT, O. A.: An introduction to medical mycology (ed. 4). Chicago: The Year Book Publishers, Inc. 1958. — LEWIS, G. M., MONTGOMERY, R. M., HOPPER, M. E.: Cutaneous manifestations of *Trichophyton purpureum* (Bang). Arch. Derm. **37**, 823 (1938). — LILLIE, R. D.: Reactions of various parasitic organisms in tissues in the Bauer, Feulgen, Gram, and Gram-Weigert methods. J. Lab. clin. Med. **32**, 76 (1947). ∼ Histopathologic technic and practical histochemistry (ed. 3). New York: McGraw-Hill Book Co., Inc. 1968. — LUSCOMBE, H. A., BINGUL, O.: Nodular granulomatous perifolliculitis caused by *Microsporum gypseum*. Arch. Derm. **89**, 162 (1964). — MACKENNA, R. N. B., CALNAN, C. D.: *Trichophyton rubrum* infection. Brit. J. Derm. **66**, 411 (1954). — MACKENZIE, D. W. R.: "Hairbrush diagnosis" in detection and eradication of non-fluorescent scalp ringworm. Brit. med. J. **2**, 363 (1963). — MAJOCCHI, D.: Sopra una nuova tricofizia (granuloma trichofitico). Studi Clinicie Micologici. Bull. R. Acad. Med. Roma **9**, 220 (1883). ∼ Contribuzione clinica istologica et micologia sul granuloma tricofitico. G. ital. Mal. vener. **61**, 397 (1920). — MALE, O., HOLUBAR, K.: Comparative studies on the enzyme-histochemical behaviour of some dermatophytes. Part 1. *In vitro* investigations (saprophytic biophase). Mycopathologia (Den Haag) **35**, 150 (1968). ∼ Comparative studies on the enzyme histochemical behaviour of some dermatophytes. Part II. *In vivo* investigations (parasitic biophase). Mycopathologia (Den Haag) **35**, 161 (1968). — MANSON-BAHR, P. H.: Manson's tropical diseases. A manual of the diseases of warm climates (ed. 15). London: Cassell & Co., Ltd. 1960. — *Manual of Histologic Staining Methods*. The Armed Forces Institute of Pathology (ed. 3). American Registry of Pathology. Ed. by L. G. LUNA. New York: McGraw-Hill Book Co., Inc. 1968. — MARPLES, M. J.: The ecology of the human skin. Springfield/Ill.: Charles C. Thomas 1965. — McCAFFREE, D. L., FETHIÉRE, A., BLANK, F.: Dermatophytic flora of Philadelphia. Dermatologica (Basel) **138**, 115 (1969). — MEHREGAN, A. H., COSKEY, R. J.: Perforating folliculitis. Arch. Derm. **97**, 394 (1968). — MEHREGAN, A. H., SCHWARTZ, O. D., LIVINGOOD, C. S.: Reactive perforating collagenosis. Arch. Derm. **96**, 277 (1967). — MERCER, E. H., VERMA, B. S.: Hair digested by *Trichophyton mentagrophytes*. An electron microscopic examination. Arch. Derm. **87**, 357 (1963). — MERWIN, C. F.: Tinea nigra palmaris. Review of the literature and case report. Pediatrics **36**, 537 (1965). — MICHALOWSKI, R., RODZIEWICZ, H.: Pityriasis versicolor in children. Brit. J. Derm. **75**, 397 (1963). — MILES, W. J., BRANOM, W. T., JR., FRANK, S. B.: Tinea nigra. Report of two cases and results of treatment with tolnaftate. Arch. Derm. **94**, 203 (1966). — MONTES, L. F.: Fungi and fungal infections. In: Ultrastructure of normal and abnormal skin. Ed. by A. S. ZELICKSON. Philadelphia: Lea & Febiger 1967. — MONTES, L. F., DOBSON, H., DODGE, B. G., KNOWLES, W. R.: Erythrasma and diabetes mellitus. Arch. Derm. **99**, 674 (1969). — MONTGOMERY, H.: Dermatopathology. New York: Harper & Row, Publ., Inc. 1967. — MOORE, M.: Radiate formation on pathogenic fungi in human tissue. Arch. Path. **42**, 113 (1946). — MOORE, M., CRATLY, R. Q., LANE, C. W.: Cicatrizing tinea capitis caused by *Trichophyton rubrum (Trichophyton purpureum)*. Arch. Derm. **66**, 363 (1952). — MUNRO-ASHMAN, D., WELLS, R. S., CLAYTON, Y. M.: Erythrasma in adolescence. Brit. J. Derm. **75**, 401 (1963). — MYERS, R. J., HAMILTON, J. B.: Regeneration and rate of growth of hairs in men. Ann. N. Y. Acad. Sci. **53**, 562 (1951). — NELSON, L. M., McNIECE, K. J.: Recurrent Cushing's syndrome with *Trichophyton rubrum* infection. Arch. Derm. **80**, 700 (1959). — NEVES, H.: Mycological study of 519 cases of ringworm infections in Portugal. Significance of multiple localizations — Tinea as a single infection. Mycopathologia (Den Haag) **13**, Fasc. 2, 121 (1960). — NEVES, J. A., COSTA, O. G.: Tinea nigra. Arch. Derm. **55**, 67 (1947). ∼ Tinea nigra. In: Handbook of tropical dermatology and medical mycology, Vol. II. Ed. by SIMONS. Amsterdam: Elsevier 1953. — NEWCOMER, V. D.: The ease of identifying superficial fungus infections. Consultant **9**, 28 (1969). — NEWCOMER, V. D., WRIGHT, E. T., STERNBERG, T. H.:

A study of the host-parasite relationship of *Trichophyton mentagrophytes* and *Trichophyton rubrum* when introduced into the granuloma pouch of rats. J. invest. Derm. **23**, 359 (1954). — PARTRIDGE, B.M.: Multiple fungous infections with special reference to their occurrence with the *Trichophyton rubrum* syndrome. Trans. St John's Hosp. derm. Soc. (Lond.) **34**, 41 (1955). — PARTRIDGE, B.M., JACKSON, F.L.: The fluorescence of erythrasma. Brit. J. Derm. **74**, 326 (1962). — PATTERSON, J.C., LAINE, S.L., TAYLOR, W.B.: White piedra. Arch. Derm. **85**, 534 (1962). — PEARSE, A.G.E.: Histochemistry theoretical and applied (ed. 2). Boston: Little, Brown & Co. 1960. — PECK, S.M.: Epidermophytosis of the feet and epidermophytids of the hands. Arch. Derm. **22**, 40 (1930). — PERCIVAL, G.H., MONTGOMERY, G.L., DODDS, T.C.: Atlas of histopathology of the skin (ed. 2). Baltimore: Williams and Wilkins Co. 1962. — PICKETT, J.P., BISHOP, C.M., CHICK, E.W., BAKER, R.D.: A simple fluorescent stain for fungi. Selective staining of fungi by means of a fluorescent method for mucin. Amer. J. clin. Path. **34**, 197 (1960). — PIPKIN, J.L.: Tinea capitis in adult and adolescent. Arch. Derm. **66**, 9 (1952). — REID, B.J., SHIMKIN, M.B., BLANK, F.: Study of tinea capitis in Philadelphia using case and control groups. Publ. Hlth. Rep. (Wash.) **83**, 497 (1968). — REISS, F.: Successful inoculations of animals with *Trichophyton purpureum*. Arch. Derm. **49**, 242 (1944). — RIDDELL, R.W.: The pathogenesis of tinea capitis. In: Modern trends in dermatology, 2nd series. Ed. by MACKENNA. New York: Paul B. Hoeber 1954. — RIPPON, J.W.: Elastase production by ringworm fungi. Science **157**, 947 (1967). — RIPPON, J.W., LORINCZ, A.L.: Collagenase activity of *Streptomyces (Nocardia) madurae*. J. invest. Derm. **43**, 483 (1964). — RIPPON, J.W., VARADI, D.P.: The elastases of pathogenic fungi and actinomycetes. J. invest. Derm. **50**, 54 (1968). — RIPPON, J.W., ENG, A., MALKINSON, F.D.: *Trichophyton simi* infection in the United States. Arch. Derm. **98**, 615 (1968). — RITCHIE, E.B., TAYLOR, T.E.: A study of tinea nigra palmaris. Report of a case and inoculation experiments. Arch. Derm. **89**, 601 (1964). — ROTHMAN, S.: Systemic disturbances in recalcitrant *Trichophyton rubrum* (*purpureum*) infection). Studies and short report on therapeutic experiments. Arch. Derm. **67**, 239 (1953). ~ Some unusual forms of cutaneous moniliasis. Arch. Derm. **79**, 598 (1959). — SABOURAUD, R.J.A.: Les Teignes. Paris: Masson et Cie. 1910. — SAFERSTEIN, H.L., BLANK, F.: Tinea corporis caused by *Trichophyton mentagrophytes* var. *granulosum*. Mycopathologia (Den Haag) **31**, 267 (1967). — SAFERSTEIN, H.L., REID, B.J., BLANK, F.: Endothrix ringworm. A new public health problem in Philadelphia. J. Amer. med. Ass. **190**, 851 (1964). — SAFERSTEIN, H.L., STRACHAN, A.A., BLANK, F., BISHOP, C.T.: *Trichophyton* activity and polysaccharides. Dermatologica (Basel) **136**, 151 (1968). — SAGHER, F.: Histologic examinations of fungous infections of the nails. J. invest. Derm. **11**, 337 (1948). — SALTON, M.R.J.: The bacterial cell wall. Amsterdam: Elsevier 1964. — SARKANY, I., TAPLIN, D., BLANK, H.: Erythrasma — common bacterial infection of the skin. J. Amer. med. Ass. **177**, 130 (1961). ~ The etiology and treatment of erythrasma. J. invest. Derm. **37**, 283 (1961). ~ Incidence and bacteriology of erythrasma. Arch. Derm. **85**, 578 (1962). ~ Organism causing erythrasma. Lancet **2**, 304 (1962). ~ Erythrasma — a bacterial disease. In: Proceedings of the XII International Congress of Dermatology, Vol. II. Ed. by PILLSBURY and LIVINGOOD. Amsterdam: Excerpta Medica Foundation, Internat. Cong. Series No. 55, 1963. — SCHREIBER, M.M., SHAPIRO, S.I., BERRY, C.Z., DAHLEN, R.F.: *Trichophyton rubrum* perifollicular granuloma of legs. Cutis **3**, 1083 (1967). — SCOTT, M.J.: Piedra. Report of a case. Arch. Derm. **64**, 767 (1951). — SEQUEIRA, J.H.: A case of trichophytic granulomata. Brit. J. Derm. **24**, 207 (1912). — SHANON, J., RAUBITSCHEK, F.: Tinea faciei simulating chronic discoid lupus erythematosus. Arch. Derm. **82**, 268 (1960). — SHELLEY, W.B., OHMAN, S.: Technique for cross sectioning hair specimens. J. invest. Derm. **52**, 533 (1969). — SIMONS, R.D.G.: Piedra and piedraia. In: Handbook of tropical dermatology and medical mycology, Vol. II. Ed. by SIMONS. Amsterdam: Elsevier 1953. — SLEPYAN, A.H., GEUTING, B.G.: Tinea nigra palmaris in the Chicago area. Arch. Derm. **76**, 570 (1957). — SMITH, J.G., JR., SAMS, W.M., ROTH, F.J., JR.: Tinea nigra palmaris. A disorder easily confused with junction nevus of the palm. J. Amer. med. Ass. **167**, 312 (1958). — STERNBERG, T.H., TARBET, J.E., NEWCOMER, V.D., WINER, L.H.: Deep infection of mice with *Trichophyton rubrum* (*purpureum*). J. invest. Derm. **19**, 373 (1952). — STRACHAN, A.A., BLANK, F.: On 1117 *Microsporum canis* infections in Montreal (1954—1961). Dermatologica (Basel) **126**, 271 (1963). — SWARTZ, J.H., CONANT, N.F.: Extensive lichenified eruption caused by *Trichophyton rubrum*. Arch. Derm. **42**, 614 (1940). — TAPLIN, D., BLANK, H.: Microscopic morphology of *Trichophyton rubrum*. J. invest. Derm. **37**, 523 (1961). — TELNER, P., BLANK, F., SCHOPFLOCHER, P.: *Trichophyton rubrum* infections of the lower legs. Canad. med. Ass. J. **77**, 1033 (1957). — TEMPLE, D.E., BOARDMAN, C.R.: The incidence of erythrasma of the toewebs. Arch. Derm. **86**, 518 (1962). — THOMPSON, K.W.: Relationship of dermatomycoses to certain peripheral vascular infections. Int. Clin. **2**, 156 (1941). ~ Skin-reacting antigen of *Trichophyton purpureum* and its relation to peripheral vascular disorders. J. invest. Derm. **5**, 475 (1942). — TOLMACH, J.A., SCHWEIG, J.: Generalized *Trichophyton purpureum* infection simulating dermatitis herpetiformis. Report of a case. Arch. Derm. **41**, 732 (1940). — VANVELSOR, H., SINGLETARY, H.: Tinea nigra palmaris. A report of 15 cases from coastal North Carolina. Arch. Derm. **90**, 59 (1964). — WAIS-

MAN, M.: *Trichophyton rubrum* infection simulating erythema perstans. J. invest. Derm. **22**, 237 (1954). — WEARY, P. E.: Pityrosporum ovale. Observations on some aspects of host-parasite interrelationship. Arch. Derm. **98**, 408 (1968). — WEARY, P. E., CANBY, C. M.: Keratinolytic activity of *Trichophyton schoenleinii*, *Trichophyton rubrum* and *Trichophyton mentagrophytes*. J. invest. Derm. **48**, 240 (1967). — WEARY, P. E., CANBY, C. M., CAWLEY, E. P.: Keratinolytic activity of *Microsporum canis* and *Microsporum gypseum*. J. invest. Derm. **44**, 300 (1965). — WEBER, W. E., ULRICH, J. A.: Kerion caused by *Trichophyton rubrum*. Report of two cases. Arch. Derm. **66**, 624 (1952). — WEINER, A. L., GOLDMAN, L.: Localized urticarial reaction associated with *Trichophyton rubrum* infections of the skin. Cutis **3**, 59 (1967). — WHITE, C. J., LAIPPLY, T. C.: Diseases of the nails. 792 cases. Clinical and microscopical findings with resume of newer therapeutic methods. Industr. Med. Surg. **27**, 325 (1958). — WILLIAMS, D. I.: Griseofulvin and *Trichophyton rubrum* infections. Arch. Derm. **81**, 769 (1960). — WILSON, J. W.: Trichophyton granuloma (tinea profunda) due to *Trichophyton rubrum*. Arch. Derm. **65**, 375 (1952). — WILSON, J. W., PLUNKETT, O. A.: The fungous diseases of Man. Berkley and Los Angeles: University of California Press 1965. — WILSON, J. W., PLUNKETT, O. A., GREGERSEN, A.: Nodular granulomatous perifolliculitis of the legs caused by *Trichophyton rubrum*. Arch. Derm. **69**, 258 (1954). — WIRTH, J. C., ANAND, S. R.: The fatty acids of *Trichophyton rubrum*. Canad. J. Microbiol. **10**, 23 (1964). — WIRTH, J. C., BEESLEY, T., MILLER, W.: The isolation of a unique sterol from the mycelium of a strain of *Trichophyton rubrum*. J. invest. Derm. **37**, 153 (1961). — WIRTH, J. C., O'BRIEN, P. J., SCHMITT, F. L., SOHLER, A.: The isolation in crystalline form of some of the pigments of *Trichophyton rubrum*. J. invest. Derm. **29**, 47 (1957). — YAFFEE, H. S., GROTS, I. A.: Tinea nigra "plantaris." Arch. Derm. **91**, 153 (1965). — YU, R. J., HARMON, S. R., BLANK, F.: Isolation and purification of an extracellular keratinase of *Trichophyton mentagrophytes*. J. Bact. **96**, 1435 (1968).

Cryptococcosis*

K. Salfelder, Mérida, Venezuela

With 68 Figures

Definition

Busse-Buschke's disease, earlier referred to also as torulosis, European blasto-mycosis, and other terms, is a deep, visceral, systemic, or generalized mycosis caused by the fungus *Cryptococcus neoformans* (Sanfelice) Vuillemin, 1901. Cryptococcosis has been reported from almost all countries of the world and is the most frequent systemic mycosis found in man in Europe (Matheis).

The incidence of cryptococcosis appears to be increasing, especially in association with malignant disorders of the lymphoreticuloendothelial system, and in patients treated with certain drugs. In man, cryptococcosis is more frequently found as a complication of other diseases than are many other systemic mycoses; and has been found in many species of domestic and wild animals.

The fungus is widespread and has been isolated from many nonliving sites, including fruit juice and milk. The infection seems to be disseminated by airborne organisms from soil, especially from soil rich in organic material. Bird excreta, particularly that from pigeons (Emmons, 1951, 1955), are often found to harbor the fungus, yet, paradoxically, the disease has not been found in these birds. Data on epidemiologic factors are so far not available.

C. neoformans is a spherical, yeastlike organism, usually single budding, which measures from 4—20 μ in tissues and cultures and is not dimorphic. Its main characteristic is a thick, mucinous capsule, a pattern unique in pathogenic fungi, but not present in all strains and occasionally seen only in a few organisms. It grows rapidly on current culture media at room temperature and at 37°C.

Several biochemical reactions distinguish this fungus from other nonpathogenic organisms.

The portal of entry is now almost unanimously believed to be the respiratory tract, from which hematogenous spread occurs. Although all organs and tissues can be involved, there is a strong neurotropic tendency, foci in the brain and especially the meninges being most frequent.

The tissue reaction is pleomorphic; grossly, gelatinous lesions or circumscribed granulomas are seen. Microscopically, in the former the solid tissue is replaced by numerous organisms forming a sort of colony. The *gelatinous aspect* is due to the mucinous capsular material of the numerous organisms also found invading the tissue. Cellular response consists principally of macrophages and scattered lympholeukocytes, with occasional giant cells. The circumscribed foci are tuberculoid granulomas generally containing fewer organisms. Marked leukocytic reaction, coagulation necrosis, and calcification do not occur. Scar formation is seen occasionally. The lack of formation of calcified residual foci does not permit

---

* The manuscript of this chapter was finished and delivered March 1968; bibliography is considered only up to this date.

clinical diagnosis of subclinical forms. The mucinous capsule is diagnostic for this fungus. Symptoms depend on organic localization. The course of disease can be of long duration and remissions occur. No drug other than amphotericin B has been found effective in therapy, although, as will be discussed later, its administration is not entirely without risk. Surgical removal of localized foci in lung, bone, skin, and brain has frequently been successful, often concomitantly with chemotherapy. Prognosis is generally better than in earlier years but is still poor when the nervous system is affected or when no treatment is given.

History

Otto Busse (Fig. 1) reported to the Greifswald Medical Society on July 7, 1894, a case of a 31-year-old woman with a leg lesion suspected to be a giant cell sarcoma. He had noticed some small, brilliant bodies in this tissue. When these bodies, at the suggestion of Grawitz, were treated with sodium hydroxide, their resistance to such treatment suggested their fungal nature and a pure culture was obtained on prune juice medium. Busse called them *Hefe* (saccharomyces), and named the disease saccharomycosis hominis. This patient died later with disseminated lesions in skin, bones, and viscera.

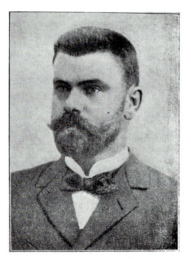

Fig. 1. Otto Busse (1867—1922) ca. 1900

Busse was at this time assistant in the Department of Pathology in Greifswald under Grawitz, himself a long-time assistant of Rudolf Virchow. While Grawitz's name is generally linked with renal cell carcinoma (Grawitz's tumor, hypernephroma), he was also much interested in bacteriologic and mycologic studies, which must have influenced Busse.

Buschke, at the same time a resident in surgery in Greifswald, also obtained cultures of these organisms. In a letter to Busse he acknowledged that his experiments were made with knowledge of Busse's original work; therefore there is no reason to consider Buschke as co-discoverer of the disease.

About this time (1894), Sanfelice isolated, from peach juice, yeastlike organisms which he called *Saccharomyces neoformans*, and was able to elicit with them experimental disease in animals. The term *neoformans* was added to *Cryptococcus* in the belief that the fungi were a possible cause of neoplasm (Sanfelice, 1898). However, as early as 1902, Nichols concluded "there is no evidence that blastomycetes have anything to do with the production of human cancers," the term blastomyces referring also to *Cryptococcus neoformans*. In spite of this statement, neoformans has been retained. The generic term *Cryptococcus* for this fungus was adopted by Vuillemin (1901), since lacking ascospores, the organisms were not true yeasts. In 1902 the fungus was isolated from a myxomatous lung lesion of a horse (FROTHINGHAM); later spontaneous disease was also proved in other species of lower animals. Soon afterwards v. HANSEMANN (1905) described the first case of cryptococcal meningitis with lesions which mimicked tuberculous meningitis and showed gelatinous cysts. Until 1914 single cases were found and diagnosed only at necropsies. VERSÉ described at this time the first human cryptococcosis of the nervous system diagnosed clinically.

Later (1916), STODDARD and CUTLER called the causative agent *Torula histolytica* because a histolytic effect of the organisms was assumed which was thought to lead to cyst formation and produce the gelatinous aspect of tissue lesions. However, it is now well known that there is no histolysis. The organisms are localized in the tissue in and outside of macrophages, forming a kind of colony when present in large numbers. The cystlike and gelatinous appearance is caused by breakdown of tissue in these areas and the great amount of mucous material in the capsules of the numerous organisms and in the spaces between them. *Cryptococcus* was early differentiated mycologically, clinically, and pathologically from the causative agents of the blastomycoses (STODDARD and CUTLER, 1916; BENHAM, 1935). Nevertheless the term European blastomycosis has been preserved by many students of the disease; actually, more cases are reported from other continents than from Europe.

The organism was first classified in 1952 as *Cryptococcus neoformans* by LODDER and KREGER-VAN RIJ; this designation has become generally accepted.

In 1954, HAUGEN and BAKER demonstrated small healing pulmonary foci in healthy persons. Successive similar findings led to the assumption of a subclinical form of the disease, a silent or asymptomatic infection, which may occur more frequently than can be definitely confirmed at this moment, since such means of proof as reliable serologic and skin tests are still not available. In addition, ZIMMERMAN and RAPPAPORT (1954) called attention to the frequent association of cryptococcosis with debilitating diseases, especially malignant disorders of the lymphatic system; this was stressed soon afterwards also by LITTMAN and ZIMMERMAN.

Although earlier monographs had dealt with cryptococcosis, the latter two authors wrote an excellent monograph (1956) with special reference to pathology and laboratory studies based on the examination of more than 100 cases and the review of more than 500 references. In this monograph, the best so far available, the respiratory system as the portal of entry of the fungus was emphasized. In the same year SEELIGER reported on the urease test for diagnostic recognition.

Incidence

The exact number of published cases of cryptococcosis is impossible to ascertain, since the same cases may be reported several times by different authors and in different papers, focusing on special points of view. Further, there are undoubtedly many unpublished cases, since in most countries, including Great Britain and the U.S.A., the disease is not notifiable. Table 1 includes published reports concerning series of more than 10 cases. A glance reveals the increasing incidence of reported cases, especially in the last 20 years. In 1925, only 15 cases were recorded; in 1956, more than 300. Fatalities in the USA alone from 1952 to 1963 totalled nearly 800; the annual occurrence of cryptococcal meningitis in the USA in 1964 was estimated at from 200—300. FETTER et al. (1967) referred to more than 500 case reports of cryptococcosis of the central nervous system. Our bibliography includes some 550 cases, representing about half of the published cases. Table 2 lists incidence by countries. There are no remarkable differences related to occupation, with the exception of pigeon breeders, who, as may be expected, are at special risk. As with other mycoses, a higher frequency of cryptococcosis is found in males than in females. The disease is more frequent in the fourth to the sixth decades of life. However, an increasing number of cases in children up to 15 years of age are reported:

Table 1. *Important casuistic reports and reviews*

Author(s), Country, Year of report	Period	Form and localiz. disease	Country occurrence	Own	No. of cases referred to
1. Shapiro and Neal, USA (1925)	—	—	—	—	15
2. Freeman, USA (1931)	up to 1931	CNS	—	—	43
3. Levin, USA (1937)	up to 1937	CNS	—	—	60
4. Binford, USA (1941)	up to 1941	CNS	—	1	70
5. Cox and Tolhurst, Australia (1946)	up to 1946	—	Australia and world	13	120
6. Mosberg and Arnold, USA (1950)	up to 1950	CNS	—	5	172
7. Collins et al., USA (1951) . .	—	—	—	—	241
8. Evans and Harrell, USA (1952)	up to 1952	—	—	—	221
9. Symmers, England (1953) . .	up to 1946	—	—	—	200
10. Zimmerman and Rappaport, USA (1954)	20 years	—	USA	60	—
11. Baker and Haugen, USA (1955)	—	—	USA	26	—
12. Jacobsen, Germany (1955) . .	—	—	Germany	—	14
13. Grasset, France (1955) . . .	—	—	—	—	350
14. Geaney et al., Australia (1956)	—	—	Australia	14	—
15. Littman and Zimmerman, USA (1956)	up to 1955	—	—	over 100	over 300
16. Plummer and Symmers, England (1957)	up to 1957	—	England	1	19
17. Wolfe and Jacobson, USA ('58)	1945—1956	—	—	21	—
18. McCullough, USA (1958) . .	annually	—	USA		50 deaths
19. Yasaki, Japan (1959)	1948—1957	—	Japan	5	24
20. Seeliger, Germany (1959) . .	—	—	—	—	500
21. Littman and Schneierson, USA (1959)	—	subclinical forms	New York City	Estimated 5000—15000	
22. Brandt, Germany (1959) . . .	up to 1959	—	Germany	1	16
23. Matheis, Germany (1960). . .	up to 1960	—	Germany Europe World	3 — —	17 107 550
24. Rook and Woods, England (1962)	up to 1962	—	England	—	21
25. Hickie and Walker, Australia (1964)	—	—	—	10	—
26. Utz et al., USA (1964)	annually	meningitis	USA	Estimated 200—300	
27. Butler et al., USA (1964) . .	1956—1962	meningitis	USA	40	—
28. Atlanta, USA (1965)	1952—1963	all fatalities	USA	—	788
29. Sauerteig, Venezuela (1966)	up to 1966	—	Venezuela	7	30[1]
30. Symmers, England (1967). . .	1947—1967	18 systemic	England	—	56[2]
31. Fetter et al., USA (1967) . .	—	CNS	—	over 500	
32. Salfelder and Schwarz, USA (1967)	—	—	USA	13	—

CNS = central nervous system.
1 Many unpublished cases.
2 Partly unpublished cases.

Baker and Haugen; Barlow; Berger et al.; Bubb; Butler et al.; Carton and Mount; Cloward; Cornish et al.; Cox and Tolhurst; D'Aunoy and Lafferty; Debré et al., 1946, 1947, 1948; Dormer et al.; Dormer and Findlay; Emanuel et al.; Fisher; Geaney et al.; Gosling and Gilmer; Greening and Menville; Hamilton and Thomson; Hickie and Walker; Hooft et al.; Hutter and Collins; Kwan; Lamardo; Lepau et al.; Longmire and Goodwin; Marshall and Teed; McMath and Hussain; Mider et al.; Monnet et al.; Nanda et al.; Reeves et al.; Sauerteig; Shah and Sharma; Siewers and Cramblett; Soysal et al.; Spicer et al.; Unat et al.; Wen et al.; Zimmerman and Rappaport.

Table 2. *Case reports of cryptococcosis from different countries*

Continent	Country	Author(s)
America	Argentina	Niño, 1934, 1938, 1947; Peroncini et al.
	Brasil	Almeida et al., 1944; Lacaz; Mendonca Cortes
	Canada	Bakerspigel et al.; Butas and Lloyd-Smith
	Chile	Vargas
	Colombia	Buitrago-Garcia and Gomez Arango
	Cuba	Curbelo et al.; Tiant and Fuentes
	Mexico	Reyes Armijo and Alamanza Velez
	Panama	Herrera et al.
	Paraguay	Riveros et al.
	Peru	Cableses-Molina et al.
	Puerto Rico	Ramos-Morales et al.
	Uruguay	Almeida, 1961
	USA	Littman and Zimmerman
	Venezuela	Sauerteig
Europe	Austria	Kohlmeier and Niel
	Belgium	Hooft et al.
	Czechoslovakia	Krejčí and Vaněček
	Denmark	Jensen
	England	Symmers, 1953; Rook and Woods; Rippey et al.
	Finland	Sonck
	France	Debré et al., 1946; Drouhet et al., 1961
	Germany	Brandt; Jacobsen; Mahnke et al.; Matheis
	Hungary	Molnar
	Italy	Reale
	Netherlands	Ruiter and Ensink
	Norway	Voss
	Poland	Zawirska and Derubska
	Spain	Rodriguez de Ledesma and Gonzalez Alguacil
	Sweden	Bergman and Linell; Frisk and Holmgren
	Switzerland	Hoigne et al.; Mumenthaler
	USSR	Chominsky
Asia	Cambodia	Brumpt and Moisant
	Ceylon	Jayewardene and Wijekoon
	China	Cheng; Kwan; Singer; Wu-Fei
	Hong Kong	Huang et al.
	India	Ahuja et al.; Aikat et al.; Anguli and Natarajan; Balkrishna and Lilauwala
	Indonesia	Soemiatno
	Israel	Brandstaetter and Levitus
	Japan	Kinoshita et al.; Mashiba et al.; Ogawa et al.
	Malaya	Lim Teong Wah and Chan Kok Ewe; Muir and Ransome
	Turkey	Soysal et al.; Unat et al.
Africa	Congo	Stijns and Royer; Vandepitte et al.
	Egypt	Cossery
	French Equatorial Africa	Ravisse et al.
	Kenya	Nevill and Cooke, Turner
	Senegal	Collomb and Cadillon
	South Africa	Dormer et al.; Bubb
Australia and Oceania	Australia	Cox and Tolhurst; Hickie and Walker
	Hawaii	Cloward
	New Guinea	Champness and Clezy
	New Zealand	Smith, F.; Willis et al.
	Philippines	Aragon and Reyes

Of the more than 50 pediatric cases reported, the youngest child was under age one (Cloward). Cases of neonatal and infantile cryptococcosis are discussed later (Pathogenesis).

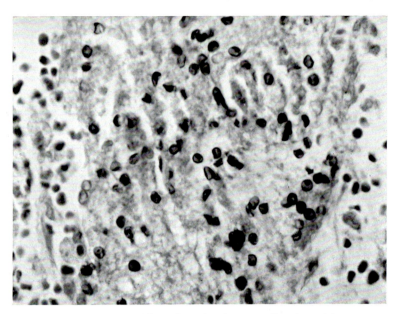

Fig. 2. Cryptococcic meningitis without lung involvement. Pauciparasitic pneumocystosis. Typical organisms filling a lung alveolus. Grocott, × 720

Associated Diseases

Coexisting disease is more frequent in cryptococcal meningitis than in pulmonary cryptococcosis (Campbell, Spickard et al.) (Fig. 2). While in many instances this may be a matter of simple coincidence, frequent coexistence of cryptococcosis and disorders of the reticuloendothelial and lymphatic systems suggests the factors of predisposition and increased susceptibility to the proliferation of the mycosis.

As will be seen in Table 3, there is a significant relationship between *cryptococcosis* and the *leucemic and lymphomatous disorders*; Hutter and Collins have reported the incidence of concomitancy to be as high as 80%.

Tissue reaction in Boeck's sarcoidosis is similar to that of cryptococcosis and other granulomatous diseases. Harris et al. (1965) reviewed 11 cases of sarcoidosis and cryptococcosis and added one of their own. The possible etiologic role of *Cryptococcus* in the production of granulomata of sarcoidosis has been suspected (Collins et al.; Fisher; Shields and discussion of three cases including one of Symmers by Littman and Zimmerman). However, to suppose that the mycosis is responsible for provoking such other nosologic entities as *sarcoidosis* seems rather hypothetical.

Shields supposes an immunoresponse to fungus invasion, perhaps modified by therapy. The morphologically minded students of diseases will reject the diagnosis of sarcoidosis when causal agents are found, reserving the denomination of sarcoidosis with misgivings for granulomatous diseases of unidentifiable etiology. This is specially indicated in cases in which diagnosis of sarcoidosis is based on examination of a single lymph node, the patient later showing lung lesions and proven cryptococcal meningitis which responded to amphotericin B therapy (Hess).

Whether the increased susceptibility to cryptococcosis is a result of *therapy* which damages the reticuloendothelial tissue is not clarified (Zimmerman and

Table 3. *Conditions reportedly coexistent with cryptococcosis*

Condition	References
Anemia, aplastic	BUTLER et al. (1 case)
Diabetes mellitus	BUTLER et al. (8 cases); COLMERS et al.; DROUHET and MARTIN; GENDEL et al.; KNUDSON et al.; RUBIN and FURCOLOW; SPICKARD et al.; ZIMMERMAN and RAPPAPORT
Fungus disease, other (candidosis, histoplasmosis, nocardiosis, coccidioidomycosis, paracoccidioidomycosis)	ANGULO ORTEGA et al.; LEOPOLD; MIDER et al.; MOSBERG and ARNOLD; RODGER et al.; ZIMMERMAN and RAPPAPORT
Hodgkin's disease[1]	BROOKS et al.; BUTLER et al.; COHEN; DEBRÉ et al. (1946, 1948); DROUHET (1964); FITCHETT and WEIDMAN; FREEMAN and WEIDMAN; GENDEL et al. (14 Hodgkins/165 crypto.); GORDON and VEDDER; HEINE et al.; HICKIE and WALKER; HOFFMEISTER; JACKSON and PARKER; JACOBSEN; LAAS and GEIGER; LITTMAN and ZIMMERMAN; MISCH; NICHOLS and MARTIN; OWEN; RODGER et al.; SALFELDER and SCHWARZ; SMITH, F.; SYMMERS (1957); SYMMERS, 1967 (8 Hodgkins/56 crypto.); TORREY; ZIMMERMAN and RAPPAPORT (18 crypto./1000 Hodgkins)
Hepatic cirrhosis	BAKER; MACGILLIVRAY; tenBERG and KUIPERS; ZIMMERMAN and RAPPAPORT
Leukemia[2, 3]	ATKINSON et al.; BUTTER et al.; GORDON and VEDDER; HERSH et al. (2 crypto./48 leuko.); HICKIE and WALKER; KURLANDER; SALFELDER and SCHWARZ; SIEWERS and FRAMBLETT; SYMMERS (1967); ZELMAN et al.; ZIMMERMAN and RAPPAPORT
Lupus erythematosus	KINOSHITA et al.; PARISER et al.; SALFELDER and SCHWARZ (2 cases); ZIMMERMAN and RAPPAPORT
Lymphoma (n.s.)	CASAZA et al. (4 crypto./139 lympho.); SYMMERS 1967 (13 crypto./1067 lympho.)
Lymphosarcoma	BRANDT; DROUHET (1964); DROUHET et al.; HAUGEN and BAKER; RUBIN and FURCOLOW; SALFELDER and SCHWARZ; SYMMERS (1953); SYMMERS, 1967 (3 lympho./56 crypto.)
Myasthenia gravis	ROWLAND et al.
Myeloma, multiple	ZIMMERMAN and RAPPAPORT
Pneumocystosis	SALFELDER and SCHWARZ (s. lung crypto. — Fig. 2); WINSLOW and HATHAWAY (c. lung crypto.)
Proteinosis, alveolar	BERGMAN and LINNEL; ROSEN et al.
Reticulum cell sarcoma	SYMMERS, 1967 (2 reticulo./56 crypto.)
Sarcoidosis	BERNARD and OWENS; BUTLER et al.; COLLINS et al.; FISHER; HARRIS et al.; HELLER et al.; HESS; McCULLOUGH et al.; PLUMMER et al.; SHIELDS; SONCK; SYMMERS, 1967 (5 sarcoid./56 crypto.)
Silicosis	BUTLER et al.; FITZPATRICK et al.
Thrombocytopenia, idiopathic	BUTLER et al. (1 case)
Thymoma	ROWLAND et al.
Tuberculosis	BUTLER et al.; CORPE and PARR; DEMME and MUMME; EMANUEL et al.; FITZPATRICK et al.; MAGRUDER; McCONCHIE; RUBIN and FURCOLOW; TABER; TÜRK; V. HANSEMANN; VERSÉ; WEBB and BIGGS; WOLFE and JACOBSON; ZIMMERMAN and RAPPAPORT

1 Reports from HORDER et al. and from TRIMBLE regarding isolation of *Cryptococcus* in 17 of 23 and in 5 of 26 cases, respectively, of Hodgkin's disease, confirmed only by culture, lack therefore proof of pathogenicity. The theories that cryptococcus, or derived products, are etiologic agents in Hodgkin's disease (BURGER and MORTON; COX and TOLHURST), and that tissue reactions are similar in cryptococcosis and Hodgkin's disease (BURGER and MORTON; COLLINS et al.; COX and TOLHURST; FITCHETT and WEIDMAN; GENDEL et al.; OWEN) have never been proved.

2 ZIMMERMAN and RAPPAPORT found 18 cases (30%) of 60 cases of cryptococcosis to be associated with leukemia or lymphomas. HUTTER and COLLINS reported that 80% of all malignancies associated with cryptococcosis belonged to the leucemic or lymphomatous group.

3 In 185 autopsies of cryptococcosis, BERGMAN found no associated malignancies.

Rappaport). X-ray, nitrogen mustard, urethan, immunorepressive drugs, and steroids are considered possible factors.

Cases of cryptococcosis after *steroid therapy* are reported by Lauze; Goldstein and Rambo; Linden and Steffen; MacGillivray; Alajouanine and Grasset; Burns; Gordon and Vedder; Hess, Ruiter and Ensink; Kalsbeek and Planteydt; tenBerg and Kuipers; Utz and Andriole. Experimentally, a negative influence of steroids has been noted (Truant and Tesluk; Levine et al., 1957; Sethi et al.; Koenigsbauer). Depletion of bone marrow was twice noted after treatment with steroids in the series of Zimmerman and Rappaport.

As associated diseases must be mentioned also secondary bacterial infections. Hickie and Walker report staphylococcal pneumonia with a case of crypto-coccosis, and coexistent bacterial pneumonia was noted in a case (Salfelder and Schwarz) in which the pneumonia had modified the inflammatory reaction in and around the cryptococcal foci.

Epidemiology

Habitat: *Cryptococcus neoformans* was isolated from juices of various fruits as early as 1894 and 1895 by Sanfelice and by Klein (1901), and later by Carter and Young from milk. It has also been found in soil (Emmons, 1951; Ajello, 1958; Frey and Durie; Silva; Kolukanow and Vojtsekhovskii (a); Sotgiu et al.), in wood (McDonough et al.; Salfelder et al.), and in exudates of mesquite in Arizona; other plants lacked the fungus (Evenson and Lamb). Emmons (1955) was the first to discover the fungus in pigeon nests and droppings. Since then it has been isolated from bird nests and excrement in many parts of the USA (Halde and Fraher; Hasenclever and Emmons; Kao and Schwarz; Littman and Schneierson; Muchmore et al.; Procknow et al.; Swatek et al.; Emmons, 1960), South America (Silva and Paula; Salfelder et al.); in Europe (Bergman; Fragner; Hajsig and Curcija; Kolukanow and Vojtsekhovskii (b); Partridge and Winner; Randhawa et al., Staib (a and e); Wiebecke and Staib); Asia (Ishida and Sato; Yamamoto et al.); and Australia-Oceania (Frey and Durie). Baum and Artis isolated two strains of *C. neoformans* from the surfaces of open caves with evidence of bat inhabitation in Israel.

A plausible explanation for the relationship between bird excreta and *C. neoformans* was provided by Staib (f), who found that only *C. neoformans*, among the *Cryptococcus* family or other yeasts, utilized creatinine as a nitrogen source. The association of bird excreta and *C. neoformans* is, however, an indirect one. Spontaneous disease has not been observed in birds, nor, apparently, do they act as carriers. The supposition is general that high body temperature of birds (e.g., pigeons 42—44°C) prevents development of the organisms in birds and in such other animals as rabbits (Kuhn). However, experimentally Littman et al. (1965) and Sethi and Schwarz (1966) succeeded in infecting pigeons, the former by the intracerebral route, the latter by intraocular injection. If organisms in excess of 30×10^6 were injected intracerebrally, dissemination to internal organs was accomplished, with recovery of the organisms from many viscera and with demonstration of tissue reaction in the form of granulomas or abscesses. In the eye, violent granulomatous response was the rule (Sethi and Schwarz, 1966). On the contrary, after feeding canaries with *C. neoformans*, Staib (d) did not succeed in obtaining infection. However, the yeasts were excreted in a viable state as long as eight days after feeding.

Transmission: Although cryptococcosis has been found as a spontaneous infection in many lower animals (Cf. chapter X), no proved cases of transmission from animal to animal or from animal to man have been reported. Theoretically there is a possibility of transmission, since the fungus has been isolated from the intestinal tract of horses, and cryptococcal mastitis in cows occurs in epidemic form in dairy herds (EMMONS, 1952; INNES et al.; POUNDEN et al.; SIMON et al.; AJELLO, 1967; SCHOLER et al.).

Infection from man to man, apparently does not occur with *C. neoformans*, for reasons not at all clear. Only one recent report could be found (HICKIE and WALKER) which mentioned a "reasonable possibility that the infection had been transmitted from patient to patient in one case" in a series of ten.

A 62-year-old female, who died from chronic lymphatic leukemia, had long been treated with steroids and developed cryptococcal meningitis. She had been hospitalized in a room separated by a narrow corridor from one in which a 57-year-old male patient had been treated two months before for pulmonary and cutaneous cryptococcosis, with many organisms in sputum and in smears from skin lesions. Both patients shared the same nursing personnel.

Sources of infection: Some human infections may be endogenous, the organisms being derived from formerly saprophytic fungi which live on or in healthy persons. Pathogenic strains of cryptococci have been isolated from different sites of human beings (BENHAM, 1935).

Nonpathogenic varieties of cryptococci have been found in large numbers on the skin and in the intestinal tract (BENHAM and HOPKINS; FELSENFELD). Some such strains are now referred to as *C. neoformans* var. innocuous (LITTMAN and ZIMMERMAN).

It is most likely that human disease occurs generally by infection from sites with heavy concentrations of fungi, as in avian habitats. In these deposits EMMONS (1962) found concentrations of 50 million viable *C. neoformans* cells per gram of dry fecal material (pigeon manure).

While the majority of investigators emphasize that the fungus occurs predominantly in dry pigeon droppings (SETHI, 1967a), GRAY and CHODOSH claim isolation also from freshly dropped feces from recently caught wild pigeons. Since the fecal material collected by pigeon breeders in the USA is considered an excellent fertilizer, this material is distributed semi-commercially, and conduces to contamination of garden soil, creating new potential sources of infection. AJELLO (1967) postulates that fungus cells from any source are carried by wind currents to avian droppings where the creatinine-rich environment favors growth and multiplication. Avian habitats become in this way prime sources of human and animal infection. This view is supported by the experience that sera from pigeon breeders are substantially more reactive to serologic antibody demonstration than controls (WALTER and ATCHISON). Circumstantial evidence has been brought forward in recent years which deals with human cases of cryptococcosis (LITTMAN, 1959). MUCHMORE et al. observed three cases of cryptococcal meningitis within a period of one year in a single small community, and were able to isolate in the environment of each of these patients *C. neoformans* from bird droppings and other material. From each of the counties of the State of Oklahoma (USA), where *C. neoformans* was cultured from soil, clinical cases were reported; 12 cases occurred in 25 years (MUCHMORE, 1967). PROCKNOW et al. report one human infection acquired by inhalation of infected pigeon excreta. Also SYMMERS (1967) calls attention to the bird excreta which existed in the neighborhood of a hospital where six cases of cryptococcosis in patients with debilitating diseases had been observed. YAMAMOTO et al. finally established a relationship between pigeon habitats and a case of pulmonary cryptococcosis in a cat.

Immunology and Serology: Reliable skin tests for *C. neoformans* are not yet available. SEELIGER (1964) states that skin tests with killed cells, filtrates, and polysaccharides of the fungus cells are questionable. BENNET et al. (1955) reported nonspecific reactions in normal patients with skin test antigens which had been considered positive by Salvin and Smith (1961).

Until recently, lack of specificity rendered serologic tests useless for diagnostic and prognostic purposes. Emmons (1960) questioned the specificity of such tests, referring especially to the case of Heller et al. Seeliger (1964) considered that the value of serologic tests remained to be explored.

However, based on the serologic behavior of capsule antigens, classification of *C.neoformans* into three capsule types (A, B and C) has been made (Evans, 1950; Evans and Kessel, 1951). Antigen has been confirmed by Neill et al. (1951) in one patient by the complement fixation test (CFT) and precipitation in spinal fluid, blood, and urine. Anderson and Beech (1958) reported a positive CFT in liquid material (capsule polysaccharides) in two cases. Seeliger and Christ in the same year confirmed antigen in the spinal fluid in one case. Seeliger (1963) stated that the confirmation of soluble antigen in spinal fluid constitutes a sensible and specific test of high diagnostic value. Abrahams et al. (1962) found antigen in infected mice. Bloomfield et al. (1963) reported antigen in serum and spinal fluid, using a latex slide agglutination test. With a modified method, these results were confirmed by Gordon and Vedder (1966) in a larger number of patients. Bennet et al. (1962) were able to prove antigens by CFT in serum and spinal fluid.

Antibodies were confirmed first by Rappaport and Kaplan (1926), who found agglutinins in serum, and agglutinins and complement fixing antibodies in the spinal fluid, and agglutinins were found in two cases in Germany by Seeliger (1960). However, Seeliger (1963) did not succeed in proving precipitating or complement fixating antibodies in eight other cases. Positive reactions were obtained in six of seven proved cases by using an indirect fluorescent antibody method (Vogel et al., 1961), but 8% of 339 sera from normal patients were also positive. In a later series, 80% of patients were positive with the indirect fluorescence antibody test (Vogel, 1966), although positivity was sometimes of a low order.

Lack of antibodies was found in several cases with exclusive central nervous system involvement. To the known serotypes A, B and C was added a new one, R, with a peculiar capsular specificity. Pollock and Ward (1962) reported hemagglutinins in sera of three patients, but sera of normal persons also reacted. Bloomfield et al. (1963) were able to confirm yeast cell agglutinin in serum and spinal fluid in three of six active cases, but weak positive reactions, presumably false, occurred also in 5 of 111 control patients.

Gordon and Vedder (1966) reported good results for antibodies with an agglutination test using formalin-killed whole yeast cells. Walter and Atchison reported recently on positive fluorescent antibody CFT. They found positive sera in 22% of 134 pigeon breeders, whereas in a group of 36 controls only 3% reacted positively.

The capsular substance is said to be serologically active and responsible for virulence (Drouhet et al., 1950). However, Littman and Tsubura stated that the degree of encapsulation is not a factor in virulence in mice.

In addition to the possible action of antibodies against *C.neoformans* in serum, human blood sera apparently have an inhibitory effect on the growth of the fungus (Allen; Baum and Artis, 1961; Baum and Artis, 1963; Howard; Igel and Bolande; Szilagyi et al.). Heating of serum for 30 min at 62°C destroyed the inhibitory effect; in addition to an iron-binding factor, other factors may be involved; the most active of which were globulins (Igel and Bolande; Szilagyi et al.).

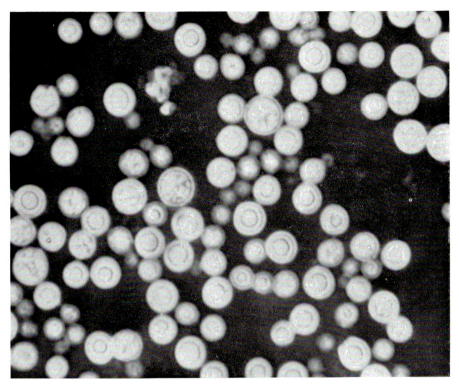

Fig. 3. India-ink suspension of *C. neoformans* from culture with encapsulated organisms. Note droplets and granules in cytoplasm. × 600

Fungicidal activity has been found also in tissue compounds derived from tissue and blood cells (GADEBUSCH, 1966) and in saliva (IGEL and BOLANDE). Immunologic studies on hypersensibility, resistance, and protection have been performed in mice (LOURIA et al.; PERCEVAL; ABRAHAMS), and in rabbits and guinea pigs by LOMANITZ and HALE.

Mycology
Terminology and classification

The generally accepted designation of the fungus involved in cryptococcosis is *Cryptococcus neoformans* (SANFELICE) VUILLEMIN (1901). Some synonyms are also used (EMMONS et al., 1963): *Saccharomyces neoformans* (SANFELICE, 1895); *Cryptococcus hominis* (VUILLEMIN, 1901); *Torula neoformans* (WEIS, 1902); *Torula histolytica* (STODDARD and CUTLER, 1916); *Debaryomyces hominis* (TODD and HERRMANN, 1936).

LODDER and KREGER-VAN RIJ (1952) listed 39 valid botanical synonyms. Taking these as a base, BENHAM (1955) added two additional species.

C. neoformans belongs to the class of *Fungi imperfecti* or *Deuteromycetes* which do not form ascospores. Asporogenous yeasts were put by LODDER and KREGER-VAN RIJ into a separate order, the *Cryptococcales*, with one family, the *Cryptococcaceae* and three subfamilies, *Trichosporoideae*, *Rhodotoruloideae*, and *Cryptococcoideae*. The latter comprehend six genera of which one is *Cryptococcus*. It is characterized by spherical or oval cells which are encapsulated, budding, forming

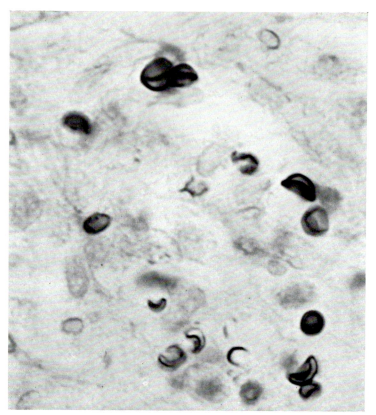

Fig. 4. Experimental cutaneous cryptococcosis in hamsters (Cincinnati 9873). Several bowl-
and half-moon-shaped cryptococci. Grocott, × 720

exceptionally pseudomycelium without ascospores, are nonfermenters, and
produce extracellular starch. The seven species of the genus *Cryptococcus* are:
C.neoformans, C.laurentii, C.luteolus, C.mucorugosus, C.albidus, C.diffluens and
C.neoformans var. innocuous. They are differentiated by size and shape of cells,
carbon and nitrogen assimilation, nonassimilation of nitrates, ability to grow at
37°C, and virulence, the last three characteristic for *C.neoformans*.

Morphology: In cultures and on direct examination of body fluids or exudates,
C.neoformans appears as a spherical to ovoid shaped yeast cell with great variation
of size, usually in the range of 4—7 *μ*, but also showing sizes of 2.5—20 *μ* in
diameter. In examining unstained smears or routinely stained preparations,
bright illumination should be reduced until structural details can be recognized.
In the cytoplasm are seen refractile granules and vacuoles which contain lipids
(FREEMAN, 1930) (Fig. 3). *C.neoformans* is said to show a more spherical structure
and a more granular aspect of cytoplasm than nonpathogenic species of *Cryptococcus* (BENHAM, 1955). Single bodies in the cytoplasm near the apex have been
mistaken for ascospores (TODD and HERRMANN); other workers have believed
these belonged to the capsule.

The wall of the fungus cells is distinctly visible but rather thin and less prominent than similar structures in *B.dermatitidis* and *Paracoccidioides brasiliensis*, for
instance. By collapse of the wall and invaginations, different shapes of the cell

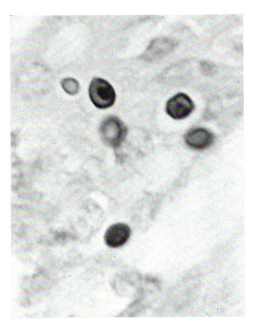

Fig. 5. Experimental cutaneous cryptococcosis in hamsters (Cincinnati 9823). Cryptococci with inner structures similar to *Pneumocystis*. Grocott, × 720

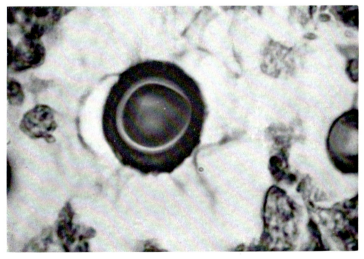

Fig. 6. Pulmonary cryptococcosis. *C. neoformans* in tissue section with broad mucicarmine-positive capsule. Mucicarmine, × 1150

may result (Figs. 4 and 5). Surrounding the wall is generally a typical capsule of variable thickness which contains muco-polysaccharide material (Fig. 6). The width of the capsule can exceed the diameter of the entire cell. In unstained preparations, the capsule can be overlooked and the fungus cell be confused with tissue or blood cells and artefacts.

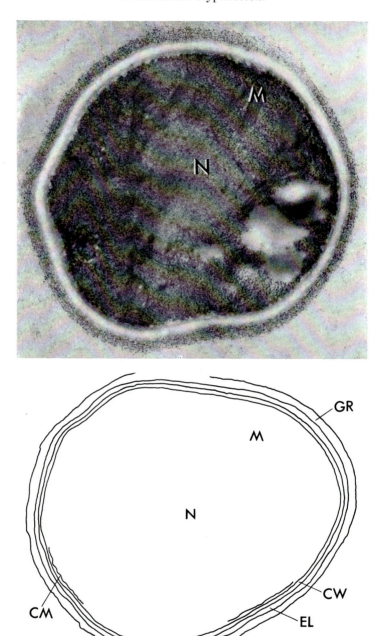

Fig. 7. *Cryptococcus neoformans*. Granular layer (GR) surrounding yeast cell represents poly-saccharide material of the mucoid capsule. Cell wall shows a nearly completely white zone, referred to by LEVINE and HIRANO as "electronlucent zone" (EL). Cell wall proper (CW) is greyish ring, immediately beneath which a fibrous or striated structure is seen under higher magnification. Next, cytoplasmic membrane (CP) can be recognized, represented by dark line, in places undulated, and most prominent where cytoplasmic contents are relatively pale in color. Nucleus (N) and mitochondria (M) are visible. × 35,100. Courtesy Drs. SEYMOUR LEVINE and ASAO HIRANO, New York

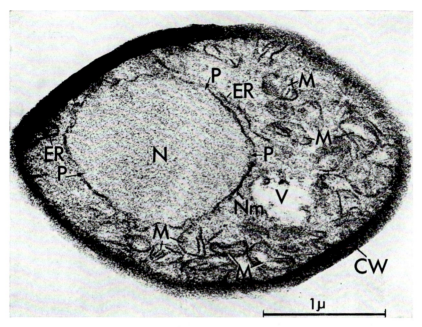

Fig. 8. Thin section through a vegetative cell of *C.neoformans* fixed in a 3% $KMnO_4$ solution for 2 hours. Cell wall (CW) is electron dense; nucleus (N) is nearly round, enclosed by a nuclear membrane (Nm), with several discontinuities termed nuclear pores (P); mitochondria (M) show varied shapes and clearly defined cristae (C). A vascular structure (V) of irregular shape is also visible. Observable in the cytoplasm are double internal membranes involved in endoplasmic reticulum (ER). Cytoplasmic membrane (CM), which is a thin membraneous structure lying just beneath cell wall, is not distinctly visualized. Courtesy Dr. TOHRU TSUKAHARA, Niigata, Japan

Most important is the fact that not all fungus cells of a given strain show the capsule and that there are entirely noncapsulated strains of *C.neoformans*. GROCOTT staining shows fungus cells nicely but the mucinous capsule is best seen in preparations with India ink (FETTER et al.) (Fig. 3), since this suspension does not penetrate into the capsule and cell and gives a uniform black background from which the organisms show distinctly as clear spots.

The capsules cannot be removed by washing in water and only partially by acid hydrolysis. Ten percent sodium or potassium hydroxide free them from adherent tissue and blood elements, alkali not having a solvent effect on the fungal organisms.

Fungus cells reproduce by budding (Fig. 4). Generally, at one point on the surface, a single and smaller daughter cell develops. Sometimes simultaneous multiple budding is observed; rarely, multiple budding gives origin to confusion with *P.brasiliensis*. The daughter cells are attached to the parent cells by a thin wall and narrow spore. Later they break free. True hyphae are not formed. However, the cells are sometimes attached to each other, forming chains, and elongated yeastlike cells present pseudohyphal structures. Only recently in the Coward strain a stable mutant with true hyphae and verticillate groups of blastospores were observed in modified Sabouraud's agar and cultured on the subsurface in pour plates. Of 34 other strains, two showed potential for hyphae production (SHADOMY and UTZ). On electronmicroscopy (Fig. 7) the mucoid capsule is seen as

a   b

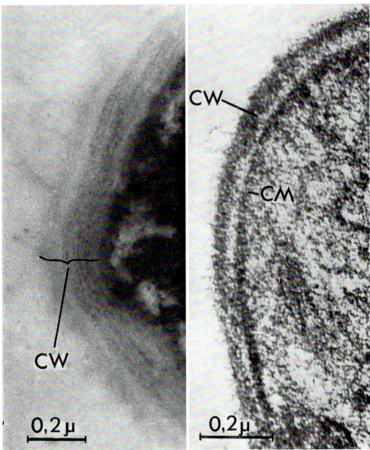

Fig. 9. Fungus cells fixed in OsO_4 (9a) and in $KMnO_4$ (9b). In the first cell (9a), lamellar structure of cell wall (CW) is demonstrated. Inner layer is divided into several layers of fibrillar electron-dense structures running longitudinally around cell body at definite intervals. In second cell (9b), cell wall (CW) consists possibly of several layers. Outer and inner layers are dense while middle layer is of lesser electron density. Courtesy Dr. TOHRU TSUKAHARA, Niigata, Japan

a granular layer. Details of the cell wall are somewhat different in Figs. 8 and 9 (9a and 9b). In Fig. 10 are seen in addition, details of nucleus and mitochondria.

Cultures: The yeast grows rapidly on almost all common culture media. Within a few days, smooth yeast colonies develop; these have at first a creamy and later a mucinous aspect which can be confused grossly with *Candida* or bacteria (Fig. 11). Cryptococcus is not dimorphic (biphasic); yeastlike fungus cells grow at room temperature and 37°C, the latter being characteristic for the species *C. neoformans*.

For isolation, 20°C Sabouraud dextrose agar or Littman's oxgall agar is recommended. In the latter the fungus develops slowly, but the medium is most useful for contaminated specimens (LITTMAN, 1947, 1948). For incubation at 37°C, brain heart infusion blood agar and Littman's liver spleen glucose blood agar (LITTMAN, 1955) are preferred. In the last-mentioned medium colonies appear generally within 24 hours. For suppression of contamination, penicillin

20 μ/ml and streptomycin 40 μ/ml should be added. Inclusion of carbohydrates in the media stimulates abundant growth; maltose is said to favor capsule formation in the fungus cells (DROUHET and COUTEAU). DEMOULIN-BRAHY and DEMOULIN-BRAHY et al. suggest other substances, to stimulate capsule formation. REID, SCHMIDT et al. and STAIB (i) recommend the addition of thiamine. For selective isolation from heavily contaminated material, a special culture medium has been

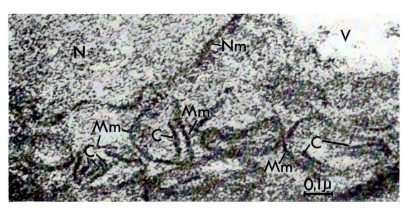

Fig. 10. Higher magnification of lower part of Fig. 8 with details of nucleus (N) and mitochondria (M). Nucleoplasm is filled with finely granular material. Nuclear membrane (NM), mitochondrial membrane (Mm), and mitochondrial cristae (C) are double membraned. Membraneous structures are reported in cells of several fungus species and other forms of life. Courtesy Dr. TOHRU TSUKAHARA, Niigata, Japan

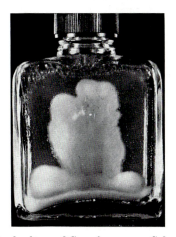

Fig. 11. Gross aspect of culture of *C. neoformans* on Sabouraud's glucose agar

recommended which contains creatinine, diphenyl, and chloramphenicol, and, as a color marker, seed extract from *Guizotia abyssinica* (AJELLO, 1966; SHIELDS and AJELLO), which elicits a brown color (STAIB (g); KREGER-VAN RIJ and STAIB; STAIB (c); STAIB (k)).

Viable cultures can be conserved by covering them with mineral oil and maintaining them at 5°C (RAPER and ALEXANDER; BUELL and WESTON; AJELLO et al., 1951; LITTMAN, 1955).

Optimal growth of *C. neoformans* is achieved at 29°C (Kuhn, 1939), although the fungus develops over a considerable range of temperatures. Unlike most cryptococci, *C. neoformans* will grow at 37°C.

Staib (Staib h) demonstrated the viability of a *Cryptococcus* strain isolated from the excreta of canaries, which had been maintained in dry sand for more than a year. Other species of *Cryptococcus* which had been kept in dry sand were resistant to dehydration. The same strain of *C. neoformans* was also resistant to heating of several hours at temperatures up to 100°C. Hitaka reported that cortisone accelerated development of *C. neoformans* in tissue cultures.

Biochemistry: Certain reactions of *C. neoformans* are of interest for taxonomic and diagnostic purposes. The fungus is aerobic (Cox and Tolhurst), but not a true fermentative yeast, insofar as it does not produce gas. It leads nevertheless to the production of acid from certain sugars (Emmons, 1951; Emmons, 1952). Assimilation of carbohydrates and nitrogenous substances has been studied by the auxanographic agar method (Beijerinck), the assimilation broth method (Wickerham and Burton), and the streak plate method for assimilation tests (Benham, 1955), all three methods giving similar results (Benham, 1955). The fungus does not use (assimilate) lactose (Lodder and Kreger-van Rij; Benham, 1955).

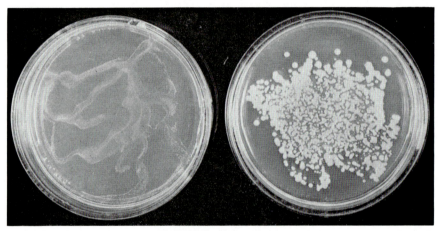

Fig. 12. *C. neoformans* does not utilize KNO_3 as the sole source of nitrogen, as can some other cryptococci. On left plate, KNO_3 as exclusive nitrogen source in culture medium

Nitrogenous substances are assimilated by all yeasts (Wickerham, 1946). Lodder and Kreger-van Rij found that nitrates are not used by *C. neoformans* (Fig. 12). *C. neoformans* is the only species which constantly assimilates creatinine (Staib, e, f, g; Kreger-van Rij and Staib). Further, better growth of *C. neoformans* was observed in sera with a higher residual N (Staib and Zissler (a and b), Staib, e).

Another useful reaction is the active production of urease (Seeliger, 1956; Lacaz et al., 1958) (Fig. 13), but in contrast to the color effect with *Guizotia abyssinica*, urease production is not species specific. Enzymes of yeasts elicit fermentation of glucose with production of alcohol. Methods for confirmation of alcohol in spinal fluid in cases of cryptococcic meningitis were reported by Tyler and by Dawson and Taghary. Since these tests apparently are not specific for *C. neoformans*, they have not been applied widely.

Studying the biochemistry of the capsule substances EINBINDER et al., (1954) and DROUHET et al. (1950), found the capsule to contain polyosid, a substance resembling hyaluronic acid. The capsule polysaccharides were studied also by infrared spectrophotometry (LEVINE et al., 1959).

In synthetic media, the fungus produces extracellular starch (ASCHNER et al.; MAGER and ASCHNER); this property was recognized by LODDER and KREGER-VAN-RIJ for definition of the genus cryptococcus. HEHRE et al. identified this substance as amylose. HIRANO et al. (1964, 1965) studied the behavior of the extracellular polysaccharid capsule material in cerebral fluid and tissue.

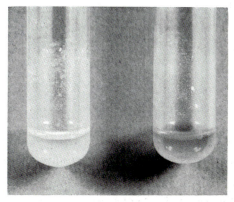

Fig. 13. Positive (pink right) urease test. SEELIGER has shown the value of this test in identification of yeasts

Pathogenesis

Exogenous or endogenous disease? The fact that cryptococcosis occurs frequently in persons debilitated by chronic diseases suggests to some that cryptococcosis is an endogenous disease, the human organism harboring strains of *Cryptococcus* (MOHR; BENHAM, 1935; RAVITS, FELSENFELD, BENHAM and HOPKINS; ZIMMERMAN and RAPPAPORT, 1954). Further studies should clarify this issue, since COLLINS et al. have brought forward controversial evidence, and RIETH in extensive studies was not able to isolate *C. neoformans* from healthy persons. It seems noteworthy that in the 13 years following this statement no further evidence has been found. EMMONS et al., 1963 consider the disease to be wholly exogenous.

Portal of Entry: General agreement does not yet exist as to the portal of entry of cryptococcosis. While it is clear that in most fungus diseases the cells are inhaled and the site of primary infection is the lung, in cryptococcosis the predominant involvement of the nervous system (COHEN and KAUFMANN) gives rise to questions.

The fact that patients with *cryptococcal meningitis* show a history of recent respiratory disease is not necessarily evidence of primary lung infection. Many patients first develop symptoms of disease of the central nervous system, and pulmonary foci are readily overlooked (FORBUS; TERPLAN) even at necropsy (HAUGEN and BAKER). Second, in cryptococcosis, calcification of residual foci in tissues does not commonly occur; hence the "healed lesions" found in tuberculosis and histoplasmosis do not seem to exist in cryptococcosis.

SHEPPE apparently first called attention to the *primary infection in the lungs* in 1924. CAMPBELL (1966) mentions more than 100 cases from the English literature which were considered as primary in the lungs. Typical case reports with clinical and surgical (anatomical) evidence of primary pulmonary cryptococcosis were published also by KATZ et al., KNUDSON et al., PROCKNOW et al., RATCLIFFE and COOK, BAHR et al. In a series of cases, HAUGEN and BAKER (1954) demonstrated small and large pulmonary lesions, generally localized in the subpleural regions, which must be considered as primary foci. Four patients were asymptomatic and in two others cryptococcal meningitis was also present.

A recent case (SALFELDER and SCHWARZ) illustrates the difficulty of pathogenic interpretation:

A middle-aged man presented a frontal skin lesion which was removed surgically and believed to be a basal cell carcinoma. Histologic examination revealed cutaneous cryptococcosis. The patient was otherwise asymptomatic and no chronic underlying disease was present. Since wo do not believe in primary skin infection, sputum and cerebrospinal fluid were examined. *C. neoformans* was recovered from both by culturing. At first attempt, no x-ray proof of lung involvement could be obtained. Only after repeated and careful radiologic lung examination, a circumscribed solitary lung focus with excavation was recognized. Consequently, the skin lesion could be interpreted as due to hematogenous spread from the lung focus resembling the asymptomatic involvement of the meninges. Pat. died 2 years later of disseminated tryptococcosis complicated by pneumocystosis.

Cryptococcal involvement of the hilar (and other) lymph nodes does occur, but is not the rule. No vascular lesions analogous to Weigert's "venous tubercles" have been found. Experimentally, primary lung infection has been successfully achieved by exposing mice to soil seeded with the fungus (SMITH et al., 1964) and the results after intranasal inoculation in mice also support the thesis that the respiratory tract is the portal of entry (RITTER and LARSH).

Meningitis has been suspected to start as an infection of the nasal and pharyngeal cavities (HIRSH and COLEMAN). In this region cryptococcal lesions have been found by COX and TOLHURST; MARSHALL and TEED; MOODY; MORRIS and WOLINSKY; TUERK. After dental extraction, NICHOLS and MARTIN and URBACH and ZACH observed cryptococcal meningitis. Without proof of any kind the tonsils were mentioned as source of infection with lymphatic spread to the meninges by FREEMAN (1930), FREEMAN (1931), LEVIN, ROYER et al. ALLEN and LOWBEER claimed a rectal ulcer with perirectal fistula as the portal of entrance for the fungus. TAKOS reported generalized disease in marmoset monkeys after feeding of the fungus. Other feeding experiments, however, failed to elicit primary intestinal cryptococcosis (POUNDEN et al.; SETHI, 1967b).

In rare cases primary infection can occur in the *skin*, especially after injury (BERGHAUSEN; BRIER et al.; DEBRÉ et al.; JOHNS and ATTAWAY; RUITER and ENSINK; SYMMERS, 1953). As a rule cryptococcal lesions in the skin or subcutaneous tissues are secondary to hematogenous spread of the fungus or involvement by contiguity from underlying tissues. Skin disease is not frequent. CAWLEY et al. found dermal foci in 13 cases of 110 patients with cryptococcal meningitis in the literature. BUREAU et al.; GANDY; and ROOK and WOODS describe cases of chronic dermal cryptococcosis which were claimed as primary, with a better prognosis than the visceral form of the disease. Also CROUNSE and LERNER and CARRIK considered the skin lesions in their cases as primary infections and stated that no other organs were affected. These patients were cured with amphotericin B. However, primary infection of skin cannot be accepted without autopsy or conclusive demonstration of the infecting "tool." An interesting case was reported lately by RUITER and ENSINK. Skin lesions developed after trauma; the patient died from shock when amphotericin B was injected; autopsy did not supposedly reveal any involvement of internal organs. In this case, with conclusive proof of skin cryptococcosis and without demonstration of fungus disease in viscera, interpretation could be of primary origin of the cutaneous lesions, although it must be objected that in the histologic examination of viscera no GROCOTT stained sections were reviewed or tissues cultured. Dissemination after subcutaneous inoculation has been achieved experimentally (LEVINE et al., 1957; SETHI et al.; BERGMAN, 1962), but this finding is no proof that in human disease the skin is generally, frequently or ever the portal of entry. Neonatal disease would point in the direction of infection by the diaplacental route or by inhalation from the genital tract at delivery. Since in generalized cryptococcosis we have also seen fungi in endometrial blood vessels, theoretic possibility of transplacental infection exists. However, conclusive cases of neonatal cryptococcosis have not been reported. The children reported by TIMMERMAN; JANSSENS and JANSSENS and BEETSTRA; NEUHAUSER and TUCKER, and OLIVEIRA CAMPOS were said to have congenital cryptococcosis but later, in personal communications to EMANUEL et al. and MATHEIS respectively, these authors reported that the children had toxoplasmosis and not cryptococcosis.

In the cases reported by NASSAU and WEINBERG-HEIRUTI; HEALTH, there is no definite proof of cryptococcosis; it is probable that mineral concretions from *Toxoplasma gondii* infections were mistaken for cryptococcosis.

Subclinical forms: While *silent infections* occur frequently in histoplasmosis and coccidioidomycosis, and presumably also in blastomycosis and paracoccidioidomycosis, confirmation of asymptomatic cryptococcosis has been scarce. HAUGEN and BAKER (1954) could demonstrate small healed pulmonary nodules in a few healthy persons. By resection of subpleural pulmonary granulomas, further asymptomatic cases have been detected and disease recognized fortuitously (BERK and GERSTL; DILLON and SEALY; HOUK and MOSER; KUYKENDALL et al.; MOSS and McQUOWN; PINNEY; WEBB and BIGGS). Lack of efficient serologic tests and skin tests impede confirmation that cryptococcosis is more common. In pigeon breeders evidence points in that direction (cf. WALTER and ATCHISON, Epidemiology). *C. neoformans* must then be looked upon as a facultative rather than an obligate pathogen, since apparently large parts of the population all over the world are exposed to the fungus; few are infected, and in the majority of infections the mammalian organism destroys the invading yeast unless unfavorable conditions, such as debilitating diseases, lead to suppression of body defenses. Also the invasiveness of *C. neoformans* is not high, if one accepts the unsuccessful (accidental) human experiment reported by HALDE. However, it is only fair to mention that a negative "take" is not synonymous with low invasiveness of a given agent.

Routes of dissemination: *Hematogenous spread* is by far the most frequent route of dissemination. It must be assumed in the great majority of cryptococcal disease of the central nervous system and also other localization of the disease. In the final stages of evolution, overwhelming hematogenous dissemination occasionally occurs without formation of tissular foci (septic form), (Fig. 14). Propagation of disease by contiguity is the second most frequent mode of dissemination. This occurs in the lung and central nervous system (invasion from the meninges to the brain with communication of brain lesions with the subarachnoidal space often in a flask-shaped form). Ascendant cryptococcosis in involvement of the spinal cord has been reported (DEMME and MUMME). Ocular disease occurs often, due to direct spread from cryptococcic meningitis or spread from focal lesions in bones, sinuses, or soft tissues to the central nervous system. Infections also may spread from bones to soft tissues (RIGDON and KIRKSEY) and skin (NIÑO, 1938) and from skin to bones (PIERS). Dermal or subcutaneous cryptococcosis has been observed after surgery of deep-seated lesions (Padberg and Martin). Lymphatic spread is not frequent. Involvement of regional lymph nodes occurs rarely. Cryptococcal lymphadenitis seems often to be the consequence of hematogenous spread. Intracanalicular dissemination has not been conclusively confirmed, although this may occur in the lungs.

Tissue reactions: The cause of the variable types of tissue lesions is unknown and speculative. Modes of tissue reactions may depend on the respective fungus strain, its virulence, number of organisms (infective dose and rate of multiplication), resistance of the host organism, or allergic reactions. It is believed that recent lesions generally show the gelatinous and older ones the granulomatous type of tissue reaction (Baker and Haugen). The tissue destruction in the gelatinous or mucinous form of cryptococcal lesions, especially in solid tissues, has been interpreted as an effect of the histolytic action of the fungus. Hence the denomination *Torula* or *Cryptococcus "histolyticus"* (Castellani and Jacono; Stoddard and Cutler). While many students of the disease (Carton and Mount; Demme and Mumme; Freeman, 1931; Freeman and Weidman; Littman and Zimmerman; Mohr; Rappaport and Kaplan) do not accept this thesis and suppose, rather, that tissue destruction is the sequence of a compression exercised by the accumulation of the fungi, Matheis strongly defends the former hypothesis, as do Conway and Brady; Schmidt et al.; Seeliger (1959). Matheis bases his opinion of the biochemical and digestive or fermentative, i.e. active role, of the fungi on the fact that signs of compression in the vicinity of brain foci, in the form of a major density of fibers or cells, could not be confirmed. On the other hand, proof of the active force of the fungus and its ability to destroy tissues, or the confirmation of a special substance which conduces to tissue destruction, has not been achieved. The fungus grown on sterile brain for weeks did not digest tissue (Freeman, 1933; Freeman and Weidman). In the light of these facts, we conceive a mechanical effect of the accumulation of numerous fungi and the extrafungal capsular substances as responsible for slow atrophy by compression of parenchyma. A comparable tissue destroying process takes place, in our opinion, in amyloidosis, in which an active role of the inert amyloid substance is not assumed. The difference between both lesions is that in the latter, spacial or spongelike patterns do not result. This could be explained by the fact that the fungi are growing and multiplying elements which can die after a certain time, leaving spaces. The extracellular mucinous substance can undergo dehydration and in this way lose volume and contribute to the formation of "spaces", in marked contrast to the tissue necroses said to be caused by such a histolytic agent as the ameba in intestine and liver! The absence or scarcity of polymorphonuclear leukocytes in the gelatinous foci of cryptococcosis (Demme and Mumme; Littman and Zimmerman) and also in amyloidosis is, in our opinion, another argument that fast tissue destruction does not occur and that an active histolytic action of the fungi is difficult to assume. It underlines the similarity of histogenesis in both otherwise different processes. The missing leukocytes parallel the lack of necrotic tissular lesions and breakdown of tissue in gelatinous cryptococcal foci. Matheis, on the contrary, supposes that the absence of leucocytic tissue reactions are due to the capsular substance of the cryptococcus. This substance impedes phagocytosis of leukocytes (Drouhet and Segretain, 1951). When necrosis, faintly similar to caseation, occurs occasionally in gelatinous lung foci, these areas are generally composed of large dead fungus cells and less of tissue debris or exudated elements. In paracoccidioidomycosis large masses of dead fungus cells form an important part of necrotic tissue areas, although there are different tissue reactions in this last-mentioned mycosis.

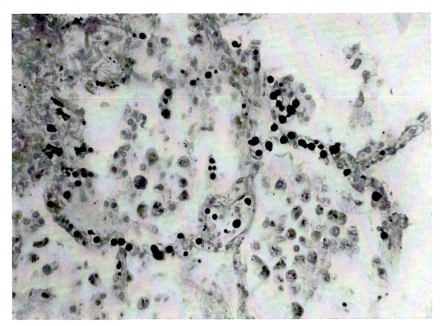

Fig. 14. Fungemia with numerous Grocott-positive (black) cryptococci in capillaries of alveolar walls. In lumina of alveoli desquamated alveolar cells (macrophages). Grocott, × 250

Pathology

Tissue reactions: Two principal types of lesions are characteristic in this mycosis: the *gelatinous* or mucinous, paucireactive lesion, with numerous fungus cells, and the *granulomatous* type, with formation of nodules and tumor-like foci. Also found is the septic form (fungemia), with abundant fungus cells in the blood vessels (Fig. 14). Less frequently are noted necrotic lesions, rarely with breakdown of tissue and formation of cavities and also, rarely, calcifications. Healing or healed fibrotic lesions also are observed exceptionally. Several of these tissue reactions may occur simultaneously in the various organs of a patient.

The *gelatinous lesions* vary in form, size, and extent. While no membrane or capsule surrounds these foci, they are nevertheless often sharply delineated from the sound tissue. Grossly their appearance is characteristically gelatinous (Fig. 15). They may be confused with myxomatous tumors. In mucosae they may be misinterpreted as pseudomembranous inflammation or mucous polyps, and in the meninges confused with an exudative meningitis. The mucinous aspect is due to the accumulation of abundant encapsulated cryptococci and of extrafungal mucinous substances derived from the capsules. Many fungi are situated inside macrophages, although this must be confirmed by close inspection. No other cellular elements or exudate except macrophages and occasional single giant cells are found. In the case of involvement of solid tissue, the parenchyma in these gelatinous foci appears rarified, with many optically empty spaces of irregular shape. The foci of spongelike appearance show as clear areas on low power in histologic sections. In the brain, the gelatinous lesions appear as perivascular cystoid formations, apparently because of shrinkage by formalin fixation.

In the *granulomatous lesions* the cellular reaction is predominant. Fungus cells are less numerous; their absence may lead to a diagnosis of sarcoidosis. Individual

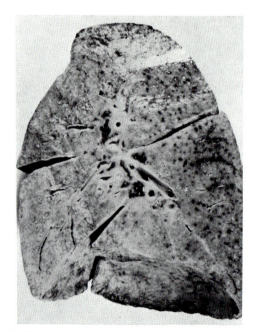

Fig. 15. Extensive gelatinous cryptococci pneumonia

granulomas may be distinguished which, by confluence, form larger nodules, or no small granulomas at all may be seen. In addition to macrophages, lymphocytes and plasma cells are visible. Giant cells are almost always present, while clear-cut epithelioid cells are infrequent. Hyperemia, edema, fibrin, and polymorpho-nuclear leukocytes are almost always absent. In the final stages of evolution, massive hematogenous spread can occur with fungus cells present in blood vessels, in capillaries of all organs and tissues. In sections stained with H and E and other routine staining methods, the often numerous fungal elements can be overlooked, while they appear distinctly in Grocott-stained preparations (Figs. 16, 17). No reactions of vascular walls or foci near the blood vessels occur in fungemic sepsis. In patients with underlying and debilitating diseases, this form of cryptococcosis occurs more frequently.

Necrosis inside cryptococcal lesions is not common. Necrotic areas outside the lesions may be due to vascular tissue loss, as occurs in the brain (Jones and Klink; Matheis; Stone and Sturdivant). If densely accumulated fungus cells die, they form foci which resemble caseating necrosis (Baker and Haugen; Sabesin et al.). Occasionally, breakdown of tissue is seen from which cavity formation may result (Littman, 1959; McCullough et al.). Infiltrates of polymorphonuclear leukocytes may be observed in these cases or as sequelae of secondary bacterial infection. In one of our cases, bacterial colonies could be observed clearly inside cryptococcal lung lesions (Salfelder and Schwarz). True abscess formation, however, is rare, although Symmers (1953) reports abscesses in human cryptococcosis and Levine et al. (1957) mention them in experiments.

Calcifications were reported exceptionally in different types of cryptococcal lesions and in different sites (Beeson; Houk and Moser; Liu; Matheis; Royer et al.; Siewers and Cramblett; Schwarz et al., 1954; Susman). They should be proved anatomically and confirmed inside of lesions due to *C. neoformans*. Small

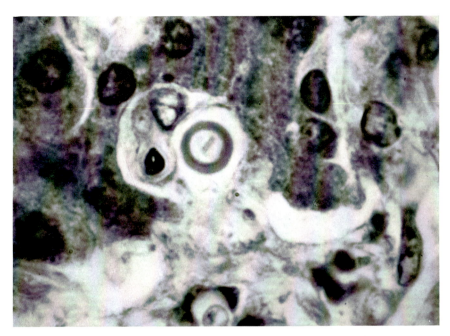

Fig. 16. Cryptococci in sinusoid capillaries of liver (fungemia). H & E, × 1100

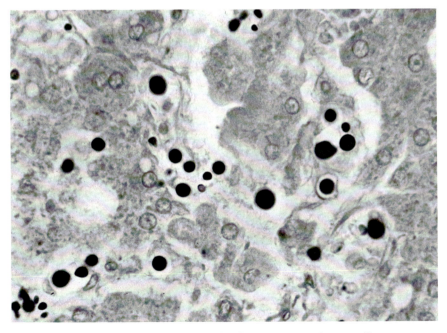

Fig. 17. Same case and organ as in Fig. 16. In this preparation fungus cells are seen more distinctly. Grocott, × 600

calcifications outside fungal lesions are without relation to disease and causal agent. Positive radiologic findings in patients with cryptococcosis are not necessarily related to this mycosis. Especially in the lungs and lymph nodes and particularly in endemic areas of histoplasmosis, the frequent calcifications occurring in the latter, as in tuberculous patients, must be ruled out. *Fibrosis and hyalinization* are unusual in cryptococcal lesions, although described in healing or healed subpleural lung lesions (Haugen and Baker), apparently of primary infection, and in surgically removed specimens. Fibrous encapsulation of healed focal lesions is not so frequent as in other fungus diseases.

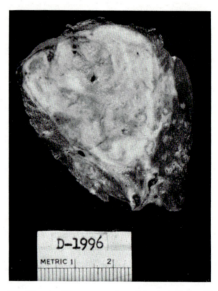

Fig. 18. Surgically removed cryptococcoma of lung

Lungs: Isolated pulmonary involvement was first reported in 1924 (Sheppe). Since then, an increasing number of similar observations have been made (Hardaway and Crawford; Sauerteig) (cf. *Pathogenesis*). Grossly, the aspect of cryptococcal lesions varies, with abundant fungi giving a mucoid and gelatinous, bland appearance of foci, or with granulomatous lesions showing a firm, grayish-white pattern which can be confused with tumorous tissue or granulomatous lesions of any origin (Fig. 18). Lung tissue, above all in disseminated disease, can be involved extensively and diffusely, with foci of different sizes and mostly of the gelatinous type. Widely disseminated miliary granulomas can, on close inspection, show a mucoid aspect and can thus be differentiated from similar foci in miliary tuberculosis and other granulomatous diseases (Fig. 19). Also multiple large foci ("pneumonic" form) are mostly of the gelatinous type. They vary in diameter from 1—7 cm, do not show a predilection for any one part of the lungs, and can easily be distinguished from caseous pneumonia. Multiple large foci can be also of the granulomatous type. However, this form occurs more frequently as localized and solitary foci, varying in size and localized more often in subpleural areas (Figs. 20 and 21). Solitary masses of either gelatinous or granulomatous nature are also denominated cryptococcomas, earlier called "torulomas", an increasing number of which have been removed surgically in recent years (cf. *Therapy*).

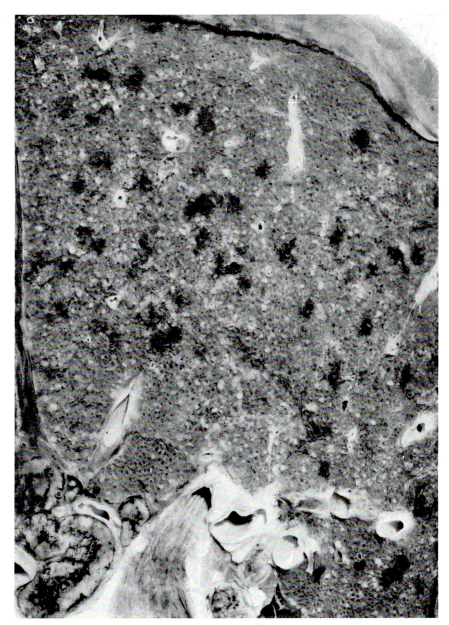

Fig. 19. Disseminated miliary cryptococcal fungi in lung parenchyma. Courtesy Dr. BERNARD F. FETTER, Dept. of Pathology, Duke University, N.C.

Cavitation in the lungs is rare; only a few cases are on record (HAWKINS; HOUK and MOSER; KRESS and CANTRELL; TILLOTSON and LERNER; SALFELDER and SCHWARZ; WOLFE and JACOBSON). They may be solitary or multiple. X-ray diagnosis alone is insufficient evidence of the cryptococcal nature of cavities. In pulmonary lesions there is an accumulation of cryptococci and mucinous material inside the alveoli (Figs. 22, 23), but the alveolar walls usually remain intact. However, in cases of overwhelming numbers of fungi and their capsular substance, the walls may rupture and give rise to formation of large "fungus lakes." In addition to the fungi, macrophages, i.e. histiocytes or alveolar cells, are present, many with engulfed fungus cells (Fig. 24). In their cytoplasm mucicarmine-positive material can also be observed. Giant cells containing fungus cells occur

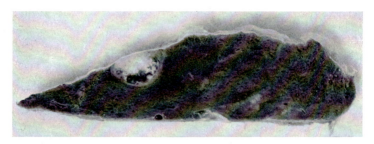

Fig. 20. Sharply circumscribed subpleural cryptococcal focus in lung with breakdown of tissue simulating tuberculoma. Courtesy Dr. Bernard F. Fetter, Dept. of Pathology, Duke University, N.C.

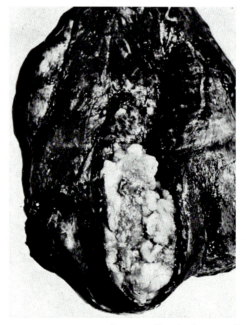

Fig. 21. Pulmonary cryptococcoma. Courtesy Dr. A. Angulo Ortega, Caracas

occasionally. Other cells are not found in the gelatinous foci. Coagulation necrosis occurs seldom (Houk and Moser). Occasionally observed areas of necrosis are composed of confluent dead fungus cells (Baker and Haugen) (Figs. 25, 26). In the granulomatous foci, the lung structure is generally indistinct (Fig. 27). The foci are sharply delimitated from the intact lung parenchyma. Fibrous tissue inside these foci is scarce and encapsulation not frequent.

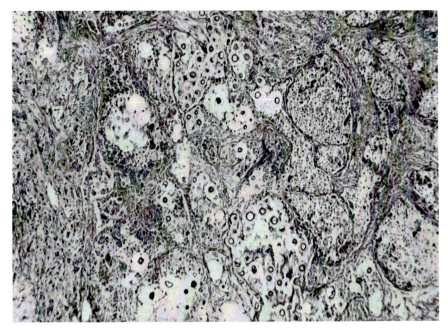

Fig. 22. Numerous fungus cells and mucinous material inside alveoli with preserved lung structure. Gelatinous form. Mucicarmine, × 172

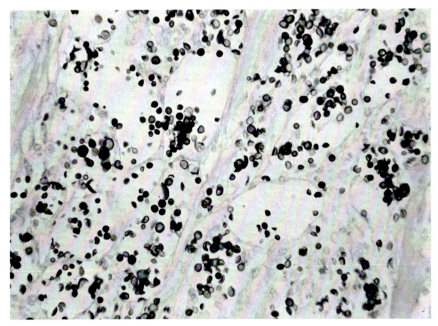

Fig. 23. Gelatinous cryptococcosis, lung. Even more fungus cells can be seen in silver-stained sections. Grocott, × 300

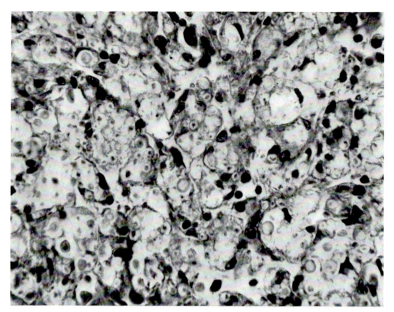

Fig. 24. Numerous cryptococci engulfed by macrophages (lung). H & E, × 450

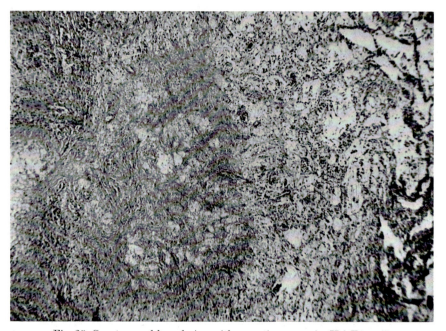

Fig. 25. Cryptococcal lung lesion with caseating necrosis. H & E, × 47

Fungi are found in macrophages and giant cells and occur also free in the tissue and in residual foci. "Burnt-out" foci of cryptococcal nature cannot be diagnosed as such in the absence of the fungus. In terminal stages of disseminated disease, fungi are found in large numbers in capillaries and in "nests" within the

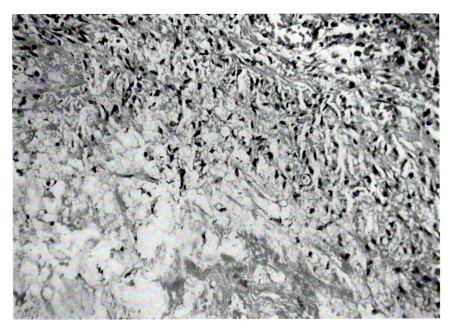

Fig. 26. In the necrotic lung lesion fungus cells are seen with difficulty. Epithelioid cell reaction in the vicinity. H & E, × 190

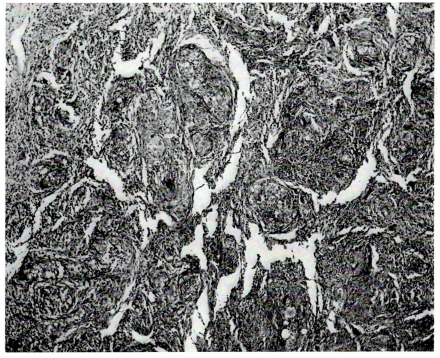

Fig. 27. Granulomatous cryptococcal lung lesion with distorted organic structure. H & E, × 47

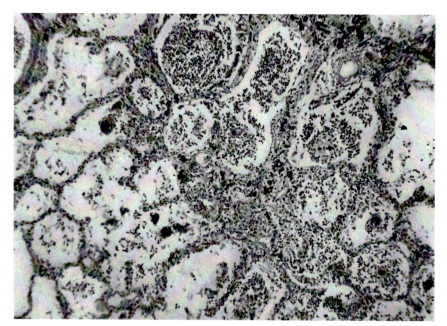

Fig. 28. Pulmonary cryptococcosis with focal bacterial pneumonia. Intraalveolar leukocytic exudate. H & E, × 72

lung tissue. Other mycoses, bacterial pneumonia, and tuberculosis elicit tissue reactions after or before development of cryptococcal disease. When leukocytes are found in a larger amount inside of cryptococcal lesions, secondary bacterial infection is possible (cf. *Pathogenesis*) (Fig. 28). In areas of coexisting or preexisting Hodgkin's disease in the lungs, Littman and Zimmerman report the fungus infecting lymphomatous areas also. We have seen cryptococcal inflammation only outside of lymphomatous lesions in the lung and in other organs.

Pleural effusion is rare, although a scarce inflammatory reaction and fibrous tissue may develop occasionally in the visceral pleura (Littman and Zimmerman, McCullough et al.; Procknow et al.; Houk and Moser; Webster; Reeves et al.; Berk and Gerstl; Gendel et al.; Webster). The finding of fungi in pleural effusions of deep mycoses is not frequent; we have observed it in only one case of paracoccidioidomycosis and rare cases of histoplasmosis and N.A. blastomycosis. Ahuja et al. reported a case with cryptococcal empyema and cryptococcoma of the posterior mediastinum. Perforations or fistula formations have not been reported.

Central Nervous System: In the cranial and spinal *meninges* cryptococcal disease is found generally in the leptomeninges. Lesions are rare in the dura mater, where only tumor-like cryptococcal granulomas occur (Bruns; Hoigne et al.; Littman and Zimmerman; Semerak). Lesions of the dura mater are more frequent in the spinal-cord canal than in the cranial cavity (Garcin et al.; Smith and Crawford). Involvement of the meninges is observed in the great majority of cases of cryptococcosis, especially in fatal ones. In 26 cases of Zimmerman and Rappaport, all but one showed meningitis. About 50% of cases of central nervous system cryptococcosis show meningeal involvement exclusively (Freeman, 1931; Gordon).

Grossly, CNS lesions may be minimal and can be overlooked; they may occur at any site but are most often found over the base of the brain and the cerebellum

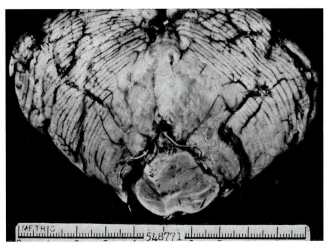

Fig. 29. Cryptococcic meningitis with gelatinous exudate (cerebellum). AFIP. 548771

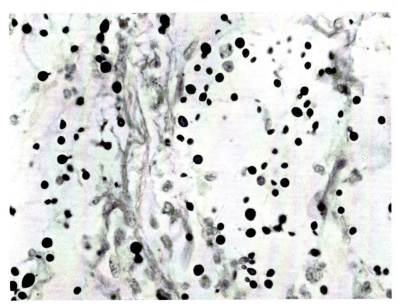

Fig. 30. Gelatinous cryptococcic meningitis with numerous fungus cells; single budding. Grocott, × 600

(Fig. 29). Leptomeningitis may be diffuse or occur in localized patches (DE BUSSCHER et al.; SHAPIRO and NEAL). The membranes are thickened and lose their transparency; details of the underlying brain tissue are often not visible. The color is grayish-white or greenish-yellow; in the gelatinous form mucinous masses are visible. Along blood vessels, chains of minute nodules may be seen. The gelatinous and the granulomatous forms do not occur exclusively but simultaneously, and one of them always predominates (MATHEIS). In the *gelatinous form* the membranes can be easily removed; in the granulomatous form and with fibrosis, especially in chronic forms, the leptomeninges adhere to the surface of the cortex

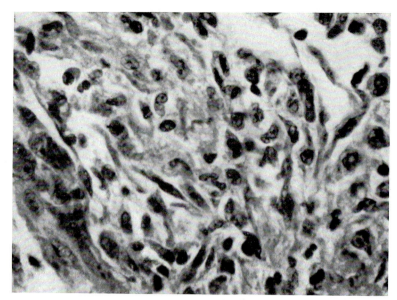

Fig. 31. Cryptococcal meningitis with granulomatous reaction, showing epithelioid cells. H & E, × 720

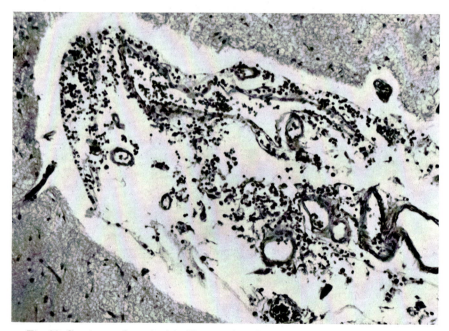

Fig. 32. Cryptococcal meningitis. Nonspecific inflammatory reaction. H & E, × 115

of the brain. Lifting the mucoid masses, or when leptomeninges are still transparent, small cystoid formations are frequently seen in the brain surface, in cases of simultaneous involvement of the brain. In the leptomeninges, tumor-like granulomas similar to those in the dura mater and in brain and spinal cord may be

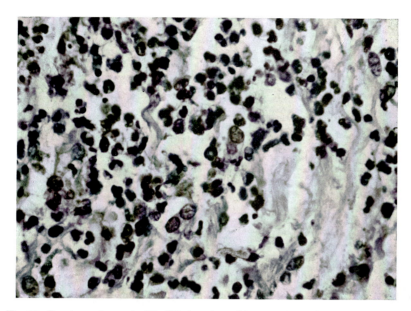

Fig. 33. Cryptococcic meningitis. Histiocytic and leucocytic exudate. H & E, × 600

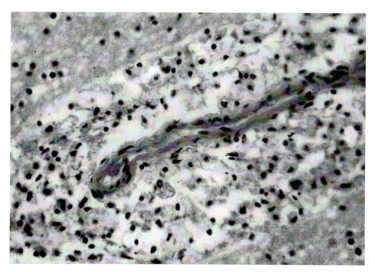

Fig. 34. Cryptococcic brain lesion; perivascular cell infiltrates. H & E, × 200

found. Microscopically, in the gelatinous form abundant fungi and a minimal cell reaction are seen in the distended subarachnoid space (Fig. 30). Adjacent lepto-meninges may be intact or show a typical granulomatous reaction of variable degree with macrophages, giant cells, and a few yeast cells (Fig. 31). In circum-scribed areas nonspecific inflammatory reactions are found, with accumulations of lymphocytes, plasma cells, some eosinophiles, and single giant cells (Fig. 32). As in cryptococcal lesions in other sites, polymorphonuclear leukocytes are generally missing, but may be present in variable amounts (Fig. 33). Their presence may

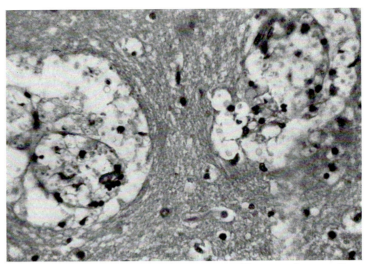

Fig. 35. Cystic cryptococcal brain lesions (gelatinous type). Numerous fungus cells can be seen.
H & E, × 200

suggest a diagnosis of suppurative meningitis of bacterial origin. In cases of chronic meningitis with fibrosis, calcifications may occur (BEESON; MATHEIS).

In the *brain* and *spinal cord* the gelatinous form often appears grossly as numerous small cysts up to 2 mm in diameter which contain a mucoid substance in fresh material (Fig. 34). They may occur in any locality but most often are found in the gray matter. Whitish granulomas are less frequent and occur predominantly in the spinal cord. Miliary granulomas are seen occasionally in the ependyma, and the choroid plexus may be firm and its volume increased. Single or multiple tumor-like lesions (cryptococcomas) of variable size are found elsewhere in the parenchyma.

The term *"cryptococcoma"* has not been clearly defined. Since the histoplasmoma (PUCKETT) is defined as a histoplasmic lesion of more than 0.5 cm in diameter, perhaps this dimension may also apply to cryptococcomas, which may bulge into the ventricles or show prominence on the surface of the brain. CARTON and MOUNT found in 1951 that one-fourth of all published cases with cryptococcosis of the nervous system showed this tumorous form, which may require surgery. Lesions of this kind were described also by CUDMORE and LISA; DILLON and SEALY; LEY et al.; LIU; MANGANIELLO and NICHOLS; MATHEIS; RAMMAMURTHI and ANGULI; SAUERTEIG; WERNER. Microscopically the cystoid lesions are found around blood vessels and show the typical "gelatinous" pattern with abundant fungus cells, polysaccharide material, and scarce cellular reaction (Fig. 35). When more macrophages or giant cells are found, the fungus elements are scarcer (Fig. 36). In the parenchyma another lesion may occur whose cryptococcal nature may be overlooked, although many fungi may be present. This lesion closely resembles encephalomalacia (LITTMAN and ZIMMERMAN) with microglial cells. Small hemorrhages may contain cryptococci (SYMMERS, 1953) and may also be seen occasionally with cryptococcomas. In the granulomatous and tumorous lesions, granulomatous tissue with cellular infiltrates and gliosis predominate with fewer fungi. Necrosis occurs infrequently. Granulomas containing giant cells are also described in the ependyma (LITTMAN and ZIMMERMAN; MATHEIS). Nests of cryptococci and an inflammatory reaction have been found also in the choroid plexus (COX and

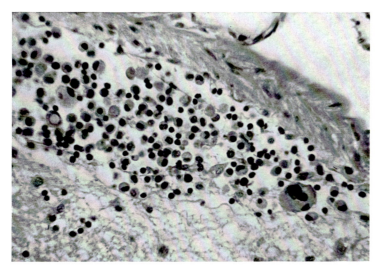

Fig. 36. Cryptococcal brain lesion with perivascular infiltrates of macrophages and scattered giant cells. Fungi are scarce in this field. H & E, × 200

Tolhurst; Champion de Crespigny; Crone et al.; Demme and Mumme; Hoigne et al.; Matheis; Mosberg and Arnold). Calcifications occur only in limited areas in cyrptococcomas (Liu; Matheis). When they are found in lesions of the central nervous system, infection with *Toxoplasma gondii* is more likely to be present than cryptococcosis. Cryptococcal neuritis and inflammatory reactions without fungi in the nerves have been reported in the cranial (Demme and Mumme; Laas and Geiger; Matheis; Monnet and Blanc) and in spinal nerves (Matheis) (cf. *Pathogenesis*, Chapter VI).

Secondary alterations may be due to the fungus or the cryptococcal lesions or be unrelated. The nerve tissue adjacent to cryptococcal lesions is generally well preserved (Littman and Zimmerman). Marked cellular lesions were reported by Atkinson et al. and interpreted as sequelae of a toxic action of *C. neoformans*. Matheis found alterations of nerve fibers in the vicinity of cryptococcal brain lesions. Necrotic foci near fungal lesions are attributed to vascular changes (Jones and Klinck; Matheis; Stone and Sturdivant). Obliterative endarteritis in the meninges is mentioned by Littman and Zimmerman; Semerak; but these are of a nonspecific nature; cryptococci were not found in the vascular wall. Obstruction of ventricular spaces by cryptococcal lesions was reported by Dandy; Matheis; Mosberg and Arnold; Stoddard and Cutler. This may lead to internal hydrocephalus, which is frequent in meningitis (Beeson). External hydrocephalus in cases of cryptococcal meningitis may produce cortical atrophy by compression (Littman and Zimmerman). Brain damage with development of scar tissue has been observed after therapy in cases of meningitis of long duration. Papilledema was reported by Freeman and Weidman and Littman and Zimmerman.

Other organs: While cryptococcal lesions are found predominantly in the lungs and central nervous system, in cases of fungemia (septic form), intravascular cryptococci are increasingly observed in other sites. One fourth of the AFIP series of 80 cases showed such lesions (Littman and Zimmerman). In the year 1965 alone, three cases of *cryptococcal prostatitis* were reported (Brooks et al.; Tillotson and Lerner; O'Connor et al.). This may be due to better diagnosis of disease. Clinical, and to some extent also anatomic, diagnosis of localized cryptococcal lesions is difficult. Only the occasional presence of mucoid masses leads to a suspicion of cryptococcosis grossly; foci or tumors of the granulomatous type can easily be misdiagnosed, since they offer grossly no diagnostic clue. Before the fungus is confirmed they may pass as neoplasms. Viscera are often not enlarged and grossly have a normal appearance. Diagnosis of cryptococcosis in kidneys, adrenals, liver, spleen, lymph nodes, and in other sites must rely therefore mostly on microscopic examination. In the large anatomically examined series of cases (BAKER and HAUGEN; COX and TOLHURST; LTTMAN and ZIMMERMAN and ZIMMERMAN and RAPPAPORT), involvement of numerous organs was found. Disseminated and localized lesions will be confirmed more often when complete autopsies are performed. The patient notes *ophthalmic* symptoms often after onset of disease in the central nervous system. These are due to direct extension of leptomeningitis to the optic nerve with cryptococcal neuritis (DE BUEN et al.; OKUN and BUTLER; WAGER and CALHOUN) or to sequelae of hematogenous spread (LITTMAN and ZIMMERMAN). In different sites multiple lesions may occur and produce cryptococcal chorioretinitis, uveitis or ophthalmitis (DE BUEN et al.; HEINSIUS; MUKHERJEA et al.; OKUN and BUTLER; WAGER and COLHOUN; WEISS et al.; ZIMMERMAN and RAPPAPORT). FAZAKAS described one case with cryptococcal keratitis. Ocular lesions in disseminated fatal disease are assumed to be more frequent, although for obvious reasons there has been no confirmation. Human ocular cryptococcosis has been confirmed anatomically.

In the *skin cryptococcal* lesions are more frequent than in the oronasal and pharyngeal mucosae. LITTMAN and ZIMMERMAN indicate that the latter are affected only about one-third as often as the skin. In a review of 120 cases of cryptococcosis (CAWLEY et al., 1950) 13 showed cutaneous manifestations. In 1952, EVANS and HARREL also reviewed the subject of cutaneous involvement. Cases with this localization were reported by BRIER et al.; BUREAU and BRONSARD; BUREAU et al. (1955); CARRICK; COLBERT et al.; DA SILVA; DEBRÉ et al.; DROUHET et al. (1961); DROUHET and MARTIN; GANDY; GEANEY et al.; GRSCHEBIN; HICKIE and WALKER; HOLTZ; KING; MAHNKE et al. (1961); McGEHEE and MICHELSON; McGIBBON and READETT; MUMENTHALER; MOORE; MOOK and MOORE; PIERS; RUITER and ENSINK; SAUERTEIG; TORREY; URBACH and ZACH; VERSÉ; WEIDMAN; WILE. Multiple foci are frequent, as are facial lesions. Grossly, acneform nodules, pustules and papules are seen; ulceration is also frequent, the latter offering the possibility of confirmation of the fungus in smears. Subcutaneous cryptococcal lesions with intact epidermis give the impression of tumors. Although pseudoepitheliomatous hyperplasia of epidermis is not as often seen as in other mycoses (N.A. blastomycosis, paracoccidioidomycosis, chromoblastomycosis) gross diagnosis of carcinoma is occasionally made. The gelatinous type of tissue reaction in cutaneous lesions may lead to gross diagnosis of myxoma or lipoma. On the other hand, the granulomatous type occurs also in the skin and mucosae.

Bone involvement has been reported in approximately the same percentage of cases of cryptococcosis as cutaneous manifestations (10%). This localization was found in 17 of 200 reviewed cases by COLLINS who added three new cases. Any bone can be involved, although there seems to be a predilection for bony prominences, cranial bones, and vertebrae (LITTMAN and ZIMMERMAN). The clinical and gross appearances often lead to an initial diagnosis of neoplasm, as in the first described classical case of cryptococcosis with lesions in the tibia (BUSSE). Only careful search for the organisms will lead to correct diagnosis, especially in cases in which no other localization of disease is manifest. The granulomatous type of tissue reaction is predominant; only rarely large foci of the gelatinous type of

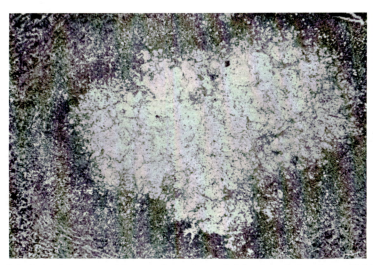

Fig. 37. Gelatinous cryptococcal focus in liver surrounded by granulation tissue. H & E, × 20

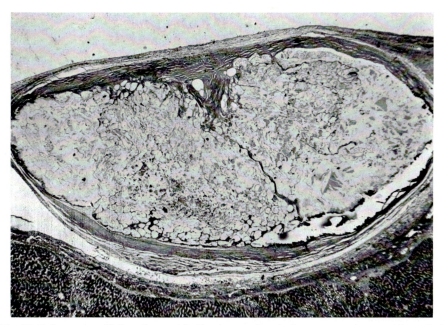

Fig. 38. Subcapsular old liver focus with fibrous capsule; single cryptococci present in central areas, not visible at this magnification. H & E, × 20

tissue reaction are seen in osseous cryptococcosis. Joints are rarely involved; no periosteal reactions have been reported. Osseous localization was described by DUCUING et al.; DROUHET and MARTIN; DURIE and McDONALD; HICKIE and WALKER; JESSE; LONGMIRE and GOODWIN; MIDER et al.; MORRIS and WOLINSKY; NICHOLS and MARTIN; RIGDON and KIRKSEY; SEMERAK; SMITH and CRAWFORD; SONCK; WIENER; WOLFE and JACOBSON. Small cryptococcal granulomas are found frequently in the bone marrow in disseminated disease.

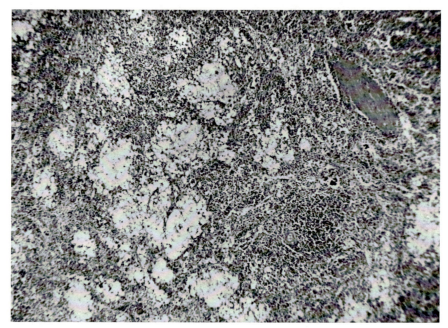

Fig. 39. Gelatinous foci of cryptococcosis in spleen. "Clear areas" at low power with numerous fungus cells visible at higher magnification. H & E, × 47

In the *cardiovascular system* cryptococcal lesions are infrequent. Anguli and Natarajan; Sabesin et al.; Zawirska and Derubska reported involvement of the myocardium with formation of cryptococcal granuloma or cryptococcoma. Fungal endocarditis has been described only twice (Colmers et al.; Lombardo et al.); the diagnosis was made in the latter case by histologic and cultural proof of the fungus in the thrombotic masses of the valve. In the case of Colmers et al., *C. neoformans* was found in blood smears and confirmed in the blood by culture. The patient was cured with amphotericin B medication; therefore anatomic proof in this case could not be obtained. Involvement of the aorta is mentioned by Longmire and Goodwin, Baker and Haugen and Rigdon and Kirksey; in the latter case a pure mycotic aneurysm was observed. Zeitlhofer reports involvement of the wall of pulmonary blood vessels. A case of chronic endarteritis in the leptomeninges was found not to be of cryptococcal nature.

Involvement of the *intestinal tract* with lesions of the granulomatous type has been observed occasionally (Allen and Lowbeer; Beck and Voyles; Flinn et al.; Linell et al.; Lippelt; Mosberg and Arnold).

In the *pancreas* cryptococcal lesions are rare. Small fungus-containing foci were seen by Zawirska and Derubska and Zimmerman and Rappaport.

In the *adrenals* small cryptococcal granulomas are found (Baker and Haugen; Bowman and Ritchey; Lombardo et al.; Nichols and Martin; Rawson et al.; Rigdon and Kirksey). Wide areas of parenchymatous destruction with caseating necrosis do not form as a rule; thus insufficiency of these organs is not a common feature, in contrast to the frequent and massive adrenal lesions in generalized histoplasmosis and paracoccidioidomycosis. Cryptococcal lesions in the *liver* occur (Baker, 1962; Gendel et al.; Kent and Leyton; Longmire and Goodwin; Misch; Procknow et al.; Symmers, 1953; Wilkins et al.; Zawirska and Derubska),

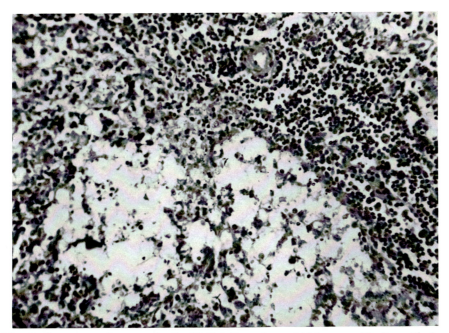

Fig. 40. Same case and organ as in Fig. 39. Gelatinous focus at higher magnification with clear spaces. H & E, × 190

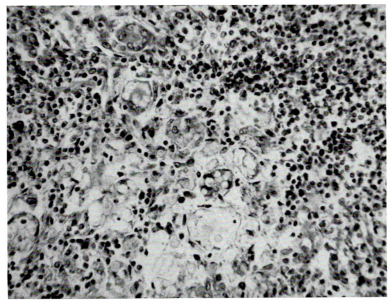

Fig. 41. Granulomatous splenic lesion of cryptococcosis. Fungus cells in histiocytes and giant cells. H & E, × 300

but are not found in all cases of generalized disease. Mostly small granulomas with organisms are observed; larger foci and the gelatinous type of tissue reaction (SABESIN et al.; SALFELDER and SCHWARZ) are exceptional findings (Figs. 37, 38).

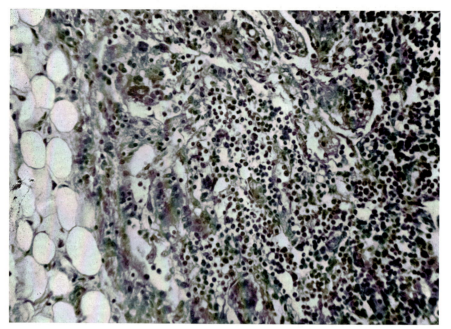

Fig. 42. Lymph node; cryptococcosis in peripheral areas. Single or accumulated giant cells containing fungus cells. H & E, × 190

In the *spleen* and *lymph nodes* cryptococcal lesions are common; but not the rule. While in the former, large areas may show the typical gelatinous type of lesions (Figs. 39, 40, 41), in the latter, granulomas, mostly of small size, are found. In cases of pulmonary cryptococcosis, hilar lymph node involvement is not an obligatory finding. Often only scattered giant cells or accumulations of such cells containing fungus cells are seen (Fig. 42). Necrotic foci and healed fibrosing granulomas (Fig. 43) are not seen, in contrast to the frequently occurring residual foci in histoplasmosis in these sites.

In the *kidneys* cryptococci are found often in glomerular loops (Fig. 44) and, less frequently, filling the lumina of tubules (Fig. 45). In such cases the fungus cells can be isolated easily from the urine. In fungemia these intravascular nests of fungus cells are a common finding also in other sites. Renal granulomatous lesions (Baker, 1952; Crone et al.; Hoigne et al.; Spivack et al.; Zimmerman and Rappaport) consist mostly of small scattered foci (Figs. 46, 47). Large areas, as in the case of Zawirska and Derubska, are not involved and gelatinous lesions do not form.

The *prostate* also can be the site of cryptococcal lesions (Baker and Haugen; Bowman and Ritchey; Brooks et al.; Cohen and Kaufmann; Dreyfuss et al.; O'Connor et al.; Sabesin et al.; Tillotson and Lerner; Voyles and Beck; Zelman et al.). Cryptococcal prostatitis is generally granulomatous; no large gelatinous lesions are found. While lesions have been detected mostly at necropsy, Dreyfuss et al.; Brooks et al.; and Tillotson and Lerner made intravitam diagnoses. Cohen and Kaufmann considered their observation (erroneously) as primary infection. The *testes* may show cryptococcal lesions (Wilson, J.W.) but no original report has been found of these or of involvement of the *parathyroid* or *pituitary* glands. Involvement of the *thymus* was reported by MacGillivray, and

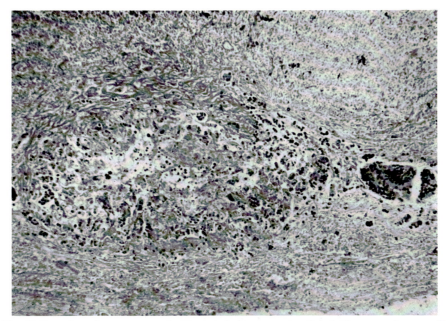

Fig. 43. Lymph node cryptococcosis. Necrotic lesions are exceptional. Numerous fungus cells in periphery of focus. H & E and Grocott, × 95

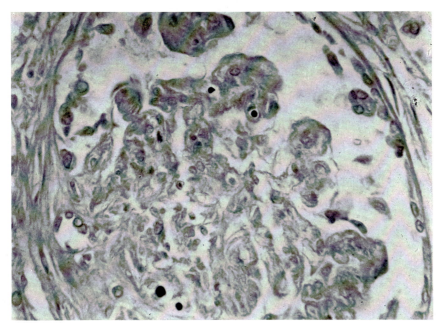

Fig. 44. Lupus erythematosus disseminatus. Single cryptococcus cells in glomerular capillaries. Grocott, × 450

small cryptococcal granulomas were reported in the *thyroid* by SABESIN et al. and were observed also in one of our cases (Fig. 48).

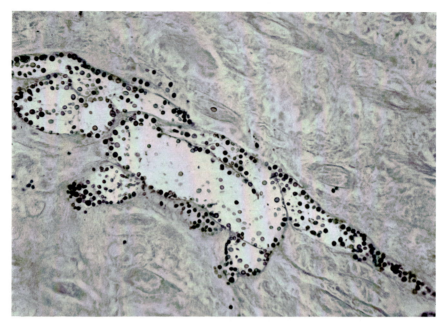

Fig. 45. Renal cryptococcosis. Numerous fungus cells filling tubules. Grocott, × 190

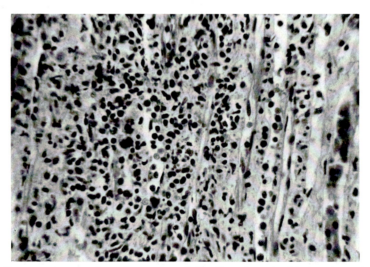

Fig. 46. Cryptococcic granuloma in renal medulla. Lymphocytic, histiocytic, and plasma-cellular infiltrate with a few leukocytes. Scarce fungus cells. H & E, × 200

Skeletal musculature, larynx, trachea, esophagus and *stomach* apparently remain free of cryptococcal invasion, as do the *female genitalia. Breast* involvement was reported by Kohlmeier and Kreitner; Symmers, and in one of our cases suffering from lupus erythematosus. Incidentally, cryptococci could be found in small blood vessels of the endometrium in one of our cases.

Fungi in tissues: While the yeastlike fungus cells stain pale-blue or pink in H and E-stained sections, many fungi do not stain with H and E, and show only

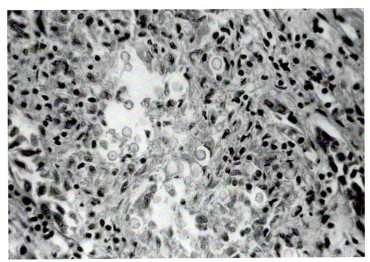

Fig. 47. Cryptococcal granuloma (kidney) with intra- and extracellular fungus cells. Macrophages and giant cells. H & E, × 200

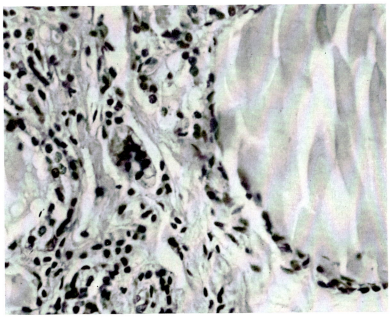

Fig. 48. Small interstitial cryptococcal granuloma in thyroid with giant cells containing poorly visible fungus cells. H & E, × 275

on Grocott staining (Figs. 49, 50), even when abundant. In tissues *C. neoformans* is generally spherical, occasionally oval (Fig. 51). Other shapes — sickle, half-moon, and bowl forms are rare and appear to correspond to degenerated fungus cells being seen after prolonged fixation in formalin and after use of fungistatics [(MATHEIS) Figs. 52, 53]. We have seen such variants in many yeasts of different species and in *Pneumocystis carinii* in tissues, mostly with the Grocott stain. The

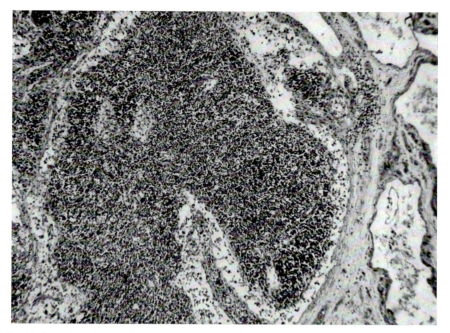

Fig. 49. Lymph node cryptococcosis. Clear marginal sinus. Also, at higher power, fungus cells are difficult to visualize in this preparation. H & E, × 55

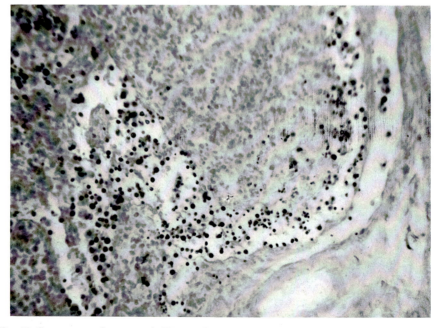

Fig. 50. Same case and organ as in Fig. 49. In the marginal sinus numerous cryptococci can be seen with this method. Grocott, × 190

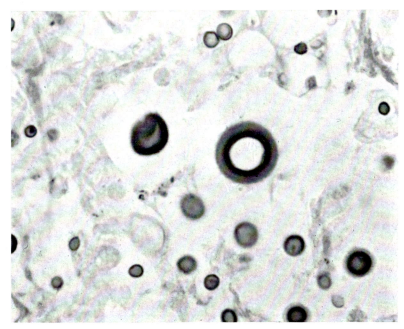

Fig. 51. Spherical fungus cells in lung alveolus. Grocott, × 720

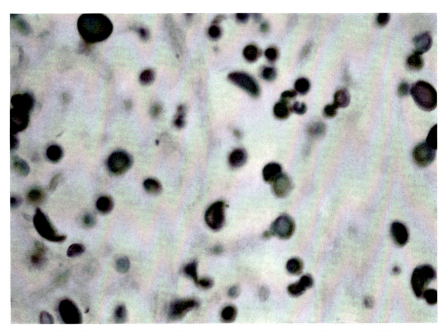

Fig. 52. Fungus cells of different shapes in lung tissue. Grocott, × 720

size of *C. neoformans* in tissues without the capsule varies considerably (Fig. 54). A diameter of 2—15 μ is the rule. MATHEIS found variations between 1—50 μ and giant forms. The fungus cells are surrounded by a thin membrane within the

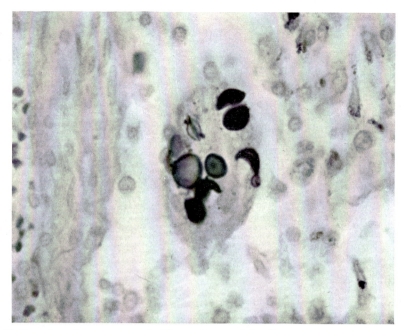

Fig. 53. Lymph node cryptococcosis. Nest of intracellular fungus cells of different shapes. Bowl, half-moon, and sickle forms. Grocott, × 720

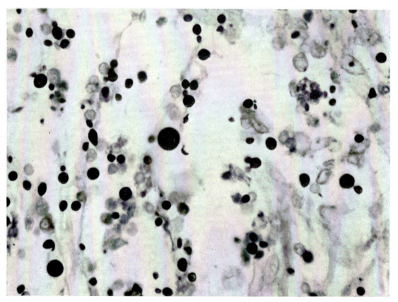

Fig. 54. Cryptococcal meningitis. Great variation in size of fungus cells. Grocott, × 720

capsule, which appears on H and E and on Grocott as a halo, often not clearly delineated. The halo has commonly a thickness of 3—5 μ; Littman and Zimmerman mention thickness as up to 7 and Fetter et al. up to 18 μ. This capsule, which contains mucopolysaccharides and appears pink with Mayer's mucicarmine,

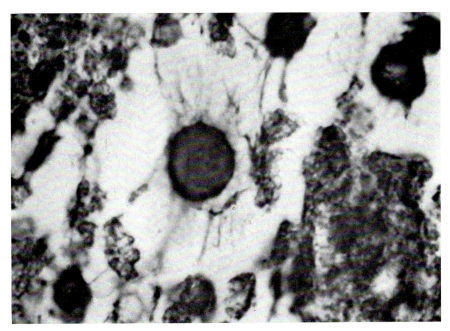

Fig. 55. Pulmonary cryptococcosis. Radiating spines of polysaccharide material surround a fungus cell. Mucicarmine, × 1500

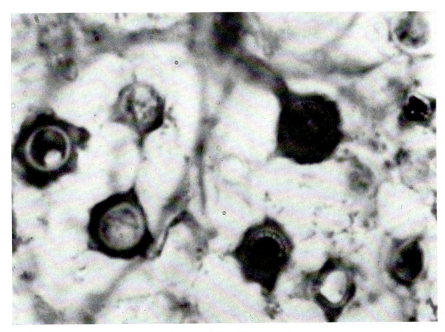

Fig. 56. Cytoplasmic structures in fungus cells of lung section; some may be artefacts from formalin fixation. H & E, × 1800

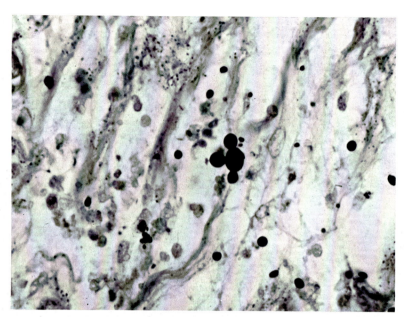

Fig. 57 Cryptococcic meningitis. Multiple budding (3 buds) of a cryptococcus cell. Exceptional finding. Grocott, × 720

Best's carmine, and the acid mucopolysaccharide method of Rinehart and Abul-Hay, is highly characteristic for *C. neoformans* and of great diagnostic value. Radiating spines, due to shrinkage of capsular material by formalin-alcohol fixation, may extend from the capsule (Fig. 55).

The whole fungus cell often appears pink when stained with mucicarmine, and fungus cell membrane and capsule are easily recognizable. Tomcsik distinguishes a mucinous halo outside the capsule and assumes a continuous transition between capsule and halo. The inner parts of the fungus cells often appear to be empty, with no internal structures visible or with only poorly defined cytoplasmic masses. However, in many organisms vacuoles and a granular material can be recognized; these are of a lipoid nature and are sudanophilic. Coarse structures which occasionally appear inside the fungus cells may be artefacts due to formalin fixation (Fig. 56). Many budding fungus cells are found in active lesions while in old foci no signs of reproduction are seen. Daughter cells are attached to parent cells by a narrow neck. Single buds are most often observed; exceptionally, double or multiple buds are seen (Caldwell and Raphael; Emmons, 1951) (Fig. 57). In cryptococcic lesions with many organisms, the fungus cells often form chains, thus giving the impression of pseudohyphae (Figs. 58, 59); true hyphal formation does not occur. The possibility of postmortem multiplication of fungus cells has been discussed (Matheis; Zeman and Bebin), but was not confirmed. The presence of granulation tissue in foci with abundant fungi clearly points to an intravital process (Matheis). In the gelatinous type of tissue reaction fungus cells with radiating spines are generally found; (De Buscher et al.); Matheis found them in both the gelatinous and granulomatous lesions. In the latter, where generally few fungi occur, they are frequently overlooked in H & E stained sections. Fungus cells are found frequently inside macrophages and giant cells. When many fungus cells are localized in macrophages with distention of cytoplasm, the

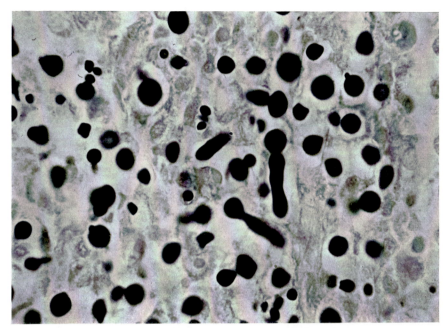

Fig. 58. Splenic cryptococcosis with numerous organisms. Elongated fungus cells forming pseudohyphae. Grocott, × 800

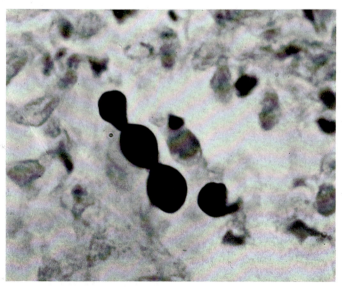

Fig. 59. Same case and organ as in Fig. 58. Three fungus cells forming chain. Grocott, × 1500

contours of tissue cells are often not visible. Besides the fungus cells in the interstices of the meshwork of gelatinous lesions, a mucicarmine-positive pink matrix of granular or homogeneous appearance is found, which derives from the capsular substance. Similar material has been found in renal tubules, forming casts when cryptococci were present in glomeruli (LITTMAN and ZIMMERMAN).

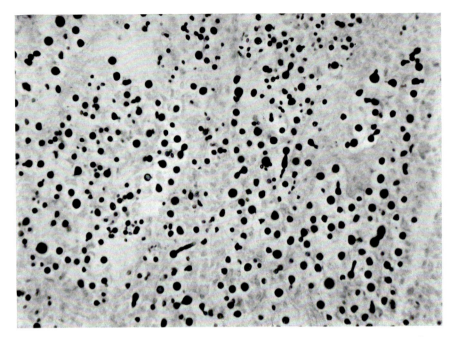

Fig. 60. Same case and organ as in Fig. 58. Numerous organisms in the tissue do not show as clearly in routinely stained tissue sections. Grocott, × 300

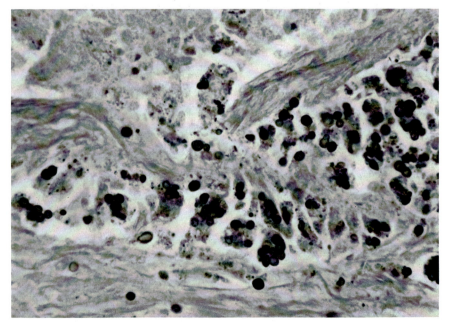

Fig. 61. Pulmonary focal cryptococcosis. In periphery of an old lesion mostly intracellular cryptococci and Grocott-positive dustlike granules. Grocott, × 450

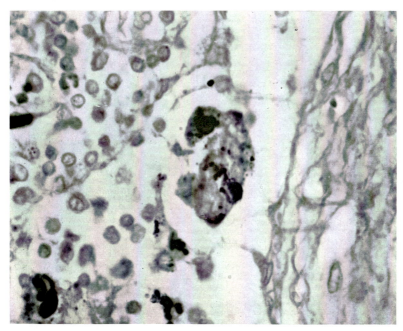

Fig. 62. Lymph node cryptococcosis. Extra- and intracellular Grocott-positive dustlike granules which must be differentiated from anthracotic pigment. This is easily done in tissues where this pigment does not occur. Grocott, × 720

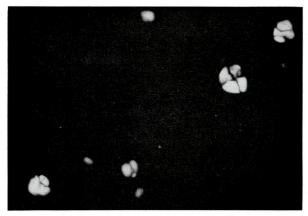

Fig. 63. Pulmonary cryptococcosis. Several of the fungus cells are optically active when observed under polarized light. Occasionally Malta crosses appear. H & E, × 700

Stains Recommended: PAS, Gridley, Gram, Hale's colloidal iron, and Bodian methods; alcian blue, toluidine blue, cresyl violet, and Sudan III have all been used successfully. Mucicarmine is best for the wall and the capsular substance.

For differential diagnosis, we prefer the Grocott method, with which all fungus cells stain black and show the extent of tissue invasion (Fig. 60), at the same time revealing single organisms. The Grocott method also shows fragmented and destroyed fungus cells with granular, dustlike elements which can be seen especially in the periphery of old lesions where numerous fungus cells accumulate (Figs. 61, 62). It is doubtful whether the Grocott-positive granular particles sometimes seen without fungus cells derive from such cells; they are similar to deposits

28*

of anthracotic pigment; similar dustlike elements have been seen in histoplasmic lesions (SALFELDER and SCHWARZ, 1967b) and paracoccidioidomycosis (unpublished data, SALFELDER and SCHWARZ).

Other methods for viewing fungus cells in tissues include use of the phase-contrast microscope (MATHEIS) and fluorescence under ultraviolet light (MOLNAR; YASAKI et al.; FETTER et al.). Under polarized light the fungus capsule gives birefringency, especially in freshly formalin-fixed tissue (MATHEIS). POTENZA and FEO, and BRASS reported this phenomenon in other mycoses with yeastlike fungus cells in tissue sections. KLATZO and GEISLER used a buffered cresyl violet technic for staining of *C. neoformans*, and observed the fungus cells with unusual clarity under polarized light. Sections from cases of paracoccidioidomycosis, coccidioidomycosis, histoplasmosis, and toxoplasmosis examined by this method failed to show anisotropic features of the organisms. Birefringency, however, is not a particularity of the fungus cells, since this phenomenon could be observed neither in mounts of fungus cells from cultures nor in frozen sections mounted in water. Parts of the fungus cells or their membranes appear birefringent when observed with crossed Nicols and show Maltese crosses (Fig. 63) only when treated with paraffin and oily substances. Maltese crosses also occur in unstained sputum and bronchial content smears, apparently representing lipoid or carbohydrate droplets; these should not be confused with fungus cells. *Cryptococcus neoformans* does not always show capsules, or they may be very thin and not visible in tissue sections (SCHOLER et al.). As mentioned earlier, India ink is the stain of choice for capsules (cf. *Mycology*, chapter V). The fluorescent antibody staining method also shows the mucicarmine-positive mucopolysaccharide capsular substance in tissue sections of formalin-fixed material (KASE and MARSHALL; MARSHALL et al., 1961). However, this is not specific for *Cryptococcus*, since *Rhinosporidium seeberi* also gives a positive antibody reaction with anticryptococcal serum.

Diagnosis and Differential Diagnosis

Clinical diagnosis is difficult and must be confirmed by identification of the fungus. While previously, postmortem diagnosis was made three times as often as intra vitam (JONES and KLINCK, 1945), conditions have changed (MATHEIS). GEANEY et al. diagnosed clinically all their series of 14 cases and BUTLER et al. all of 40 cases.

In pulmonary involvement, all kinds of infectious or malignant diseases, especially metastatic carcinoma, must be excluded (LOURIA). The lack of specific radiographic signs makes radiologic diagnosis difficult (DICK), and small radiologic foci may be overlooked, in both pulmonary and osseous disease. Bacterial meningitis, meningeal carcinomatosis, and sarcoidosis must be ruled out in cases of cryptococcic meningitis and especially of tuberculous meningitis. Cerebrospinal fluid sugar values are not necessarily low in cryptococcal meningitis, as was believed earlier. Cryptococcomas in the brain and meninges produce a clinical pattern similar to that of space-occupying tumors. Hematologic data are not characteristic. Duration of disease gives certain clues for diagnosis, as also chronic diseases of the lymphatic system, malignant lymphomas, and Hodgkin's disease. In cases of localized nodular lesions in lung, bones, central nervous system, and occasionally other sites, and in cases of cryptococcomas, diagnosis is made more frequently after exploratory surgery, which often simultaneously constitutes effective therapy.

In clinical material *C. neoformans* can be proved without great difficulty, but several pitfalls should be considered before a definite diagnosis is made. The presence of encapsulated yeast cells of 5—10 μ in smears of spinal fluid (Fig. 64) should always be considered an alarming finding, but diagnosis in the laboratory should be made only if lymphocytes are found simultaneously. We have twice found encapsulated yeast cells in spinal fluid without pleocytosis and have assumed that they came from the glassware, which was bacteriologically sterile but not microscopically clean. Leucocytes in spinal fluid often show a halo phenomenon when suspended in India-ink preparations and must be differentiated from yeast cells by demonstration of the nucleus and the absence of the easily visible bubbles of lipid in the yeast. Once yeast cells are accepted, cultures should be initiated according to the following routine procedure.

Cultures should be made on Sabouraud's glucose agar (with and without actidione) at room temperature and at 37°C. Growth only on media *without* actidione gives strong tentative evidence for *Cryptococcus*. If the organisms grow on media incubated at 37°C, further evidence for *C.neoformans* is established. A selective or differential culture medium has lately been recommended by STAIB (k); WIEBECKE and STAIB, and SHIELDS and AJELLO. The next step is a positive urease test, which rules out the genus *Candida* and establishes the identity of the *Cryptococcus*. If the organism has been found in spinal fluid from a case of mening-itis, further identification for clinical purposes is rarely necessary. If there is

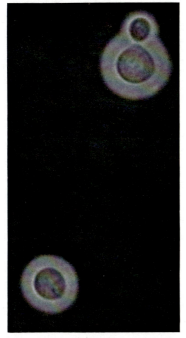

Fig. 64. India-ink preparation from sediment of spinal fluid in a case of cryptococcal meningitis.
× 1000
The capsules in mounts from human or animal material often show wider capsular envelopes than in culture mounts

another source, such as sputum or urine or pus from peripheral sites, assimilation tests should be carried out. *C.neoformans* does not assimilate potassium nitrate as the sole source of nitrogen, nor lactose as the sole source of carbohydrate. The intracerebral injection of culture material into mice is proof conclusive of patho-genicity (Fig. 65) when lesions are produced, and rules out other *Cryptococci*. But this can take as long as eight weeks and may not always result in lesions in all mice (KAO and SCHWARZ). In tissues, solitary yeast cells can produce serious diagnostic problems, especially if no extra material is available for special stains. *C.neofor-mans* usually stains selectively with mucicarmine, but often only a few cells will take the stain, the majority remaining unstained. In instances where the capsule is very prominent, capsular stain can be obtained with mucicarmine. Sometimes only radial fibers stain pink or red, producing a confusing picture, simulating even

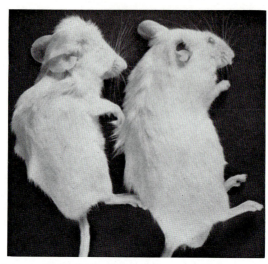

Fig. 65. Result of intracerebral injection of *C. neoformans*. The mouse on the left shows loss
of weight and dome-shaped elevation of skull

the multiple buds of *Paracoccidioides brasiliensis*. Often one sees great variation
from field to field, in the thickness of the capsule in the same section, and the
corresponding morphology of "holes" in the tissue becomes dubious.

C. neoformans is intensely stained by the Grocott procedure, but this alone
lacks specificity, as do the Gridley and PAS stains. Rhodamin, acridine orange and
other fluorochrome procedures bring the organisms out in great contrast but
contribute little toward selective diagnostic recognition. Fluorescent antibody
stains have been tried successfully, but it has to be remembered that the fluorescent antibody methods (EVELAND et al.; MARSHAL et al., 1958, 1959, 1961; SMITH
et al., 1959), work capriciously on formalin fixed material. They do not stain some
strains and the method needs to be extensively evaluated as a diagnostic tool
(KAUFMAN, 1965). From the point of view of differential diagnosis in tissue sections, several other fungi must be excluded. *B. dermatitidis* generally shows a
thicker wall. Its bud has a broad base, while the neck of the bud in *C. neoformans*
is narrow. No capsule is seen in *B. dermatitidis*, but it can also be minimal or even
absent in *C. neoformans*. *Paracoccidioides brasiliensis* is as a rule somewhat larger,
and if multiple budding can be demonstrated in several instances, the differentiation is definitive. Double or multiple buds in *C. neoformans* are rare. The spherules
of *Coccidioides immitis* with endospores cannot be confused with *C. neoformans*.
Isolated endospores can simulate *C. neoformans* in size and shape but lack budding
and a capsule. *Histoplasma capsulatum* and *H. duboisii* are not easily confused
with *C. neoformans*; the former is smaller and is not often seen in H & E preparations, although it comes out distinctly with Grocott; however, small and recently
formed yeast cells of *C. neoformans* are of the same size and shape. In one case of
HOUK and MOSER *H. capsulatum* was diagnosed in a specimen which cultured as
C. neoformans. The larger *H. duboisii* can be mistaken more easily for *C. neoformans*,
but the fungus cells show a more compact aspect and lack the capsule. Recently
we have seen a case of Lobo's disease in which the fungus cells showed broad halos,
in H & E sections so that diagnosis of *C. neoformans* was briefly considered. On
Grocott, however, the typical localization of fungus cells in chains led to a correct
diagnosis. *Candida* cells are only rarely mistaken for *C. neoformans*.

The outstanding "practical" differentiation is the selective staining of *C. neoformans* with mucicarmine. While *Rhinosporidium seeberi* is also mucicarmine positive its morphology is so different that this fungus does not form part of the organisms considered in differential diagnosis. In addition to other fungi, certain structures in tissue sections show features which may lead to misdiagnosis of *C. neoformans*. These include, in granulation tissue, large tissue cells, hydropic inflammatory cells, Russell bodies, and even erythrocytes; also mineral concretions or corpora amylaceae in the lungs. However, these show structural details which are not present in *C. neoformans* and in addition do not have the staining properties of the fungus cells. The concentric layers or laminated appearance of these structures may sometimes simulate a capsule.

In brain tissue the corpora amylaceae also show Grocott positivity, are similar to *C. neoformans* in size and shape, and may even show pseudobudding (FETTER et. al.). However, they stain dark in H & E and have no capsule. SEGRETAIN and COUTEU recommend staining with iodine. MATHEIS and HOIGNE et al. discuss the difficulty of distinguishing corpora amylacea from *C. neoformans* in cases in which both elements occur together in cryptococcal lesions. Also in brain tissue the sickle, half moon, lemon and bowl forms of *Toxoplasma gondii* may lead to false diagnosis of *C. neoformans* (MATHEIS) (cf. *Cryptococcosis of the Newborn*). Tissue reaction in the presence of single suspicious elements does not always help in diagnosis. In unstained smears from brain tissue, fat droplets, air bubbles and myelin globules may easily simulate the shape of fungus cells and suggest *Cryptococci* (Borelli). In urinary sediment, erythrocytes have been mistaken for yeast cells (FITZPATRICK et al.). *C. neoformans* var. innocuous can be tentatively differentiated from *C. neoformans* by the more spherical shape and granular aspect of the cytoplasm of the latter.

Torulopsosis: Finally, infection with *Torulopsis glabrata* must be differentiated from cryptococcosis. This rare mycosis, whose infective agent was formerly considered as nonpathogenic, does not present serious diagnostic problems, since the fungus has the morphology and dimensions of *H. capsulatum*. The agent was first described in 1917 in human beings (ANDERSON). It was examined mycologically and experimentally by LODDER and DE VRIES; LOPEZ FERNANDEZ and ARTAGEREYTIA-ALLENDE. A few fatal cases have been reported and a septic form is known (BLACK and FISHER; GRIMLEY et al.; LOURIA et al., 1961; MINKOWITZ et al.; PLAUT).

Clinical Aspects

Symptoms and signs of cryptococcic disease vary considerably, according to organic involvement. It is not unusual to find fungi or cryptococcal lesions at necropsy, in individuals who showed no symptoms of cryptococcosis intra vitam. In many cases, symptoms of associated diseases overshadow the fungal disease; when cryptococcic infection occurs secondarily, its manifestations may be difficult to differentiate from remissions and relapses of the basic disease.

Of characteristic signs and symptoms of cryptococcosis only those involving the central nervous system, especially the meninges, are patent. Of these, the major symptom is headache. Pulmonary symptoms are rarely observed; cases like those of SHEPPE with manifest pulmonary disease, are the exception. LITTMAN and ZIMMERMAN give five *radiologic characteristics of lung involvement:* 1. Predilection for the lower half of the lung fields. 2. Rare cavitation. 3. Minimal or absent fibrosis or calcification. 4. Inconspicuous hilar lymphadenopathy. 5. Infrequency of massive pulmonary collapse.

Ocular cryptococcosis rarely causes blindness. Polyarthritic symptoms, as reported by SHIELDS in a case with associated sarcoidosis, are exceptional. Bone involvement produces pain, suggestive of any osseous lesion. In two cases of endocarditis, symptoms of valve disease with fever suggested endocarditis lenta. Hepatic symptoms have been recorded only in the cases of SABESIN et al. and PROCKNOW et al., and renal insufficiency only in the observation of ZAWIRSKA and DERUBSKA.

The course of the disease is capricious and unpredictable. Periods of remission and relapse are common in untreated cases. PALMROSE and LOSLI report the death of a patient from cryptococcosis 3 years after resection of a pulmonary lesion. BEESON describes a patient who experienced several remissions and died 16 years after the onset of cryptococcosis, showing chronic meningitis and hydrocephalus. Others (REEVES et al.; VOYLES and BECK; WIENER) report cases of several years' duration. Fulminant infections, with cryptococcal meningitis, which terminate fatally within a few weeks (ROANTREE and DUNKERLEY) are rare. Single localized and small lesions of the lung and the skin of the subclinical form or when clinically apparent may occasionally heal without therapy. (BONMATI et al.; HARDAWAY and CRAWFORD; HOUK and MOSER; KUYKENDALL et al.; McCULLOUGH et al.; STODDARD and CUTLER; WEBSTER). Surgical resection of skin, bone, central nervous system, and lung lesions have been performed successfully and there has been also a surgical indication in liver disease (PROCKNOW et al.), but surgical extirpation is most often associated with pulmonary lesions, and was suggested by TABER as early as 1937. Surgically treated cases are described by BERK and GERSTL; CORNISH et al.; DORMER et al.; DORMER and SCHER; FROIO and BAILEY; HAWKINS; HICKIE and WALKER; KATZ et al.; KUYKENDALL et al.; McCONCHIE; POPPE; SCHEPEL and CARSJENS; SUSMAN; WEBSTER; WHITE and ARANY; WOLFE and JACOBSON.

In addition to the report of their own cases, KNUDSON et al., in 1963, reviewed more than 50 cases with resected pulmonary lesions. Previously, CARTON and MOUNT (1951) had reviewed more than 40 operated cases of central nervous system lesions. DILLON and SEALEY, KRAINER et al. and LEY et al. published reports of cured cases after surgery.

Cure of osseous cryptococcosis (WOLFE and JACOBSON; LEOPOLD) by resection is less frequent (COLLINS). Surgical procedures are now generally accompanied by medical treatment and prognosis is improved (WEBSTER; KATZ et al.). Localized cryptococcal lesions, above all in the lung, should be resected even though there is also central nervous system disease (FETTER et al.). Before the use of amphotericin B, many drugs were tried in the medical therapy of cryptococcosis. These have been summarized and discussed exhaustively by LITTMAN and ZIMMERMAN, who also stated that there is no convincing evidence of the effectiveness of heat therapy. Only one report of favorable results with sulfadiazine has been found (SIEWERS and CRAMBLETT). The *drug of choice* clearly appears to be *amphotericin B*, given intravenously; this is also the only effective drug in some other deep mycoses (ANDRIOLE and KRAVETZ; FURCOLOW; LITTMAN, 1962; NEWCOMER et al.; RUBIN et al.; SEABURY and DASCOMB; SEABURY). There should no longer be disputes about the efficacy of amphotericin B in the treatment of cryptococcal meningitis. Improvement and apparent cures have been reported in single cases and also in larger series of patients (APPELBAUM and SHTOKALKO; BARRASH and FORT; BEER; BUTAS and LLOYD-SMITH; BUTLER et al.; DROUHET, 1961—1964; EMANUEL et al.; FITZPATRICK et al.; FITZPATRICK and POSER; FRISK and HOLMGREN; GETTELFINGER; HELLER et al.; HESS; HICKIE and WALKER; KATZ et al.; SMITH, 1958; SMITH et al., 1960; SPICKARD et al.). In the recent series of BUTLER et al. (40 cases),

1-year survival was observed in more than 50% of the patients given this drug; three were free of disease after 5 years.

The unfavorable side-effects and complications of amphotericin B, however, cannot be ignored. Above all, its nephrotoxicity requires expert management (BUTLER et al. (b); BELL et al.); CARNECHIA and KURTZKE reported on anatomically proved liver and renal damage in one case of cryptococcosis. HILL et al. reported renal histopathology in man and dog; and RHOADES et al. studied renal function in man after amphotericin B treatment. Neurologic and hematologic complications were mentioned by HABER and JOSEPH and BRANDRISS et al., respectively. A patient of RUITER and ENSINK, with extensive cutaneous cryptococcosis, died in shock during injection with amphotericin B. Only HOUK and MOSER question the value of this treatment, at least in certain cases, and speak against its routine use. In their 6 cases, improvement was observed without amphotericin B; in 5 cases, lung lesions had been resected. Two cases were followed for more than 10 years and two for more than 6 years. It is possible that cases with self-limited lesions have a benign evolution, although the final evaluation can be made only after long-term followup.

Prognosis was originally desperate. Only 25% of patients with meningitis survived the first year of illness (FETTER et al.) without the therapy now available. The outlook was better in cases of isolated disease in the lung and other sites, in which remissions might be hoped for. While surgery and amphotericin B treatment have improved the prognosis considerably, the situation still remains dangerous when the central nervous system is involved or when associated debilitating diseases influence the course of disease.

The disappearance of fungi from clinical material indicates improvement. GORDON and VEDDER lately attribute value also to the latex slide agglutination test in controlling the course of evolution.

Animals

Spontaneous cryptococcosis occurs in a large variety of domestic, wild, and laboratory animals. It has been found in many countries and can be of economic importance in dairy herds. The fungus was isolated from the tissue of an ox as early as 1895 by SANFELICE. VUILLEMIN reported pulmonary cryptococcosis in a pig in 1901 (LITTMAN and ZIMMERMAN), although subsequently no reports of the disease in this species could be found. FROTHINGHAM detected cryptococcosis in a horse in 1902. Cryptococcosis in these animals must be distinguished from the epizootic lymphangitis caused by *Histoplasma farciminosum*. BARRON; LITTMAN and ZIMMERMAN; AJELLO, 1967 reviewed the subject of cryptococcosis in lower animals. Table 4 brings the bibliographic data up to date.

The largest number of cases have been reported in dairy cattle in which cryptococcal mastitis is often self-limited. In bovine mastitis, infection apparently can enter through the teats; in other animals the portals of entry of the fungus are varied but have no proved significance for human disease. Gross pathology, histology, and localization of lesions are similar to those in human cryptococcosis. No evidence has been brought forward to suggest animals as a source of human infection. It is worthy of repetition to note that spontaneous disease has not been found in birds.

Much work in *experimental* animal cryptococcosis has been done in recent years. LITTMAN and ZIMMERMAN summarized the results of studies of virulence in mice, rats, guinea pigs, rabbits, and chick embryos up to 1956. BERGMAN in 1961 undertook extensive experimental studies on more than 1000 mice.

Table 4. *Spontaneous cryptococcosis in animals*

Animals	Author(s) and year of report
cat	Curtis, 1951; Holzworth, 1952; Holzworth and Coffin, 1953; McGrath, 1954; Littman and Zimmerman, 1956; Trautwein and Nielson, 1962.
cattle	Madsen, 1942; Innes et al., 1952; Pounden et al., 1952; Emmons, 1952; Simon et al., 1953; Galli, 1954; Ajello, 1958; Scholer et al., 1961.
Miscellaneous data:	*Cryptococcus neoformans* in milk from apparently healthy cows: Klein, 1901; Carter and Young, 1950.
civet cat	Littman and Zimmerman (Eyestone), 1956.
dog	Helmboldt and Jungherr, 1952; Seibold et al., 1953; McGrath, 1954; Smith, D.L.T., et al., 1955; Trautwein and Nielson, 1962
ferret	Skulski and Symmers, 1954
fox	Littman and Zimmerman (Eyestone), 1956
gazelle	Saez, 1965
goat	Sutmoeller and Poelma, 1957; Dacorso and Chagas, 1957
guinea pig	Dezest, 1953; Bertschinger and Scholer, 1965
horse	Frothingham, 1902; Meyer, 1914; Kikuchi, 1923; Schellner, 1935; Bennett, 1944; Alajouanine et al., 1953; Herin and Dormal, 1962
Miscellaneous data:	*Cryptococcus* in equine intestinal tract: van Uden et al., 1958
koala	Backhouse and Bolliger, 1960; Bolliger and Finckh, 1962, 1962
leopard	Saunders, 1948; Weidman and Ratcliffe, 1954
monkey	Takos and Elton, 1953 (Marmoset); Littman and Zimmerman (Eyestone), 1956 (Mangabey)
mouse	Sacquet et al., 1959
mink	Trautwein and Nielson, 1962
wallaby	Saez, 1965

The most widely used animal is the white mouse. It has been used especially for studies of *pathogenicity* because of its susceptibility to *C.neoformans*. To confirm the presence of this fungus and to rule out nonpathogenic cryptococci, the intracerebral route of inoculation is preferred and is frequently lethal, unlike injection of other yeasts (Emmons, 1952). The fungus can be recovered in smears from the mouse brain; typical cryptococcic lesions also can be found in this organ histologically. Not all animals die, however, after intracerebral inoculation; neither do all rapidly develop tissue lesions. Formation of lesions can take up to eight weeks (Kao and Schwarz). Death should not be considered as conclusive proof of pathogenicity without positive histologic confirmation. Other routes of inoculation in the mouse may lead to disseminated disease, but the intracerebral route is the most certain. Rats and hamsters must be inoculated by other routes, since their skulls are too thick for injection without trepanation. Disease can easily be elicited in these animals.

In guinea pigs, varied results have been observed. Some die after inoculation; in others injection has no observable effect. Rabbits rarely develop infection (because of their high body temperature ?). Also chick embryos inoculated intravenously are not animals of choice for pathogenicity studies, since only fungemia, without inflammatory tissue reactions, are observed in this species (Kligman et al., 1951); the high mortality rate (Kligman and Weidman, 1949) can be due to other causes.

Virulence in mice has been studied by Hasenclever and Mitchell; Hasenclever and Emmons; Vanbreuseghem. After serial passage through mice, virulence can be enhanced (Littman and Zimmerman). Birds are not *hosts* of the fungus and show low pathogenicity. After feeding canaries with the fungus

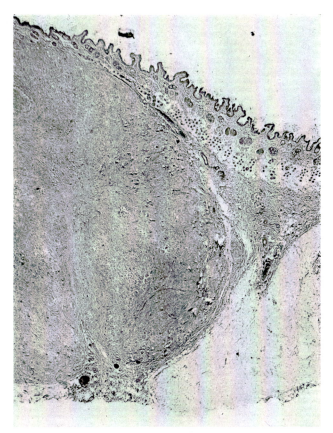

Fig. 66. Part of a huge granuloma 15 days after subcutaneous injection of a highly concentrated inoculum of *C. neoformans* in hamster. H & E, × 50

(Staib d), the organisms could be recovered from the intestinal passage, but no disease developed. Littman et al. (1965) were able to elicit cerebral disease and dissemination in pigeons after intracerebral inoculation; Sethi and Schwarz produced ocular disease in pigeons and, in more than 10%, disseminated disease after intraocular inoculation. Basu Mallik et al. obtained lesions in the lung and brain of mice by intranasal infection of the organisms. Herrold observed disease in hamsters first in the nasal cavity and paranasal tissues and cavities and later direct extension to the central nervous system. Ritter and Larsh produced primary lung infection. Inhalation of seeded soil conduced to pulmonary and disseminated disease in mice (Smith et al., 1964). After intratracheal inoculation, Wade and Stevenson achieved visceral cryptococcosis without involvement of the central nervous system.

Local infection and dissemination after subcutaneous inoculation has been studied in mice (Bergman, 1961; Binford; Cox and Tolhurst; Khan et al.; Levine et al., 1957; Wade and Stevenson; Staib b); in guinea pigs (Binford; Bureau et al., 1955; Cox and Tolhurst; Freeman, 1931); in rats (Cox and Tolhurst; Levine et al., 1957); in rabbits (Levine et al., 1957); in monkeys (Debré et al., 1947); and in hamsters (Sethi et al., 1965) (Fig. 66). The intestinal route of infection was studied by feeding the fungus to canaries (Staib d); to

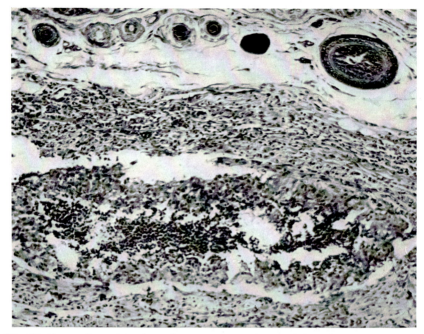

Fig. 67. Abscess formation after subcutaneous inoculation of *C.neoformans* in hamster.
H & E, × 100

hamsters and mice (Sethi b); to a calf (Pounden et al.); and to marmoset monkeys (Takos), only the last-mentioned reporting positive results. Other routes of
inoculation were the intraocular (Weiss et al.; Kligman and Weidman in rabbits);
intraperitoneal (Fazekas and Schwarz in mice; Staib b in mice; Mahnke in
mice; Subramanian et al. in mice; Kligman and Weidman in mice; Cox and
Tolhurst in mice; Hale and Lomanitz in mice; Lutzky and Brodish in dogs;
Stoddard and Cutler in rats; Sethi et al. in hamsters); intravenous (Littman
and Zimmerman in mice; Staib b in mice; Lutzky and Brodish in dogs); intrathecal (Lutzky and Brodish in dogs); intratesticular (Sethi et al., 1965 in
hamsters; Bergman, 1966 in rabbits); intrapleural (Stoddard and Cutler in
rats); and intracardiac (Stoddard and Cutler in rats). As routes of dissemination
the hematogenous is currently seen in experimental disease. Lymphatic spread, as
regional lymph node involvement as part of the primary complex, has been confirmed only occasionally (Sethi et al., 1965).

Immunologic studies have been done mostly in mice (Louria et al., 1963;
Levine et al., 1957; Perceval; Abrahams and Gilleran; Bergman and
Stormby; Hoff; Louria, 1960; Gadebusch, 1958; Neill and Kapros), in
hamsters (Sethi et al., 1965), and in rabbits and guinea pigs (Lomanitz and Hale).
The achieved protection or acquired resistance was, however, of a low degree. No
clear-cut and usable results have yet been obtained.

Mycologic studies have revealed differences of virulence in certain strains of the
fungus (Benham, 1950; Levine et al., 1957; Sethi et al., 1965). Cryptococcus
does not alter in virulence on growth in culture media (Littman and Zimmerman).
Degrees of enhancement of encapsulation and virulence were studied by Littman
and Tsubura (1959) and Scholer et al. (1961) in mice. In tissue explants few
cytologic variations could be observed in comparison with dimorphic fungi

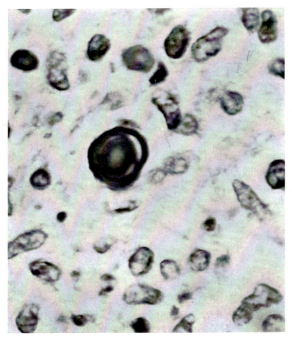

Fig. 68. Schaumann body around *C. neoformans* cell in cryptococcal granuloma 32 days after s.c. inoculation. H & E, × 1200

(GOLDMAN and SCHWARZ, 1966). *Pathology* in animals shows a few notable features. The histology of cryptococcal disease in mice was exhaustively studied by FAZEKAS and SCHWARZ; LEVINE et al. (1957); BERGMAN (1961). In contrast to human cryptococcosis, leukocytic exudation and abscess formation were observed in mice and hamsters (LEVINE et al., 1957; BERGMAN, 1961; SETHI et al., 1965) (Fig. 67). In hamsters, formation of Schaumann bodies around yeast cells (SETHI et al., 1965) (Fig. 68) occurred as in other experimental mycoses in this species (OKUDAIRA et al.). Cryptococcic lesions in the skeletal muscle of the mouse were described by STAIB (b). Phagocytosis of *C. neoformans* in anemic mice was studied by GADE-BUSCH (1959). Of the *factors influencing infection* in animals, the importance of thiamine was noted by GADEBUSCH and GIKAS and of anemia in mice by GADEBUSCH (1959). HALE and LOMANITZ observed that the onset of death was significantly enhanced in mice when, in addition to i.p. inoculation with *C. neoformans*, the animals were given serum from patients with Hodgkin's disease or leukemia. X-ray irradiation enhanced experimental cryptococcal infection (LEVINE et al., 1957), and corticosteroids produced a more severe infection in mice, rats, rabbits, and hamsters (LEVINE et al., 1957; SETHI et al., 1965). *Amphotericin B treatment* has been found effective in experimental animals by LOURIA et al. (1957) and GORDON and LAPA. The latter also injected gamma globulin, in addition to amphotericin B, into mice.

References

ABRAHAMS, I.: Further studies on acquired resistance to murine cryptococcosis. Enhancing effect of *Bordetella pertussis*. J. Immunol. **96**, 525—529 (1966). — ABRAHAMS, I., GILLERAN, T.G.: Studies on actively acquired resistance to experimental cryptococcosis in mice. J. Immunol. **85**, 629—635 (1960). — ABRAHAMS, I., GILLERAN, T.F., WEISS, C.B.: Quantitative studies on reverse cutaneous anaphylaxis in mice with progressive cryptococcosis. J. Immunol. **89**, 684—690 (1962). — Agustoni, C. B., Vivot, N. A., Marini, L. C.: Criptococcosis (torulosis) cerebromeningea. Estudio clínico y anatomopatológico. Prens. méd. argent. **37**, 1055—1059 (1950). — Ahuja, M. M., Nayak, N. C., Bhargava, S.: Clinicopathological conference A.I.I.M.S. (a fatal case of cryptococcosis). J. Indian med. Ass. **42**, 474—478 (1964). — Aikat, B. K., Chatterjee, B. D., Banerjee, P. L.: The rising incidence of cryptococcosis. Indian. J. med. Res. **55**, 43—46 (1967). — Aitken, G. W., Symonds, E. M.: Cryptococcal meningitis in pregnancy treated with amphotericin B. A case report. J. Obstet. Gynaec. Brit. Comm. **69**, 677—679 (1962). — Ajello, L.: Occurrence of *Cryptococcus neoformans* in soils. Amer. J. Hyg. **67**, 72—77 (1958). ~ Medium for selective isolation of *Cryptococcus neoformans*. U.S. Department of Health, Education and Welfare, Communicable Disease Center, Atlanta, Georgia **151**, 208—209 (1966). ~ Comparative ecology of respiratory mycotic disease agents. Bact. Rev. **31**, 6—24 (1967). — Ajello, L., Grant, V.Q., Gutske, M.A.: The effect of tubercle bacillus concentration procedures on fungi causing pulmonary mycoses. J. Lab. clin. Med. **38**, 486—491 (1951). — Alajouanine, Th., Grasset, A.: La cryptococcose (torulose) de systeme nerveux central. Sem. Hôp. Paris **33**, 3575—3585 (1957). — Alajouanine, Th., Houdart, R., Drouhet, E.: Les formes chirurgicales spinales de la torulose torulome de la queue de cheval. Revue Neurol. **88**, 153—163 (1953). — Alderman, L.W.: Report of a case of cerebrospinal meningitis due to *Cryptococcus neoformans (Torula hominis)*. Med. J. Aust. **2**, 914—916 (1949). — Allen, W.P.: An investigation of the anticryptococcal properties of normal serums. Doctoral Dissertation, University of Michigan. Michigan: Ann Arbor 1955. — Allen, V.K., Lowbeer, T.: Rectal ulcera with perirectal fistula as a port of entrance for torula (histolytica) encephalitis. Sth. med. J. **38**, 565—569 (1945). — Allende, G.: Meningitis a torula. Prens. méd. argent. **27**, 816—818 (1940). — Almeida, F.: Algunos datos sobre la criptococcosis en América del Sur. Mycopathologia (Den Haag) **15**, 389—393 (1961). — Almeida, F., Lacaz da Silva, C., Monteiro Salles: Blastomicose do tipo Busse-Buschke (granulomatose criptococcia. Torula infection, Torulosis). Segundo caso observada en São Paulo. An. Fac. Med. Univ. São Paulo **20**, 115—139 (1944). — Amorim, F. de, Pascualucci, E.A.: Natureza das lesoes do sistema nervoso central na torulose. Rev. lat.-amer. Anat. pat. **2**, 41—50 (1958). ~ Die Art der Schäden des ZNS bei Torulosis. Rev. lat.-amer. Anat. pat. **2**, 41—50 (1958) [Portugiesisch, mit englischer Zusammenfassung]. — Anderson, H.W.: Yeast-like fungi of human intestinal tract. J. infect. Dis. **21**, 341—385 (1917). — Anderson, K., Beech, M.: Serological tests for the early diagnosis of cryptococcal infection. Med. J. Aust. **45**, 601—602 (1958). — Andre, L., Desausse, P., Moncourrier, L., Billiotter, J., Deletraz, R.: Un cas mortel de blastomycose thoracique avec envahissement du canal medullaire. Bull. Soc. méd. Hôp. Paris **66**, 1046—1049 (1950). — Andriole, V.T., Kravetz, H.M.: The use of amphotericin B in man. J. Amer. med. Ass. **180**, 269—272 (1962). — Aneck-Hahn, H.G.L.: Blastomycosis of the central nervous system. S. Afr. med. J. **7**, 369—370 (1933). — Anguli, V.C., Natarajan, P.: Systemic cryptococcosis with a toruloma of the left ventricle. Case report. Indian. J. Path. Bact. **4**, 179—182 (1961). — Angulo Ortega, A., Rodriguez, C., Garcia Galindo, G.: Cryptococcosis in Venezuela. Mycopathologia (Den Haag) **15**, 367—388 (1961). — Appelbaum, E., Shtokalko, S.: Cryptococcus meningitis arrested with amphotericin B, a new fungicidal agent. Ann. intern. Med. **47**, 346—351 (1957). — Aragon, P.R., Reyes, A.C.: Cryptococcus neoformans infection of the brain-laboratory studies. Acta med. philipp. **16**, 23—30 (1959). — Artagereytia-Allende, R.C.: Contribución al conocimiento de Torulopsis glabrata (Anderson 1917) Lodder y de Vries 1938. An. Fac. Med. Montevideo **37**, 467—469 (1952). — Arzt, L.: Zur Klinik und Pathologie der Sproßpilzerkrankungen. Arch. Derm. Syph. (Berl.) **145**, 311—312 (1924). — Aschner, M., Mager, J., Leibowitz, J.: Production of extracellular starch in cultures of capsulated yeasts. Nature (Lond.) **156**, 295 (1945). — Atkinson, J.B., Delaney, W.E., Miller, F.R.: *Cryptococcus* meningitis in a case of congenital hemolytic anemia. Ann. intern. Med. **44**, 1015—1019 (1956). — *Atlanta:* Morbidity and Mortality Weekly Report, Communicable Disease Center, Atlanta, Ga.; Annual Suppl. Vol. 11, 16, Sept. 1963; Vol. 13, 30, Sept. 1965. — Bacon, A.E., Jr., Scott, E.G., Huntington, P.W.: Meningoencephalitis due to Cryptococcus neoformans (Torula histolytica). Delaware med. J. **26**, 3—8 (1954). — Backhouse, T.C., Bollinger, A.: Cryptococcosis in the Koala (*Phascolarctos cinereus*). Aust. J. Sci. **23**, 86—87 (1960). — Bahr, R.D., Satz, H., Purlia, V.L.: Primary pulmonary cryptococcosis. Case report. Amer. J. Roentgenol. **87**, 859—864 (1962). — Baker, R.D.: Resectable mycotic lesions and acutely fatal mycoses. J. Amer. med. Ass. **150**, 1579—1581 (1952). ~ Leukopenia and therapy in leukemia as factors predisposing to fatal mycoses. Amer. J. clin. Path. **37**, 358—373 (1962). — Baker, R.D., Haugen, R.K.: Tissue changes and tissue diagnosis in cryptococcosis. Study of 26 cases. Amer. J. clin. Path. **25**, 14—24 (1955). — Bakerspigel, A., Campsall, E.W.R., Hession, B.L.: A case of cryptococcal meningitis in South Western Ontario. Canad. med. Ass. J. **79**, 998—1002 (1958). — Balkrishna, Rao, B.N., Lilauwala, N.F.: Cryptococcosis of the central nervous system with report of a case. Indian J. Surg. **14**, 10—19 (1952). — Ball, H.A.: Human torula infections: review; report of cases. Calif. west. Med. **32**, 338—346

(1930). — Barbeau, A., Gagnon, J.: La torulose cerebrale. Un. méd. Can. **93**, 1374—1381 (1964). — Barlow, D. L.: Primary blastomycotic meningitis occurring in a child. Med. J. Aust. **2**, 302—304 (1923). — Barnard, P. J. J.: Meningitis due to Torula histolytica. Proc. Transv. Mine med. Offrs' Ass. **25**, 92—94 (1945). — Barrash, M. J., Fort, M.: Amphotericin B therapy in torula meningitis. Arch. intern. Med. **106**, 271—274 (1960). — Barron, C. N.: Cryptococcosis in animals. J. Amer. vet. med. Ass. **127**, 125—132 (1955). — Basu Mallik, K. C.: An epidemiological study of cryptococcosis in Calcutta area. Indian J. med. Res. (1967). — Basu Mallik, K. C., Banerjee, P. L., Chatterjee, B. D., Pramanick, M.: An experimental study of the course of infection in mice after intranasal insufflation with Cryptococcus neoformans. Indian J. med. Res. **54**, 608—610 (1966). — Baum, G. L., Artis, D.: Growth inhibition of Cryptococcus neoformans by cell free human serum. Amer. J. med. Sci. **241**, 97—100 (1961). ~ Characterization of the growth inhibition factor for *Cryptococcus neoformans* in human serum. Amer. J. med. Sci. **246**, 87—91 (1963). ~ Isolation of fungi from Judean Desert soil. Mycopathologia (Den Haag) **29**, 350—354 (1966). — Bazex, A., Dupre, A., Parant, M., Lucioni: La cryptococcose (etude, clinique, biologique, anatomo-pathologique et therapeutique). Toulouse méd. **58**, 111—146 (1957). — Bazex, A., Bouisson, H., Salvador, R., Dupre, A., Parant, M., Fabre, J.: Cryptococcose. Suites evolutives et aspects anatomiques. Bull. Soc. franç. Derm. Syph. **70**, 298—301 (1963). — Beck, E. M., Volyes, C. Q.: Systemic infection due to torula histolytica (Cryptococcus hominis). II. Effect of chemotherapeutic agents (potassium iodide, sulfadiazine, and sulfonamide) in experimentally produced infections. Arch. intern. Med. **77**, 516—525 (1946). — Beer, K.: Über Torulose. Schweiz. Z. allg. Path. **19**, 534—539 (1956). — Beeson, P. B.: Cryptococcic meningitis of nearly sixteen years duration. Arch. intern. Med. **89**, 797—801 (1952). — Beijerinck, M. V.: L'auxanographie, ou la methode de l'hydrodiffusion dans la gelatine appliquee aux recherches microbiologiques. Arch. neerl. dsc. exactes **23**, 367—372 (1889). — Bell, N. H., Andriole, V. T., Sabesin, S. M., Utz, J. P.: On the nephrotoxicity of amphotericin B in man. Amer. J. Med. **33**, 64—69 (1962). — Benda, C.: Fall von Blastomycosis cerebri. Dtsch. med. Wschr. **13**, 945—946 (1907). — Benham, R. W.: Cryptococci — their identification by morphology and by serology. J. infect. Dis. **57**, 255—274 (1935). ~ The terminology of the cryptococci with a note on Cryptococcus mollis. Mycologia **27**, 496—502 (1935). ~ Cryptococcosis and blastomycosis. Ann. N. Y. Acad. Sci. **50**, 1299—1314 (1950). ~ The genus Cryptococcus. The present status and criteria for identification of species. Trans. N. Y. Acad. Sci. (Ser. II) **17**, 418—429 (1955). — Benham, R. W., Hopkins, A. M.: Arch. Derm. Syph. (Chic.) **28**, 532—543 (1933). — Bennett, S. C. J.: Cryptococcus infections in equidae. J. roy. Army vet. Cps **16**, 108—118 (1944). — Bennett, J. E. Tines, B. S. Hasenclever, H. F.: A complement-fixing antigen test for cryptococcal meningitis. Clin. Res. **10**, 213 (1962). — Bennett, J. E., Hasenclever, H. F., Baum, G. L.: Evaluation of a skin test for cryptococcosis. Amer. Rev. resp. Dis. **91**, 616 (1965). — Bennett, J. E., Hasenclever, H. F., Tynes, B. S.: Detection of cryptococcal polysaccharide in serum and spinal fluid. Value in diagnosis and prognosis. Trans. Ass. Amer. Phycns. **77**, 145—150 (1964). — Berg, J. A. G. ten, Kuipers, F. C.: Generaliseerde toroulosis bij sen patiente met levercirrhose van Laennec. Ned. T. Geneesk. **106**, 2429—2434 (1962). — Berger, H., Bianchetti, B., Kuersteiner, W., Widmer, R., Stricker, E., Gloor, F.: Diagnostic difficulties in a fatal infection with Cryptococcus neoformans in a child. Ann. paediat. (Basel) **199**, 315—346 (1962). — Berghausen, O.: Torula infection in man. Ann. intern. Med. **1**, 235—240 (1927/1928). — Bergman, F.: Pathology of experimental cryptococcosis. A study of course and tissue response in subcutaneously induced infection in mice. Acta path. microbiol. scand. **147**, 1—163 (1961). ~ Occurrence of *Cryptococcus neoformans* in Sweden. Acta med. scand. **174**, 651—655 (1963). ~ Effect of temperature on intratesticular cryptococcal infection in rabbits. Sabouraudia **5**, 54—58 (1966). — Bergman, F., Linell, F.: Cryptococcosis as a cause of pulmonary alveolar proteinosis. Acta path. microbiol. scand. **53**, 217—224 (1961). — Bergman, F., Stormby, C.: A study of white blood cell and antibody response in mice infected subcutaneously with *Cryptococcus neoformans*. Sabouraudia **4**, 107—111 (1965). — Berk, M., Gerstl, B.: Torulosis (Cryptococcosis) producing a solitary pulmonary lesion. Report of 4 year cure with lobectomy. J. Amer. med. Ass. **149**, 1310—1312 (1952). — Bernard, L. A., Owens, J. C.: Isolated cryptococcosis associated with Boeck's sarcoid. Arch. intern. Med. **106**, 101—111 (1960). — Bernhardt, R., Zalewski, G., Burawski, J.: Generalisierte Torulose (Europäische Blastomykose). Arch. Derm. Syph. (Berl.) **173**, 78—90 (1935). — Bertrand, I., Mollaret, H.: Etude histo-pathologique d'un cas d'envahissement des centres nerveux et des viscères par torula histolytica, 1916 (Cryptococcus neoformans, 1949). Rev. neurol. **97**, 241—250 (1957). — Bertschinger, H. U., Scholer, H. J.: Spontaneous cryptococcosis in guinea pigs. Path. et Microbiol. (Basel) **28**, 12—20 (1965). — Bettin, M. E.: Report of case of torula infection. Calif. west. Med. **22**, 98—101 (1924). — Biddle, A., Koenig, H.: An agent effective against cryptococcosis of the central nervous system. Arch. intern. Med. **102**, 801—805 (1958). — Binford, C. H.: Torulosis of central nervous system. Review of recent literature and report of case. Amer. J. clin. Path. **11**, 242—251 (1941). — Black, R. A., Fisher, C. V.: Cryptococci bronchopneumonia. Amer. J. Dis. Child.

54, 81—88 (1937). — Blair, D.: Torulosis of central nervous system. J. ment. Sci. **89**, 42—51 (1943). — Blanc, P. E.: Contribution à l'étude des Cryptococcose humaines. A propos d'une observation anatomo-clinique d'infestation par un „Torula stricto sensu". Lyon: Université Faculté mixte de med. et de pharm. 1954. — Bloomfield, N., Gordon, M. A., Elmendorf, D. F., Jr.: Detection of *Cryptococcus neoformans* antigen in body fluids by latex particle agglutination. Proc. Soc. exp. Biol. (N.Y.) **114**, 64—67 (1963). — Börner, P.: Eine viscerale Torulopsis neoformans-Infektion. Zbl. allg. Path. path. Anat. **107**, 257—260 (1965). — Boj, E., Wojcik, B.: A case of European torulosis of the central nervous system. Pol. Tyg. lek. **19**, 958—959 (1964). — Bolliger, A., Finckh, E. S.: Cryptococcosis in the koala (*Phascolarctoscinereus*). Further observations. Aust. J. Sci. **24**, 325—326 (1962). ~ The prevalence of cryptococcosis in the koala. Med. J. Aust. **1**, 545—547 (1962). — Bonmati, J., Rogers, J. V., Jr., Jopkins, W. A.: Pulmonary cryptococcosis. Radiology **66**, 188—194 (1956). — Borelli, D.: Ventajas y peligros del examen directo en fresco en el diagnóstico de la blastomicosis sudamericana. VI. Congreso Venezolano de Ciencias Medicas. **IV**, 2159—2174 (1955). — Boshes, L. D., Sherman, I. C., Hesser, C. J., Milzer, A., MacLean, M.: Fungus infections of the central nervous system. Experience in treatment of cryptococcosis with cycloheximide (Actidione). Arch. Neurol. Psychiat. (Chic.) **75**, 175—197 (1956). — Bowman, H. E., Ritchey, J. O.: Cryptococcosis (torulosis) involving brain, adrenal and prostate. J. Urol. (Baltimore) **71**, 373—378 (1954). — Brandriss, M. W., Wolff, S. M., Moores, R., Stohlman, F., Jr.: Anemia induced by amphotericin B. J. Amer. med. Ass. **189**, 663—666 (1964). — Brandstaetter, S., Levitus, Z. A.: Torula meningitis. J. med. Ass. Israel. **4**, 18 (1949). — Brandt, M.: Zur pathologischen Anatomie der Meningoencephalitis (ME) cryptococcica (Torulosis). Zbl. allg. Path. path. Anat. **99**, 113—120 (1959). ~ Über Meningoencephalitis cryptococcica (Torulosis). Ärztl. Wschr. **13**, 995—1000 (1958). — Brandt, N. J., Sturup, H.: Kryptokokmeningitis behandlet med amphotericin B. Et tilfaelde hos en patient med histologisk diagnosticeret Boecks sarkoid. Ugeskr. Laeg. **121**, 1132—1134 (1959). — Brewer, G. E.: A case of blastomycosis. Proc. N.Y. path. Soc. **7**, 54—57 (1907). — Brewer, G. E., Wood, F.C.: Blastomycosis of the spine. Double lesion. Two operations. Recovery. Ann. Surg. **48**, 889—896 (1908). — Brier, R. L., Coleman, M., Stone, J.: Cutaneous cryptococcosis. Presentation of a case and a review of previously reported cases. Arch. Derm. **75**, 262—263 (1957). — Brooks, M. H., Scheerer, P., Linman, J. W.: Cryptococcal prostatitis. J. Amer. med. Ass. **192**, 143—145 (1965). — Brumpt, V., Moisant, P.: Premiere observation de cryptococcose neuromeningee au Cambodge. Bull. Soc. Path. exot. **57**, 12—16 (1964). — Bruns, G.: Generalisierte Torulose (mit Befall der Dura mater). Zbl. allg. Path. path. Anat. **87**, 360—364 (1951). — Bubb, H.: *Cryptococcus neoformans* infection in bone. S. Afr. med. J. **29**, 1259—1261 (1955). — Buckle, G., Curtis, D. R.: Therapy of human torulosis with Actidione and "Contramine". A report on two cases. Med. J. Aust. **2**, 854—859 (1955). — Brass, K.: Fortschritte in der histologischen Diagnostik der Pilzerkrankungen. Verh. dtsch. Ges. Path. **38**, 260—265 (1954). — Buell, C. B., Weston, W. H.: Application of the mineral oil conservation method to maintaining collections of fungous cultures. Amer. J. Botany **34**, 555—561 (1947). — Buitrago-Garcia, E., Gomez-Arango, S.: Comprobación de un caso de criptococosis. Caldas méd. **1**, 5—16 (1960). — Bureau, Y., Bronsard, M.: Blastomycose cutanée à "torula histolytica" ou "torulopsis neoformans". Bull. Soc. franç. Derm. Syph. **61**, 175 (1954). — Bureau, Y., Barriere, H., Trichereau, R.: La torulose cutanée. Ann. Derm. Syph. (Paris) **82**, 484—509 (1955). — Bureau, Y., Trichereau, R., Barriere, H.: Un cas de torulose cutanée. Bull. Soc. franç. Derm. Syph. **62**, 28 (1955). — Burger, R. E., Morton, C. B.: Torula infection. Surgery **15**, 312—325 (1944). — Burns, R. E.: Fungus disease as a complication of steroid therapy. Arch. Derm. Syph. (Chic.) **77**, 686—689 (1958). — Burrows, B., Barclary, W. R.: Combined cryptococcal and tuberculous meningitis complicating reticulum cell sarcoma. Amer. Rev. Tuberc. **78**, 760—768 (1958). — Burton, R. M.: Lead encephalopathy complicating torula infection. West Virg. M.T. **37**, 212—214 (1941). — Buschke, A.: Über eine durch Coccidien hervorgerufene Krankheit des Menschen. Dtsch. med. Wschr. **21**, 14—22 (1895). — Busse, O.: Über parasitäre Zelleinschlüsse und ihre Züchtung. Cbl. Bakt. **16**, 175—180 (1894). — Butas, C. A., Lloyd-Smith, D. L.: Cryptococcal meningitis treatment with amphotericin B. Canad. med. Ass. J. **87**, 558—591 (1962). — Butler, W. T., Alling, D. W., Spickard, A., Utz, J. P.: Diagnostic and prognostic value of clinical and laboratory findings in cryptococcal meningitis. New Engl. J. Med. **270**, 59—67 (1964). — Butler, W. T.: Nephrotoxicity of amphotericin B. Early and late effects in 81 patients. Ann. intern. Med. **61**, 175—187 (1964). — Cableses-Molina, F., Ravens, J. R., Eidelberg, E.: Meningitis por Torula histolytica (presentación de un caso clinico). Rev. Neuro-psiquiat. **14**, 90—103 (1951). — Caldwell, D.C., Raphael, S.S.: A case of cryptococcal meningitis. J. clin. Path. **8**, 32—37 (1955). — Campbell, G. D.: Primary pulmonary cryptococcosis. Amer. Rev. resp. Dis. **94**, 236—243 (1966). — Carnecchia, B.M., Kurtzke, J.F.: Fatal toxic reaction to amphotericin B in cryptococcal meningoencephalitis. Ann. intern. Med. **53**, 1027—1036 (1960). — Carrick, L.: Cutaneous cryptococcosis. Report of a case treated with potassium iodide and X-ray therapy. Arch.

Derm. Syph. (Chic.) **76**, 777—778 (1957). — CARTER, H.S., YOUNG, J.L.: Note on the isolation of Cryptococcus neoformans from a sample of milk. J. Path. Bact. **62**, 271—273 (1950). — CARTON, C.A.: Treatment of central nervous system cryptococcosis. Ann. intern. Med. **37**, 123—154 (1952). — CARTON, C.A., LIEBIG, L.S.: Treatment of central nervous system cryptococcosis and laboratory studies. Arch. intern. Med. **91**, 773—783 (1953). — CARTON, C.A., MOUNT, L.A.: Neurosurgical aspects of cryptococcosis. J. Neurosurg. **8**, 143—156 (1951). — CASAZZA, A.R., DUVALL, C.P., CARBONE, P.P.: Infection in lymphoma. Histology, treatment, and duration in relation to incidence and survival. J. Amer. med. Ass. **197**, 118—124 (1966). — CASTELLANI, A.: Balanoposthitis chronica ulcerative cryptococcica. Dermatol. Trop. **2**, 137—147 (1963). — CASTELLANI, A., JACONO, I.: Manuale di Clinica Tropicale. Torino: Rosenberg & Sellier 1937. — CASTELLANO, T.: Estudio clinico y anatomopatológico de un caso de torulosis meningeoencefálica y pulmonar. Rev. Asoc. méd. argent. **58**, 1051—1055 (1944). — CAWLEY, E.P., GREKIN, R.H., CURTIS, A.C.: Torulosis. A review of the cutaneous and adjoining mucous membrane manifestations. J. invest. Derm. **14**, 327—344 (1950). — CHAMPION DE CRESPIGNY, C.T.: Torula infection of the central nervous system. Med. J. Aust. **31**, 605—615 (1944). — CHAMPNESS, L.T., CLEZY, J.K.: Torulosis in Papua and New Guinea. Med. J. Aust. **49**, 560 (1962). — CHENG, W.F.: Cryptococcosis. Report of a case. Chin. med. J. (Peking) **74**, 374—386 (1956). — CHIARI, H.: Zur Pathologie und Histologie der generalisierten Torulose (Blastomykose). Arch. Derm. Syph. (Berl.) **162**, 422—435 (1930). — CHOMINSKIJ, B.S.: K patomorfologii mikozow centralnoj nierwnoj sistemy. Arch. Patologii **18**, 43—50 (1956). ∼ Arch. Pat. (Moskwa) **18**, 4—43 (1956). — CLELAND, J.B.: A case of systemic blastomycosis with formation of a myxomatous-looking tumor-like abscess. Med. J. Aust. **1**, 337—340 (1927). — CLOWARD, R.B.: Torula meningitis. First case to be reported in Hawaii. Hawaii med. J. **7**, 377—381 (1948). — COHEN, M.: Binocular papilledema in a case of torulosis associated with Hodgkin's disease. Arch. Ophthal. **32**, 477—479 (1944). — COHEN, J.R., KAUFMANN, W.: Systemic cryptococcosis. Report of case with review of literature. Amer. J. clin. Path. **22**, 1069—1076 (1952). — COLBERT, J.W., JR., STRAUSS, M.J., GREEN, R.H.: The treatment of cutaneous blastomycosis with propamidine. Preliminary report. J. invest. Derm. **14**, 71—73 (1950). — COLLOMB, H., PHILIPPE, Y., CADILLON, J.: Cryptococcose meningocerebrale (a propos d'un cas observé au Senegal). Bull. Soc. Path. exot. **57**, 105—110 (1964). — COLMERS, R.A., IRNIGER, W., STEINBERG, D.H.: Cryptococcus neoformans endocarditis cured by amphotericin B. J. Amer. med. Ass. **199**, 762—764 (1967). — COLLINS, V.P.: Bone involvement in cryptococcosis (torulosis). Amer. J. Roentgenol. **63**, 102—112 (1950). — COLLINS, V.P., GELLHORN, A., TRIMBLE, J.R.: The coincidence of cryptococcosis and disease of the reticuloendothelial and lymphatic systems. Cancer **4**, 883—889 (1951). — CONWAY, W.J., BRADY, T.: Mechanism of high acid production by yeast; bearing on hydrochloric acid formation in stomach. Nature (Lond.) **159**, 137—138 (1947). — COOK, A.W.: Cryptococcus (torula) meningitis. Report of 2 cases. J. Amer. med. Ass. **146**, 1105—1107 (1951). — CORNISH, A.L., BALOWS, A., CHIPPS, D.H., HOLLOWAY, J.B., JR.: Isolated pulmonary cryptococcosis. Arch. intern. Med. **99**, 285—289 (1957). — CORPE, R.F., PARR, L.H.: Pulmonary torulosis complicating pulmonary tuberculosis treated by resection. J. thorac. Surg. **27**, 392 (1954). — COSSERY, G.N.: Blastomycetic meningitis. J. Egypt. med. Ass. **13**, 198—206 (1930). — COX, L.B., TOLHURST, J.C.: Human Torulosis. Melbourne: University Press 1946. — CRONE, J.T., DEGROAT, A.F., WAHLIN, J.G.: Torula infection. Amer. J. Path. **13**, 863—879 (1937). — CROTTY, J.M.: Systemic mycotic infection in Northern Territory aborigines. Med. J. Aust. **1**, 184—186 (1965). — CROUNSE, R.G., LERNER, A.B.: Cryptococcosis. Arch. Derm. **77**, 210—215 (1958). — CRUICKSHANK, D.B., HARRISON, G.K.: Case of pulmonary cryptococcosis. Thorax **7**, 182—184 (1952). — CUDMORE, J.H., LISA, J.R.: Torula meningo-encephalitis. Case report. Ann. intern. Med. **11**, 1747—1752 (1938). — CURBELO, A., MARQUEZ, V., PALACIN, A., VELASCO, R., LEDO, E.A.: Septicemia y meningitis a *Cryptococcus neoformans*. Arch. Hosp. univ. (Habana) **9**, 324—327 (1957). — CURTIS, A.C.: Society Transactions. March 27, 1940. Arch. Derm. Syph. (Chic.) **62**, 330—331 (1950). — CURTIS, A.J.: A case of torulosis in a domestic cat. Aust. J. Med. Technol. **1**, 71 (1951). — DACORSO, P., CHAGAS, W.A.: Criptococcose pulmonar em caprino. An. col. anat. bras. **3**, 55—70 (1957). — DANDY, W.E.: Hirnchirurgie. Leipzig: Ambrosius Barth 1938. — DANIEL, P.M., SCHILLER, F., VOLLUM, R.L.: Torulosis of the Central nervous System. Report of 2 cases. Lancet **1949**, 53—56. — Da SILVA, N.N.: Criptococose cutanea (Cutaneous cryptococcosis). Hospital (Rio de J.) **44**, 375—381 (1953). — D'AUNOY, R., LAFFERTY, C.R.: Torula meningitis in child. Amer. J. clin. Path. **9**, 236—238 (1939). — DAWSON, D.M., TAGHAVY, A.: A test for spinal-fluid alcohol in torula meningitis. New Engl. J. Med. **269**, 1423—1424 (1963). — DEBRÉ, R., LAMY, M., GRUMBACH, M., NORMAND, E.: Development d'une meningite a Torula histolytica chez un enfant de douze ans atteint de lymphogranulomatose maligne. Bull. Acad. Méd. (Paris) **150**, 443—449 (1948). — DEBRÉ, R., LAMY, M., LEBLOIS, C., NICK, J., GRUMBACH, M., NORMAND, E.: Sur la torulose. Etude clinique et expérimentale. A-propos d'un cas observé chez un enfant atteint de lymphogranulomatose maligne. Bull. Acad. Méd. (Paris) **130**, 443—449 (1946). ∼ Sur la torulose. Etude clinique et expérimentale. A-propos d'un cas observé chez un enfant atteint de lymphogranulomatose maligne. Ann. paediat. (Basel) **168**, 1—33 (1947). — De Buen, S., Zimmerman, L.E., Foerster, H.C.: Patologia ocular en la Criptococcosis. Rev. Inst. Salubr. Enferm. trop. (Méx.) **14**, 163—178 (1954). — De Busscher, J., Scherer, H.J., Thomas, F.: La meningite a Torula (contribution à l'étude des localisations nerveuses des infections a pseudolevures). Rev. neurol. **70**, 149—168 (1938). — DeLedesma, J.P.R., Alguacil, D.C.G.: Torula histolitica cerebral. Rev. clin. esp. **46**, 106—108 (1952). — Demassieuz, J.L., Grasset, A., Mollaret, H., Bejot, J., Lacret, P., Safavian, A.: Septicemie a Cryptococcus neoformans. Presse méd. **71**, 1297—1299 (1963). — Demme, H., Mumme, C.: Blastomykose des Zentralnervensystems. Dtsch. Z. Nervenheilk. **127**, 1—26 (1932). — Demoulin-Brahy, L.: Study of the influence of the culture medium on the formation of the capsule in Cryptococcus neoformans. Ann. Soc. belge Méd. trop. **43**, 35—46 (1963). — Demoulin-Brahy, L., Feyen, M., Kellens, M.R.: The capsule of Cryptococcus neoformans. Ann. Soc. belge Méd. trop. **44**, 641—651 (1964). — Despeignes, M., Battesti, M.R., Viala, J.: Diagnostique de laboratoire de la cryptococcose meningee. Lyon méd. **212**, 1079—1087 (1964). — De Wan, C.H., Leffler, R.J., Collette, T.S.: Case report of cryptococcus meningitis. Guthrie Clin. Bull. (Sayre) **19**, 75—80 (1949). — Dezest, K.G.: Torulose spontanee chez le cobaye. Ann. Inst. Pasteur **85**, 131—133 (1953). — Dick, R.: The cryptococcus reviewed. J. Coll. Radiol. Aust. **9**, 212—219 (1965). — Dickmann, G.H., Veppo, A.A., Negri, T.: Torulopsis del sistema nervioso central (cerebelo) de forma tumoral. Rev. neurol. B. Aires **7**, 347—360 (1942). — Dienst, R.B.: *Cryptococcus histolyticus* isolated from subcutaneous tumor. Arch. Derm. Syph. (Chic.) **37**, 461—464 (1938). — Dillon, M.L., Sealy, W.C.: Surgical aspects of opportunistic fungus infections. Lab. Invest. **11**, 1231—1236 (1962). — Dimond, A.H.: Cryptococcal meningoencephalitis. J. roy. Army med. Cps **109**, 174—177 (1963). — Dintaman, P.G.: Cryptococcosis — apparent cure by use of amphotericin B. J. Indiana med. Ass. **55**, 317—321 (1962). — Dormer, B.A., Friedlander, J., Wiles, F.J., Simson, F.W.: Tumor of the lung due to Cryptococcus histolyticus (blastomycosis). J. thorac. Surg. **14**, 322—329 (1945). — Dormer, B.A., Scher, P.: Tumor of the lung due to Cryptococcus histolyticus. Clin. Proc. **6**, 269—273 (1947). — Dormer, B.A., Findlay, M.: Generalized cryptococcosis with osseous involvement. S. Afr. med. J. **34**, 611—613 (1962). — Dosa, A.: Ein Fall von Blastomycosis purulenta profunda (Busse-Buschke). Arch. Derm. Syph. (Berl.) **176**, 742—746 (1938). — Dreyfuss, M.L., Simon, S., Sommer, R.I.: Granulomatous prostatitis due to *Cryptococcus neoformans* (Torula) with disseminated cryptococcosis and meningitis. N.Y. J. Med. **61**, 1589—1592 (1961). — Drouhet, E.: Action de l'amphotericine B dans les mycoses profondes. Etude mycologique, clinique et therapeutique de 15 observations. Sem. Hôp. Paris **37**, 101—121 (1961). ~ Therapeutique de la cryptococcose. Ann. Soc. belge Méd. trop. **44**, 673—690 (1964). — Drouhet, E., Segretain, G., Aubert, J.P.: Polyoside capsulaire d'un champignon pathogene Torulopsis neoformans. Relation avec la virulence. Ann. Inst. Pasteur **79**, 891—900 (1950). — Drouhet, E., Couteau, M.: Sur les variations sectorielles des colonies de Torulopsis neoformans. Ann. Inst. Pasteur **80**, 456—457 (1951). — Drouhet, E., Segretain, G.: Inhibition de la migration leucocytaire *in vitro* par un polyoside capsulaire de Torulopsis (Cryptococcus) neoformans. Ann. Inst. Pasteur **81**, 674—676 (1951). — Drouhet, E., Martin, L., Brumpt, L., Debray, J.: Cryptococcose cutanée, meningée et viscerale associée a une reticulose maligne. Presse méd. **69**, 1983—1986 (1961). — Drouhet, E., Martin, L.: Cryptococcose cutanée et osseuse chez une diabetique agée. Traitement par l'amphotericine B. Bull. Soc. franç. Derm. Syph. **69**, 25—29 (1962). — Ducuing, J., Bassal, L., Miletsky, O.: Tumeur osseuse de l'orbite a allure cancereuse determinée par le Torulopsis neoformans. Bull. Ass. franç. Cancer **26**, 580—584 (1937). — Durant, J.R., Epifano, L.D., Eyer, S.W.: Pulmonary cryptococcosis. Treatment with amphotericin B. Ann. intern. Med. **53**, 534—547 (1960). — Durie, E.B., MacDonald, L.: Cryptococcosis (torulosis) of bone. Report of case. J. Bone Jt Surg. **43**, 68—70 (1961). — Einbinder, J.M., Benham, R.W., Nelson, C.T.: Chemical analysis of the capsular substance of *Cryptococcus neoformans*. J. invest. Derm. **22**, 279—283 (1954). — Eisen, D., Shapiro, I., Fischer, J.B.: Case of cryptococcosis with involvement of lungs and spine. Canad. med. Ass. J. **72**, 33—35 (1955). — Elkins, C.W., Fonseca, J.E.: Ventriculovenous anastomosis in obstructive and acquired communicating hydrocephalus. J. Neurosurg. **18**, 139—144 (1961). — Emanuel, B., Ching, E., Lieberman, A.D., Goldin, M.: *Cryptococcus* meningitis in a child successfully treated with amphotericin B. J. Pediat. **59**, 577—591 (1961). — Emmons, C.W.: Isolation of *Cryptococcus neoformans* from soil. J. Bact. **62**, 685—690 (1951). ~ The isolation from soil of fungi which cause disease in man. Trans. N.Y. Acad. Sci., Ser. II, **14**, 51—54 (1951). ~ *Cryptococcus neoformans* strains from a severe outbreak of bovine mastitis. Mycopathologia (Den Haag) **6**, 231—234 (1952). ~ Saprophytic sources of *Cryptococcus neoformans* associated with the pigeon (Columbia livia). Amer. J. Hyg. **62**, 227—232 (1955). ~ Prevalence of *Cryptococcus neoformans* in pigeon habitats. Publ. Hlth. Rep. (Wash.) **75**, 362—365 (1960). ~ Natural occurrence of opportunistic fungi. Lab. Invest. **11**, 1026—1032 (1962). — Emmons, C.W., Binford, C.H., Utz, J.P.: Medical Mycology. Philadelphia: Lea & Febiger 1963. — Erbsloh, F., Wolfer, E.: Zur Pathogenese der chronischen diffusen Meningopathien. Dtsch. Z. Nervenheilk. 167, 51—73 (1951). — ERIKSEN, K.R., JENSEN, E., RESKE-NIELSE, E., STENDERUP, A., VIDEBAEK, A.: Et tilfaelde af kryptokokkose (Torulose). A case of cryptococcosis (torulosis). Ugeskr. Laeg. 121, 1127—1131 (1959). — ERIKSEN, K.R., ERICHSON, I.: Isolation of pathogenic yeast Cryptococcus neoformans from pigeon droppings. Ugeskr. Laeg. 124, 1878—1880 (1962). — EVANS, E.E.: The antigenic composition of Cryptococcus neoformans. I. A serologic classification by means of the capsule agglutination reactions. J. Immunol. 64, 423—430 (1950). — EVANS, E.E., KESSEL, J.F.: The antigenic composition of Cryptococcus neoformans. II. Serologic studies with the capsular polysaccharide. J. Immunol. 67, 109—114 (1951). — EVANS, E.E., HARRELL, E.R., JR.: Univ. Mich. med. Bull. 18, 43—63 (1952). — EVANS, N.: Torula infection. Report of two cases. Calif. Med. 20, 383—385 (1922). — EVELAND, W.C., MARSHALL, J.D., SILVERSTEIN, A.M.: Rapid identification of pathogenic microorganisms using fluorescent antibodies of contrasting colors. VIIth Intern. Congr. Microbiol., p. 313 (1958). — EVENSON, A.E., LAMB, J.W.: Slime flux of mesquite as a new saprophytic source of Cryptococcus neoformans. J. Bact. 88, 542 (1964). — FARRER, R.: Torula meningitis. Roy. Melb. Hosp. clin. Rep. 12, 31—32 (1941). — FAZAKAS, S.: Report on oculomycoses due to the fungus flora of human eyes. Ophthalmologica (Basel) 121, 249—258 (1951). — FAZEKAS, G., SCHWARZ, J.: Histology of experimental murine cryptococcosis. Amer. J. Path. 34, 517—529 (1958). — FELDMAN, R.: Cryptococcosis (torulosis) of the central nervous system treated with amphotericin B during pregnancy. Sth. med. J. (Bgham, Ala.) 52, 1415—1417 (1959). — FELSENFELD, O.: Yeast-like fungi in the intestinal tract of chronically institutionalized patients. Amer. J. med. Sci. 207, 60—63 (1944). — FETTER, B.F., KLINTWORTH, G.K., HENDRY, W.S.: Mycoses of the Central Nervous System. Baltimore: Williams and Wilkins 1967. — FINGERLAND, A., VORTEL, V., DVORAK, J., ZDRAHAL, L.: Generalisovana kryptokokkosa (torulosa). Čas. Lék. čes. 93, 809—816 (1954). — FISHER, A.M.: Clinical picture associated with infections due to Cryptococcus neoformans (Torula histolytica). Report of three cases with experimental studies. Bull. Johns Hopk. Hosp. 86, 383—414 (1950). — FITCHETT, M.S., WEIDMAN, F.D.: Generalized torulosis associated with Hodgkin's disease. Arch. Path. 18, 225—244 (1934). — FITZPATRICK, M.J., RUBIN, H., POSER, C.M.: The treatment of cryptococcal meningitis with amphotericin B, a new fungicidal agent. Ann. intern. Med. 49, 249—259 (1958). — FITZPATRICK, M.J., POSER, C.M.: Management of cryptococcal meningitis. Arch. intern. Med. 106, 261—270 (1960). — FLINN, L.B., HOOKER, J.W., SCOTT, E.G.: Torula histolytica (Cryptococcus hominis) infection. Report of a case refractory to sulfonamides. Delaware med. J. 18, 141—147 (1946). — FLU, P.C., WOENSDREGT, M.M.C.: Een geval van blastomycose van het centraatzenuwstelsel. Mededel. Geneesk. Nederl. Indie 3, 1—36 (1918). — FORBUS, W.D.; in discussion, TERPLAN, K.: Pathogenesis of cryptococcic (Torula) meningitis. Amer. J. Path. 24, 711—712 (1948). — FORTUNE, C., DONNAN, G., COLEBATCH, J., LUBBE, T.: Torulosis. Med. J. Aust. 2, 199—204 (1955). — FRAGNER, P.: Parasitische Pilze beim Menschen. Prag: Verlag der Tschechoslowakischen Akademie der Wissenschaften 1958. — FREEMAN, W.: Torula infection of the central nervous system. J. Psychol. Neurol. (Lpz.) 61, 236—345 (1931). ~ Torula meningo-encephalitis. Comparative histopathology in 17 cases. Trans. Amer. neurol. Ass. 56, 203—217 (1930). ~ Fungus infections of the central nervous system. Ann. intern. Med. 6, 595—607 (1933). — FREEMAN, W., WEIDMAN, F.D.: Cystic blastomycosis of the cerebral gray matter. Arch. Neurol. Psychiat. (Chic.) 9, 589—603 (1923). — FREY, D., DURIE, E.B.: The isolation of Cryptococcus neoformans (Torula histolytica) from soil in New Guinea and pigeon droppings in Sydney, New South Wales. Med. J. Aust. 25, 947—949 (1964). — FRISK, Å., HOLMGREN, B.: Amphotericin B vid cryptococcusmeningit. Nord. méd. 61, 927—929 (1959). — FROIO, G.F., BAILEY, C.P.: Pulmonary cryptococcosis. Report of case with surgical cure. Dis. Chest. 16, 354—359 (1949). — FROTHINGHAM, L.: A tumor-like lesion in the lung of a horse caused by a blastomyces (Torula). J. med. Res. 3, 31—43 (1902). — FURCOLOW, M.L.: The use of amphotericin B in blastomycosis, cryptococcosis and histoplasmosis. Med. Clin. N. Amer. 47, 1119—1130 (1963). — FURTADO, T.A.: Cryptococcosis, 6 first cases observed in Minas Gerais and treatment of 2 cases with amphotericin B. Hospital (Rio de J.) 62, 151—164 (1962). — GADEBUSCH, H.H.: Phagocytosis of Cryptococcus neoformans in anemic mice. J. Bact. 78, 259—262 (1959). — GADEBUSCH, H.H.: Active immunization against Cryptococcus neoformans. J. infect. Dis. 102, 219—226 (1958a). ~ Passive immunization against Cryptococcus neoformans. Proc. Soc. exp. Biol. (N.Y.) 98, 611—614 (1958b). ~ On the mechanisms of cytotoxicity by cationic tissue proteins for Cryptococcus neoformans. Z. Naturforsch. 21b, 1048—1051 (1966). — GADEBUSCH, H.H., GIKAS, P.W.: Natural host resistance to infection with Cryptococcus neoformans. The influence of thiamine on experimental infection in mice. J. infect. Dis. 112, 125—133 (1963). — GADEBUSCH, H.H., JOHNSON, A.G.: Natural host resistance to infection with Cryptococcus neoformans. IV. The effect of some cationic proteins on the experimental disease. J. infect. Dis. 116, 551—565 (1966). ~ Natural host resistance to infection with Cryptococcus neoformans. V. The influence of cationic tissue proteins upon phagocytosis and on circulating antibody synthesis. J. infect. Dis. 116, 566—572 (1966). — GALINDO, D.L., BOHLS, S.W.: Combined pulmonary and central nervous system cryptococcosis. A case report. Milit. Surg. **113**, 403—413 (1953). — Galli, G.: Osservazioni e studi su casi di mastite micotica bovina. Vet. ital. **5**, 587—604 (1954). — Gandy, W.M.: Primary cutaneous cryptococcosis. Arch. Derm. Syph. (Chic.) **62**, 97—104 (1950). — Gantz, J.A., Nuetzel, J.A., Keller, L.B.: Cryptococcal meningitis treated with amphotericin B. Arch. intern. Med. **102**, 795—800 (1958). — Garcin, R., Gruner, J., Valmas, T.: Sur un cas de mycose vertebrale et epidurale ayant simule une tuberculose verticale posterieure (cryptococcose prealable). Sem. Hôp. Paris **33**, 2281 (1957). — Garin, J.P., Humbert, G., Yongui: Un cas de meningite a Cryptococcus neoformans. Soc. fr. mycol. med. Lyon, 25 mai. 1963. — Gaspar, I.: Blastomycotic meningo-encephalitis. Report of a case. Arch. Neurol. Psychiat. (Chic.) **22**, 475—486 (1929). — Geaney, B., Horsfall, W.R., Neilson, G.: Torulosis in Queensland. Report of 14 cases. Med. J. Aust. **2**, 378—382 (1956). — Geever, E.F., Carter, H.R., Neubuerger, K.T., Schmidt, E.A.: Roentgenologic and pathologic aspects of pulmonary tumors probably alveolar in origin. With report of 6 cases, one of them complicated by torulosis of the central nervous system. Radiol. **44**, 319—327 (1945). — Gendel, B.R., Ende, M., Normal, S.L.: Cryptococcosis. A review with special reference to apparent association with Hodgkin's disease. Amer. J. Med. **9**, 343—355 (1950). — Genevray, Bablet: Sur un cas de blastomycose meningée a saccharomyces tumefaciens observé au Tonkin. Arch. Inst. Pasteur Indochine **1930**, 33—44. — Geraci, J.E., Donoghue, F.E., Ellis, F.H., Jr.: Focal pulmonary cryptococcosis. Evaluation of necessity of amphotericin B therapy. Proc. Mayo Clin. **40**, 552—559 (1965). — Germain, A., Morvan, A.: A-propos du diagnostic du rhumatisme cerebral: meningoencephalite aigue a Torulopsis histolitica. Bull. Soc. Méd. Paris **54**, 231—234 (1938). — Gerstenbrand, F., Weingarten, K.: Torulose des Nervensystems. Wien. klin. Wschr. **69**, 278—280 (1957). — Gettelfinger, W.C.: *Cryptococcus* meningitis. J. Kentucky State Med. Ass. **56**, 1112—1113 (1958). — Gifford, H., Hullinghorst, R.L.: Streptomycin in cryptococcosis. Calif. Med. **69**, 279—282 (1948). — Gill, W.D.: Torula mycosis in man with special reference to involvement of upper respiratory tract. Trans. Amer. laryng. rhin. otol. Soc. **40**, 247—262 (1934). ~ Torula mycosis in man with special reference to involvement of the upper respiratory tract, with case reports. Ann. Otol. Rhinol. Laryngol. **44**, 702—718 (1935). — Globus, J.H., Gang, K.M., Bergmann, P.S.: Torula meningo-encephalitis. J. Mt Sinai Hosp. **16**, 14—34 (1949). ~ Torula meningo-encephalitis. J. Neuropath. exp. Neurol. **10**, 208—228 (1951). — Goldberg, F.A.: Torula meningitis. Memphis med. J. **23**, 129—130 (1948). — Goldberg, L.H.: Torula infections of central nervous system. J. Lab. clin. Med. **26**, 299—301 (1940). — Goldman, J.N., Schwarz, J.: Cytology of four yeastlike organisms in tissue explants. Mycopathologia (Den Haag) **24**, 161—167 (1966). — Goldstein, E., Rambo, O.N.: Cryptococcal infection following steroid therapy. Ann. intern. Med. **56**, 114—120 (1962). — Gonzalez, A., Fuentes, E., Perez-Tamayo, R.: Cryptococcosis generalizada. Presentación de un caso. (Disseminated cryptococcosis. Report of a case.) Prens. méd. mex. **24**, 373—378 (1959). — Goodhart, S.E., Davison, C.: Torula infection of the central nervous system. Arch. Neurol. Psychiat. (Chic.) **37**, 435—438 (1937). — Gordon, J.J.: Torulose. Med. Klin. **26**, 74 (1948). — Gordon, M.A., Lapa, E.: Synergistic action of immune globulin with amphotericin B in cryptococcosis. Ann. Rep. Div. Lab. Res. Albany **1961**, 70—80. ~ Serum protein enhancement of antibiotic therapy in cryptococcosis. J. infect. Dis. **114**, 373—377 (1964). — Gordon, M.A., Vedder, D.K.: Serologic tests in diagnosis and prognosis of cryptococcosis. J. Amer. med. Ass. **197**, 961—967 (1966). — Gosling, H.R., Gilmer, W.S., Jr.: Skeletal cryptococcosis (torulosis). Report of case and review of literature. J. Bone Jt Surg. **38-A**, 660—668 (1956). — Goto, K.: Über Blastomycetenmeningitis. Mitt. med. Fak. Tokyo **15**, 75—101 (1915). — Grasset, A.: La cryptococcose (torulose) du systeme nerveux central. These (Paris) 1955. — Gray, F.C.: Two cases of torula meningitis with special reference to laboratory findings. S. Afr. med. J. **14**, 65—70 (1940). — Gray, J.B., Chodosh, S.: Mycoses in New England. New Engl. J. Med. **276**, 62 (1967). — Greenfield, J.G., Martin, J.P., Moore, M.T.: Lancet **1938 II**, 1154—1157. — Greening, R.R., Menville, L.J.: Roentgen findings in torulosis. Report of 4 cases. Radiol. **48**, 381—388 (1947). — Gridley, M.F.: A stain for fungi in tissue sections. Amer. J. clin. Path. **23**, 303—307 (1953). — Grimley, P.M., Wright, L.D., Jr., Jennings, A.E.: *Torulopsis glabrata* infection in man. Amer. J. clin. Path **43**, 216—223 (1965). — Grocott, R.G.: A stain for fungi in tissue sections and smears. Using Gomori's methenamine-silver nitrate technic. Amer. J. clin. Path. **25**, 975—979 (1955). — Grschebin, S.: Ein Fall von tiefer primärer Blastomykosis der Haut (Busse-Buschke). Derm. Wschr. **85**, 1049—1055 (1927). — Haber, R.W., Joseph, M.: Neurological manifestation after amphotericin B therapy. Brit. med. J. **5273**, 230—231 (1962). — Hagen, W.S.: *Torula histolytica* meningoencephalitis. Report of a case; spinal fluid studies and autopsy report. Milit. Surg. **94**, 29—35 (1944). — Hajsig, M., Curcija, Z.: Kriptokoki u fekalijama fazana golubova s osvrtom na nalaze *Cryptococcus neoformans*. Vet. Arch. **35**, 115—118 (1965). — Hale, J.M., Lomanitz, R.: Enhanced dissemination of experimental murine cryptococcosis with Hodgkin's serum. J. Okla. med. Ass. **57**, 104—108 (1964). — Halde, C.: Percutaneous *Cryptococcus neoformans* inoculation without infection. Arch. Derm. **89**, 545 (1964). — Halde, C., Fraher,

M.A.: *Cryptococcus neoformans* in pigeon feces in San Francisco. Calif. Med. **104**, 188—190 (1966). — HALL, G.W., HIRSCH, E.F., MOCK, H.E.: *Torula histolytica* meningoencephalitis. Arch. Neurol. Psychiat. (Chic.) **19**, 689—694 (1928). — HALPERT, B., WHITCOMB, F.C., McROBERTS, C.C., CARTON, C.A.: Systemic and central nervous system involvement in cryptococcosis and coccidioidomycosis. Sth. med. J. (Bgham, Ala.) **47**, 633—642 (1954). — HAMILTON, J.B., TYLER, G.R.: Pulmonary torulosis. Radiol. **47**, 149—155 (1946). — HAMILTON, L.C., THOMPSON, P.E.: Treatment of cryptococcic meningitis with penicillin. Report of a case. Amer. J. Dis. Child. **72**, 334—342 (1946). — HAMMERSCHLAG, E.: Zur Kasuistik und experimentellen Pathologie der generalisierten Blastomykose. Wien. klin. Wschr. **46**, 43—46 (1933). — HANSEMANN, D. v.: Über eine bisher nicht beobachtete Gehirnerkrankung durch Hefen. Verh. dtsch. Ges. Path. **9**, 21—24 (1905). — HANSMANN, G.H.: Torula infection in man. Report of a case. Boston med. surg. J. **190**, 917—919 (1924). — HARDAWAY, R.M., CRAWFORD, P.M.: Pulmonary torulosis. Report of a case. Ann. intern. Med. **9**, 334—340 (1935). — HARLAND, W.A.: Cryptococcosis. Report of 5 cases. Canad. med. Ass. J. **83**, 580—584 (1960). — HARRIS, T.R., BLUMENFELD, H.B., CRUTHIRDS, T.P., McCALL, C.B.: Coexisting sarcoidosis and cryptococcosis. Arch. intern. Med. **115**, 637—643 (1965). — HASENCLEVER, H.F., MITCHELL, W.O.: Virulence and growth rates of *Cryptococcus neoformans* in mice. Ann. N.Y. Acad. Sci. **89**, 156—162 (1960). — HASENCLEVER, H.F., EMMONS, C.W.: The prevalence and mouse virulence of *Cryptococcus neoformans* strains isolated from urban areas. Amer. J. Hyg. **78**, 227—231 (1963). — HASPEL, R., BAKER, J., MOORE, M.B., JR.: Disseminated *Cryptococcus neoformans*. New Orleans med. surg. J. **101**, 573—575 (1949). — HASSIN, G.B.: Torulosis of the central nervous system. J. Neuropath. exp. Neurol. **6**, 44—60 (1947). — HAUGEN, R.K., BAKER, R.D.: The pulmonary lesions in cryptococcosis with special reference to subpleural nodes. Amer. J. clin. Path. **24**, 1381—1390 (1954). — HAWKINS, J.A.: Cavitary pulmonary cryptococcosis. Amer. Rev. resp. Dis. **84**, 579—581 (1961). — HEALTH, P.: Massive separation of retina in full term infants and juveniles. J. Amer. med. Ass. **144**, 1148—1154 (1950). — HEHRE, E.J., CARLSON, A.S., HAMILTON, D.M.: Crystalline amylose from cultures of a pathogenic yeast (Torula histolytica). J. biol. Chem. **177**, 289—293 (1949). — HEINE, J., LAUER, A., MUMME, C.: Generalisierte Blastomykose und Lymphogranulomatose. Beitr. path. Anat. **104**, 55—75 (1940). — HEINRICHS, H.: Beitrag zur Pathologie der Blastomykose. Zbl. Path. **53**, 422—428 (1932). — HEINSIUS, E.: Augenbeteiligung bei Blastomykose. Ber. dtsch. ophthal. Ges. **55**, 358—362 (1949). — HELLER, S., McLEAN, R.A., CAMPBELL, C.G., JONES, I.H.: A case of coexistent non-meningitic cryptococcosis and Boeck's sarcoid. Amer. J. Med. **22**, 986—994 (1957). — HELMBOLDT, C.F., JUNGHERR, E.L.: Case 5, Seminar, Amer. Coll. Vet. Path., Chicago, Nov. 29. 1952. — HERIN, V., DORMAL, R.: Un cas de cryptococcose equine cerebrale en Leopoldville. Ann. Soc. belge Méd. trop. **42**, 865—870 (1962). — HERMS, G.: Morphologie der generalisierten Kryptokokkose. Gegenbauers morph. Jb. **109**, 85—90 (1966). — HERRERA, J.M., BRICEÑO, C.E., SOUZA, O.E.: Blastomicosis generalizada por Cryptococcus neoformans. Primer caso mortal estudiado en Panama. Arch. méd. panameñ. **5**, 105—125 (1956). — HERSH, E.M., BODEY, G.P., NIES, B.A., FREIREICH, E.J.: Causes of death in acute leukemia. J. Amer. med. Ass. **193**, 105—109 (1965). — HESS, R.: Cryptococcosis. A case report and review. Southwestern Med. **47**, 266—269 (1966). — HICKIE, J.B., WALKER, T.: Cryptococcosis (torulosis). Some problems in diagnosis and management. Aust. Ann. Med. **13**, 229—240 (1964). — HILL, G.J., BUTLER, W.T., WERTLAKE, P.T., UTZ, J.P.: The renal histopathology in amphotericin B toxicity in man and dog. A study of biopsy and post-mortem specimens. Clin. Res. **10**, 249 (1962). — HIRANO, A., ZIMMERMAN, H.M., LEVINE, S.: The fine structure of cerebral fluid accumulation. III. Extracellular spread of cryptococcal polysaccharides in the acute stage. Amer. J. Path. **45**, 1—19 (1964). ~ The fine structure of cerebral fluid accumulation. IV. On the nature and origin of extracellular fluid following cryptococcal polysaccharide implantation. Amer. J. Path. **45**, 195—207 (1964). ~ The fine structure of cerebral fluid accumulation. V. Transfer of fluid from extracellular to intracellular compartments in acute phase of cryptococcal polysaccharide lesions. Arch. Neurol. (Chic.) **11**, 632—641 (1964). ~ The fine structure of cerebral fluid accumulation. VI. Intracellular accumulation of fluid and cryptococcal polysaccharide in the oligodendroglia. Arch. Neurol. (Chic.) **12**, 189—196 (1965). ~ The fine structure of cerebral fluid accumulation. VII. Reactions of astrocytes to cryptococcal polysaccharide implantation. J. Neuropath. exp. Neurol. **24**, 386—397 (1965). — HIRSH, E.F., COLEMAN, G.H.: Acute miliary torulosis of lungs. J. Amer. med. Ass. **92**, 437—438 (1929). — HITAKA, O.: The growth of *Cryptococcus neoformans* in tissue culture. Jap. J. med. Mycol. **5**, 154—169 (1964). — HOCHSTETTER, W.: Rare infection simulating expanding intracranial lesions. Proc. R. Virchow Med. Soc. N.Y. **10**, 71—72 (1951). — HOFF, C.L.: Immunity studies of *Cryptococcus hominis (Torula histolytica)* in mice. J. Lab. clin. Med. **27**, 751—754 (1942). — HOFFMEISTER, W.: Die Torulosis neoformans-Infektion. Beitrag zur Differentialdiagnose der Meningoencephalopathie, Lymphogranulomatose und pneumonischen Infiltrationen. Klin. Wschr. **29**, 301—307 (1951). — HOGEN, W.S.: *Torula histolytica* meningoencephalitis. Report of case; spinal fluid studies and autopsy report. Milit. Surg. **94**, 29—35 (1944). — HOIGNE, R., BEER, K., COTTIER, H.: Über

Torulose. Schweiz. med. Wschr. **1957**, 97—101. — Holmes, S.J., Hawks, G.H.: Torulosis of the central nervous system. Canad. med. Ass. J. **68**, 143—146 (1953). — Holt, R.A.: Identification of *Blastomycoides histolytica* in 3 infections of central nervous system. J. Lab. clin. Med. **27**, 58—62 (1941). — Holtz, K.H.: Torulosis (cryptococcosis) with skin involvement. Report of case treated with amphotericin B. Arch. klin. exp. Derm. **211**, 347—350 (1960). — Holzworth, J.: Cryptococcosis in a cat. Cornell Vet. **42**, 12—15 (1952). — Holzworth, J., Coffin, D.L.: Cryptococcosis in a cat. A second case. Cornell Vet. **43**, 546—550 (1953). — Hooft, C., Pintelon, J., Callens, J.: Meningite a cryptococcus. Acta paediat. belg. **9**, 152—168 (1955). — Hooper, K.H., Wannan, J.S.: Torulosis in Queensland. Med. J. Aust. **2**, 669—671 (1941). — Houk, V.N., Moser, K.M.: Pulmonary cryptococcosis. Must all receive amphotericin B? Ann. intern. Med. **63**, 583—596 (1965). — Howard, D.H.: Some factors which affect the initiation of growth of *Cryptococcus neoformans*. J. Bact. **82**, 430—435 (1961). — Howe, G.W.: An atypical case of meningoencephalitis due to *Cryptococcus neoformans* (Torula histolytica). Sth. med. J. (Bgham, Ala.) **43**, 649—651 (1950). — Huang, P.T.: A case of cryptococcal meningitis. Acta paediat. Sinica **4**, 270—273 (1963). — Huant, C.T., Wong, P.C., Chan-Tesh, C.H.: Cryptococcal meningitis in Hong Kong. J. clin. Path. **26**, 464—469 (1963). — Hubschmann, K., Trapl, J., Fragner, P.: Zum Problem der Diagnostik und Pathogenese der Kryptokokkose. Hautarzt **10**, 534—539 (1959). — Hutter, R.V.P., Collins, H.S.: The occurrence of opportunistic fungus infections in a cancer hospital. Lab. Invest. **11**, 1035—1045 (1962). — Igel, H.J., Bolande, R.P.: Humoral defense mechanisms in cryptococcosis. Substances in normal human serum, saliva, and cerebrospinal fluid affecting the growth of *Cryptococcus neoformans*. J. infect. Dis. **116**, 75—83 (1966). — Innes, J.R.M., Seibold, H.R., Arentzen, W.P.: The pathology of bovine mastitis caused by *Cryptococcus neoformans*. Amer. J. vet. Res. **13**, 469—475 (1952). — Ishida, K., Sato, A.: Isolation of *Cryptococcus neoformans* from pigeon droppings in Japan. In: Recent Advances in Botany, pp. 326—330. Toronto: University of Toronto Press 1961. — Jackson, H., Parker, F.: Hodgkin's disease and allied disorders (p. 177). New York: Oxford University Press 1947. — Jacobs, L.G.: Pulmonary torulosis. Radiol. **71**, 398—403 (1958). — Jacobsen, J.: Zur Kenntnis der Torulopsis-neoformans-Infektion. Frankfurt. Z. Path. **66**, 135—141 (1955). — Janssens, J.: Torulosis bij een zwangere vrouw, met lokalisatie in de longen. Ned. T. Geneesk **101**, 824—826 (1957). — Janssens, J., Beetstra, A.: Torulose bei einer schwangeren Frau (Lokalisation in der Lunge). Geburtsh. u. Frauenheilk. **19**, 892—899 (1959). — Jayewardene, R.P., Wijekoon, W.B.: Cryptococcosis of the nervous system. Postgrad. Med. **39**, 546—547 (1963). — Jensen, K.: Cryptococcosis. Oversigt of et pulmonalt tilfaelde. (Cryptococcosis. A survey and a report of a case with pulmonary involvement; First case in Denmark.) Nord méd. **60**, 1722—1725 (1958). — Jesse, C.H.: *Cryptococcus neoformans* infection (torulosis) of bone. Report of a case. J. Bone Jt Surg. **29**, 810—811 (1947). — Johns, F.M., Attaway, C.L.: Torula meningitis. Report of a case and summary of literature. Amer. J. clin. Path. **3**, 459—465 (1960). — Johnson, G.F., Saichek, H.B., James, L.R.: Pulmonary cryptococcosis. Neb. St. med. J. **46**, 146—150 (1961). — Jones, E.L.: Torula infection of the nasopharynx. Sth. med. J. (Bgham, Ala.) **20**, 120—126 (1927). — Jones, S.H., Klinck, G.H., Jr.: *Torula histolytica* (*Cryptococcus hominis*) meningitis. A case report and therapeutic experiments. Ann. intern. Med. **22**, 736—745 (1945). — Kalsbeek, F., Planteyde, H.T.: Cryptococcosis tijdens behandeling met cortison en breedspectrum antibiotica. Geneesk. Gids **36**, 150—152 (1958). — Kao, C.J., Schwarz, J.: The isolation of *Cryptococcus neoformans* from pigeon nests. Amer. J. clin. Path. **27**, 652—663 (1957). — Kase, A., Marshall, J.D.: A study of *Cryptococcus neoformans* by the fluorescent antibody technique. Amer. J. clin. Path. **34**, 52—56 (1960). — Katz, R.I., Birnbaum, H., Eckmann, B.H.: Resection of pulmonary cryptococcosis associated with meningitis. Amer. resp. Dis. **84**, 725—729 (1961). — Kaufman, L.: The application of fluorescent antibody techniques for the detection and identification of mycotic disease agents. Mycopathologia (Den Haag) **26**, 257—263 (1965). — Kent, T.H., Layton, J.M.: Massive pulmonary cryptococcosis. Amer. J. clin. Path. **38**, 596—604 (1962). — Khan, M.J., Myers, R., Koshi, G.: Pulmonary cryptococcosis. A case report and experimental study. Dis. Chest **36**, 656—660 (1959). — Kikuchi, K.: Über einen Fall von Blastomykose beim Pferd. J. Jap. Soc. Vet. Sci. **2**, 4—5 (1923). — King, R.H.: Torulosis. Aust. J. Derm. **6**, 303—310 (1962). — Kinoshita, Y., Sasagawa, T., Nakana, S., Arakawa, M., Morita, A., Niwayama, A.: A case of systemic lupus erythematodes associated with cryptococcosis. J. Jap. Soc. Int. Med. **51**, 38—43 (1962). — Kisszekelyi, O., Trencseni, T.: Acut szakban felismert *Cryptococcus neoformans* altal okozott meningoencephalitis hazai esete (Hungarian case of meningoencephalitis caused by Cryptococcus neoformans and diagnosed in the acute phase). Orv. Hetil. **1957**, 1110—1112. — Klatzo, I., Geisler, P.H.: Demonstration of *Cryptococcus neoformans* in polarized light. Stain Technol. **33**, 55—56 (1956). — Klein, E.: Pathogenic microbes in milk. J. Hyg. (Lond.) **1**, 78—95 (1901). — Kligman, A.M., Crane A.P., Norris, R.F.: Effect of temperature on survival of chick embryos infected intravenously with *Cryptococcus neoformans*. Amer. J. med. Sci. **221**, 273—278 (1951). — Kligman, A.M., Weidman, F.D.: Experimental cryptococcosis (Torulosis). Arch. Derm. **60**, 726—741 (1949). — KLOOS, K., BÜSING, C.W.: Mesenchymreaktionen bei Cryptococcose des Menschen. Berl. Med. **13**, 287—293 (1962). — KNUDSON, R.J., BURCH, H.B., HATCH, H.B.: Primary pulmonary cryptococcosis. J. thorac. cardiovasc. Surg. **45**, 730—740 (1963). — KOHLMEIER, W.: Torulose der Nasennebenhöhlen. Zbl. allg. Path. path. Anat. **93**, 92 (1955). — KOHLMEIER, W., KREITNER, H.: Blastomykose der Mamma. Wien. klin. Wschr. **65**, 13—15 (1953). — KOHLMEIER, W., NIEL, K.: Über einen Fall von Torulose, europäischer Blastomykose. Wien. klin. Wschr. **62**, 97—98 (1950). — KOLUKANOV, I.E., VOJTSEKHOVSKII, B.L.: On the isolation of cryptococci and keratinolytic fungi from the soil. Mycological studies. Proc. Sci. Mycol. Congr., 6th, Leningrad, 106—108 (1965a). ~ On the evaluation of pigeons as a source of environment infection. Mycological studies. Proc. Sci. Mycol. Congr., 6th, Leningrad, 108—110 (1965b). — KÖNIGSBAUER, H.: Über die Wirkung von Corton auf die experimentelle Torulose und Chromoblastomykose. Zbl. Bakt., I. Abt. Orig. **160**, 637—643 (1954). — KOSHI, G., SUDERSANAM, D., SELVAPANDIAN, A.J., MYERS, R.: Cryptococcosis "masquerading" as tuberculosis of the spine. Indian J. Path. Bact. **7**, 264—271 (1964). — KOVI, J.: Mycoses associated with leukemia. Orv. Hetil. **105**, 1175—1179 (1964). — KRAINER, L., SMALL, J.M., HEWLITT, A.B., DENESS, T.: A case of systemic torula infection with tumor formation in the meninges. J. Neurol. Neurosurg. Psychiat. **9**, 158—162 (1946). — KREGER-VAN-RIJ, N.J.W., STAIB, F.: The utilization of creatine and creatinine by some debaryomyces species. Arch. Mikrobiol. **45**, 115—118 (1963). — KREJČI, D., VANEČEK, R.: Cryptococcal meningoencephalitis unsuccessfully treated with amphotericin B. Čas. Lek. Česk. **102**, 910—914 (1963). — KREJČI, O., VYSOKÁ, B., HANZAL, F., ŘEHÁNEK, L., MANYCH, J.: Generalizovana kryptokokoza (Toruloza) Generalized cryptococcosis [Torulosis]). Čas. Lek. Česk. **100**, 484—492 (1961). — KRESS, M.B., CANTRELL, J.R.: Pulmonary and meningeal cryptococcosis. Successful treatment of the meningitis with lateral cerebral intraventricular injection of amphotericin B. Arch. intern. Med. **112**, 386—392 (1963). — KRUYT, R.C.: Torulosis van het centrale zenuwstelsel behandeld met amfotericine B (Torulosis of the central nervous system treated with amphotericin B). Ned. T. Geneesk. **104**, 1370—1373 (1960). — KUHN, L.R.: Growth and viability of *Cryptococcus hominis* at mouse and rabbit body temperatures. Proc. Soc. exp. Biol. (N.Y.) **67**, 539—541 (1939). — KUO, D.: A case of torulosis of the central nervous system during pregnancy. Med. J. Aust. **1**, 558—560 (1962). — KURLANDER, G.J.: X-ray film of the month. Dis. Chest. **39**, 549—550 (1961). — KURUP, P.V., PANIKAR, C.K.J.: Pulmonary cryptococcosis. Mycopathologia (Den Haag) **21**, 129—134 (1963). — KUYKENDALL, S.J., ELLIS, F.H., JR., WEED, L.A., DONOGHUE, F.E.: Pulmonary cryptococcosis. New Engl. J. Med. **257**, 1009—1016 (1957). — KWAN, W.Y.: Mycotic meningitis. Report of a case. Chung Nan Med. J. **2**, 472 (1952). — LAAS, E., GEIGER, W.: Blastomykose bei Lymphogranulomatose. Dtsch. Z. Nervenheilk. **159**, 314—331 (1948). — LACAZ DA SILVA, C., PEREIRA, O.A., DE CASTRO FERNANDES, J., MATTOS ULSON, C.: Contribução para o estudo da prova de urease na identicião do Cryptococcus neoformans. Med. Cirurg. Farm. 262/263 (1958). — LACAZ DA SILVA, C.: Manual de Micologia Medica. 3a. edicao. Rio de Janeiro/Sao Paulo, 1960. — LAMARDO, M.R.: Cryptococcosis. Arch. venez. Pueric. **29**, 404—407 (1966). — LAMERSON, O.P.: Cryptococcus infections in man. Delaware med. J. **30**, 70—72 (1958). — LAPORTE, A., HOUDART, R., CALDERA, R., MANIGAND, G.: La meningite a *Cryptococcus neoformans*. Un nouveau cas d'evolution rapide. Presse méd. **62**, 44—47 (1954). — LAUMEN, F.: Cryptococcal infection as an apparent cause of exudative pleuresy and meningoencephalitis. Prax. Pneumol. **18**, 234—243 (1964). — LAUZE, S.: Infection a Torula chez un individu traite aux antibiotiques et a la cortisone. Union Med. Canada **81**, 935—940 (1952). — LEITHOLD, S.L., REEDER, P.S., BAKER, L.A.: Cryptococcal infection treated with 2-Hydroxystilbamidine in a patient with Boeck's sarcoid. Arch. intern. Med. **99**, 736—743 (1957). — LEOPOLD, S.S.: Pulmonary moniliasis and cryptococcal osteomyelitis in the same patient. Med. Clin. N. Amer. **37**, 1737—1746 (1953). — LEPAU, H., RUBINSTEIN, L., COHN, F., SHANDRA, J.: A case of *Cryptococcus neoformans* meningoencephalitis complicating Boeck's sarcoid. Pediatrics **19**, 377—386 (1957). — LESTER, J.P., LANE, J.C., KERN, W.H., JONES, J.C.: The surgical treatment of isolated pulmonary cryptococcosis. J. thorac. cardiovasc. Surg. **44**, 207—215 (1962). — LEVIN, E.A.: Torula infection of the central nervous system. Arch. intern. Med. **59**, 667—684 (1937). — LEVINE, S., ZIMMERMAN, H.M., SCORZA, A.: Experimental cryptococcosis (torulosis). Amer. J. Path. **33**, 385—409 (1957). — LEVIN, S., EVANS, E.E., KABLER, P.W.: Studies of cryptococcus polysaccharides by infrared spectrophotometry. J. infect. Dis. **104**, 269—273 (1959). — LEVI-VALENSI, A., SARFATA, E., COHEN-ADAD, F., LORENTE, P.: Maladie de Hodgkin associée a une tuberculose ganglionaire et compliquée de torulose a forme meningée. Arch. franç. Pediat. **14**, 225—233 (1957). — LEWIN, W., ROUX, P.: Torula infection of the central nervous system. Four recent cases. S. Afr. med. J. **20**, 2—5 (1946). — LEY, A., JACAS, R., OLIVERAS, C.: Torula granuloma of cervical spinal cord. J. Neurosurg. **8**, 327—335 (1951). — LIM TEONG WAH, CHAN KOK EWE: Observations on the laboratory diagnosis of cerebral torulosis (cryptococcosis). Med. J. Malaya **16**, 193—205 (1962). — LINDEN, I.H., STEFFEN, C.G.: Pulmonary cryptococcosis. Amer. Rev. Tuberc. **69**, 116—120

(1954). — Line, F.G.: A case of cryptococcus (torula) meningitis treated with ethyl vanillate. J. Tenn. med. Ass. **47**, 292—294 (1954). — Linell, F., Magnusson, B., Nordén, A.: Cryptococcos (torulos), ett fall med sympton fran hud, lungor och centrala nervsystemet. (Kryptokokkose [Torulose]. Ein Fall mit Symptomen an Haut, Lungen und zentralem Nervensystem.) Nord. Med. **46**, 1195—1199 (1951). ∼ Cryptococcosis. Review and report of a case. Acta derm. venereol. (Stockh.) **33**, 103—122 (1953). — Lippelt, H.: Zur Pathogenität der Blastomyzeten. Zbl. Bakt., I. Abt. Orig. **140**, 116—118 (1937). — Littman, M.L.: A culture medium for the primary isolation of fungi. Science **106**, 109—111 (1947). ∼ Growth of pathogenic fungi on a new culture medium. Amer. J. clin. Path. **18**, 409—420 (1948). ∼ Liver-spleen glucose blood agar for *Histoplasma capsulatum* and other pathogenic fungi. Amer. J. clin. Path. **25**, 1148—1159 (1955). ∼ Cryptococcosis (torulosis). Current concepts and therapy. Amer. J. Med. **27**, 976—998 (1959). ∼ Therapy of cryptococcosis. In: Fungi and Fungal Diseases, pp. 292—306. Springfield/Ill.: Ch.C. Thomas 1962. — Littman, M.L., Zimmermann, L.E.: Cryptococcosis, Torulosis or European blastomycosis. New York and London: Grune & Stratton 1956. — Littman, M.L., Schneierson, S.S.: *Cryptococcus neoformans* in pigeon excreta in New York City. Amer. J. Hyg. **69**, 49—59 (1959). — Littman, M.L., Tsubura, E.: Effect of degree of encapsulation upon virulence of Cryptococcus neoformans. Proc. Soc. exp. Biol. (N.Y.) **101**, 773—777 (1959). — Littman, M.L., Borok, R., Dalton, T.J.: Experimental avian cryptococcosis. Amer. J. Epidem. **82**, 197—207 (1965). — Liu, C.T.: Intracerebral cryptococcic granuloma. Case report. J. Neurosurg. **10**, 686—689 (1953). — Lodder, J., DeVries, N.F.: Some notes on *Torulopsis glabrata* (Anderson) nov. comb. Mycopathologia (Den Haag) **1**, 98—103 (1938). — Lodder, J., Kreger-van Rij, N.J.W.: The Yeasts. A Taxonomic Study. Amsterdam: North-Holland Publishing 1952. — Lomanitz, R., Hale, J.M.: Production of delayed hypersensitivity to *Cryptococcus neoformans* in experimental animals. J. Bact. **86**, 505—509 (1963). — Lombardo, T.A., Rabson, A.D., Dodge, H.T.: Mycotic endocarditis. Report of a case due to *Cryptococcus neoformans*. Amer. J. Med. **22**, 664—670 (1957). — Longmire, W.P., Jr., Goodwin, T.C.: Generalized Torula infection. Case report and review with observations on pathogenesis. Bull. Johns Hopk. Hosp. **64**, 22—43 (1939). — Lopez Fernandez, J.R.: Acción patógena experimental de la levadura *Torulopsis glabrata* (Anderson, 1917) Lodder y de Vries 1938 productora de lesiones histopatológicas, semejantes a las de la histoplasmosis. An. Fac. Med. Montevideo **37**, 470—483 (1952). — Louria, D.B.: Specific and non-specific immunity in experimental cryptococcosis in mice. J. exp. Med. **111**, 643—665 (1960). ∼ In: Baum, G.L.: Textbook of Pulmonary Diseases. Boston: Little, Brown and Co. 1965. — Louria, D.B., Feder, N., Emmons, C.W.: Amphotericin B in experimental histoplasmosis and cryptococcosis. Antibiotics. Ann. 1956—1957, New York Med. Encyclopedia, Inc., p. 870, 1957. — Louria, D.B., Greenberg, S.M., Molander, D.W.: Fungemia caused by certain nonpathogenic strains of family cryptococcaceae. Report of 2 cases due to rhodotorula and Torulopsis glabrata. New Engl. J. Med. **263**, 1281—1284 (1961). — Louria, D.B., Kaminski, T., Finkel, G.: Further studies on immunity in experimental cryptococcosis. J. exp. Med. **117**, 509—520 (1963). — Lutsky, I., Brodish, J.: Experimental canine cryptococcosis. J. infect. Dis. **114**, 273—276 (1964). — Lynch, F.B., Jr., Rose, E.: Torula meningitis. Report of an additional case. Ann. clin. Med. **4**, 755—760 (1926). — MacGillivray, J.B.: Two cases of cryptococcosis. J. clin. Path. **19**, 424—428 (1966). — Madsen, D.E.: Some studies of three pathogenic fungi isolated from animals. Cornell Vet. **32**, 383—389 (1942). — Magarey, F.R., Denton, P.H.: Brit. med. J. **116**, 1082—1083 (1948). — Mager, J., Aschner, M.: Starch reaction as aid in identification of causative agent of European blastomycosis. Proc. Soc. exp. Biol. (N.Y.) **62**, 71—72 (1946). — Magruder, R.G.: A report of three cases of Torula infection of the central nervous system. J. Lab. clin. Med. **24**, 495—499 (1939). — Mahnke, P.-F.: Experimentelle Cryptococcose der Maus. Zbl. allg. Path. path. Anat. **103**, 447—454 (1962). — Mahnke, P.-F., Schimpf, A., Schönborn, Ch., Dieckmann, U.: An cryptococcosis with skin involvement. Frankfurt. Z. Path. **71**, 383—397 (1961). — Manfredi, R.A.: Cryptococcal meningitis. Proc. Inst. Med. Chic. **25**, 160 (1964). — Manganiello, L.O.J., Nichols, P., Jr.: Intraventriuclar torula granuloma. J. Neurosurg. **12**, 306—310 (1955). — Markham, J.W., Alcott, D.L., Manson, R.M.: Cerebral granuloma caused by *Cryptococcus neoformans*. Report of a case. J. Neurosurg. **15**, 562—568 (1958). — Marshall, T.M.: Torular meningoencephalitis. J. Ky med. Ass. **50**, 292—297 (1952). — Marshall, M., Teed, R.W.: *Torula histolytica* meningoencephalitis. Recovery following bilateral mastoidectomy and sulfonamide therapy. J. Amer. med. Ass. **120**, 527—529 (1942). ∼ Ann. intern. Med. **34**, 1277—1279 (1951). — Marshall, J.D., Eveland, W.C., Smith, C.W.: Superiority of fluorescein isothiocyanate (Riggs) for fluorescent antibody technique with modification of its application. Proc. Soc. exp. biol. (N.Y.) **98**, 898—900 (1958). — Marshall, J.D., Iverson, L., Eveland, W.C., Kase, A.: Comparison of fluorescent antibody staining and special histologic stains for the identification of *Cryptococcus neoformans*. Amer. J. Path. **35**, 684—685 (1959). ∼ Application and limitations of the fluorescent antibody stain in the specific diagnosis of cryptococcosis. Lab. Invest. **10**, 719—728 (1961). — Martin, H., Padberg, F.: Torulosis of the brain. Arch. Neurol. Psychiat.

(Chic.) **62**, 679—680 (1949). — Martin, W.J., Nichols, D.R., Svien, H.J., Ulrich, J.A.: Cryptococcosis. Further observations and experience with amphotericin B. Arch. intern. Med. **104**, 4—15 (1959). — Mashiba, H., et al.: Case of cryptococcosis. Nika **13**, 777—782 (1964). — Massee, J.C., Rooney, J.S.: Meningitis due to *Torula histolytica*. Report of a case. J. Amer. med. Ass. **94**, 1650—1653 (1930). — Matheis, H.: Die Cryptococcose (Torulose) des Nervensystems. Dtsch. Z. Nervenheilk. **180**, 595—639 (1960). — Matras, A., Tappeiner, S.: Über eine tödlich verlaufende generalisierte Blastomykose der Haut und der inneren Organe. Arch. Derm. Syph. (Berl.) **181**, 444—450 (1940). — May, J., Afed-Kamiuska, M., Zgorzelski, S.: Torulosis (cryptococcosis) zomowieniem wtasnego przypadku. Pol. Tyg. lek. **13**, 480—484 (1958). — McConchie, I.: Torula granuloma of the lung. Med. J. Aust. **38**, 685—686 (1951). — McConchie, I.H., Hayward, J.I.: Torula histolytica (*Cryptococcus neoformans*) granuloma of the lung treated by pulmonary resection. Postgrad. med. J. **34**, 190—194 (1958). — McCullough, N.B., Louria, D.B., Hilbish, T.F., Thomas, L.B., Emmons, C.: Cryptococcosis. Clinical staff conference at the National Institutes of Health. Ann. intern. Med. **49**, 642—661 (1958). — McDonough, E.S., Ajello, L., Ausherman, R.J., Balows, A., McClellan, J., Brinkman, S.: Amer. J. Hyg. **73**, 75—83 (1961). — McGehee, J.L., Michelson, I.D.: Torula infection in man. Report of a case. Surg. Gynec. Obstet. **42**, 803—808 (1926). — McGibbon, C., Readett, M.: Torulosis presenting in a skin department. Brit. J. Derm. **72**, 430—433 (1960). — McGrath, J.T.: Cryptococcosis of the central nervous system in domestic animals. Amer. J. Path. **30**, 651 (1954). — McKendree, C.A., Cornwall, L.H.: Meningo-encephalitis due to torula. Arch. Neurol. Psychiat. (Chic.) **16**, 167—181 (1926). — McMath, W.F.T., Hussain, K.K.: Cryptococcal meningoencephalitis. Brit. med. J. **4244**, 91—93 (1961). — Mello, R.P., Teixera, G. de A.: Cryptococcosis in the initial phase of dissemination. Hospital (Rio de J.) **61**, 355—361 (1962) [Portuguese]. — Mendonca Cortez, J.: Criptococcose pulmonar (Blastomicose europeia). An. paul. Med. Cirurg. **58**, 315 (1949). — Mezey, C.M., Fowler, R.: Torula cerebro-spinal cryptococcosis (due to *Cryptococcus* or *Torula histolytica*). J. Amer. med. Ass. **132**, 632—634 (1946). — Meyer, K.F.: A pathogenic blastomyces from the horse. Proc. path. Soc. Philad. **16**, 28 (1914). — Mider, G.B., Smith, F.D., Bray, W.E., Jr.: Systemic manifestations with *Cryptococcus neoformans (Torula histolytica)* and *Histoplasma capsulatum* in the same patient. Arch. Path. **43**, 102—110 (1947). — Miller, J.M., et al.: Treatment of infection due to cryptococcosis with stilbamidine. Antibiot. and Chemother. **2**, 444—446 (1952). — Minkowithz, S., Koffler, D., Zak, F.G.: *Torulopsis glabrata* septicemia. Amer. J. Med. **34**, 252—255 (1963). — Misch, K.A.: Torulosis associated with Hodgkin's disease. J. clin. Path. **8**, 207—210 (1955). — Mitchell, L.A.: Torulosis. J. Amer. med. Ass. **106**, 450—542 (1936). — Mohr, W.: Die Mykosen. In: Handbuch der inneren Medizin, Bd. II, S. 825—937. Berlin-Göttingen-Heidelberg: J.F. Springer 1952. — Mollaret, P., Reilly, J., Bastin, R.: La forme ganglionaire localisée de la cryptococcose. Lyon méd. **1**, 71—84 (1960). — Molnar, J.: Torulosis. Orv. Hetil. **96**, 685 (1955). ∼ Meningo-encephalitis caused by *Cryptococcus neoformans*. Acta morph. Acad. Sci. hung. **6**, 233—239 (1955). — Monnet, P., Blanc, P.: Les cryptococcoses humaines. Sem. Hôp. Paris **31**, 3851—3862 (1955). — Monnet, P., Coudert, J., Berthenod, M., Blanc, P.E.: Meningo-encephalite a Torula chez un nourrisson. Lyon méd. **193**, 377—388 (1955). — Moody, A.M.: Asphyxial death due to pulmonary cryptococcosis. A case report. Calif. Med. **67**, 105—106 (1947). — Mook, W.H., Moore, M.: Cutaneous torulosis. Arch. Derm. Syph. (Chic.) **33**, 951—962 (1936). — Moore, M.: Cryptococcosis with cutaneous manifestations. J. invest. Derm. **28**, 159—182 (1957). — Morris, E., Wolinsky, E.: Localized osseous cryptococcosis. A case report. J. Bone Jt Surg. **47**, 1027—1029 (1965). — Mosberg, W.H., Jr., Alvarez-DeChoudens, J.A.: Lancet **1951**, 1259—1260. — Mosberg, W.H., Jr., Arnold, J.G., Jr.: Torulosis of the central nervous system. Ann. intern. Med. **32**, 1153—1183 (1950). — Moss, E.M., McQuown, A.L.: Atlas of Medical Mycology. Baltimore: Williams & Wilkins 1960. — Muchmore, H.G., Rhoades, E.R., Nix, G.E., Felton, F.G., Carpenter, R.E.: Occurrence of *Cryptococcus neoformans* in the environment of three geographically associated cases of cryptococcal meningitis. New Engl. J. Med. **268**, 1112—1114 (1963). — Muchmore, H.G.: Meeting. Amer. Soc. Mycol. ,New Orleans 1967. — Muir, C.S., Ransome, G.A.: *Cryptococcus neoformans* meningitis. Med. J. Malaya **14**, 125—134 (1959). — Mukherjea, A.K., Sengupta, M., Roy, H.N.: Retinal cyst due to *Cryptococcus neoformans*. Bull. Calcutta Sch. trop. Med. **9**, 106—107 (1961). — Muller, E., Schaltenbrandt, G.: Coccidiose der Meningen. Nervenarzt **19**, 327—333 (1948). — Muller, E., Hilscher, W.M.: Zur Frage der generalisierten Blastomykose und ihrer Beziehungen zur Lymphogranulomatose. Zbl. allg. Path. path. Anat. **92**, 331—338 (1954). — Mumenthaler, M.: Meningoencephalitis durch *Cryptococcus neoformans*. Schweiz. med. Wschr. **90**, 386—391 (1960). — Mumme, C., Lippelt, H.: Zur Pathogenität der Blastomyceten. Z. klin. Med. **135**, 187—197 (1938). — Muslow, F.W., Lindley, E.L.: *Cryptococcus neoformans* meningoencephalitis. A case report. J. Iowa St. med. Soc. **47**, 579—580 (1957). — Nanda, S.P., Kass, I., Cohn, M., Dressler, S.H.: Coexistence of tuberculous and cryptococcal meningitis. Pediatrics **20**, 45—52 (1957). — Nassau, E., Weinberg-Heiruti, C.: Torulosis of the newborn. Harefuah **35**, 50—51 (1948). —

Negroni, P., Briz-de Negroni, C.: Manifestaciones cutaneomucosas de la blastomicosis europea. A proposito de una nueva observacion. Rev. argent. Dermatosif. **34**, 228—232 (1950). — Neill, J. M., Kapros, C. E.: Serological tests on soluble antigens from mice infected with *Cryptococcus neoformans* and *Sporotrichum schenckii*. Proc. Soc. exp. Biol. (N.Y.) **73**, 557—559 (1950). — Neill, J. M., Sugg, J. Y., McCauley, D. W.: Serologically reactive material in spinal fluid, blood, and urine from a human case of cryptococcosis (Torulosis). Proc. Soc. exp. Biol. (N.Y.) **77**, 775—778 (1951). — Neuhauser, E. B. D., Tucker, A.: The Roentgen findings produced by diffuse torulosis in the newborn. Amer. J. Roentgenol. **59**, 805—815 (1948). — Nevill, L. M. B., Cooke, E. R. N.: Human cryptococcosis in Kenya. E. Afr. med. J. **36**, 209—219 (1959). — Newcomer, V. D., Sternberg, T. H., Wright, E. T., Reisner, R. M., McNall, Sorensen, L. J.: The treatment of systemic fungus infections with amphotericin B. Ann. N.Y. Acad. Sci. **89**, 221—239 (1960). — Nichols, E. H.: The relation of blastomycetes to cancer. J. med. Res. **7**, 312—359 (1902). — Nichols, I. C.: Torula meningoencephalitis. Report of a case. R. I. med. J. **24**, 221—222 (1941). — Nichols, D. R., Martin, W. J.: Cryptococcosis. Clinical features and differential diagnosis. Ann. intern. Med. **43**, 767—780 (1955). — Nicod, J. L.: Un cas autochthone de Blastomycose des meninges. Schweiz. med. Wschr. **68**, 234—237 (1938). — Niño, F. L.: Blastomycosis humana generalizada por Cryptococcus (n. sp.). Estudio clínico, parasitológico, anatomopatológico y experimental. Sexta Reunión Soc. Arg. Path. Geog. del Norte. Univers. Buenos Aires 1934. ~ Contribución al estudio de las blastomicosis en la República Argentina. Capitulo V. Granuloma criptococcico. Estudio de un nuevo caso argentino. Bol. Inst. Clín. quir. (B. Aires) **14**, 656—755 (1938). — Niño, F. L., Marano, A.: Blastomicosis a focos multiples por Cryptococcus neoformans (Sanfelice). Arch. Soc. argent. Anat. **9**, 307—318 (1947). — Norris, J. C., Armstrong, W. B.: Membraneous cryptococcic nasopharyngitis (Cryptococcus neoformans). Arch. Otolaryng. **60**, 720—722 (1954). — O'Connor, F. J., Foushee, J. H. S., Jr., Cox, C. E.: Prostatic cryptococcosis. J. Urol. (Baltimore) **94**, 160—163 (1965). — O'Donoghue, J. G.: A case of blastomycotic meningitis. Med. J. Aust. **1**, 118 (1933). — Ogawa, K., Uejima, A., Inohara, T., Kuroda, K., Murase, J., Kanamoto, A.: Cryptococcosis. Pathological observations of 5 autopsy cases and one biopsy case. Acta Med. Okayama **13**. 319—347 (1959). — Okudaira, M., Schwarz, J., Adriano, S. M.: Experimental production of Schaumann bodies by heterogenous microbial agents in the golden hamster. Lab. Invest. **10**, 968—982 (1961). — Okun, E., Butler, W. T.: Ophthalmologic complications of cryptococcal meningitis. Arch. Ophthal. **71**, 52—57 (1964). — Oliveira Campos, J. de: Congenital meningo-encephalitis due to *Torulopsis neoformans* (cryptococcosis). Rev. clín. Inst. matern. Lisboa **87**, 92 (1954). ~ Preliminary report. Congenital meningoencephalitis due to *Torulopsis neoformans* (cryptococcosis). Bol. clin. Hosp. Lisboa **18**, 609—618 (1954). — O'Neill, F. J., Newcomb, A., Nielsen, C. S.: Cryptococcus meningitis. U.S. nav. med. Bull. **49**, 300—305 (1949). — Owen, M.: Generalized cryptococcosis simulating Hodgkin's disease. Tex. St. J. Med. **35**, 767—771 (1940). — Padberg, F., Martin, J.: Torulosis of the brain. J. Neurosurg. **9**, 307—309 (1952). — Palmrose, E. C., Losli, E. J.: Cryptococcus meningitis. Report of two cases. Northw. Med. (Seattle) **51**, 121—126 (1952). — Pariser, S., Littman, M. L., Duffy, L.: Cryptococcal meningo-encephalitis associated with systemic lupus erythematosus. J. Mt Sinai Hosp. **28**, 550—561 (1961). — Partridge, B. M., Winner, H. I.: *Cryptococcus neoformans* in bird droppings in London. Lancet **1965 I**, 1060—1062. — Perceval, A. K.: Experimental cryptococcosis: hypersensitivity and immunity. J. Path. Bact. **89**, 645—655 (1965). — Peroncini, J., Bence, A. E., Vaccarezza, D. A., Aguero, J. G.: Torulosis bronquial y meningica. Medicina (B. Aires) **9**, 363—370 (1949). — Perruchio, P., Bruel, R., Lagarde, C., Delpy, J.: Le torulome bronchectasiant. Une nouvelle forme clinique de la torulose respiratoire. Presse méd. **67**, 387—390 (1959). — Piers, F.: Torulosis, Cryptococcosis (European Blastomycosis, Buschkes disease). R. D. Simons Medical Mycology, pp. 254—260. Amsterdam: Elsevier 1952. — Pierson, P. H.: Torula in man. Report of a case with necropsy findings. J. Amer. med. Ass. **69**, 2179—2181 (1917). — Pinney, C. T.: Solitary circumscribed lesion of the lung due to *Cryptococcus neoformans*. Amer. Rev. Tuberc. **74**, 441—444 (1956). — Piontek, J., Pulverer, G., Walter, H. T.: Cryptococcose bei Lymphogranulomatose. Medizinische **1959**, 1373—1379. — Piper, J. E.: Torulosis of cerebrospinal type. Case report. Med. J. Aust. **31**, 441 (1944). — Plaut, A.: Human infection with *Cryptococcus glabratus*. Report of a case involving uterus and Fallopian tubes. Amer. J. clin. Path. **20**, 377—380 (1950). — Plummer, N. S., Symmers, W. St. C., Winner, H. I.: Sarcoidosis in identical twins with torulosis as a complication in one case. Brit. med. J. **2**, 599—603 (1957). — Pollock, A. Q., Ward, L. M.: A hemagglutination test for cryptococcosis. Amer. J. Med. **32**, 6—16 (1962). — Poppe, J. K.: Cryptococcosis of the lung. Report of two cases with successful treatment by lobectomy. J. thorac. Surg. **27**, 608—613 (1954). — Potenza, L., Benaim, H.: Observación de dos casos con torulopsis (*Cryptococcus neoformans*) en el sistema nervioso central. Arch. venez. Pat. trop. **1**, 236—263 (1949). — Potenza, L., Feo, M.: Use of polarized light in diagnosis of mycotic infections. Tech. Bul. Amer. Soc. Clin. Path. **26**, 91—99 (1956). — Potenza, L., Rodriguez, C., Feo, M.: *Torulopsis neoformans* pleural. Estudio clinico, patológico y micológico del primer caso observado en Venezuela. Rev. Sanid. Asist. soc. 16, 195—213 (1951). — POUNDEN, W. D., AMBERSON, J. M., JAEGER, R. F.: A severe mastitis problem associated with *Cryptococcus neoformans* in a large dairy herd. Amer. J. vet. Res. 13, 121—128 (1952). — PROCKNOW, J. J., BENFIELD, J. R., RIPPON, J. W., DIENER, F., ARCHER, L.: Cryptococcal hepatitis presenting as a surgical emergency. J. Amer. med. Ass. 191, 93—98 (1965). — PUCKETT, T. F.: Pulmonary histoplasmosis. Study of 29 cases with identification of *H. capsulatum* in resected lesions. Amer. Rev. Tuberc. 67, 453—476 (1953). — PUND, E. R., VAN WAGONER, F. D.: Torula meningitis. Report of case. J. med. Ass. Ga 25, 48—50 (1936). — QUODBACH, K.: Ein Beitrag zur Pathologie der Blastomykosen des Zentralnervensystems. Zbl. allg. Path. path. Anat. 69, 227—231 (1938). — RAMMAURTHI, B., ANGULI, V. C.: Intramedullary cryptococcic granuloma of the spinal cord. J. Neurosurg. 11, 622—624 (1954). — RAMOS-MORALES, F., DEJESUS, M. A., DETORREGROSA, M. V., DIAZ RIVERA, R. S.: Cryptococcal (Torula) meningitis. Case report. Bol. Asoc. méd. P. Rico 52, 121—130 (1960). — RANDHAWA, H. S., CLAYTON, Y. M., RIDDELL, R. W.: Isolation of *Cryptococcus neoformans* from pigeon habitats in London. Nature (Lond.) 208, 801 (1965). — RAPER, K. B., ALEXANDER, D. F.: Preservation of molds by the lyophil process. Mycologia 37, 499—525 (1945). — RAPPAPORT, B. Z., KAPLAN, B.: Generalized torula mycosis. Arch. Path. 1, 720—741 (1926). — RATCLIFFE, H. E., COOK, W. R.: Cryptococcosis. U.S. armed Forces med. J. 1, 957—967 (1950). — RAVISSE, P., REYNAND, R., DEPOUX, R., SALLES, P.: Sur le premier cas de cryptococcose decouvert en A.E.F. Presse méd. 67, 727—728 (1959). — RAVITS, H. G.: Cutaneous cryptococcosis. A survey of cryptococcosis on normal and pathologic skin. J. Invest. Derm. 12, 271—284 (1949). — RAWSON, A. J., COLLINS, L. H., JR., GRANT, J. L.: Histoplasmosis and torulosis as causes of adrenal insufficiency. Amer. J. med. Sci. 215, 363—371 (1948). — REALE, E.: Un caso di meningite da torula histilitica. Morgagni 73, 66—68 (1931). — REEVES, D. L., BUTT, E. M., HAMMACK, R. W.: Torula infection of the lungs and central nervous system. Arch. intern. Med. 68, 57—79 (1941). — REICHEL, R.: Über Blastomykose des Gehirns, der Hirnhäute und der Lunge. Klin. Wschr. 1939, 1468—1471. — REID, J. D.: The influence of the vitamin B complex on the growth of *Torulopsis* (*Cryptococcus*) *neoformans* on a synthetic medium. J. Bact. 58, 777—782 (1949). — REILLY, E. B., ARTMAN, E. L.: Cryptococcosis. Report of a case and experimental studies. Arch. intern. Med. 81, 1—8 (1948). — REVOL, L., GARIN, J. P., MOREL, P. L.: Hepatosplenomegalie febrile mortelle. Association cryptococcosetoxoplasmose. Soc. Fr. Mycol. Med. Lyon, 25 mai. 1963. — REYBELLET, J.: Les mycoses des systeme nerveux central. Rev. méd. Suisse rom. 83, 734—748 (1963). — REYES ARMIJO, E., ALAMANZA VELEZ, R.: Comunicacion preliminar sobre cuatro casos de torulosis del sistema nervioso central. Rev. méd. Hosp. gen. (Méx.) 27, 293—300 (1964). — RHOADES, E. R., GINN, H. E., MUCHMORE, H. G., SMITH, W. O., HAMMARSTEN, J. F.: Effect of amphotericin B upon renal function in man. Clin. Res. 8, 232 (1960). — RIETH, H.: Untersuchungen zur Hefediagnostik in der Dermatologie. Arch. klin. exp. Derm. 207, 413—430 (1958). — RIGDON, R. H., KIRKSEY, O. T.: Mycotic aneurysm (cryptococcosis) of the abdominal aorta. Amer. J. Surg. 84, 486—491 (1952). — RINEHART, J. F., ABUL-HAJ, S. K.: Improved method for histologic demonstration of acid mucopolysaccharides in tissues. Arch. Path. 52, 189—194 (1951). — RING, E. D., WILLIAMS, T. H.: Torulosis. Canad. med. Ass. J. 67, 360—361 (1952). — RIPPEY, J. J., ROBER, W. A. G., JEANES, A. L., BRIGHT, M. V.: Cryptococcal meningo-encephalitis. J. clin. Path. 18, 296—300 (1965). — RISGAARD PETERSEN, B.: Cryptococcosis. Ugeskr. Laeg. 128, 1060—1061 (1966). — RITTER, R. C., LARSH, H. W.: The infection of white mice following an intranasal instillation of *Cryptococcus neoformans*. Amer. J. Hyg. 78, 241—246 (1963). — RIVEROS, M., BOGGINO, J., MAYOR, V.: Sobre un caso blastomicosis a Torula histilitica. Rev. méd. Parag. 3, 95—102 (1946). — ROANTREE, W. B., DUNKERLEY, G. E.: Meningoencephalitis due to *Cryptococcus neoformans*. Report of a case. Lancet 1952, 1274—1278. — ROBERTSON, H. C., JR., MOSELEY, V.: Cryptococcus meningitis. Ann. intern. Med. 36, 1538—1540 (1952). — ROBERTSON, W. E., ROBERTSON, H. F., RIGGS, H. E., SCHWARTZ, L.: Torulosis involving human cerebrum. J. Amer. med. Ass. 113, 482—484 (1939). — RODGER, R. C., TERRY, L. L., BINFORD, C. H.: Histoplasmosis, cryptococcosis and tuberculosis complicating Hodgkin's disease. Report of a case. Amer. J. clin. Path. 21, 153—157 (1951). — RODRIGUEZ DE LEDESMA, J. P., GONZALEZ ALGUACIL, C.: Torula histilitica cerebral. Rev. clín. esp. 46, 106—108 (1952). — RODRIGUEZ PEREZ, J., SUQUET, M.: Blastomicosis de los centros nerviosis. Vida nueva 28, 452—461 (1931). — ROGER, H., POURSINES, Y.: La meningoencephalite a Torula. Marseille-méd. 80, 24—42 (1943). — ROGER, H., POURSINES, Y., PITOT, TEMPIER: Etude anatomo-clinique d' une meningoencephalite a Torula a forme d' hypertension intracranienne aigue. Rev. neurol. 74, 333—334 (1942). — ROOK, A., WOODS, B.: Cutaneous cryptococcosis. Brit. J. Derm. 74, 43—49 (1962). — ROSE, F. CL., GRANT, H. C., JEANES, A. L.: Torulosis of the central nervous system in Britain. Brain 81, 542—555 (1958). — ROSEN, S. H., CASTLEMAN, B., LIEBOW, A. A.: Pulmonary alveolar proteinosis. New Engl. J. Med. 258, 1123—1142 (1958). — ROSS RUSSEL, R. W., DEAN, D.: Torula meningitis in Malaya. Brit. med. J. 5045, 627 (1957). — ROWLAND, L. P., GRIFFITHS, C. D., KABAT, E. A.: Myasthenia gravis, thymoma and cryptococcal meningitis. New Engl. J. Med. 273, 620—627 (1965). —

Royer, P.J., Delville, P., Mairlot, F.: Observations d'un cas de torulose meningée et pulmonaire. Ann. Soc. belge Méd. trop. **34**, 229—232 (1954). — Rubin, H., Furcolow, M.L.: Promising results in cryptococcal meningitis. Neurology (Minneap.) **8**, 590—595 (1958). — Rubin, H., Lehan, P.H., Fitzpatrick, M.J., Furcolow, M.L.: Amphotericin B in the treatment of cryptococcal meningitis. Antibiot. Ann. 1957—1958, Medical Encyclopedia, Inc., New York, pp. 71—74, 1958. — Ruiter, M., Ensink, G.J.: Acute primary cutaneous cryptococcosis. Dermatologica (Basel) **128**, 185—201 (1964). — Rusk, G.Y.: A case of pulmonary cerebral and meningeal blastomycosis. Proc. N.Y. path. Soc. **10**, 48—50 (1910/1911). — Rusk, G.Y., Farnell, F.J.: Systemic oidiomycosis. A study of 2 cases developing terminal oidiomycetic meningitis, with clinical notes. Univ. Calif. Publ. Path. **2**, 47—58 (1912). — Sabesin, S.M., Fallon, H.F., Andriole, V.T.: Hepatic failure as a manifestation of cryptococcosis. Arch. intern. Med. **111**, 661—669 (1963). — Sacquet, E., Drouhet, E., Vallee, A.: Un cas spontanée de cryptococcose (Cryptococcus neoformans) chez le souris. Ann. Inst. Pasteur **97**, 252—253 (1959). — Saez, H.: Etude de 29 souches de cryptococcus isolées en cinq ans chez des mammiferes et des oiseaux. Rev. Mycol. **30**, 57—73 (1965). — Sagi, T., Feherpataky, J.: Torulom des Zentralnervensystems. Path. et Microbiol. (Basel) **23**, 3—9 (1960). — Salfelder, K., Schwarz, J.: Thirteen cases of cryptococcosis in Cincinnati. Unpublished data (1967a). — Histoplasma capsulatum and chickens. Mykosen **10**, 337—350 (1967b). — Salfelder, K., Schwarz, J., Romero, A., de Liscano, T.R., Zambrano, Z., Diaz, P.I.: Habitat de Nocardia asteroides, Phialophora pedrosoi y Cryptococcosus neoformans en Venezuela. Mycopathologia (Den Haag) (1967) [in press]. — Salveraglio, F.J., Mackinnon, J.E., Cantonnet-Blanch, P., Canzani, R., Cantoni de Anzalone, H., Fazzio-Montans, H., Conti-Diaz, I.A.: Caso autóctono de criptococosis en el Uruguay. An. Fac. Med. Montevideo **47**, 25—32 (1962). — Salvin, S.B., Smith, R.F.: Mechanism of fungus pathogenicity. 4. Delayed hypersensitivity and cryptococcosis. Mycopathologia (Den Haag) **14**, 232 (1961). ~ An antigen for detection of hypersensitivity to Cryptococcus neoformans. Proc. Soc. exp. Biol. (N.Y.) **108**, 498—501 (1961). — Sanfelice, F.: Sull'azione patogena de blastomiceti como contributo alla etiologia dei tumori maligni. Nota preliminare. II. Policlinico, Sez. chir. **2**, 204—211 (1895). ~ Sull'azione patogena dei blastomiceti. Ann. d'Igiene **5**, 239—262 (1895). ~ Über einen neuen pathogenen Blastomyceten, welcher innerhalb der Gewebe unter Bildung kalkartig aussehender Massen degeneriert. Zbl. Bakt., I. Abt. Orig. **18**, 521—526 (1895). ~ Contributo alla morfologia e biologia dei blastomiceti che si sviluppano nei succhi di alcuni frutti. Ann. d'Igiene **4**, 463—465 1895—1899). ~ Ein weiterer Beitrag zur Ätiologie der bösartigen Geschwulste. Zbl. Bakt., I. Abt. Orig. **24**, 155—158 (1898). — Sampson, B.F., Farren, J.E.: Another case of torula meningitis. S. Afr. med. J. **16**, 245—247 (1942). — Sandhu, R.S., Jaggi, O.P., Randhawa, H.S., Sandhu, D.K., Gupta, I.M.: Isolation of Cryptococcus neoformans from a patient without clinical signs of infection. A case report. Indian J. Chest Dis. **6**, 93—97 (1964). — Sanz, J., Gomez, J., de Cisneros, J.M.: Torulosis pulmonar de forma diseminada. Rev. clin. esp. **70**, 303—309 (1958). — Sauerteig, E.: Beitrag zur Kenntnis der Torulopsis neoformans. Infektion des Menschen. Z. Tropenmed. Parasit. **17**, 109—123 (1966). — Saunders, L.Z.: Systemic fungus infections in animals. A review. Cornell Vet. **38**, 213—238 (1948). — Sawers, W.C., Thomson, E.F.: Torulosis with a report of a case of meningitis due to Torula histolytica. Med. J. Aust. **2**, 581—593 (1935). — Schellner: Über eine beim Pferde durch Hefezellen verursachte Geschwulst in der Nasenhöhle und deren Nebenhöhlen. Z. Vet. **47**, 111—116 (1935). — Schepel, J.A.C., Carsjens, F.W.: Torulosis with pulmonary localization; case. Ned. T. Geneesk. **97**, 2723—2726 (1953). — Schmidt, E.G., Álvares-de Choundens, J.A., McElvain, N.F., Beardsley, J., Tawab, S.A.A.: A microbiological study of Cryptococcus neoformans. Arch. Biochem. **26**, 15—24 (1950). — Scholer, H.J., Schneider, P.A.: Nachweis von Cryptococcus neoformans und anderen Hefen aus Milch von Kühen mit Mastitis. Path. et Microbiol. (Basel) **24**, 803—818 (1961). — Schwarz, J., Baum, G.L.: Pioneers in the discovery of deep fungus diseases. Mycopathologia (Den Haag) **25**, 73—81 (1965). — Schwarz, J., Schornagel, H.E., Straub, M.: Ein Fall von Torulosis; Pilzkrankheiten und Tuberculose, ihre Ähnlichkeit und Unterschiede. Docum. Med. geogr. trop. (Amst.) **6**, 69—75 (1954). — Sciortino, A.L., MacHaffie, R.H., Alliband, G.T., Zaayer, R.: Cryptococcosis. Arch. intern. Med. **102**, 451—458 (1958). — Seabury, J.F.: Experience with amphotericin B. Chemotherapia (Basel) **3**, 81—94 (1961). — Seabury, J.H., Dascomb, H.E.: Experience with amphotericin B (Fungizone) for treatment of systemic mycoses. Arch. intern. Med. **102**, 960—976 (1958). ~ Experience with amphotericin B. Ann. N.Y. Acad. Sci. **89**, 202—220 (1960). — Seeliger, H.P.R.: Use of a urease test for the screening and identification of cryptococci. J. Bact. **72**, 127—131 (1956). ~ Das kulturell-biochemische und serologische Verhalten der Cryptococcus-Gruppe. Ergebn. Mikrobiol. **32**, 23—72 (1959). ~ Les phenomenes d'immunité dans les mycoses. Path. et Biol. **8**, 297—306 (1960). ~ Immunbiologisch-serologische Nachweisverfahren bei Pilzerkrankungen. In: Handbuch der Haut- und Geschlechtskrankheiten, Bd. IV, S. 605—734. Berlin-Göttingen-Heidelberg: J.F. Springer 1963. ~ Use of serological methods for the diagnosis of cryptococcosis. A review. Ann. Soc. belge Méd. trop. **44**, 657—668

(1964). — SEELIGER, H.P.R., CHRIST, P.: Zur Schnelldiagnose der Cryptococcus-Meningitis mittels der Liquorpräcipitation. Mykosen 1, 88—92 (1958). — SEGRETAIN, G., COUTEAU, M.: Differentation entre Torulopsis (Cryptococcus) neoformans et corps amyloides du systeme nerveux central. Ann. Inst. Pasteur 88, 128—132 (1955). — SEIBOLD, H.R., ROBERTS, C.S., GORDON, E.M.: Cryptococcosis in a dog. J. Amer. vet. med. Ass. 122, 213—215 (1953). — SEILER, S.: Beitrag zur Klinik der Blastomykose. Beitr. klin. Chir. 156, 609—624 (1932). — SEMERAK, C.B.: Torula leptomeningitis. Arch. Path. 6, 1142—1145 (1928). — SETHI, K.K.: Pigeons and mycoses. New Engl. J. Med. 276, 62 (1967a). ~ Attempts to produce experimental intestinal cryptococcosis and sporotrichosis. Mycopathologia (Den Haag) 31, 245—250 (1967b). — SETHI, K.K., SALFELDER, K., SCHWARZ, J.: Experimental cutaneous primary infection with Cryptococcus neoformans (Sanfelice) Vuillemin. Mycopathologia (Den Haag) 27, 357—368 (1965). — SETHI, K.K., SCHWARZ, J.: Experimental ocular cryptococcosis in pigeons. Amer. J. Ophthal. 62, 95—98 (1966). — SHADOMY, H.J., UTZ, J.P.: Preliminary studies on a hypha-forming mutant of Cryptococcus neoformans. Mycologia 98, 383—390 (1966). — SHAH, P.M., SHARMA, K.D.: Cryptococcosis. A report of a case with review of the literature. Indian J. Pediat. 1, 181—189 (1964). — SHAPIRO, L.L., NEAL, J.B.: Torula Meningitis. Arch. Neurol. Psychiat. (Chic.) 13, 174—190 (1925). — SHEPPE, W.M.: Torula infection in man. Amer. J. med. Sci. 167, 91—108 (1924). — SHIELDS, L.H.: Disseminated cryptococcosis producing a sarcoid type reaction. Arch. intern. Med. 104, 736—770 (1959). — SHIELDS, A.B., AJELLO, L.: Medium for selective isolation of Cryptococcus neoformans. Science 151, 208—209 (1966). — SIEWERS, C.M.F., CRAMBLETT, H.G.: Cryptococcosis (torulosis) in children. A report of 4 cases. Pediatrics 34, 393—400 (1964). — SILVA, M.E.: Ocorrencia de Cryptococcus neoformans e Microsporum gypseum em solos da Bahia, Brasil. Bol. Fund. G. Moniz 17, 1—14 (1960). — SILVA, M.E., PAULA, L.A.: Isolation of Cryptococcus neoformans from excrement and nests of pigeons (Columba livia) in Salvador, Bahia (Brasil). Rev. Inst. Med. trop. S. Paulo 5, 9—11 (1963). — SIMON, S.L.: Pulmonary moniliasis and cryptococcal osteomyelitis in the same patient. Med. Clin. N. Amer. 37, 1737—1746 (1953). — SIMON, J., NICHOLAS, R.E., MORSE, E.V.: An outbreak of bovine cryptococcosis. J. Amer. vet. med. Ass. 122, 31—35 (1953). — SINGER, E.: Two cases of fungus infection. China med. J. 66, 85—89 (1949). — SINHA, G.B., BARUA, D.: Cerebral cryptococcosis. Bull. Calif. Sch. Trop. Med. 8, 140 (1960). — SKULSKI, G., SYMMERS, W. ST. C.: Actinomycosis and torulosis in the ferret (Mustela puro). J. comp. Path. 64, 306—311 (1954). — SMITH, G.W.: The treatment of Torula meningo-encephalitis with amphotericin B. J. Neurosurg. 15, 572—575 (1958). — SMITH, F.B., CRAWFORD, J.S.: Fatal granulomatosis of the central nervous system due to a yeast (Torula). J. Path. Bact. 33, 291—296 (1930). — SMITH, F.: Cryptococcosis and associated Hodgkin's disease. N.Z. med. J. 59, 285—288 (1960). — SMITH, D.L.T., FISCHER, J.B., BARNUM, D.A.: Generalized Crypto-coccus neoformans infection in a dog. Canad. med. Ass. J. 72, 18—20 (1955). — SMITH, C.W., MARSHALL, J.D., JR., EVELAND, W.C.: Use of contrasting fluorescent dye as counter stain in fixed tissue preparations. Proc. Soc. exp. Biol. (N.Y.) 102, 179—181 (1959). — SMITH, G.W., KEMP, J.A., FARRAR, W.E., JR., KEMBLE, J.W., PHILPOT, D.F., JR.: Cryptococcosis of central nervous system. Four cases treated with amphotericin B. Sth. med. J. (Bgham, Ala.) 53, 305—311 (1960). — SMITH, C.D., RITTER, R., LARSH, H.W., FURCOLOW, M.L.: Infection of white swiss mice with airborne Cryptococcus neoformans. J. Bact. 87, 1364—1368 (1964). — SOEMIATNO: Meningitis disebabkan oleh Debaryomyces (Cryptococcus) neoformans dan sum-bangan pen getahuan tentang „Blastomycetes"-Djamur Jang pathogen bagimanusia. J. In-dones. med. Ass. 3, 137—149 (1953). — SONCK, C.E.: Kryptokokkose mit Knochenmetastase. Mykosen 10, 319—324 (1967). — SOTGIU, G., MAZZONI, A., MANTOVANI, A., AJELLO, L., PAL-MER, J.: Survey of soils for human pathogenic fungi from the Emilia Romagna region of Italy. II. Isolation of Allescheria boydii, Cryptococcus neoformans, and Histoplasma capsulatum. Amer. J. Epidemiol. 83, 329—337 (1966). — SOYSAL, S.S., UNAT, E.K., TAHSINOGLU, M.: Un cas de cryptococcose. Arch. franç. Pédiatr. 11, 246—260 (1954). — SPIVACK, A.P., NADEL, J.A., EISENBERG, G.M.: Cryptococcus renal infection. Report of case. Ann. intern. Med. 47, 990—1002 (1957). — SPICER, C., HIATT, W.O., KESSEL, J.F.: Candida albicans and Crypto-coccus neoformans occurring as infective agents in an 8-year-old boy. J. Pediat. 33, 761—769 (1948). — SPICKARD, A., BUTLER, W.T., ANDRIOLE, V.T., UTZ, J.P.: The improved prognosis of cryptococcal meningitis with amphotericin B therapy. Ann. intern. Med. 58, 66—83 (1963). — STAIB, F. (a): Vorkommen von Cryptococcus neoformans im Vogelmist. Zbl. Bakt., I. Abt. Orig. 182,562—563(1961). ~ (b): Cryptococcus neoformans im Muskelgewebe. Zbl. Bakt., I. Abt. Orig. 185, 135—144 (1962). ~ (c): Cryptococcus neoformans und Guizotia abyssinica (syn. G. oleifera D.C.). Z. ges. Hyg. 148, 466—475 (1962). ~ (d): Cryptococcus neoformans beim Kanarienvogel. Zbl. Bakt., I. Abt. Orig. 185,129—134(1962). ~ (e): Zbl. Bakt., I. Abt. Orig. 186,233—247(1962). ~ (f): Zbl. Bakt., I. Abt. Orig. 186, 274—275 (1962). ~ (g): Zur Kreatinin-Kreatin-Assimila-tion in der Hefepilzdiagnostik. Zbl. Bakt., I. Abt. Ref. 191,429—432 (1963). ~ (h): Zur Wider-standsfähigkeit von Cryptococcus neoformans gegen Austrocknung und hohe Temperaturen. Arch. Mikrobiol. 44, 323—333 (1963). ~ (i): The importance of thiamin (vitamin B_1) for the assimilation of creatinine by Cryptococcus neoformans. Zbl. Bakt., I. Abt. Orig. **190**, 115—131 (1963). ~ (k): Membranfiltration und Negersaat (Guizotia abyssinica). Nährboden für den *Cryptococcus neoformans*-Nachweis (Braunfarbeffekt). Z. ges. Hyg. **149**, 329—335 (1963). ~ (l): Saprophytic life of *Cryptococcus neoformans*. Its relation to low molecular nitrogen substances in nature and the human. Ann. Soc. belge Méd. trop. **44**, 611—615 (1964). ~ (m): Zur Cryptococcose bei Mensch und Tier unter besonderer Berücksichtigung des Vorkommens von *Cryptococcus neoformans* im Vogelmist. Tierärztl. Umsch. **19**, 69—72 (1964). — Staib, F., Zissler, J. (a): Sproßpilze, insbesondere *Cryptococcus neoformans* und menschliches Serum. Z. Haut- u. Geschl.-Kr. **35**, 145—148 (1963). ~ (b): The possibility of utilization of rest nitrogen substances of human sera by *Cryptococcus neoformans*. Zbl. Bakt., I. Abt. Orig. **189**, 117—119 (1963). — Starr, K.W., Geddes, B.: Pulmonary torulosis. Aust. N.Z.J. Surg. **18**, 212—214 (1949). — Stein, J.M., Burdon, P.J.: *Cryptococcus neoformans* infection of the central nervous system. A case treated by amphotericin B with postmortem examination. Ann. intern. Med. **52**, 445—453 (1960). — Stenvers, H.W.: Torula-infectie van het centrale zenuwstelsel. Ned. T. Geneesk. **78**, 3361—3366 (1934). — Stevenson, L.D., Vogel, F.S., Williams, V.: Cryptococcosis of the central nervous system and incidental cryptococcic granuloma. Arch. Path. **49**, 321—332 (1950). — Stiefel, E., Andreu Urra, J., Lazaro, J.: La criptococcosis pulmonar. Rev. clín. esp. **49**, 293—300 (1953). — Stijns, J., Royer, P.: Un cas de meningite a torulosis au Congo belge. Ann. Soc. belge Méd. trop. **33**, 483—486 (1953). — Stiles, W.W., Curtiss, A.N.: Torula meningoencephalitis. Observations of cerebrospinal fluid. J. Amer. med. Ass. **116**, 1633—1635 (1941). — Stoddard, J.L., Cutler, E.G.: Torula Infection in Man. Rockefeller Inst. Med. Res. Monograph No. 62, pp. 1—98 (Jan. 31) 1916. — Stone, W.J., Sturdivant, B.F.: Meningoencephalitis due to Torula histolytica. Arch. intern. Med. **44**, 560—575 (1929). — Stypulkowski, C., Maciejewska, G., Nowak, J.: Intra vitam diagnosis of cryptococcal septicemia involving especially the central nervous system during the course of lymphatic leukemia. Pol. Tyg. lek. **19**, 104—107 (1964). — Subramanian, S., Sivaraman, K., Prabhaker, R.: Cultivation and animal pathogenicity of Cryptococcus neoformans isolated from a case of meningitis. Ind. J. Microbiol. **5**, 61—64 (1965). — Susman, M.P.: Torula (cryptococcus) infection of the lung. Aust. N.Z.J. Surg. **23**, 296—299 (1953—1954). — Sutmoller, P., Poelma, F.G.: Cryptococcus neoformans infection (torulosis) of goats in the Leeward Islands region. W. Indian med. J. **6**, 225—228 (1957). — Swanson, H.S., Smith, W.A.: Torula granuloma simulating cerebral tumor. Report of two cases. Arch. Neurol. Psychiat. (Chic.) **51**, 426—431 (1944). — Swatek, F.E., Becker, S.W., Wilson, J.W., Omieczynski, D.T., Kazan, B.H.: A new method for the direct isolation of Cryptococcus neoformans from the soil. Proc. 7th Intern. Congr. Trop. Med. Malaria **3**, 122—124 (1964). — Swift, H., Bull, L.B.: Notes on a case of systemic blastomycosis. Blastomycotic cerebrospinal meningitis. Med. J. Aust. **2**, 265—267 (1917). — Symmers, W.St.C.: Torulosis. A case mimicking Hodgkin's disease and rodent ulcer, and a presumed case of pulmonary torulosis with acute dissemination. Lancet **1953**, 1068—1074. ~ Torulosis and Hodgkin's disease. Brit. med. J. **1**, 459—460 (1957). ~ Torulosis. Lancet **1959**, 943—944. ~ Cryptococcus neoformans in bird droppings. Letters. Lancet (January 21) **1967**, 159—160. — Szilagyi, G., Reiss, F., Smith, J.C.: The anticryptococcal factor of blood serum. A preliminary report. J. invest. Derm. **46**, 306—308 (1966). — Taber, K.W.: Torulosis in man. Report of a case. J. Amer. med. Ass. **108**, 1405—1406 (1937). — Takos, M.J.: Experimental cryptococcosis produced by the ingestion of virulent organisms. New Engl. J. Med. **254**, 598—601 (1956). — Takos, M.J., Elton, N.W.: Spontaneous cryptococcosis of marmoset monkeys in Panama. Arch. Path. **55**, 403—407 (1953). — Taylor, W.A.: Demonstration at 96th meeting of Pathological Society of Gt. Britain and Ireland in London. Cited by Symmers, p. 1068 (1953). — Terplan, K.: Pathogenesis of cryptococcic (Torula) meningitis. Amer. J. Path. **24**, 711—712 (1948). — Thiers, H., Coudert, J., Pelloux, H., Fayolle, J., Colomb, D., Joud, R.: Un cas de cryptococcose osseuse et pulmonaire. Bull. Soc. franç. Derm. Syph. **67**, 127—128 (1960). — Thomas, R.C., McClenathan, J.E., Osborne, D.P.: Pulmonary cryptococcosis. Report of three cases. Med. Ann. D.C. **31**, 77—80 (1962). — Tiant, F.R., Fuentes, C.A.: Cryptococcosis de localización cutánea. Bol. Soc. cuba. Derm. Sif. **15**, 65—72 (1958). — Tillotson, J.R., Lerner, A.M.: Prostatism in an 18-year-old boy due to infection with Cryptococcus neoformans. New Engl. J. Med. **273**, 1150—1152 (1965). — Timmermann, H.J.: Fatal case of yeast meningitis in pregnancy. Amer. J. Obstet. Gynec. **31**, 686—688 (1936). — Tinney, W.S., Schmidt, H.W.: Torula infection. Med. Clin. N. Amer. **28**, 950—956 (1944). — Todd, R.L., Herrmann, W.W.: The life cycle of the organism causing yeast meningitis. J. Bact. **32**, 89—103 (1936). — Tomcsik, J.: Die Struktur der Bakteriengrenzflächen. In: Ergebnisse der medizinischen Grundlagenforschung, p. 1—56. Stuttgart: Georg Thieme 1956. — Toone, E.C., Jr.: Torula histolytica (Blastomycoides histolytica). Report of case with recovery. Virginia med. Mth. **68**, 405—407 (1941). — Torrey, F.A.: Cutaneous cryptococcosis in a patient with Hodgkin's disease. Arch. Derm. Syph. (Chic.) **55**, 738—739 (1947). — Trautwein, G., Nielson, S.V.: Cryptococcosis in 2 cats, a dog and a mink. Amer. Vet. Med. Ass. **140**, 437—442 (1962). — Truant, J.P., Tesluk, H.: The effect of cortisone upon experimental cryptococcosis. Bact. Proc. **87**, 1 p. (1956). — TURK, W.: Ein Fall von Hefeinfektion (Saccharomykose) der Meningen. Arch. Klin. Med. **90**, 335—366 (1907). — TURNER, P.P.: A case of cryptococcosis with choroidal torulomata. E. Afr. med. J. **36**, 220—223 (1959). — TYLER, R.: Spinal fluid alcohol in yeast meningitis. Amer. J. med. Sci. **232**, 560—561 (1956). — UNAT, E.K., PARS, B., KOSYAK, J.P.: A case of cryptococcosis of the colon. Tip. Fak. Mec. (Istanbul) **22**, 1327—1330 (1959). ~ A case of cryptococcosis of the colon. Brit. med. J. **2**, 1501—1502 (1960). — URBACH, E., ZACH, F.: Generalisierte Torulosis. Arch. Derm. Syph. (Chic.) **162**, 401—421 (1930). — UTZ, J.P., ANDRIOLE, V.: Analysis of amphotericin treatment failures in the systemic fungal diseases. Ann. N.Y. Acad. Sci. **89**, 277—282 (1960). — UTZ, J.P., BENNETT, J.E., BRANDRISS, M.W., BUTLER, W.T., HILL, G.S.: Amphotericin B toxicity. Combined clinical staff conference at the National Institutes of Health. Ann. intern. Med. **61**, 334—354 (1964). — UTZ, J.P., BUTLER, T.: Cryptococcus Meningitis. Neuere Beobachtungen zur Erkennung und Therapie. Dtsch. med. Wschr. **90**, 941—943 (1965). — VANBREUSEGHEM, R.: Torulose et Torulopsis neoformans. Ann. Soc. belge Méd. trop. **33**, 495—501 (1953). ~ Cryptococcose chez la souris blanche. Bull. Soc. franç. Mycol. Med. **8**, 1964. — VANDEPITTE, J., COLAERT, J., LIEGEOIS, A.: Leptomeningite aigue a Torulopsis neoformans. Seconde observation congolese. Ann. Soc. belge Méd. trop. **33**, 503—509 (1953). — VARGAS, A.: Cryptococcosis (o torulosis) pulmonar (con excepcional reacción hemática); 1. Sección estudio clínico. Rev. méd. Valparaíso **3**, 42—52 (1950). — VARMA, R.M., SRIRAMACHARI, S., PILLAI, K.M., SRIDHARA RAMA RAO, B.S., RAMANANDA RAO, R., SIRSI, M.: A case report of cryptococcal infection of the brain. Trans. All India Inst. Ment. Hlth. **1**, 63—73 (1960). — VASSILIADIS, P., DEANTAS, V.: Nouveau cas de cryptococcosis au Congo belge. Ann. Soc. belge Méd. trop. **39**, 753—758 (1959). — VERSÉ, M.: Über einen Fall von generalisierter Blastomykose beim Menschen. Verh. dtsch. path. Ges. **17**, 275—278 (1914). — VIALA, J.J., FAITH, A., RACLE, P.: Cryptococcose cerebro-meningee et hemopathie maligne a-propos de deux observations. Lyon méd. **212**, 1059—1077 (1964). — VOGEL, R.A.: The indirect fluorescent antibody test for the detection of antibody in human cryptococcal disease. J. infect. Dis. **116**, 573—580 (1966). — VOGEL, R.A., SELLERS, T.F., JR., WOODWARD, P.: Fluorescent antibody techniques applied to the study of human cryptococcosis. J. Amer. med. Ass. **178**, 921—923 (1961). — VOSS, J.A.: Generalized blastomycosis with clinical picture of meningitis. Norsk Mag. Laegevidensk. **84**, 550—560 (1923). — VOYLES, G.Q., BECK, E.M.: Systemic infection due to Torula histolytica (Cryptococcus hominis). I. Report of four cases and review of literature. Arch. intern. Med. **77**, 504—515 (1946). — VUILLEMIN, P.: Les blastomycetes pathogenes. Rev. Gen. Sci. **12**, 732—751 (1901). — WADE, L.J., STEVENSON, L.D.: Torula Infection. Yale J. Biol. Med. **13**, 467—476 (1941). — WAGER, H.E., CALHOUN, F.P.: Torula uveitis. Trans. Amer. Acad. Ophthal. **58**, 61—67 (1954). — WALTER, J.E., ATCHISON, R.W.: Epidemiological and immunological studies of Cryptococcus neoformans. J. Bact. **92**, 82—87 (1966). — WARVI, W.N., RAWSON, R.W.: Torula meningitis. Arch. intern. Med. **69**, 90—98 (1942). — WATTS, J.W. Torula infection. Amer. J. Path. **8**, 167—192 (1932). — WEBB, W.R., BIGGS, R.H.: Pulmonary cryptococcosis. Dis. Chest **30**, 659—668 (1956). — WEBER: Sitzungsbericht. Zbl. inn. Med. **24**, 96 (1903). — WEBSTER, B.H.: Bronchopulmonary cryptococcosis. Dis. Chest **43**, 513—518 (1963). — WEGMANN, T.: Blastomykose und andere Pilzerkrankungen der Lunge. Dtsch. Arch. klin. Med. **199**, 192—205 (1952). — WEIDMAN, F.D.: Cutaneous torulosis. Sth. med. J. (Bgham, Ala.) **26**, 851—863 (1933). — WEIDMAN, F.D., RATCLIFFE, H.L.: Extensive generalized torulosis in a chetah or hunting leopard. Arch. Path. **18**, 362—369 (1934). — WEIS, J.D.: Four pathogenic torulae (blastomycetes). J. med. Res. **2**, 280—311 (1902). — WEISS, C., PERRY, I.H., SHEVKY, M.C.: Infection of the human eye with Cryptococcus neoformans (Torula histolytica). Arch. Ophthal. **39**, 739—751 (1948). — WELSH, J.D., FOERSTER, D.W., CAMP, W.A., RHOADES, E.R.: Torula meningitis treated with amphotericin B. J. Okla. med. Ass. **52**, 683—687 (1959). — WEN, S.F., YANG, S.P., LU, H.C., LU, C.H.: Cryptococcosis. A report of 4 additional cases with review of 11 cases found in Taiwan. J. Formosa Med. Ass. **60**, 861—867 (1961). — WERNER, W.A.: Pulmonary and cerebral cryptococcosis without meningitis. Amer. Rev. resp. Dis. **92**, 476—478 (1965). — WETTINGELD, R.F., SCHMIDT, E.C., NAEGELE, C.F., DOERNER, A.A.: Systemic cryptococcosis without central nervous system involvement. A case report. Ann. intern. Med. **44**, 1259—1264 (1956). — WHITE, E.C.: A case of meningo-encephalitis due to Torula. U.S. nav. med. Bull. **28**, 615—618 (1930). — WHITE, M., ARANY, L.S.: Resection in pulmonary cryptococcosis (torulosis). J. thorac. Surg. **35**, 402—410 (1958). — WHITEHILL, M.R., RAWSON, A.J.: Treatment of generalized cryptococcosis with 2-hydroxystilbamidine. Report of a case with apparent cure. Virginia med. Mth. **81**, 591—594 (1954). — WICKERHAM, L.J.: A critical evaluation of the nitrogen assimilation tests commonly used in the classification of yeasts. J. Bact. **52**, 293—301 (1946). — WICKERHAM, L.J., BURTON, K.A.: Carbon assimilation tests for the classification of yeasts. J. Bact. **56**, 363—371 (1948). — WIEBECKE, B., STAIB, F.: Generalisierte Cryptokokkose. Münch. med. Wschr. **107**, 361—365 (1965). — WIENER, M.F.: Generalized torulosis with bone involvement. Arch. intern. Med. **87**, 713—726 (1951). — WILE, U.J.: Cutaneous torulosis. Arch. Derm. Syph. (Chic.) **31**, 58—66

(1935). — Wilhelmj, C. M.: The primary meningeal form of systemic blastomycosis. Amer. J. med. Sci. 169, 712—721 (1925). — Wilkins, R. H., Bennett, J. E., Wertlake, P. T., West, J. T.: Mesenchymoma and visceral cryptococcosis. Report of a case. Arch. Surg. 88, 761—767 (1964). — Willis, J. D., Marples, M. J., Dihanna, M. E., Rodda, R., Pullar, T. H.: Cryptococcal (Torula) meningitis in New Zealand. A report of four cases. N.Z. med. J. 56, 99—109 (1957). — Wilson, H. M., Duryea, A. W.: Cryptococcus meningitis (torulosis) treated with a new antibiotic, Actidione. Arch. Neurol. Psychiat. (Chic.) 66, 470—480 (1951). — Wilson, J. W.: Cryptococcosis (torulosis, European blastomycosis, Busse-Buschke's disease). J. chron. Dis. 5, 445—459 (1957). — Wilson, L. L.: Cryptococcosis (torulosis). A report of 9 cases. Aust. Ann. Med. 7, 276—285 (1958). — Winslow, D. J., Hathaway, B. M.: Pulmonary pneumocystis and cryptococcosis. Amer. J. clin. Path. 31, 337—342 (1959). — Wolfe, J. N., Jacobson, G.: Roentgen manifestations of torulosis. Amer. J. Roentgenol. 79, 216—227 (1958). — Wortis, S. B., Wightman, H. B.: A case report of Torula meningitis. Bull. N.Y. Acad. Med. 4, 531—536 (1928). — Wu-Fei, C.: Cryptococcosis. Report of a case. China med. J. 74, 374—384 (1952). — Yamamoto, S., Ishida, K., Sato, A.: Isolation of Cryptococcus neoformans from pulmonary granuloma of a cat and from pigeon droppings. Jap. J. vet. Sci. 19, 179—191 (1957). — Yasaki, Y., Miyake, M., Okudaira, M., Toriumi, J., Inoue, T., Nakajima, S.: A new histological method for the detection of Cryptococcus neoformans and its histopathological study. Acta path. jap. 9, 351—360 (1959). — Zappoli, R., et al.: On 2 cases of cerebral mycosis caused by Torula histolitica (Cryptococcus neoformans). Riv. Pat. nerv. ment. 86, 135—151 (1965). — Zawirska, B.: Mitteilung über 4 Fälle von Torulose des Zentralnervensystems. Pat. pol. 8, 305—316 (1957). — Zawirska, B., Bratter, J.: Case of cryptococcosis of the central nervous system diagnosed as progressive paralysis. Neurol. Neurochir. Psychiat. pol. 5, 627 (1958). — Zawirska, B., Derubska, A.: Diagnostische Schwierigkeiten in einem seltenen Falle generalisierter Torulosis. Zbl. allg. Path. path. Anat. 102, 178—188 (1961). — Zeitlhofer, J.: Torulopsis neoformans-Infektion des Menschen; „Torulom" der Cauda equina. Frankfurt. Z. Path. 69, 324—335 (1958). — Zelman, S., O'Neil, R. H., Plaut, A.: Disseminated visceral torulosis without nervous system involvement. With clinical appearance of granulocytic leukemia. Amer. J. Med. 11, 658—664 (1951). — Zeman, W., Bebin, J.: Zur pathologischen Anatomie der Torula-Meningoencephalitis. Dtsch. Z. Nervenheilk. 168, 406—417 (1952). — Zimmerman, L. E.: Etiology of so-called pulmonary tuberculoma. Med. Ann. D.C. 23, 423—427 (1954). — Zimmerman, L. E., Rappaport, H.: Occurrence of cryptococcosis in patients with malignant disease of reticuloendothelial system. Amer. J. clin. Path. 24, 1050—1072 (1954).

North American Blastomycosis

E. W. CHICK, Lexington/Kentucky, USA

With 40 Figures

Definition

North American Blastomycosis is a disease of protean manifestations caused by the fungus *Blastomyces dermatitidis*. Blastomycotic infections may be benign and self-limiting or progressive with involvement of virtually any organ of the body by dissemination from a primary pulmonary focus. Lesions may be exudative, suppurative, or granulomatous. Historical highlights are listed in Table 1.

Table 1. *Historical Highlights of Blastomycosis*

1894	GILCHRIST	Presented report of first case.
1896	GILCHRIST and STOKES	Reported first case.
1898	GILCHRIST and STOKES	Named fungus *Blastomyces dermatitidis*.
1901	RICKETTS	Reported 15 cutaneous cases. Studied mycelial phase growth. First use of agglutination tests.
1902	WALKER and MONTGOMERY	Report of first systemic case.
1902	MONTGOMERY	First successful use of x-ray in treatment.
1907	HAMBURGER	Demonstrated diphasic growth patterns.
1907	HEKTOEN	Extended epidemiologic and pathologic aspects.
1908	MONTGOMERY	First use of potassium iodide in treatment.
1914	STOBER	Studies on pathogenesis and clinical aspects. Demonstration of fungus (?) on decaying wood.
1916	STODDARD and CUTLER	Clarified differences between *B. dermatitidis* and other fungi.
1916	WADE and BEL	Review of 49 cases. Limited infection to North America.
1934	BENHAM	Demonstrated identity of *Blastomyces* isolates.
1939	CONANT	Demonstrated identity of *Blastomyces* isolates.
1935	MARTIN	First use of complement fixation test.
1939	MARTIN and SMITH	Comprehensive review of 347 cases. Indicated role of allergy in pathogenesis and usefulness of antibody determinations in prognosis.
1942 BAKER		
1947 BAKER	Detailed tissue responses.	
1949	MANWARING	Demonstrated small forms of *B. dermatitidis*.
1949	SMITH	Classification of disease by immunologic types.
1950	COLBERT et al.	Use of propamidine in treatment.
1951	SCHOENBACH et al.	Use of stilbamidine in treatment.
1951	SCHWARZ and BAUM	Postulated basic respiratory route of infection.
1952	HOPKINS and MURPHY	First clinical use of undecylenic acid.
1952	RAMSEY and CARTER	Canine cases found in areas where human cases occur.
1953	SNAPPER and McVAY	Use of 2-hydroxystilbamidine in treatment.
1955	WILSON et al.	Report of four cases of primary cutaneous inoculation.
1955	SMITH et al.	Reported first epidemic.
1957	HARRELL and CURTIS	Use of amphotericin B in treatment.
1961	DENTON et al.	Report of isolation from soil.
1967	McDONOUGH	Isolation and identification of perfect stage of *B. dermatitidis* (*Ajellomyces dermatitidis*).

Epidemiology

a) Geographic of Distribution

α) Cases from North America (USA and Canada)

Most of the cases of *B. dermatitidis* infection have occurred in the USA. A review of 735 cases reported in the literature (CHICK et al., 1960) indicated most cases occurring east of the Mississippi River, as shown in Fig. 1. In a more recent study BUSEY et al. (1968) have compiled the distribution of human and canine cases of blastomycosis in North America. These cases include 1,244 human and 305 dog cases in which the etiology has been confirmed by culture or histopathology, and in which there was sufficient data to localize the case by county. A similar general distribution was found (Fig. 2), but with notable increases in the numbers of cases in states with previously unreported cases. The high areas, as indicated, are unique in their band-like character, but at this point no associated demographic, climatic, or geographic conditions are known to explain the distribution.

Occasional cases of blastomycosis have been reported from Canada (GILLIES, 1933; POIRIER, 1955; SCHWARZ and FURCOLOW, 1955; SOLWAY et al., 1939; STARRS and KLOTZ, 1948; WATSON et al., 1958). AJELLO (1967) quotes GRANDBOIS (1963) as compiling 114 cases of blastomycosis in Canada between 1906 and 1963. It is somewhat surprising, in view of the number of cases reported in some states in the northernmost U.S., that even more cases have not been reported from Canada, particularly the southern portions.

It is unfortunate that extensive skin test surveys for blastomycosis have not been undertaken as have been for tuberculosis, histoplasmosis and coccidioidomycosis. This is due in large part to the lack of a good specific antigen. When such an antigen is developed, skin test surveys may further elucidate the geographic distribution of infections due to *B. dermatitidis*, as well as to determine the prevalence of inapparent infections, if such occur.

β) Cases Outside North America

Until a few years ago it was generally believed that *Blastomyces dermatitidis* infections were confined to the North American Continent, as implied by the name North American Blastomycosis. It is now been documented repeatedly that *B. dermatitidis* infections do occur in other parts of the world.

Cases are reported in South Africa and in Uganda by EMMONS et al. (1964), in the Congo (GATTI et al., 1964, 1968), and in Mulago (JELLIFFE et al., 1964). POLO et al. (1954) reported a case in Venezula. AJELLO (1967) and GATTI et al. (1968) quote the cases of Arias LUZARDO (1962) and DE MONTEMAYOR (1954) as apparently autochthonous.

The case in Tunis reported by BROC and HADDAD (1952), by HADDAD (1952), and by VERMEIL et al. (1954) is felt by GATTI et al. (1968) to be inconclusive, since cultures failed to sporulate and could not be converted to intracellular form. WEGMAN (1952) reported a patient in Zurich, Switzerland with a positive skin test and complement fixation titer, although *B. dermatitidis* was not cultured from sputum. This patient worked in a tobacco factory which processed tobacco from the United States. DOWLING and ELSWORTHY (1926) reported a case in England with smears and cultures apparently positive for *Blastomyces dermatitidis*; this patient also had a history of close contact with materials shipped from the U.S.

A number of cases have been reported from Europe and South America but these have either had direct contact with the U.S., are inconclusive culturally, or represent infections by other fungi (CHICK et al., 1960; CHICK, 1961; AJELLO, 1967).

b) Age Distribution

Blastomycosis occurs over a wide age range, cases having been reported from the age of 5 months (ACREE et al., 1954; SMITH et al., 1955) to the ninth decade of

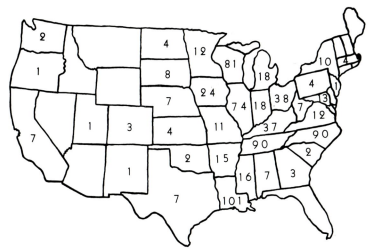

Fig. 1. Distribution of 735 reported cases of North American blastomycosis

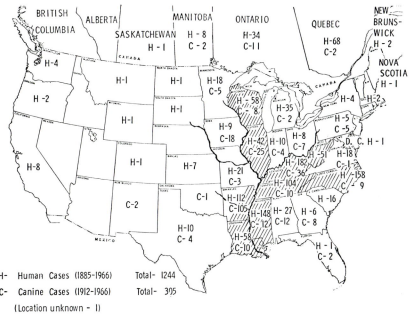

H- Human Cases (1885-1966)   Total- 1244

C- Canine Cases (1912-1966)   Total- 305

(Location unknown - 1)

Fig. 2. Distribution of human and canine cases of infection with *Blastomyces dermatitidis* in North America. |///////| High Area in the United States (States with 50 cases or more)

life (SCHWARZ and BAUM, 1951). There is, however, a marked increase in the number of cases occurring in certain age groups, varying somewhat with the series reported.

MARTIN and SMITH (1939) found 50% of their cases between 20 and 40 years of age with a range from 6 months to over 70 years. STARRS and KLOTZ (1948) found somewhat less than 50% between the ages of 20—40 years, and 50% in the group of over 40 years. In the series of KUNKEL et al. (1954) the average age was 46.6

30*

years, and a peak incidence occurred between 40 and 49 years. SCHWARZ and
GOLDMAN (1955) found 49% of their patients over 50 years of age and 40%
between the ages of 30 and 49. Similarly, CHERNISS and WAISBREN (1956) found
75% of patients over 30 years of age with 50% between the ages of 40 and 60.
CHICK et al. (1956) found 23% of their patients less than 30 years of age, 43%
between 31 and 50, and 34% over 50 years. The largest 10 year grouping was
30.2% in the 26—35 year group. In patients in Veterans Administration Hospitals
BUSEY et al. (1964) found an age range from 19—69 years in their series of 198
patients. Eighty percent were over 30, with a mean age of 42 years.

Thus, although blastomycosis may occur at almost any age, there is a marked
increase in the number of cases occurring between 30 and 50 years of age. This is
the period associated with more intensive productive livelihood. The importance
of this age incidence becomes of more interest in relation to sex and occupational
distribution and to the natural habitat of the fungus.

c) Sex Distribution

A preponderance of males is found among patients with blastomycosis. In
most series of patients (CHERNISS and WEISBREN, 1956; CHICK et al., 1956;
MARTIN and SMITH, 1939; SCHWARZ and GOLDMAN, 1955) the ratio of males to
females is 8 or 9 to 1, although in one series (SCHWARZ and BAUM, 1951) a ratio of
15 to 1 was found. In the epidemic studied by SMITH et al. (1955) an unexpected
1 to 1 ratio was found. Some differences in the male to female ratio have been
found when the cases are divided into systemic or cutaneous involvement. One of
the more striking differences was reported by KUNKEL et al. (1954) who found a
ratio of 5 males to 1 female in systemic cases and 10 to 1 in cutaneous cases,
giving an overall ratio of 7 to 1.

d) Racial Distribution

In the various series of cases reported in the U.S. the racial distribution has
usually reflected the population characteristics of the area from which the patients
are drawn. Thus, in the northern areas of the country the race has been predominately white (86—93%) (CHERNISS and WAISBREN, 1956; KUNKEL et al., 1954;
SCHWARZ and GOLDMAN, 1955) whereas in the southern areas the proportion of
Negro patients increases (HOWLES and BLACK, 1953; MARTIN and SMITH, 1939;
BUSEY et al., 1964), one series reporting 69% Negro patients (CHICK et al., 1956).

e) Occupation

There have been frequent attempts to correlate blastomycosis to occupations
or living conditions which are closely associated with nature. CHICK et al. (1956)
found that 33% of their patients were laborers, 17% were agricultural workers,
13% were "white collar" workers, and in 37% the occupation was unknown.
SCHWARZ and GOLDMAN (1955) found a similar occupational distribution with
46 patients in the "dust-exposed" group (farmers, laborers, construction workers,
carpenters, and miners) and 36 patients who were not "dust-exposed" (housewives,
bankers, veterinarians, teachers, cooks, etc.). Even more striking was the finding
that 47 out of 58 patients with cutaneous blastomycosis seen in New Orleans gave
some form of manuel labor as their occupation (HOWLES and BLACK, 1953).
STARRS and KLOTZ (1948) emphasized a correlation between this disease and
persons who worked or lived in damp, wooded, or dirty areas. Many of Stober's
(1914) patients lived in damp surroundings, often with dirt floors and rotting wood
walls. KUNKEL et al. (1954), however, could find no special relationship with

occupation. CHERNISS and WAISBREN (1956) found that of their 40 patients 21 were outdoor workers and 19 were indoor workers. In an attempt to define any suggestive contacts, they found an association with soil or vegetation in 13 patients, with animals in 5, and with no suggestive contact in the remaining 22 patients. All of the 198 patients in the Blastomycosis Cooperative Study of the Veterans Administation were characterized as having contact with soil to a greater or lesser degree (BUSEY et al. ,1964).

No definitive correlation has yet been demonstrated, since in each series there is always some proportion of the patients who appear to have no contact with soil or soil products. However, it should be kept in mind that many of these people work in their yards or gardens, go on picnics, or walk in the fields or woods occasionally, or drive through the country for business or pleasure. Such activities often are not considered in an epidemiologic history. The potential importance of this is apparent by analogy to coccidioidomycosis. Persons are known to have been infected with *C.immitis* by merely riding through an endemic area in a car or train without having stopped to get out of their vehicle (SMITH, 1955). Another factor which is not often considered is that blastomycosis is notorious for its chronicity. A small focus of infection may apparently smoulder for months or years before becoming severe enough to be clinically apparent.

f) Epidemics

The first culturally documented epidemic of North American blastomycosis was reported by SMITH et al. (1955). This epidemic occurred over a period of a few months in a small rural North Carolina town and involved 10 persons, ranging in age from 5 months to 77 years. All of the patients had pulmonary lesions. One had, in addition, a local skin lesion. It was thought that a respiratory mode of transmission was operative in this epidemic. Extensive culturing of soil samples from this area failed to reveal *B.dermatitidis*. Following the first report of this epidemic, there were several additional cases from this area.

Two other smaller epidemics of blastomycosis have been studied by the author in collaboration with Dr. M.L. FURCOLOW and other personnel of the Communicable Disease Center, U.S. Public Health Service. The first of these epidemics involved four negro males living on farms in close proximity in Boliver County, Mississippi. All four developed blastomycosis within a period of some months. A detailed epidemiological study did not reveal an indication of the source of infection, except that all had close contact with soil or soil products. Samples of soil from the suspected areas were negative for *B.dermatitidis*.

The second epidemic occurred in a rural community in southern Arkansas and involved a white male farmer and 12 dogs. Pulmonary blastomycosis was diagnosed following resection of the lung lesion. He had been asymptomatic following treatment with potassium iodide. Twelve of the dogs on his farm had evidence of pulmonary infections: many of them died. After the diagnosis of the farmer's pulmonary lesion had been established, two of the remaining ill dogs were examined and found to be infected with *B.dermatitidis* by culture and histopathologic techniques. The significant epidemiologic feature was that the dogs, many of them puppies, stayed chiefly under the house which was elevated by low brick pillars. The man had been under the house on two occasions to do repair work in the 6 months prior to the onset of his illness. A search for the organism in soil and timber under the house and about the farm was unsuccessful. It is interesting that two other human cases are known to have occurred in this area within a period of 2 or 3 years of this epidemic.

g) Natural Occurrence of Organism

There are no verified instances of human to human, animal to animal, or animal to human transmission of the organism. Procknow (1966) has reported an instance of presumed human to human transmission.

Epidemiologic considerations have provided an insight in means of transmission. Patients with blastomycosis are usually males who are in the active productive period of life, that is, the 30—50 year age group. Their occupation is frequently that of farmer, common laborer, or an occupation that entails work out-of-doors, or work with materials freshly obtained from natural sources (for example, wood, plants, soil, etc.). The age, sex, and occupational distributions all seem to indicate that the infection is acquired through contact with nature, especially soil or soil products.

Such a conclusion is in keeping with two other fungus diseases, coccidioidomycosis and histoplasmosis, which have many features similar to blastomycosis. The etiologic agents of these two diseases, *Coccidioides immitis* and *Histoplasma capsulatum*, are known to exist in the soil, and infections occur by inhalation of spores from infected soil or soil products. A variety of pathogenic or potentially pathogenic fungi which occur in the soil have been listed by Ajello (1956, 1967). The cycle of infection and the relation to soil or soil products has been demonstrated for many of these organisms.

That *Blastomyces dermatitidis* may follow this pattern is evidenced by the fact that the organism can be grown on sterilized soil or tree bark in the laboratory (Emmons, 1949; Menges et al., 1952). Stober (1914) examined the home conditions of a number of his patients and found a fungus growing on wet and decaying wooden walls. This fungus culturally resembled *Blastomyces dermatitidis*. He conservatively did not specifically so designate this fungus, but called attention to its similiarity. It is regrettable that he did not do animal inoculations, since this may have shown conclusively the nature of this fungus.

Denton et al. reported in 1961 the first isolation of *Blastomyces dermatitidis* from soil taken from a barn near Lexington, Kentucky. It is interesting that a dog had died of blastomycosis in this barn. In a subsequent study of 365 soil specimens taken near Augusta, Georgia, Denton and DiSalvo (1964) cultured *B. dermatitidis* from 10 samples taken at 5 sites. All sites were within a 1.8 mile radius and included an unused cattle ramp, old chicken houses and rabbit pen, a mule stall, and an abandoned kitchen. Repeated culturing of the original samples and of the sites covered in both reports were negative. Ajello (1967) has reviewed the chemical and biological factors of soil which might relate to the frustrating inability to culture repeatedly from the soil and concludes that "through diligent field and laboratory work its natural habitat will eventually be discovered".

Mycology

α) Cultural Characteristics

Blastomyces dermatitidis is a diphasic fungus occurring as mycelial growth in its saprophytic phase and as yeast in its tissue phase (Conant et al., 1954; Ajello et al., 1962). Although the use of the genus *Blastomyces* has been questioned for this organism, consensus and tradition by usage will probably maintain this designation. The synonymy of *B. dermatitidis* is listed in Table 2.

In the saprophytic or mycelial phase *B. dermatitidis* grows on a variety of common laboratory media at room temperature. Sabouraud's dextrose agar is most commonly used in clinical laboratories. The mycelial phase is usually slow-

Table 2. *Synonymy of Blastomyces dermatitidis*

Blastomyces dermatitidis, GILCHRIST and STOKES	1898
Oidium dermatitidis, RICKETTS	1901
Cryptococcus gilchristi, VUILLEMIN	1902
Zymonema gilchristi, BEURMANN and GOUGEROT	1909
Cryptococcus dermatitidis, BRUMPT	1910
Mycoderma gilchristi, JANNIN	1913
Mycoderma dermatitidis, BRUMPT	1913
Glenospora gammeli, POLLACCI and NANNIZZI	1927
Acladium gammeli, OTA	1928
Blastomycoides tulanensis, CASTELLANI	1928
Blastomycoides dermatitidis, CASTELLANI	1928
Endomyces capsulatus, DODGE and AYERS	1929
Geotrichum dermatitidis, BASGAL	1931
Monosporium tulanense, AGOSTINI	1932
Aleurisma tulanense, OTA and KAWATSURE	1933
Glenospora brevis, CASTELLANI	1933
Torulopsis dermatitidis, ALEMEIDA	1933
Endomyces capsulatus, var. *isabellinus*, MOORE.	1933
Endomyces dermatitidis, MOORE	1933
Gilchristi dermatitidis, REDAELLI and CIFERRI	1934
Zymonema dermatitidis, DODGE	1935
Aleurisma breve, DODGE	1935
Zymonema capsulatum, DODGE	1935
Trichosporium gammeli, DODGE	1935

growing with 2—5 weeks required for adequate growth for identification. Colony growth may be noted first as growth close to the surface of the agar. At this stage the colony may be rather colorless and waxy or exhibit some degree of aerial white mycelia. Microscopic examination at this stage reveals broad, thick-walled, closely septate hyphae which may superficially resemble *Geotrichum*: With subsequent growth the colony may develop a "prickly stage". At this point the colonies appear heaped-up with excrescences and projections (Fig. 3). This phase should arouse strong suspicion that the colony is *B.dermatitidis*, although other fungi may sometimes give this appearance. The "prickly phase" rather quickly passes into the more characteristic aerial mycelial colony. There is usually abundant cottony growth which is white initially and gradually becomes buff to brown with age (Fig. 3). Frequently an accentuated pattern of concentric ringed growth may be noted (Fig. 4). Again, this appearance should arouse suspicion that the colony is *B.dermatitidis*. Microscopically the colony is composed of narrow branching septate hyphae which range 1—3 microns in diameter. Numerous small round, oval, or pyriform conidia (3—5 m) are borne on short lateral conidiophores (Fig. 5). With age intercalary and terminal chlamydospores may be present.

To verify the identification of the mycelial colony it should be converted to the yeast phase. The yeast phase may be cultivated at 37 °C on brain-heart infusion blood agar or similiar enriched media. After inoculation of the media with a small portion of the mycelial growth, the colony develops slowly, becoming visable in 4—7 days (occasionally 14 or more days). The colony is initially white but rapidly becomes darker by accumulation of blood pigments from the medium (Fig. 3). Microscopically, the colony is composed of rounded, thick-walled yeast cells which range from 8—10 microns in diameter although they may occasionally be as large as 20 microns (AJELLO et al., 1962). The thick hyaline wall often gives the fungus a "double-contoured" appearance. BUDDING is common; the single bud connected with the parent cell by a broad base (Fig. 6) rather than the "pinched"

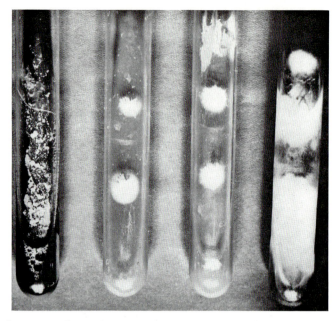

Fig. 3. The three types of growth of *B.dermatitidis* are shown. The tube on the left contains the yeast-phase grown at 37° C. The other 3 tubes were maintained at room temperature. The middle two tubes contain colonies in the "prickly" stage of growth. The tube on the right contains the more characteristic white cottony growth

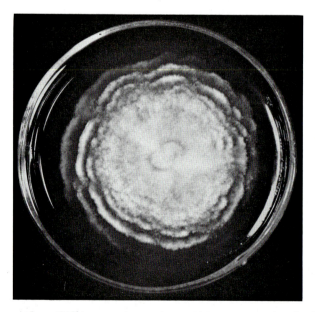

Fig. 4. *Blastomyces dermatitidis* grown at room temperature may vary in color from cream to buff or tan. The concentric ring pattern is characteristic

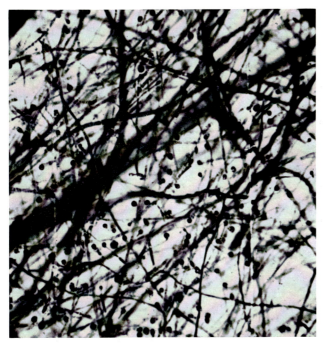

Fig. 5. A lactophenol cotton blue preparation of the mycelial growth reveals septate hyphae producing small round and pyriform conida

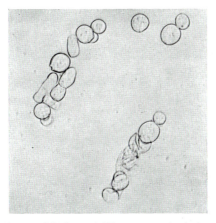

Fig. 6. Examination of cultures of *B.dermatitidis* grown on brain-heart infusion glucose blood agar at 37° C reveals round, budding yeasts similar to those seen in exudates. Oval or elongated forms may sometimes be present and represent attempts of the organism to form mycelia

appearance of buds with many other yeasts. Initial hyphal fragments may still be present. Many of the yeast cells may have an elongated appearance giving rise to abortive germ tubes as reversion to the mycelial phase. Repeated passage on fresh media at 37°C may be required to obtain colonies of predominately yeast cells. Occasionally animal passage is necessary to obtain the yeast phase.

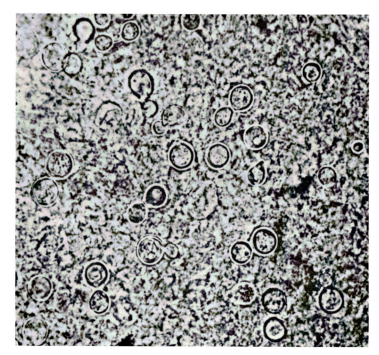

Fig. 7. This picture illustrates well the appearance of *B.dermatitidis* in pus following clearing with potassium hydroxide. The thick wall, sometimes referred to as "doubly-refractile", is clearly apparent. The budding forms are characteristic, especially the flattening of the area of attachment of the bud to the parent cell

β) Clinical Specimens

Clinical specimens, such as pus, discharges, exudates, transudates, sputum, urine, etc., should be examined directly under the microscope and cultured. The characteristic yeasts may be quite numerous in the specimen, but not uncommonly diligent search is needed to find even a single organism. Subdued lighting (by reducing substage illumination) is often helpful by making the thick hyaline walls of the yeast more refractile and therefore more obvious.

Where leukocytes and other cellular materials are present to an extent to interfer with search for the yeast forms, treatment of the specimen with potassium hydroxide may be beneficial. Material to be examined is placed on a slide and covered with a drop of 10—20% KOH under a cover slip. The preparation is heated gently and then examined microscopically. The KOH "clears" the preparation by disrupting leukocytes and other cells leaving an amorphous residue in which the yeasts still maintain typical morphology (Fig. 7).

Clinical materials should be cultured on appropriate media at both room temperature and 37°C. Since other organisms may be present in these specimens, antibiotics (penicillin and streptomycin, or chloramphenicol) are often incorporated in the media to inhibit growth of bacteria. Similarly, cyclohexamide (actidione) may be incorporated in agar used for mycelial growth to inhibit saprophytic fungal growth (Ajello et al., 1962).

Occasionally in clinical laboratories the clinical specimen is cultured on blood plates for bacterial growth, and only subsequently is the possibility of fungus raised. Such blood agar plates may yield fungal growth even in the presence of extensive bacterial growth. After 3—4 days incubation at 37°C., the plates are sealed and allowed to incubate at room temperature. After several days the plates are examined daily for evidence of mycelial growth. If such occurs, a portion of the mycelial growth should be subcultured on antibiotic media and suitable cultures may be obtained for identification.

γ) Animal Inoculation

Animals may be inoculated with clinical specimens or with mycelial cultures. In either event the yeast phase of *B.dermatitidis* will be recovered. Swiss albino mice are most commonly used for such inoculations, but hamsters may be equally suitable. Guinea pigs appear somewhat more resistant to infection. The inoculations may be intraperitoneal or intravenous; the latter appears to provide more consistant results (DENTON et al., 1961). The mice should be killed at 3—4 weeks after inoculation. Lungs, liver, spleen, kidneys, and lymph nodes inoculated animals should be cultured for the fungus on appropriate media. All specimens should be examined microscopically as well as being cultured.

Pathogenesis and Immunology

Epidemiologic studies have repeatedly pointed to soil or soil products as the natural habit of *Blastomyces dermatitidis*. The isolation of *B.dermatitidis* by DENTON et al. (1961, 1964) reinforces this association. Man or other animals may be infected by inhalation of fungus particles which are present in soil or substances contaminated by soil. The primary lesion of blastomycosis appears to be in the lung (SCHWARZ and BAUM, 1951, 1953). Most cases appear to progress slowly with extension of pulmonary disease and/or spread to other organs. A few cases are known to have healed spontaneously. It may be that as better antigens for skin testing and serologic studies are developed, blastomycosis may be found to follow the pattern of histoplasmosis and coccidioidomycosis and that a significant proportion of *B.dermatitidis* infections will be asymptomatic and benign. At the present state of knowledge, the presence or absence of such asymptomatic infections is a moot point.

A very few cases are acknowledged to be the result of primary cutaneous inoculation. (WILSON et al., 1955). These cases occurred during autopsy procedures in which the individuals injured themselves with contaminated instruments. Lesions from such inoculation differ from those usually seen in blastomycosis with skin lesions secondary to a pulmonary focus. Other types of cutaneous inoculation may possibly occur (SMITH, 1966).

SMITH (1966) in comparing pathogenesis of blastomycosis with tuberculosis, histoplasmosis, and coccidioidomycosis has emphasized some interesting differences in infections due to *B.dermatitidis*. Reinfection of the upper lobes has not been observed. Enlargement of regional lymph nodes commonly seen in the above diseases is rare in blastomycosis. Localized areas of calcification following the primary infection are not seen as in the other diseases. He related this to a lack of caseation as a result of the development of only a mild degree of tuberculintype allergy.

This low degree of tuberculin-type allergy is reflected also in the use of skin tests and serologic tests in blastomycosis, and further complicated by the lack of suitable antigens for *B.dermatitidis*. As in histoplasmosis and coccidiodomycosis a positive titer to a serologic test indicates active infection. A rising titer reflects progressing disease, whereas a declining titer indicates improvement. Unlike histoplasmosis, coccidioidomycosis, and tuberculosis skin test reactivity appears to be erratic and transitory.

Serologic tests generally appear to be less uniform in producing results than similiar tests in histoplasmosis and coccidioidomycosis (CAMPBELL, 1967). Some patients may have demonstrable titers, while other patients with similar disease do not. Indeed there are often unaccountable fluctuations in titers during the course of an individual patient's disease.

Serologic tests and skin tests will cross-react with antigens of other fungi. Heterologous reactions are most common with *Histoplasma capsulatum*, but also occur with *Coccidioides immitis*, *Candida albicans*, *Blastomyces brasiliensis*, and others. These cross-reactions have been noted in most of the methods used and with antigens prepared from both the mycelial and yeast phases of *B.dermatitidis*. Appropriate absorptions may remove the cross-reactivity and provide relatively specific antigen-antibody reactions, however.

SALVIN (1963) and CAMPBELL (1967) have recently reviewed the literature regarding the agglutination, precipitation, complement-fixation, hemagglutination, and collodion agglutination tests and skin tests. The recently developed agar-gel precipitation test for blastomycosis appears to be more useful in diagnosis than complement-fixation test, but even so it is emphasized that culture of the organism is needed for verification (ABERNATHY and HEINER, D.C., 1961; BUSEY, J.F., and HINTON, P.E., 1967).

Pathology

a) General Pathology

North American blastomycosis is a disease of protean manifestations (BAKER, 1942, 1947, 1953, 1957; FORBUS, 1943; KUNKEL et al., 1954; CHICK, 1961; BUSEY et al., 1964). Lesions have occurred in virtually every organ of the body except stomach and hair (Fig. 8). The reaction which is produced by the presence of *Blastomyces dermatitidis* in tissue may be quite varied. The type of tissue reaction may vary from a purely suppurative one to a fibrosing granulomatous process, or may exhibit varying degrees of the two extremes. There may be very little tissue response to the presence of numerous organisms, or there may be a marked reaction to the presence of only a few organisms.

In many of the earlier publications, and indeed, even in the recent literature, blastomycosis is considered primarily as a granulomatous disease, such as exemplified by tuberculosis. However, in the study of large numbers of cases, or reports of such cases, a similarity to tuberculosis becomes more distant. In general, the *polymorphonuclear leukocyte is found to be the prominent reaction cell type*. These cells may appear as conglomerates forming *abscesses*, or they may be diffusely scattered through the area of inflammation. Even where tubercle formation is prominent, leukocytes are often present *in the central portions of the tubercle*, a finding which is rare in tuberculosis. It is of interest, however, that most of the early pathologic descriptions comparing blastomycosis to tuberculosis were based on the study of lung lesions, since these lesions are the ones which more closely resemble tuberculosis than lesions in other parts of the body. Abscesses are common in blastomycosis, but are relatively uncommon in tuberculosis.

Eosinophilic polymorphonuclear leukocytes may sometimes be prominent in blastomycotic lesions, but in most instances they are not impressive in their numbers. Macrophages, epithelioid cells, lymphocytes, and plasma cells appear in varying degrees depending upon the type of tissue reaction. Multinucleated giant cells can be found in almost every case, but they are sometimes very rare, at other times quite numerous. When the type of tissue reaction is granulomatous, numerous mononuclear inflammatory cells may be found forming the lesion. These may occur as large aggregates of cells, or may be more diffusely scattered through the remaining parenchymal structures. Usually there is some degree of tubercle formation. This may be abortive with only scattered, poorly formed accumulations of histiocytes and epithelioid cells. More often tubercles are well-formed and consist of an outer collar of lymphocytes, an intermediate concentric ring of

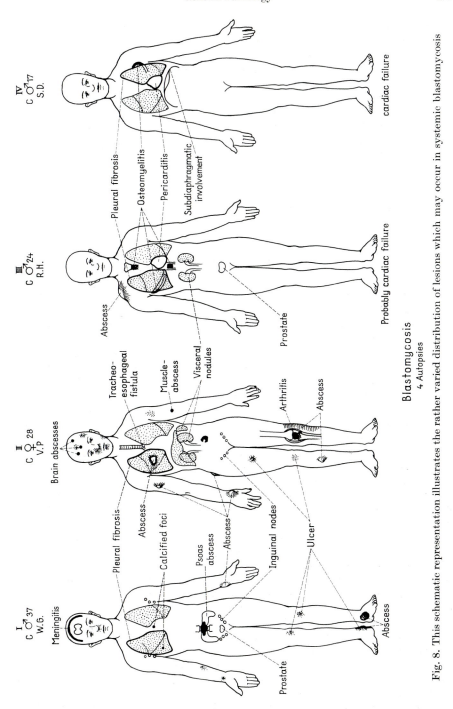

Blastomycosis
4 Autopsies

Fig. 8. This schematic representation illustrates the rather varied distribution of lesions which may occur in systemic blastomycosis

epitheloid cells and macrophages, and an inner zone containing *multinucleated giant cells.* As mentioned previously, in this inner zone polymorphonuclear leukocytes may be an important feature. Necrosis is rather common, and varies

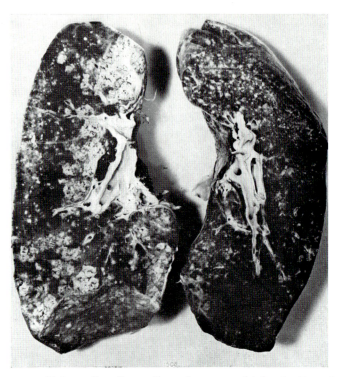

Fig. 9. There are multiple small, rather uniform abscesses and tubercles throughout the left lung. Similar lesions are also present in the right lung, but in addition there are multiple confluent areas of caseous pneumonia

from slight disintegration of inflammatory and tissue cells to a caseous-like necrosis. It appears that much of the material making up areas of caseous-like necrosis is composed of dead organisms (Baker, 1942). Fibrosis may be found to some degree in virtually every case and is frequently prominent in the tissue response. This tendency to heal by fibrosis is quite evident in pulmonary lesions, and is apparent in almost any tissue which is chronically infected.

Organisms may occur in almost any area of the lesion. When the reaction is of the suppurative type, they may be found in large numbers in abscesses. If the lesion is more granulomatous in character, organisms may be found contained within the cytoplasm of multinucleated giant cells or within the inner zone of tubercles. Organisms may also be found in large aggregates with little or no inflammatory reaction secondary to their presence.

Although in many cases it may be possible to distinguish to some degree between blastomycosis and tuberculosis on morphological grounds, it cannot be emphasized too strongly that it is often impossible to make this differentiation or to differentiate blastomycosis from other fungus diseases. This is especially true of histoplasmosis and coccidioidomycosis. Definitive diagnosis is dependent upon demonstration of the organisms.

B.dermatitidis is one of the few fungi which may be readily identified in hematoxylin and eosin stained sections. Occasionally however special stains may be required. The Grocott methenamine silver technique is quite useful, however *B.dermatitidis* often stains very intensely and structure may be difficult to

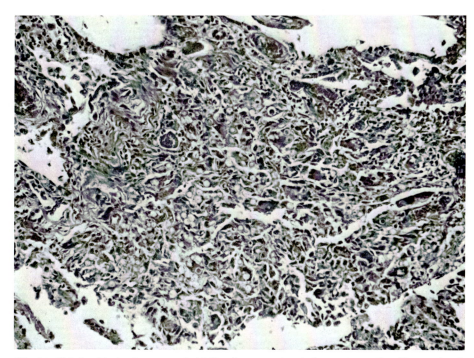

Fig. 10. This focal lesion is composed chiefly of mononuclear inflammatory cells with occasional multinucleated giant cells. Organisms are quite numerous. × 180

determine. The PAS and Gridley fungus stains tend to give somewhat better delineation of structure. Their chief disadvantage is in their staining of background tissue, lacking the contrast of the methenamine silver method.

b) Special Pathology

Lung

According to the present concept of this disease, pulmonary lesions occur in virtually every case of blastomycosis, the exception being the extremely rare true primary cutaneous type of involvement. Lesions in the lungs may range from a very small, almost insignificant focus to an extensive pneumonic process which may involve most of the parenchyma of both lungs. The type of reaction may run the gamut from an acute exudative one to fibrosis and scarring (SCHWARZ and BAUM, 1951).

Single or multiple small lesions may be found in one or both lungs. Such lesions may vary in size from a millimeter or so up to several centimeters (Fig. 9). These lesions are often tubercle-like in appearance, with concentrically arranged epithelioid cells, central multinucleated giant cells, and sometimes peripheral lymphocytic accumulation. Organisms are not common in this type of lesion, and are usually found within giant cells. Occasionally there may be a central accumulation of polymorphonuclear leukocytes in tubercles. In other areas there may be collections of mononuclear cells without tubercle formation (Fig. 10).

A type of pulmonary involvement may be found which resembles the Ghon (*primary*) *complex* of tuberculosis, histoplasmosis, and coccidioidomycosis. There may be a small peripherally-located parenchymal nodule composed chiefly of

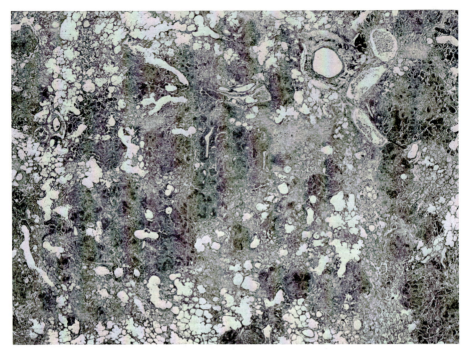

Fig. 11. This type of reaction may occur in acute blastomycosis. There are multiple focal and confluent lesions composed of polymorphonuclear leukocytes, mononucleated inflammatory cells, and multinucleated giant cells. × 8

fibrous scar tissue. Organisms are not usually found in this type of lesion. There may or may not be an associated and corresponding lesion of the hilar lymph nodes draining this area.

The nodular lesions may coalesce to form larger lesions, or areas of pneumonia may occur, *per se*. Confluent lesions are frequently granulomatous in character with numerous macrophages, giant cells, and epithelioid cells filling alveolar spaces. Areas of pneumonic involvement arising "de novo" are often exudative or suppurative in character. Alveolar spaces are filled with myriades of polymorphonuclear leukocytes and distinctly lesser numbers of chronic inflammatory cells (Fig. 11). Organisms are usually much more common in the suppurative type of lesion than in the granulomatous type.

Involvement of small bronchi or bronchioles is a common, if not usual occurrence. This may occur by extension from alveoli opening into the bronchiole, or by extension through the wall from an adjacent lesion. Microscopically there is usually a prominent inflammatory response in the sub-epithelial tissue, often with varying degrees of ulceration of the epithelium. Blastomycotic bronchitis may occur without involvement of the lung parenchyma (SCHWARZ and BAUM, 1951).

Necrosis may be entirely absent in pulmonary lesions, or there may be gradations in the amount present up to the formation of rather large abscesses. According to some authors caseation as exhibited in tuberculosis is not common, if it does occur (KUNKEL et al., 1954; SCHWARZ and BAUM, 1951, 1953; STARRS and KLOTZ, 1948), and in that of others (BAKER, personnal communication; LEWIS et al., 1958) caseation does not appear to be uncommon. *Cavitation* (Fig. 12) is not infrequent in pulmonary blastomycosis, occurring in 25% of pulmonary cases in the Veterans

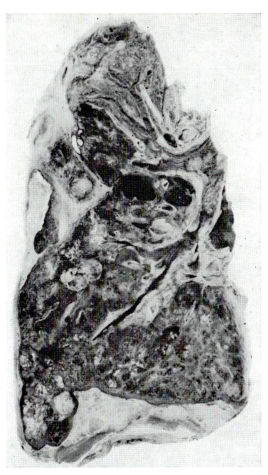

Fig. 12. Pulmonary blastomycosis. There is a diffuse, nodular, and interstitial infiltrate throughout the lung. Multiple cavities have been formed in the upper half of the lung. There is also an extensive organizing pleural reaction which had obliterated the thoracic cavity

Administration series (BUSEY et al., 1964). Although it is usually stated that the cavities are small, ACREE et al. (1954) cite a case of a cavity which measured 7 centimeters in diameter. Blastomycotic cavities are usually thick-walled; fibrosis is often a predominant component of the histologic appearance (Fig. 13).

Blastomycotic pleuritis is common with pulmonary lesions. This may be manifested by an adhesive fibrinous exudate, or in older lesions by firm fibrous adhesions. In the early stages the reaction may be somewhat granulomatous with rather numerous histiocytes and giant cells, but this is soon replaced by granulation tissue. At this stage organisms are often quite rare. Thick fibrous scarring is the usual end result.

Skin

Primary Cutaneous Lesions: WILSON et al. (1955) described four patients with a primary type of cutaneous lesion. Each of these patients developed an infection with *B. dermatitidis* by minimal trauma to the hand or arm while working with infected tissue in the autopsy room. The pattern of the resulting disease was

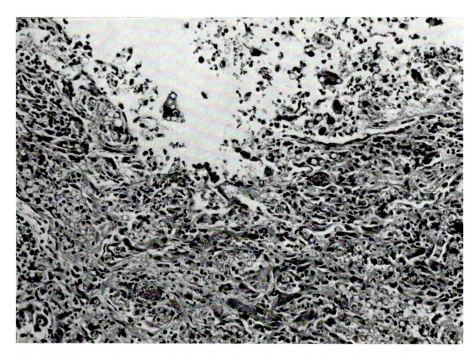

Fig. 13. Pulmonary blastomycosis. A section through the wall of a small cavity illustrates the chronic nature of the inflammatory reaction. Organisms are easily found both in the wall and within the lumen of the cavity. × 184

strikingly different from the cutaneous lesions usually associated with cutaneous blastomycosis, and complemented the somewhat earlier reports of Schwarz and Baum (1951, 1953). From a careful study of a number of cases and in so-called cutaneous cases were identical in appearance, they postulated that such skin lesions must be due to hematogenous spread from a focus elsewhere in the body.

Wilson et al. (1955) have described the pathogenesis as follows. Following direct inoculation of *B.dermatitidis* into the skin, the initial traumatic injury tends to heal uneventfully. However, in about a week a reddened papule develops at this site. This papule gradually enlarges and tends to ulcerate, formig a chancre-like lesion. During this time lymphangitis and lymphadenitis becomes apparent. Frequently there will be multiple tender nodules along the course of lymphatics draining the primary lesion. These lesions do not exhibit a tendency to ulcerate. Epitrochlear and axillary lymph nodes are often involved and may attain the size of a hen's egg.

The primary lesion is rather small and discrete (Fig. 14). Microscopically, there is usually one or more areas of dermal perivascular inflammation composed of large numbers of polymorphonuclear leukocytes and lymphocytes. Organisms are numerous in these foci. The overlying epidermis may be intact in the early stages, or ulcerated in later stages. There may be slight acanthosis. The lymphatics draining this area are filled with an inflammatory infiltrate of mixed cell type with numerous organisms. The involved lymph nodes are enlarged by an acute granulo-matous reaction. Giant cells are numerous and contain organisms.

This type of chancriform syndrome is also seen in other diseases where intra-cutaneous inoculation of organisms occurs, namely, tuberculosis, syphilis, yaws,

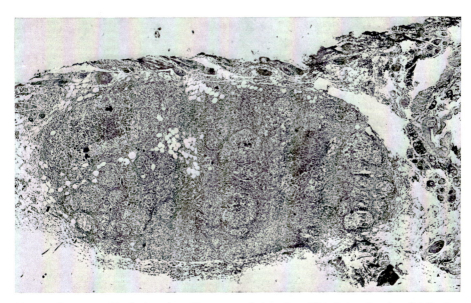

Fig. 14. Cutaneous North American blastomycosis in a dog. This lesion developed following the direct inoculation of organisms into the skin of a dog. The lesion is localized within the dermis, and there is none of the epidermal alteration usually associated with skin lesions of blastomycosis. This type of lesion has also been observed in several human cases following the direct inoculation of organisms into the skin as, a result of trauma during an autopsy. Usually there is an associated lymphangitis and lymphadenitis. × 38

espundia, and sporotrichosis (WILSON et al., 1955). This syndrome has also been observed in coccidioidomycosis (WILSON et al., 1953).

Secondary or Hematogenous Skin Lesions: Striking differences are found in secondary skin lesions as compared to the primary cutaneous lesions. The secondary skin lesions are usually first noted as a papular or nodular swelling which may or may not be slightly tender. These lesions may be either subcutaneous or dermal in location. In either event, the lesion progresses through a pustular stage and ruptures through the epidermis, allowing a mixture of tissue fluid and pus to exude out to the surface. This fluid material soon becomes crusted and heaped-up. The lesion progresses by marginal extention producing a gradually expanding type of involvement. Minute abscesses are present in the verrucous heaped-up margins. There is a striking tendency toward central healing, leaving thin atrophic scar tissue surrounded by a violaceous active margin; although occasionally central healing does not occur, resulting in a continuous large heaped-up lesion. Lesions may progress to form large cauliflower-like areas of involvement covering 10 or more square centimeters (Fig. 15). Involvement of lymphatics is strikingly absent.

Histopathologically, in the earliest stages before ulceration has occurred, there is a granulomatous reaction of the dermis or subcutaneous layer. Numerous polymorphonuclear leukocytes, lymphocytes, and mononuclear inflammatory cells are seen. A somewhat more extensive picture is present after the lesion has progressed to the expanding, ulcerative stage; this is the stage most often attained at the time medical advice is sought by the patient. At this time at the periphery of the lesion there is a pronounced pseudo-epitheliomatous hyperplasia and acanthosis alternating with areas of atrophic epidermis. In many of the areas of epidermal hyperplasia, and in the intervening dermal areas, there are minute micro-abscesses

31*

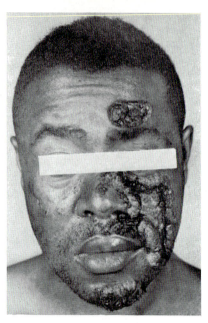

Fig. 15. Cutaneous North American blastomycosis

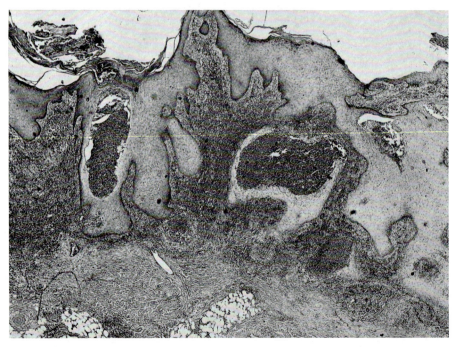

Fig. 16. Cutaneous North American blastomycosis. The characteristic pseudoepitheliomatous hyperplasia and microabscesses of skin lesions are apparent in this section. There is a diffuse infiltration of mononuclear inflammatory cells throughout the dermis. A rather unusual amount of hyperkeratosis is present. × 31

composed largely of leukocytes. There is usually a rather extensive mononuclear inflammatory cell infiltration through the underlying dermis (Fig. 16). Cellular arrangements resembling tubercles may or may not be present. Multinucleated giant cells are often common. In distinction to the numerous organisms found in the primary skin lesion, *organisms* may be *exceedingly sparce* and require a diligent search on the part of the pathologist to locate even one. The central portion of the lesion may be ulcerated and similar to the reaction at the periphery, or may be composed of scar and granulation tissue with atrophy of the epidermis and dermis. Among diseases to be considered in the differential diagnosis of this type of lesion are coccidioidomycosis, chromoblastomycosis, maduromycosis, and bromoderma (CHICK and LEHAN, 1957).

Bone

Although bone lesions are quite common in blastomycosis, it is surprising how few good pathologic studies are available. Skeletal lesions occur in about two-thirds of the cases of disseminated disease. Vertebra, rib, skull, tibia, and tarsus are sites which are frequently involved (REEVES and PEDERSON, 1954; CARNESDALE and STEGMAN, 1956; RHANGOS and CHICK, 1964). Blastomycosis of bone often presents an area of inflammation with prominent osteolysis. The borders of such lesions are usually sharp; there is a sharp junction between the area of involvement and normal bone. In contrast, tuberculous lesions have rough irregular borders and often demineralization of adjacent bony structures. At times the above picture of blastomycotic lesions may resemble an area of infarction, particularly in the long bones (JONES and MARTIN, 1941). In long bones lesions are often found in the subepiphyseal or subarticular regions. There may or may not be a corresponding periosteal reaction. Rupture or extension of such a lesion into the joint space leads to involvement of the joint.

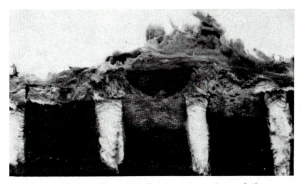

Fig. 17. Blastomycotic periostitis and osteitis. Large retroperitoneal abscesses were also present

Vertebral lesions due to *B. dermatitidis* may, on occasion, create a difficult diagnostic problem as regards the possibility of tuberculosis. Usually blastomycosis of the spine is characterized by a marked destruction of bone with little associated proliferation. Narrowing of the disc spaces may occur, but collapse of vertebral bodies is not common as with tuberculosis (Fig. 17). Several vertebrae and ribs may be involved simultaneously. Any one or all of the components of a vertebra may be involved. Paravertebral or psoas abscesses may occur as a result of extension of the bony lesions. Draining sinuses from blastomycotic bone lesions are not common (KUNKEL et al., 1954). The bone marrow may be involved

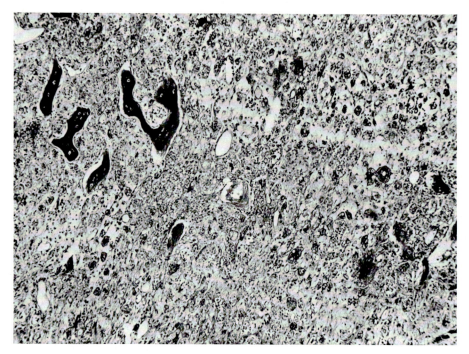

Fig. 18. North American blastomycosis of the spine. The vertebral bone marrow has been replaced by the massive proliferation of organisms. There is a relative paucity of inflammatory cells in relation to the large number of organisms. × 94

extensively (Fig. 18) or may contain only a few focal lesions. It has been suggested that the bone marrow may be a good site to culture or to demonstrate organisms morphologically (SCHWARZ and BAUM, 1951).

Genitourinary Tract

Epididymis and Testes: Blastomycotic involvement of the epididymis and testes may range from a small circumscribed lesion to a diffuse reaction involving virtually the entire parenchyma of one or both organs. With minor degrees of involvement there may be one or several firm, yellowish nodules which are homogeneous in appearance (Fig. 19). The nodules may be sharply circumscribed but are not encapsulated (HERBUT, 1952). With more extensive involvement there may be marked enlargement of the epididymis and/or testis (HERBUT, 1952) which appear nodular and indurated (Fig. 20). In other instances there are multiple, often confluent abscesses. Involvement of the scrotal wall may lead to a scrotal ulcer or draining sinus (KUNKEL et al., 1954).

Prostate — Varying degrees of prostatic involvement by *B. dermatitidis* may be found, from one or more small foci to extensive, almost complete involvement (Fig. 21). Usually the prostate is enlarged and may exhibit either a generalized increased firmness or an irregular nodular appearance with some degree of fluctuation (HERBUT, 1952). Large amounts of green yellow pus may be expressed from the gland (BURR and HUFFINESS, 1954). The appearance of the cut surface is one of single or multiple abscesses of varying size.

Organisms are usually found in abundance within the areas of necrosis or in giant cells about the periphery of the lesions (Fig. 22). It is interesting that

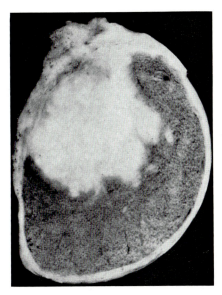

Fig. 19. North American blastomycosis of the testis. This lesion occupies about one-third of the testis. The lesion is rather soft, yellow, and bulges above the adjacent normal tissue. The epididymis is also involved

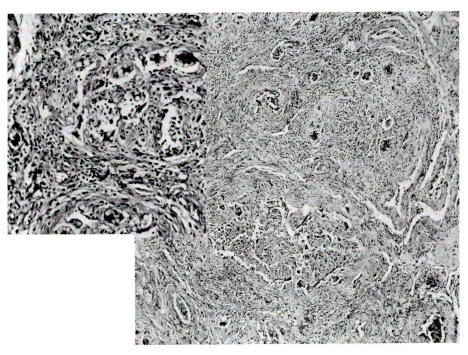

Fig. 20. North American blastomycosis of the testis. An extensive granulomatous inflammatory reaction has replaced the normal architectural pattern of the testis. A tendency toward tubercle formation is apparent. Many of the giant cells contain organisms. × 70

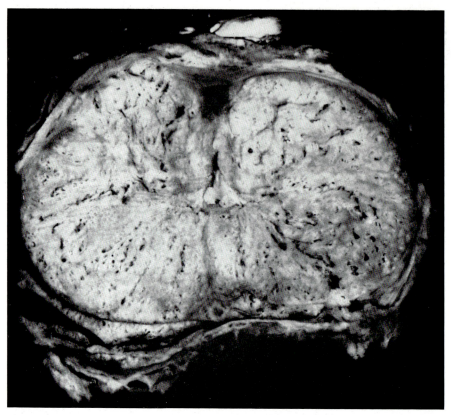

Fig. 21. North American blastomycosis of the prostate. The prostate is greatly enlarged and contains multiple scattered and confluent green-yellow abscesses

occasionally the reaction appears to be restricted to the glandular portion, histologically; indeed, one may find dilated glands containing myriads of organisms and a virtual abscence of inflammatory reaction.

Kidney — Blastomycosis appears to involve the cortical area of the kidney more than the medullary portion (Schwarz and Baum, 1951). The degree of involvement may range from one or more small isolated foci (Fig. 23) to large areas of tissue destruction. Any portion of the nephron or of the interstitial tissue may be involved; the infection is usually bilateral.

Certain specific lesions are of interest. Occasionally one may find inflammation in and about a glomerulus, giving the appearance of embolic glomerulitis and periglomerulitis. Large numbers of organisms may occasionally be found within the lumen of a tubule, forming a "cast".

Although the usual histopathological features indicate that the hematogenous route of spread is primary in the pathogenesis of renal infections due to *B. dermatidis*, Schwarz and Baum (1951) mention one case (Case No. 10), however, in which there was ulceration of the calyces and a marked exudative reaction in the interstices of the medulla. The cortex was involved to a much lesser degree. This was described as associated with "ascending infection".

Seminal Vesicles — Involvement of the seminal vesicles may occur by direct extension from the adjacent infected prostate, or may occur by hematogenous

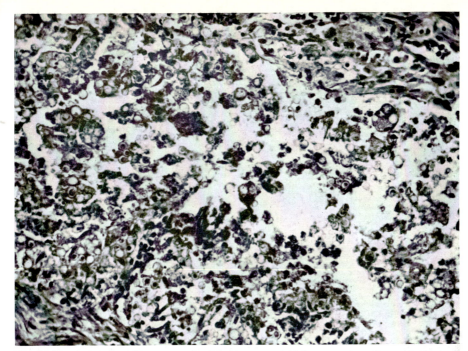

Fig. 22. North American blastomycosis of the prostate. A high power view of a prostatic gland containing numerous organisms. There is some necrotic debris, but the relative paucity of inflammatory cells is apparent. In other areas there were dense accumulations of inflammatory cells in glands and overt focal abscesses of the parenchyma. × 180

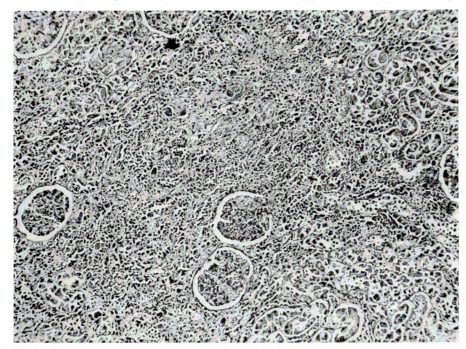

Fig. 23. North American blastomycosis of the kidney. This focal lesion has destroyed the architectural pattern of the kidney locally. The cellular reaction is predominately mononuclear with rare multinucleated giant cells. Organisms may or may not be common in this type of lesion. × 101

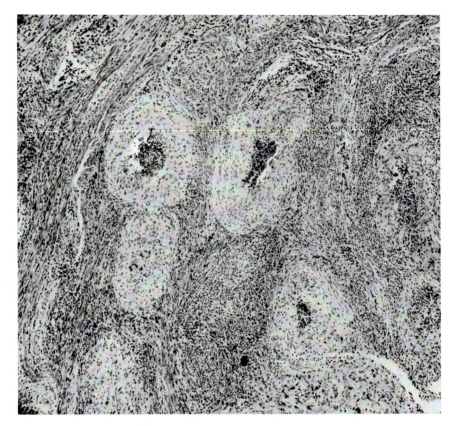

Fig. 24. North American blastomycosis of the uterus. There is a diffuse mononuclear inflammatory cellular response throughout the myometrium of the uterus. Tubercle formation is prominent. The centrally located abscess in the tubercle is a common feature in blastomycosis.
Multinucleated giant cells are not common in this section. × 69

inoculation in the absence of prostatic involvement. The reaction is usually one of
abscesses or foci of necrosis with myriads of polymorphonuclear leukocytes.
Varying degrees of granulomatous inflammation may also occur.

Bladder — Lesions in the urinary bladder usually consist of areas of mucosal
ulceration with varying degrees of inflammatory cells in the base of the ulcer and
the underlying muscularis. Organisms can usually be found in such areas.

Female Reproductive Organs — The classic report of Hamblen et al. (1935)
serves as the basis for the descriptions in this group of organs.

Uterus — The uterus may be of normal size or slightly enlarged with focal
lesions apparent on the serosal surface. The cut surface of the uterus may appear
normal grossly, or there may be minute abscesses or nodules. Microscopically,
there are scattered tubercles with central giant cells in the endometrium and
myometrium (Fig. 24). Occasionally there is central necrosis of the tubercles.
Organisms can usually be demonstrated in such lesions. A scattering of acute and
chronic inflammatory cells may also occur.

Fallopian tubes — The Fallopian tubes may show varying degrees of enlargement. The serosal surface may be roughened, red, and covered with granular or
taglike excrescences. The wall of the tube is usually thickened and indurated,

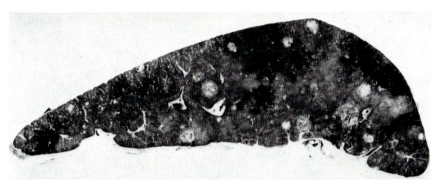

Fig. 25. North American blastomycosis of the spleen. Scattered firm nodules are present throughout the spleen. These nodules vary in size up to one centimeter in diameter

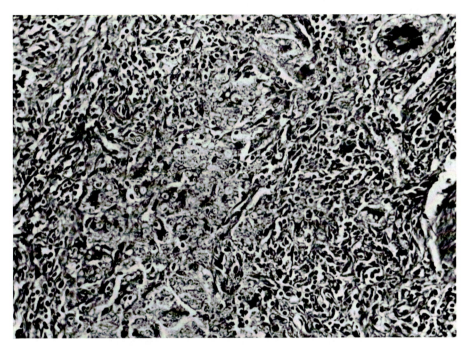

Fig. 26. North American blastomycosis of the spleen. In this area of the spleen there is a massive proliferation of yeasts. The multinucleated giant cells contain many organisms. × 180

sometimes discolored and friable. The tubal cavity may contain large amounts of thick pus.

Ovary — Ovarian involvement is quite rare, and no reports are known to the author.

Liver and Spleen

Lesions of the liver and spleen may occur, usually associated with extensive disseminated disease. There may be few or numerous small nodules (Fig. 25) or there may be somewhat larger areas of necrosis. It is interesting that, in comparison to hematogenous miliary tuberculosis, hepatic and splenic involvement occurs rather infrequently (SCHWARZ and BAUM, 1951). This may be related to the

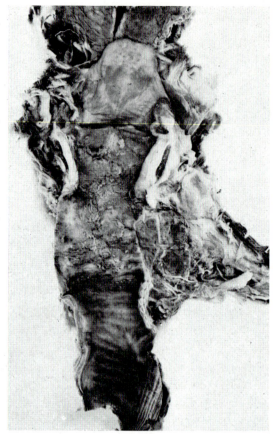

Fig. 27. North American blastomycosis of the larynx and trachea. The ulceration of the laryngeal wall extends into the upper trachea. The vocal cords have been destroyed. This lesion may
be mistaken for carcinoma clinically and in biopsy sections

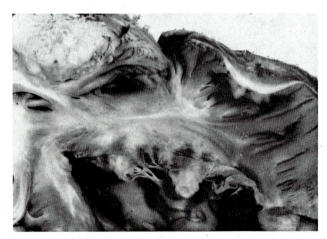

Fig. 28. North American blastomycosis of the heart. An extensive fulminating hematogenous
spread of organisms may occur from heart lesions such as the one shown in the wall of the auricle

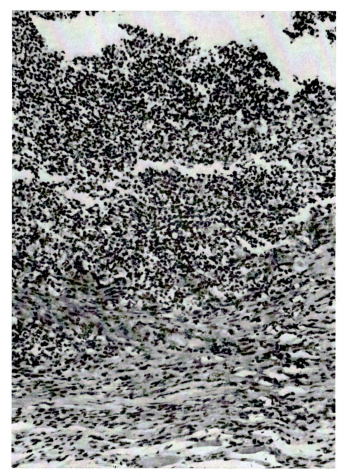

Fig. 29. North American blastomycosis of the heart. This section is taken through the edge of a large abscess of the myocardium. There is destruction of myocardial fibers. Organisms are not visible. × 184

absence of gastrointestinal lesions in blastomycosis. Lesions may be granulomatous with tubercle formation, but suppurative reactions appear to be relatively more common. Organisms may be quite numerous (Fig. 26).

Other Organs

1. Larynx. Blastomycotic involvement of the larynx may be considered in two stages, the inflammatory and the fibrotic (RANIER, 1951). Early in the inflammatory stage the vocal cords and adjacent larynx appear edematous and nodular. The nodules are usually minute in size and may be gray to yellow. Ulceration is often a prominent feature (Fig. 27). This may or may not be associated with a thin membrane which leaves a raw inflamed surface when peeled away.

Microscopic examination usually reveals a marked acanthosis and pseudoepitheliomatous hyperplasia of the squamous epithelium, which may be mistaken for carcinoma. Microabscesses composed largely of polymorphonuclear leukocytes are common. The subepithelial tissues contain a rather dense accumulation of

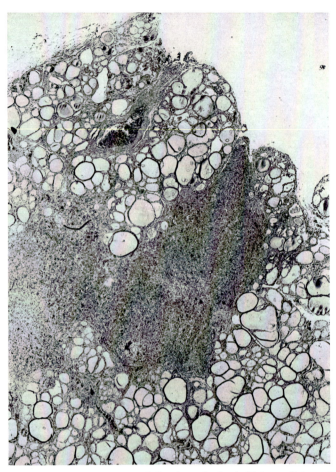

Fig. 30. North American blastomycosis of the thyroid gland. This small irregular nodule in the thyroid was caused by *B.dermatitidis*. There is a preponderance of macrophages and numerous multinucleated giant cells. × 28

inflammatory cells. Caseation may occur (Lester et al., 1958). Organisms may be found within giant cells or scattered in areas of inflammatory cells.

With progression of time fibrosis may occur and produce a fixation of the vocal cords. Stenosis of the glottis may follow. Discharging fistulas and communicating abscesses of the neck are sometimes seen (Ranier, 1951).

2. Heart. Lesions of the heart due to *B.dermatitidis* may occur by extension from lesions in adjacent lung or pericardium, or by localization via the hematogenous route (Baker and Brian, 1937; Hurley, 1916; Pond and Humphreys, 1952). Where direct extension from a lung lesion has occurred, there will usually be continuity between the lung, pericardium, and heart wall. Occasionally the pericardial space alone may be involved. The pericardial space may contain varying amounts of fluid ,which may or may not be purlent in character. Occasionally in older lesions there can be fibrosis and obliteration of the pericardial space. Spread to the heart wall may be expressed in various ways, whether the lesion is in the epicardium, myocardium, or endocardium, or combinations of these struc-

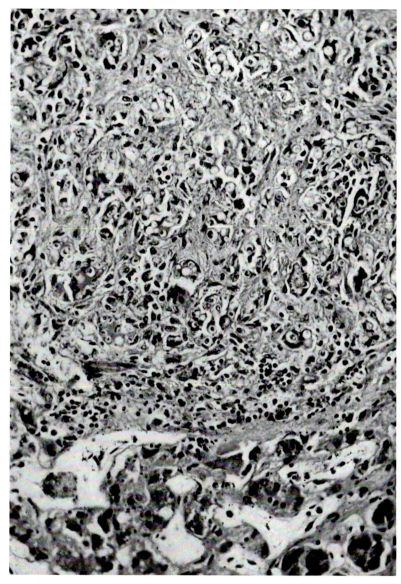

Fig. 31. North American blastomycosis of the adrenal gland. Organisms are numerous. The cellular reaction is chronic, with numerous multinucleated giant cells. There is a fibroblastic proliferation. × 180

tures. Firm nodules may be found which are solid throughout, or which have soft necrotic centers (Fig. 28). There may be ulceration of such lesions when on the epicardium or endocardium. Areas of necrosis or focal abscesses of varying size may be found within the heart wall (Fig. 29). Extension of the inflammatory process into the great vessels may occur. In some cases only small focal lesions may be found in the heart wall without evidence of pericardial disease. Such lesions probably represent hematogenous dissemination. Vegetative lesions may occur

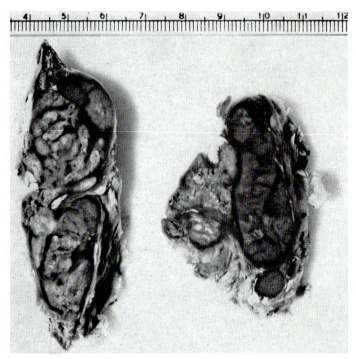

Fig. 32. North American blastomycosis of lymph nodes. Lymph nodes in many areas of the body may be enlarged. These nodes contain multiple yellow caseous and firm, gray nodules

along the endocardial surface irrespective of pathogenesis. Such vegetations may serve to seed the blood stream with organisms.

Histologically the lesions may be suppurative or granulomatous. Tubercle formation is rather common. Organisms may be numerous, particularly within multinucleated giant cells.

3. Endocrine Glands. The endocrine glands may contain lesions as a result of extensive dissemination of *B.dermatitidis* in the body. Such lesions are usually small and are relatively inconspicuous in regard to both symptoms and pathologic manifestations, in contrast to the extensive lesions elsewhere in the body (Fig. 30).

Adrenal involvement warrants further comment in view of the current interest in adrenal necrosis due to infections organisms, in particular tuberculosis, histoplasmosis, and coccidioidomycosis. Blastomycosis of the adrenal glands is not common. It is interesting that most of the reported cases have also had involvement of the genitourinary system. Lesions in the adrenals may range from a single small focus to almost complete destruction of both glands (Fig. 31). Addison's disease due to *B.dermatitidis* has been reported (Abernathy and Melby, 1962; Kent and Collier, 1965).

4. Gastrointestinal Tract. If one ignores lesions of the oral cavity and the rectum, which are uncommon and may be grouped with the skin in regard to type of reaction, infections of the gastrointestinal tract due to *B.dermatitidis* are virtually non-existent. Kunkel et al. (1954) mention one case in which there was an annular granuloma in the upper third of the esophagus. This case may be related to laryngeal lesion, although the author did not so specify. Occasionally there may be direct extension from the lung or trachea to the esophagus.

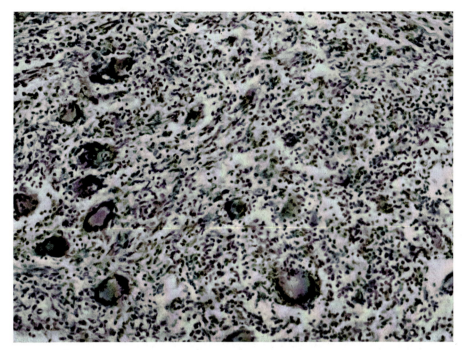

Fig. 33. North American blastomycosis of a lymph node. A focal lesion. An occasional giant
cell contains organisms. × 192

5) Other Tissues — Other tissue masses, such as muscle, tendons, etc., may
contain lesions to a varying extent. Such lesions are almost always secondary to
extensive disseminated disease, and as such assume a role of minor importance in
most cases (Figs. 32, 33).

Central Nervous System

Involvement of the central nervous system is not uncommon in blastomycosis
and has been expressed as meningitis, meningo-encephalitis, brain abscess, and
dural abscess. In various autopsy series of cases of blastomycosis involvement has
ranged from 6% (CHICK et al., 1956) to 33% of cases (CHERNISS and WEISBREN,
1956; D'AUNOY and BEVEN, 1930; LEVITAS and BAUM, 1953; LEWIS, 1917;
MARTIN and SMITH, 1939; WADE and BEL, 1916). The various case reports have
been reviewed in some detail in CHICK et al. (1960) and in FETTER et al. (1967).

Meningitis is common (Fig. 34). This may be exudative, purulent or fibrinopurulent, or granulomatous, and involve focal areas, or it may be diffuse. This may
be associated with osseous, extradural, or cerebral abscesses. Thickening and
fibrous adhesions may result. Microscopically the lesions may be predominately
polymorphonuclear leukocytic or may be histiocytic (Fig. 35).

The *cerebrum, cerebellum* (Fig. 36), basal ganglia, and *spinal cord* may be the
site of single or multiple lesions. Overt abscess formation may occur (Fig. 37) or
the lesion may be hard and tumor-like (blastomycoma). Lesions in the pituitary
have been described by SCHWARZ and BAUM (1951) and by WATSON et al. (1958).
Peripheral nerve involvement has been reported (SCHWARZ and BAUM, 1951).

Lesions in the eye are rare. Cases have been reported by SCHWARZ and BAUM
(1951), STOBER (1914), KUNKEL et al. (1954), CASSADY (1946), SINSKEY and

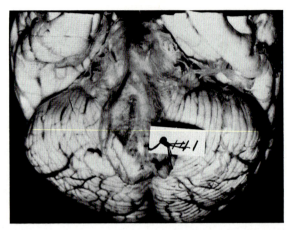

Fig. 34. Meningeal North American blastomycosis. Over the base of the brain the meninges are cloudy and contain opaque patches

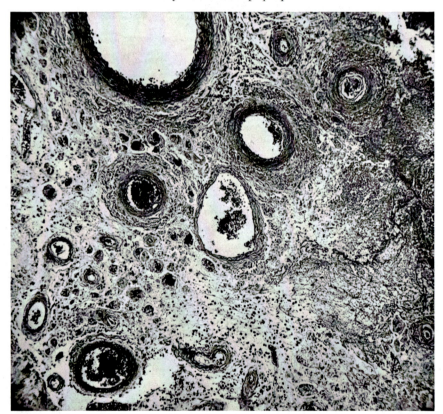

Fig. 35. Meningeal North American blastomycosis. Two types of reaction in the meninges are illustrated. To the left giant cells. To the right there is abscess. × 69

Anderson (1955), and Font et al. (1967). These cases have included iridocylitis, iritis with hypopion, bilateral posterior uveitis, endophthalmitis, and panophthalmitis.

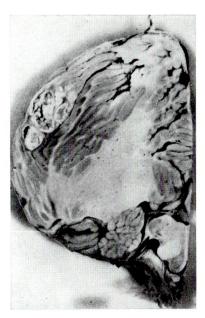

Fig. 36. Cerebellar abscesses in North American blastomycosis. Two small abscesses. It is easy to see how a meningitis could develop with extension of such lesions

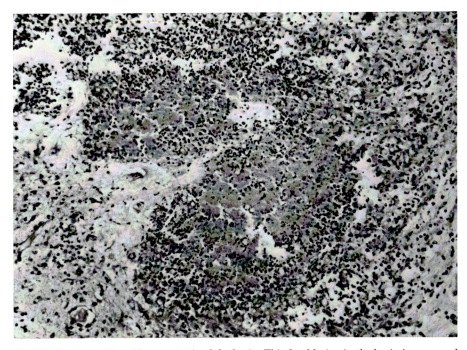

Fig. 37. North American blastomycosis of the brain. This focal lesion in the brain is composed of a central area of necrosis with a peripheral cuffing of inflammatory cells, chiefly polymorpho-nuclear leukocytes. Organisms are numerous. $\times$ 166

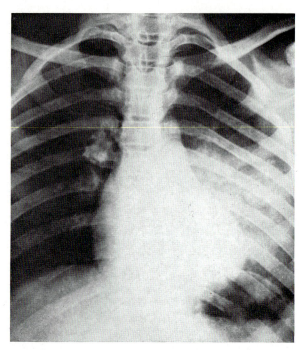

Fig. 38. North American blastomycosis of left lung. 13 yr. C.M. admitted for evaluation of chest lesion. Film showed rt hilar calcification and infiltrate on left, thought to be tuberculous pneumonia secondary to breakdown of calcified focus. AFB studies all negative, then fungus infection consided and *B.dermatititis* found

Clinical Features

Blastomycosis may present clinically with a variety of signs and symptoms (ABERNATHY, 1959; BUSEY et al., 1964; CHERNISS and WEISBREN, 1956; CHICK et al., 1956; EMMONS et al., 1963; KUNKEL et al., 1954; WALKUP and MOORE, 1964). This is not surprising when consideration is given to the fact that virtually every organ of the body may be involved, although some organs are more often involved than others (Table 3). In a comparison of the clinical demonstration of organ or system involvement with autopsy studies, percentage differences may be noted. For example, in autopsy studies the lungs are involved in 95% of the cases (EMMONS et al., 1963). Other lesions in the body may be either asymptomatic or masked by more prominent symptoms and signs.

Table 3. *Distribution of organ or organ system involvement in series of cases of blastomycosis in the literature*

	Martin and Smith, 1939	Kunkel et al., 1954	Chick et al., 1956	Cherniss and Weibren, 1956	Busey et al., 1964
Number of cases	347	90	86	40	198
Pulmonary	95%	25%	57%	70%	60%
Cutaneous	80%	60%	50%	75%	60%
Osseous	50%	31%	23%	48%	23%
Reticuloendothelial	—	—	17%	13%	8%
Central Nervous System	5%	4%	4%	10%	5%
Genitourinary . . .	—	9%	11%	28%	16%

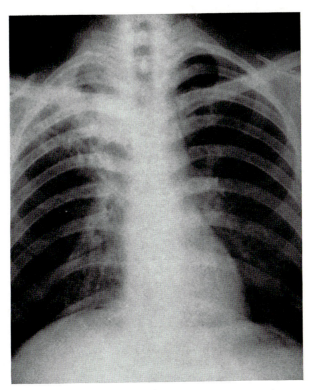

Fig. 39. Pulmonary North American blastomycosis. 36 yr. W.M. diabetic with cough, chest pain, and weakness. Skin tests: 2nd strength PPD+, histo, blasto, and cocci negative. Smears and cultures neg. for AFB. Bronchoscopy smears positive for *B.dermatitidis*, cultures of sputum positive. Treated with 2 courses of oral amphotericin B, 1 course of iv. amphotericin B, and 2-hydroxystilbamidine and lobectomy with final good results. (Neg. DVAH No. 5229-609)

Signs and symptoms referrable to the chest and lung are most common. Cough may be dry and nonproductive or productive of varying amounts of sputum. Hemoptysis may occur. Chest pain is not an uncommon complaint. Dyspnea may be prominent on occasion. Radiologic findings may be quite variable (Figs. 38 and 39).

Skin lesions are equally common as presenting signs and symptoms. These lesions occur most often on the exposed surfaces of the body. The usual course is a subcutaneous nodule which gradually ulcerates and progresses to form a verrucous, heaped up, scaling lesion. Peripheral extension with central healing is common.

Non-specific signs and symptoms are often present. Chills, fever, and night sweats may be pronounced or may be minimal. Malaise, easy fatigability, and various nondescript "aches and pains" may be marked. Localized swellings, draining sinuses, genito-urinary complaints, hoarseness, painful joints, neurologic disturbances, and dysphagia may occur in relation to specific organ involvement (Fig. 40).

With such protean manifestations, it is imperative that one maintain a high index of suspicion that a patient's disease may be caused by *B.dermatitidis*. Without such suspicion appropriate diagnostic studies cannot be undertaken to demonstrate the correct etiology.

When blastomycosis is suspected, serum should be collected for serologic tests before a skin test is done. This will preclude the possibility of a possible amnestic

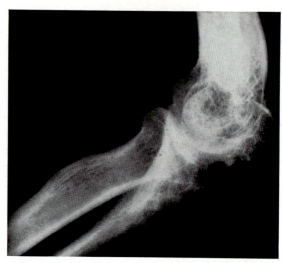

Fig. 40. North American blastomycosis of bone. Numerous punctate osteolytic lesions are present in the proximal ulna. Blastomycotic lesions of bone radiographically usually have a sharp border between the lesion and normal bone; in long bones there may also be a resemblance to infarction

boost in the titer. Unfortunately the skin test and the complement fixation tests for blastomycosis are not as reliable as those for histoplasmosis, coccidioidomycosis, or tuberculosis. A negative result in either the skin test or complement-fixation reaction does not rule out the possibility of blastomycosis, since false negative reactions are common. Conversely, a positive reaction in either instance does not verify the diagnosis, since these may be cross-reactions with a variety of other fungi. A positive test in these instances should lead to increased diligence to demonstrate the causative organism. The agar-gel precipitin test appears to be of higher accuracy than the complement fixation test.

The diagnosis of blastomycosis is verified by demonstration of the organism. The yeast phase of *B.dermatitidis* is characteristic enough in appearance to allow diagnosis by histopathologic or clinical microscopic techniques. However, cultural verification should always be sought in every case. All clinical materials possible should be cultured and examined directly under the microscope. The specimen may be examined directly, after treatment with KOH, by drying and staining with the usual histologic staining methods, or by fluorescent microscopy (Pickett et al., 1960; Chick, 1965; Kaplan and Kaufman, 1963).

Therapy

A variety of chemotherapeutic agents, potassium iodide, fatty acids, undecylenic acid, vaccines, propamidine, stilbamidine, 2-hydroxystilbamidine, and amphotericin B, as well as roentgen therapy have been used in the treatment of blastomycosis (Smith, D.T., 1954; Utz and Treger, 1959; Wilson, 1961; Walkup and Moore, 1964; Busey et al., 1964; Utz, 1965). Amphotericin B and 2-hydroxystilbamidine are the two antifungal agents most commonly used in blastomycosis at this time. Results of treatment with either drug are remarkably similiar (Busey et al., 1964; Seabury and Dascomb, 1964; Lockwood et al., 1962; Abernathy and Jansen, 1960; Furcolow, 1963; Wood, 1968; Pickar and Walker, 1968; Parker et al., 1968). Sixty to eighty percent of patients treated have had cures with either drug. Some patients have relapsed with either 2-hydroxystilbamidine or amphotericin B, but retreatment with the same or opposite antifungal agent has frequently resulted in cure. As a result of the use of these agents, the mortality of 90% reported by Martin and Smith in 1939 has been reduced to only a small percentage today.

Toxic manifestations of amphotericin B sometimes complicate treatment. Chills, fever, muscle aches, anemia, and renal impairment may occur. Reactions to 2-hydroxystilbamidine are much less common and milder. A new polypeptide antifungal agent, x-5079 C appears encouraging in the treatment of blastomycosis (UTZ et al., 1961; WITORSCH et al., 1966; PROCKNOW, 1966).

References

ABERNATHY, R.S.: Clinical manifestations of pulmonary blastomycosis. Ann. intern. Med. **51**, 707—727 (1959). — ABERNATHY, R.S., JANSEN, G.T.: Therapy with amphotericin B in North American blastomycosis. Ann. intern. Med. **53**, 1196—1203 (1960). — ABERNATHY, R.S., HEINER, D.C.: Precipitation reactions in agar in North American blastomycosis. J. Lab. clin. Med. **57**, 604—611 (1961). — ABERNATHY, R.S., MELBY, J.C.: Addison's disease in North American blastomycosis. New Engl. J. Med. **266**, 552—554 (1962). — ACREE, P.W., DeCAMP, P.T., OCHSNER, A.: Pulmonary blastomycosis. A critical analysis of medical and surgical therapies, with a report of six cases. J. thorac. cardiovasc. Surg. **28**, 175—193 (1954). — AJELLO, L.: Soil as the natural reservoir for human pathogenic fungi. Science **123**, 876—879 (1956). ~ Soil as the natural reservoir for human pathogenic fungi. In: Therapy of fungus disease, edited by T. H. STERNBERG and V. D. NEWCOMER. Boston: Little Brown & Co. 1956. — AJELLO, L., GEORG, L.K., KAPLAN, W., KAUFMAN, L.: Laboratory manual for medical mycology. 2nd edition. Communicable Disease Center, U.S. Public Health Service, Atlanta, Georgia 1962. — AJELLO, L.: Comparative ecology of respiratory mycotic disease agents. Bact. Rev. **31**, 6—24 (1967). — ARIAS LUZARDO, J.J.: Micosis profundas mas frequentes en Mexico. Thesis. Universidad Nacional Autonoma de Mexico, Escuela Nacional de Medicina, 1962. — BAKER, R.D.: Personal communication. ~ Experimental blastomycosis in mice. Amer. J. Path. **18**, 463—477 (1942). ~ Tissue reactions in human blastomycosis. Analysis of tissue from 23 cases. Amer. J. Path. **18**, 479—497 (1942). ~ Tissue changes in fungous disease. Arch. Path. **44**, 459—466 (1947). ~ Fungus infections. In: W.A.D. ANDERSON, Pathology, 2nd edition, pp. 340—346. St. Louis: C.V. Mosby Co. 1953. ~ The diagnosis of fungus diseases by biopsy. J. chron. Dis. **5**, 552—570 (1957). — BAKER, R.D., BRIAN, E.W.: Blastomycosis of the heart. Report of two cases. Amer. J. Path. **18**, 139—148 (1937). — BAKER, R.D., WARRICK, G.W., NOOJIN, R.O.: Acute blastomycotic pneumonia. Arch. intern. Med. **90**, 718—724 (1952). — BENHAM, R.W.: Fungi of blastomycosis and coccidioidal granuloma. Arch. Derm. **30**, 385—400 (1934). — BROC, R., HADDAD, N.: Tumeur bronchique a „scopulariopsis Amaericana" determination precoce d'une malaidie de Gilchrist. Bull. Soc. méd. Hôp. Paris **68**, 679—682 (1952). — BRODY, M.: Blastomycosis, North American type. A proved case from the European Continent. Arch. Derm. Syph. (Chic.) **56**, 529—531 (1947). — BURR, A.H., HUFFINESS, R.: Blastomycosis of the prostate with miliary dissemination treated by stilbamidine. J. Urol. (Baltimore) **71**, 464—468 (1954). — BUSEY, J.F., BAKER, R.D., BIRCH, L., BUECHNER, H., CHICK, E.W., JUSTICE, F.K., MATTHEWS, J.H., McDEARMAN, S., PICKAR, D.N., SUTLIFF, W.D., WALKUP, H.E., ZIMMERMAN, S.: Blastomycosis. 1. A review of 198 collected cases in Veterans Administration Hospitals. Amer. Rev. resp. Dis. **89**, 659—672 (1964). — BUSEY, J.F., HINTON, P.F.: Precipitins in blastomycosis. Amer. Rev. resp. Dis. **95**, 112—113 (1967). — BUSEY, J.F., CHICK, E.W., MENGES, R., FURCOLOW, M.L.: The distribution of human and canine blastomycosis in the United States. Amer. Rev. resp. Dis. **98**, 137 (abstr.) (1968). — CAMPBELL, C.C.: Serology in the respiratory mycoses. Sabouraudia **5**, 240—259 (1967). — CANELAS, H.M., LIMA, F.P., BITTENCOURT, J.M.T., ARAUJO, R.P., ANGHINAH, A.: Blastomykose des Nervensystems. Arch. Neuro-psiquiat. (S. Paulo) **9**, S. 203—222, mit englischer Zusammenfassung (1951) [Portugiesisch]. — CARNESDALE, P.L., STEGMAN, K.F.: Blastomycosis of bone. Report of four cases. Ann. Surg. **144**, 252—257 (1956). — CASSADY, J.V.: Uveal blastomycoses. Arch. Ophthal. **35**, 84—97 (1946). — CHERNISS, E.I., WAISBREN, B.A.: North American blastomycosis. A clinical study of 40 cases. Ann. intern. Med. **44**, 105—123 (1956). — CHICK, E.W., SUTLIFF, W.D., RAKICH, J.H., FURCOLOW, M.L.: Epidemiological aspects of cases of blastomycosis admitted to Memphis/Tennessee hospitals during the period of 1922—1954. A review of 86 cases. Amer. J. med. Sci. **231**, 253—262 (1956). — CHICK, E.W., LEHAN, P.H.: Diagnostic aspects of bromoderma and blastomycosis. Gen. Pract. Clin. **16**, 104—107 (1957). — CHICK, E.W., PETERS, H.J., DENTON, J.F., BORING, W.D.: Die Nordamerikanische Blastomykose. Ergebn. allg. Path. path. Anat. **40**, 3, 34—98 (1960). — CHICK, E.W.: North American blastomycosis. Rec. Adv. Bot., p. 273—277. Univ. Toronto Press (1961). ~ Pulmonary fungal infections simulating and misdiagnosed as other diseases. Amer. Rev. resp. Dis. **85**, 702—707 (1962). ~ Fluorescence microscopy and other special procedures for diagnosis and study of mycotic infections. Amer. Rev. resp. Dis. **92**, 175—179 (1965). — COLBERT, J.W., STRAUSS, M.J., GREEN, R.H.: The treatment of cutaneous blastomycosis with propamidine. A preliminary report. J. invest. Derm. **14**, 71—73 (1950). — CONANT, N.F.: Laboratory study of *Blastomyces dermatitidis* GILCHRIST and STOKES, 1898. Proc. Sixth Pacific Science Congr. **5**,

853—862 (1939). — CONANT, N.F., SMITH, D.T., BAKER, R.D., CALLOWAY, L.J., MARTIN, D.S.: Manual of clinical mycology, second edition. Philadelphia: W.B. Saunders Co. 1954. — COUPAL, J.F.: Report of six cases of blastomycosis. Int. Clin. 4, 1—14 (1924). — CSILLAG, A., BRANDSTEIN, L.: The role of a blastomyces in the aetiology of interstitial plasmocytic pneumonia of the premature infant. Acta microbiol. Acad. Sci. hung. 2, 179—190 (1954). ~ The role of a blosomyces species in the genesis of interstitial pneumonia of the premature infant. A prelminiary report. Acta microbiol. Acad. Sci. hung. 1, 525—529 (1954). — D'AUNOY, R., BEVEN, J.L.: Systemic blastomycosis. J. Lab. clin. Med. 16, 124—130 (1930). — DeMONTE-MAYOR, L.: Blastomyces dermatitidis — GILCHRIST & STOKES 1898 en Venezuela. Nota Previa. Gac. méd. Caracas 62, 675—689 (1954). — DENTON, J.F., McDONOUGH, E.W., AJELLO, L., AUSHERMAN, R.J.: Isolation of Blastomyces dermatitidis from soil. Science 133, 1126—1127 (1961). — DENTON, J.F., DiSALVO, A.F.: Isolation of Blastomyces dermatitidis from natural sites in Augusta, Georgia. Amer. J. trop. Med. Hyg. 13, 716—722 (1964). — DOWLING, G.B., ELSWORTHY, R.R.: Case of blastomycetic dermatitidis (GILCHRIST). Proc. roy. Soc. Med. 19, 4 (1926) (Derm. Sect.). — EMMONS, C.W.: Isolation of Histoplasma capsulatum from soil. Publ. Hlth Rep. (Wash.) 64, 892—896 (1949). — EMMONS, C.W., OLSON, B.J., ELDRIDGE, W.W.: Studies of role of fungi in pulmonary disease; cross reactions of histoplasmin. Publ. Hlth Rep. (Wash.) 64, 892—896 (1949). — EMMONS, C.W., BINFORD, C.H., UTZ, J.P.: Medical mycology. Philadelphia: Lea and Febiger 1963. — EMMONS, C.W., MURRAY, I.G., LURIE, H.I., KING, M.H., TULLOCH, J.A., CONNOR, D.H.: North American blastomycosis. Two authochthouous cases from Africa. Sabouraudia 3, 306—311 (1964). — FAVA, NETTO, C., de BRITO, T., da SILVA LACAZ, C.: Experimental South American blastomycosis of the guinea pig. An immunologic and pathologic study. Path. et Microbiol. (Basel) 24, 192—206 (1961). — FERNÁNDEZ GARCIA, E., RODRIGUEZ DE LEDESMA, J.: Consideraciones clinicas sobre un caso de blastomicosis verrucosa de Gilchrist, en su forma generalizada. Rev. clin. esp. 50, 56—59 (1953). — FETTER, B.F., KLINTWORTH, G.K., HENDRY, W.S.: Mycoses of the central nervous system. Baltimore: Williams and Wilkins Co. 1967. — FIALHO, A.: Die pathologische Anatomie der südamerikanischen Blastomykose (Lutzsche Krankheit). Ergebn. allg. Path. path. Anat. 40, 99—138 (1960). — FONT, R.L., SPAULDING, A.G., GREEN, W.R.: Endogenous mycotic panophthalmitis caused by Blastomyces dermatitidis. Arch. Ophthal. 77, 217—222 (1967). — FORBUS, W.D.: Reaction to injury. Vol. I, pp. 735—740. Baltimore: William and Wilkins Co. 1943. — FURCOLOW, M.L.: The use of amphotericin in blastomycosis, cryptococcosis, and histoplasmosis. Med. Clin. N. Amer. 47, 1119—1130 (1963). — GATTI, F., RENOIRTE, R., VANDEPITTE, J.: Premier cas de blastomycose Nord-Americaine observe au Congo (Leopoldville). Ann. Soc. belge Méd. trop. 44, 1057—1066 (1964). — GATTI, F., DeBROE, M., AJELLO, L.: Blastomyces dermatitis infection in the Congo. Report of a second autochthouous case. Amer. J. trop. Med. Hyg. 17, 96—101 (1968). — GILCHRIST, T.C.: A case of blastomycetic dermatitis in man. Rep. Johns Hopk. Hosp. 1, 269—283 (1896). — GILCHRIST, T.C., STOKES, W.R.: The presence of an oidium in the tissues of a case of pseudo-lupus vulgaris. Bull. Johns Hopk. Hosp. 7, 129—133 (1896). — GILLES, M.: A case of blastomycosis. Canad. med. Ass. J. 29, 183—185 (1933). — GRANDBOIS, J.: La blastomycose Nord-Americaine au Canada. Loval Med. 34, 714—731 (1963). — HADDAD, N.: Mycose viscerale metastique mortelle due a Scopulariopsis americana. These. Faculte mixte de medicine et de pharmacie de Lyon. 1952. — HAMBLEN, E.C., BAKER, R.D., MARTIN, D.S.: Blastomycosis of the female reproductive tract with report of a case. Amer. J. Obstet. Gynec. 30, 345—356 (1935). — HAMBURGER, W.W.: A comparative study of four strains of organisms isolated from four cases of generalized blastomycosis. J. infect. Dis. 4, 201—209 (1907). — HARRELL, E.R., CURTIS, A.C.: The treatment of North American blastomycosis with amphotericin B. Arch. Derm. 76, 561—569 (1957). — HEINSIUS, E.: Augenbeteiligung bei Blastomykose. 55. Zusammenkunft Heidelberg, 26.—28. IX. 1949; Ber. dtsch. ophthal. Ges. 1950, S. 358—362. — HEKTOEN, L.: Systemic blastomycosis and coccidioidal granuloma. J. Amer. med. Ass. 49, 1070—1077 (1907). — HERBUT, P.A.: Urological pathology. Philadelphia: Lea & Febiger 1952. — HOPKINS, J.E., MURPHY, J.D.: Pulmonary resection and undecylenic acid in systemic blastomycosis. J. thorac. Surg. 23, 409—418 (1952). — HOWLES, J.K., BLACK, C.I.: Cutaneous blastomycosis. A report of 58 unpublished cases. J. La med. Soc. 105, 72—73 (1953). — HOWELL, A., JR.: Studies of fungus antigens. I. Quantitative studies of cross-reactions between histoplasmin and blastomycin in guinea pigs. Publ. Hlth Rep. (Wash.) 62, 631—651 (1947). — HURLEY, T.D.: Blastomycosis, an unique lesion of the heart in systemic blastomycosis. J. med. Res. 33, 499—501 (1916). — JELLIFFE, D.B., HUTT, M.S.R., CONNOR, D.H., KING, M.H., LUNN, H.F.: Report of a clinico-pathological conference from Mulago, July 30, 1963. E. Afr. med. J. 41, 79—87 (1964). — JONES, R.R., JR., MARTIN, D.S.: Blastomycosis of bone. Surgery 10, 931—938 (1941). — KAPLAN, W., KAUFMAN, L.: Specific fluorescent antiglobulin for the detection and identification of Blastomyces dermatitidis yeast phase cells. Mycopathologia (Den Haag) 19, 173—180 (1963). — KENT, D.C., COLLIER, T.M.: Addison's disease associated with North American blastomycosis, A case report. J. clin. Endocr. 25, 164—169 (1965). — KÖHLMEIER, W., KREIT-

NER, H.: Blastomykose der Mamma. Wien. klin. Wschr. **1953**, 13—15. — KUNKEL, W. M., JR., WEED, L. A., McDONALD, J. R., CLAGETT, O. T.: Collective review; North American blastomycosis — Gilchrist's disease. Clinicopathologic study of ninety cases. Int. Abstr. Surg. **99**, 1—26 (1954). — LAAS, E., GEIGER, W.: Blastomykose bei Lymphogranulomatose. Dtsch. Z. Nervenheilk. **159**, 314—331 (1948). — LESTER, G. F., CONRAD, F. G., ATWELL, R. J.: Primary laryngeal blastomycosis. Review of the literature and presentation of a case. Amer. J. Med. **24**, 305—309 (1958). — LEVITAS, J. R., BAUM, G. L.: Surgical aspects of blastomycosis. Surgery **33**, 93—101 (1953). — LEWIS, P.: Blastomycosis and sporotrichosis. Surg. Clin. (Chic.) **1**, 1125—1138 (1917). — LEWIS, G. M., et al.: An introduction to medical mycology. 4th edition. Chicago/Ill.: Year Book Publ. Inc. 1958. — LOCKWOOD, W. R., BUSEY, J. F., BATSON, B. E., ALLISON, F., JR.: Experiences in the treatment of North American blastomycosis with 2-hydroxystilbamidine. Ann. intern. Med. **57**, 553—562 (1962). — LUGER, A., NEUHOLD, R.: Systematische Blastomykose. Hautarzt **13**, 160—168 (1962). — MANWARING, J. H.: Unusual forms of *Blastomyces dermatitidis* in human tissues. Arch. Path. **48**, 421—425 (1949). — MARTIN, D. S.: Complement-fixation in blastomycosis. J. infect. Dis. **57**, 291—295 (1935). ~ Practical applications of immunologic principles in the diagnosis and treatment of fungus infections "Medical Mycology". Ann. N.Y. Acad. Sci. **50**, 1376—1379 (1950). ~ Serologic studies on North American blastomycosis. Studies with soluble antigens from untreated and sonic-treated yeast-phase cells of *Blastomyces dermatitidis*. J. Immunol. **71**, 192—201 (1953). ~ Evaluation of skin tests and serologic methods in fungus infections. J. chron. Dis. **5**, 580—591 (1957). — MARTIN, D. S., SMITH, D. T.: The laboratory diagnosis of blastomycosis. J. Lab. clin. Med. **21**, 1289—1296 (1936). ~ Blastomycosis (American blastomycosis, Gilchrist's disease). I. Review of literature. Amer. Rev. Tuberc. **39**, 275—304 (1939). ~ Blastomycosis (American blastomycosis, Gilchrist's disease). II. A report of 13 new cases. Amer. Rev. Tuberc. **39**, 488—515 (1939). — MARTINEZ, BAEZ M., REYES, A. MOTA, GONZALES OCHOA, A.: Blastomycosis Norteamericana en Mexico. Rev. Inst. Salubr. Enferm. trop. (Méx.) **14**, 225—232 (1954). — MENGES, R. W., FURCOLOW, M. L., LARSH, H. W.: Laboratory studies on histoplasmosis. I. The effect of humidity and temperature on the growth of *Histoplasma capsulatum*. J. infect. Dis. **90**, 67—70 (1952). — MONTGOMERY, F. H.: A brief summary of the clinical, pathologic, and bacteriologic features of cutaneous blastomycosis (Blastomycetic dermatitis of Gilchrist). J. Amer. med. Ass. **39**, 1486—1493 (1902). — MONTGOMERY, F. H., ORMSBY, O. S.: Systemic blastomycosis. Arch. intern. Med. **2**, 1—41 (1908). — MÜLLER, E., HILSCHER, W. M.: Zur Frage der generalisierten Blastomykose und ihrer Beziehungen zur Lymphogranulomatose. Zbl. allg. Path. path. Anat. **92**, 331—338 (1954). — PARKER, J. D., DOTO, I. L., TOSH, F. E.: Amphotericin B in the treatment of blastomycosis. A National Communicable Disease Center Cooperative Mycoses Study. Amer. Rev. resp. Dis. **98**, 120 (1968) (Abstr.). — PICKAR, D. N., WALKER, R.: Therapy of blastomycosis. A twenty-year study. Amer. Rev. resp. Dis. **98**, 119—120 (1968) (Abstr.). — PICKETT, J. P., BISHOP, C. M., CHICK, E. W., BAKER, R. D.: A simple fluorescent stain for fungi. Selective staining of fungi by means of a fluorescent method for mucin. Amer. J. clin. Path. **34**, 197—202 (1960). — POIRIER, P.: Blastomycose Nord-Americaine (Maladie de Gilchrist). Un. méd. Can. **84**, 287 (1955). — POLO, J. F., BRASS, K., DeMONTEMAYOR, L.: Enfermeded de Gilchrist en Venezuela. Primer case; estudio clinico; comprobacion histologica; aislamiento y determinacion de la primera cepa Suramericana de *blastomyces dermatitides*. Rev. San. (Caracas) **19**, 217—235 (1954). — POND, N. W., HUMPHREYS, R. J.: Blastomycosis with cardiac involvement and peripheral embolization. Amer. Heart J. **43**, 615—620 (1952). — PROCKNOW, J. J.: Disseminated blastomycosis treated successfully with the polypeptide antifungal agent x-5079C. Evidence for human to human transmission. Amer. Rev. resp. Dis. **94**, 761—772 (1966). — RAMSAY, F. K., CARTER, G. R.: Canine blastomycosis in the U.S. J. Amer. vet. med. Ass. **120**, 93—98 (1952). — RANIER, A.: Primary laryngeal blastomycosis. A review of the literature and report of a case. Amer. J. clin. Path. **21**, 444—450 (1951). — RAVOGLI, A.: Blastomycosis. Acta derm.-venereol. (Stockh.) **6**, 281—289 (1925). — REEVES, R. T., PEDERSEN, R.: Fungus infection of bone. Radiology **62**, 55—69 (1954). — RHANGOS, W. C., CHICK, E. W.: Mycotic infections of bone. Sth. med. J. (Bgham, Ala.) **57**, 664—674 (1964). — RICKETTS, H. T.: Oidiomycosis of the skin and its fungi. J. med. Res. **6**, 373—547 (1901). — SALVIN, S. B.: Immunologic aspects of the mycoses. Progr. Allergy **7**, 213—331 (1963). — SCHOENBACH, E. B., GREENSPAN, E. M.: The pharmacology, mode of action and therapeutic potentialities of stilbamidine, and other aromatic diamidines. A review. Medicine (Baltimore) **27**, 327—377 (1948). — SCHOENBACH, E. B., MILLER, J. M., GINSBERG, M., LONG, P. H.: Systemic blastomycosis treated with stilbamidine. J. Amer. med. Ass. **146**, 1317—1318 (1951). — SCHWARZ, J., BAUM, G. L.: Blastomycosis. Amer. J. clin. Path. **21**, 999—1029 (1951). ~ North American blastomycosis. Geographic distribution, pathology and pathogenesis. Docum. Med. geogr. trop. (Amst.) **5**, 29—41 (1953). — SCHWARZ, J., FURCOLOW, N. L.: Some epidemiologic factors and diagnostic tests in blastomycosis, coccidioidomycosis and histoplasmosis. Amer. J. clin. Path. **25**, 261—265 (1955). — SCHWARZ, J., GOLDMAN, L.: Epidemiologic study of North American blastomycosis. Arch. Derm. Syph. (Chic.)

71, 84—88 (1955). — Seaburg, J.H., Dascomb, H.E.: Results of the treatment of systemic mycoses. J. Amer. med. Ass. 188, 509—513 (1964). — Sinskey, R.M., Anderson, W.B.: Miliary blastomycosis with metastatic spread to posterior uvea of both eyes. Arch. Ophthal. 54, 602—604 (1955). — Smith, D.C., Turner, H.C., Sanderson, E.S.: Systemic blastomycosis, with report of fatal case. Brit. J. Derm. 40, 344—359 (1928). — Smith, D.T.: Immunologic types of blastomycosis. A report on 40 cases. Ann. intern. Med. 31, 463—469 (1949). ~ Therapy for the systemic fungus infections. N.Y. St. J. Med. 54, 2303—2309 (1954). ~ Problems in the diagnosis of pulmonary mycoses. Tex. St. J. Med. 51, 787—792 (1955). ~ Primary and secondary blastomycosis of the lungs and skin. Lancet 86, 499—502 (1966). — Smith, J.G., Jr., Harris, J.S., Conant, N.F., Smith, D.T.: An epidemic of North American blastomycosis. J. Amer. med. Ass. 158, 641—646 (1955). — Snapper, I., Scheid, B., McVay, L., Lieben, F.: Pharmacology and therapeutic value of diamidine derivatives, particularly of 2-hydroxystilbamidine. Trans. N.Y. Acad. Sci. 14, 269—271 (1952). — Snapper, I., McVay, L.V., Jr.: The treatment of North American blastomycosis with 2-hydroxystilbamidine. Amer. J. Med. 15, 603—623 (1953). — Solway, L.J., Kohan, M., Pritzker, H.G.: A case of disseminated blastomycosis. Canad. Med. Ass. J. 41, 331—336 (1939). — Spaccarelli, G., Callieri, B.: Le blastomatosi diffuse delle leptomeningi. Recenti Progr. Med. 10, 17—41 (1951). — Stampfl, B.: Über einen eigenartigen Fall von Blastomykose. 33. Tagung, Kiel, 7.—10. VI. 1949; Verh. dtsch. Ges. Path. S. 187—191 (1950). — Starrs, R.A., Klotz, M.O.: North American blastomycosis (Gilchrist's disease). I. A study of diseases from a review of the literature. Arch. intern. Med. 82, 1—28 (1948). ~ North American blastomycosis (Gilchrist's disease). II. Analysis of Canadian reports and description of a new case of the systemic type. Arch. intern. Med. 82, 29—53 (1948). — Stober, A.M.: Systemic blastomycosis. Arch. intern. Med. 13, 509—556 (1914). — Stoddard, J.L., Cutler, E.C.: Torula infection in man. Rockefeller Institute for Medical Research. Monograph 6, New York 1916. — Utz, J.P., Treger, A.: The current status of chemotherapy of systemic fungal diseases. Ann. intern. Med. 51, 1220—1229 (1959). — Utz, J.P., Andriole, V.T., Emmons, C.W.: Chemotherapeutic activity of X-5079C in systemic mycoses of man. Amer. Rev. resp. Dis. 84, 514—528 (1961). — Utz, J.P.: Antimicrobial therapy in systemic fungal infections. Amer. J. Med. 39, 826—830 (1965). — Vermeil, C., Gordeeff, A., Haddad, N.: Sur un cas Tunesien de mucose generalisee mortelle. Ann. Inst. Pasteur 86, 636—646 (1954). — Wade, H.W., Bel, G.S.: A critical consideration of systemic mycosis. Arch. intern. Med. 18, 103—130 (1916). — Walker, J.W., Montgomery, F.H.: Further report of a previously recorded case of blastomycosis of the skin; systemic infection with blastomycoses. Death, autopsy. J. Amer. med. Ass. 38, 867—871 (1902). — Walkup, H.E., Moore, J.A.: North American blastomycosis. In: Steele, J.D.: The treatment of mycotic and parasitic diseases of the chest, pp. 3—30. Springfield/Ill.: Ch. C. Thomas 1964. — Watson, S.H., Moore, S., Blank, F.: Generalized North American blastomycosis. Canad. med. Ass. J. 78, 35—38 (1958). — Wegmann, T.: Blastomykose und andere Pilzerkrankungen der Lunge. Dtsch. Arch. klin. Med. 199, 192—205 (1952). — Wegmann, T., Zollinger, H.U.: Tuberkuloide Granulome in Mundschleimhaut und Halslymphknoten. Südamerikanische Blastomykose. Schweiz. med. Wschr. 89, 1151—1153 (1959). — Wilson, J.W., Smith, C.E., Plunkett, O.A.: Primary cutaneous coccidioidomycosis. The criteria for diagnosis and a report of a case. Calif. Med. 79, 233—239 (1953). — Wilson, J.W., Cawley, E.P., Weidman, F.D., Gillmer, W.S.: Primary cutaneous North American blastomycosis. Arch. Derm. Syph. (Chic.) 71, 39—45 (1955). — Wilson, J.W.: Therapy of systemic fungous infections in 1961. A Symposium. Arch. intern. Med. 108, 292—316 (1961). — Wilson, R.P.: Blastomycosis of the conjunctiva. Bull. ophthal. Soc. Egypt 28, 99—103 (1935). — Witorsch, P., Andriole, V.T., Emmons, C.W., Utz, J.P.: The polypeptide antifungal agent (X-5079C). Further studies in 39 patients. Amer. Rev. resp. Dis. 93, 876—888 (1966). — Witorsch, P., Utz, J.P.: North American blastomycosis. Study of 40 patients. Medicine (Baltimore) 47, 169 (1968). — Wood, W.B.: North American blastomycosis. Efficacy of dihydroxystilbamidine. Amer. Rev. resp. Dis. 98, 119 (1968) (Abstr.). — Zawirska, B.: Südamerikanische Blastomykose des Wurmfortsatzes (Lutz-Splendorede Almeida Krankheit). Zbl. allg. Path. path. Anat. 99, 593—600 (1959).

Fig. 1, Fig. 3 through 37 and Fig. 40 reprinted from Chick, E.W., Peters, H.J., Denton, J.F., and Boring, W.D.: Die Nordamerikanische Blastomykose. Ergebn. allg. Path. path. Anat. 40, 34—98 (1960). — Fig. 3 and 5 courtesy of Dr. N.F. Conant. — Fig. 4 and 6 courtesy of Dr. J.F. Denton. — Fig. 7, 21 and 28 courtesy of Dr. W.D. Forbus. — Fig. 8 from Baker. Amer. J. Path. 18. — Fig. 11, 24, 33 courtesy of Dr. Dr. R.D. Baker. — Fig. 14 courtesy of Dr. J. Schwarz. Fig. 40 courtesy of Dr. D.S. Martin. — Fig. 2 modified from Busey, J.F., Chick, E.W., Menges, R., Furcolow, M.L.: The distribution of human and canine blastomycosis in the United States. Amer. Rev. resp. Dis. 98, 137 (1968). — Fig. 38 and 39 reprinted from Chick, E.W.: Pulmonary fungal infections simulating and misdiagnosed as other diseases. Amer. Rev. resp. Dis. 85, 702—707 (1962).

Paracoccidioidomycosis

ALBERTO ANGULO O. and LADISLAO POLLAK, Caracas/Venezuela

With 70 Figures

Synonyms: South American Blastomycosis; Brazilian Blastomycosis; Tropical Granulomatous Blastomycosis; Paracoccidioidal Granuloma; Paracoccidioidal Granulomatosis; Lutz' Disease; Lutz-Splendore-Almeida's Disease; Almeida's Disease.

Definition: Paracoccidioidomycosis is a chronic, progressive and granulomatous disease that mainly attacks the lungs, mucosa of the mouth and nose, and neighboring teguments, with frequent spread to the lymph nodes, adrenal glands and other viscera.

History

The disease was discovered by LUTZ (1908) in Brasil. He observed lesions of the mucosa and was able to culture the fungus. Later, *Splendore* (1910—1912) studied several cases, confirming the presence of mucosal lesions and the culture characteristics as described by LUTZ, and in 1912 proposed the name *Zymonema brasiliensis* to designate the fungus that produced the disease. Between 1908 and 1915, as this new entity became known, many cases were reported by different Brazilian authors (CARINI, LINDENBERG, RABELLO, PEREIRA and GASPAR VIANA, MONTENEGRO, CASTRO CARVALHO, DIAZ DA SILVA, GOMEZ DE CRUZ, PORTUGAL and KEHL). During the first years the fungus was mistaken for *Coccidioides immitis*. ALMEIDA (1927) demonstrated that the fungus cultured by LUTZ was a different one and in 1930 he created the new genus *Paracoccidioides*, keeping, however, Splendore's term *brasiliensis* for the species. Eleven years later, CONANT and HOWELL (1941) proposed the name *Blastomyces* to designate the genus and *dermatitidis* and *brasiliensis* for the two species. However, the genus *Blastomyces* is not acceptable, as CONSTANTIN and ROLAND (1888) had already proposed this name for a saprophytic fungus which was completely different from the causal agent of North and South American Blastomycosis. Finally ALMEIDA (1946) suggested, as the most logical solution, the acceptance of the genus *Paracoccidioides* with the species *dermatitidis* and *brasiliensis*. Since the designation of the name *Paracoccidioides* (1930) was prior to CONANT and HOWELL's proposal (1941) and, moreover, the genus *Blastomyces* has been reserved for another fungus, we accept the term *Paracoccidioides brasiliensis*. (SPLENDORE, 1912; ALMEIDA, 1930). OLIVEIRA RIBEIRO (1940) was the first to introduce sulfas for the treatment of the disease.

After the Brazilian publications, the disease began to be found in other Latin American countries: Argentina (LLAMBIAS et al., 1930); Colombia (MÉNDES-LEMAITRE, 1950); Costa Rica (CHAVARIO et al., 1949); Ecuador (RODRÍGUEZ, 1953); Guatemala (TEJADA et al., 1960); Honduras (FERNÁNDEZ, 1961); México (GONZÁLEZ OCHOA, 1950); Paraguay (BOGGINO, 1935, 1938); Perú (WEISS and ZABALETA, 1937); Uruguay (FREIJO, 1940); Venezuela (O'DALY, 1937) etc.

Etiology

Etiologic agent: *Paracoccidioides brasiliensis* (Splendore) Almeida, 1930.

Synonyms: *Zymonema brasiliense* SPLENDORE, 1912; *Mycoderma brasiliensis* BRUMPT, 1912; *Mycoderma histosporocellularis* NEVEU-LEMAIRE, 1921; *Monilia*

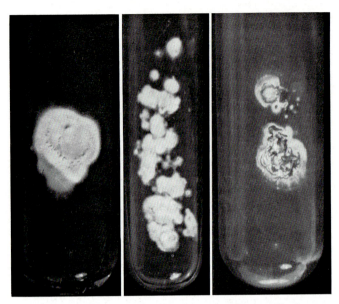

Fig. 1. Left: *P. brasiliensis*, mycelial phase of culture on Sabouraud's glucose agar, 30 days at room temperature; middle: *P. brasiliensis*, mycelial phase on Sabouraud's glucose agar 30 days at room temperature; right: *P. brasiliensis*, mycelial phase on Sabouraud's glucose agar, 50 days, room temperature

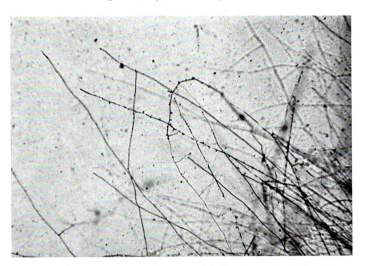

Fig. 2. *P.brasiliensis*, mycelial phase with aleuriospores, slide culture

brasiliensis VUILLEMIN, 1922; *Coccidioides brasiliensis* ALMEIDA, 1929; *Coccidioides histosporocellulares* FONSECA, 1932; *Paracoccidioides cerebriformis* MOORE, 1935; *Paracoccidioides tenuis* MOORE, 1935; *Lutziomyces histosporocellularis* FONSECA FILHO, 1939; *Blastomyces brasiliensis* CONANT and HOWELL, 1941; *Aleurisma brasiliensis* AROEIRA NEVES and BOGLIOLO, 1951.

    P.brasiliensis is a dimorphic fungus. In the mycelial phase at 30°C it grows slowly in about 20—30 days. The macroscopic appearance is variable. White

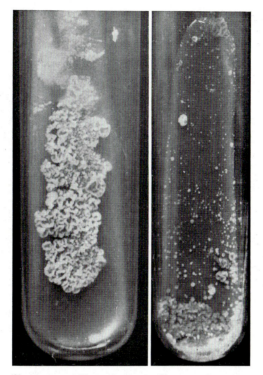

Fig. 3. Left: *P. brasiliensis*, yeast-like culture on Thompson's medium, 14 days at 37° C; right: *Paracoccidioides brasiliensis* yeast-like culture on Thompson's medium 6 days, at 37° C

colonies with short aerial hyphae were the most frequent finding (Fig. 1). With time the central part of the colony rises, and ruptures. Sometimes, no aerial hyphae are seen, or there may be very short and delicate ones on the surface of cerebriform or membranous colonies that can be either flat, or wrinkled. The latter are cinnamon or brown in color. These variations do not justify the creation of new species (*P.cerebriformis* MOORE, 1939). Microscopic examination reveals branched or septate hyphae with chlamydospores. Oval or round conidia are rare or are not produced at all. Under special culture-conditions, aleuriospores develop (NEVES BOGLIOLO, 1951; BORELLI, 1956; POLLAK, 1967) (Fig. 2).

The fungus grows faster at 35°—37°C, developing cerebriform yeast-like colonies in 5—10 days (Fig. 3). The color of these colonies varies according to the culture medium used. In media containing blood they are brown, whereas in Sabouraud's medium they are ivory.

Microscopic examination reveals round or oval yeast-like cells, with a rigid cell wall, that can be up to 30 microns in diameter and sometimes up to 50—60 microns. Cultures in active growth display small forms 2—3 microns in diameter. The fungus reproduces itself by single or multiple budding, the latter form being the characteristic one (Fig. 4). At times, the mother cell is completely covered with small daughter cells. In young cultures, budding is so intense that several generations of cells can be seen. The daughter cell is attached to the mother cell by a narrow neck. As observed with electron microscopy (CARBONELL and POLLAK, 1963) there is no endosporulation (Ciferri's cryptosporulation). When the fungus is cultured at room temperature, the yeast phase is transformed into the mycelial

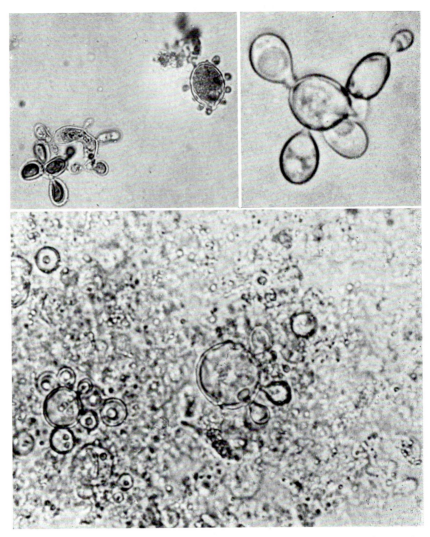

Fig. 4. Upper left: *P. brasiliensis*, multiple budding cells from Thompson's medium at 35° C, Lactophenol cotton blue; upper right: *P. brasiliensis*, multiple budding cell from Thompson's medium at 35° C; lower: *P. brasiliensis*, multiple budding cells in sputum

phase. The mycelial phase can be reconverted into a yeast form if it is transferred to fresh medium and incubated at 37 °C. The yeast phase is the tissue form of the fungus. The fungus shows the same form in tissue as in culture.

By means of *electron microscopy*, it has been demonstrated that the cell wall of the yeast form has an average thickness of 179 milimicrons. It has a cytoplasmic membrane with pinocytic activity, multiple nuclei, 40—50 mitochondria (in actively growing forms), and little endoplasmic reticulum. There are also vacuoles with a content of high electronic density which has been identified as lipids and myelinic figures, which apparently are intimately related to the osmiophilic vacuoles. *P. brasiliensis* is intensely osmiophilic in young forms, but this osmiophilic

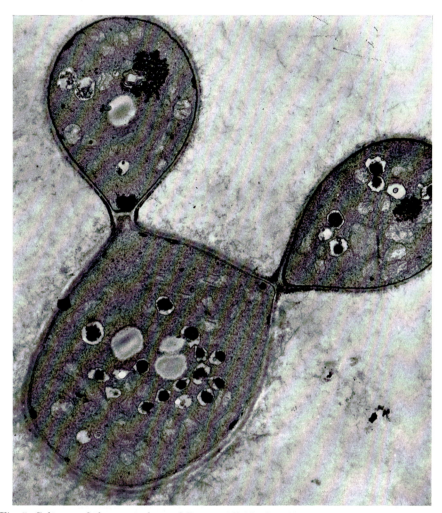

Fig. 5. Cultures of the yeast phase of *Paracoccidioides brasiliensis*. Note that the budding is almost completed. Budding occurs in this fungus with an increase in the optical density of the cell wall at the narrow neck between the two cells. ×11000
(Courtesy of Dr. L. M. CARBONELL)

density decreases with the beginning of budding. Thereafter, a central granular zone appears that continues growing until it covers the whole fungus in its old forms (CARBONELL and POLLAK, 1962, 1963) (Fig. 5).

Epidemiology

Paracoccidioidomycosis is a disease of New World origin (Fig. 6). It is found from Mexico to Argentina (with the exception of Chile, El Salvador and Panama), and is the mycosis most frequently encountered in South American countries, especially in Brazil, Venezuela and Colombia. According to its known distribution to date it should be called Latin American blastomycosis. Cases reported in countries outside of the American continent have a history of residence in the aforementioned endemic areas. Reports of South American blastomycosis in

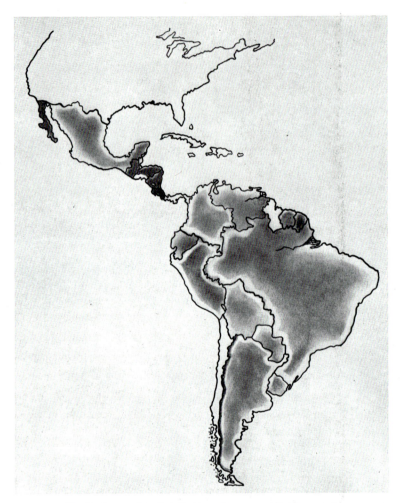

Fig. 6. Geographic distribution of paracoccidioidomycosis

Portugal, Spain and other European countries, as well as in the United States, involve persons that lived in endemic Latin American zones for some time.

The natural habitat of *P. brasiliensis* is unknown. It is suspected that it lives in the soil or in vegetation. Plants could play a role as intermediate hosts for human infection (Lacaz, 1967). Such an assumption is based on the fact that there is a higher frequency of the disease among farmers and inhabitants of rural zones.

Until the present, however, the search for the fungus in nature has proven unsuccessful. Chaves Batista (1962) reported that he had cultured *P. brasiliensis* from the soil, but this finding has not been confirmed. Man is the only known host. So far, the fungus has never been found in domestic animals but, logically, there must be an extrahuman reservoir, since the transmission of the disease from person to person is unknown. Grose and Tamsitt (1965) reported the finding of *P. brasiliensis* in the intestinal contents of 3 bats (*Artibeus lituratus*).

P. brasiliensis is found in almost all Latin American countries. According to Borelli (1961), it is found in areas with tropical or subtropical climates, located between the 23°N and 30°S, parallels where the annual average temperatures range from 17° to 24°C.

Paracoccidioidomycosis can affect persons of all ages, but it is more frequent between 25 and 45 years. It is rare in children and adolescents.

In Venezuela, the disease does not seem to predominate in any particular race. On several occasions, we have observed serious disseminated paracoccidioidomycosis in European immigrants. In Brazil, however, it predominates in the white race, secondly in Japanese immigrants and lastly among Negroes and mulattos.

In our material (Instituto Nacional de Tuberculosis) the female to male ratio is 1:20, LACAZ in Brazil reports 1:12 and RODRÍGUEZ in Ecuador 1:27 (1959).

According to RODRÍGUEZ et al. (1959), two thirds of the patients were farmers; Lacaz's statistics on 2,902 cases demonstrated that 1,024 were rural workers.

Currently an intensive search is being made to obtain a specific and standardized antigen for intradermic use in epidemiological surveys. FAVE NETTO and RAPHAEL (1961) in Brazil, and RESTREPO et al. (1968) in Colombia, among others, have carried out surveys with paracoccidioidin in order to demonstrate paracoccidioidomycois.

Portal of Entry

The portal of entry of *P.brasiliensis* is still under discussion. It is generally thought that the fungus penetrates the buccal, pharyngeal or nasal mucosa, producing different types of lesions, and then is carried to the lymph glands, lungs and other viscera, via the lymph channels or the bloodstream. According to some authors, the buccal mucosa is favored as the portal of entry because of the habit that farmers have of using chips of wood or thorns as toothpicks, and of chewing leaves or bark from trees. These objects can easily inflict wounds in the mouth that facilitate the entry of the fungus. Nevertheless, *P.brasiliensis* has never been isolated from plants nor from the soil. Less frequently cited as portals of entry are the laryngeal and rectal mucosa and the ocular conjuntiva. Several Brazilian authors point to the ano-rectal mucosa as the site of primary lesions in cases of farmers that often employ the leaves of plants, stones, etc., for their anal "toilette".

Primary cutaneous lesions are observed only exceptionally. As in other systemic mycoses, the lungs might be considered as a possible portal of entry due to inhalation of the infecting agent. There are clinical reports of cases with lesions of the lungs that never presented mucosal lesions or in which the latter appeared a long time after the former. MACKINNON et al. (1959), injected cultures of *P. brasiliensis* into the hearts of guinea pigs and rabbits and obtained pulmonary lesions first, and lesions of the mouth, nose, and rectum secondarily. According to MACKINNON, the mucosal lesions represented secondary spread of the granulomatous myositis previously induced through the blood stream. Since the buccopharyngeal region is rich in striated muscle, lesions of the mucosa appear more frequently in this area.

After inoculating rats intracutaneously, TEXEIRA et al. (1965) did not observe a local response, but found pulmonary lesions after 60 days.

In over 200 cases examined by us, the majority (90%) of the patients showed simultaneous muco-cutaneous and pulmonary lesions, but we could not determine which of the two appeared first. Cases with only mucosal lesions and no apparent pulmonary or visceral findings represented a scant 6% of our material.

In summary, it can be said that, in the light of current observations, both the mucosal and pulmonary routes are feasible. Research is at present being carried out in order to clarify this question.

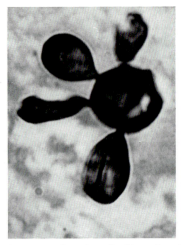

Fig. 7. *P. brasiliensis* in a lesion of a lymph node. Note the 4 large buds. GMS × 1200

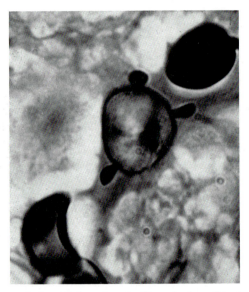

Fig. 8. *P. brasiliensis* in a lesion of a lymph node. Note the 3 small buds on the central fungal cell, the single small bud on the upper right fungal cell, and the fungal cell in the left lower corner, apparently without buds. GMS × 1200

Histopathology

The histopathologic reaction to *P. brasiliensis* is granulomatous (this disease is also called paracoccidioidal granuloma and paracoccidioidal granulomatosis). In ulcerated muco-cutaneous lesions, and in lesions infected secondarily, there is also a pyogenic inflammatory reaction. This type of tissue reaction is not characteristic of this disease, as it is common to other mycoses and to diseases produced by other etiologic agents. In order to verify morphologically the etiology of a paracoccioidal lesion, it is necessary to find the fungus in its characteristic form, that is, as a

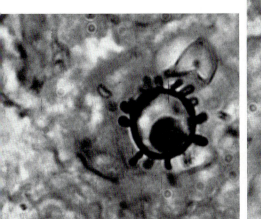

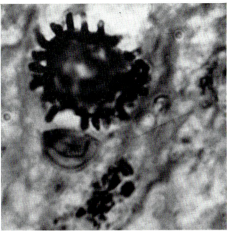

Fig. 9   Fig. 10

Fig. 9. *P. brasiliensis* in a lesion of a lymph node. Note the 14 minute buds, and the retraction of the central material of the fungal cell away from the wall. GMS × 1200

Fig. 10. *P. brasiliensis* in a lesion of a lymph node. Note more than a score of minute buds protruding from the wall of the large fungal cell. GMS × 1200

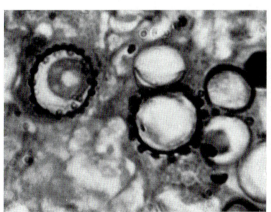

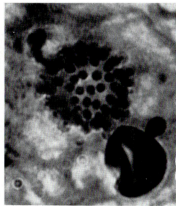

Fig. 11   Fig. 12

Fig. 11. *P. brasiliensis* in a lesion of a lymph node. Two of the fungal cells show numerous small buds. GMS × 1200

Fig. 12. *P. brasiliensis* in a lesion of a lymph node. The central fungal cell is studded with small buds, whereas the cell in the right lower corner of the illustration has a single, medium-sized bud. GMS × 1200

spherical or oval cell (mother cell) which varies between 10 and 60 microns in size (usually between 10 and 20) and displays multiple small buds (daughter cells) on its periphery, which give the fungus an "airplane motor" or "ship's helm" appearance (Figs. 7—12). This multibudding form in tissue is characteristic of *P. brasiliensis*. The mother cell may be empty or may contain a protoplasmic body susceptible to retraction with tissue-fixation methods, causing the appearance of a light space between the protoplasmic body and the cell wall (Fig. 13). At a given phase in their evolutive cycle, the cells show a chromatic mass which is finely

33*

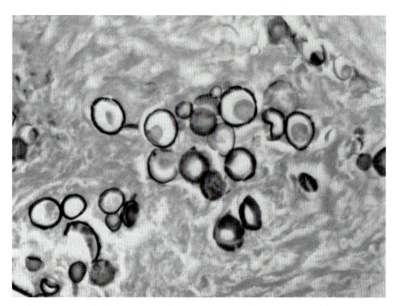

Fig. 13. *P.brasiliensis*. The fungi seen either empty or with retraction of the protoplasm. GMS method, ×320

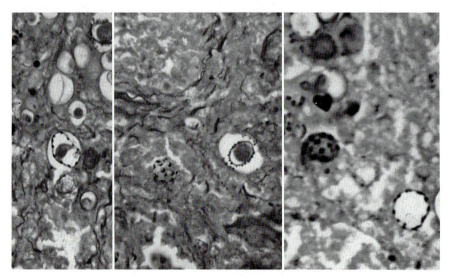

Fig. 14. *P.brasiliensis*. Fragments of chromatic mass located next to the cell wall. GMS method, ×320

divided into small fragments and distributed throughout the cytoplasm or located at the periphery (Fig. 14), under the cell wall, having carried with them a small portion of the cytoplasm. The buds or daughter cells are almost always multiple, identical or unequal in size, with a range of 1—5 microns. They may be either rounded or pyriform and are attached to the mother cell by a neck that generally is narrow.

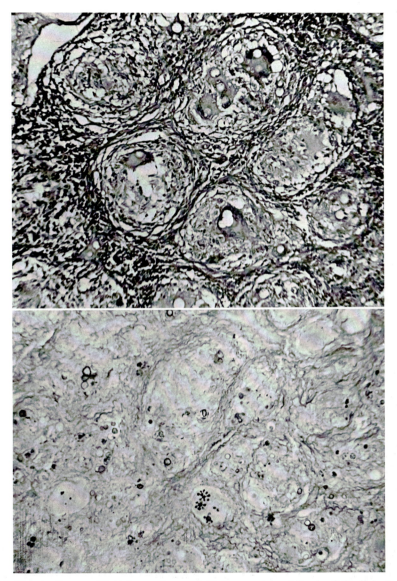

Fig. 15. Upper: *Paracoccidioidal granuloma*. Multiple granulomas. Some of the "giant cells" contain "vacuoles" which were identified as fungus cells. Lymph node section. H&E, ×200; lower: Another field of the same section with some typical forms of *P. brasiliensis*. GMS, ×150

The granulomas have a varied appearance. In the absence of secondary infection, the nodule is formed by epithelioid cells, Langhans or foreign body giant cells, plasmocytes, lymphocytes, etc. (Figs. 15, 16).

The fungi are generally observed inside the giant cells or mixed with inflammatory cells (Fig. 17). The nodules may be necrotic in their center in which case their appearance is very similar to that of a tubercle (Fig. 18) with which they may be easily mistaken unless a special stain is employed. At other times, the epithelioid nodules are not necrotic, the giant cells are scarce and the fungi are

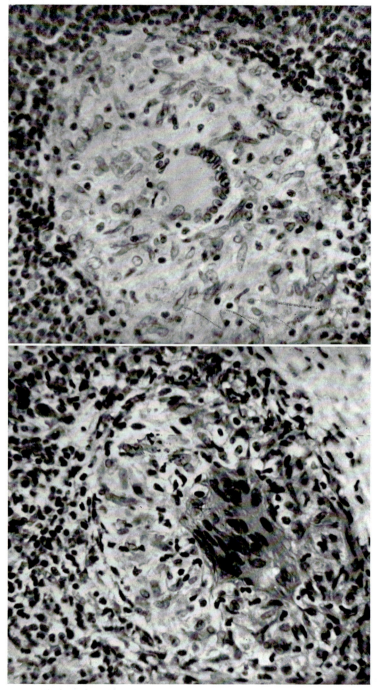

Fig. 16. Upper: Epithelioid nodule with LANGHANS giant cell similar to a tubercle. No fungi are seen in this lymph gland section. H&E, ×320; lower: Epithelioid nodule with foreign body giant cell. No fungi are visible. H&E, ×320

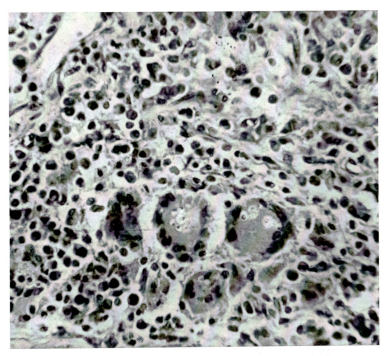

Fig. 17. Paracoccidioidal granuloma. Observe the fungi within the giant cells. H & E, ×320

very difficult to recognize. This histological picture is very similar to that of sarcoidosis (Fig. 19). These epithelioid nodules, either spontaneously or due to the drugs employed, may present regressive changes and become partially or totally fibrotic or hyalinized (Fig. 20). Even in these cases, however, it is possible to recognize the fungi or their remains. In muco-cutaneous lesions the tissue reaction is almost always of a mixed type, granulomatous and pyogenic with microabscesses. The same phenomenon occurs in pulmonary lesions infected secondarily where the fungi are seen mixed with polymorphonuclear leucocytes. Rarely, the inflammatory reaction is completely diffuse, without nodule formation, and with an infiltrate composed mainly of lymphocytes, plasmacytes, histiocytes and a few giant cells.

Generally it may be said that *P. brasiliensis* is easy to recognize with H & E in fresh, active lesions. In granulomas, however, its recognition is not always easy, either because the fungus is not present in the section examined, or because it is not present in its characteristic form. In the former case it becomes necessary to prepare sections cut in series, and in the latter, to stain sections with GMS (Gomori's methenamine-silver nitrate; Grocott's stain modified for fungi), PAS or Gridley. In recent necrotic lesions, the fungi may be identified with H & E, but in old, encapsulated, necrotic foci it is necessary to use GMS. The systematic study of smears is highly recommended for any lesion in which a mycotic etiology is suspected, as they are a valuable diagnostic aid.

In histologic sections *P. brasiliensis* is not always seen in its characteristic multiple budding form: consequently it must be distinguished from other fungi.

A. *Small forms* (3—4 micra), seen infrequently, may be confused with *H. capsulatum*, especially when they are intracellular. In this case, a GMS stain must

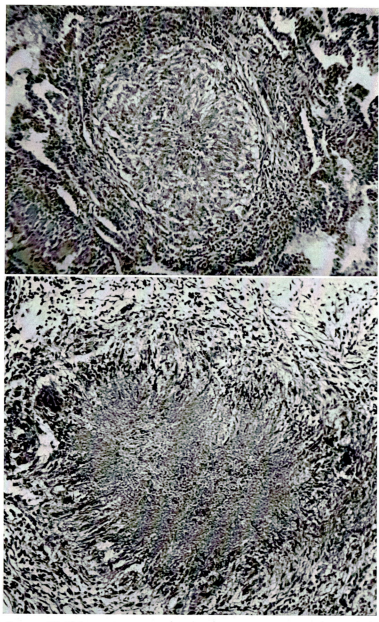

Fig. 18. Paracoccidioidal granuloma (lung). Epithelioid nodules with slight (upper) and extensive (lower) central necrosis, similar to tubercles. No fungi are visible. H&E, ×150 and ×320

be made; if it is *P. brasiliensis*, the yeast-like elements are not so uniform in size as with *H. capsulatum*, and, on examination of many sections in series, a few large elements, with or without buds, may be found (Fig. 21). This difficulty is confronted more frequently in old, encapsulated, necrotic foci. In these latter cases, the distribution of the fungi is helpful for orientation. In cases of paracoccidioi-

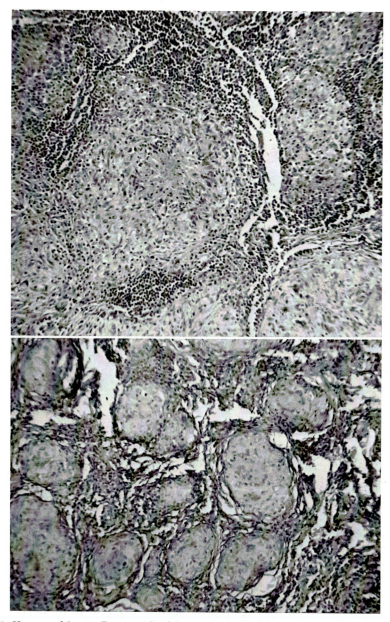

Fig. 19. Upper and lower: Paracoccidioidal granuloma. Nodules similar to those observed in
sarcoidosis (without caseous necrosis). No fungi are visible. H&E, ×150

domycosis the fungi are located in the periphery of the focus as well as in its
center (Fig. 22), and principally in the limit between the capsule and the necrotic
area, while in histoplasmosis the distribution is more central than peripheral.

B. The *medium-sized forms* may be confused with *C. neoformans* in encapsulated
necrotic lesions. Here the distinction is easier; using Mayer's mucicarmin or a PAS
stain, the mucinous capsule of this fungus is made visible.

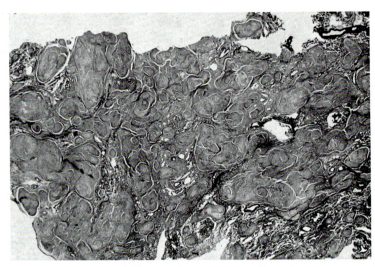

Fig. 20. Multiple nodules, almost all of which are hyalinized. Pulmonary paracoccidioidomycosis treated with sulfadiazine. No fungi are seen. H & E, ×45

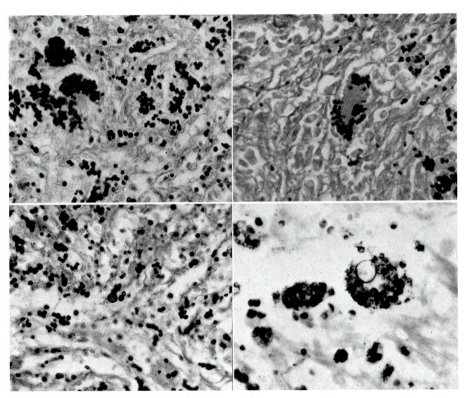

Fig. 21. Small forms of *P. brasiliensis* (positive culture) similar to *H. capsulatum*. GMS, ×360.
Upper left: In an encapsulated, necrotic focus; upper right: In a granulomatous lesion: some
fungi inside a giant cell; lower left: Observe the varying size of the fungi; lower right: Many
small elements and one large one are seen inside a giant cell

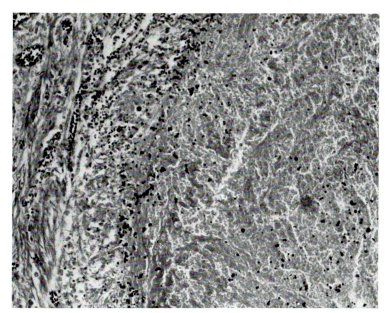

Fig. 22. *P.brasiliensis* (positive culture). Observe the distribution of the fungi in the periphery and in the center of an encapsulated necrotic focus, ×150. GMS.

C. The *large, empty forms* without budding may be mistaken for empty elements of *C.immitis*, in encapsulated, necrotic foci. Serial sections, using a GMS stain, may unmask the endosporulation of this latter fungus or the multiple-budding appearance of *P.brasiliensis*. Also a knowledge of the geographic distribution of these two mycoses, so well defined, is helpful for orienting the diagnosis.

D. Confusion with *B.dermatitidis* is improbable from a practical point of view, since the geographic distribution of both fungi is well known. (Only one case of North American blastomycosis in South America is known, diagnosed in Venezuela by POLO and collaborators in 1954). From a morphologic point of view, *B.dermatitidis* has well-defined characteristics, such as a thick wall, budding with stems, etc.

When a mycotic lesion is suspected, it is always advisable to systematically practice a culture, a smear, and histopathologic examination of the material.

The different nature of the lesions will be described for each organ in particular.

Clinical Forms

Paracoccidioidomycosis, a disease that poses many unanswered questions, has been considered progressive and fatal if not treated promptly and adequately. Nevertheless, tests with paracoccidioidin carried out by LACAZ et al. (1959), FAVA-NETTO and RAPHAEL (1961), RESTREPO et al. (1968), and others, have demonstrated positivity in persons without apparent manifestations of the disease. LACAZ (1967) studied serologic reactions of paracoccidioidin-positive persons, with or without clinical and radiological manifestations of the disease, using complement-fixation and precipitin tests, and obtained positive reactions. In two autopsied cases of persons that died of other diseases, we found pulmonary calcifications in which we were able to demonstrate *P.brasiliensis* in its characteristic form (Fig. 23). These observations lead one to believe in the existence of a subclinical form of paracoccidioidomycosis.

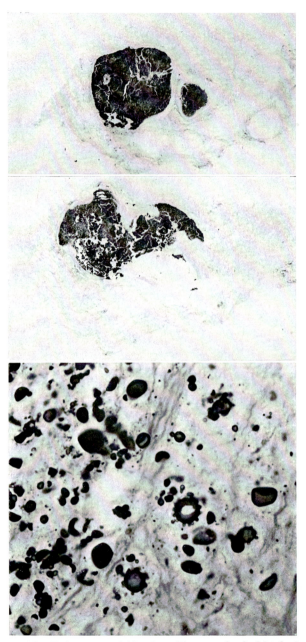

Fig. 23. Top and middle: Pulmonary calcifications. Photograph of a histologic section stained by v. Kossa's method for the demonstration of calcium; lower: *P. brasiliensis* stained with GMS in the calcified focus seen in top figure

Cases of paracoccidioidomycosis described in Europe or in North America in persons who developed the disease 10, 20, 30 or more years after having left endemic Latin American regions show that there are asymptomatic or subclinical infections that may remain dormant or latent for many years and later become active when the patient is exposed to unfavorable conditions. The length of time between the infection and the appearance of clinical manifestations is, therefere, not known.

Brazilian authors have classified the anatomicoclinical manifestations of the disease in the following manner:

1. Tegumentary forms (mucocutaneous).
2. Lymphadenoid forms.
3. Visceral forms.
4. Mixed forms.

This classification may be accepted on a provisional basis. Until we clarify the unknown factors of the disease and learn more about its evolution it is arbitrary to subdivide it into static forms. There are indications of the existence of subclinical paracoccidioidomycosis, and in a few cases spontaneous cicatrization of super-ficial ulcerations has been observed clinically. This does not signify cure since the granulomatous lesion may persist underneath. However, the disease is considered in the majority of cases to have a chronic, progressive and fatal evolution.

Because of the lack of knowledge of certain aspects of the disease, it is pre-ferable to describe the lesions according to the different organs and systems in which they occur, with the pertinent observations, rather than to describe definite anatomicoclinical forms which may be modified when the portal of entry of the fungus is known with certainty.

The description of the lesions is based on the study of 204 biopsies from various sites, predominantly mucous membrane, and 33 autopsies, 24 of which were performed and studied by the author. Table 1 indicates the organ and tissue involvement of the autopsies by lesions of paracoccidioidomycosis. Histopatho-logical examination of all the organs was performed in the period between 1954 and 1968.

Table 1. *Lesions of paracoccidioidomycosis noted in the organs and tissues of 33 autopsied cases*

	1937 – 1948 Autopsies: 11 Cases Nos. of Case	1954 – 1968 Autopsies: 22 Cases Nos. of Cases
Mouth and Pharynx	5	16
Larynx	3	12
Lungs	9	22
Trachea	2	4
Stomach and intestines	5	7
Esophagus	0	1
Liver	5	17
Lymph Nodes	9	22
Spleen	3	18
Adrenals	5	21
Kidneys	2	3
Testicles	2	1
Aorta	2	3
Central Nervous System	1	3
Bone	0	5
Skin	4	12

Mucocutaneous Lesions

Research on mucocutaneous lesions has been reported by Brazilian authors, AGUIAR PUPO and CUNHA MOTTA (1936), OLIVEIRA RIBERO (1942), and others.

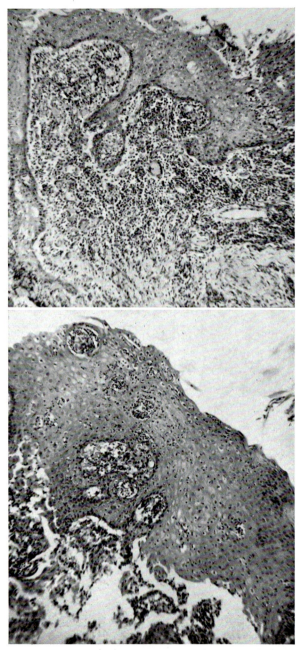

Fig 24. Pseudo-epitheliomatous hyperplasia with diffuse, chronic inflammation of the dermis. Observe the giant cells of the Langhans type. H&E, ×45; lower: Intra-epithelial abscesses with fungus. H&E, ×150

Lesions of the mucosa are the most frequent, and are located in the mouth, nose, larynx and anorectal regions. Pure cutaneous lesions are rare; they are generally a consequence of the spread of mucosal lesions and are located around the natural orifices.

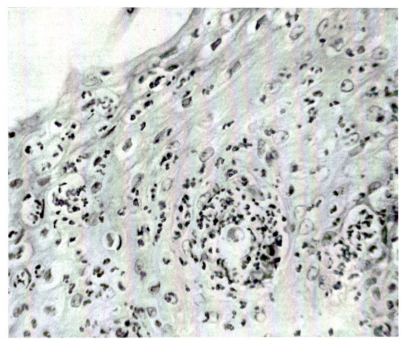

Fig. 25. Detail of the previous photograph. Observe an abscess with a fungus in the center.
H & E, ×150

a) Mucosal Lesions

Mucosal lesions appear as superficial ulcerations with poorly defined borders. They bleed little, are often painless and show a pink granular base with yellow spots (abscesses). Occasionally, they are penetrating lesions, which may reach neighboring osseous structures.

1. The buccal mucosa is most frequently affected. The lesions are located in the gums, lips, cheeks, pharynx, tonsils, tongue, and angles of the lips. The patients report varied symptoms, such as discomfort upon opening the mouth or when chewing or swallowing, a burning sensation or pain, edema, sialorrhea and loose teeth. At times the ulcerations are asymptomatic and appear after extraction of decayed teeth. Periodontitis has also been reported; *P. brasiliensis* has been found in dental apical granulomas with or without ulceration of the gums. Destructive lesions may appear in the soft palate, pillars of the tonsils and uvula and may spread to the hypopharynx. The tonsils may also become ulcerated. RAPHAEL DA NOVA (1940) described the so-called "hidden paracoccidioidal tonsillitis" in which the macroscopic appearance does not raise the suspicion of mycotic lesions. Almost always these mucosal lesions are accompanied by satellite adenitis, which may be evident in some cases and barely noticeable in others.

The histopathological characteristic of lesions of the buccal mucosa and, in general, of any mucosal lesion produced by *P. brasiliensis* is a pseudo-epitheliomatous hyperplasia combined with purulent and granulomatous inflammation (Figs. 24, 25). Frequently there are intraepithelial abscesses which drain on the surface. In this type of lesion, in addition to the epithelioid granulomas with giant cells and polymorphonuclear neutrophilic leucocytes, there is frequently diffuse

plasmacytic and lymphocytic infiltration. The fungi are easily seen to be intra-
and extracellular. Etiologic diagnosis of mucosal lesions is not difficult. It is only
necessary to scrape the lesion and place the material obtained together with a drop
of water between a glass slide and a coverslip, and to observe the fresh preparation
under the microscope. With experience, the multiple budding cell of the fungus

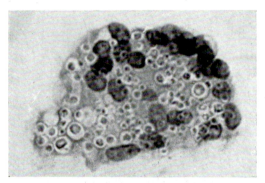

Fig. 26. Giant cell with many *P. brasiliensis* cells. Smear from ulcerative lesion in the mouth.
H & E, ×320

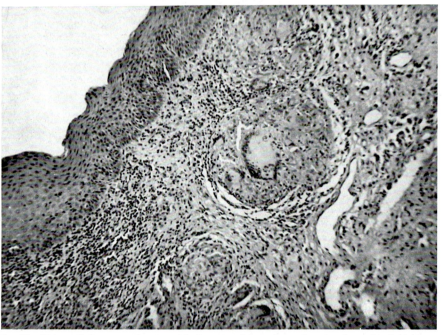

Fig. 27. Giant-cellular granulomatous lesions in the corium of a vocal cord; there is no
ulceration. H & E, ×150

can be easily recognized. Smears of ulcerous lesions can also be made; they should
be fixed by heat or ether-alcohol and stained with H & E.; the fungus, in its
characteristic form, can then be recognized within the giant cells (Fig. 26).

Clinically, it has been observed that small, superficial ulcerations may heal
spontaneously, but that the granulomatous lesion remains in the corium (Fig. 27).

2. The nasal mucosa is frequently affected. The lesions may be ulcerous or polypoid, and sometimes destroy the cartilage. The lesions may simulate epitheliomas.

3. Lesions of the laryngeal mucosa may be congestive, granulomatous, ulcerated or pseudo-tumoral and are located in the epiglottis, vocal chords or, arytenoids. Frequently there is destruction of the epiglottis, sometimes causing stenosis. Patients complain of dysphonia and sore throat.

4. Lesions of the tracheal and bronchial mucosa are not frequent. In rare cases, we have observed deep ulcerations with destruction of cartilage in the lower third of the trachea with a diffuse mediastinitis.

5. The anorectal mucosa has been reported as a portal of entry for *P.brasiliensis* (Sodre and Cerruti, 1930; Monteiro and Fialho, 1937). Proliferative lesions resembling polyps or condylomas and ulcers have been described (Fig. 28).

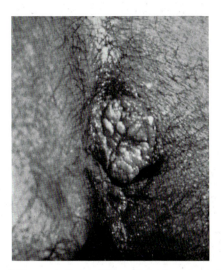

Fig. 28. Lesions of the anus of a cauliflower type (courtesy of Dr. H. Garcia)

b) Cutaneous Lesions

Primary cutaneous lesions are rare; almost always they are a propagation of contiguous mucosal lesions, and frequently appear in the mouth or nose (Figs. 29, 30). Isolated cutaneous lesions located on the eyelids, chest, back, perianal region, or back of the hand, can be explained by autoinoculation of pre-existing small wounds which are contaminated secondarily. Cutaneous manifestations are polymorphous. They may be papular, nodular, ulcerous, ulcerous with crusts, warty, or vegetative. Brazilian authors have described these lesions at length and have named them according to their macroscopic appearance. Silva-Lacaz (1967) summarizes them as follows:

Papular dermo-epidermal
Papulopustular dermo-epidermal
Tuberous dermo-epidermal
Dermo-epidermal of ulcerous crusty type
Vegetative dermo-epidermal
Tuberculoid dermo-epidermal
Scrofulodermal

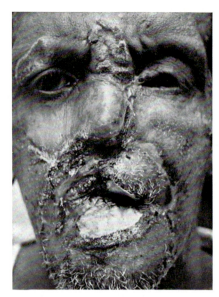

Fig. 29. Muco-cutaneous ulcerative lesions of the mouth, nose, eyelids and eyebrows (courtesy of Dr. Dante Borelli)

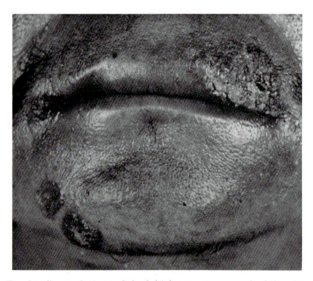

Fig. 30. Crusty lesions of the labial commissure and of the chin

Many of these lesions are mucocutaneous and not simply cutaneous. There are also secondary cutaneous lesions after softening and fistulization of affected lymph nodes or of subcutaneous abscesses.

The histopathologic lesions are the same as those described for the mucosal forms, that is, pseudo-epitheliomatous hyperplasia of the epidermis with multiple intraepithelial abscesses and diffuse granulomatous and purulent inflammation of the dermis. The fungi can be easily recognized in smears of the lesions and examination is made in the same way as for the mucosal lesions.

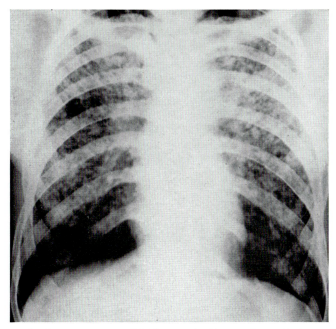

Fig. 31. Advanced pulmonary paracoccidioidomycosis. Observe the similarity of the lesions on both sides and the hypertransparency of the lung bases

Pulmonary Lesions

Pulmonary lesions are very frequent. FIALHO (1947) found them in 84% of cases; ANGULO (1948) in 81.81%; and BRASS (1966) in 72.7%. In 204 cases of paracoccidioidomycosis that we have diagnosed by biopsy (fragments of oral mucosa, lymph nodes, etc.) 90%, at some time in the course of their disease, presented radiological shadows in the lungs attributable to paracoccidioidomycosis. In 33 cases of autopsies which we have performed or observed, 31 (93.93%) were found to have pulmonary lesions of one form or another. From 1954 until the present, all of the autopsies with paracoccidioidomycosis (22 of the 33 cases) which we have observed had pulmonary lesions.

There is no radiographic finding in the lung characteristic of the disease. The shadows observed may be: a) nodular (small, medium-sized or large) b) trabecular, or c) trabeculo-nodular. The latter are the most frequent. In the majority of cases, the lesions are bilateral, with a tendency toward symmetry and with a predominance in the middle and lower fields (Figs. 31, 32, 33). In the milder forms, the lesions are more pronounced in the upper lung fields. Moderate and advanced forms are accompanied by increased radiolucency in the lower fields due to emphysema. Shadows of consolidation of the pneumonic type are rare. Cavities are infrequent, and are observed in advanced cases of confluent trabeculo-nodular lesions and in pneumonic and bronchopneumonic forms (Fig. 34). They may have an irregular or a circular shape with sharp borders as in tuberculous cavities. In the last few years we have seen some cases of pneumonic lesions in patients treated for supposed tuberculosis who had received steroids as well as anti-tuberculous therapy. In children and young adults, large mediastinal adenopathies with slight pulmonary participation, similar to those observed in lymphomas and Hodgkin's disease, are a common finding (Fig. 35).

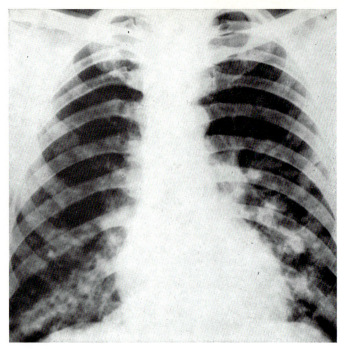

Fig. 32. Pulmonary paracoccidioidomycosis: Predominantly basal lesions (moderately advanced case)

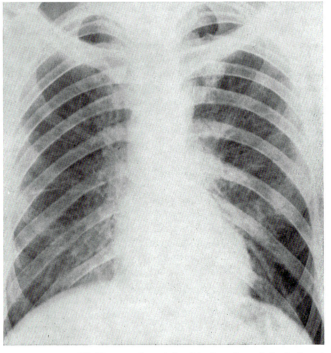

Fig. 33. Pulmonary paracoccidioidomycosis: minimal trabeculo-nodular lesions in a case with muco-cutaneous lesions (etiology confirmed by open-chest lung biopsy)

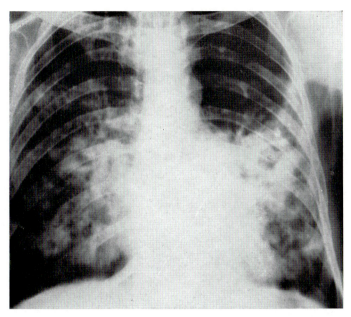

Fig. 34. Pulmonary paracoccidioidomycosis: confluent para-cardiac lesions in both bases with "cavitary" shadows. Hypertransparency of the upper left lobe due to bullous emphysema

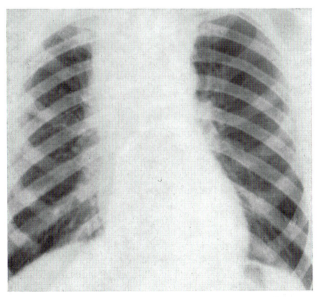

Fig. 35. Mediastinal widening due to enlarged lymph nodes. Minimal lesions in the lungs. Clinical suspicion of Hodgkin's disease

The symptomatology is that which is common to other respiratory diseases: cough, almost always a dry one, and dyspnea on exertion; hemoptysis is infrequent. In many cases the slight symptomatology contrasts markedly with the wide extension of the pulmonary lesions, as shown in the radiographic findings.

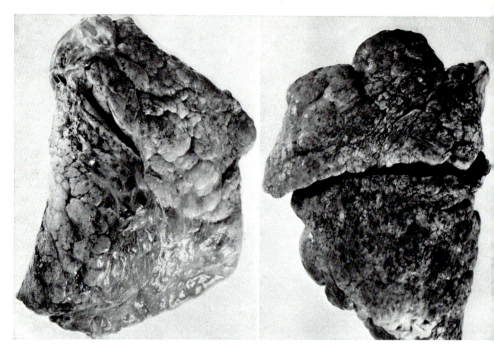

Fig. 36. External appearance of the lung in paracoccidioidomycosis. Observe the surface irregularity and the focal thickening of the pleura (left), and particularly the emphysema (right)

Grossly, the lungs show chronic, advanced, or disseminated lesions in some cases. In other cases there is pronounced pulmonary fibrosis with cor pulmonale. On a few occasions we have observed minimal or discrete pulmonary lesions in cases of accidental death or during exploratory thoracotomies for diagnostic purposes.

In advanced cases, the lungs show, exteriorly, a discrete or moderate thickening of the visceral pleura, with a surface that is very irregular due to depressions and projections, the former corresponding to areas of fibrosis and the latter to areas of emphysema (Fig. 36). The emphysema, a constant finding in paracoccidioidomycosis, may be bullous or diffusely alveolar of a pan-acinar type. Rupture of the bullae may cause spontaneous pneumothorax, a not infrequent complication of this disease (Figs. 37, 38). In contrast to other chronic pulmonary inflammations, pleural adhesions or obliteration of the pleural cavity is infrequent.

The appearance of the cut surface of the lung is variable. The interstitial form is characterized grossly by thickening of the interlobular septa, and a net-like appearance due to dilated alveoli (Fig. 39). The thickening in the para-hilar regions decreases progressively as the septa approach the surface of the lung. This *interstitial form*, which corresponds radiologically to the trabecular shadow, is accompanied by a diffuse pan-acinar emphysema and generally does not contain either nodules or cavities. Those cavities that may be found eventually are emphysematous, intra-parenchymal bullae. Microscopically, the thickening of the interlobular and alveolar septa is due to collagen fibers, with or without remnants of granulomatous lesions. The alveoli are usually free of exudate and the blood vessels show marked intimal proliferation which may obliterate their lumina.

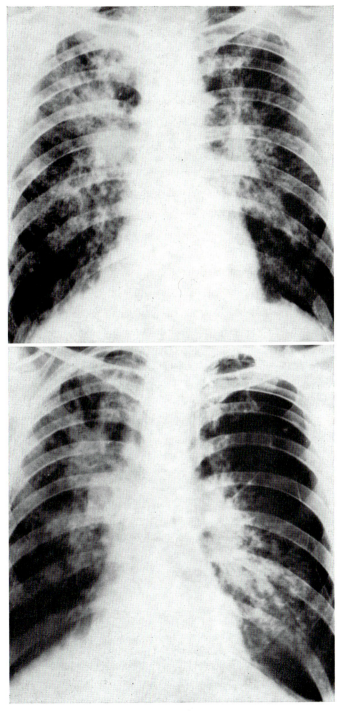

Fig. 37. Top: Pulmonary paracoccidioidomycosis; bottom: the same case with left spontaneous pneumothorax

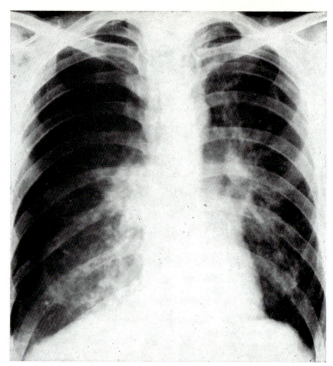

Fig. 38. The same case with bilateral spontaneous pneumothorax

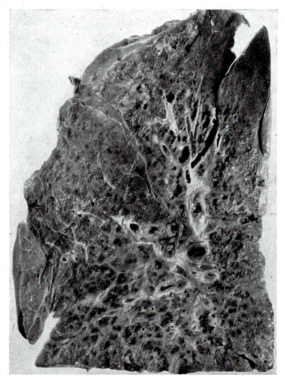

Fig. 39. Pulmonary paracoccidioidomycosis, interstitial form

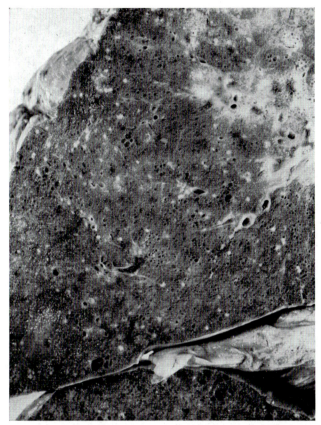

Fig. 40. Pulmonary paracoccidioidomycosis: miliary form

Rarely, intravascular granulomas may be recognized. This interstitial form is associated with hypertrophy of the right side of the heart.

In the *nodular form*, the appearance of the cut surface of the lung is variable. The nodular lesion may be: a) of small granules (Fig. 40), miliary, (1—2 millimeters in diameter); b) of large granules (4 or more millimeters); c) acinous; and d) acino-nodular (Fig. 41). Grossly the nodules are grayish white or yellowish white. The first two forms are rounded and the last two are lobulated, and either isolated or confluent, giving the impression, in the latter case, of pneumonic or bronchopneumonic consolidation. In the miliary and non-miliary nodular forms, the similarity of the lesions in both lungs, their distribution, and their uniformity suggest the possibility of hematogenous dissemination from an extra-pulmonary source. In these cases, the finding of fungi in the blood capillaries is the rule. Microscopically the miliary nodules are constituted of epithelioid cells with or without LANGHANS giant cells or foreign body giant cells, and without lymphocytes. They are similar to tubercles, and like them, may become necrotic (Fig. 42). They may soften and form microcavities. These miliary nodules are located in the septa and open into the alveolar spaces.

The larger, non-miliary nodules, are almost always necrotic with a peripheral epithelioid cell reaction and a more or less pronounced fibrous reaction, for the lesions are almost always chronic and of long evolution.

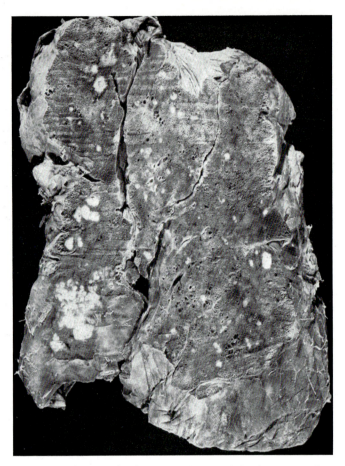

Fig. 41. Pulmonary paracoccidioidomycosis: large nodular form, partially confluent

In the case of acinous and acino-nodular lesions, we may observe also histiocytes, plasmacytes and polymorphonuclear neutrophils in the alveoli, with the formation of micro-abscesses. All these lesions may become softened and give rise to cavities. In acinous and acino-nodular lesions it is easy to find the fungus when a sputum smear is examined; the opposite occurs with miliary nodules. Emphysema, in one or another of its forms, is almost always present.

The *cavitary forms* are not frequent, as they are in tuberculous lesions. They are usually circular with an inner, necrotic surface and an external granulomatous reaction with slight fibrosis, with a somewhat elastic wall, similar to tuberculous cavities that are inflated by a valvular mechanism (Fig. 43). On other occasions the cavities have an external fibrous layer, as in very chronic, fibroulcerative tuberculosis (Fig. 44). There may be bronchopneumonic dissemination, but this never has the extent or the frequency that it does in cavitary tuberculosis.

The *condensed pneumonic or confluent bronchopneumonic forms* with an acute or sub-acute evolution are exceptional. Only in cases of pulmonary paracoccidioidomycosis treated with steroids as supposed cases of tuberculosis, and treated also with specific anti-tuberculous therapy, were the acute excavated pneumonic

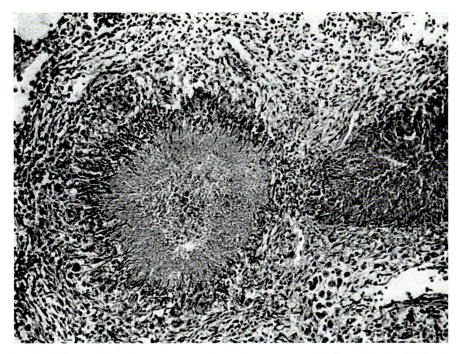

Fig. 42. Miliary nodule with central necrosis: no fungi are seen. H & E, ×320. The GMS stain was positive

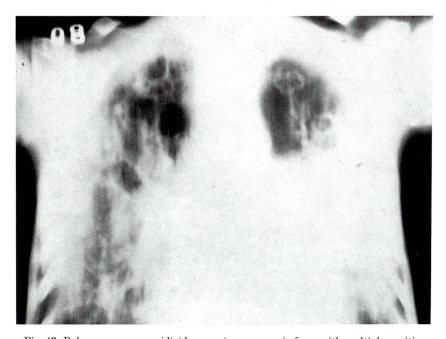

Fig. 43. Pulmonary paracoccidioidomycosis: pneumonic form with multiple cavities

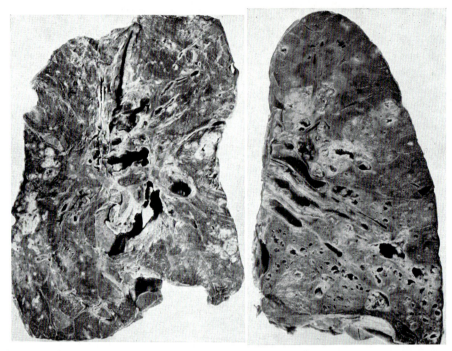

Fig. 44. Left: Pulmonary paracoccidioidomycosis: observe the cavity in the middle right field, and miliary and acinous nodules; right: Pulmonary paracoccidioidomycosis: large nodules partially softened and forming cavities. Bronchiectasis

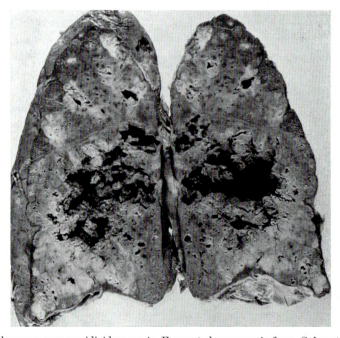

Fig. 45. Pulmonary paracoccidioidomycosis. Excavated pneumonic form. Subacute evolution

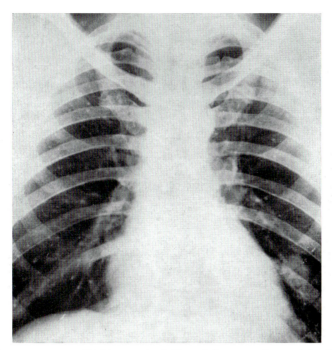

Fig. 46. Pulmonary paracoccidioidomycosis. Solitary left paracardiac nodule. (The calcified small nodules correspond to a residual histoplasmosis)

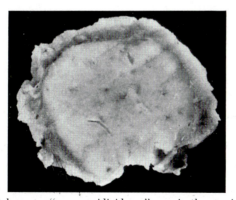

Fig. 47. Pulmonary "paracoccidioidoma" seen in the previous X-ray

forms present, similar to ulcerated caseous pneumonias (Fig. 45) or to abscessed pneumonias.

All forms of pulmonary paracoccidioidomycosis were found to have lesions of the hilar or mediastinal lymph nodes, either in the form of granulomatous adenitis, abscessed adenitis or caseous adenitis, focal or diffuse.

The *solitary nodular form*, of the coin-lesion type, frequent in histoplasmosis and coccidioidomycosis, has not been described in paracoccidioidomycosis. In our material we have observed two cases, one in an autopsy, and the other in a segmental resection (Fig. 46), each with a round, solitary nodule, grossly composed of a rounded, pneumonic focus (Fig. 47), well limited, and grayish white. Micro-

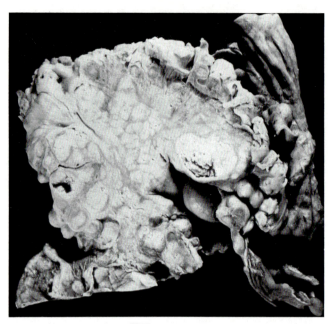

Fig. 48. Caseous mesenteric lymph nodes, similar to those observed in intestinal tuberculosis

scopically there was granulomatous pneumonitis with numerous fungi. In neither of these two cases could the existence of a regional caseous adenitis be confirmed, which would have represented the lymph node focus of a bipolar complex, not yet described in paracoccidioidomycosis.

The lesions of the larynx, trachea and bronchi were mentioned earlier in the section dealing with lesions of the mucous membranes.

The pulmonary lesions have been studied by Basgal (1931), Cunha Motta (1946), Padilha Goncalves and Bardy (1946), Santos Silva (1946), Fialho (1946) and Machado Filho (1960).

Lesions of Lymph Nodes

Lesions of lymph nodes are almost as frequent as are mucocutaneous and pulmonary ones. Usually they are manifested by a slight increase in the size of the cervical lymph nodes when the lesions are located in the mouth or neighboring regions. The adenopathy may be solitary or multiple, isolated or confluent, elastic or hard, and usually painless. The glands may soften, form abscesses or phlegmons, usually cold ones, that terminate by fistulization.

In the thick or thin greenish-yellow pus, numerous parasites are often easily observed when the material is examined between a slide and a coverslip, whether in a fresh preparation or in a smear stained with hematoxylin and eosin or other stain.

Sometimes, for example with superficial ulcerative lesions of the oropharynx and perhaps with recent muco-cutaneous lesions, the adenopathies may pass unnoticed during a most careful clinical examination. In cases of bilateral pulmonary lesions without apparent muco-cutaneous ones, enlarged mediastinal lymph nodes may be observed in the chest films. It is possible, in these cases, to make a histopathologic diagnosis of the lesions by examining the pre-scalen fat, even when lymph nodes are not palpated.

On the contrary, in the true lymphadenoid form, common in young adults and children, and in the progressive visceral forms of the disease, the lymph nodes are greatly increased in size, either soft or hard, and almost always necrotic. In the young adult and in children, these lesions of lymph nodes may be confused clinically and radiologically with lymphomas (Fig. 35), and anatomically with the caseous lymph nodes of primary tuberculosis (Fig. 48). In these predominantly lymph node forms, all the lymph node groups may be affected, and especially the cervical, mediastinal and abdominal ones. In these cases the pulmonary and mucous membrane participation is very limited.

The adenopathies may have a regional character, cervical with oropharyngeal lesions or inguinal with rectal lesions, or they may be generalized, in which case their appearance may be simultaneous or progressive. The softening and fistulization of superficial adenopathies may give rise to subcutaneous abscesses, and the same process in the deeper ones may cause them to perforate into the natural cavities or into thoracic or abdominal organs.

The histopathologic reaction is generally a granulomatous one with or without necrosis as has already been described. In rare cases a tuberculoid reaction may be seen, similar to that in sarcoidosis, with or without parasites that are sometimes difficult to identify. At other times the appearance of blastomycotic adenitis is that of a massive caseation similar to that of primary tuberculous adenitis, with little or no granulomatous reaction in its periphery.

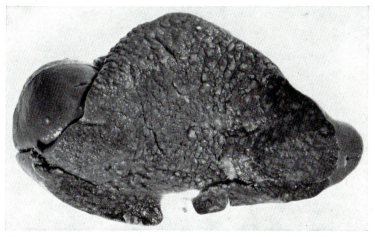

Fig. 49. Multiple nodules in the spleen similar to those observed in miliary tuberculosis. (Child, 9 years old)

Lesions of the Spleen

According to Cunha Motta (1938), the spleen is affected in 98% of cases of paracoccidioidomycosis, with a high frequency of splenomegaly.

Grossly the lesions have a nodular character, either miliary or with larger nodules similar to those observed in splenic tuberculosis (Fig. 49). These necrotic, grayish white or yellowish nodules may be confluent, giving the spleen the appearance that is described in Hodgkin's disease. Many times the spleen is of normal size and without lesions grossly, but the histologic examination demonstrates the presence of granulomas of different stages. In our material, cases with conspicuous gross lesions always coincided with a severe involvement of the lymph nodes and

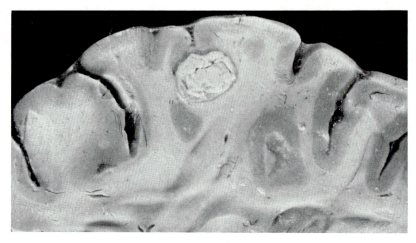

Fig. 50. "Paracoccidioidoma" of the cerebral cortex

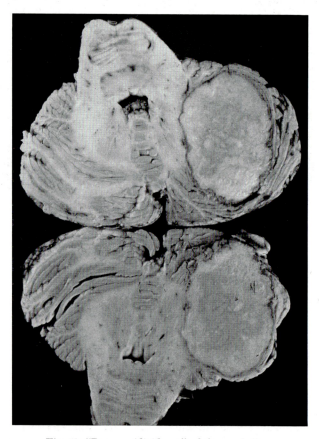

Fig. 51. "Paracoccidioidoma" of the cerebellum

showed a preference for children and young adults. Thromboangiitis of the splenic vessels has also been found, rich in fungi and coinciding with severe lesions of the organ (O'DALY, 1937). Also, traumatic rupture of the spleen has been documented in cases of paracoccidioidomycosis (DIEZ, 1951). Splenomegaly is rare in our material.

Lesions of the Nervous System

Lesions of the central nervous system in paracoccidioidomycosis are infrequent. They are found, principally, in two forms: A) the pseudotumorous form, the so-called "blastomycoma" or "paracoccidioidoma" and B) the meningitic form. The first form, which is the most frequent, manifests itself clinically as a space-occupying lesion and anatomically as a necrotic nodule. These nodules are well circumscribed, similar to "tuberculomas", of a size which varies from several millimeters to several centimeters (Figs. 50, 51), usually solitary, although there may be several, and preferentially situated in the cerebral cortex, in the cere-

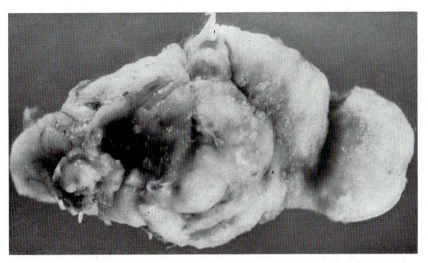

Fig. 52. "Paracoccidioidoma" of the dura mater

bellum, or in the basal ganglia. The histopathological reaction is similar to that in other organs; nevertheless, the lesions are more necrotic and are accompanied by arteritis and by granulomatous phlebitis. The second form, the meningitic, has as a morphological basis a predominantly basal, granulomatous meningitis, similar to the tuberculous one, although diffuse forms may also be observed. These meningeal lesions are propagated to the cerebral substance via the VIRCHOW-ROBIN spaces, especially at the level of the hypothalamus and of the lateral fissure. We have seen pseudotumorous forms in the dura mater with clinical characteristics of meningiomas (Fig. 52). Lesions of the spinal cord are very rare.

Lesions of the Cardiovascular System

The cardiac muscle is not a favored site for *P. brasiliensis*. CUNHA MOTTA (1948) described a case of granulomatous myocarditis and pericarditis. The few cases of myocardial lesions that have been described correspond to miliary hematogenous

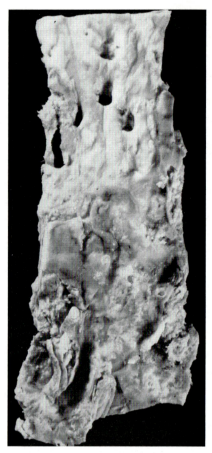

Fig. 53. Paracoccidioidomycosis of the abdominal aorta

dissemination and the lesions were found to be histiocytic or epithelioid granulomas with giant cells. In our material we have found only one case; one with a granulomatous myocarditis that coincided with a miliary pulmonary form, but we were not able to identify the fungus despite a careful examination of many histologic sections. BRASS (1966) found also only one case in his material. In the bibliography that we have consulted, we found no cases of blastomycotic endocarditis. Endocarditis has been described in other mycoses, for example, in histoplasmosis.

Paracoccidioidomycosis of the Aorta. In contrast to the heart, the aorta and its main branches are affected in the course of generalized paracoccidioidomycosis. GUERRA (1940) and ANGULO (1948) published the first cases of this curious localization. It is noteworthy that an organ that is seldom damaged, except by arteriosclerosis and syphilis, should be affected by this disease with relative frequency. In our five cases, the lesions were limited to the abdominal aorta, with or without participation of the iliac, renal, mesenteric or celiac arteries. In all of these cases there was a severe, ulcerated and thrombosed arteriosclerosis, and it was the microscopic examination that revealed the presence of numerous fungi, not only in the thrombi but also in granulomatous lesions within the arterial walls.

Grossly, there are no characteristic lesions; the appearance is simply that of a severe arteriosclerosis (Fig. 53) which is ulcerated and thrombosed, at times to the extent of obliteration of the arterial lumen with the production of ischemic changes in the lower extremities. BRASS (1966), in his material of 33 autopsies, found 3 cases of blastomycotic aortitis. We have also observed a case of granulomatous arteritis of the renal artery, and another with similar involvement of the splenic artery. Our impression is that these arterial lesions are secondary, favored by the pre-existent arteriosclerosis. We know that in critical, generalized cases the fungi are present in the blood stream, and from there they may penetrate the vascular wall through the intimal lesions. The abundance of fungi in the thrombi and the many different growth forms they present lead us to believe that the thrombi make as excellent a culture medium as do purulent foci. Within the thrombi small abscesses may also be observed.

Nevertheless, the arterial lesions are not limited to the larger arteries. In miliary forms, we have seen endarteritis and panarteritis of the small pulmonary vessels. In necrotic cerebral foci a diffuse arteritis is also frequent. Rarely we have seen a granulomatous, circumscribed, nodular endarteritis (Fig. 54).

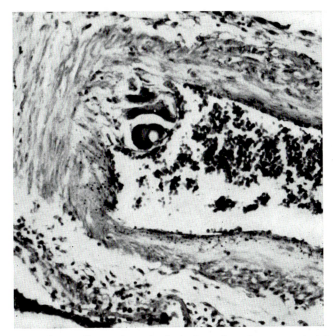

Fig. 54. Giant cell granuloma in the intima of a pulmonary arteriole

Lesions of the Digestive System

The lesions of the oral mucosa were described with the muco-cutaneous lesions. Both the mucous and the cutaneous lesions are less serious and less extensive in those patients who inhabit regions near the equator. In our material, cases similar to those observed, for example, in the state of Sao Paulo (Brazil) are rare. Lesions of the buccal mucosa are mainly ulcers of the lips, gums, palate, tonsils. They are superficial with a smooth or granular base and usually with exudate (Fig. 55). Seldom do they spread in depth and damage the bone.

Lesions of the *tongue* (Fig. 56) are ulcers located on the borders or on the anterior half of the dorsal surface. Sometimes they simulate carcinomas.

Lesions of the *pharynx* are almost always extensions from the buccal mucosa. The *esophagus* is affected only exceptionally in paracoccidioidomycosis: in the literature we found no references to it. In our material we observed one case of an ulceration located in its middle third (Fig. 57) which originated by propagation from a blastomycotic, mediastinal, caseous adenitis which perforated into the lumen of the esophagus, and whose borders were infiltrated by granulomatous lesions.

The stomach is rarely affected in this disease. In only one case in our material did we find ulcerations in the gastric mucosa but it was not possible to identify fungi. SANTOS and ALMEIDA (1932) described a case of perforation of a blasto-mycotic gastric ulcer.

Intestine: The various portions of the small and large intestine may be affected in paracoccidioidomycosis, and the preferred sites are the ileum, ileocecal region and appendix. The lesions are ulcers, separated from one another by a distance of from several millimeters to two or three centimeters, or they may be confluent and give the appearance of a diffuse lesion (Fig. 58). They may penetrate in depth,

35*

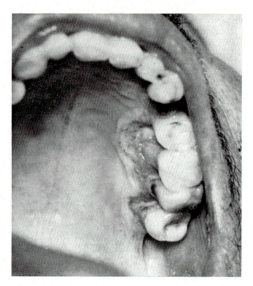

Fig. 55. Ulcerative lesions of the roof of the mouth

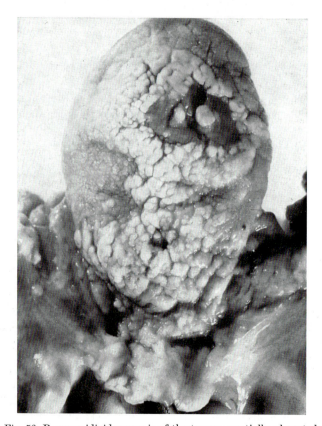

Fig. 56. Paracoccidioidomycosis of the tongue, partially ulcerated

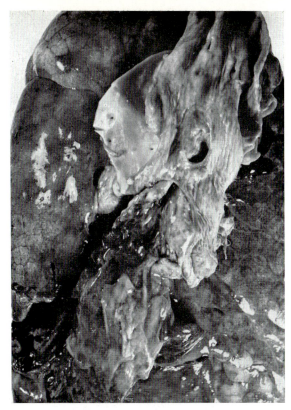

Fig. 57. Paracoccidioidomycosis of the esophagus. Perforated ulcer in the middle third

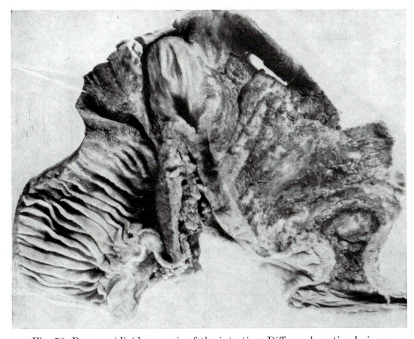

Fig. 58. Paracoccidioidomycosis of the intestine. Diffuse ulcerative lesions

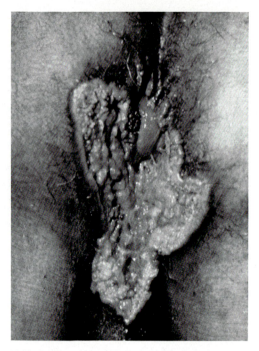

Fig. 59. Extensive ulceration of the perianal region

perforate into the peritoneal cavity and give origin to a blastomycotic peritonitis. We share the opinion of Cunha Motta (1945) that the intestinal lesions are produced by hematogenous or lymphatic dissemination, as we have sometimes observed granulomatous lesions in the lymph follicles with integrity of the intestinal mucosa, which at a later date may ulcerate. The more serious cases of intestinal lesions in our material coincided with extensive necrosis of superficial and deep lymph nodes, especially in children or young adults. Using our cases as a basis for an opinion, it is difficult to conceive of the intestine as a portal of entry of the organism.

The rectum is a relatively frequent site of ulcers and some consider it a portal of entry; from the rectum the lesions may spread to the anus and to the peri-anal region (Fig. 59). Mackinnon (1961) has produced rectal lesions in guinea pigs after inoculation through the intracardiac route. Yarzabal (1962) produced proctitis experimentally.

Hepatic Lesions

Hepatic lesions are frequent in generalized cases, almost always being histologic findings which are represented by miliary nodules formed by histiocytes, epithelioid cells, lymphocytes and Langhans or foreign body giant cells in whose interior the fungi are seen (Fig. 60); there may be necrosis or not. Usually these lesions are not noticed grossly, which explains the infrequency in the literature. Sometimes there is clinical hepatomegaly and the diagnosis may be made by biopsy. Cases of obstructive jaundice have been cited (Lacaz, 1967) due to granulomatous lesions of the common duct or to extrinsic compression by enlarged lymph glands (Almeida, 1948).

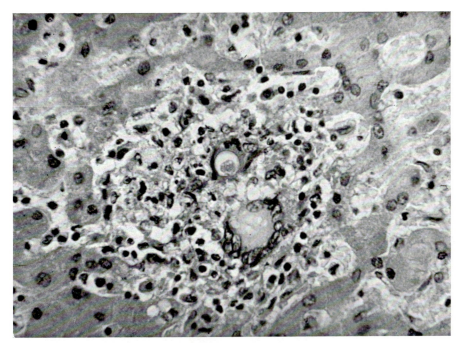

Fig. 60. Miliary dissemination in the liver. Observe the fungi within the giant cells. H & E, ×320

Pancreatic Lesions

Several authors, among them Mosto (1933), Marengo (1934) and Forattini (1946, 1947) have described pancreatic lesions. They may be caused by hematogenous spread or by extension from neighbouring blastomycotic adenitis.

Lesions of Endocrine Glands

Endocrine glands may be affected in cases of paracoccidioidomycosis, and among them, the most frequently affected are the adrenals. These lesions are not only important pathologically but also clinically, because of the clinical manifestations. (Azevedo, 1934; Prado, 1944; Silva, 1952).

The incidence of the localization of *P. brasiliensis* in the adrenals is high, as is demonstrated by statistical studies. In our second series of autopsies, between 1954 and 1968, the incidence was 95.4%. Brass (1966) found 81.8%. Del Negro (1961), in 53 cases of paracoccidioidomycosis, found adrenal lesions to be in third place, after pulmonary and lymph node lesions. Mackinnon (1959) has confirmed this high frequency experimentally.

The gross appearance (Figs. 61, 62) of the adrenal lesions may vary from one or several necrotic or granulomatous foci of several millimeters in diameter to a diffuse necrosis of all or almost all the gland, unilateral or bilateral, with a considerable increase in its weight and size. In our material each has weighed as much as 50 grs. The necrotic foci may be located in the cortex or in the medulla. When the necrosis is diffuse, compact, and yellowish white, the appearance is that of a caseous tuberculosis; at other times, when the necrosis is soft and greenish in color, the appearance is more like that of an abscess. In these advanced cases, the glands are adherent to neighboring tissues.

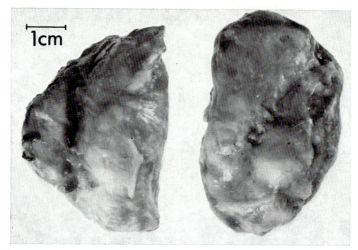

Fig. 61. Paracoccidioidomycosis of the adrenal gland. External appearance

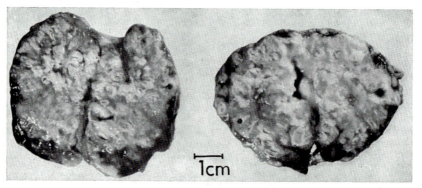

Fig. 62. Paracoccidioidomycosis of the adrenal gland. Cut surface; observe the extensive necrosis

Sometimes these cases with advanced adrenal lesions show an absence of grossly significant foci in other organs. In three of our cases severe lesions of the adrenals coincided with interstitial lesions of the lungs (Fig. 39), which simulated a diffuse fibrosis and which only upon microscopic examination revealed the existence of granulomas, not only in the septa but also intravascularly. In smears prepared from necrotic adrenal tissue or in histologic sections, one's attention is called to the polymorphism of the fungus as to size, appearance and form, and one may even see segmented "germinating tubes" (Fig. 63).

Del Negro (1961) studied the functional disturbances of the adrenal glands in generalized paracoccidioidomycosis and found diverse degrees of insuffiency, from a "diminished adrenocortical reserve", without symptomatology or clinical signs, to an Addison's syndrome with all its signs and symptoms. Marsiglia (1966) also found signs of adrenal insufficiency in generalized paracoccidioidomycosis.

There is no satisfactory explanation for the frequency of the adrenal lesions. Experimentally, Mackinnon (1960) observed in rats that the organs most frequently affected were those of lower temperature. Brass (1966) thinks that the frequency may be related to steroid production.

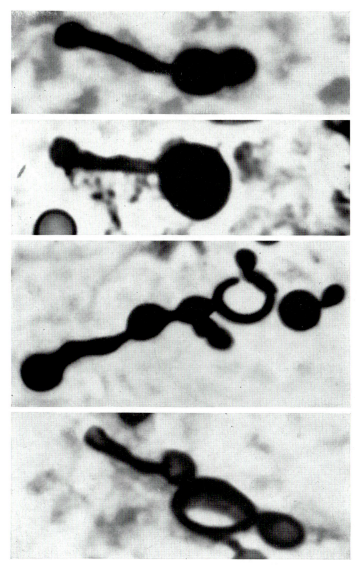

Fig. 63. Histologic section of the adrenal gland. Observe the elongated forms of *P.brasiliensis*. The "germinating tubes" show transverse segmentation. GMS, ×450

Lesions of the *thyroid gland*, on the other hand, are rare (FLAVIANO SILVA, 1936; FIALHO A., 1960). When present, they almost always take the form of miliary nodules in generalized cases. At other times, as in the case of FIALHO, the lesion is a necrotic focus of approximately 1 cm in diameter, propagated directly from a lymph node.

Neither in our material nor in the literature did we find lesions of the *parathyroid glands*.

Freire, cited by FIALHO (1960), found a case with necrosis of the *pituitary gland*, with numerous fungi. In our material we found no pituitary lesions.

Urinary Tract

Renal lesions are infrequent. In 5 cases of generalized paracoccidioidomycosis we found lesions composed of small, necrotic or granulomatous nodules from 1 to 2 millimeters in diameter, which were isolated, located in the cortex, and simulated small abscesses or a miliary tuberculosis. One case was associated with a blasto-mycotic arteritis of the renal artery, and the granulomatous foci were disseminated in the cortex and in the medulla. There are no data as to localization in the renal pelvis, ureters or bladder.

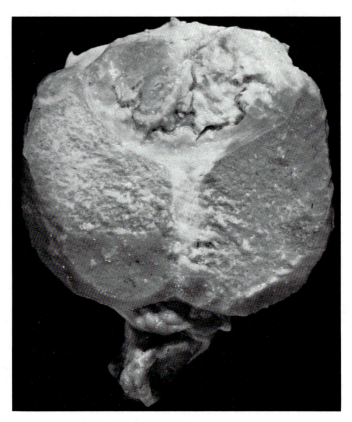

Fig. 64. Caseous epididymitis caused by *P.brasiliensis*

Lesions of the Genital System

The male genital organs may be affected in generalized cases of paracoccidioi-domycosis, although such involvement is rare. Fialho (1960) cites some cases with ulcerations of the skin of the penis and others with granulomatous pros-tatitis. In our material, we found only three cases, two of the testicle and one of the epididymis (Fig. 64), always in the form of circumscribed, necrotic foci between 0.4 and 1.2 cm in diameter. The lesions of the epididymis are very similar to the tuberculous ones. Neither in our material nor in the literature consulted by us did we find lesions in female genital organs.

Osteoarticular Lesions

Osseous lesions are found relatively frequently during the course of generalized paracoccidioidomycosis. Nogueira DA SILVA (1933), LIMA FILHO (1944), TOBÍAS (1944), BARROS (1944), LACAZ (1945), CERRUTI (1948), and FIALHO (1960), published cases of paracoccidioidomycosis with osseous manifestations. MARCANO (1963) observed the case of a child with multiple lesions in the bones of the extremities, thorax, and cranium, and with spontaneous fractures. These lesions may be solitary or multiple, and are constituted of isolated, osteolytic foci (Fig. 65)

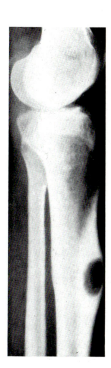

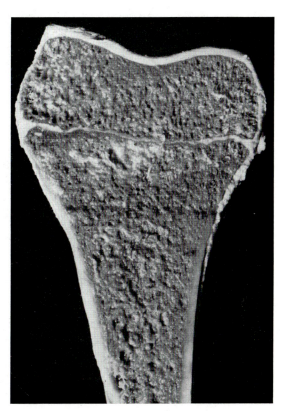

Fig. 65. Paracoccidioidomycosis. Osteolytic lesion

Fig. 66. Paracoccidioidomycosis of the tibia

or of a diffuse osteomyelitis (Figs. 66, 67) with invasion of neighboring soft tissue and formation of subcutaneous abscesses rich in fungi. The bones most frequently affected are the clavicle, the ribs, the vertebrae, and those of the extremities. Our impression is that the involvement of bone by *P. brasiliensis* is more frequent than that indicated in the statistical analyses and that more cases will be recognized by routine X-ray examination. We have seen the osseous lesions in the forms of the disease that are predominantly in lymph nodes, in children and young adults. These lesions improve and heal by scarring to a surprising degree with sulfa treatment.

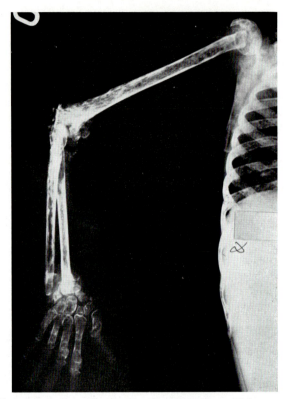

Fig. 67. Osteolytic lesions in the entire upper extremity with multiple, spontaneous fractures

Paracoccidioidomycosis in Association with other Diseases

Paracoccidioidomycosis is found in association with other diseases that frequently attack the lungs, such as tuberculosis (Almeida and Lacaz, 1938; Silva, 1941; Goncalves, 1946; Louzada, 1954 etc.), other mycoses, bronchogenic cancer.

A. Association with mycobacteria. This association is the most frequent. Pollak and Angulo, O. (1966) found 41 cases (35.65%), in a total of 113 cases of paracoccidioidomycosis studied both by culture and by histopathologic methods, in association with mycobacteria. Of these 41, 32 (27.82%) of the 113 cases were *M.tuberculosis* and 9 (7.83%) were atypical mycobacteria. Fialho (1946) shows 12% in association with tuberculosis.

This high frequency of coexistence of these two diseases must be kept in mind. We have seen cases of patients whose mycotic lesions, not previously suspected, were reactivated and aggravated during the course of a treatment which combined steroids with triple, antituberculous therapy.

B. Association with other mycoses. In our autopsy and biopsy material we have been able to confirm by culture and histopathology paracoccidioidomycosis in association with histoplasmosis, crytococcosis (Angulo et al., 1961) and aspergillosis.

C. Association with other diseases. Paracoccidioidomycosis has also been found in association with bronchogenic cancer and Hodgkin's disease (Lacaz et al., 1948).

Immunology

Hypersensitivity: Since 1927 many investigators, particularly in Brazil and Uruguay, have tested various antigens in order to study hypersensitivity in paracoccidioidomycosis. They have used filtered cultures of *P. brasiliensis*, suspensions of tle yeast phase of the fungus, and dilute pus (FONSECA FILHO and AREA LEAO, ALMEIDA and LACAZ in Brazil; MACKINNON and ARTAGAVEYTIA-ALLENDE in Uruguay). These antigens have been tested in small numbers of patients, and most of them have not been standardized, so that definite criteria as to their usefulness cannot be formulated. Recently, RESTREPO prepared two antigens from filtered cultures of the mycelial and yeast forms after extraction with ethanol. It is assumed that the active part of these antigens is a glucopeptide. Restrepo applied the antigen to 20 patients with verified paracoccidioidomycosis, 15 of whom reacted to the extract of mycelial phase and 10 to the extract of the yeast phase. Eight patients also had positive reactions to histoplasmin. The health of nine of the patients was severely impaired; of these nine, six had a positive reaction to the antigen prepared from the mycelial phase and three to that from the yeast phase.

RESTREPO et al. (1968) made a survey among 3,938 persons with their two antigens and obtained 9.6% positive reactions to the mycelial paracoccidioidin and 6.4% to the extract from the yeast phase. Cross reactions were observed with *H. capsulatum*.

Circulating antibodies: The complement fixation and precipitin tests are being used in serologic studies of paracoccidioidomycosis.

The most important studies on the serology of paracoccidioidomycosis were done by FAVA-NETTO (1965), who used the complement fixation test with polysaccharides of the yeast phase of *P. brasiliensis* as antigens as well as the precipitin test in tubes. LACAZ et al. and RESTREPO have studied immunodiffusion.

FAVA-NETTO found that the complement fixation and precipitin tests revealed the presence of circulating antibodies in 94.8% of the patients. Precipitins are the first antibodies to appear and also the first to disappear from the circulation. Sometimes they are the earliest indication of a relapse when they reappear.

A negative reaction to the complement fixation test, following positive ones, is considered to be the certain indication of cure. After effective treatment a low titer of complement fixation may be observed, which FAVA-NETTO called a "serologic scar". Cross reactions of complement fixation with histoplasmin and blastomycin are frequent, and are less so with coccidioidin.

The double diffusion test in agar gel is a simple and practical procedure. In our laboratory, 44% of the positive reactions were in cases in which paracoccidioidomycosis had not been verified by culture. Some of these patients presented enlarged hilar nodes or small parenchymatous lesions, with all bacteriological and mycological tests negative. In 6.5% of the cases, cross reactions with histoplasmin occurred. Double and triple precipitation lines may be observed.

Laboratory Tests

Direct examination: Direct examination of ulcerated mucosal or muco-cutaneous lesions, and of suppurative lymph glands, is simple and the results are satisfactory. Material scraped from ulcers or pus from lymph nodes is mixed with a drop of physiologic saline solution or with 10% sodium hydroxide and examined with the microscope. Smears may be made from biopsy material taken from the lesions, which are then fixed and stained. The material can be fixed by heat or in equal amounts of ether-alcohol for a few minutes and then stained with routine or special procedures. Hematoxylin-eosin gives very good results and the fungi may be easily seen inside the giant cells (Fig. 26). This is a simple and very useful method, particularly in rural zones where other resources are not available.

Culture: The material is cultured on Sabouraud's medium with or without antibiotics, according to whether the material is contaminated or not. Sabouraud's or other similar medium may be used with penicillin, streptomycin and cyclohexamide or with chloramphenicol and cyclohexamide. When incubated at room temperature, the mycelial phase with white colonies and short aerial hyphae is obtained. The colonies appear from the 15th to the 25th day.

In order to obtain the yeast form, the material is cultured in blood agar, brain and heart infusion with penicillin and streptomycin, and it is incubated at 37°C. Rough colonies are obtained in 8—10 days. Microscopically, multiple budding yeast-like cells will be seen. These cells have rigid walls and a diameter of approximately 30 microns.

Inoculation: This method is little used, being employed especially with contaminated material. Intratesticular inoculation in guinea pigs produces orchiepididymitis and the fungus can be observed in the pus in its characteristic tissue form. Mice and hamsters may be inoculated intraperitoneally, with the latter being more sensitive to infection by *P.brasiliensis*.

Treatment

According to Sampaio (1960), the history of the therapy of South American blastomycosis has two periods. The first begins with Lutz' publication which individualizes the disease and ends with the introduction of sulfonamide compounds by Ribeiro (1940). The second period begins with the use of these drugs.

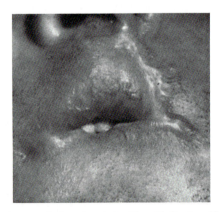

Fig. 68. Scarred mucocutaneous lesions treated with sulfadiazine. Note the narrowed buccal orifice

According to Lacaz (1956), before the use of sulfonamide preparations, patients with South American blastomycosis were condemned to death within a more or less variable length of time, depending on their organic resistance and the anatomicoclinical form of their infection.

According to Borelli (1967), sulfonamides are the drugs of choice and should be administered without interruption for a period of 3 years.

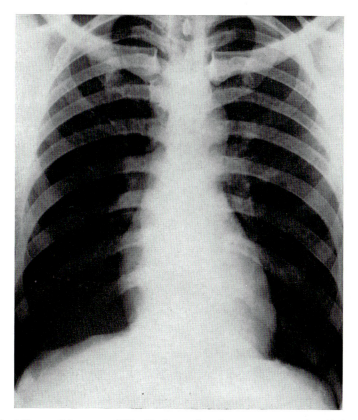

Fig. 69. Chest X-ray of the case of Fig. 31, 7 months after treatment with sulfadiazine. Note the resolution of the lesions

Sulfonamide compounds act as fungistatics and the most often used are sulfadiazine (3—4 grs. daily), sulfamethoxipyridoxine (0.5—1 grs. daily), sulfisoxazole (6—8 grs. daily), and tri-sulfas. There is general agreement that they should be administered for a long period (1—2—3 years) and preferably in a sustained manner with the object of preventing relapses, since patients have the tendency to abandon treatment when they feel better. According to GONCALVES (1946) a sulfonemia of 5 mgs. per 100 ml. of blood guarantees an efficacious effect, *in vivo*, on *P.brasiliensis*.

These drugs, in general, are well tolerated and act rapidly. Superficial ulcerations heal by scarring (Fig. 68), the exudate in the lung is reabsorbed (Fig. 69) and the enlarged lymph nodes diminish in size, although more slowly.

Among the complications of sulfonamide therapy in the treatment of patients with pulmonary lesions, a diffuse fibrosis is the most frequent and the most important one, due to the production of cor pulmonale. The most severe cardiac hypertrophy observed on the autopsy table is that seen in cases of paracoccidioidomycosis treated with sulfas and in cases of pulmonary bilharziosis. Grossly, the lungs at autopsy show a diffuse fibrosis similar to that observed in the Hamman-Rich syndrome. Microscopically a diffuse fibrosis is seen, with or without granulomatous remains, and with severe intimal sclerosis of the arterioles which may cause their complete obliteration. The granulomas may heal in the form of hyaline

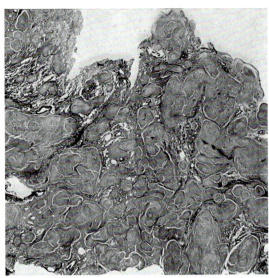

Fig. 70. Hyaline pulmonary nodules. H&E ×150. Case treated with sulfadiazine. No fungi were seen

nodules (Fig. 70) or may present as encapsulated, necrotic foci, in which fungi may still be seen, although generally they are no longer viable in culture.

Lacaz (1967), Sampaio (1960), Miranda and Machado (1957) and many other authors have been using Amphotericin B for more than 10 years with excellent results in the treatment of paracoccidioidomycosis. Sampaio (1960) recommends doses that vary from 2,000 to 8,500 mgs., administered within a period of 30—90 days, depending on the clinical form and the extension of the lesions. The drug is administered slowly, intravenously, in 5% dextrose solution. Due to the toxicity of the drug, adequate controls must be carried out.

Whether the treatment used be sulfas or Amphotericin B, it is recommended that complement fixation reactions and investigation of precipitins be practiced before, during and after treatment. An elevation of the titer or the appearance of precipitins after treatment makes necessary a resumption of drug therapy (Lacaz, 1967; Sampaio, 1960). Also it is recommended that, during treatment, a general, periodic clinical examination with a biopsy of superficial lesions, and blood sedimentation tests be carried out.

References

Aberastury, M.: Blastomicosis. A propósito de un caso con lesiones cutáneas y poligang-lionares. Bol. Inst. Med. exp. Cancer (B. Aires) 3, 885 (1926). ∼ A propósito de un caso de Blastomicosis. "Tercer Congreso Nacional de Medicina", t. IV, p. 938, 1927 (Argentina).— Adrianza, M., Recagno, A., Ascanio, R.: La función ventilatoria en paracoccidioidomicosis de localización pulmonar. IV Cong. Venz. de Tisiologia y Neumonología. Mycopathologia (Den Haag) 15, 163 (1961). — Aleixo, H.: Estudo de um caso de blastomicose. S. Paulo méd. 18, 411 (1945). ∼ Sobre um caso de blastomicose. An. bras. Derm. Sif. 21, 263 (1946). — Aleixo, J.: Estudo clínico terapéutico de blastomicose brasileira. II Reunião anual dos dermato-sifilógrafos brasileiros. Belo Horizonte, 1945. — Aleixo, J., Furtado, T.A.: Micose de Lutz de inicio possivelmente dentario. (Relato de cinco casos). Brasil-méd. 62, 265 (1948). — Almeida, F.P.: Lesões cutáneas da blastomycose en cobayos experimentalmente infectados, An. Fac. Med. S. Paulo 3, 59 (1928). ∼ Sobre a localização cutánea da "blastomicose" em uma cobaya inoculada experimèntalmente no testículo. Sci. med. 6, 173 (1928). ∼ Aspectos histo-lógicos dos casos de blastomicose verificados em São Paulo. Brasil-méd. 43, 485 (1929a). ∼ Blastomicose experimental. Bol. biol. (S. Paulo) 15, 20 (1929b). ∼ Incidéncia da blastomicose no Brasil. Bol. biol. (S. Paulo) **15**, 23 (1929c). ∼ Estudo comparativo do granuloma cocci-dióidico nos Estados Unidos e no Brasil. An. Fac. Med. S. Paulo **4**, 91 (1929d). ∼ Estudos sôbre o parasito do granuloma coccidiódico (nota prévia). Bol. biol. (S. Paulo) **15**, 97 (1929e). ∼ Em tôrno do problema da blastomycose brasileira. Bol. Soc. Med. Cirug. (S. Paulo) **14**, 373 (1930a). ∼ Estudos comparativos do granuloma coccidióidoco nos Estados Unidos e no Brasil. Novo género para o parasito brasileiro. An. Fac. Med. S. Paulo **5**, 125 (1930b). ∼ Dife-renças entre o agente etiológico do granuloma coccidióidico dos Estados Unidos e do Brasil. Um novo genero para o cogumelo brasileiro. Rev. biol. hig. **2**, 179 (1930c). ∼ Granuloma para-coccidióidico. Bol. Soc. Med. Cirurg (S. Paulo) **15**, 216 (1931). ∼ Contribuicão para o estudo da morfología do Coccidioides immitis nos tecidos parasitados. An. Fac. Med. S. Paulo **7**, 117 (1932a). ∼ Epidemiologia da blastomicose brasileira (granuloma paracoccidioidico) no Brasil. An. paul. Med. Cirurg. **23**, 191 (1932b). ∼ As blastomycoses no Brasil. An. Fac. Med. S. Paulo **9**, 69 (1933a). ∼ Blastomycoses em geral e sua classificação. Definição e classificação das blastomycoses. Rev. paul. Med. **3**, 270 (1933b). ∼ Notas sobre a morfologia do Paracocci-dioides brasiliensis nos tecidos parasitados. Rev. biol. hig., **4**, 3 (1933c). ∼ The influence of temperature upon the aspect of the culture of the Paracoccidioides brasiliensis. Rev. biol. hig., **4**, 107 (1933d). ∼ Nota sôbre uma denominação genérica. Rev. biol. hig., **2**, 68 (1934a). ∼ Formações radiadas da membrana dos cogumelos parasitos. An. Fac. Med. S. Paulo **10**, 163 (1934b). ∼ Contribuição para o estudo dos agentes etiológicos das blastomicoses brasileiras. Rev. Soc. Med. Cirurg. (Rio de J.) **48**, 281 (1934c). ∼ Le blastomicosi nel Brasile. Folia clin. biol. (S. Paulo) **6**, 1 (1934d). ∼ Ação do mel sôbre as culturas do Paracoccidioides brasiliensis. An. Fac. Med. S. Paulo **11**, 291 (1935a). ∼ Considerações em tôrno dos agentes etiológicos das Blastomycoses. An. paul. Med. Cirug. **29**, 11 (1935b). ∼ Considerações sobre a inoculação cardíaca do Coccidioides immitis e Paracoccidioides brasiliensis. Folia clin. biol. (S. Paulo) **8**, 67 (1936a). ∼ Granuloma paracoccidióidico e sua localisação bucal. Rev. Otolaryng (S. Paulo) **4**, 679 (1936b). ∼ Granuloma paracoccidióidico. Sua distribuição no Brasil e particularmente em São Paulo. An. Fac. Med. (S. Paulo) **12**, 403 (1937). ∼ Vacina contra o granuloma paracocci-dioides cerebriformes, Moore, 1935 (Nota 1). An. Fac. Med. S. Paulo **14**, 235 (1938). ∼ Myco-logia Médica. Estudo das mycoses humanas e de seus cogumelos. São Paulo: Melhoramentos 1939. ∼ A blastomicose no Brasil e seus cogumelos. Arch. Biol. (S. Paulo) **26**, 179 (1942). ∼ Micoses e sua importancia prática. Fichário Med. Terap. Labofarma (S. Paulo) **7**, 3 (1945a). ∼ Contribuição para o estudo da morfologia do Coccidioides immitis nos tecidos parasitados. Rev. Sudamer. Morf. **3**, 103 (1945b). ∼ Blastomycoses e Paracoccidioides. An. Fac. Med. (S. Paulo) **22**, 61 (1946). ∼ Micoses pulmonares. Resen. clin.-cient. **17**, 457 (1948a). ∼ Sôbre um caso de blastomicose ganglionar determinando compressões das vias biliares. Rev. paul. Med. (S. Paulo) **32**, 157 (1948b). ∼ Consideracões sobre a blastomicose sul-americana em sua forma queloi-deana. Rev. Inst. A. Lutz **10**, 31 (1950). ∼ South American Blastomycosis. In "Clinical Tropical Medicine", de Gradwohl, R.B.H. St. Louis: Mosby Co. 1951. — ALMEIDA, F.P., FERNANDES, M.: Isolamento rápido do Paracoccidioides brasiliensis. An. Fac. Med. S. Paulo **20**, 155 (1944). — ALMEIDA, F.P., LACAZ, C.S.: Breves considerações sobre tuberculose ganglionar e blastomicose. Rev. biol. hig. **9**, 139 (1938). ∼ Considerações em torno das mico-ses cirúrgicas. Arq. cir. clin. exper. **3**, 133 (1939a). ∼ Considerações sobre um caso de blasto-micose cutáneo-mucosa. An. paul. Med. Cirurg., **38**, 285 (1939b). ∼ Sôbre um caso de granu-loma paracoccidióidico, com curiosos aspectos morfológicos do parasito, nos tecidos. Folia clin. biol. (S. Paulo) **12**, 11 (1940a). ∼ Procesos pulmonares mixtos, com especial referencia a associação tuberculomicótica. An. paul. Med. Cirurg., **39**, 357 (1940b). ∼ I — Intradermo-reação com paracoccidioidina no diagnostico do granuloma paracoccidióidico. II — A reação de Montenegro no granuloma paracoccidióidico. Folia clin. biol. (S. Paulo) **13**, 177 (1941). ∼ Notas a propósito dos blastomicoses pròpriamente ditas. Rev. Med. Cirug. (S. Paulo) **26**, 27 (1942a). ∼ Micoses bronco-pulmonares. São Paulo: Melhoramentos 1942b. ∼ Considerações em torno de um cogumelo isolado de um caso de blastomicose. Folia clin. biol. (S. Paulo) **14**, 25 (1942a). ∼ A reação de Montenergo no granuloma paracoccidióidico (Nota previa) Rev. paul. Med. **20**, 158 (1942b). ∼ Valor das intradermo-reações no diagnóstico das micoses. An. Fac. Med. S. Paulo **18**, 125 (1942c). ∼ Conceito atual da blastomicose. Rev. paul. Med. **20**, 46 (1942d). ∼ Estudos sôbre a blastomicose brasileira: a) Dados estatísticos. b) Resistencia do Paracoccidioides brasiliensis nos tecidos parasitados. c) Notas terapêuticas. Rev. paul. Med. **22**, 178 (1943a). ∼ A blastomicose brasileira, com especial referência do Paracoccidioides brasiliensis. Rev. paul. Med. **23**, 57 (1943b). ∼ Notas sobre algumas questões micologicas. Arch. Biol. (S. Paulo) **28**, 57 (1944). ∼ Blastomicose "tipo Jorge Lobo". An. Fac. Med. S. Paulo **24**, 5 (1948). — ALMEIDA, F.P. LACAZ, C.S., COSTA, O.: Dados estatísticos sôbre as principais micoses humanas observadas em nosso meio. An. Fac. Med. S. Paulo **24**, 39 (1948, 1949). — ALMEIDA, F.P., LACAZ, C.S., CUNHA, A.: Estudos sôbre a blastomicose brasileira. Rev. paul. Med. **24**, 189 (1944.) — ALMEIDA, F.P., LACAZ, C.S., CUNHA, A.C.: Intradermo-reação para o diagnóstico da blastomicose sul-americana (granulomatose paracoccidióidica). Arch. bras. Med. **35**, 267 (1945a). ∼ Hemossedimentação na granulomatose paracoccidióidica (blastomicose sul-americana). Rev. med. (S. Paulo) **29**, 505 (1945b). ∼ Anatomía patológica da granulomatose paracoccidióidica (blastomicose sul-americana) II — Reunião dos dos dermato-sifilógrafos brasileiros. Belo Horizonte, 1945c. ∼ Provas de função hepática na granulomatose paracoccidiódica (blastomicose sul-americana) II — Reunião anual dermato-sifilógrafos brasileiros. Belo Horizonte, 1945d. ∼ A terapéutica da blastomicose sul-americana e seu contrôle de cura. Rev. bras. Med. **3**, 187 (1946a). ∼ Dados estatísticos sôbre o granulomatose paracoccidióidica. (Blastomicose sul-americana ou paracoccidioidose). Rev. bras. Med. **3**, 91 (1946b). — Almeida, F. P., Lacaz, C. S., Fava Netto, C.: Dados estatísticos sôbre o granuloma paracoccidiódico no Brasil. (Importancia de seu estudo). An. Fac. Med. S. Paulo **18**, 137 (1942). — Almeida, F. P., Lacaz, C. S., Fernandes, M.: Temperatura e meio de cultivo como fâctores de modificações das culturas do Paracoccidioides brasiliensis. Arch. Derm. Sif. S. Paulo **10**, 5 (1946a). ∼ Resistencia do Paracoccidioides brasiliensis, mantido em culturas, em relação do tempo. Arch. bras. Med. **36**, 31 (1946b). ∼ Ação do Yatren e do Merthiolate, "in vitro" sôbre o Paracoccidioides brasiliensis. Arch. bras. Med. **36**, 41 (1946c). — Almeida, F. P., Lacaz, C. S., Forattini, O. P.: Ação da sulfanilamida e seus derivados, "in vitro", sobre o Paracoccidioides brasiliensis. Resen. clin.-cient. **15**, 113 (1946). — Almeida, F. P., Lacaz, C. S., Junqueira, L. C., Melo, F. F.: Ação de algumas substancias "in vitro" sôbre o crescimento de cogumelos. Rev. Med. (S. Paulo) **27**, 11 (1943). — Almeida, F. P., Moura, R. A. A., Monteiro, E. V. L.: Granuloma paracoccidioidico. Breves considerações sobre a morfologia macroscópica de culturas do Paracoccidioides brasiliensis. Rev. Inst. A. Lutz (S. Paulo) **10**, 53 (1950). — Almeida, F. P., Ribeiro, D. O., Ashcar, H., Lacaz, C. S., Sampaio, S. A. P.: I. Ação da penicilina "in vitro" sobre o Paracoccidioides brasiliensis. — II. Resultados obtidos com a administração dêsse antibiotico no tratamento da blastomicose sul-americana. Hospital (Rio de J.) **29**, 109 (1946). — Almeida, F. P., Santos, L. F.: Sôbre um caso de blastomycose pulmonar. An. Fac. Med. S. Paulo **2**, 221 (1927). — Alvarez, C. J., Leone, G.: Histoplasmosis y Blastomicosis Sul-americana. Gaceta Médica (Ecuador) IX, **3**, 283 (1954). — Alvarez, P. J., Barnola, J.: Paracoccidioidomicosis en un niño de 6 años. Arch. venez. Pueric. **21**, 57 (1958). — Americo, J., Picena, J. P., Ameriso, A. M., Rodriguez, A. D. F.: A propósito de micosis y otras parasitosis faringolaringeas. Rev. Otorrinolaring. (del Litoral, Rosario) **3**, 170 (1944). — Andrade, L. C.: Sôbre um caso de blastomicose. An. Hosp. Exérc. (Rio de J.) **3**, 5 (1938). — Angulo, O. A.: La Paracoccidioidosis en el Servicio de Anatomía Patológica en el Hospital Vargas de Caracas. Rev. Sudamer. Morf. **6**, 145 (1948). ∼ Paracoccidioimicosis. Bol. Hosp. Hosp. (Caracas) **57**, 19 (1958). ∼ Paracoccidioidomicosis. Cartilla Micológica, Publ. Comisión Coordinadora del Estudio Nacional de las Micosis, Fund. Eugenio Mendoza, p. 21, 1959 (Caracas). ∼ Las micosis bronco-pulmonares en el Departamento de Anatomía Patológica del Instituto Nacional de Tuberculosis. Rev. Tisiol. Neumonol. **1**, 101 (1959). ∼ Valor del frotis tisular en el diagnóstico de las micosis. Rev. Tisiol. Neumonol. **1**, (1959). ∼ Paracoccidioidomicosis en niños. VI Cong. Latino-americano de Patología, San Juan (Puerto Rico) 47, Dic. 1967. ∼ Consideraciones sobre la Patogenia de la Paracoccidioidomicosis en base a observaciones clínico-patológicas, VI Cong. Latino-americano de Patolog. San Juan (Puerto Rico) 52, Dic. 1967. — Angulo, O. A., Carbonell, L.: Labor realizada en el campo Anatomo-Patológico. Vol. XV, p. 61 Mycopathologia (Den Haag) 1961. — Annes Diaz, H.: Blastomicose generalizada simulando o mal de Hodgkin. Med. Cirurg. Farm. 1937, Set/Out. — Arantes, A.: Linfogranuloma maligno de origen "coccidioide". S. Paulo, Tese, 1921. — Aranz, S. L., Steinberg, J. R., Carlone, M. F.: Blastomicosis extensiva de origen Velo-palatino y tuberculosis pulmonar. Sem. med. (B. Aires) **2**, 1576 (1942). — Artagaveytia-Allende, R. C.: Some biological characteristics of the pathogenic fungi named Paracoccidioides brasiliensis and Paracoccidioides cerebriformes. J. dent. Res. **28**, 242 (1949). — Artagaveytia-Allende, R. C., Garcia-Zorron, N.: Las espécies del género Paracoccidioides, Almeida 1930. An. Inst. Hig. Montevideo, **2**, 69 (1948). — Artagaveytia-Allende, R. C., Montemayor, L.: Estudio comparativo de várias cepas de Paracoccidioides brasiliensis y especies afines. An. Inst. Hig. Montevideo **2**, 129 (1948). ∼ Estudio comparativo de varias cepas de Paracoccidioides brasiliensis y especies afines. Mycopathologia (Den Haag) **4**, 356 (1949). — Arauz, S. L., Steinberg, I. R., Carlone, M. F.: Blastomicosis extensiva a origen velopalatino y tuberculosis pulmonar. Sem. méd. (B. Aires) **2**, 1 (1942). — Azevedo, A. P. P.: Blastomicose da glandula suprarrenal por Coccidioides immitis, sem lesões linfáticas e com focos de fibrose nos pulmoes. Mem. Inst. Osw. Cruz **29**, 189 (1934). — Azevedo, A. P.: Lesões do sistema nervoso central na doença de Lutz (Blastomicose brasileira). Hospital (Rio de J.) **36**, 465 (1949). — Azevedo, P. C.: Considerações sôbre a agente etiológica da blastomicose sul-americana. Pará-Med. **11**, 11 (1950). — Azulay, R. D.: Um caso de blastomicose brasileira (comunicação casuistica). Com. Cient. Wander, Janeiro-Marco, 1950. ∼ Contribuição ao estudo da micose de Lutz. Rio de Janeiro: Tese 1950. ∼ Dois casos de micose de Lutz (blastomicose brasileira) submetidos á traqueotomia. Hospital (Rio de J.) **42**, 923 (1952). ∼ Amigdalitis paracoccidióidica. Arch. argent. Derm. **3**, 1 (1953). — Azulay, R. D., Feldeman, J., Azulay, J. D.: Caso de micose de Lutz (Blastomicose sul-americana) de localização ganglionar.

Hospital (Rio de J.) **48**, 309 (1955). — BAKER, R.D.: Tissues changes in fungus diseases. Arch. Path. **44**, 459 (1947). — BALAKANOV, K.V.A., BALABANOFF, ANGELOV, N.: Blastomycosis Sudamericaine Chez un laboureur bulgare revenu depuis 30 ans de Brésil. Mycopathologia (Den Haag) **24**, 264 (1964). — BALDO, J.I.: Paracoccidioidomicosis pulmonar. Rev. Sanid. Asist. soc. **18**, 163 (1953). — BARBOSA, J.E.R.: Estatística dos casos blastomicose nasobuco-laringéa observados no servicio de Otorino-laringologiada Santa Casa de São Paulo. Rev. Otolaring. (S. Paulo) **4**, 715 (1936). — BARBOSA, F.A.S.: Em tôrno de uma questão de nomen-clatura botanica medica: Paracoccidioides brasiliensis (Splendore, 1912) (Almeida 1930), o agente etiologico da forma brasileira da "blastomicose" (granuloma paracoccidióidico). J. Med. Pernambuco, **36**, 429 (1940). — BARBOSA, J.F.: Um caso de blastomicose ganglionar com lesões nasais e faringeas. Tratamento e cura. Rev. bras. Otorinolaring. **14**, 53 (1946). — BARBOSA, J.E.R., DIAS, M.C., SOUZA.: A.C.T.H. e blastomicose das mucosas. Com. Depto. de O.R.L. da A.P.M. Sessão de 17/8/1953. — BARDY, C.: Sinais radiológicos pulmonares de Blastomicose-sul-americana. J. Bras. Med. **6** (4), 484 (1962). — BARRETO. M.: Sôbre um caso de blastomicose ganglionar (sindrome de Hodgkin de causa blastomicótica). Rev. med. Minas Gerais, **4**, 7 (1936). — BARRETO, P.M., LACAZ, C.S.: Aspectos clínicos de paracoccidioidomiciase pulmonar. Rev. paul. Med. **32**, 177 (1948). — BARROS, J.H.: Acerca de la primera comuni-cación sobre paradentosis paracoccidióidica. Venez. odont. **16**, 39 (1951). ~ Estudio general de la Paracoccidioidosis brasiliensis. Su importancia en Odontología. Bol. Clin. L. Rasetti **16**, 493 (1952). ~ Tratamiento de la Paracoccidioidosis brasiliensis. Rev. Soc. Odontol. de la Cruz Roja Venez. **1**, 22 (1953). — BARROS, O.M.: Blatomicose com localisações ósseas múlti-plas. Rev. paul. Med. **25**, 110 (1944). ~ Sur la maladie de Lutz, Splendore et Almeida. Bull. Soc. Path. exot. **43**, 114 (1950). — BASGAL, W.: Contribuição ao estudo das blastomicosis pulmonares. Rio de Janeiro: Tese 1931. — BATISTA, L., BELLIBONI, N.: Paracoccidioidose sistémica (blatomicose sul-americana) simulando eritematodes. Rev. Hosp. Clin. Fac. Med. S. Paulo **10**, 134 (1955). — BATISTA, A.C., SHONE S.K., MARQUES DOS SANTOS F.: Patho-genicity of Paracoccidioides brasiliensis isolated from soil. Publiçaço N° 373. Inst. de Mico-logía, Univ. do Recife, Brasil 1962. — BELFORT, E.: Paracoccidioidomicosis: diagnóstico mediante inoculación a Proechimys guayanensis. Dermat. Venez. **3**, 91 (1961). — BELFORT, F.: Um caso de blastomicose conjuntival. S. Paulo Med. **2**, 777 (1930). — BENAIM PINTO, H.: Contribución al estudio de la Paracoccidioidosis brasiliensis en Venezuela. Arch. venez. Pat. trop. **2**, 183 (1950). ~ Ensayo de las pentamidinas en el tratamiento de la Paracoccidioidosis brasiliensis. Acta méd. venez. **3**, 82, (1955) ~ La paracoccidioidomicosis brasiliensis como enfermedad sistémica. Comentarios a la casuística venezolana. IV Congreso Venezolano de Tisiología y Neumonología, Valencia, 1959. Mycopathologia, (Den Haag) **15**, 90 (1961). — BENAIM PINTO, H., COLL, E.: Paracoccidioidosis forma mucosa-ganglionar asociada a tuber-culosis extrapulmonar y hepatitis en sujeto con miocarditis crónica. Acta méd. venez. **2**, 153, (1954). — BERTACCINI, G.: Contributo allo studio della cosidetta "Blastomicosi aul-ameri-cana" G. ital. Derm. Sif. **75**, 783 (1934). — BIOCCA, E., LACAZ, C.S.: Açáo "in vitro" do ácido para-amino-benzóico sobre o Paracoccidioides brasiliensis e o Actinomyces brasiliensis, Arch. Biol. (S. Paulo) **29**, 151 (1945). — BITTENCOURT, H.: Sôbre um caso de Blastomicose pulmonar. Bol. Soc. Med. Hosp. (Bahia) **20**, 20 (1937). — BOCALANDRO, I., ALBUQUERQUE, F.J.M.: Icterícia a comprometimento hepático na blastomicose sul-americana. Rev. paul. Med. **53**, 350 (1960). — BIOGGINO, J., INSAURRALDE, C., e PRIETO, R.: Tercer caso nacional de granuloma paracoccidiódica. An. Fac. Cienc. méd. Paraguay **11**, 21 (1938). — BOGLIOLO, L.: Contribuição ao conhecimento da morfología do agente da moléstia de Lutz, em seu ciclo parasitário (Primeira nota) Rev. bras. Biol. **5**, 321 (1945). ~ Contribuição ao conhecimento da morfología do agente causal da moléstia de Lutz, (Segunda nota) Rev. bras. Biol. **6**, 61 (1946). ~ Granuloma apical dentário por Paracoccidioides brasiliensis (Splendore) Almeida, 1930. Brasil-méd. **60**, 341 (1946). ~ Terceira contribuição ao conhecimento da morfología do agente da moléstia de Lutz, nos tecidos humanos parasitados. Rev. bras. Biol. **6**, 181 (1946). ~ Sulla morfologia a sul modo di riproduzione del Paracoccidioides brasiliensis (Splendore) Almeida, 1930. Pathologica, **39**, 1 (1947). ~ Contribuição á patogenia da doença de Lutz. Brasil-méd. **63**, 1 (1949). ~ South American Blastomycosis (Lutz's disease): contribution to knowledge of its pathogenesis. Arch. Derm. Syph. (Chic.) **61**, 470 (1950). ~ About the morphology and mode of reproduction of "Aleurisma brasiliensis" Aroeira Neves and Bogliolo, 1950, in human tissues. Rev. Ass. méd. Minas Gerais **1**, 253 (1950). ~ Contribuição ao conhecimento da patogenia da doença de Lutz. Actualidades Odontol. **9**, 23 (1954). — BONIFACIO FONSECA, Jr.: Blastomicose sul-americana. Lesões dentárias e paradentarias. São Paulo: Tese de lione docencia 1957. — BORELLI, D.: Las aleurias de Paracoccidioides brasiliensis. IV Cong. Venez. Cienc. Méd. **4**, 2, 241 (1955). ~ Ventajas y peligros del examen directo en fresco en el dia-gnóstico de las blastomicosis sudamericana. Memorias VI Cong. Venez. Cienc. Méd. **IV**, 2159 (1955). ~ Modelos isotérmicos para la parasitología experimental: Paracoccidioidosis en Echimys, Proechimys y Heteromys. Dermat. Venez. **3**, 98 (1961). ~ Hipótesis sobre ecología de paracoccidioides, Dermat. Venez. **3**, 130 (1961b). ~ Concepto de reservarea. La reducida reservarea de la paracoccidioidosis. Dermat. Venez. **4**, 71 (1964). ~ Tratamiento de la micosis. Comunicación al VII Cong. Venez. de Cienc. Méd. Memorias VII Cong. Venez. Cienc. Méd. (en prensa) 1967. — Borrero, J., Restrepo, A., Robledo, M.: Blastomicosis Suramericana de forma pulmonar pura. Antioquia méd. **15**, 503 (1965). — Brass, K.: Las micosis Profundas. Estudio comparativo del material autópsico y biópsico del Servicio de Anatomía Patológica del Hospital Central de Valencia durante los años 1951—1966. Valencia, Venezuela. (En prensa.). — Bruni-Celli, B., Martinez Coll, A., Perret Gentil, R.: Aclaratoria sobre "Paracoccidioidosis del sistema nervioso central del Dr. Armando Domínguez". Gac. méd. Caracas LXX (1—2), 143 (1962). — Bungeler, W.: Brazilian blastomycosis and the histological demonstration of Paracoccidioides brasiliensis. Virchows Arch. path. Anat. **309**, 76 (1942); Biol. Abt. **24**, (19850) (1950). — Bustus, F.M.: Blastomicosis visceral e puerta de entrada broncofaringea. Bol. trab. Acad. argent. cir. **29**, 523 (1945). — Calvo, A., Merenfeld, R.: Algunas consideraciones sobre micosis de la boca vistas en el Servico de Oncología del Hospital Vargas. Venez. odont. **16**, 24 (1952). — Camargo, J.M., Carvalho, J.G.: Blastomicose localisada. Abcesso de Brodie. Rev. paul. Med. **18**, 319 (1941). — Campins, H.: Micosis profundas endémicas en Venezuela. Mem. VI Cong. Venez. Cienc. Méd. **5**, (2) 786 (1955). — Campins, H., Scharyi, M.: El polimorfismo clínico de la micosis de Lutz. Nueva casuística venezolana (Granuloma paracoccidióidico). II Jornadas Venezolanas de Dermatol. Venerol. Leprol. **501**, 1952. — Campos, E.S.: Blastomycosis. Coccidioidic and paracoccidioidic granuloma. Lecture before the Japan Medical Association, 1935. — Campos, E.S., Almeida, F.P.: Contribuição para o estudo das "blastomycoses" (granulomas coccidioides, observados em São Paulo). An. Fac. Med. S. Paulo **2**, 203 (1927). — Campos, E.C.: Sôbre dois casos de granuloma paracoccidióidico no Rio Grande do Sul. Arq. Est. Saúde Rio Grande do Sul, **3**, 71 (1942). ~ A propósito de um caso de blastomicose de Lutz. An. bras. Derm. Sif. **22**, 205 (1947). ~ Noticia histórica sôbre a blastomicose de Lutz no Brasil. Rev. Med. (Rio Grande do Sul) **5**, 53 (1948). ~ Micose de Lutz (Blastomicose sul-americana). Contribuição ao seu estudo no Estado do Rio Grande do Sul. Tese. de Livre-docencia. Porto Alegre 1960. — Campos, J.A.: Resumo estatístico dos casos de blastomicose naso-buco-faringea, observados no Servicio de Otorrinolaringología da Santa Casa de São Paulo nos anos de 1939 a 1944. II Reunião anual dos dermato-sifilógrafos brasileiros. Belo Horizonte 1945. — Canelas, H.M., Lima, F.P., Bittencourt, J.M., Araujo, R.P., Anghinah, A.: Blastomicose do sistema nervoso. Arch. Neuropsiquiat. (S. Paulo) **9**, 203 (1951). — Cancela-Freijo, J.: Paracoccidioidomicosis (tres nuevos casos encontrados en el Uruguay). Hoja tisiol. **8**, 89 (1948). — Carbonell, L.M.: Cell wall changes during the budding process of Paracoccidioides brasiliensis and Blastomycoses dermatitidis. J. Bact. **94** (1), 213 (1967). ~ Glycogen in yeast form of Paracoccidioides brasiliensis. Nature (Lond.) **208** (5011), 686 (1965). — Carbonell, L.M., Castejon, H., Pollak, L.: Cytochemistry of Paracoccidioides brasiliensis. I. Cytochemistry of cytoplasmic polyssaccharides in yeast form cultures with light microscope. J. Histochem. Cytochem. **12**, 413 (1964). — Carbonell, L.M., Kanetsuna, F.: Nature of intrinsic factore which reduced tetra-zolium salt in the histochemical demostration of dehydrogenases in the fungus. Paracoccidioides brasiliensis. Ann. Histochim. **11**, 375 (1966). — Carbonell, L.M., Pollak, L.: Ultraestructura de Paracoccidioides brasiliensis en cultivos. Rev. lat.-amer. Anat. pat. **5**, 26 (1961). ~ "Myelin figures" in yeast cultures of Paracoccidioides brasiliensis. J. Bact. **83**, 1356 (1962). ~ Ultraestructura del Paracoccidioides brasiliensis en cultivos de la fase levaduriforme. Mycopathologia (Den Haag) **19**, 184 (1963). ~ Ultraestructura de los hongos especialmente patógenos. Acta cient. venez. **1**, 174 (1963). — Carbonell, L.M., Rodriguez, J.: Transformation of mycelial and yeast forms of Paracoccidioides brasiliensis in cultures and in experimental inoculations. J. Bact. **90** (2), 504 (1965). — Cardoso da Cunha, A., Col.: O hemograma e o mielograma na granulomatose paracoccidióidica (Blastomicose sul-americana). An. Fac. Med. S. Paulo **24**, 155 (1948, 1949). — Carini, A.: Um caso de blastomicose com localisação primitiva na mucosa da boca. Rev. Soc. Cient. (S. Paulo) **3**, 120 (1908). ~ Um caso de blastomicose peritoneal. An. paul. Med. Cirurg. **5**, 142 (1915). ~ Um caso de blastomicose curada com aplicações de azul de metileno. Bol. Soc. Med. Cirug. (S. Paulo) **1**, 26 (1918). — Carneiro, J.F.: Enfisema intersticial e Pneumatorax Espontaneo NA Paracoccidioidose. XII Congreso Panamericano de tuberculose, pgs. 32—34. Bahia 1960. — Carvalho, A.: Sôbre o emprêgo de paracoccidioidina na cidade do Rio de Janeiro (primeiros resultados baseados no estudo de 475 individuos). Rev. bras. Tuberc. **21**, 73 (1953). ~ Sôbre o uso Intradérmico de Paracoccidioidina (filtrado e suspensão) como Meio Auxiliar Diagnóstico na Doença de Lutz. Monografía N° 2 do Servicio Nacional de Tuberculose. 54 pgs. Rio de Janeiro 1958. — Carvalho, J.C.F.: Sobre uma forma rara de blastomycose. Tese. Rio de Janeiro: Typ. Alexandre Borges 1911. — Casiello, A., Klass, R.L.: A propósito de una blastomicosis paracoccidioide a forma de granulia pulmonar y meningea. Rev. méd. Rosario **37**, 748 (1947). — Casteran, E.: Dos casos de micosis laríngea. Rev. Asoc. méd. argent. **43**, 475 (1930). — Castro, M., Defina, A., Cypis, J., Carvalhais, L.: Blastomicose brasileira (considerações sobre um caso observado). Gaz. clin. (S. Paulo) **40**, 43 (1942). —

CASTRO, M.B., BORGES, S.J.P., PACHECO, J.S.: Blastomicose .Gaz. clin. (S. Paulo) **41**, 199 (1943). — CASTRO, O., BOGLIOLO, O., BERGO, L.M.: Um caso de micose de Lutz. An. bras. Derm. Sif. **23**, 64 (1948). — CASTRO, O., BERGO, M.: Blastomicose com regressão pelo azul de metileno e sulfas. An. bras. Derm. Sif. **24**, 92 (1949). — CELIS-PÉREZ, A.: Las localizaciones buco-rino-faringo-la-ringeas del granuloma Paracoccidioides. Rev. Policlin. Valencia **1** (1), 25 (1941). ~ Micosis de la laringe. Memorias II Congreso Latino-americano (Caracas) p. 651—681. ORL (1954). — CELLIS-PERÉZ, A., GONZALEZ. C.: Un caso de Paracoccidioidosis primitiva de la laringe. Bol. Ser. ORL. Hosp. Central Valencia **2**, 53 (1952). — CERRUTI, H., ZAMITH, V.A.: Blastomicose sul-americana. Estudo de seu tratamento e de alguns aspectos mas interesantes. Monografía (S. Paulo) 1948. — CERRUTI, H., ZAMITH, V. A., FORATTINI, O.P.: Dados estatisticos sobre 300 casos de blastomiciase sul-americana internados na 4a. M. H. da Santa Casa de São Paulo, no periodo de 1915 a 1948. Rev. paul. Med. **34**, 213 (1949). — CERRUTI, H., ZAMITH, V. A., MELO FILHO, A.: Auto-inoculação experimental na blastomiciase sul-americana. Rev. paul. Med. **32**, 164 (1948). — CEZAR PINTO: Blatomicose de Adolfo Lutz. Rev. bras. Tuberc. **23**, 91 (1955). — CHAROSKY, L., VIVOLO, D., INK, J.: Sobre un caso de paracoccidioidosis buco-linguo-laringeo con propagación broncopulmonar. Pren. méd. argent. **32**, 2182 (1945). — CHIRIFE, A.: La paracoccidioidosis en el Paraguay. An. Fac. Cienc. méd. Paraguay **4**, 9 (1944). — CHIRIFE, A.V., DEL RIO, C.A.: Geopatología de la Blastomicosis Suramericana. Pren. méd. argent. **52**, 54 (1965). — CIFERRI, R., REDAELLI, P.: Coccidioides immitis et Paracoccidioides brasiliensis comme producteurs d'ammoniaque aux dépens des substances organiques azotées. Boll. Sezione Ital. Soc. intern. Microbial. **6**, 126 (1934). ~ Paracoccidioidaceae, n. fam. istituida per l'agente del "Granuloma Paracoccidioide" (Paracoccidioides brasiliensis) Boll. Ist. Sieroter. milan. **15**, 97 (1936). — CLAUSELL, D.T.: Estudo micológico e experimental de trés casos de granuloma paracoccidióidica. Arq. Depto. Est. Saúde Rio Grande da Sul. **3**, 81 (1942). — COELHO, B.: Sôbre um caso de blastomicose. An. Fac. Med. Recife N° 4/5, 5 (1937, 1938). — CONANT, N.F., HOWELL, A.: Etiological agents of North and South American Blastomycosis. Proc. Soc. exp. Biol. (N.Y.) **46**, 426 (1941). ~ The similary of the fungi causing South American Blastomycosis (Paracoccidioidal granuloma) and North American Blastomycosis (Gilchrist's Disease) J. invest. Derm. **5**, 353 (1942). — CONANT, N.F., MARTIN, D.S., SMITH, D.T., BAKER, R.D., CALLAWAY, J.L.: Manual of Clinical Mycology. Philadelphia: Saunders 1944. — CONSTANTIN and ROLAND, cit. p. DODGE (loc. cit.) — CONTI-DIAZ, I.A., YARZABAL, L.A., MACKINNON, J.E.: Lesiones cutáneas orofaríngeas, rectales y musculares por inoculación intracardíaca de Paracoccidioides brasiliensis en cobayo y el conejo. An. Fac. Med. Montevideo **44**, 601 (1959). — CONTI-DIAZ, A.: Lesiones oculares en la blastomicosis sudamericana. Hospital (Rio de J.) **58**, 903 (1960). — CORDERO, A.: Blastomicosis Sudamericana. Pren. méd. argent. **43**, 913 (1956). — COSTA, A.F. Jr.: Granuloma coccidióidico. Ensaio terapéutico pelos sais se auto. Brasil-méd. **43**, 1400 (1929). — COSTA, E.D.: Blatomicose (forma linfogranulomatoide) An. bras. Derm. Sif. **17**, 503 (1942). — CRUZ, G.: Das blasomicoses. (Rio de Janeiro): Tese 1913. — CUNHA, A.C.: Ação "in vitro" de algumas sulfas sobre o crecimento de Paracoccidioides brasiliensis. Rev. Med. Cirug. S. Paulo **28**, 399 (1944). — CUNHA, A.C., ALMEIDA, F.P., LACAZ, C.S.: O hemograma e o mielograma na granulomatose paracoccidióidica (Blastomicose sul-americana) An. Fac. Méd. S. Paulo **24**, 155 (1948, 1949). — CUNHA, A.R.: Blastomicose (dermo-epidermite papulo pustulosa e tuberculosa). II Reunião anual dos dermato-sifilógrafos brasileiros. Belo Horizonte 1945. ~ Blastomicose brasileira: dermoepidermite tuberosa simulando altamente a lepra lepramatosa. An. bras. Derm. Sif. **21**, 262 (1946). — CURBAN, G.V.: Blastomicose brasileira experimental. Contribuição para o estudo da evolução no cabaio. Rev. paul. Méd. **36**, 145 (1950). — DECOURT, L.V., ALMEIDA, F.P., ROMERO NETO, M.M., LACAZ, C.S.: Possibilidades terapéuticas na blastomicose sul-americana. (Considerações sobre um caso de forma cutánea-visceral) Rev. Hosp. Clin. Fac. Med. S. Paulo **1**, 247 (1946). — DEL NEGRO, G.: Blastomicose sul-americana. Rev. Med. Cirug. S. Paulo **38**, 143 (1954). ~ Tratamento da blastomicose sul-americana. Pinheir. ter. **7**, 1 (1955). ~ Localização Supra-Renal da Blastomicose Sul-Americana, Thesis, Univ. of S. Paulo School of Medicine, Brazil, 1961. — DEL NEGRO, G., FARIA, J.L.: Reação á paracoccidioidina em cobaios. Rev. Ass. méd. bras. **1**, 156 (1954). — DEL NEGRO, G., LACAZ, C.S., BOLOGNANI FILHO, H.: Açáo "in vitro" da auremicina, terramicina e claranfenicol sôbre o Paracoccidioides brasiliensis. Rev. Hosp. Clin. Fac. Med. S. Paulo **10**, 74 (1955). — DEL NEGRO, G., MELO e ALBUQUERQUE, F.L., CAMPOS, E.P.: Localização nervosa da blastomicose sul-americana. Rev. Hosp. Clin. Fac. Med. S. Paulo **9**, 64 (1954). — DEL NEGRO, G., WAJCHENBERG, B.L., PEREIRA, V.G., SHNAIDER, J., CINTRA, A.B.U., ASSIS, L.M., SAMPAIO, S.A.P.: Addison's Disease Associated with South American Blastomycosis. Ann. intern. Med. **54**, 189 (1961). — DIAS, H.A.: Blastomicose generalisada simulando mal de Hodgkin. Med. Cirurg. Farm. **6**, 47 (1937). ~ Blastomycose generalisada. Liçóes clin. Med. **6**, 299 (1938). ~ Doença de Lutz (granulomatose blastomicóide neotropical). Liçóes clin. Med. **8**, 249 (1942). — DIEZ, A.: Paracoccidioidomicosis esplénica primitiva. Bol. Soc. venez. Cirug. **4**, 137 (1951). — DILLON, N.L., MENEZES NETO, J.R., SAMPAIO, S.A.P.: Moléstia de Addison na blastomicose sul-americana. Apresentação de um caso com comprovação anátomo-patológica. Rev. paul.

Med. **56** (2), 164 (1960). — Dodge, D.W.: Medical Mycology. Saint Louis: The C.V. Mosby Co. 786 (1935). — Dominguez, C.: Paracoccidioides del sistema nervioso central. Gac. méd. Caracas LXX (7—9), 377 (1961). — Donati, A.: Ação dos Coccidioides immitis sobre os tecidos cultivados "in vitro" Bol. Soc. méd. Cirurg. (S. Paulo) **3**, 292, (1920, 1921). — Donati, A., Manginelli, L.: Ricerche batteriologiche sullo "Zymonema brasiliense" Atti. Ars Médica, **1**, 97 (1924). — Dowding, E.S.: Histoplasma and Brazilian Blastomyces. Mycología **42**, 668 (1950). — Drouhet, E., Zapater, R.C.: Phase levure et phase filamenteuse de Paracoccidioides brasiliensis; Etude des noyaux. Ann. Inst. Pasteur **87**, 396 (1954). — Dueñas, V.H., Garcia Cortes, C., Mora Ramirez, J.M.: South American blastomycosis in Colombia. An. Soc. Biol. Bogotá **7**, 1 (1951). — Dueñas, V., Garcia, C., Ramirez, J.: Contribución al estudio de la blastomicosis Suramericana en Colombia. An. Soc. Biol. Bogotá, **7**, 1 (1955). — Elmore, T., Eguren, L., Paccini, J.: Consideraciones sobre un caso de Paracoccidioidosis, Rev. Sanid. milit. Peru **79**, 29 (1955). — Escomel, E.: Leishmaniosis y Blastomicosis en América. Lima: Imprenta Americana 1922. ～ Blastomicosis secundaria nasal incipiente. Rev. Soc. argent. Pat. Reg. Norte **6**, 109 (1931). — Farah, C.: Considerações sobre um caso de blastomicose. Pediat. prát. (S. Paulo) **10**, 207 (1939). — Faria, L., Veiga, A.: Blstomicose cutánea. Brasil-méd. **24**, 114 (1910). — Fava Netto, C.: Estudos quantitativos sôbre a fixação do complemento na blastomicose sul-americana con antigeno polissacarídico. São Paulo: Tese 1955. ～ Contribuição para o estudo imunológica da blastomicose sul-americana. São Paulo: Tese de livre-docencia, 1960. ～ Contribuição para o estudo imunológico da blastomicose de Lutz. (Blastomicose sul-americana) Rev. Inst. A. Lutz (S. Paulo) **21**, 99 (1961). ～ The immunologic of South American blastomycosis. Mycopathologia (Den Haag) **26**, 349 (1965). — Fava Netto, C., Brito, T., Lacaz, C.S.: Experimental South American blastomycosis of the guinea pig: an immunologic and pathologic study. Path. et Microbiol. (Basel) **24**, 192 (1961). — Fava Netto, C., Del Negro, G.: Localização testiculo-epididimaria da blastomicose sul-americana. Rev. Ass. méd. bras. **1**, 210 (1954). — Feijo, E.J., Viano, F.J., Dargoltz, E.: Nuevos casos de blastomicosis en Santiago del Estero. Octava reunión de la Soc. argent. Pat. Norte **8**, 324 (1933). — Ferguson, R., Upton, M.F.: The isolation of Paracoccidioides brasiliensis from a case of South American blastomycosis. J. Bact. **53**, 376 (1947). — Fernandes, R., Mendes, W.: Localização pulmonar da doença de Lutz. Clin. tisiol. **6**, 211 (1951). ～ Localizações pulmonares da "micose de Lutz". Clin. tisiol. **8**, 1 (1953). — Fialho, A.: Blastomicose. Coloração de cortes histológicos. An. bras. Derm. Sif. **7**, 126 (1932). ～ Um caso de blastomicose com lesões ósseas articulares, ganglionares erraticas. An. bras. Derm. Sif. **9**, 34 (1934). ～ Coloração dos blastomicetos nos tecidos. An. bras. Derm. Sif. **11**, 34 (1936). ～ Localizaçóes pulmonares da "blastomicose brasileira" Bol. Acad. nac. Med. (Rio de J.) **115**, 35 (1944). ～ Localizações pulmonares da micose de Lutz, Anatomia patológica e patogenia. Tese (Rio de Janeiro) Tip. Jornal do Comércio 1946. ～ Patogenia da blastomicose pulmonar. Rev. méd. munic. (Rio de J.) **10**, 79 (1947). ～ Die pathologische Anatomie der Südamerikanischen Blastomykose (Lutzsche Krankheit). Ergeb. Path. path. Anat. **40**, 101 (1960). — Fialho, F.: Localizações viscerais da micose de Lutz. J. Brasil.-méd. **6** (4) 458 (1962). — Fialho, F., Gonçalves, A.P.: Contribuição no estudo da blastomicose brasileira. Estudo experimental desta micose no cobaio. Hospital (Rio de J.) **30**, 397 (1946). — Figueiredo, M.A.: Formas pequenas da blastomicetos em lesões humanas. Rev. paul. Med. **45**, 178 (1954). — Fonseca, J.B.: Blastomicose sul-americana. Estudo das lesões dentárias e paradentárias sob o ponto de vista clínico e histopatológica. Tese. á Faculdade e Odontologia da Univ. São Paulo: Estab. Gráfico Politipo Ltda. 1957. — Fonseca, O.: Ensayo de revisión de las blastomicosis Sudamericanas. Pren. med. argent. **15**, 512 (1928). — Fonseca Filho, O., Leao, A.E.A.: Diagnóstico differencial entre as formas brasileiras de blastomycose. Sci. Med. **5**, 615 (1927). — Fonseca Filho, O.O.R.: Ensayo de revisión de las blastomicosis sudamericanas. 4a. Reunião Soc. Argent. Pat. Reg. Norte (Santiago del Estero) **4**, 469 (1928). ～ Sôbre o agente etiológico da granulomatose blastomicóide néotropical. An. bras. Derm. Sif. **14**, 85 (1939). — Forattini, O.P.: Um caso de blastomicose com localização pancreática. Rev. Med. Cirug S. Paulo **30**, 515 (1946). ～ Blastomicose da região pancreática. Rev. paul. Med. **31**, 165 (1947). — Freijo, J.C., Zelada, L.A.: Granuloma paracoccidióidico. Primer caso autoctono observado en el Uruguay. An. Oto-rino-laring. Urug. **10**, 175 (1940). — Freire, A., Pelegrino, L.A.: Ação da sulfamida e derivados no "Paracoccidioides brasiliensis". An. bras. Derm. Sif. **21**, 270 (1946). — Fried, C.: Nossa contribuição á roentgenterapia na blastomicose. II Reunião anual dermato-sifilógrafos brasileiros. Belo Horizonte 1945. — Friedman, L., Conant, N.F.: Immunologic studies on the etiologic agents of North and South American blastomycosis. I Comparison of hypersensivity reactions. Mycopathologia (Den Haag), **6**, 310 (1953). — Furtado, T.A.: Comprometimento pulmonar na blastomicose sul-americana. Rev. Ass. méd. Minas Gerais **3**, 49 (1952). ～ Localizações ganglionares de Blastomicose brasileira. J. bras. Med. **6**, (4), 468 (1962). ～ Mechanisms of infection in South American Blastomycosis. Derm. Trop. **2**, 27 (1963). — Furtado, T.A., Aleixo, J.: Doença de Lutz, com inicio possivelmente por um agressão do tecido dentário ou peridentário. An. bras. Derm. Sif. **23**, 63 (1948). —

References567

FURTADO, T.A., LOPEZ, ALMEIDA, C.F., Jr., MOREIRA FILHO, J.A., PIMENTA, L.G.: Tratamento da blastomicose sul-americana pela anfotericina B. Hospital (Rio d. Je) **56**, 1001 (1959). — FURTADO, T.A., PELLEGRINO, J.: A terapéutica da blastomicose sul-americana. Ensaios "in vitro" com a estreptomicina Brasil-méd. **62**, 54 (1948). — FURTADO, T.A., WILSON, J.W., PLUNKETT, O.A.: South American blastomycosis or Paracoccidioidomycosis. Arch. Derm. Syph. (Chic.) **70**, 166 (1954). — GARCIA CARDENAS, H.: Localización ano-rectal de la Paracoccidioidomicosis. Mycopathologia (Den Haag) **XV**, 139 (1961). — GARZON, R., FERRARIS, L.V.: Una nueva observación de granuloma paracoccidióidico. Rev. Fac. Cienc. méd. Univ. Córdoba **8**, 161 (1950). — GIL YEPEZ, C., LIMA GOMEZ, O., PUIGBO, J.J., FERNANDEZ, P., WUANI, H.: Corazón pulmonar crónico por Paracoccidioides brasiliensis. Rev. Policlin. Caracas **XXV**, 117 (1957). — GOMES, J.M.: Um caso de granuloma coccidióide. Bol. Soc. Méd. Cirurg. (S. Paulo) **3**, 329 (1920). — GOMES, O., PEREIRA, R.: Blastomicose pulmonar (Sóbre um caso pulmonar de micose de Lutz). Rev. bras. Tuberc. **13**, 13 (1944). — GONÇALVES, A.P.: Um caso de blastomicose. An. bras. Derm. Sif. **17**, 49 (1942). ~ Da frequencia do aspecto de queilite glandular simples na blastomicose brasileira. II — Reunião anual dos dermatosifilógrafos brasileiros. Belo Horizonte 1945b. ~ Associação de blastomicose brasileira e tuberculose em lesões ganglionares. II — Reunião dos dermato-sifilografos brasileiros. Belo Horizonte 1945. ~ Estudo das concentrações sanguíneas das sulfonamidas no decurso do tratamento da blastomicose brasileira. Hospital (Rio de J.) 29—875 (1946a). ~ Da frequencia do aspecto da queilite ganglionar na blastomicose brasileira. An. bras. Derm. Sif. **21**, 133 (1946b). ~ Caso de blastomicose brasileira com presença de Paracoccidioide nas fezes. An. bras. Derm. Sif. **21**, 85 (1946c). ~ Associação da blastomicose brasileira e tuberculose em lesões ganglionares. Rev. bras. Med. **3**, 525 (1946d). ~ Aspectos clínicos e radiológicos da lesões ganglionares. Rev. bras. Med. **3**, 525 (1946d). ~ Blastomicose braileira em criança. An. bras. Derm. Sif., **22**, 195 (1947a). ~ Tentativa de tratamento da blastomicose brasileira pela vitamina D2. An. bras. Derm. Sif., **22**, 144 (1947b). ~ Queilite glandular simples e blastomicose brasileira. An. bras. Derm. Sif. **23**, 51 (1948). ~ Paradoxo terapéutico na blastomicose sul-americana pulmonar. An. bras. Derm. e Sif. **25**, 107 (1950). — GONÇALVES, A.P., BARDI, C.: Aspectos clínicos e radiológicos da blastomicose brasileira pulmonar. II — Reunião dos dermatosifilografos brasileiros. Belo Horizonte 1945a. ~ Aspectos clínicos e radiológicos da blastomicose brasileira pulmonar. Hospital (Rio de J.) **30**, 1021 (1946). ~ GONÇALVES, G., BOGGINO, J.: Para la casuística de las formas meningoencefalicas de la enfermedad de Lutz-Splendore-Almeida (granuloma paracoccidioidico). An. Fac. Cienc. méd. Paraguay **4**, 66 (1944). — GONÇALVES, A.P., FIALHO, F.: Contribuição do estudo da blastomicose brasileira experimental do cobaio. An. bras. Derm. Sif. **21**, 260 (1946). — GONZALEZ OCHOA, A., DOMINGUEZ, L.: Blastomicosis sudamericana. Casos mexicanos. Rev. Inst. Salubr. Enferm. trop. (Méx.) **17**, 97 (1957). — GONZALEZ OCHOA, A., ESQUIVEL, E.: Primer caso de granuloma paracoccidioideo (Blastomicosis sud-americana) en México. Rev. méd. Hosp. Gral. **13**, 159 (1950). — GRECO, N.V.: Origine des tumeurs et obsérvations de mycoses (blastomycoses etc.) Argentines. Buenos Aires, ed. "La Semana Médica", 1916. — GRIEGO, V., LOBO, J.I.: Sóbre um caso de blastomycose pulmonar. Rev. paul. Med. **8**, 225 (1936). — GROSE, E., TAMSITT, J.R.: *Paracoccidioides brasiliensis* recovered from the intestinal tract of three bats (Artibeus lituratus) in Colombia. S.A. Sabouraudia **4**, 124 (1965). — GUERRA, P.: El granuloma paracoccidióidico, su importancia en patología pulmonar. (Resumo) Trop. Dis. Bull. **38**, 353 (1941). — GUIMARÃES, F.N.: Infecção do Hamster (Cricetus auratus Water-house) pelo agente da micose de Lutz (blastomicose sul-americana) Hospital (Rio de J.) **40**, 515 (1951). — GUIMARÃES, F.N., MACEDO, D.G.: Contribuição ao estudo das blastomicosis na Amazonia (Blastomicose queloideana e blastomicose sul-americana). Hospital (Rio de J.) **38**, 223 (1950). — GUIMARÃES, F.: Infecção do Hamster (Cricetus auratus Water-house) pelo agente da micose de Lutz (Blastomicose Sul-Americana) Hospital (Rio de J.) **40**, 515 (1951). ~ Inoculações en Hamster da blastomicose sulamericana (doença de Lutz) da blastomicose queloidiforme (doença de Lobo) e da blastomicose dos indios de Tapajos-Xingu, Hospital (Rio de J.) **66**, 581 (1964). — GUIMARÃES, N.: Micose de Lutz na Bahia. A propósito de um novo caso Hospital (Rio de J.) **38**, 639 (1950). — GUNCHE, F.F., Mosto, D., LAPALUCCI, L.: Granuloma paracoccidiioide (blastomicosis) de Almeida. Rev. Asoc. méd. argent. **52**, 166 (1938). — GUNCHE, F.F., RADICE, J.C., FEOLI, L.S.: Blastomicosis primitiva de boca. (Paracoccidioides brasiliensis) Sem. méd. (B. Aires) **55**, 866 (1948). — GURGEL, L.N.: Blastomicose generalizada. Brasil-méd. **34**, 540 (1920). — HABERFELD, W.: Granuloma ganglionar maligno de origem "blastomycética". (Monografia). Secção de obras "O Estado de São Paulo", 1919. ~ Nova contribuição ao estudo da blastomicose interna. Rev. Med. Cirurg. S. Paulo **3**, 5 (1920). ~ Observações sôbre a blastomicose. Atti. Ars. Med. **1**, 135 (1924). — HABERFELD, W., HABERFELD, A.: Blastomicose de localização abdominal e um caso desta moléstia combinado com dysenteria amoebiana. Arch. bras. Med. **5**, 107 (1915). — HABERFELD, W., LORDY, C.: Forma visceral primária da blastomicose. 1° Congresso Médico Paulista São Paulo 1916. — HENRICI, A.T.: South American blastomicosis. In "Molds, yeast and actinomycetes". p. 186, 2a. ed. New York: J. Wiley

1947. — Iriarte, D.R., Rodriguez, C.: Un caso de granulomatosis Paracoccidióidica o Blastomicosis brasiliensis. Rev. Clin. L. Razetti **II** (4), 209 (1939). — Iriarte, D.R.: Granulomatosis paracoccidióidica ó Blastomicosis brasilera. Mem. ler. Congr. Sudam. de Orl, 1940. Consideraciones sobre Paracoccidioidosis. Bol. Lab. Cl. L. Razetti. **VI** (16): 277 y Arch. Venz. Orl. oft Neurol. **V** (3), 136 (1944). — Jervis, O.: Blastomicosis Sudamericana observada en Guayaquil II. Aspecto clínico. Rev. ecuat. Ent. Parasit. **1** (2), 44 (1953). — Jordan, J.W., Weidman, F.D.: Coccidioidal granuloma: comparison of the North and South American diseases with special reference to Paracoccidioides brasiliensis. Arch. Derm. Syph. (Chic). **33**, 31 (1936). — Joseph, E.A., Mare, A., Irving, W.R.: Oral South American blastomycosis in the United States of America. Oral Surg. **21**, 732 (1966). — Juca, W.: Forma pulmonar da doença de Lutz no Ceará. Med. Farm. **174**, 470 (1950). — Kehl, R.F.: Blastomycose. Tese. Rio de Janeiro. Typ. Jornal do Comércio e Cia. 1915. — Kletter, G., Winckel, W.E.F., Collier, W.A.: A case of South American blastomicosis in Surinam. Docum. Med. geogr. trop. (Amst.) **5**, 25 (1953). — Lacaz, C.S.: O iodo no tratamento das micoses. An. paul. Med. Cirurg. **39**, 379 (1940). ~ Formas pulmonares da blastomicose brasileira. Rev. paul. Med. **24**, 197 (1944). ~ Intradermoreações para o diagnóstico da granulomatose paracoccidióidica (Blastomicose brasileira). Rev. paul. Med. **26**, 303 (1945a). ~ Contribuição para o estudo das micoses com lesões ósteo-articulares. São Paulo: Edigraf Ltda. 1945b. ~ Contribuição para o estudo dos actinomicetos produtores de micetomas. Tese. São Paulo: Ed. Rosollilo 1945c. ~ Contribuição brasileira para o estudo da blastomicose sul-americana. (granulomatose para-coccidióidica). Hospital (Rio de J.) **28**, 249 (1945d). ~ A reação de fixação do complemento na blastomicose sul-americana. An 2° Cong. Med. Paulista **2**, 927 (1945e). ~ Contribuición brasileña para el estudio de la "blastomicosis sud-americana" (granulomatosis paracocci-dióidica). Arch. urug. Med. **27**, 167 (1945f). ~ Aspectos atuais da epidemiología, diagnóstico e terapéutica da blastomicose brasileira. Rev. paul. Med. **29**, 146 (1946a). ~ Etiología da blastomicose brasileira. An. bras. Derm. Sif. **21**, 260 (1946b). ~ Ação "in vitro" de diversas substancias químicas e antibioticas sôbre o Paracoccidioides brasiliensis. Rev. paul. Med. **32**, 150 (1948a). ~ Blastomicose sul-americana. An. Inst. Pinheiros **11**, 23 (1948b). ~ Blastomicose sul-americana. Reações intradérmicas com a paracoccidioidina e blastomicetina. Rev. Hosp. Clin. Fac. Med. S. Paulo **3**, 11 (1948c). ~ Micoses pulmonares. Seu conceito atual. Hospital (Rio de J.) **35**, 97 (1949a). ~ Dosagem de sulfa no sangue em pacientes portadores de blastomicose. Rev. paul. Med. **34**, 214 (1949b). ~ Novos dados em relação a blastomicose sul-americana e seu agente etiologico. Rev. Med. Cirug. S. Paulo **9**, 303 (1949)c. ~ Associação de sulfadiazina e sulfamerazina no tratamento da blastomicose sul-americana. Niveis san-guíneos obtidos. Profilaxia dos acidentes sulfamidicos. Hospital (Rio de J.) **37**, 689 (1950). ~ Lesões pulmonares na blastomicose sul-americana. Inquerito preliminar realizado com a paracoccidioidina. Hospital (Rio de J.) **39**, 405 (1951a). ~ Notas sôbre a denominação genérica e específica do agente da blastomicose sul-americana. Comentarios sobre uma questão de nomenclatura botanica medica. Mycopathologia (Den Haag) **6**, 38 (1951b). ~ Manual de Micología Médica. São Paulo: Ed. Irmaos Dupont 1953a. ~ South American blastomycosis. A review. Mycopathologia (Den Haag) **6**, 241 (1953b). ~ Ação "in vitro" do antimoniato de N-metilglucamina sôbre o sporotrichum schenkii e o Paracoccidioides brasiliensis. Folia clin. biol. (S. Paulo) **21**, 229 (1954). ~ South American Blastomycosis. Vd. XXIX., 1—120. An. Fac. Med. S. Paulo (1955, 1956). ~ Manual de Micologia Médica, 3a. Rio de Janeiro: Edição Revista e ampliada, Livraria Atheneu S/A, 1960. ~ Blastomicose sul-americana. Ficháico Medico-Terapéutico. Jan.-Feb.-March. 1—6 (1961). ~ Compendio de Micologia Médica, Sarvier Editora da Universidade de São Paulo Brasil 1967. — Lacaz, C.S., Ashcar, H., Costa, O., Viotti, M.R.: Ação da estreptomicina "in vitro" sobre o "Paracoccidioides brasiliensis" Ensaio terapéutico na blastomicose sul-americana. Hospital (Rio de J.) **33**, 693 (1948). — Lacaz, C.S., Assis, J.L., Bittencourt, J.M.T.: Micoses do sistema nervoso. Arch. Neuro-psiquiat. (Habana) **5**, 1 (1947). — Lacaz, C.S., Azevedo, P.C., Bolognani Filho, H.: Novos meios de cultivo para o "Paracoccidioides brasiliensis". Arch. bras. Med. **34**, 423 (1944). — Lacaz, C.S., Cruz, R.V.: Blastomicose sul-americana. Referencias bibliográficas. Hospital (Rio de J.) **46**, 393 (1954). — Lacaz, C.S., Cerrutti, H.: Mielocultura na granu-lomatose paracoccidioidica (blastomicose sul-americana). Folia clin. biol. (S. Paulo) **21**, 327 (1954). — Lacaz, C.S., Faria, J.L., Moura, R.A.A.: Blastomicose sul-americana associada a molestia de Hodgkin. Hospital (Rio de J.) **34**, 313 (1948). — Lacaz, C.S., Ferreira, M.: Ensaios experimentais com um soro anti-Paracoccidioides brasiliensis. Rev. paul. Med. **34**, 209 (1949). — Lacaz, C.S., Iara, S.T., Ferreira, M., Martins, A.A., Vega, V.S.: Blastomi-cose experimental (nota preliminar). Hospital (Rio de J.) **36**, 341 (1949). — Lacaz, C.S., Minami, P.S., Fernandes Ramos, W.: Aspectos morfológicos do Paracoccidioides brasiliensis em vioa parasitária, Rev. Hosp. Clin. Fac. Med. S. Paulo **18**, 273 (1963). — Lacaz, C.S., Oliveira, E.: Blastomicose da região ano-retal. Considerações sobre dois casos. Hospital (Rio de J.) **33**, 845 (1948). — Lacaz, C.S., Ribeiro, D.O., Sampaio, S.A.P., Zamith, V.A.: A intradermo-reação de Frei na blastomicose sul-americana e na leishmaniose tegumentar. Rev. Med. Cirug. S. Paulo **29**, 455 (1945). — LACAZ, C.S., PEREIRA, U.G., SAMPAIO, S.A.P.: Blastomicose generalizada con lesões cutáneas de tipo psoriasiforme: considerações sôbre um caso. Rev. Hosp. Clin. Fac. Med. S. Paulo **12**, 451 (1957). — LACAZ, C.S., SAMPAIO, S.A.P.: Tratamento da blastomicose sul-americana con anfotericina B. Resultados preliminares. Rev. paul. Med. **52**, 443 (1958). — LACAZ, C.S., SAMPAIO, S.A.P., ULSON, C.M.: Ação in vitro da anfotericina B. sôbre o Paracoccidioides brasiliensis. Rev. paul. Med. **54**, 357 (1959). — LACAZ, C.S., SAMPAIO, S.A.P., DEL NEGRO, G.: Atividade de duas diamidinas aromáticas na blastomicose sul-americana. Hospital (Rio de J.) **48**, 163 (1955). — LACAZ, C.S., STERMAN, L., MONTEIRO, E.V.L., PINTO, D.C.: Blastomicose queloideana. Comentários sobre novo caso. Rev. Hosp. Clin. Fac. Med. S. Paulo **10**, 254 (1955). — LACAZ, C.S., SILVA, M.S., FERNANDES, M.: Ação da tirotricina "in vitro" sobre o Paracoccidioides brasiliensis. Ensãio terapêutico na blastomicose sul-americana. Rev. bras. Med. **3**, 356 (1946). — LAPORT, F., FIALHO, A.: Um caso de blastomicose. Rev. méd. munic. (Rio de J.) **3**, 60 (1942). — LEAO, A.E.A.: Blastomicose. A contribuição de Adolfo Lutz. An. bras. Derm. Sif. **20**, 125 (1945). — LEAO, A.E.A., GOTO, M.: Lutz disease (paracoccidioidal granuloma, South American blastomycosis). Pathogenesis of the disease to the types of multiplication of its agent in the tissues. Quinto Cong. Intern. Microbiol., Rio de Janeiro, 1950 (Resumos dos trabalhos, pág. 129). — LEITAO, J. MARIA, MARIA ESTER.: Sôbre um caso de blastomicose brasileira ganglionar. — O Hospital — Vol. **64**—**6**, 1963. — LEITE, A.S.: Alguns casos de blastomicose sul-americana em Porto Velho, Território Federal de Guaparé. Rev. bras. Med. **9**, 491 (1952). — LEITE, A.S., RE, L.: Aspectos do Paracoccidioides brasiliensis e do P. cerebriformis em seprofitismo. An. Inst. méd. Trop., **8**, 27 (1951). — LEON, G.S.: Granuloma Paracoccidioidico endolaríngeo. sem. méd. (B. Aires) **59**, 276 (1952). — LEVY, J.A., DILLON, N., MENEZES NETO, J.B., SAMPAIO, S.A.P.: Meningite na blastomicose sul-americana. Rev. paul. Med. **55**, 519 (1959). — LIMA, F.X.P.: Contribuição ao estudo clínico e radiológico da blastomicose pulmonar. Tese. (São Paulo) 1952a. ~ Contribuição do estudo clínico e terapêutico da blastomicose sul-americana visceral. Tese. (São Paulo) 1952b. — LIMA, H.R.: Histopathologie der exostischen blastomykosen. Verhandlungen der Deutschen Pathologischen Gesellschaft. 20. Tagung. Würzburg 1925. — LIMA, O.F.: Sôbre um caso de blastomicose (granuloma paracoccidioide) curada pela sulfanilamida. An. paul. Med. Cirurg. **44**, 51 (1942). — LIMA FILHO, R.: Estudo radiológico das manifestações ósseas da granulomatose paracoccidióidica. Rev. paul. Med. **25**, 111 (1944). — LLAMBIAS, J., TOBIAS, J.W., NIÑO, F.L.: Blastomicosis cutáneomucosa de la boca, terminada por una forma granúlica pulmonar. Quinta Reunión de la Soc. Argent. Pat. Reg. Norte **1**, 240 (1930). — LOBO, J.: Um caso de blastomicose. Brasil-méd. **44**, 746 (1930). ~ Um caso de granuloma de origem coccidióide. Publ. méd. (S. Paulo) **1**, 3 (1930). ~ Contribuição ao estudo das blastomicoses. An bras. Derm. Sif. **8**, 43 (1933). ~ Contribuição ao estudo das blastomicoses. Tese. Recife 1933. ~ Contribuição ao estudo das blastomicoses. An. Fac. Med. Recife N° 4/5, 39 (1937, 1938). ~ Blastomicoses. Arch. Med. Cirurg. Pernambuco **1**, 3 (1949). — LONDERO, A.T., FISCHMAN, O. y RAMOS, C.: A critical review of medical mycology in Brazil, 1946—1960. Mycopathologia (Den Haag) **18**, 293 (1962). — LONDOÑO, F.: La blastomicosis Suramericana en Colombia. Rev. Fac. méd. Univ. Nal. **25**, 101 (1957). — LONDOÑO, R., BLAIR, J.: Comentarios sobre un caso de blastomicosis Suramericana.Anot. pediát. **1**, 153 (1954). — LOPEZ, H.H., HURTADO, CORREA, G.: Las micosis profundas en el Hospital S. Juan de Dios. El Médico, **10**, 20—27 (1965). — LOPES, O.S.S.: Descrição de uma técnica de concentração para pesquisa do Paracoccidioides brasiliensis no escarro. Hospital (Rio de J.) **47**, 557 (1955). — LOUZADA, A.: Blastomicose e tuberculose. Med. Cirurg. **16**, 38 (1954). — LUNA, D.F., CASET, I.E., ABBATE, E.A.: Nueva observación de Paracoccidioidomicosis (forma buco-laringo-pulmonar) Rev. Asoc. méd. argent. **61**, 571 (1947). ~ Blastomicose sudamericana. Compendio Méd. **46**, 4 (1947). — LUTZ, A.: Uma micose pseudococcidica localisada na bocca e observada no Brasil. Contribuição ao conhecimento das hyfoblastomicosis americanas. Brasil-méd. **22**, 121 (1908). — LYTHOTT, G.I., EDGCOME, J.H.: The Occurrence of South American Blastomycosis in Accra, Ghana. Lancet **1964 I**, 916. — MACCLURE, E., PAIS LEME, M.A.: Considerações em torno de um caso de blastomicose pulmonar tratada. II Congreso Latino Americano de Anatomía Patológica, Sao Paulo, 1958. — MACHADO, O.: Cogumelos das blastomicoses. Rev. Flumin. Med. **3**, 169 (1938). — MACHADO FILHO, J., CARVALHO, M.C.M.: Considerações em torno das localizações pulmonares da paracoccidioidose brasileira. Rev. bras. Tuberc. **20**, 503 (1952a). ~ Cortisone em paracoccidioidose brasileira. Rev. paul. Tisiol. **13**, 157 (1952b). — MACHADO FILHO, J., MIRANDA, J.L.: Considerações em torno da blastomicose sul-americana. Localizações, sintomas iniciais, vias de penetração e disseminação em 313 casos consecutivos. O Hospital **58** (1), 99 (1960). ~ Considerações relativas a blastomicose sul-americana. Da participação pulmonar entre 338 casos consecutivos. O Hospital **58** (3), 432 (1960b). — MACHADO FILHO, J., MIRANDA, I.R.R.A. Considerações relativas a Blastomicose sulamericana. Evolução, resultados terapéuticos e moléstias associadas em 394 casos consecutivos. O Hospital **6** (4), 372 (1961). — MACHADO FILHO, J., RIBEIRO, G., DE ABREU, M.: Rev. paul. Tisiol. **11**, N° 3, 147 (1945). — MACKINNON, J.E.:

Naturaleza o significados de la forma en "rueda de timón" de Paracoccidioides brasiliensis. An. Fac. Méd. Montevideo **35**, 653 (1950). ~ Amfotericina B en la blastomicosis sudamericana experimental. An. Fac. Méd. Montevideo **43**, 201 (1958). ~ Blastomicosis sudamericana experimental evolutiva obtenida por vía pulmonar. An. Fac. Méd. Montevideo **44**, 355 (1959). ~ Miositis en la blastomicosis sudamericana experimental. An. Fac. Méd. Montevideo **44**, 149 (1959a). ~ Pathogenesis of South American blastomycosis. Trans. roy. Soc. trop. Med. Hyg. **53**, 487 (1959b). ~ Miositis en la Blastomicosis Sudamericana y en la histoplasmosis. Mycopathologia (Den Haag) **XV**, 171 (1961). ~ Ambient temperature and some deep mycoses. Recent. Progress in Microbiology **8**, 662 (1962). ~ Revisión sobre observaciones experimentales y humanas demostrativas del efecto de la temperatura en algunas micosis. El Tórax, Vol. XIII, N° 3 y 4, p. 266 (1964). — Mackinnon, J. E., Artagaveytia-Allende, R. C., Arroyo, L.: Sobre la especifidad de la intrademorreación con paracoccidioidina. An. Fac. Méd. Montevideo, **38**, 363 (1953). — Mackinnon, J. E., Conti-Diaz, I. A., Yarzabal, L. A., Tavella, N.: Temperatura ambiental y blastomicosis sudamericana. An. Fac. Méd. Montevideo **45**, 310 (1960). — Mackinnon, J. E., Gurri, J.: Morfologia y mecanismo de multiplicación de Paracoccidioides brasiliensis, en su forma parasitaria, estudiada por el método del carbonato de plata. An. Fac. Méd. Montevideo **35**, 1033 (1950). — Mackinnon, J. E., Montemayor, L., Vinelli, H.: Observaciones personales sobre la morfología del "Paracoccidioides brasiliensis" en los tejidos. An. Inst. Hig. Montevideo **2**, 131 (1948). ~ Observaciones personales sobre la morfologia de Paracoccidioides brasiliensis en los tejidos. An. Fac. Méd. Montevideo **34**, 453 (1949). — Mackinnon, J. E., Vinelli, H.: Observaciones sobre la forma multibrotante de "Paracoccidioides brasiliensis" en los cultivos. An. Inst. Hig. Montevideo **2**, 133 (1948). ~ Caracteres diferenciales de Paracoccidioides brasiliensis y Blastomices dermatitidis en los tejidos. An. Fac. Med. Montevideo **35**, 299 (1950). — Madeira, J. A., Lacaz, C. S.: Forattini, O. P., Considerações sobre um caso de blastomicose (granulomatose paracoccidioidica) generalizada com o isolamento do "Paracoccidioides brasiliensis" a partir do sangue circulante. Hospital (Rio de J.) **31**, 845 (1947). — Madureira, P.: Human and experimental histopathology of the keloid form of Lutz' disease (Lobo's syndrom, gleonosporellosis). Quinto Cong. Intern. Microbiol., Rio de Janeiro, 1950 (Resumos dos trabalhos, pags. 128). — Maeckelt, G. A.: Estudio sobre el valor de antígenos de Histoplasma capsulatum y Paracoccidioides brasiliensis para el serodiagnóstico de estas micosis. Arch. venez. Med. trop. **III** (2), 149 (1961). — Maffei, W. E.: Micoses do sistema nervoso. An Fac. Med. S. Paulo **19**, 297 (1943). — Magarinos Torres, C., Duarte, E., Guimaraes, J. P. Moreira, L. P.: Destructive lesion of the adrenal gland in South American blastomycosis (Lutz' disease). Amer. J. Path. **28**, 145 (1952). — Malfatti, M. G., Zapater, R. C.: Consideraciones sobre la evolution y morfologia del Paracoccidioides brasiliensis que resultan de la observación electrónica. Pren. méd. argent. **41**, 534 (1954). — Manzoli, J.: Contribuição ao estudo da blastomicoses. Tese. (Rio de Janeiro) 1928. — Marano, A., Niño, F.: Localización ganglionar del Paracoccidioides brasiliensis. Rev. Asoc. méd. argent. **61**, 570 (1947). — Marcano-Coello, H., Hernandez, S., Cabrera, C.: Paracoccidioidosis brasiliensis infantil de evolución poco común. Rev. Tisiol. Neumonol. **5** (1), 87 (1963). — Marengo, R., Caldas, E. A., Raffo, J. M.: Granuloma paracoccidioide con localización pancreática. Sem. méd. (B. Aires) **41**, 975 (1934). — Marin, J. V., Zelarrayan, L. M., Luppi, J. E.: Paracoccidioidosis pulmonar a forma granúlica. Rev. méd. Rosario **34**, 850 (1944). — Marsiglia, I., Pinto, J.: Adrenal cortical insufficiency associated with paracoccidioidomycosis (South American Blastomycosis). Report or four patients. J. clin. Endocr. **26**, 1109 (1966). — Martin, D. S., Jones, R. R., Jr.: Systemic blastomycosis. Surgery **10**, 939 (1941). — Martinez-Coll, A., Bruni-Celli, B., Perret Gentil, R.: Granuloma Paracoccidioidósico operado con diagnóstico ventriculográfico de tumor del vermis cerebeloso. Arch. Hosp. Vargas **2** (3), 353 (1960). — Mazza, S., Niño, F. L., Nicolini, R.: Blastomicosis de la mucosa labiogeniana. 5a. Reunión de la Soc. Argent. Pat. Reg. Norte **1**, 231 (1930). — Mazza, S., Palamedi, B.: Caso mortal de blastomicose cutáneomucosa. 7a. Reunión de la Soc. Argent. Pat. Reg. Norte **7**, 424 (1932). — Mazza S., Parodi, S.: Una micosis chaqueña de la laringe causada por un nuevo tipo de hongo. 4a. Reunión de la Soc. Argent. Pat. Reg. Norte **1**, 213 (1930). — Medina, H.: Lesões histopatológicas em trés casos de granuloma paracoccidióidico. Est. Saúde Rio Gr. Sul **3**, 99 (1942). — Medina, H., Bodziak, C., Jr.: Contribuição ao conhecimento do ciclo extra-parasitário do Paracoccidioídes brasiliensis (Almeida, 1931). (Nota previa). Arq. Biol. Tecnol. **3**, 95 (1948). ~ Contribuição ao conhecimento do ciclo extra-parasitário do Paracoccioides brasiliensis (Almeida, 1931). Rev. méd. Paraná **18**, 145 (1949a). ~ Contribuição ao conhecimento do ciclo do P. brasiliensis (Almeida, 1930). Arq. Biol. Tecnol. **4**, 3 (1949b). — Mendez, L. A.: Blastomicosis Suramericana y otras micosis en Colombia. Rev. Hosp. Samarit. (Bogotá) **1**, 3 (1950). — Mendez, L. A., Garcia, C.: Blastomicosis Suramericana en Colombia. Med. Cir. **15**, 215 (1951). — Michalany, J.: Corpos asteroides nas lesões granulomatosas, com especial referencia a blastomicose ou doença de Jorge Lobo. Rev. Ass. méd. bras. **2**, 61 (1955). — Miranda, J. L., Machado Filho, J.: Considerações em torno da blastomicose sul-americana. Sôbre a ação da anfotericina B. Hospital (Rio de J.) 56, 93 (1959). — MIRANDA, R. N.: Blastomicose sulamericana Sulfametazina "Ciba". Ciencia Med. 19, 36 (1950). — MONCADA-REYES, F., SALFELDER, K., HARTUNG, M.: Comentarios a cerca de un caso de Blastomicosis Sud-americana. Rev. Col. Méd. Mérida VII (21—22), 369 (1966). — MONTEIRO, A., FIALHO, A.: Sôbre um caso de blastomicose perineo-ano-rectal. Rev. bras. Cirurg. 6, 177 (1937). ∿ Blastomicose perineoano-rectal, cura. Hospital (Rio de J.) 17, 931 (1940). — MONTEIRO, A., APRIGLIANO, F.: Blastomicose primitiva do laringe. Rev. bras. Oto-rino-laring. 22, 13 (1954). — MONTEIRO, E. V. L., ALMEIDA, F. P., MOURA, R. A.: Conjunto alantocorial no estudo de agentes infecciosos. I- Obtenção experimental da Granulomatose paracoccidioidica (Blastomicose sul-americana) em ovos embrionados. Folico clin. Biol., 16, 96 (1950). — MONTENEGRO, B.: Blastomicose. Arch. Soc. Med. Cirurg. S. Paulo 2, 324 (1911). — MONTENEGRO, J.: Acerca da inoculabilidade da blastomicose no Brasil. Brasil-méd. 41, 808 (1927). — MORAL, G. J. L.: Aspecto anatomopatológico de la Blastomicosis Sudamericana. Memorias de las Segundas Jornadas del Capítulo de Guayaquil de la Asoc. Med. Panamericana 317, 231 (1958). — MORALES, J., ROMERO, O.: Cinco nuevos casos de Blastomicosis sudamericana diagnosticados en Lima. Arch. peru. Pat. Clin. IX, N° 1 (1955). — MOORE, M.: A new species of the Paracoccidioides Almeida (1930). P. cerebriformis Moore. Rev. Biol. Hig. 6, 148 (1935). ∿ La blastomicosis y la cromomicosis de la América del Norte y del Sud. Sem. méd. (Habana) 43, 43 (1936a). ∿ Un nuevo tipo de blastomicosis producido por Paracoccidioides cerebriformes n.sp. Arch. urug. Med. 8, 224 (1936b). ∿ Blastomycosis coccidioidal granuloma and paracoccidioidal granuloma. Comparative study of North American and European organisms and clinical types. Arch. Derm. Syph. (Chic.) 38, 163 (1938). ∿ Mycotic granulomata of North and South America. Prac. Sixth Pacific. Sci. Cong. 5, 821 (1939). ∿ South American blastomycosis in "Clinical Tropical Medicine", p. 711. New York: P. B. Hoeber 1944. — MOSES, A.: Fixação do complemento no blastomicose. Mem. Inst. Osw. Cruz. 8, 68 (1916). — MOSTO, D.: Blastomicosis generalizada con localización pancreática. Hospital (Rio de J.) 4, 417 (1933). ∿ Granuloma paracoccidioides. Quinto Cong. Nac. Med. 3, 704 (1934). — MOSTO, D., JARICCI, V.: Presentación de un caso de granuloma por Paracoccidioides brasiliensis. Rev. méd. argent. 59, 826 (1945). — MOTTA, L. C.: Granulomatose paracoccidióidica, "blastomicose brasileira". An. Fac. Med. S. Paulo 11, 293 (1935a). ∿ Granulomatose paracoccidióidica. An. Fac. Med. S. Paulo 11, 293 (1935b). ∿ Granulomatose paracoccidióidica (Blastomicose brasileira) An. Fac. Med. S. Paulo 12, 407 (1936). ∿ Granulomatose paracoccidióidica (blastomicose brasileira). An. Fac. Med. S. Paulo 13, 239 (1937a). ∿ Granulomatose paracoccidióidica. An. Fac. Med. S. Paulo 13, 239 (1937b). ∿ Granulomatose oaracoccidióidica (Baco). An. Fac. Med. S. Paulo 14, 333 (1938a). ∿ Granulomatose paracoccidióidica (blastomicose brasileira). An. Fac. Med. S. Paulo 14, 333 (1938b). ∿ Granulomatose paracoccidióidica (blastomicose brasileira). An. Fac. Med. S. Paulo 18, 145 (1942). ∿ Granulomatose paracoccidióidica (Blastomicose brasileira). An. Fac. Med. S. Paulo 21, 205 (1945). ∿ Paracoccidioidal granulomatosis. Cardiac localization in a case of generalized form. Amer. J. Path. 24, 323 (1948). ∿ Granulomatose paracoccidióidica. Forma orgánica isolada. Rev. Hosp. Clin. Fac. Med. S. Paulo 11, 353 (1956). — MOTTA, L. C., PUPO, J. A.: Granulomatose paracoccidióidica. An. Fac. Med. S. Paulo 12, fasc. 3 (1936). — MOYSES, J.: Blastomicose pulmonar. Brasil méd. cirurg. 10, 497 (1948). — NEGRONI, P.: Estudo micologico sobre 50 casos de micosis observados en la ciudad de Buenos Aires. Tese. Fac. Med. (Buenos Aires) 1931. ∿ Micosis cutáneas y viscerales. Buenos Aires: El Ateneo 1944. ∿ Sobre el tratamiento de la blastomicosis sudamericana. A propósito de dos nuevas observaciones. Rev. argent. Dermatosif. 30, 223 (1946). — NEGRONI, P., BASOMBRIO, G., BONFIGLIOLI, H.: Revisión del granuloma paracoccidioidal en Argentina a propósito de una observación. Rev. argent. Dermatosif. 21, 484 (1937). — NEGRONI, P., DAGLIO, C. A. N.: Sobre la flora micológica de los esputos y su interpretación. Pren. méd. argent. 35, 450 (1948). — NEGRONI, P., GATTI, J. C., CARDAMA, J. E., BALIÑA, L. M.: La blastomicosis sudamericana en la Argentina. A propósito de una observación. Rev. argent. Dermatosif. 35, 221 (1951). — NEGRONI, P., NEGRONI, R.: Nuestra experiencia de la blastomicosis sudamericana en la Argentina. Mycopathologia (Den Haag) 26, 264 (1965). — NEVES, J. A., BOGLIOLO, L.: Researches on the etiological agents of the American Blastomycosis. I. — Morphology and systemic of the Lutz's disease agent. Rev. argent. Dermatosif. 36, 269 (1952). — NICHO, A.: Contribución al estudio de las micosis profundas en el Perú. Arch. peru. Pat. Clin. II, N° 4 (1948). — NIÑO, F. L.: Ulceración blastomicética cutáneomucosa del labio inferior (Consideraciones acerca de su diagnóstico etiológico) 5ª: Reunion de la Soc. Argent. Pat. Reg. Norte, 1, 213 (1930). ∿ Aspectos microscópicos de los granulomas llamados blastomicóticos. Pren. méd. argent. 25, 203 (1938a). ∿ Contribución al estudio de las blastomicosis en la República Argentina. Bol. Inst. Clin. quir. (B. Aires) 14, 591 (1938b). ∿ Granuloma paracoccidióidico con localización bucal. Contribución al estudio de las blastomicosis en la República Argentina. Biol. Inst. Clín. quir. (B. Aires) 14, 905 (1938c). ∿ Estudio de las lesiones producidas en el sistema ganglionar linfático por el "Paracoccidioides brasiliensis". Rev. Asoc. méd. argent. 53, 995 (1939a). ∿ Nueva observación de granuloma paracoccidióidico en la

República Argentina. (Forma linfático-tegumentaria). Estudio clínico y micologico. Bol. Inst. Clín. quir. (B. Aires) **15**, 459 (1939b). ~ Nueva observación de granuloma paracoccidióidico en la República Argentina (forma linfático-tegumentária). Estudio clínico y micológico. Mycopathologia (Den Haag) **3**, 51 (1941). ~ Granuloma paracoccidióidico. Estudio de una nueva observación en la República Argentina. Rev. Asoc. méd. argent. **59**, 830 (1945). ~ Granuloma paracoccidióidico (Estudio clínico-micológico). Bol. Inst. Clín. quir. (B. Aires) **22**, 209 (1946a). ~ Granuloma paracoccidióidico curado con sulfadiazina.Bol. Inst. Clín. quir. (B. Aires) **22**, 7 (1946b). ~ El granuloma paracoccidioidico en la República Argentina (Sintesis de nuestros conocimientos actuales). Bol. Inst. Clín. quir. (B. Aires) **22**, 335 (1946c). ~ Consideraciones sobre algunas micosis de interés médico-quirúrgico. Bol. Inst. Clín. quir. (B. Aires) **23**, 110 (1947a). ~ Granuloma paracoccidióidico (estudio clínico-micológico). Bol. Inst. Clín. quir. (B. Aires) **22**, 209 (1947b). ~ Granuloma paracoccidióidico. (Forma linfático-tegumentaria curada con sulfadiazina). Bol. Inst. Clín. quir. (B. Aires) **24**, 114 (1948a). ~ Granuloma paracoccidióidico. (Forma generalizada tratada con sulfadiazina). Arch. Soc. argent. Anat. **10**, 284 (1948b). ~ Siete nuevas observaciones de granuloma paracoccidióidico en la República Argentina. Bol. Inst. Clín. quir. (B. Aires) **26**, 272 (1950a). ~ La paracoccidioidomicosis en la República Argentina. Quinto Cong. Intern. Microbiol., Río de Janeiro, 1950b (Resumos dos trabalhos, pag. 127). ~ Frequencia de las localizaciones pulmonares en la paracoccidioidomicosis. Quinto Cong. Intern. Microbiol., Río de Janeiro, 1950c (Resumos dos trabalhos, pag. 124). — Niño, F.L., Latienda, R., Volpii, J.P.: Granuloma paracoccidióidico ganglionar en cavidad abdominal. Rev. Sanid. milit. **45**, (1), 290 (1964). — Niño, F.L., Perez, B.: Blastomicosis de la mucosa gingivo-geniana. 7: Reunión de la Soc. Argent. Pat.Reg.Norte **7**, 413 (1932). — Niño, F.L., Pons, L.M., Gay, A.E.: Granuloma paracoccidióidico de localización laringea. Pren. méd. argent. **28**, 445 (1941). — Niño, F.L., Risolia, A., Ferrada, U.L.: Nueva observación de paracoccidioidomicosis en la República Argentina. Bol. Inst. Clín. quir. (B. Aires) **26**, 71 (1950). — Nova, R.: Formas oto-rino-laringológicas das blastomicoses. Primeiro Congresso Sul-Americano de Otorrinolaringología. Buenos Aires 1940. ~ O tratamento sulfamídico da blastomicose brasileira. An. paul. Med. Cirurg. **41**, 532 (1941a). ~ A blastomicose brasileira no dominio da Otorrinolaringología. Rev. paul. Med. **18**, 132 (1941b). — Nuñez Montiel, J.T., Wenger, F.: Sobre un caso de Paracoccidioidosis brasiliensis linfática. Bol. Soc. venez. Cirurg. **11**, 47, 487 (1957). — O'Daly, J.A.: Las blastomicosis en Venezuela. Bol. Hosp. (Caracas) N° 3 (1937). ~ Paracoccidioidosis. Tract. Oto-rhino-laring. **5**, 144 (1943). — Oliveira, E.: Blastomicose da recto. An. paul. Med. Cirurg. **49**, 451 (1950). — Oliveira, L.C.: Cáncer da língua. Hospital (Rio de J.) **33**, 257 (1948). — Ortega Ch., A., Arguello, A.: Paracoccidioidomicosis con localización laríngea y pulmonar. Rev. de Radiolog. y Fisoter. **1**, 636 (Incluída en Gaceta Médica, X, 4) (1955). — Paixao, U., Guimaraes, N.A.: Lesões ósseas de blastomicose sul-americana. O Hospital **65**, (6) 1253 (1964). — Pardo-Castello, V.: Dermatología y Sifilografía 3a. ed. La Habana, Cultural S/A, 1945. — Parodi, S.: Blastomicosis primitiva de la mucosa nasal. Rev. Soc. Argent. Reg. Norte **6**, 112 (1931). — Paula, D.De.: O pulmao na blastomicose brasileira. J. bras. Med. **6** (4), 480 (1962). — Pedroso, A.M.: Algunas considerações sôbre Coccidioides. An. paul. Méd. Cirurg. **10**, 193 (1919). — Peisojovich, A., Nusimovich, B., Vargas, H.: Granuloma paracoccidioidico brasiliensis. Sem. Méd. (B. Aires) **103**, 424 (1953). — Pellegrino, J.: Ação "in vitro" da sulfanilamida e derivados sôbre o desenvolvimento do "Paracoccidioides brasiliensis" Almeida, 1.929 II-Reunião dos Dermato-Dermato-sifilógrafos brasileiros. Belo Horizonte, 1945a. ~ Ação "in vitro" do cloreto de tetrametiltionina (Azul de metileno) no desenvolvimento do Paracoccidioides brasiliensis, Almeida, 1929. Arch. Biol. **30**, 93 (1945b). ~ Ação "in vitro" da sulfanilamida e derivados sôbre o desenvolvimento do Paracoccidioides brasiliensis Almeida 1929. Rev. bras. Biol. **6**, 73 (1946). ~ Influencia do azul de metileno na ação da sulfadiazine "in vitro" sôbre o desenvolvimento do "Paracoccidioides brasiliensis" (Splendore), Almeida 1929. Hospital (Rio de J.) **31**, 867 (1947). — Pena Chavarria, A.: Algunas consideraciones sobre la blastomicosis de la mucosa bucco-faríngea, fundados en observaciones hechas en varios países de la América Latina. Rev. Med. lat.-amer. **13**, 1290 (1928). — Pena Chavarria, A., Aguilar Bonilla, M., Fallas Dias M. e Castro Jenkins, B.A.: Apuntes sobre un nuevo caso de granuloma paracoccidioides en Costa Rica. Rev. méd. C. Rica **8**, 369 (1949). — Pena Chavarria, A., Rotter, W.: Consideraciones anatomopatológicas y clínicas de la blatomicosis en Costa Rica. Rev. Med. lat.-amer. **19**, 1113 (1934). — Peña, C.: Deep Mycotic infections in Colombia. A. clinicopathological study of 162 cases. Amer. J. clin. Path. **47**, 505 (1967). — Pereira, C.: Blastomicose brasileira curada pela sulfamida Rev. bras. Tuberc. **11**, 147 (1942). — Pereira, A.C.: Sobre un caso de blastomicose de localização multipla. II. Reunião anual dos dermato-sifilógrafos brasileiros. Belo Horizonte 1945. — Pereira Filho, M.J.: Aspectos macro e microscópicos das culturas do agente da blastomicose sul-americana. Algumas fases do seu ciclo evolutivo. Rev. Med. Rio Grande do Sul **4**, 277 (1948a). ~ Nótulas sobre o ciclo evolutivo do agente da blastomicose sul-americana. Localizações pulmonares. Administração prolongada da sulfamerazina. Rev. Med. Rio Grande do Sul **4**, 205 (1948b). ~

References 573

Estudos do agente etiológico da blastomicose sul-americana. Rev. Med. Rio Grande do Sul 5,
188 (1949a). ~ Sobre o saprofitismo do agente da blastomicose sul-americana (nota previa).
An. bras. Derm. Sif. 24, 299 (1949b). ~ Morfologia e modo reprodução do agente da blastomicose sul-americana. Pat. e Clin. 1, 5 (1951a). ~ Estudos do agente etiológico da blastomicose
sul-americana. An. Cinqüentenario Fac. Med. de Porto Alegre 2, 111 (1951b). — PERYASSU, D.:
Ensaio clínico e experimental sobre a ação de sulfamida derivados na blastomicose brasileira.
An. bras. Derm. Sif. 17, 261 (1942). ~ O sistema reticulo-endotelial na blastomicose brasileira
experimental do cobaio. II Reunião anual dos dermato-sifilógrafos brasileiros. Belo Horizonte
1945. ~ O sistema reticulo-endotelial na blastomicose brasileira experimental do cobaio. Rev.
bras. Biol. 6, 265 (1946). — PERRY, H.O., WEDD, L.A., KIERLAND, R.R.: South American
Blastomycosis. Arch. Derm. Syph. (Chic.) 70, 477 (1954). — PERUZZI, M.: Sulle cellule giganti
intraepitaliali della blastomicosi brasiliana di Splendore. Ricerche istologiche. Ann. Med. nav.
colon. 33, 3 (1927). — PICADO, F., AVILA-GIRON, CARVALLO, E.: Consideraciones sobre un
caso de absceso cerebeloso por Paracoccidioides brasiliensis. Gac. méd. Caracas LXXV (7—12),
371 (1967). — PIERINI, L.E.: Un caso de blatomicosis. Rev. argen. Dermatosif. 17, 179 (1933).
— PINTO, C.: Sinopse das doenças parasitárias do homem. Porto Alegre, Tip. Gundlach 1942.
— POLLAK, L.: El cultivo de hongos de material contaminado. Bol. Hosp. (Caracas) 57, 83—90
(1957). — POLLAK, L., ANGULO ORTEGA, A.: Diagnóstico patológico y micológico de la Blastomicosis suramericana (Trabajo presentado al IV Congreso Internacional de Enfermedades del
Tórax, Viena, 1959). ~ Asociación de micobacterias con Paracoccidioides brasiliensis. Derm.
Venez. 5 (3) 4, 149 (Resumen) (1966). ~ Las micosis broncopulmonares en Venezuela, Tórax 16
(3), 135 (1967). — POLLAK, L., GARCIA LOPEZ, J.: Paracoccidioides brasiliensis en el granuloma
dental apical (trabajo presentado en el IV Congreso Venezolano d Tisiología y Neumonología,
Valencia 1959). Mycopathologia (Den Haag) XV, 156 (1961b). — POLLAK, L., RODRIGUEZ, C.:
Una nueva posibilidad de diagnóstico de Blastomicosis suramericana. Algunas hipótesis de su
patogenia. Bol. Hosp. 57, 31—36 (1957). — PORTO, J.A., RODRIGUES DA SILVA, J.: Micose de
Lutz (Blastomicose sul-americana) Considerações a propósito da manifestação inicial e do
compromeitmento visceral. J. bras. méd. 6 (2), 192 (1962). — PORTUGAL, O.P.: Blastomicose
(dissertação) Tese. Rio de Janeiro, Tip. Aurora 1914. — PORTUGAL, O.: Tratamento da
blastomicose (n. pr.) Bol. Soc. méd. Cirurg. S. Paulo, 17, 264 (1934). — POTENZA, L., LARES-
CAMPOS, C., FEO, M.: Paracoccidioidosis infantil en Venezuela. Aspecto del parásito a la luz
polarizada. Arch. venez. Pueric. 16, 7—22 (1953). — POTENZA, L., DE FEO, M.: Use of polarized
light in diagnosis of mycotic infections. Amer. J. clin. Path. 26, 543 (1956). — PRADO, A.A.:
A contribuição paulista ao estudo dos linfogranulomas. S. Paulo méd. 3, 209 (1929). ~ Blastomicose dos pulmoes e das suprarrenais. Sindrome de cardíaco negro. An. Fac. Med. S. Paulo
20, 215 (1944). ~ Retrospecto evolutivo da clínica médica no Brasil. In "Estudos Médicos"
Sao Paulo 1947. — PRADO, J.M., INSAUSTI, T., MATERA, R.F.: Contribución al estudio de las
coccidio y paracoccidioimicosis del sistema nervioso. Arch. Neurocirug. 3, 90 (1946). —
PUPO. J.A.: Dois casos de blastomicose. An. paul. Med. Cirurg. 5, 148 (1915). ~ Um caso de
blastomicose. An. paul. Med. Cirurg. 6, 8 (1916). ~ Das blastomycoses e seu tratamento pelas
materias corantes antisépticas (Azul de methyleno e trypaflavina) S. Paulo méd. 1, 434
(1928); Rev. Terap. 9, 364 (1929). — QUEIROZ, S.: Blastomicose palpebral. Bol. Soc. méd.
Cirurg. Campinas 3, 130 (1943). — QUIROGA, M., NEGRONI, P., CORDERO, A.: Resultado de la
terapéutica sulfamídica asociada a la vacunoterapia específica en la blastomicosis sudamericana. Rev. argent. Dermatosif. 31, 566 (1947). — RABELLO, E.: Blastomicoses e Esporotricoses. Arch. bras. Med. 2, 358 (1912). ~ Blastomicose. An. bras. Derm. Sif 8, 36 (1933). —
RABELLO, E., RABELLO, F.E., Jr., BOAS, V., PORTUGAL, H.: Considerações em torno de um
caso de coccidioide com estrutura sarcoide. An. bras. Derm. Sif. 9, 34 (1934). — RABELLO,
F.E., Jr.: Coccidioidina como tratamento de blastomicose. An. bras. Derm. Sif. 9, 34 (1934). ~
Natureza e freqüencias das lesões pulmonares na micose de Lutz. An. bras. Derm. Sif. 17, 299
(1942). ~ Aspectos internísticos da dermatología .Arch. Derm. Sif. (S. Paulo) 7, 22 (1943). ~
Micose de Lutz (A. Lutz, 1908) An. bras. Derm. Sif. 20. 121 (1945). — RABELLO, F.E., Jr.,
PORTUGAL, H., ANTUNES, A.G., ROCHA, G.L.: A micose de Lutz.-Seus caracteres biológicos e
clínicos. II Reunião anual dos dermato-sifilógrafos brasileiros. Belo Horizonte 1945. —
RADICE, J.C., KAPLEN, S.: Blastomicosis por Paracoccidioides brasiliensis. Estudio anatomo-
patológico y coloración fluorescente del parásito. Rev. Asoc. Méd. argent. 63, 61 (1949). —
RADICE, J.C., NEGRONI, P.: Coloración fluorescente mediante la primulina. Estudio histo-
lógico em diversas micosis. Arch. Soc. argent. Anat. 9, 80 (1947). — RAMOS, J.A., ORIA, J.,
SILVA, M.P.: Alterações do sangue periférica e dos órgaos hematopoiéticos em portadores de
blastomicose externa com repercussão visceral. Folia clin. biol. (S. Paulo) 11, 129 (1939). —
RAMOS E SILVA, J.: Blastomicose sul-americana. O Hospital 65 (1), 53 (1964). — REDAELLI, P.:
L'attuale sistemazione delle cosidetti "Blastomicosi" Rass. clin.-sci. Ist. biochem. ital. 19, 85
(1936). ~ A sistematização actual das chamadas blastomicoses. Resen. clin.-cient. 6, 60 (1937).
— REDAELLI, P., CIFERRI, R.: Morfología biológica sistemática di Paracoccidioides brasiliensis (Splendore) Almeida (Fam. Paracoccidioidaceae) con notizie sul granuloma para-

coccidioide. Mem. Cl. Sci. Fis. Nat. Reale Accad. d'Italia, **8**, 559 (1937). ∼ Le granulomatosi fungine dell' uomo nelle regioni tropicalli e subtropicalli. In "Trattato de micopatología umana" p. 263. Firenze: Sansoni Ed. Scientifiche 1942. — Restrepo, A.: Comportamiento inmunológico de 20 pacientes con paracoccidioidomicosis. Antioquia méd. **17**, 211—230 (1967). — Restrepo, A., Calle, G., Restrepo, M.: Contribución al estudio de la blastomicosis Suramericana en Colombia. Antioquia méd. **13**, 26—41 (1963). — Restrepo, A., Calle, G., Sanchez, J., Correa, A.: A review of Medical Mycology in Colombia. S.A. Mycopathologia (Den Haag) **12**, 93—102 (1962). — Restrepo, A., Espinal, L.S.: Algunas consideraciones sobre la Paracoccidioidomicosis en Colombia. Antioquia méd. **18**, (6), 433 (1968). — Restrepo, A., Robledo, M., Ospina, S., Restrepo, M., Correa, L.: Distribution of paracoccidioidin sensitivity in Colombia. Amer. J. Trop. Med. Hyg. **17**, 25 (1968). — Retamoso, B.: Blastomicosis Suramericana. Rev. Soc. méd. quir. (Atlántico) **9**, 91 (1965). — Ribeiro, E.B.: Blastomicose da lingua. Bol. Sanat. São Lucas, **1**, 38 (1939). ∼ Blastomicose da lingua. In "Estudos cirúrgicos". São Paulo 1940. — Ribeiro, D.O.: Nova terapéutica para a blastomicose. Publ. méd. (S. Paulo) **12**, 36 (1940). ∼ Nova terapéutica da blastomicose. An. paul. Med. Cirurg. **41**, 64 (1941a). ∼ Um caso de blastomicose das mucosas e das ganglios curado pelos derivados sulfamidicos (nota previa). Nova terapéutica da blastomicose. Rev. paul. Med. **18**, 272 (1941b). ∼ Tratamento da blastomicose pela sulfamido-crisoidina. Rev. paul. Med. **19**, 172 (1941c). ∼ Forma clínica rara (forma tuberculóide) de blastomicose cutánea. Rev. paul. Med. **21**, 303 (1942a). ∼ Tratamento da blastomicose pelo derivado acetilado das sulfamidas (Albucid). Rev. paul. Med. **20**, 392 (1942b). An. paul. Med. Cirurg. **44**, 249 (1942b). ∼ Estado actual da tratamento sulfanilamidico da blastomicose. Rev. paul. Med. **23**, 56 (1943). — Ribeiro, D.O., Lacaz, C.S., Elejalde, G.: Blastomicose pulmonar pelo Paracoccidioides brasiliensis. Rev. paul. Med. **20**, 390 (1942). — Ribeiro, D.O., Sampaio, S.A.P.: Hemossedimentação na blastomicose sul-americana. An. bras. Derm. Sif. **23**, 255 (1948). — Ritter, F.H.: Tumor cerebral granulomatose por paracoccidioide. A propósito de dois casos operados. Arch. Neuropsiquiat. (Habana) **6**, 352 (1948). — Rizzo, V.F., Arzube, R.M.: Blastomicosis Sudamericana Tratamento de un caso con Sulphamethoxypyridacina y plástia quirúrgica de la cicatriz. Rev. ecuat. Hig. **14**, (4) 7 (1957). — Robledo, M.: Paracoccidioidomicosis. Antioquia méd. **15**, 364—365 (1965). — Rocha, G., Roca, R., Lacerda, P.R., Barbosa, M., Lima, E.F.: Blastomicose sul-americana ganglionar primitiva com calcificações abdominais. O Hospital, **70**, N° 6, 195 (1967). — Rocha, M.: Micoses em oftamologia. Arch. Inst. P. Burnier **9**, 28 (1952). — Rodriguez, C., Martin Piñate, F.: La Paracoccidioidosis brasiliensis en Venezuela. Estudio de 120 casos. Observaciones clínicas. Gac. méd. Caracas. LXXIV (1—6), 101 (1966). — Rodriguez, C., Rincon, N.L.: Contribución al estudio de la Paracoccidioidosis brasiliensis en Venezuela. Publ. Cent. Méd. Caracas **1** (12) 9 (1957). — Rodriguez, C., Rincon, N.L., Troconis, G.: Contribución al estudio de la Paracoccidioidomicosis brasiliensis en Venezuela. Consideraciones sobre 62 casos estudiados con especial referencia a las localizaciones respiratorias. Mycopathologia (Den Haag) **XV**, 115 (1961). — Rodriguez, J.D.: Revisión crítica de investigaciones y literatura Micológicas durante los años 1950—1960 en Ecuador Mycopathologie (Den Haag) **17**, 185—202 (1962). — Rodriguez, M.J.D.: A propósito de un caso de Blastomicosis Sudamericana observado en Guayaquil. Rev. ecuat. Ent. Parasit. **1** (2), 39 (1953). ∼ A propósito de un caso de Blastomicosis Sudamericana procedente de la Provincia de Loja. Rev. ecuat. Hig. **14** (4), 11 (1957). ∼ Revisión de las micosis profundas en el Ecuador. Rev. ecuat. Hig. **15** (4), 177 (1958). — Rosa, M.M.: Aspectos clínico e radiológico da forma pulmonar da blastomicose de Lutz. Arq. Dpto. Saúde Rio Gr. Sul **6**, 101 (1945). — Rosenfeld, G.: Presença do Paracoccidioides brasiliensis no Sangue circulante. Rev. Clin. (S. Paulo) **7**, 197 (1940). — Rubinstein, P.: Micosis broncopulmonares. Buenos Aires: Ed. Beta. 1954. — Sadek, H.M., Vasconcellos, E.: Blastomicose periana. Arch. Cir. Clin. exp. **16**, 11 (1953). — Sahione, F.C.: Tratamento de um caso de blastomicose sul-americana ou doença de Lutz. Rev. méd. munic. (Rio de J.) **4**, 495 (1942). — Salfelder, K., Schwarz, J., Johnson, Ch.: Experimental cutaneous South American Blastomycosis in Hamsters. Arch. Derm. **97**, 69 (1968). — Salman. L., Sheppard, S.M.: South American Blastomycosis Oral. Surg. **15**, 671 (1962). — Sammartino, R.: Abscesso cerebelar por Paracoccidioides brasiliensis. Arch. Soc. argent. Anat. **9**, 360 (1947). — Sampaio, A.A.P., Almeida, F.P.: O vanilato de etila no tratamento de algumas micoses. Arch. Hig. Suáde Púb. **18**, 285 (1953). — Sampaio, J.M.: Doença de Lutz. Arch. Inst. Biol. Exérxito. **9**, 56 (1948). — Sampaio. S.A.P.: Tratamento da Blastomicose Sulamericana com Anfotericina B. Tese. de professorado. São Paulo 1960. — Sampaio, S.A.P., Alayon, F.: Caso atípico de blastomicose sul-americana. An. bras. Derm. Sif. **26**, 99 (1951). — Sampaio, S.A.P., Lacaz, C.S., Bolognani Filho, H.: Ação do Sulfisoxazol na Blastomicose Sul-americana. Rev. Assoc. méd. bras. **2**, 33 (1955). — Sanson, R.D.: Sôbre um caso de blastomicose das cordas vocais tratado pela electrocoagulação através de uma laringo-fissura. Rev. Oto-laring (S. Paulo) **4**, 689 (1936). ∼ Sôbre um caso de blastomicose das cordas vocais tratado pela eletrocoagulação através de uma laringofissura. Bol. Acad. Nac. Med. (Rio de J.) **108**, 951 (1937). ∼ Das localizações otorrinolaringológicas das blastomicoses. Bol. Acad. Nac. Med. (Rio de J.) **112**, 42 (1940). — SEIJAS, O.: Contribución al estudio de la Paracoccidioidomicosis ósea. Gac. méd. Caracas. LXIII (3—5), 235 (1956). — SERRA, O., AZULAY, R.: Micose de Lutz: forma tegumentaria primitiva solitária. An bras. Derm. Sif. **21**, 161 (1946). — SEVA, O.A.: Blastomicose generalizada. Bol. Soc. Med. Cirurg. Campinas **3**, 39 (1942). ~ Sulfanilamidas e vacina na blastomicose de forma cutánea-ganglionar. Bol. Soc. Med. Cirurg. Campinas 3, 92 (1943). — SILVA, F.: Blastomicose generalizada. Brasil-méd. **42**, 1108 (1928). ~ Comentários em torno de alguns casos de blastomicose por Paracoccidioides observados na Bahia. Brasil-méd. **50**, 706 (1936). ~ Blastomicose (Paracoccidioidease) associada a tuberculose pulmonar. Rev. méd. Bahia **9**, 296 (1941). ~ Contribuição ao estudo blastomicoses na Bahia. II — Reunião anual dos dermato-sifilógrafos brasileiros. Belo Horizonte 1945. ~ Lesões pulmonares da blastomicose de Lutz-Splendore-Almeida. Arch. Univ. Bahía **1**, 321 (1946). ~ Granuloma paracoccidioide. An. bras. Derm. Sif. **24**, 293 (1949). — SILVA, F., ARAUJO, E.: Blastomicose na Bahia. Brasil-méd. **40**, 53 (1926). — SILVA, J.R.: Sôbre a forma puramente cutánea de inicio da blastomicose brasileira. Hospital (Rio de J.) **22**, 737 (1942). ~ Estatistica da blastomicose de 1938—1945. An. bras. Derm. Sif. **21**, 257 (1946). — SILVA, J.R., FIALHO, A.: Dermatite blastomicética. An. bras. derm. Sif. **12**, 73 (1937). — SILVA, M.P.: Duas observações de "Exascose" (ex-blastomicose na Bahia) Rev. Med. (S. Paulo) ns. **13/14**, 7 (1919). ~ Contribuição para o estudo da punção ganglionar como meio semiótico. Arch. Cir. Clin. Exp. **7**, 71 (1943). ~ La blastomycose. Son diagnostic por la punction ganglionaire. Sang. **21**, 537 (1950). ~ Tratamento da blastomicose sul-americana. (granulomatose paracoccidioidica ou moléstia de Lutz, Splendore e Almeida, blastomicose brasileira). Rev. bras. Med. **2**, 918, (1945a). ~ Tratamento da blastomicose brasileira. Rev. bras. Med. **2**, 34 (1945b). ~ Blastomicose pulmonar (Paracoccidioideose pulmonar). Rev. bras. Med. **3**, 723 (1946a). ~ Considerações sôbre a blastomicose. Rev. bras. Med. **3**, 14 (1946b). ~ Afecções da boca. Pub. Odontol. **1**, 3 (1947). ~ Sessão clínico-patológica n. °5. Rev. bras. Tuberc. **21**, 863 (1953). — SILVA, M.S., LACAZ, C.S.: Ação do éter "in vitro" sôbre o Paracoccidioides brasiliensis. Ensaio terapêutico na blastomicose sul-americana. An. bras. Derm. Sif. **21**, 210 (1946). — SILVA, N.N.: Intradermo-reação para o diagnóstico de blastomicose de Lutz. Arch. Depto. Est. Saúde Río Gr. Sul **6**, 127 (1945). — SILVA, N.N., CAMPOS, E.C.: A blastomicose de Lutz no Rio Grande do Sul. Arch. Depto. Saúde Rio Gr. Sul **6**, 81 (1945). Est. — SILVA, N.N., ROSA, M.M.: Forma pulmonar primitiva da blastomicose. An. Cinqüentenário Fac. Med. de Porto-Alegre. **2**, 95 (1951). — SILVA, P.D.: Sôbre um caso de blastomicose humana (Contribuição ao estudo das exacoses) Tese. Rio de Janeiro, 1912a. ~ Blastomicose humana. Tese. São Paulo, Tip. Mendes 1912b. ~ Contribuição ao estudo das blastomicoses tegumentares. Tese. São Paulo, Graf. Universal 1914. — SILVA, P.D., CAMPOS, E.S.: Sôbre dois casos de blastomicose hépato-espleno-ganglionar. Rev. Med. (S. Paulo) **5/6**, 305 (1917a). ~ Sôbre mais um caso de blastomicose hépato-espleno-ganglionar. Rev. Med. (S. Paulo) ns 5/6, 346, 1917b). ~ Nota preliminar sobre seis casos de blastomicose ultimamente observados no Hospital da Santa Casa de Misericordia de Sao Paulo. Rev. Med. (S. Paulo) ns **9/10**, 38 (1918a). ~ Blastomicose hépato-espleno-ganglionar (peritonite blastomicética). Bol. Soc. Med. Cirug. (S. Paulo) **1**, 61 (1918b). — SILVA, P.N.: Algumas notas para o estudo da blastomicose. Tése. São Paulo, 1931. — SILVA, U.A., MONTENEGRO, M.R., INAGVE, T.: Doença de Addison de origen blastomicótica. Rev. paul. Med. **41**, 258 (1952). — SIMAS, F.: Sôbre dois casos de granuloma paracoccidióidico observados em Curitiba. Pub. Med. **15**, 11 (1944). ~ Mais alguns casos de blastomicose sul-americana observados em Curitiba. Rev. méd. Parana **18**, 395 (1949). — SOARES FILHO, F.P., MEDINA, H.: Contribuição ao conhecimento das espécies do género Paracoccidioides (Almeida, 1930). Arch. Biol. Tecnol. **5/6**, 39 (1950, 1951). — SODRE, L.A., CERRUTTI, H.: Retite blastomicósica. Bol. Soc. Med. Cirug. (S. Paulo) **14**, 167 (1930). — SOUZA, B.P.: Um caso de blastomicose cutánea tratada com salicilato de sódio. Rev. Med. (S. Paulo) **15**, 203 (1931). — SPLENDORE, A.: Sôbre um novo caso de blastomycose generalizada. Rev. Soc. Cient. S. Paulo **4**, 52 (1909). ~ Blastomicoses americanas. Brasil-méd. **24**, 153 (1910). ~ Bouba. Blastomycose. Leishmaniose. Nota sobre afecções framboesidas observadas no Brasil. Imp. Med. **19**, 1 (1911a). ~ Bouba. Blastomicosi. Leishmaniosi. Nota sopra alcune affezione framboesiche osservate nel Brasile. Policlinico **28**, C, 3 (1911b). ~ Un affezione micotica con localizzazione nella mucosa della bocca osservata in Brasile, determinate da funghi apparteneti alla tribú degli Exiascei Zymonema Brasiliense n. sp.) Extraído do volume "in onore del Prof. Angelo Celli nel 25° anno di insegnamento", Roma, Tip. di G. Bertero E.C., 1912. ~ Zymonematosi con localizzazione nella cavitá della bocca, osservata in Brasile. Bull. Soc. Path. Exot. **5**, 313 (1912). ~ Blastomiosi-sporotricosi e rapporti con processi affini. 7° Cong. Int. Dermat. e Sif. Roma, 1912. — STACHOWSKY, L., YESPICA, V., POLLAK, L., WINKLER, O.: Un caso de Paracoccidioidomicosis primitiva de la laringe, tratado con la estilbamidina. Mem. III Congreso Latinoamaricano de O.R.L., 745—756, 1954. — SUAREZ, H.A.: Blastomicossi boliviana. Tese (La Paz) 1936. — TAIANA, J.A., BORAGINA, R.C., NINO, F.L.: Granuloma paracoccidióidico. Laringobronscopia en dos casos. Rev. Asoc. méd. argent. **59**, 1356 (1945). — TALICE, R.V., MACKINNON, J.E.: Primer caso de blastomicosis (Tipo

Gilchrist) observado en Uruguay. Arch. urug. Med. **3**, 177 (1933). — Taves, J.N., Beolchi, E.A.: Sobre um caso de blastomicose ganglionar generalizado. Rev. Med. (S. Paulo) **27**, 40 (1943). — Teixeira, R.: O problema da blastomicose sul-americana na Bahia. Med. Cir. Farm. **304**, 115—120 (1963). — Texeira, G.A., Machado, J. Miranda, J.L.: Blastomicose sul-americana experimental: Estudo experimental em tatos com considerações relatives a patogenia des lesões, Hospital (Rio de J.) **68**, 1081 (1965). — Tella, R.: Blastomicoses tegumentares. Tese (Rio de Janeiro) 1925. — Terra, F.S.: Tres casos de Blastomicose. Brasil-méd. **32**, 41 (1923). — Terra, F.S., Barreto, B.: Blastomicose cutáneo-mucosa. An. Fac. Med. (Rio de J.) **3**, 78 (1919). — Tobias, J.W.: Granuloma paracoccidioidal de forma sépticopiohemia con extensas lesiones óseas. Pren. méd. argent. **31**, 1164 (1944). — Tobias, J.W., Niño, F.L.: Estudio de una nueva observación de granuloma paracoccidiódico (forma linfático visceral) Pren. méd. argent. **25**, 232 (1938). — Torres, L.A.M.: Blastomicose da criança. Rev. med. munic. (Rio de J.) **5**, 383 (1943). — Torres, C.M., Duarte, E. Guimaraes, J.P., Moreira, L.F.: Lesão destrutiva da suprarrenal na blastomicose sul-americana (Doença de Lutz). Amer. J. Path. **28**, 145 (1952). — Torres, E.T.: Blastomicose. Bol. Centro de Estudos Hosp. Serv. Estado **6**, 321 (1954). — Trejos, A., Romero, A.: Contribución al estudio de las blastomicosis en Costa Rica. Rev. Biol. Trop. **1**, 63 (1953). — Urdaneta, E., Belfort, E.: Micosis sistémicas en el niño. II. Paracoccidioidomicosis. Arch. venz. Pueric. **29** (4), 390 (1966). — Vargas, C., Soto, R.: Dos nuevos casos de Paracoccidioidomicosis. Rev. Univ. Zulia **10** (38), 37 (1967). — Veronesi, R., Mello, F.J., Del Negro, G., Macedo Soares, J.C., Jr.: Blastomicose retal primitiva (Revisão da literatura e apresentação de um caso). Rev. Hosp. Clin. Fac. Med. S. Paulo **9**, 327 (1954). — Versiani, O.: Blastomicose. Rev. bras. Biol. **5**, 37 (1945). ~ Blastomicose sul-americana. Teste cutáneo com coccidiodin. Rev. bras. Biol. **6**, 211 (1946). — Versiani, O., Bogliolo, L.: Lutz's disease (South American blastomycosis). Proc. Fourth Intern. Cong. on Trop. Med. and Malaria **2**, 1287 (1948). — Viana, G.O.: Moléstia de Posadas. Wernicke, nas lesões apendiculares. Tese (Rio de Janeiro) 1913. — Vinelli, H.: Estudio de la membrana de blastomyces dermatitidis y de paracocci- dioides brasiliensis en cultivos levaduriformes. An. Fac. Med. Montevideo **35**, 497 (1950). — Wegman, T., Zollinger, H.U.: Tuberkuloide Granulome in Mundschleimhaut und Hals- lymphknoten: Südamerikanishe Blastomykose. Schweiz. med. Wsch. **89**, 1151 (1959). — Weiss, Pedro, Zavaleta, Teodoro.: Sôbre un caso de linfogranulomatosis micósica causada por Blastomyces brasiliensis, encontrado en Lima. Actualid. méd. peru. **XI.**, p. 442 (1937). — Weiss, P., Flores, L.: Nuevos casos de Linfogranulomatosis micósica encontrados en Lima. Rev. Med. Exp. Vol. VII, 1, 2, 3, 4, 1—14, 1948. — Weiss, P., Aguilar, P.: Casos de micosis profundas encontrados en el Perú. Rev. Med. Per. Año X, N° 227, Lima, 1947. — Wenger, F.: Las micosis profundas en el material de anatomía patológica de Maracaibo. Mem. VI Cong. Venez. Ciencias Med. **5**, 2887 (1955). — Yarzabal, L.A.: Rectitis y lesiones perianales en la blastomicosis sudamericana experimental. G. E. N. (Caracas) 1—10 (1961). — Zerpa-Morales, J.R.: Blastomicosis del ciego. G. E. N. (Caracas) V (1—2), 41 (1950).

Lôbo's Disease (Keloidal Blastomycosis)

JAN P. WIERSEMA, Washington/D.C.*, USA

With 13 Figures

Definition

Lôbo's disease is a chronic infection of the skin caused by *Blastomyces Lôboï*, and characterized by very slowly growing tumors of the dermis, which are composed of granulomatous inflammatory tissue with numerous spherical fungal cells.

History

JORGE LÔBO presented, in 1931, at a meeting of the Medical Society of Pernambuco, the history of a 52-year-old resident of Amazonas who had keloidal lesions on the skin of his back for 23 years. The lesions were composed of granulomatous inflammatory tissue that contained numerous spherical budding fungi. The disease of this patient was considered a mild form of South American blastomycosis; therefore it was named *keloidal blastomycosis*. The causative fungus was thought to be a new species because it neither grew on ordinary fungal media nor produced infection in laboratory animals. Seven years later, AMADEU FIALHO reported, in a 55-year-old resident of Amazonas, a tumorous lesion of the right auricle (the external ear) that had existed for 12 years. Histopathologic examination revealed a similar granuloma. FIALHO expressed the opinion that the chronic fungal infection of his patient had much in common with that of Lôbo's patient and that both differed widely from South American blastomycosis; therefore, he recognized the infection as a new disease, naming it Lôbo's disease.

Altogether 53 cases of Lôbo's disease were reported in the literature through 1965. The first nine cases were reported in Brazil between 1931 and 1951 (LÔBO, 1931; FIALHO, 1938; ALMEIDA, 1949; GUIMARAES, 1950). The tenth case was reported in Costa Rica (TREJOS, 1953). From 1955 until 1966, one case was reported in Panama (HERRERA, 1955), three in Venezuela (CONVIT, 1961; REYES, 1961), three in Colombia (CORREA, 1958; VILLEGAS, 1965; MARTINEZ, 1965), five in French Guiana (FONTAN, 1960; SILVERIE, 1963; DESTOMBES, 1964), and thirteen in Surinam (WIERSEMA, 1965). In the meantime the number of cases reported in Brazil increased to a total of twenty-seven. (LÔBO, 1955; LACAZ, 1955; SILVA, 1957; AZULAY, 1957; FIALHO, 1958; MORAES, 1962a, b; MICHELANY, 1963).

Geographical Distribution; Incidence; Epidemiology

The geographical distribution of 53 cases reported in the literature is demonstrated in Fig. 1.

All patients were adults at the time the disease was recognized. Forty-eight were men, and five were women. The ages of forty-nine patients were mentioned; they varied from 18—85 years and averaged 50 years. The duration of the disease was mentioned in the reports of forty-two patients; it varied from 1—41 years and averaged 15 years. Subtraction of the disease's duration from the patient's age revealed that the age of the onset varied from 1—70 years and averaged 38 years. Three patients claimed that their first lesions developed during childhood at ages

---

* Address at time of printing: Good Samaritan Hospital, 1425 West Fairview Ave., Dayton, Ohio 45406 USA.

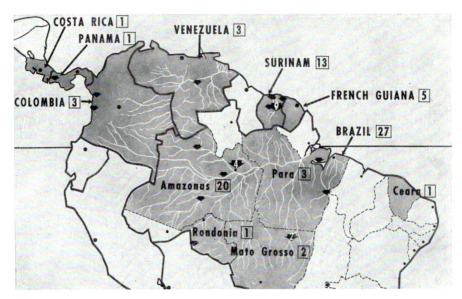

Fig. 1. Lôbo's disease. Map of tropical South and Central America. Demonstrated in grey color is the geographical distribution of Lôbo's disease according to the 53 cases reported in the literature from 1931—1966. The numbers within the rectangles are the number of cases reported in each country (capitalized) and in each state of Brazil (not capitalized). Arrows indicate areas where 28 patients contracted the disease; a small arrow represents one; a large arrow, two or more patients, as indicated by a number on the arrow.
(Prepared by the Medical Illustration Service, A.F.I.P., Washington, D.C.)

1, 7, and 13 years; at the time of diagnosis, their first lesions were 40, 23, and 5 years old respectively. All patients were natives of South or Central America. The colors of their skin varied from white to black; comprising those of Creoles, Mestizoes, Mulattoes, American Indians and Negroes.

Lôbo's disease occurred in the rural people who frequently traveled or lived permanently in the forest, often under primitive conditions. Several patients stated that their first lesions developed in a superficial wound of the skin caused by trauma, or at the site of the bite of an insect. Spontaneous transmission of the disease to humans or domestic animals was not observed. All cases were isolated infections that apparently had been contracted from an unknown source in the tropical forest of South and Central America. Although the total number of cases was very small in respect to the total population of the endemic area, Lôbo's disease was reported to be the most frequently occurring deep fungal infection in certain parts of Brazil, in Surinam and in French Guiana.

Clinical Picture

A typical case of Lôbo's disease was that of a 42-year-old woman who lived in the forest of Surinam. Figure 2 demonstrates a large irregularly-shaped, flat tumor on the skin of her right arm near the elbow. Three small nodules are situated close to the median border of the large lesion. According to the patient's information, a small lesion was noticed when she was about 1 year old. During her life it slowly increased in size and similar lesions developed in the same area of the skin. After many years, several lesions blended and formed the large flat tumor that is shown in the photograph. The lesions were freely movable with the skin. Further examination of the skin and superficial lymphnodes was unremarkable. The patient did not have any particular complaints about the lesions of her arm and her general health condition had always been excellent.

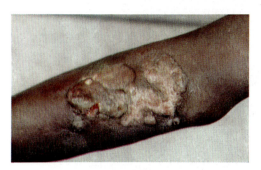

Fig. 2. Lôbo's disease. Lesion on the right arm of a 42-year-old Surinam woman. The gap in the lower margin is the site where a biopsy was taken

Figure 3 demonstrates disseminated lesions of the skin in a 60-year-old man with Lôbo's disease of thirty years' duration. The first lesion developed on his left shin, after it was wounded. At that time he worked and lived in the forest of Surinam. Gradually, lesions developed in other areas of the skin, often initiated by a superficial wound. The patient complained about itching of the lesions stating that he used to scratch them frequently. It is likely that the infection was spread by scratching because all of the involved parts of the skin were within easy reach of his hands, whereas those parts of the back beyond reach were spared; besides, an extensive clinical examination, including x-ray photographs, failed to produce evidence that internal organs, bones, or lymph nodes were involved. The general health of the patient was unaffected.

The clinical picture of Lôbo's disease is characterized by very slowly growing skin tumors, usually located in one area, as in the first patient; but sometimes, in the course of years, the infection spreads to other areas of the skin, as in the second patient.

In forty-nine of the cases reported in the literature, the locations of the first lesions were mentioned. They were as follows: leg, 19; auricle, 14; arm, 9; face, 4; neck, 1; gluteal region, 1; and lumbo- sacral region, 1. The number and the distribution of the lesions varied. In patients who had the disease for more than five years, there were usually multiple distinct lesions restricted to one area of the skin. Often one or two large lesions were surrounded by a number of small lesions as demonstrated in Fig. 2. In some patients, lesions spread along draining lymphatics. Frank disseminated lesions of the skin did occur in ten patients. The locations of the first lesions in these ten patients were: leg, 7; arm, 1; auricle, 1; and unknown, 1.

Involvement of regional lymph nodes was observed in six patients. In fourteen patients, the regional lymph nodes were reported normal. Involvement of mucous membranes, internal organs or bones was not noted in any patient, and the general well-being of the patients was not affected.

With regard to treatment, no benefit was reported from the administration of drugs at that time available for treatment of fungal diseases. Surgical excision of the skin lesions cured several patients but in others recurrence was reported in the surgical scars.

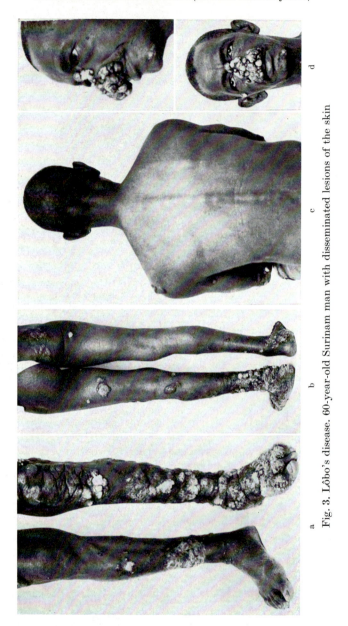

Fig. 3. Lôbo's disease. 60-year-old Surinam man with disseminated lesions of the skin

Macroscopic Pathology

All lesions of the skin that have been reported in Lôbo's disease can be described as tumors of the dermis. Young tumors are usually flat with a smooth, shiny epidermal surface, devoid of hairs, and sometimes hypopigmented. Such lesions resemble keloids in areas of the skin with a flat surface. Old, flat tumors often have a dull, scaly surface. Flat keloidal lesions with a shiny surface and flat lesions with a dull and scaly surface are demonstrated in Fig. 2. In two patients with disseminated lesions of the skin, some originally flat, smooth tumors changed after many years into verrucous plaques that resembled lesions of chromoblastomycosis. An example of such verrucous lesions, found on the legs, is demonstrated in Fig. 3. In a substantial number of patients, the tumors were not flat, but they projected more in the center than at the periphery. Such tumors were particularly common on the auricles. They also occurred in other areas of the skin where its surface is not flat but curved. Figure 3 demonstrates projecting nodules of the skin of the nose. Finally, it must be mentioned that, in four patients, lesions of Lôbo's disease did present as ulcerating tumors. An example is shown in Fig. 4.

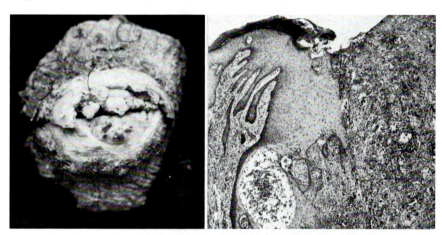

Fig. 4. Lôbo's disease. A single ulcerating lesion removed from the thigh of a 20-year-old Surinam man under the presumptive diagnosis of skin carcinoma. Microscopically there is marked pseudoepitheliomatous hyperplasia of the epidermis at the edge of the ulcer

On the cut surface, the lesions reveal a yellowish-gray, homogeneous, fairly well-circumscribed tumor in the dermis that often projects for a short distance into subcutaneous tissue, but never invades muscle, bone or cartilage. The tumor has an elastic consistency.

Microscopic Pathology

Histopathologically, the lesions are highly characteristic. The epidermis may be normal, stretched and atrophic or sometimes hypertrophic. All variations are often represented in different areas of the same lesion. Where the epidermis is changed, there is usually hyperkeratosis and sometimes focally parakeratosis (Figs. 5, 6). Pseudoepitheliomatous hyperplasia may be conspicuous at the borders of ulcerating lesions (Fig. 4).

The tumor itself is a histiocytic granuloma that replaces most dermal tissues, including epidermal appendages. The granuloma is characterized by an abundance of giant cells, histiocytes and fungal cells, whereas necrosis, suppuration and frank fibrosis are absent (Figs. 6, 7). The giant cells are of irregular shape with a diameter of 40—80 microns. Two to forty nuclei are usually located in the periphery of the cell and if numerous, often in two separate groups. The cytoplasm of the giant cells is eosinophilic and reveals a fine reticular pattern. One or two asteroid bodies are observed in about 1% of the giant cells. The histiocytes are about 20 microns in diameter. The cytoplasm reveals the same reticular pattern as that of the giant cells. Occasionally, a histiocyte in mitosis is observed. The

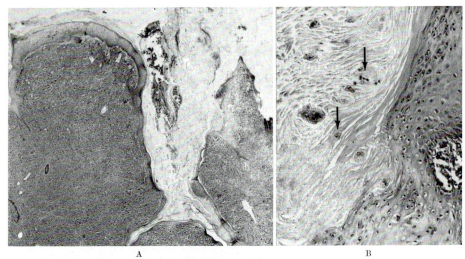

Fig. 5. Lôbo's disease. Pseudo-verrucous lesion of the left foot of the patient in Fig. 3, revealing hypertrophic epidermis that is covered with crusts. Several fungal cells are present in the crusts; shown by the arrows. — A. Gridley-fungus stain, ×15; A.F.I.P. No. 66-13387. — B. Gridley-fungus stain, ×70; A.F.I.P. No. 66-13382

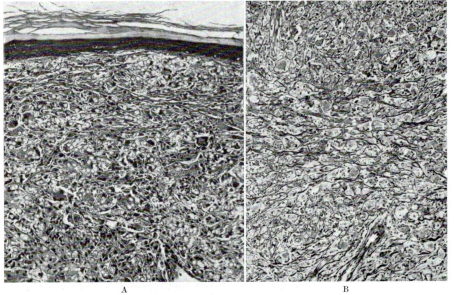

Fig. 6. Lôbo's disease. A tumor of the nose of the patient in Fig. 3. — A. Hematoxylin-eosin stain, ×40; A.F.I.P. No. 66-13311. — B. Reticulum stain, ×40; A.F.I.P. No. 66-13310

giant cells and histiocytes are supported by a meshwork of reticular fibers and irregularly distributed strands of collagenous fibers (Fig. 6).

The abundance of fungal cells is best demonstrated in sections stained with silver. Several fungal cells are connected with each other and appear as beaded strings. The majority of fungal cells are surrounded by giant cells or histiocytes. Light microscopy is unable to elucidate whether the fungal cells are located

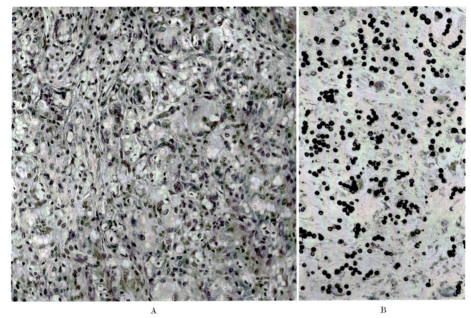

A   B

Fig. 7. Lôbo's disease. A tumor of the nose of the patient in Fig. 3. Histiocytic granuloma with giant cells and numerous fungal cells. — A. Hematoxylin-eosin stain, ×100; A.F.I.P. No. 66-9094. — B. Gomori's methenamine Silver method, ×100; A.F.I.P. No. 66-9097

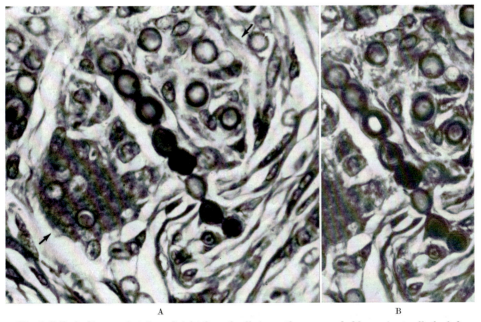

A   B

Fig. 8. Lôbo's disease. A string of eight fungal cells is partly surrounded by a giant cell, the left lower and right upper borders of which are shown with arrows. Most nuclei of the giant cell are located in the left lower part. The third fungal cell of the string, counted from the upper end, contains a double refractile body. B shows the same string of fungal cells photographed with partly crossed polarizer and analyzer. Gridley-fungus stain, ×700; A.F.I.P. No. 66-9101, and 66-9102

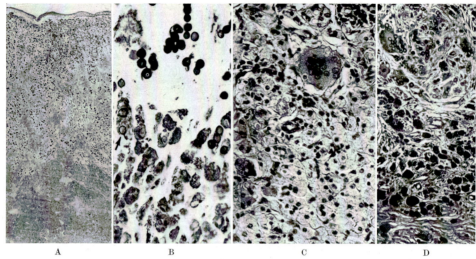

A   B   C   D

Fig. 9. Lôbo's disease. A tumor of the nose of the patient in Fig. 3. — A. Low magnification of silver stained section shows the fungal cells in the superficial part, but no fungal cells in the lower part of the tumor. — B. High magnification of the border zone reveals strings of fungal cells in the upper part and grey cells with a few remnants of fungal cells (arrow) in the lower part of the photograph. — C. and D. Hematoxylin-eosin and P.A.S. stained sections of border zones. — A. Gomori's methenamine silver method, ×14; A.F.I.P. No. 66-9088. — B. Gomori's methenamine silver method, ×265; A.F.I.P. No. 66-9100. — C. Hematoxylin-eosin stain, ×210; A.F.I.P. No. 66-13314. — D. P.A.S. stain, ×115; A.F.I.P. No. 66-13312

within the cytoplasm or surrounded by cytoplasm and separated from it by the cell wall. The latter relationship appears to exist in the case of long strings of fungal cells (Fig. 8). Fungal cells also occur in between collageneous fibers, particularly at the borders of the granulomas and in epidermal crusts (Fig. 5b).

In many, if not all, lesions, accumulations of peculiar mononuclear cells occur at the borders of the granuloma (Fig. 9). The mononuclear cells resemble those of a granular cell myoblastoma. Their cytoplasm reacts with P.A.S. and with fat stains. They do not contain fungal cells. In sections stained with silver, however, it appears that remnants of fungal cells are present in some, which indicates that fungal cells have been destroyed. A substantial part of some granulomas is occupied by these cells. If a small punch biopsy is taken from such a part for histopathologic examination, the mycotic nature of the lesion my be overlooked. Several small groups of similar cells are frequently dispersed in the granuloma between giant cells, histiocytes, and connective tissue fibers.

Plasma cells and lymphocytes are usually present, always in small numbers, and eosinophilic leucocytes and neutrophilic leucocytes are never missing; but in comparison with most other granulomas caused by fungi, that of Lôbo's disease stands out by cellular homogeneity of all parts: either giant cells and histiocytes with numerous fungal cells (Fig. 7), or peculiar mononuclear cells with remnants of fungal cells (Fig. 9).

The surface of the ulcerating lesions consists of non-specific granulation tissue without fungal cells. Underneath this layer of granulation tissue, the granuloma does not differ, essentially, from that of closed lesions; with the exception of the border zone where polymorphonuclear leucocytes are interspersed with giant cells and histiocytes. The epidermis at the edge of ulcerating lesions is usually hyperplastic, sometimes to the extent of pseudoepitheliomatous hyperplasia (Fig. 4).

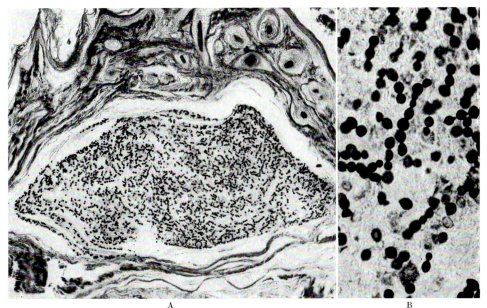

A   B

Fig. 10. A lesion in the hind foot of a golden hamster, eight months after inoculation with a suspension of fungal cells prepared from a biopsy of a skin lesion of the patient in Fig. 3. — A. Silver stain, ×63; A.F.I.P. No. 66-13302. — B. Silver stain, ×359; A.F.I.P. No. 66-13304

The infrequent occurrence of ulceration in such long-standing granulomas and the absence of necrosis and suppuration in the depth of ulcerating lesions, suggest that ulceration is a complication caused, perhaps, by trauma and secondary infection.

Mycology

It was reported in the literature that specimens from twenty-two patients were used for inoculation of fungal media. In 1940, Fonseca Fialho and Area Leao claimed to have isolated and grown, on a particular medium, a fungus from the lesions of Lôbo's first patient. The fungus was named *Glenosporella lôboï*. A similar fungus was later isolated from two other patients of Brazil. Successful cultivation was also reported from the lesions of one patient in Venezuela (Convit, 1961) and one patient in French Guiana (Destombes, 1964). None of these isolated fungi were proven to be pathogenic for man or for animals. Furthermore, cultivation efforts were reported unsuccessful with fungal suspensions prepared from lesions of sixteen patients, although many different media were inoculated and incubated at room temperature and at 37 °C, in several instances, for many months. It is therefore understandable that *Glenosporella lôboï* was generally not accepted as the fungus that causes Lôbo's disease.

Several authors reported that they inoculated laboratory animals with suspensions of fungal cells prepared from the lesions of their patients. Most inoculations were performed according to the technique that is used for the transmission of South American blastomycosis. These animal transmission efforts were reported unsuccessful. Inoculation of the foot-pads of golden hamsters (Wiersema, 1965) resulted in granulomatous lesions with numerous typical fungal cells eight months after inoculation (Fig. 10).

Dante Borelli (1961) inoculated a patient with Lôbo's disease in the healthy skin of the knee with a fungal suspension prepared from a spontaneous lesion. A

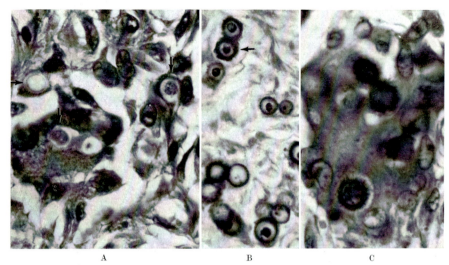

A　　　　　　　　　B　　　　　　　　　C

Fig. 11. Lôbo's disease. A. A tumor of the nose of the patient in Fig. 3. A giant cell and a histiocyte contain fungal cells with cytoplasm (vertical arrows). Another fungal cell is apparently empty (horizontal arrow). — B. Ulcerating lesion of Fig. 4. Some fungal cells are surrounded by P.A.S.-positive capsular material. — C. A tumor of the patient in Fig. 3. It shows a giant cell with three fungal cells which are surrounded by capsular material. Irregular P.A.S.-positive particles are present in the lower fungal cell. — A. Hematoxylin-eosin stain, ×1000; A.F.I.P. No. 66-9105. — B. P.A.S. — light-green stain, ×650; A.F.I.P. No. 67-1556. — C. P.A.S. — hematoxylin stain, ×1000; A.F.I.P. No. 66-9106

typical nodule developed at the site of inoculation. Four years later, it had reached the size of 33 mm.

In tissue sections, the fungi appear as spherical cells that vary little in size. The average diameter of the fungal cells is 9—10 microns. Since this exceeds the thickness of the tissue sections, many of the fungal cells must have been cut. The relatively large size of the fungal cells requires focusing of the microscope at different levels in order to examine their structure. The wall of each fungal cell is approximately one micron thick and is not stained by hematoxylin-eosin (Fig. 11A). With P.A.S. and with Gridley's fungus stain, the wall turns red (Fig. 8) and with Gomori's methenamine silver stain it becomes grey or black (Fig. 13), depending on the time of exposure to the silver solution. A thin irregular capsule is observed around some fungal cells (Figs. 11B, C). The capsular material reacts with stains for acid mucopolysaccharides. Within the cell wall, a cytoplasmic mass may be noticed in hematoxylin-eosin or P.A.S. stained sections (Fig. 11). but often the majority of fungal cells do not reveal any stained contents whatsoever. In the cytoplasm, that is often retracted from the cell wall, high magnification reveals small basiphilic dots, sometimes as many as eigth, which apparently are the nuclei of the fungal cells. Other cells contain only a P.A.S. positive mass, which does not reveal any structure. In a small number of fungal cells, a double refractile body is often the only visible content (Fig. 8).

In silver stained sections, many fungal cells appear to be connected by narrow, short tubes that contain two small bodies, each shaped as a sandglass (Fig. 13 B). Several fungal cells connected in a row appear as a beaded string (Fig. 12A). Such strings have one or more short side branches. The occurrence of several strings in a microscopical field raises the question of how many of the apparently isolated cells really belong to strings that were not in the plane of the section. In addition, one

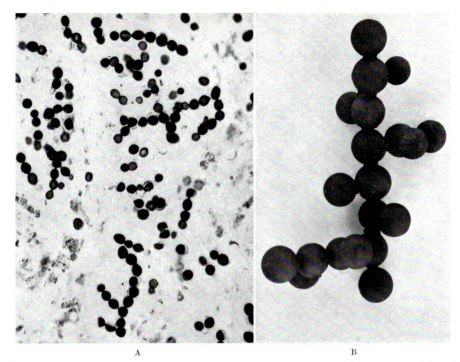

A   B

Fig. 12. Lôbo's disease. A. Selected microscopical field shows several long strings of fungal cells. Gomori's methenamine silver stain, ×265; A.F.I.P. No. 66-9099. — B. A three-dimensional model of a complex of twenty fungal cells as it may, in reality, exist in the granulomas. The main string is eight cells long

C

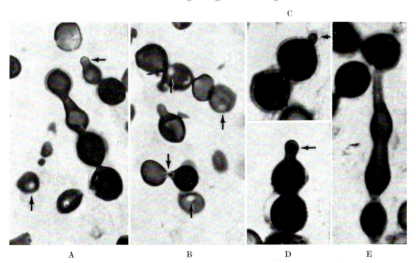

A   B   D   E

Fig. 13. Lôbo's disease. The vertical arrow, pointing down, in B., indicates a tube with two small sandglass-shaped bodies that connect fungal cells. The vertical arrows, pointing up, indicate small holes in the walls of the fungal cells where connecting tubes were cut. The hole in A. is in focus; the rings at the periphery represent the inner and outer borders of the cell wall; the small dot in the center of the hole is the thin part of a sandglass-shaped body. Horizontal arrows indicate buds. A pseudohypha is shown in E. — A. Silver stain, ×1000; A.F.I.P. No. 66-9107. — B. Silver stain, ×1000; A.F.I.P. No. 66-9108. — C. Silver stain, ×1190; A.F.I.P. No. 66-13306. — D. Silver stain, ×1190; A.F.I.P. No. 66-13305. — E. Silver stain, ×1000; A.F.I.P. No. 66-9103

may wonder if the number of side branches of a string is not much greater than it appears, since random distribution would locate very few in the plane of the section. Careful examination of apparently isolated fungal cells reveals, in many of them, remnants of connecting tubes (Figs. 13A, B). This indicates that such cells were parts of strings. Counts of the number of connections produced evidence that the majority of fungal cells is connected in units of at least twenty cells (Fig. 12B), and that branching occurs frequently (Wiersema, 1965).

In hematoxylin-eosin stained sections, it is evident that the cytoplasm of those cells connected by short tubes, is completely separated. Single budding is shown by very few cells, never more than 2%. A bud may appear at the end of a string or project sidewards from it. A bud may also occur within the row of fungal cells that form a string (Fig. 13). The occurrence of short pseudo-hyphae is very spasmodic (Fig. 13E).

Differential Diagnosis

A long-lasting skin granuloma, composed of giant cells, histiocytes and a tremendous number of spherical fungal cells, from which several appear as parts of branching strings in silver stained sections, is so highly characteristic for Lôbo's disease, that it will be recognized without difficulty; and can hardly be mistaken for any other fungal infection.

References

Almeida, F., Lacaz, C. da S.: Blastomicose "Tipo Jorge Lôbo". Ann. Fac. Med. S. Paulo 24, 5 (1949). — Azulay, R. D., Miranda, J., Azulay, J. D.: Doenca de Jorge Lôbo. O Hospital 51, 685 (1957). — Borelli, D.: Lobomicosis experimental. Dermat. Venez. 3, 72 (1961, 1962). — Convit, J., Borelli, D., Albornoz, R., Rodriguez, G., Hómez, J. Ch.: Micetomas, Cromomicosis, Esporotricosis y enfermedad de Jorge Lôbo. Mycopathologia (Den Haag) 15, 394 (1961). — Correa, P.: Blastomicosis queloidiana. Rev. lat.-amer. Anat. pat. 2, 139 (1958). — Destombes, P., Ravisse, P.: Etude histologique de 2 cas Guyanais de Blastomycose Chéloidienne (Maladie de J. Lôbo). Bull. Soc. Path. exot. 57, 1018 (1964). — Fialho, A.: Blastomicose du tipo "Jorge Lôbo". O Hospital 14, 903 (1938). — Fialho, F.: Dois Casos de Micose de Jorge Lôbo. Rev. bras. Cirurg. 35, 567 (1958). — Fonseca Filho, O., Area Leao, A. E.: Contribuicao para o comhecimento das granulomatoses blastomicoides, o agente etiologico da micose de Jorge Lobô. Rev. méd.-cirurg. Brasil 3, 147 (1940). — Fontan, R.: Premier cas de maladie de Lôbo observé en Guyane Française. Arch. Inst. Pasteur Guyane franç. 21, 1 (1960). — Guimaraes, F. N., Macedo, D. G.: Contribuicao ao Estudo das Blastomicoses na Amazonia. O Hospital 38, 224 (1950). — Herrera, J. M.: Paracoccidioidosis Brasiliense. Estudio del primer caso observado en Panamá de Blastomicosis suramericana en su forma cutanea queloidiana o Enfermedad de Lôbo y propuesta de una variante técnica para la impregnación argéntica del parásito. Arch. méd. panameñ. 4, 209 (1955). — Lacaz, C. da S., Sterman, L., Monteiro, E. V. L., Pinto, D. O.: Blastomicose Queloideana. Comentarios sôbre novo cazo. Rev. Hosp. Clin. Fac. Med. S. Paulo 10, 254 (1955). — Lôbo, J.: Um caso de blastomicose produzido por uma especie nova encontrado em Recife. Rev. méd. Pernambuco 1, 763 (1931). ~ Blastomycoses. Ann. Derm. Syph. (Paris) 4, 382 (1955). — Martinez, F. A., Hoffmann, E.: Blastomicosis Queloidiana. Antioquia méd. 15, 417 (1965). — Michalany, J., Lagonegro, B.: Corpos Asteroides na Blastomicose de Jorge Lôbo. A proposito de um novo caso. Rev. Inst. Med. trop. S. Paulo 5, 33 (1963). — Moraes, M. A. P.: Blastomicose tipo Jorge Lôbo. Seis casos novos encontrados no Estado do Amazonas, Brasil. Rev. Inst. Med. trop. S. Paulo 4, 187 (1962). — Moraes, M. A. P., Oliveira, W. R.: Novos casos da micose de Jorge Lôbo encontrados em Manaus, Amazonas Rev. Inst. Med. trop. S. Paulo 4, 403 (1962). — Reyes, O., Goihman, M., Goldstein, C.: Blastomicosis Queloidiana o Enfermedad de Jorge Lôbo. Dermat. Venez. 2, 245 (1961). — Silva, D.: Sur un nouveau cas de la mycose de Jorge Lôbo Arch. belges Derm. 13, 26 (1957). — Silverie, Ch. R., Ravisse, P., Vilar, J. P., Moulins, C.: La blastomycose cheloidienne ou maladie de Jorge Lôbo en Guyane Française. Bull. Soc. Path. exot. 56, 29 (1963). — Trejos, A., Romero, A.: Contribución al estudio de las blasto-micosis en Costa Rica. Rev. Biol. trop. (S. José) 1, 63 (1953). — Villegas, M. R.: Enfermedad de Jorge Lôbo (Blastomicosis queloidiana). Presentación de un nuevo caso colombiano. Mycopathologia (Den Haag) 25, 373 (1965). — Wiersema, J. P., Niemel, P. L. A.: Lôbo's disease in Surinam patients. Trop. geogr. Med. 17, 89 (1965).

Mycetoma[1]

Donald J. Winslow[2], [3], Bay Pines/Florida, USA

With 24 Figures

Historical

The early history of mycetoma has been outlined by Hirsch (1886), Chalmers and Archibald (1916) and Boyd and Crutchfield (1921). The term "mycetoma" was introduced by Vandyke Carter (1860) for a disease which Gill (1842) had recognized as a clinical entity while working at the Madura Dispensary in southern India. This disease, which usually affected the feet of barefoot native workers, was characterized by progressive tumefaction, formation of multiple fistulas and sinuses, and deformity with loss of function. In the serosanguineous or seropurulent discharges from the fistulas there were peculiar grains or granules, soft or hard, 1—2 mm in diameter, with a smooth or rough surface. Colebrook (1846), who succeeded Gill at the Madura Dispensary, confirmed Gill's observations and stated that the term "Madura foot" was commonly being used to designate the disease prevalent in southern India. Carter classified the cases of Madura foot according to the color of the grains which were present in the lesions and discharges. He noted that there were black, red and yellow varieties, and from the tissue he cultured a fungus which the mycologist Berkeley called *Chynonyphe carteri*. Carter named the disease "mycetoma" to indicate that it was a tumefaction caused by a fungus. He believed at first that the disease was caused by a single type of fungus and that yellow grains were produced by degenerative changes in black grains. Boyce and Surveyor (1894), however, reported that the yellow and black grains of mycetomas represented entirely different groups of microorganisms. Cultural studies resulted in the isolation of actinomycetes from the yellow grains and true fungi from black grains. Pinoy (1913), in France, subdivided mycetoma into two types: (1) actinomycosis, caused by actinomycetes, and (2) true mycetoma, caused by true fungi. Chalmers and Archibald (1916) revised this terminology, calling the true mycetoma "maduromycosis", a term that has generic and geographic implications which subsequent investigations have proved inaccurate. Fungi other than those belonging to the genus *Madurella* are now known to be causative agents of mycetoma, and the disease has been recognized in many parts of the world far removed from Madura.

Gammel (1927) has reviewed later progress in the investigations of mycetoma. Vincent (1894) isolated *Streptothrix (Streptomyces) madurae* from a patient in Algiers. Wright (1898)

1 Material for this study from the files of the Armed Forces Institute of Pathology includes case material from the military, Veterans Administration, and civilian sources.

2 Infectious Disease Branch, Armed Forces Institute of Pathology, Washington, D.C. 20305.

3 The author expresses his appreciation to Dr. Chester W. Emmons, formerly Chief, Medical Mycology Section, Laboratory of Infectious Diseases, National Institute of Allergy and Infectious Diseases, National Institutes of Health, and to Dr. Chapman H. Binford, Medical Director, Leonard Wood Memorial, and Chief, Special Mycobacterial Diseases Branch, Armed Forces Institute of Pathology, Washington, D.C., for their review of this manuscript and helpful suggestions.

isolated a hyphomycete from a black-grain-mycetoma in Boston. LAVERAN (1902) studied the black-grain-mycetoma previously reported by CHABANEIX et al. (1091), and he named the fungus *Streptothrix mycetomi (Madurella mycetomi)*. BOUFFARD (1906) isolated *Actinomyces (Streptomyces) somaliensis* from a white-grain-mycetoma. BRUMPT (1906) proposed the generic name *Madurella* for the hyphomycete from black-grain-mycetomas and changed the name *Streptothrix mycetomi* to *Madurella mycetomi*.

YAZBEK (1920) observed *Actinomyces bovis (israelii)* in 3 mycetomas in Brazil. LOVEJOY and HAMMACK (1925) found *Actinomyces mexicanus (Nocardia brasiliensis)* in a mycetoma in Los Angeles. MUSGRAVE and CLEGG (1907) observed *Actinomyces (Nocardia) asteroides* in a typical Madura foot in the Philippines. PELLETIER and THIROUX (1912) found *Actinomyces (Streptomyces) pelletieri* in red-grain-mycetomas in India, Egypt and Senegal.

The actinomycetes have been classified as higher bacteria (BREED et al., 1957) and included as causative agents of mycetoma. The classification of PINOY and of CHALMERS and ARCHIBALD did not include other bacteria as possible causative agents of mycetoma. Botryomycosis is a disease caused by certain bacteria which form grains in suppurative foci. BOLLINGER (1870) discovered this disease in horses, and RIVOLTA (1884) gave it the name botryomycosis. OPIE (1913) published the first report of human botryomycosis in the United States, and this was also the first account of visceral involvement. There are now published reports of about 50 cases of human botryomycosis. Most of these have been regional integumentary infections, but some have been of the disseminated visceral type.

LIGNIERES and SPITZ (1903) isolated *Actinobacillus* from some cases of "lumpy jaw" in cattle. The bacteria were present in grains. ARCHIBALD (1910) described a number of cases of mycetoma in which the grains contained cocci rather than hyphae. MAGROU (1919) proved that botryomycosis of the type seen in horses and described by BOLLINGER could be caused by *Staphylococcus*. The lesions with suppurative foci and sinuses containing pale yellow grains simulated mycetoma and actinomycosis. MAGNUSSON (1928) showed that the so-called actinomycosis of the cow's tongue or soft tissues of the jaw was often caused not by *Actinomyces bovis* but by *Actinobacillus lignieresi*, a Gram negative bacillus, and that many granular infections in the udders of cows and pigs were caused by staphylococci rather than *Actinomyces bovis*. BEAVER and THOMPSON (1933) reported a fatal human infection by *Actinobacillus lignieresi* and described grains that were present in the lesions. BERGER et al. (1936) reported a patient with genital botryomycosis in which the grains contained both *Staphylococcus* and *Escherichia coli*. FINK (1941) described a patient with fatal visceral botryomycosis of the lung and liver, and the etiologic agent was proved to be *Staphylococcus aureus*. AUGER (1948) reported 4 cases of botryomycosis, one of which was fatal, involved the kidneys, and was caused by *Actinobacillus lignieresi*. WINSLOW (1959) reported 6 patients with botryomycosis, one of which was of the fatal visceral type and caused by a *Proteus* microorganism. The other 5 patients had integumentary lesions most of which were caused by staphylococci and all of which had been previously mistakenly diagnosed as actinomycosis or mycetoma. WINSLOW and CHAMBLIN (1960) reported visceral botryomycosis probably caused by *Pseudomonas aeruginosa*. GREENBLATT et al. (1964) reported a patient with botryomycosis of the lower lobe of the left lung. The grains contained chains of Gram positive cocci, and cultures grew a microaerophilic nonhemolytic *Streptococcus*. Following resection of involved segments of the lung the patient was apparently cured.

Terminology

The characteristic lesions of mycetoma can be produced not only by true fungi but also by filamentous bacteria-like fungi and by true bacteria. To the pathologist, the microscopic appearance of such lesions is quite similar; and to the clinician, the gross appearance and behavior of such lesions are often similar. Mycetoma is not restricted to the foot or to one geographic area as was suggested by the original term "Madura Foot." In fact it has become increasingly evident that the concept of mycetoma must be expanded to include morphologically characteristic lesions in any part of the body, and the location of such lesions may vary according to the habitat, occupation or habits of the patient, as well as the etiologic agent.

It is possible to create some order in the classification of mycetoma by determining the specific etiologic agent and classifying the lesions according to botanical terminology. Since mycetoma is essentially a tumor due to mycetes, we can divide the mycetomas into three groups as shown in Table 1.

Table 1. *Classification and Examples of Causative Agents of Mycetomas*

I. *Eumycetoma* ("true mycetoma", "mycetoma vera", "Maduro-mycosis"): caused by true fungi, the Eumycetes.
   1. *Madurella mycetomi*
   2. *Madurella grisea*
   3. *Monosporium apiospermum (Allescheria boydii)*
   4. *Cephalosporium sp. (falciforme, recifei*; possibly others)
   5. *Phialophora jeanselmei*
   6. *Pyrenocheata romeroi*
   7. *Leptosphaeria senegalensis*
   8. *Neotestudina rosatii*

II. *Actinomycetoma* ("actinomycotic mycetoma", "actinomy-cosis"): caused by higher bacteria (lower fungi), the Actino-mycetes.
   1. *Nocardia brasiliensis*
   2. *Nocardia asteroides* (? *Nocardia caviae*)
   3. *Actinomyces israelii (bovis)*
   4. *Streptomyces madurae*
   5. *Streptomyces pelletieri*
   6. *Streptomyces somaliensis*

III. *Botryomycosis* ("actinophytosis", "bacterial pseudomycosis"): caused by true bacteria, the Eubacteriales, classified by Bergeys' manual under Schizomycetes, the fission fungi.
   1. *Micrococcus pyogenes*
   2. *Escherichia coli*
   3. *Actinobacillus lignieresi*
   4. *Proteus sp.*
   5. *Pseudomonas aeruginosa*
   6. *Streptococcus* (nonhemolytic)

Definition

A *mycetoma* (Figs. 1, 2, 3) is a chronic suppurative, more or less granulamotous infection by fungi or bacteria usually beginning as a nodule in the soft tissues of the integument and progressing locally by destruction of all types of contiguous tissue, including muscles and bones. The mycetoma is characterized by tumefaction and derformity, multiple sinus formation and fistulous tracts which usually communicate with one another, with deep abscesses, and with ulcerated areas of the skin. Within the tissues, especially in foci of suppuration, the fungi or bacteria form characteristic grains or granules (Fig. 4) which are composed of colonies embedded in and surrounded by an eosinophilic, somewhat hyaline material, the exact nature of which is not known. This material may form a smooth shell around the colonies, but it is often knobby, irregular, or in the form of club-like or ray-like extensions from the periphery of a colony. It probably represents part of the host reaction rather than an integral part of the fungus.

For purposes of differential diagnosis if for no other reason, *disseminated actinomycosis* and *disseminated botryomycosis* as well as the *regional integumentary forms* of these two types of infection should be included in the classification of mycetomas. Since the lesions contain grains in suppurative foci and may be associated with sinus and fistula formation, they are histologically similar to other mycetomas. Moreover, the integumentary forms of botryomycosis may simulate actinomycetomas and eumycetomas. GONZALES OCHOA (1962) stated that when the lungs or abdominal viscera are involved by extension of nocardial mycetomas of the thoracic or abdominal wall, the clinical and pathologic picture simulates visceral actinomycosis which has invaded the body wall.

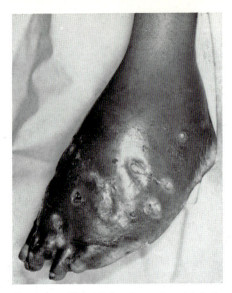

Fig. 1. Mycetoma pedis, showing swelling, deformity and multiple fistulas. *Nocardia asteroides* was cultured and the grains contained Gram positive branching filaments. Photographed by Dr. DANIEL H. CONNOR. Case contributed to the Armed Forces Institute of Pathology by Dr. Connor and the Makerere Medical College, Uganda, East Africa. AFIP Acc. No. 1040116

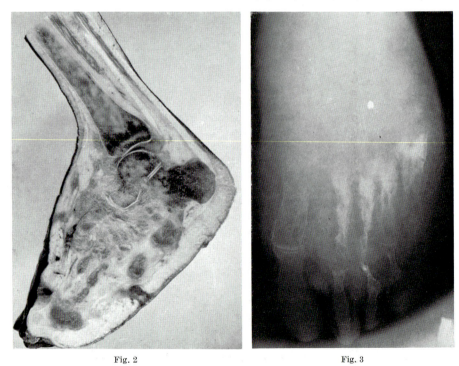

Fig. 2   Fig. 3

Fig. 2. Mycetoma pedis. Same case as shown in Fig. 1. Hemisection showing destruction of deep tissues including bone. Photographed by Dr. DANIEL H. CONNOR

Fig. 3. Mycetoma pedis. Case as shown in Fig. 1. Photograph of roentgenogram of foot contributed by Dr. DANIEL H. CONNOR. Note marked destruction of bones of feet

Infections which do not form grains are not classified under the mycetomas. Thus granuloma pyogenicum and mycotic granuloma are not included when grain formation is absent. To some investigators this may seem to be an artificial separation of no great importance, but the histologic picture and clinical behavior are not the same as those of mycetoma. Fungus balls in the respiratory passages, such as aspergillomas, are not included here under mycetomas although such infestations are frequently referred to in the literature as pulmonary mycetomas. In our experience these have not shown characteristic grain and sinus formation. Pulmonary actinomycosis and pulmonary botryomycosis, however, cause lesions which are similar to each other and may be classified as pulmonary mycetomas histologically.

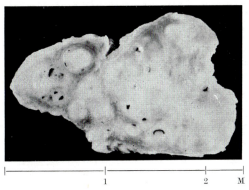

|———————————|———————————|——————|
1   2   M

Fig. 4. Gross photo of tissue excised from a mycetoma pedis. Black grains can be seen in some of the abscesses. Morphologically the grains were consistent with those of *Phialophora jeanselmei*. AFIP Neg. 58-9383

The definition of mycetoma refers to progressive tissue involvement and sinus formation even though early mycetomas begin before any grains or sinuses have formed. Very early mycetomas may therefore be difficult to diagnose as such. This difficulty is rarely if ever a practical problem.

The definition of mycetoma which is used here is broader than that generally used. Usually only the eumycetomas, the nocardial mycetomas and the streptomycetomas are included in the whole group of mycetomas. It must be remembered, however, that actinomycosis of the jaw, neck or other parts of the integument, even if secondary to visceral actinomycosis, may appear clinically and pathologically similar to nocardial mycetoma or streptomycetoma. Also, botryomycosis of the integument can simulate nocardial mycetoma, streptomycetoma or even eumycetoma.

Etiology and Pathogenesis

A large number of different types of fungi, actinomycetes and bacteria have been named as causative agents of eumycetoma, actinomycetoma and botryomycosis. Some have been isolated by cultural methods without comparison with the microscopic appearance of the grains in tissue sections. Since the agents are ubiquitous in nature, (Ajello, 1962) it is possible to isolate contaminants which are not causally related to the lesions. In addition, many of the agents are difficult to classify, and different names have been given to similar fungi by different investigators. On the basis of present knowledge concerning the role of fungi and bacteria in the etiology of human mycetomas, the causative agents which are representative and most important are shown in Table 1.

As seen microscopically in tissue sections, the real causative agents of mycetomas are the grains and not individual elements of fungi or bacteria. In most
mycetomas, the bacteria or fungi are usually not found outside of grains. This is
perhaps the fundamental difference between mycetomas and other types of
infection.

The earliest beginning of mycetoma is considered to result from entrance of
certain fungi or bacteria through a break in the skin or mucosa. Actinomycosis
starts within the oral, respiratory or gastrointestinal tract as an endogenous
infection by *Actinomyces israelii* which is frequently a part of the oral or pharyngeal natural flora. Botryomycosis may originate from outside sources through a
break in the skin or mucosa, or it may begin as an infection of the genitourinary
tract or respiratory tract. Other mycetomas, which are localized to the integument
and underlying tissues, originate from outside sources. These include the eumycetomas, nocardial mycetomas and streptomycetomas. For example, GONZALEZ
OCHOA (1962) isolated *Nocardia brasiliensis* from the soil in Mexico and stated that
the predominant site of mycetoma there is on the foot and back of Mexicans
because of their custom of going barefoot and often carrying soil-contaminated fiber sacks on their back.

Once the bacteria or fungi have gained entrance into the tissues, a period of
growth and multiplication results in the formation of a colony or perhaps more
than one colony. This phenomenon of *colonization* may be necessary to the survival
of these agents which are mostly saprophytic and of low virulence. The local
reaction between the colony and the host consists of a surrounding zone of polymorphonuclear neutrophilic leukocytes and an intervening barrier of eosinophilic material, the so-called clubs, rays or shells. The exact nature of this material
is not known but its staining reactions suggest it is proteinaceous, and it may
contain antigenantibody complexes.

Beyond the zone of polymorphonuclear neutrophiles there is chronic granulation tissue and more or less granulomatous inflammation, sometimes with multinucleated giant cells. Lymphocytes, plasma cells and epithelioid cells are usually
present in varying proportions outside the zone of acute reaction. In the chronic
lesions fibrosis is prominent and may seal up some sinuses and fistulas.

One of the mysteries of the pathogenesis of mycetomas has to do with the
method of *spread* and *invasion of contiguous tissue*. There is no satisfactory experimental data to solve this problem, and the following suggested explanation is
made from clinical and histologic observations. It is known that the grains cause
necrosis, abscesses, intercommunicating sinuses and fistulas. For parasite survival,
these grains do well to escape with discharges into the external environment
where they may continue to live on decaying organic material. The fungi and
bacteria which compose the grains are not well adapted to the human or animal
host, and their survival in tissues apparently requires a special form of adaptation,
the formation of colonies. At the periphery of each colony there is an intense host-
parasite reaction which results in necrosis of tissue and the formation of sinuses
and fistulas. This reaction even dissolves bone, producing osteitis and osteomyelitis.

There is also an effect on the colony or grain (DESTOMBES and PATOU, 1964).
If the grain is composed of *Actinomyces israelii* or certain bacteria, some organisms
may leave the colony and enter lymphatics or capillaries, escaping from the local
intense host-parasite reaction and disseminating to regional lymph nodes or other
parts of the host. If the grain is large and composed of higher fungi (*Eumycetes*)
with broad hyphae there is little tendency to invade lymphatics and capillaries.
Instead, the hyphae tend to form thick-walled spherical chlamydospores especially

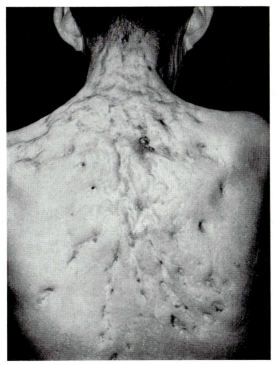

Fig. 5. Clinical photograph of a patient with thoracopulmonary mycetoma caused by *Nocardia brasiliensis*. (Courtesy of Dr. A. REYES, Jefe del Servicio de Anatomia Patológia. Centro Anticanceroso y Hospital O'Horan, Mérida, Yuc., México)

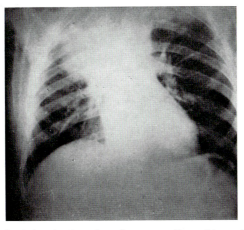

Fig. 6. Radiogram of chest showing invasion of upper portions of lungs by thoracopulmonary mycetoma caused by *Nocardia brasiliensis*. Same case as Fig. 5. (Courtesy of Dr. A. REYES)

near the periphery of the grains. In addition, fragments of the colony break away from the mother colony and start fresh growth in contiguous sites. By this means, numerous grains are formed, and these increase in number as the mycetoma advances. Small grains composed of actinomycetes or bacteria may also multiply

38*

in a similar manner, but individual organisms may break away from the mother colony and start new colonies. Nocardial mycetomas and streptomycetomas occasionally metastasize to regional lymph nodes. Direct extension from thoracic wall to lungs is common in Mexico. REYES (1963) has reported finding grains in the sputum of a patient with thoracopulmonary mycetoma caused by *Nocardia brasiliensis* (Figs. 5, 6). This patient developed hemoptysis from pulmonary invasion and died. Autopsy showed wide spread visceral dissemination of nocardial mycetoma. In addition to the lung there was involvement of pancreas, spleen, liver, kidney and thyroid. These disseminated lesions contained characteristic grains and cultures grew *Nocardia brasiliensis*. In a personal communication Dr. REYES stated that he believed nocardial mycetomas may spread not only by extension but via the blood stream as shown in the above patient. This patient also had several subcutaneous abscesses on different parts of the body presumably as the result of the blood stream dissemination.

Geographic Distribution and Prevalence

Mycetomas may occur in any part of the world, but they more commonly occur in tropical or subtropical climes, especially in the lower extremities of individuals who walk barefooted. The greatest number of cases has been reported from Africa, India, Mexico and South America.

Mycetoma is sporadic in the United States but has been reported from at least 20 states, mostly from the southwest (GREEN et al., 1964). It has occurred mostly in negroes who labor out-of doors. About 30 acceptable cases of eumycetoma and 33 cases of actinomycetoma are reported to have originated in the USA.

The geographic distribution of the different etiologic types of mycetoma is not well known but some of the available data is shown in Table 2. F. MARIAT (1963) has presented data from a world wide survey of 854 mycetomas. He found 40% caused by true fungi and 60% by actinomycetes. This survey indicated the predominant etiologic types of mycetoma and their relative frequency. There were 159 mycetomas caused by *Madurella mycetomi*, 28 by *M. grisea*, 45 by *L. senegalensis*, 29 by *A. boydii* or *Monosporium apiospermum*, 66 by *Streptomyces madurae*, 63 by *S. somaliensis*, 268 by *Nocardia asteroides* and *N. brasiliensis*, and 81 by *S. pelletieri*. MARIAT lists these as the principal agents of mycetoma, indicating that other microorganisms have been much less frequently and/or less precisely documented. He also concludes that the geographic distribution of the various etiologic agents is dependent on climatic factors. LATAPI (1959) has stated that 90% of mycetomas in Mexico are caused by *Nocardia brasiliensis*. In the Sudan, most mycetomas are caused by *Madurella mycetomi*, *Streptomyces somaliensis* or *Streptomyces pelletieri*. *Madurella mycetomi* has been reported also from West Africa and from India, Venezuela, Curacao, Brazil, Peru and Argentina.

BAYLET et al. (1961) stated that white grain mycetomas constitute only a minority in West Africa. They isolated 3 strains of *Cephalosporium sp.* from mycetomas in Senegal. Two were closely related to *C. falciforme* and the third to *C. recifei*. The majority of mycetomas studied in West Africa (REY, 1961) have been caused by *Madurella mycetomi*, *Madurella grisea*, *Streptomyces somaliensis*, *Streptomyces pelletieri*, *Leptosphaeria senegalensis* or *Pyrenochaeta romeroi*.

WILSON (1965) reported in Uganda that histological and cultural studies of 8 mycetomas at Mulago Hospital, Kampala, demonstrated that 6 were caused by *Nocardia asteroides*, 1 by *Nocardia brasiliensis* and 1 by *Cephalosporium* sp. WILSON found that Uganda has relatively few cases of mycetoma and that most of them are caused by actinomycetes.

ORIO et al. (1963) reviewed 50 mycetomas occurring in the French Somali Coast where thorny bush is very common and trauma is a frequent part of the clinical history. The agent isolated from 23 mycetomas was *Streptomyces somaliensis*; from 20, *Madurella mycetomi*; from 4, *Streptomyces madurae*; and histopathologic diagnosis was made on one mycetoma caused by *Leptosphaeria senegalensis* and one by *Pyreuochaeta romeroi*.

GAIND et al. (1962) reported the isolation of a new species of *Cephalosporium*, *C. infestans* sp. nov., from a mycetoma in a soldier in India. This species developed black grains in the host. Four species of *Cephalosporium* have been reported as causal agents of mycetoma; *C. falciforme*, *C. receifei*, *C. granulomatis* and *C. madurae*. *C. falciforme* and *C. recifei* are reported to

Table 2. *Geographic Distribution of some Etiologic Types of Mycetoma*

Etiologic Type	Geographic Areas*
Madurella mycetomi	2, 3, 8, 10, 12
Madurella grisea	3, 8, 10, 11, 12
Monosporium apiospermum . .	2, 3, 4, 6, 7, 8, 9, 11, 12, 14
Cephalosporium sp.	1, 3, 8, 12, 13,
Phialophora jeanselmei	8
Pyrenochaeta romeroi	3
Leptosphaeria senegalensis . . .	3
Neotestudina rosatii	3
Nocardia brasiliensis	9, 12
Nocardia asteroides	3, 9, 12
Streptomyces madurae	2, 3, 8, 9, 12
Streptomyces pelletieri	3, 9, 12
Streptomyces somaliensis	3, 9

* 1 Japan, 2 India, 3 Africa, 4 Italy, 5 Portugal, 6 Germany, 7 Canada, 8 USA, 9 Mexico, 10 Netherlands Antilles, 11 British West Indies, 12 South America, 13 Puerto Rico, 14 Cuba

Source References:

REIFFERSCHIED and SEELIGER (1957)
MACKINNON and ARTAGAVEYTIA-ALLENDE (1956)
LATABI and ORTIZ (1963)
ROSATI et al. (1961)
LACAZ and BELFORT (1961)

MACKINNON (1954)
BAYLET et al. (1959)
REY (1961)
MACKINNON (1963)
LAVALLE (1966)
GONZALEZ OCHOA (1962)

Note: KLOKKE, A. H. (1964) isolated *Nocardia brasiliensis* from a farmer in India and stated that this was the first reported isolation of this microorganism from mycetoma in Asia. KLOKKE also referred to rare isolations of *N. brasiliensis* from mycetomas in Uganda, the Congo and South Africa.

produce white grains. *C. madurae* and *C. granulomatis* are said to produce black grains (TWINING et al., 1946). Various species of *Cephalosporium*, however, are common contaminants, and well documented reports of mycetomas proved to be caused by *Cephalosporium* are rare.

In the United States *Monosporium apiospermum* has been the cause of a majority of reported cases of mycetoma, (GAY and BIGELOW, 1930; FIENBERG, 1944), but this fungus has also been found in mycetomas occurring in Canada (SHAW and MacGREGOR, 1935) and other areas of the world. A black mycetoma caused by *Madurella ikedae (Madurella mycetomi)* was reported by THOMPSON and IKEDA (1928). The patient was a 39-year old negro who injured his foot while employed as a laborer on a farm in Texas.

The importance of mycetomas as a health problem in certain parts of the world is indicated by estimates of the prevalence. In Mexico, LAVALLE et al. (1963) stated that mycetomas and sporotrichosis constitute the most frequent deep mycoses and that mycetomas are the more important and more difficult to treat. In the Sudan, SLADE et al. (1956) reported 1729 hospital attendances for mycetoma in the year 1951, and ABBOTT (1956) stated that 1231 cases were reported as hospital admissions in a $2^1/_2$ year period. EMMONS (1965) stated that mycetoma presents the most severe mycological health problem in Africa.

The occurrence of actinomycosis and botryomycosis is world-wide and not of great regional frequency. Intrinsic host factors are of more importance in determining the prevalence of the disseminated infections, but regional integumentary botryomycosis is related to trauma and chance inoculation with causative bacteria.

Clinical Features

Lynch (1964), reported from the Sudan on 325 cases of black mycetoma caused by *Madurella mycetomi* and 214 cases of yellow mycetoma caused by *Streptomyces somaliensis*. He stated that he had not seen mycetomata in different anatomic sites at the same time, but 6 patients gave a history of mycetoma affecting another site. The intervals between the 2 mycetomata ranged from 3—30 years. Yet mycetoma tends to involve contact or pressure points of feet, hands, legs, trunk, thighs, arms and head. Following inoculation, a small nodule develops and grows in the subcutaneous tissue. Later, after a few or many months, blebs or blisters may appear on the skin surface. These rupture and through these ulcerated areas there is discharged an oily, seropurulent or bloody fluid containing grains. The grains, 0.5 to 2 mm. in size, contain fungi or bacteria and are diagnostic if studied for intrinsic color, microscopic structure and cultural characteristics.

The eumycetomas produce marked tumefaction, deformity, destruction of tissues including bone, and functional loss. There is rarely any lymphatic spread to regional lymph nodes, and visceral dissemination does not occur. There is however, regional extension to contiguous tissues. The patient usually has no pain, unless there is secondary bacterial infection with a more acute inflammatory reaction.

The actinomycetomas may usually be separated clinically from actinomycosis since the latter begins within the oral cavity, intestinal tract or respiratory tract. On some occasions, however, the presenting lesions of actinomycosis may be in the integument of the neck, thorax, abdomen or extremity. There may then be a problem of differentiating lesions caused by anerobic *Actinomyces israelii* from those produced by aerobic *Nocardia* or *Streptomycetes*. The regional actinomycetomas tend to be more rapidly aggressive than the eumycetomas but they usually do not metastasize to the viscera or other anatomic sites as do actinomycosis and disseminated botryomycosis. Rarely the actinomycetomas spread to regional lymph nodes, and in contrast to eumycetomas some of them have a tendency to invade fascial sheaths rather than just spread between them (Lynch, 1964). Therefore the regional extension of actinomycetomas is apt to be more rapid than that of eumycetomas, and there may be pain and redness around the lesions. In Mexico actinomycetomas of the thoracic or adbominal wall often extend into the viscera (Gonzalez Ochoa, 1962) and there may rarely be dissemination by blood stream. (Personal communication from Dr. Reyes-Perez, Hospital O'Horan, Merida, Yuc., Mexico).

Primary mycetoma of the patella has been reported by Majid et al. (1964) in Poona, India. The etiologic agent was *Madurella mycetomi*. A cystic lesion was present in the patella, and a soft-tissue swelling presented just below this. The main mass of grains was present in the bone. The patient, a 13-year-old boy, had fallen on his knee 6 months prior to hospitalization. The authors suggest that the fungus made its way into the bone by direct implantation. Complete excision of the mycetoma was possible in this case by resection of the patella, prepatellar bursa and the infrapatellar fat pad. Primary mycetoma of bone is rare and this is the first reported primary mycetoma of the patella.

Chadfield (1964) reported an unusual mycetoma of the foot in a 51-year-old native of Grenada (Windward Islands, West Indies). According to the history the mycetoma probably began when the patient injured his foot at the age of 31. Yet examination 20 years later revealed swelling and deformity but no sinuses or bony involvement. Nodular lesions contained grains identified morphologically and culturally as those of *Madurella grisea*. The diagnosis was therefore established and the disease was easily differentiated from tuberculosis, syphilis, elephantiasis, neoplasia, leprosy, yaws, blastomycosis, chromoblastomycosis, sporotrichosis and coccidioidomycosis. This case demonstrates another unusual but definite mycetoma of the eumycetoma type.

Mycetomas involving a foot often invade the bones and they may extend up the leg. By the time medical advice is sought the only practical treatment may be amputation. When the mycetoma involves the scalp, the orbit, the neck, and other hazardous locations, complete excision may be impossible. Without adequate treatment the disease progresses, the patient finally succumbing to secondary infection or some other disease.

Pathology

By using a purified polysaccharide from *Nocardia brasiliensis*, BOJALIL and ZAMORA (1963) were able to detect precipitins in the sera of patients with mycetoma caused by this microorganism. At the present time, however, diagnostic antigenic material from the various causative agents of mycetoma is not available for routine testing of patients.

Although clinical, radiologic and immunologic studies may be of some aid the most important method of diagnosis consists of a combination of histologic and mycologic examination (EMMONS et al., 1963; WINSLOW and STEEN, 1964). The mycologic examination is not sufficient by itself because of the difficulty of excluding contaminants, and the histologic method requires mycologic support for identification of different causative agents.

If grains are present in the discharges of a draining mycetoma, microscopic examination of these will furnish information as to whether they contain bacteria, actinomycetes or eumycetes. Some of the grains can then be washed in sterile saline, crushed and cultured on appropriate media.

Table 3. *Color of Grains in Unstained Tissue Sections*

White to Yellow	Brown to Black
Monosporium apiospermum	*Madurella mycetomi*
(Allescheria boydii)	*Madurella grisea*
Cephalosporium falciforme	*Phialophora jeanselmei*
Cephalosporium recifei	*Pyrenochaeta romeroi*
Neotestudina rosatii	*Leptosphaeria senegalensis*
Streptomyces madurae	
Nocardia asteroides	
(? Nocardia caviae)	
Nocardia brasiliensis	
Actinomyces israelii	
Botryomycotic granules	
Red to Pink	Yellow to Brown
Streptomyces pelletieri	*Streptomyces somaleinsis*

Mycetomas which have not perforated the skin and are not discharging grains should be excised or biopsied, and multiple sections should be prepared for histologic examination. Gram stains are useful for staining actinomycetes or bacteria within grains. The periodic acid-Schiff and Gomori methenamine-silver methods (Armed Forces Institute of Pathology, 1960) are excellent for staining eumycetes. Unstained thick (15 micra) sections may be mounted in the usual mounting medium, covered with a cover slip and examined under the microscope with reflected light. The natural intrinsic color of the grains can be seen by this method and offers a clue as to the causative agent (Table 3).

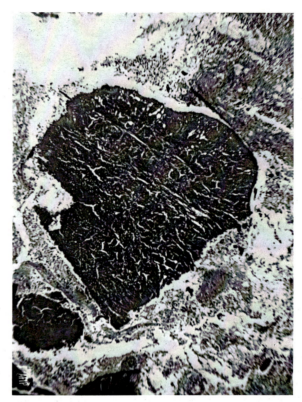

Fig. 7. Photomicrograph showing grain characteristic of *Madurella mycetomi*. H & E, ×100, AFIP Neg. 63-2350

The appearance of the different types of grains as seen in tissue sections stained with hematoxylin and eosin may be correlated with the microorganismal component and the cultural findings. With experience it is then possible to recognize some grains by their morphologic appearance.

The excellent studies of MACKINNON (1954, 1962, 1963), REY (1961), REY et al. (1962), CAMAIN et al. (1957), BAYLET et al. (1959), EMMONS et al. (1963) and LATAPI (1959) have aided greatly in establishing morphologic criteria based on cultural findings.

Madurella mycetomi: The grains tend to be large, brown in color, irregular in outline and easily fractured (Figs. 7, 8). The matrix is stained by brown interstitial pigment originating from the fungus. The grains are morphologically characteristic and a presumptive diagnosis of the species can be made without cultures.

Madurella grisea: The peripheral part of the grain is deep brown due to intrinsic pigment in the chlamydospores and hyphae (Fig. 9). The central portion of the grain is composed of loosely arranged hyphae with much less pigment giving the appearance of a hollow grain. These grains may be as large or larger than those of *Madurella mycetomi*. They do not have the interstitial pigment seen in grains of *M.mycetomi*. Morphologic differentiation from grains of *Leptosphaeria senegalensis* and *Pyrenochaeta romeroi* may be difficult and cultures are necessary.

Monosporium apiospermum: The grains are quite large, or become so, and are non-pigmented (Fig. 10). They are somewhat similar to grains of *Cephalosporium*

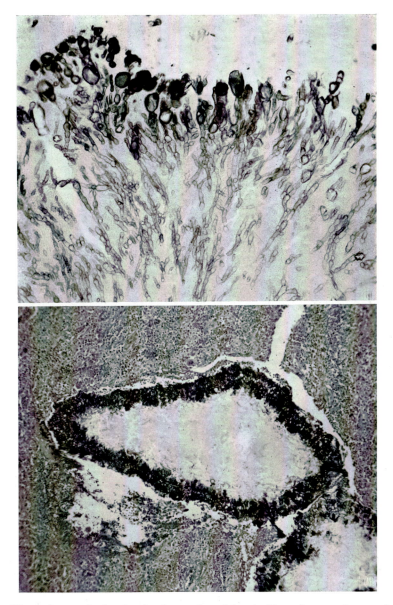

Fig. 8. Photomicrograph showing hyphae and peripheral chlamydospores in a grain of a eumycetoma caused by *Madurella mycetomi*. Gridley Fungus stain, ×305, AFIP Neg. 62-1295

Fig. 9. Photomicrograph showing grain characteristic of *Madurella grisea*. H & E, ×100, AFIP Neg. 63-2348

sp. but may have more chlamydospores around the periphery and a thick knobby eosinophilic shell. Cultures are necessary to confirm the etiologic diagnosis. EMMONS (1944) has shown that *Allescheria boydii* is the perfect or ascocarpic form of *Monosporium apiospermum*.

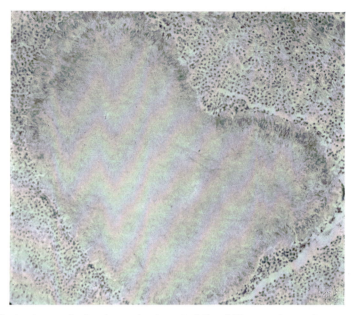

Fig. 10. Photomicrograph showing grain characteristic of *Monosporium apiospermum*. H & E,
×100, AFIP Neg. 57-18240

Cephalosporium sp.: The grains grow to a rather large size but some may be quite small. They are non-pigmented and the edges may be composed mostly of tangled hyphae (Fig. 11). There may be relatively little tendency to form an eosinophilic shell, the edges of the colony being immediately surrounded by polymorphonuclear neutrophiles. Cultures are necessary.

Phialophora jeanselmei: The grains are usually smaller than those of *Madurella grisea* but have somewhat similar brownish rinds and "hollow" centers (Fig. 12). The rind is often incomplete, having a curved linear arrangement. Cultures are necessary.

Pyrenochaeta romeroi: The moderate-sized brown grains with hollow centers have no interstitial pigment and have a resemblance to *Madurella grisea* and *Leptosphaeria senegalensis* (Fig. 13). Cultures are necessary.

Leptosphaeria senegalensis: The grains are moderate in size, brown, with "hollow" centers, simulating grains of *Madurella grisea* and *Pyrenochaeta romeroi* (Fig. 14). Cultures are necessary.

Neotestudina rosatii: The grains are moderately large, non-pigmented, composed largely of numerous thick-walled chlamydospores embedded in an abundant eosinophilic matrix and may be surrounded by adherent foreign body giant cells with focal intervening collections of polymorphonuclear neutrophiles (Fig. 15). According to ROSATI et al. (1960), the matrix or cement is formed by the hyphae of the fungus, is homogenous, reacts negatively to the periodic acid-Schiff reaction, contains no stainable mucin, and is stained intensely violet by the Gram method.

Nocardia brasiliensis: The grains are small or of moderate size, non-pigmented, irregular in shape but with rounded edges. They stain poorly with hematoxylin and eosin, appearing slightly amphophilic (Fig. 16). Special stains are necessary to demonstrate the gram positive branching filaments, 0.5—1 micra in diameter, in the grains. The organisms can be demonstrated as acid-fast in tissue sections

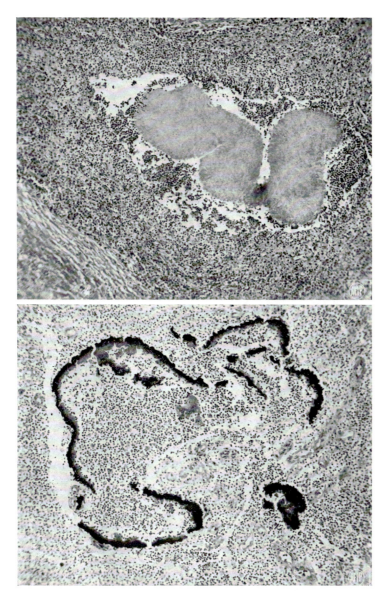

Fig. 11. Photomicrograph showing grain characteristic of *Cephalosporium sp.* H & E, ×100, AFIP Neg. 63-2337

Fig. 12. Photomicrograph showing grain characteristic of *Phialophora jeanselmei.* H & E, ×100, AFIP Neg. 63-2343

using a special staining method for *Nocardia* (EMMONS et al., 1963, p. 366). Cultures are necessary.

Nocardia asteroides: According to DESTOMBES et al. (1961) the grains are non-pigmented, small, rounded, oval or irregular in shape. Much of the grain fails to stain with hematoxylin eosin, but a layer of filaments near the edge of the grain is often stained well by hematoxylin, and many of the branching filaments can be

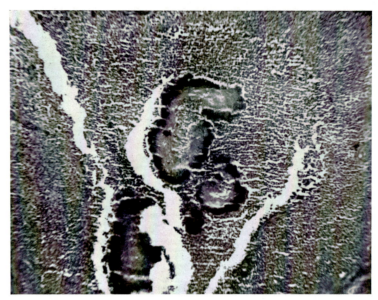

Fig. 13. Photomicrograph showing grain characteristic of *Pyrenochaeta romeroi*. H & E, ×100, AFIP Neg. 62-2342

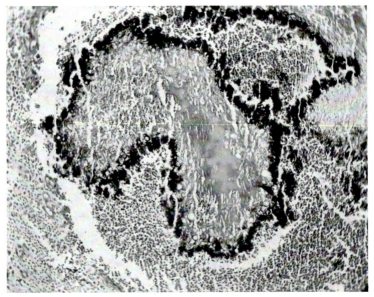

Fig. 14. Photomicrograph showing grain characteristic of *Leptosphaeria senegalensis*. H & E, ×100, AFIP Neg. 66-9315

seen in such preparations (Fig. 17). They are about 0.5—1 micron in diameter. The organisms can be demonstrated as acid-fast in tissue sections using a special staining method for *Nocardia*. Cultures are necessary and differentiation from *Nocardia caviae* may be difficult (GORDON and MIHM, 1962; EMMONS et al., 1963). In AFIP cases of pulmonary or disseminated nocardiosis caused by *Nocardia*

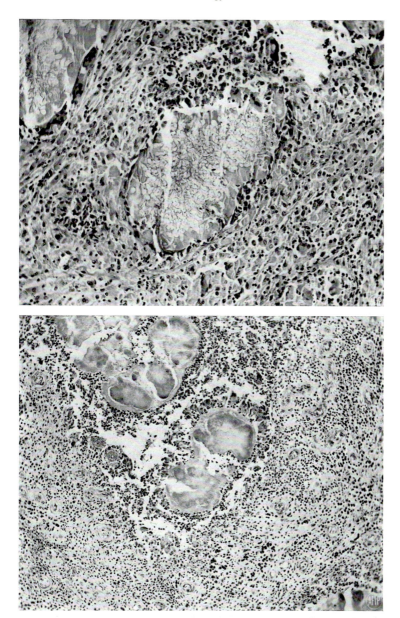

Fig. 15. Photomicrograph showing grain characteristic of *Neotestudina rosatii*. H & E, ×150,
AFIP Neg. 66-9320

Fig. 16. Photomicrograph showing grain characteristic of *Nocardia brasiliensis*. H & E, ×100,
AFIP Neg. 58-7236

asteroides, grain formation has not been observed and there is yet doubt about the
etiologic role of this organism in mycetomas.

MACOTELA and MARIAT (1963) examined the grains produced in experimental
infections of different animals by subcutaneous and intraperitoneal inoculation of

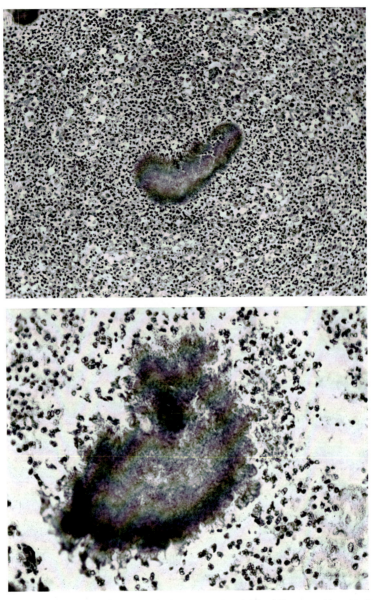

Fig. 17. Photomicrograph showing grain characteristic of *Nocardia asteroides*, (? *N.caviae*). H & E, ×150, AFIP Neg. 66-9314

Fig. 18. Photomicrograph showing grain characteristic of *Actinomyces israelii*. H & E, ×400, AFIP Neg. 57-18215

Nocardia asteroides and *N.brasiliensis*. They concluded that these grains possessed no specific differential characteristics and that their variable morphologic features depended on the host reaction. The grains produced by either microorganism were small, as in human lesions, and were partially acid-fast, Gram positive, and reacted positively when stained by the periodic acid-Schiff method.

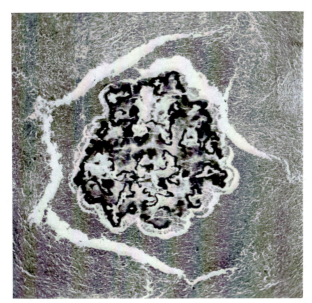

Fig. 19. Photomicrograph showing grain characteristic of *Streptomyces madurae*. H & E, ×42, AFIP Neg. 66-9318

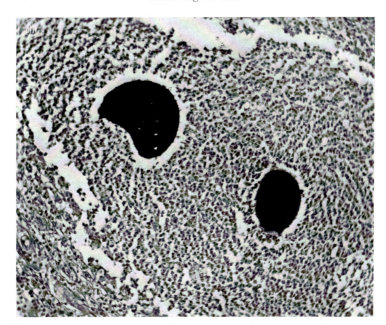

Fig. 20. Photomicrograph showing grain characteristic of *Streptomyces pelletieri*. H & E, ×165, AFIP Neg. 66-7426

Actinomyces israelii (bovis): It is doubtful if *Actinomyces israelii* is essentially different than *Actinomyces bovis* (Fig. 18) (EMMONS et al., 1963). Anaerobic cultures are important to differentiate *A.israelii* from aerobic *Nocardia* and *Streptomyces*. The grains are non-pigmented, small, and they usually have promi-

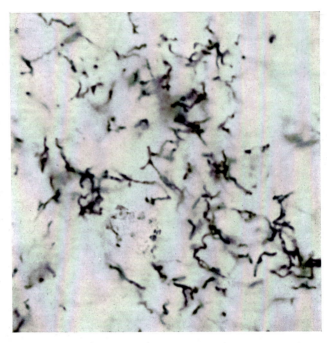

Fig. 21. Photomicrograph showing Gram positive branching filaments in a grain of an actino-mycetoma caused by *Streptomyces pelletieri*. BROWN and BRENN Gram stain, ×1900, AFIP Neg. 66-7414

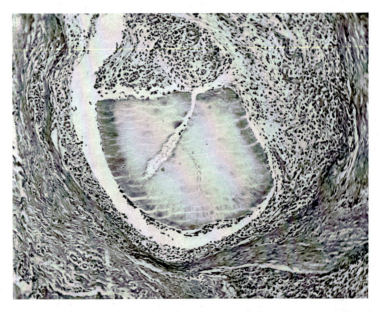

Fig. 22. Photomicrograph showing grain characteristic of *Streptomyces somaliensis*. H & E, ×100, AFIP Neg. 66-9317

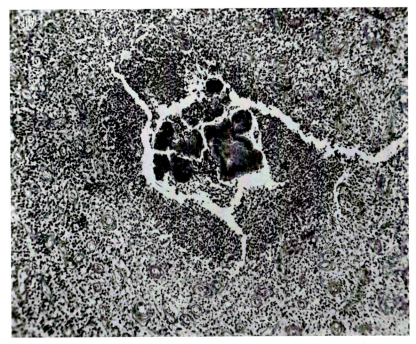

Fig. 23. Photomicrograph showing grain characteristic of botryomycosis caused by *Staphylococcus*. H & E, ×100, AFIP Neg. 63-2560

nent eosinophilic rays or clubs at the periphery. The shape of the grains is rounded or irregular, and beneath the periphery of each grain the filaments which measure about 0.5—1 micron in diameter, are stained prominently by hematoxylin. A presumptive diagnosis can be made from the appearance of the grains and is supported by clinical or pathologic evidence of an internal or disseminated infection.

Streptomyces madurae: The grains become quite large and consist of rounded or oval colonies with a wavy or variegated intertwining layer of hematoxylin-stained filaments, 0.5—1 micron in diameter, throughout each grain (Fig. 19). There is little shell or club formation. Such grains are morphologically characteristic and a presumptive diagnosis can be made without cultures.

Streptomyces pelletieri: The grains are small, often rounded or semicircular and homogeneously deeply stained by hematoxylin (Fig. 20). Individual filaments, 0.5—1 micron in diameter, are difficult to detect except at the periphery of the grain (Fig. 21). There is little if any shell, ray or club formation. Unstained thick sections examined microscopically by reflected light reveal a pink or reddish intrinsic pigmentation of the grains. The morphologic appearance, staining qualities and natural pink color of the grains allow a presumptive diagnosis without cultures.

Streptomyces somaliensis: The grains are rounded, oval or irregular and may grow to moderate size. They usually appear non-pigmented or faint yellow in unstained sections. The grains are not stained well by hematoxylin but faintly stained parallel crowded strands of thin hyphae, 0.5—1 micron in diameter, extend from the center to the periphery of many of the grains (Fig. 22). There is little if any shell, ray or club formation. The ends of the filaments at the periphery of the grain may be swollen and rounded. Cultures are necessary.

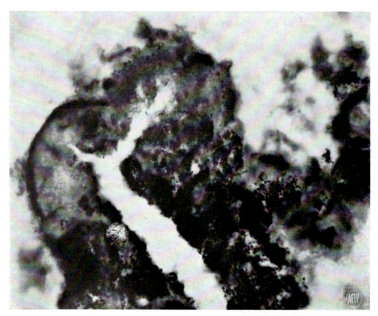

Fig. 24. Photomicrograph showing Gram positive cocci in a grain of botryomycosis caused by *Staphylococcus*. Brown and Brenn Gram stain, ×975. AFIP Neg. 63-2561

Micrococcus pyogenes: The grains are small, rounded or irregular in shape, non-pigmented and they frequently have scalloped or grape-like margins with a surrounding eosinophilic shell (Figs. 23, 24). Some grains stain well with hematoxylin, especially in areas where masses of cocci are present. Many cocci fail to stain with hematoxylin or Gram stains, presumably because of degeneration. Oil immersion examination reveals some cocci dividing by fission. We have seen one case in which some of the cocci were arranged in chains and cultures grew alpha streptococcus.

Other bacteria: The grains have an appearance similar to those containing micrococci, except that gram negative bacilli and cocco-bacilli are difficult to demonstrate unless special stains such as Giemsa, Brown and Brenn and Goodpasture-MacCallum are used. Cultures are important for identification of agents of botryomycosis.

Secondary bacterial infection: Although various bacteria may gain a superficial foot-hold in ulcerated areas and fistulas, it is remarkable how rarely secondary bacterial invasion of the deep tissues can be demonstrated by bacterial stains. In rare cases bacteria associated with grains of a eumycetoma or actinomycetoma may indicate a true mixed infection. The apparent rarity of this occurrence suggests that the fungi or bacteria causing the mycetoma exert a deep anti-microbial effect against secondary invaders.

The pathologic features of mycetoma may be summarized as follows:

1. Mycetoma produces multiple abscesses, intercommunicating sinuses and draining fistulas with more or less surrounding chronic granulomatous inflammation. Considerable fibrosis occurs, and some sinuses and fistulas may be periodically sealed off while others open to permit passage of exudate and grains.

2. There is usually regional extension and eventual destruction of deep tissues, including bone, but this evolution may require many months or years and occa-

sionally, even then, there is no bone destruction. Nerves and tendons survive the longest.

3. Actinomycosis and disseminated botryomycosis may spread via the blood stream to widely separated parts of the body, but both may also be regional and localized to the integument and deep structures.

4. Eumycetomas, nocardial mycetomas and streptomycetomas have a localized distribution in one part of the body such as an extremity, the buttocks, wall of the abdomen or thorax, the neck and the scalp. *Nocardia asteroides* (or *Nocardia caviae*) has been isolated from a few regional mycetomas. *Nocardia asteroides* may also, in different patients, produce pulmonary or disseminated nocardiosis, in which there is a diffuse distribution of Nocardia in the lesions without grain formation. GONZALEZ OCHOA (1962) found that mycetoma caused by *Nocardia brasiliensis* frequently invades the thoracic or abdominal wall and involves the viscera. There was pulmonary involvement in 25% of Mexican patients with thoracic mycetoma. Rarely there may be dissemination by blood stream probably as the result of direct invasion of visceral blood vessels. (Personal communication from DR. REYES-PEREZ, Hospital O'Horan, Merida, Yuc., Mexico).

5. By studying isolated grains or tissue sections containing grains in focal suppurative or granulomatous areas it is possible to differentiate eumycetomas, actinomycetomas and botryomycosis. In eumycetomas the grains contain elements of higher fungi (eumycetes), usually broad hyphae and chlamydospores. In actinomycetomas, the grains contain thin branching hyphae, 0.5—1 micron in diameter. In botryomycosis, the grains contain bacteria, most commonly cocci. The thin hyphae of actinomycetes may be fragmented and the fragments can resemble bacteria. Special stains and the examination of a number of grains will usually allow differentiation of actinomycetoma from botryomycosis.

6. Careful cultures of the deep lesions and washed grains is always desirable, but a detailed histologic examination combined with clinical information will frequently allow a presumptive etiologic diagnosis in mycetomas caused by *Madurella mycetomi*, *Madurella grisea*, *Monosporium apiospermum* or *Cephalosporium sp.*, *Neotestudina rosatii*, *Actinomyces israelii*, *Streptomyces madurae*, *Streptomyces pelletieri* and *Micrococcus sp.*

Treatment

The treatment of mycetoma as of other infections is most effective when given early. If cultures can be obtained and sensitivity to chemotherapeutic or antibiotic agents determined, a rational approach to medical treatment is possible. Many of the actinomycetes and bacterial agents are sensitive to antibiotics or sulfonamides. SEABURY et al. (1959) recommended penicillin for infections with *Actinomyces bovis (israelii)* and sulfadiazine for nocardial infections. Surgical drainage and local instillation of drug or isolated limb perfusion (FONKALSRUD et al., 1961) may be helpful. ZIPRKOWSKI et al. (1957) reported successful treatment with streptomycin of infections caused by *Streptomyces somaliensis*.

Early mycetomas may be completely excised and, where necessary, skin grafts can be used to cover defects. In advanced mycetomas of an extremity, amputation is often necessary.

Unfortunately some eumycetomas of the scalp and orbit (HICKEY, 1956) may be so far advanced that complete excision is not feasible. At the present time there is also no proved effective drug for these patients.

COCKSHOTT and RANKIN (1960) made a plea for a more optimistic outlook in the treatment of mycetoma. They treated patients with mycetoma in Ibadan with a preliminary course of a wide-spectrum antibiotic to eradicate the almost invariable secondary infection and then followed this with a long course of dapsone (diaminodiphenylsulfone). When feasible the affected part was immobilized. Dapsone 100 mg. twice daily, was given orally over many months, up to 2 years. Eight of a group of 18 patients responded to medical treatment. The high dosage of dapsone, however, the long period of treatment and the lack of evidence of effectiveness against Eumycetes must be considered in evaluating each patient to be treated.

References

AJELLO, L.: Epidemiology of Human Fungous Infections. Fungi and Fungous Diseases. Edited by GILBERT DALLDORF Springfield Ill.: Thomas. N.Y. Academy of Medicine, Sec. of Microbiology, Symposia, No. 11. 1. Fungi, 2. Mycoses, p. 69 (1962). — ARCHIBALD, R.G.: Human Botryomycosis. Brit. med. J. 2, 971 (1910). — Armed Forces Institute of Pathology, Manual of Histologic and Special Staining Technics, 2nd Ed., The Blakiston Division, Mc McGRAW-Hill Book Co., Inc., N.Y. 1960. — ARREDONDO, H.G., CEBALLOS, J.L.: Unusual Location of Mycetoma. Radiology 78, 72 (1962). — AUGER, C.: Human actinobacillary and staphylococcic actinophytosis. Amer. J. clin. Path. 18, 645 (1948). — BAYLET, J., CAMAIN, R., SEGRETAIN, G.: Identification Des Agents Des Maduromycoses Du Senegal Et De La Mauritanie. Description D'Une Espece Nouvelle. Bull. Soc. Path. exot. 52, 448 (1959). — BAYLET, R., CAMAIN, R., BEZES, H., REY, M.: Mycetomes A Cephalosporium Au Senegal. Bull. Soc. Path. exot. 54, 802 (1961). — BEAVER, D.C., THOMPSON, L.: Actinobaciliosis of man; report of a fatal case. Amer. J. Path. 9, 603 (1933). — BERGER, L., VALLEE, A., VEZINA, C.: Genital staphylococcic actinophytosis (botryomycosis) in human beings. Arch. Path. 21, 273 (1936). — BERKELEY: cited by HIRSCH (1886). — BOJALIL, L.F., ZAMORA, A.: Precipitin and skin tests in the diagnosis of Mycetoma due to Nocardia brasiliensis. Proc. Soc. exp. Biol. (N.Y.) 113, 40 (1963). — BOLLINGER (1870): cited by OPIE (1913). — BOUFFARD (1906): cited by GAMMEL (1927). — BOYCE, SURVEYOR (1894): cited by CHALMERS and ARCHIBALD (1916). — BOYD, M.F., CRUTCHFIELD, E.D.: A Contribution to the Study of Mycetoma in North America. Amer. J. trop. Med. 1, 214 (1921). — BREED, R.S., MURRAY, E.G.D., SMITH, N.R., (E.D.S.): Bergey's Manual of Determinative Bacteriology, 7th Ed., p. 33, 281. Baltimore: Williams & Wilkins Co. 1957. — BRUMPT, E.: Les Mycetomas. Arch. Parasit. 10, 489 (1906). — CAMAIN, R.; SEGRETAIN, G., NAZIMOFF, O.: Les mycetomes du Senegal et de la Mauritanie: apercu epidemiologique et etude histopathologique. Sem. Hop. Paris 33, 771 (1957). — CARTER, H., VANDYKE (1860): cited by CHALMERS and ARCHIBALD (1916). — CHABANEIX et al. (1901: cited by GAMMEL (1927). — CHADFIELD, H.W.: Maduromycosis. Proc. roy. Soc. Med. 57, 103 (1964). — CHALMERS, A.J., ARCHIBALD, R.G.: A Sudanese maduromycosis. Ann. trop. Med. Parasit. 10, 169 (1916). — COCKSHOTT, W.P., RANKIN, A.M.: Medical Treatment of Mycetoma. Lancet 1960 II, 1112. — COLEBROOK (1846): cited by CHALMERS and ARCHIBALD (1916). — DESTOMBES P., MARIAT, F., NAZIMOFF, O., SATRE, J.: A propos des mycetomes a Nocardia. Sabouraudia 1, 161 (1961). — DESTOMBES, P., PATOU, M.: Morphology of Mycetoma granules due to Nocardia or Cephalosporium, reconstituted by the method of serial histologic sections. Bull. Soc. Path. exot. 57, 393 (1964). — EMMONS, C.W.: Allescheria Boydii and Monosporium Apiospermum. Mycologia 36, 188 (1944). ∼ Mycoses in Africa. Intern. Path. 6, 33 (1965). — EMMONS, C.W., BINFORD, C.H., UTZ, J.P.: Medical Mycology, p. 305. Philadelphia: LEA & FEBIGER 1963. — FIENBERG, R.: Madura foot in a native American. Amer. J. clin. Path. 14, 239 (1944). — FINK, A.A.: Staphylococcic actinophytotic (botry-o mycotic) abscess of the liver with pulmonary involvement. Arch. Path. 31, 103 (1941). — FONKALSRUD, E.W., SHINER, J., HAAN, R., MARABLE, S.A., NEWCOMER, V., ROCHLIN, D.C.: Experimental studies and clinical experience with isolated limb perfusion of fungicidal drugs. Surg. Gynec. Obstet. 113, 306 (1961). — GAIND, M.L., PADHYE, A.A., THIRUMALACHAR, M.J.: Madura foot in India caused by Cephalosporium infestans sp. nov. Sabouraudia 1, 230 (1962). — GAMMEL, J.A.: Etiology of maduromycosis, with mycologic report on two new species observed in United States. Arch. Derm. Syph. (Clin.) 15, 241 (1927). — GAY, D.M., BIGELOW, J.B.: Madura foot due to Monosporium apiospermum in a native American. Amer. J. Path. 6, 325 (1930). — GILL (1842): cited by CHALMERS and ARCHIBALD (1916). — GONZALEZ OCHOA, A.: Mycetomas caused by Nocardia brasiliensis; with a note on the isolation of the causative organism from soil. Lab. Invest. 11, 1118 (1962). — GORDON, R.E., MIHM, J.M.: Identification of Nocardia caviae (Erikson) nov. comb. Ann. N.Y. Acad. Sci. 98, 628 (1962). — GREEN, W.O., Jr., ADAMS, T.E.: Mycetoma in the United States; a review and report of seven additional cases. Amer. J. clin. Path. 42, 75 (1964). — GREENBLATT, M., HEREDIA, R., RUBENSTEIN, L., ALPERT, S.: Bacterial pseudomycosis ("botryomycosis").

Amer. J. clin. Path. **41**, 188 (1964). — HICKEY, B. B.: Cranial Maduramycosis. Trans. roy. Soc. trop. Med. Hyg. **50**, 393 (1956). — HIRSCH, A.: Handbook of Geographical and Historical Pathology. London: Sydenham Society's Translation **3**, 700 (1886). — LACAZ, C. DA S., BELFORT, E. A.: Maduromycosis of the foot with black granules, caused by *Madurella grisea.* Hospital (Rio de J.) **60**, 367 (1961). — LATAPI, F.: Micetoma Analisis De 100 Casos Estudiados En La Ciudad De Mexico. Memorias. III Congreso Ibero Latino Americano De Dermatologia, p. 203 (1959). — LATAPI, F., ORTIZ, Y.: Los Micetomas En Mexico, Memorias Del Primer Congreso Mexicano De Dermatologia, pp. 126—144 (1963). — LAVALLE, P.: Nuevos datos sobre la etiologia del micetoma en Mexico y sobre su patogenia. Gac. méd. Méx. **96**, 545 (1966). — LAVALLE, P., SAUL, A., PENICHE, J.: La sulfadimetoxipiridazine en el tratamiento de los micetomas. Memorias Del Primer Congreso Mexicano De Dermatologia, pp. 525—535 (1963). — LAVERAN (1902); cited by GAMMEL (1927). — LIGNIERES, J., SPITZ, G.: Contribution a l'etude des affections connues sous le nom d'actinomycose. Arch. Parasitol. **7**, 428 to 479 (1903). — LOVEJOY, HAMMACK (1925): cited by GAMMEL (1927). — LYNCH, J. B.: Mycetoma in the Sudan. Ann. roy. Coll. Surg. Engl. **35**, 319 (1964). — MACKINNON, J. E.: A Contribution to the Study of the Causal Organisms of Maduromycosis. Trans roy. Soc. trop. Med. Hyg. **48**, 470 (1954). ~ Mycetomas as opportunistic wound infections. Lab. Invest. **11**, 1124 (1962). ~ Agentes de Maduromicosis En La Region Neotropical. An. Fac. Med. Montevideo **48**, 453 (1963). — MACKINNON, J. E., ARTAGAVEYTIA-ALLENDE, R. C.: The Main Species of Pathogenic Aerobic Actinomycetes Causing Mycetomas. Trans. roy. Soc. trop. Med. Hyg. **50**, 31 (1956). — MACOTELA-RUIZ, E., MARIOT, F.: On the production of experimental mycetomas by *Nocardia brasiliensis* and *Nocardia asteroides.* Bull. Soc. Path. exot. **56**, 46 (1963). — MAGNUSSON, H.: The commonest forms of actinomycosis in domestic animals and their etiology. Acta. path. microbiol. scand. **5**, 170 (1928). — MAGROU, J.: Les formes actinomycotiques du staphylocoque. Ann. Inst. Pasteur **33**, 344 (1919). — MAJID, M. A., MATHIAS, P. F., SETH, H. N., THIRUMALACHAR, M. J.: Primary mycetoma of the patella. J. Bone Jt. Surg. **46**, 1283 (1964). — MARIAT, F.: On the geographic distribution and incidence of mycetoma agents. Bull. Soc. Path. exot. **56**, 35 (1963) (Fr.). — MUSGRAVE, CLEGG (1907): cited by GAMMEL (1927). — OPIE, E. L.: Human botryomycosis of the liver. Arch. intern. Med. **11**, 425 (1913). — ORIO, J., DESTOMBES, P., MARIOT, F., SEGRETAIN, G.: Mycetoma in the French Somali Coast. Review of 50 cases observed between 1954 and 1962. Bull. Soc. Path. exot. **56**, 161 (1963) (Fr.). — PELLETIERI, THIROUX (1912): cited by GAMMEL (1927). — PINOY, E.: Actinomycoses et Mycetomes. Bull. Inst. Pasteur **11**, 977 (1913). — REIFFERSCHEID, M., SEELIGER, H.: Monosporiosis and Maduromycosis. Germ. med. Mth. **2**, 139 (1957). — REY, M.: Les Mycetomes Dans L' uest Africain. Paris: Imprimerie, R. FOULON and Cie 1961. — REY, M., BAYLET, R., CAMAIN, R.: Current data on mycetoma, Appros of 214 cases in Africans. Ann. Derm. Syph. (Paris) **89**, 511 (1962). — REYES, A.: Examen Histologico De Esputos Metodo Auxiliar En El Diagnostico De Las Micosis Pulmonares, Dermatologia. Rev. mex. **7**, 29 (1963). — RIVOLTA (1884): cited by BERGER, VALLEE and VEZINA (1936). — ROSATI, L., DESTOMBES, P., SEGRETAIN, G., NAZIMOFF, O., ARCOUTEIL, A.: Sur Un Nouvel Agent De Mycetome Isole En Somalia. Bull. Soc. Path. exot. **54**, 1265 (1961). — SEABURY, J. H., KROLL, V. R., LANDRENEAU, R.: A Conservative Method of Treatment for Maduromycosis. Sth med. J. (Bgham, Ala.) **52**, 1176 (1959). — SHAW, R. M., MacGREGOR, J. W., Maduromycosis: With the Report of a Case Due to *Monosporium Apiospermum.* Canad. med. Ass. J. **33**, 23 (1935). — SLADE, P. R., HASEEB, M. A., MORGAN, H. V.: Oxytetracycline in treatment of Maduromycosis. J. trop. Med. Hyg. **59**, 262 (1956). — THOMPSON, H. L., IKEDA, K.: Maduromycosis. Arch. Surg. **16**, 764 (1928). — TWINING, H. E., DIXON, H. M., WEIDMAN, F. D.: Penicillin in Treatment of Madura Foot. U. S. nav. med. Bull. **46**, 417 (1946). — VINCENT (1894): cited by GAMMEL (1927). — WILSON, A. M.: The aetiology of mycetoma in Uganda compared with other African countries. E. Afr. med. J. **42**, 182 (1965). — WINSLOW, D. J.: Botryomycosis. Amer. J. Path. **35**, 153 (1959). — WINSLOW, D. J., CHAMBLIN, S. A.: Disseminated Visceral Botryomycosis. Amer. J. clin. Path. **33**, 43 (1960). — WINSLOW, D. J., STEEN, F. J.: Considerations in the histologic diagnosis of Mycetoma, Amer. J. clin. Path. **42**, 164 (1964). — WRIGHT (1898): cited by GAMMEL (1927). — YAZBEK (1920): cited by GAMMEL (1927). — ZIPRKOWSKI, L., ALTMANN, G., DALITH, F., SPITZ, U.: Mycetoma Pedis. Arch. Derm. **75**, 855 (1957).

Sporotrichosis

HARRY I. LURIE, Richmond/Virginia, USA

With 22 Figures

Sporotrichosis is a chronic, usually benign, infection caused by the fungus *Sporotrichum*. It most commonly involves the skin and subcutaneous tissues, but occasionally the musculoskeletal tissues, mucous membranes and viscera are affected.

Mycology

The *Sporotrichum* is a genus of the order Hyphomycetales which is a division of the class Fungi Imperfecti. It is characterized by the presence of septate, repent, irregularly branched hyphae. There are no well-differentiated conidiophores; the spores are borne laterally or terminally, singly or in groups. They are sessile, or on short sterigmata, pyriform, ovoid or spherical in shape, usually small, hyaline or lightly colored.

As long ago as 1809 LINK described eleven species of *Sporotrichum*, most of them found on decaying wood. Probably the first description of a pathogenic *Sporotrichum* was that of MONTAGUE in 1844; the fungus was isolated by GRUBLER and WEIS from a case of bronchomycosis and therefore named *S. bronchiole*. In 1898 SCHENCK reported the first case of what is now known as the typical lymphangitic type of sporotrichosis. With the assistance of E. F. SMITH he described the fungus in great detail; they concluded that it belonged to the genus *Sporotrichum* but that it did not conform exactly with any of the 100 or more species tabulated in Saccardo's Syllage Fungorum. In the following year BRAYTON described the second case of a similar type. One year later (in 1900) HEKTOEN and PERKINS published the third case and named the fungus *Sporothrix Schenckii*. In 1903 DE BEURMANN and RAYMOND reported the first case in France. The fungus isolated from their case was studied by MATRUCHOT and RAYMOND who named it *Sporotrichum Beurmanni*, maintaining that it differed from the American strain and was therefore a new species. In 1906 DE BEURMANN and GOUGEROT referred to the American strain as *Sporotrichum Schenckii* (pp. 993—1006) and in 1910 MATRUCHOT officially reported it as a separate species.

Subsequently many more "new species" were described, for example: *S. asteroides*, SPLENDORE 1909; *S. equi*, CAROUGEAU 1909; *S. Jeanselmei*, BRUMPT and LANGERON 1910; *S. Carougeaui*, LANGERON 1913; *S. Councilmanni*, WOLBACH, SISSON and MEIER 1917; *S. lipsiense*, BENEDEK 1926; *S. epigoeum* (Brunaud), ASCHIERI 1929; *S. anglicum*, CASTELLANI 1937; *S. tropicale*, PANJA, DEY and GHOSH 1947. Several of these have since been removed from the genus of Sporotrichum and the others, including *S. Beurmanni*, have been shown to be identical with *S. Schenckii*, or merely variants of this fungus which do not warrant separation into new species. Most mycologists now accept only one valid species and give priority to the name of Schenckii.

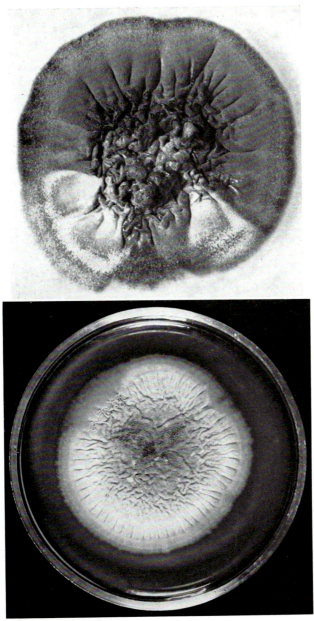

Fig. 1. *Sporotrichum Schenckii*. Growth on Sabouraud's glucose agar, pigmented (above) and unpigmented (below)

Sporotrichum Schenckii

When grown on Sabouraud's glucose agar at room temperature a recognizable growth usually appears in 3—5 days. The colonies are at first small, white and discrete, resembling yeast colonies, with no visible aerial mycelium. As growth increases the colonies enlarge, their surface becoming wrinkled and folded until they eventually coalesce to form a moist-looking wrinkled membrane on the surface of the medium. Later it appears more dry and leathery. The color may vary from white, through cream, tan and brown to black, depending on the medium, the strain of the fungus and probably on other as yet unknown factors (Fig. 1).

Microscopically it consists of very delicate, branching, septate, hyaline hyphae measuring 1.5—2 μ in thickness (Fig. 2). The conidia are borne laterally on the hyphae or in clusters at the ends of lateral branches. They vary in shape depending on the age of the culture, the medium and the strain; in some cultures they are pyriform, in others they are ovoid or spherical. In several instances triangular or conical spores have been described (BROWN et al.; MARIAT et al.), and in older cultures they tend to become round and thick-walled. Their size varies from 2—4 μ by 2—6 μ. In most cultures they appear hyaline but in darkly pigmented cultures they are lightly colored; the hyphae, however, never show pigment. Chlamydospores, usually intercalary, sometimes terminal or lateral, may appear in older cultures (D. J. DAVIS, 1914).

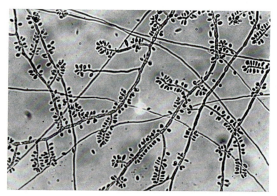

Fig. 2. *Sporotrichum Schenckii*. Microscopic appearance of growth on Sabouraud's glucose agar, × 600

When the fungus is grown on Francis' glucose cystine blood agar or on brain-heart infusion agar at 37°C, the tissue or yeast phase is obtained. The colonies resemble those of bacteria; they are soft, and greyish-yellow in color. Microscopically the growth is seen to consist of spindle-shaped, elliptical or ovoid bodies which reproduce by budding. A few short pseudohyphae are usually present.

The carbohydrate and nitrogen metabolism are of no value in the differentiation of the species or even in separating strains (MEYER and AIRD; LURIE, 1950, 1951). However NORDBRING found that the presence of thiamine in the medium has a pronounced influence on the growth of the fungus, and BURKHOLDER and MOYER showed that it was in fact essential for growth. DROUHET and MARIAT found that pyrimidine is the only growth factor required by *S. Schenckii* and MARIAT et al. demonstrated that the requirement for growth of the pyrimidine fraction of thiamine is specific for *S. Schenckii*.

GOUGEROT and BLANCHETIERE (1909) proved the presence of a strong endotoxin and a weak exotoxin. SALVIN confirmed the presence of an endotoxin.

Geographical Distribution

During 1907 and 1908 DE BEURMANN and GOUGEROT published numerous articles on sporotrichosis, following which, reports of further cases in other provinces of France appeared. Knowledge of the disease spread and soon cases were being recognized in other parts of the world. By 1912 about 200 cases had been reported and in that year DE BEURMANN and GOUGEROT accumulated all the known facts about the disease in their brilliant monograph "Les Sporotrichoses". Case reports followed in rapid succession from various countries. The disease apparently is world-wide in distribution, except in areas north of the 50th latitude above the equator and south of the 50th latitude below the equator.

The references listed under the geographical distribution include only those of the earliest or latest reports, review articles or single cases from areas where the disease is uncommon; it is not intended in this work to make reference to every publication on sporotrichosis.

North America. Since the first case reported in the United States of America by SCHENCK in 1898, the second by BRAYTON and the third by HEKTOEN and PERKINS, there have been many cases reported from that country (FOERSTER, 1924; EVERETT). The disease appears to be most prevalent in the Missouri Valley and in the Mississippi basin (SUTTON, 1914; GASTINEAU et al.) and least prevalent in the Western states of Washington, Oregon, Nevada, Idaho, Wyoming, Utah, Arizona and New Mexico.

There have been a few cases in Canada (FISCHER and MARKKANEN; LEARMONTH; BURGESS; HAWKS) but no cases have been seen in Alaska (DUNN).

Central America. It is fairly prevalent in Central America and in the Caribbean Islands, with the highest incidence in Mexico (SANCHEZ MARROQUIN and GONZÁLEZ; GONZÁLEZ OCHOA and GONZÁLEZ MENDOZA; ACEVES ORTEGA et al.; LATAPÍ, 1963).

Cases have been reported from Guatemala (MORALES), from Costa Rica (BOLAÑOS and TREJOS; SOLANO, 1965), from Panama (CALERO and TAPIA), from Salvador (LLERENA), from Cuba (DUQUE; MENOCAL; GONZÁLEZ BENAVIDES, 1956; PARDO COSTELLO and TRESPALACIOS), from Puerto Rico (KESTEN et al.) and from the West Indies (AUDEBAUD et al.).

South America. On this continent the disease is extremely prevalent in Brazil (LUTZ and SPLENDORE; LINDENBERG; DE REZENDE; DE AGUIAR PUPO; O.G. COSTA; PADILHA GONÇALVES and PERYASSU; DE ALMEIDA et al.; SAMPAIO and DA SILVA LACAZ; RAMOS E. SILVA, 1963; ROTBERG et al.). It is also fairly common in Uruguay (GRECO, 1908; BORDES et al.; MAY; SILVA CORREA; ERRECART; MACKINNON, 1949a, b). Cases have been reported from Colombia (POSADA BERRIO; SILVA; GONZALO CALLE and ANGELA RESTREPO; POSADA TRUJILLO et al.; PEÑA), from Venezuela (JIMINEZ-RIVERO and BRICEÑO-IRAGORRI; DE MONTEMAYOR), from Guiana (HENRY; LEFROU; SILVERIE and RAVISSE), from Peru (ESCOMEL) and from Argentina (BALIÑA and MARCÓ DEL PONT; DE GREGORIIS; QUIROGA; GAVIÑA ALVARADO et al.; PESTANA et al.; ROMAÑA and UGHETTI).

Europe. After DE BEURMANN and RAYMOND reported the first case from France in 1903 there were innumerable cases in that country, many having been reported by DE BEURMANN and GOUGEROT with various co-authors. Within the first decade there were about 100 cases, most of them reported as isolated occurrences; but in recent years the disease has become very rare in that country, only occasional cases having been reported (MERKLEN et al.; BESSIERE). It has always been uncommon in the rest of Europe. However cases have been seen in England (VON OFENHEIM; WALKER and RITCHIE; GREIG; GRAY and BAMBER; RIDDELL), in Ireland (BEATTY), in Germany (ARNDT; FIELITZ; WOLFF; HUGEL; JUNG), in Belgium (LERAT; DOCKX), in Holland (KEHRER; VAN DIJK and DER KINDERIN), in Switzerland (STEIN; BLOCH; JADASSON; DU BOIS), in Austria-Hungary (KREN and SCHRAMEK; HECHT), in Jugoslavia (SLAMJER), in Bulgaria (BALABANOFF; DESPOTOV and SHIK), in Rumania (CÁPUŞAN et al.), in Italy (STANCANELLI; CAMPANA; VIGNOLO-LUTATI; CURCIO; SEGRE; DEL GUASTA; CAMPANELLA; CALIFANO), in Portugal (ALVARES and PRAZERES; NEVES and NAVARRO DA SILVA; NAVARRO DA SILVA et al.), in Spain (DE OYARZABAL; PEYRE; NOGUER MORÉ and DAUSÁ; ALVAREZ PUEYO and DE ARMAS), in Norway (BOECK; WIDIRØE; VOSS; NORDEN, 1951, 1952) and in Finland (HELVE et al.).

Asia. The first case in the Union of Soviet Socialist Republics was reported as early as 1907 by MESCHTSCHERSKI, and during the next few years several more cases were reported (ZELENEFF; PERKEL; PESHKOVSKI; BREMENER). In the last three decades the disease has become much less common, the more recent cases having been seen by BRODSKYI and MITZENMACHER, ARAVYSKY and ARIYEVICH, and by RAPPAPORT and MEKLER. Cases have been reported in Turkey (HODARA and BEY; RICHTER and ERBAKAN), in Israel (ZIPRKOWSKI et al.), in India (GHOSE; PANJA et al.; DAS-GUPTA et al.; DEY), in China (TYAU; LIU; LÜ; SUN and CHÜ), in Vietnam (SEQUIN), in Indonesia (TEN BRINK, 1916, 1918), in Japan (KOBAYASHI; TAKAHASHI; FUKUSHIRO and KAGAWA; FUKUSHIRO et al.) and in the near and middle East (MUMFORD).

Africa. The first evidence of sporotrichosis on the African continent was found in horses in Algeria by BRIDRÉ et al. in 1912. Human cases were reported by CATANEI and by MONTPELLIER et al. Cases were found in Liberia by the Harvard African Expedition in 1926—1927;

in Egypt by EL-MOFTY and NADA; in Nigeria by SHRANK and HARMAN; in Mozambique by SALAZAR LEITE and DA LUZ; in South Africa by PIJPER and PULLINGER; DANGERFIELD and GEAR; DU TOIT and HELM and BERMAN.

In Madagascar, too, the disease was first recognized in horses (CAROUGEAU, 1909a) and soon thereafter in man (CAROUGEAU, 1909b). Further cases were reported by FONTOYNONT and by FONTOYNONT and CAROUGEAU (1922).

Australia. The disease has been reported from Australia (ROBINSON and ORBAN; BARRACK and POWELL; MINTY et al.; MEAD and RIDLEY; BARRACK; DURIE et al.; O'DONNELL) and from the Pacific Islands (MUMFORD and MOHR; CAMPBELL).

The areas of greatest prevalence appear to have changed on at least two occasions. At the beginning of the century it was most prevalent in France and in the United States of America, but some cases were also seen in South America, Europe, Russia and in the Far East. Between 1930 and 1940 relatively few cases were seen anywhere in the world, but in the 1940's an epidemic of about 3,000 cases occurred in South Africa. In more recent times the disease has been most common in Central and South America, with the greatest prevalence in Brazil, while a moderate number of cases is still being seen in the United States of America, South Africa and Japan. However the disease has almost entirely disappeared from the European scene. No cases at all have been seen at the St. Louis Hospital in Paris during the last 5 years (DEGOS), and during the last 30 years the disease has become a rarity in the Soviet Union (ARAVYSKY).

Etiology

Saprophytism: The *Sporotrichum Schenckii* normally exists as a saprophyte in nature. DE BEURMANN and GOUGEROT (1907 f) isolated the fungus frow straw, leaves, grains of wheat, fruits, bark, wood, thorn bushes, tilled earth, dead insects and their larvae, caterpillars and living flies. They also recovered it from beech bark, horsetail fern (*Equisetum*) and dried out grains of oats (1908 b). SARTORY found it on the husks of blighted wheat and DOMINGUEZ found the fungus growing on tobacco leaves. Both EMMONS (GASTINEAU et al.) and D'ALESSIO et al. recovered it from sphagnum moss. BROWN et al. found profuse growths on the timber in the gold mines of the Witwatersrand. In addition to the above sources the fungus has been recovered from a rose plant (BROOKS); from soil in the USA (EMMONS, 1952; DEAN and HALEY) and in Brazil (ROGERS and BENEKE); from dust, litter, animal and bird excreta (EMMONS, 1954); from soil, marine animals, algae, feathers and bird droppings on beaches (DABROWA et al.); from used bedding material (COOKE and FOTER) and from reeds — *Arundo donax* (HARANT et al.). HARSH and ALLEN found *Sporotrichum* spores in the atmosphere in San Diego and RICHARDS isolated them from the air over Britain. BROWN et al. reported that on one occasion only *S. Schenckii* was isolated from the atmosphere in a gold mine in which there was an epidemic of sporotrichosis. However a more recent report from the Transvaal and Orange Free State Chamber of Mines suggests that airborne spores play no part in the spread of the disease.

Both the geographical distribution and the epidemiology of the disease suggest that the weather, atmospheric temperature and relative humidity, influence the growth of the fungus in its saprophytic state (MACKINNON, 1949 c, d). SINGER and MUNCIE are also of the opinion that the humidity plays a significant role. HELM and BERMAN, MEAD and RIDLEY and LLERENA found a distinct seasonal incidence with most cases occurring in the warmer and more humid months of the year. On the contrary, however, GONZÁLEZ OCHOA (1965) found that in Mexico 37% of cases occurred in winter, 34% in autumn, 15% in summer and 12% in spring. LONDERO et al. (1963) attributed most of their 57 cases in Argentina both to climatic factors and to the proximity of the people to vegetation,

Occupation: As the fungus responsible is primarily a saprophyte growing on vegetation and in the soil, it is understandable that certain occupations which involve close contact with these infected materials would predispose to infection. Such occupations include florists (GASTINEAU et al.; GREENBURG), workers in plant or tree nurseries (FOERSTER, 1924, 1926; BLAIR and YARIAN; CREVASSE and ELLNER; HAYES; SCHNEIDAU et al.; D'ALESSIO et al.), horticulturists (MASON et al.), farmers and farm laborers (HAMBURGER; RUEDIGER; FOERSTER, 1926; COSTA and JUNQUEIRA), bulb farmers (SINGER and MUNCIE; CIPOLLARO), berry pickers (STOUT), professional gardeners (FOERSTER, 1926; GASTINEAU et al.), miners (PIJPER and PULLINGER; DANGERFIELD and GEAR; DU TOIT; HELM and BERMAN) and general laborers (GASTINEAU et al.). Vendors of fresh vegetables and chefs who handle these vegetables are sometimes infected (DE BEURMANN and GOUGEROT, 1907 f).

Among florists and nursery employees the infection is contracted by handling the sphagnum moss (GASTINEAU et al.; CREVASSE and ELLNER; HAYES; D'ALESSIO et al.). Florists, horticulturists and gardeners, both professional and amateur, are frequently infected as a result of being pricked by the thorns of barberry bushes, *Berberis thunbergii* (DE BEURMANN and SAINT-GIRONS; FOERSTER, 1924, 1926; CARTER; BLAIR and YARIAN; FLO and SMITH; MASON et al.) or by the thorns of rose bushes (NETHERTON and CURTIS; COLE and LOBITZ; DURIE et al.; GIROUX and PERRY). Three cases resulted from pricks by cactus thorns (LEHMAN and PIPKIN; LEWIS and CUDMORE; RIORDAN). Bulb farmers contract the disease by contact with salt hay mulch, sometimes called salt marsh grass, *Spartena patens* (SINGER and MUNCIE; CIPOLLARO). Farmers and farm laborers probably contract the disease from the soil or, rarely, from tobacco leaves. Several cases have been reported to follow injury while peeling potatoes (RITCHIE; RUEDIGER; DOMINICI and RUBENS DUVAL; LUDWIG), and one case from handling garden manure (ROBINSON and ORBAN).

Rather unexpected occupations associated with sporotrichosis are packers on brick yards and pottery works where the products are packed in straw (DE ALMEIDA et al.; LYONS) or in zocate (forage) grass (GONZÁLEZ BENAVIDES, 1956, 1959; GARRETT and ROBINS; GONZÁLEZ OCHOA, 1965). SILVA and GUIMARÃES reported four cases in a family who contracted the disease from straw used for packing domestic utensils. Another such occupation is the gathering of reeds, *Arundo donax*, used in the manufacture of paper (HARANT et al.).

Many other occupations are listed in the literature, the majority of which appear to be completely unrelated to one another and to the disease process: merchant, druggist, insurance agent, clerk, teacher, etc.

In addition to these saprophytic sources of infection, many cases have resulted from trauma involving wire, nails, wood, etc.

Bites of Insects and Animals: Many cases have been attributed to bites, which include:

insect bite (SKEER), mosquito bite (MOORE and MANTING; MIKKELSEN et al.), bee sting (BAUCKUS), bite of a field mouse (MOORE and DAVIS), rat bite (ANDERSON and SPECTOR; JEANSELME and CHEVALIER, 1911; RUGIERO et al.; SOLANO, 1965), bite of a boa constrictor (GRAY and BAMBER), hen bite (SUTTON, 1910; SOLANO, 1965), parrot bite (ROUSLACROIX; WYSE-LAUZUN), dog bite (ROUSLACROIX), horse bite (RISPAL and DALOUS), bite of a bat (SOLANO, 1965) and the bite of a fish (DE MAGALHAES).

In the cases cited above there was no direct evidence that the insects or animals actually carried the fungus. It is therefore possible that the skin of the patient may have been contaminated with infected soil or other material, and that the bite merely introduced the fungus into the skin. However DE BEURMANN and GOU-

GEROT (1907 f) have cultured the fungus from dead insects. It is of interest to note that in South America the facial lesions in infants are attributed to insect bites (MARIAT et al.). The *Sporotrichum* has been isolated from the fur of rats, rabbits and cats living in stables of infected horses (DE BEURMANN and GOUGEROT, 1906), from the mouth and fur of healthy rats (LUTZ and SPLENDORE), from the mouth and coats of horses (MEYER). The fungus has never been found in fish but DABROWA et al. found it in marine animals and algae, and DE MONTEMAYOR and HEREDIA DE GAMERO recovered it from shrimps. The boa constrictor died of a "canker" of the mouth (GRAY and BAMBER).

Contact with infected animals: Many cases of spontaneous, naturally occurring sporotrichosis have been observed in a variety of wild and domestic animals. These include rats and mice (LUTZ and SPLENDORE, 1907 a, b; PRINGUALT and VIGNE), rabbits (LUTZ and SPLENDORE, 1907 b, p. 631), dogs (GOUGEROT and CARAVEN; SOUZA; COLLES; GUILHON and OBRY; LONDERO et al., 1964), cats (LUTZ and SPLENDORE, 1907 b, p. 631; SINGER and MUNCIE), horses (CAROUGEAU, 1909 a; PAGE et al.; MEYER; BRIDRE et al.; ROBINSON and PARKIN; JONES and MAURER; THOROLD; PEPPLER and TWIEHAUS; DAVIS and WORTHINGTON), mules (PIRATININGA; SALIBA et al.), donkeys (WENDT; ALBORNOZ) and in cattle (HUMPHREYS and HELMER).

In a few instances human infection has occurred as a result of handling animals known to be infected.

These include handling gophers (OLSON), skinning rabbits (MADDEN), handling green hides (ARMSTRONG; STICKNEY), handling an infected cat (SINGER and MUNCIE), an infected dog (SHERWELL) and a heifer (QUAINE, 1911), riding an infected horse (BEINHAUER). Veterinary surgeons have contracted the disease from an infected mule (CAROUGEAU, 1909a, p. 148) and from treating a horse with hives (MEYER).

Contact with Human Cases and Iatrogenic: Accidental infection has occurred in the laboratory (BERTIN and BRUYANT; FIELITZ; WILDER and McCULLOUGH; MEYER; FOERSTER, 1924; MIKKELSEN et al.). Infection of the eye has followed a cataract operation (FRANÇOIS et al.). Four cases of cutaneous lesions followed injections with contaminated hypodermic syringes (JEANSELME et al., 1928 a, b). The disease has been transmitted from one person to another by way of infected dressings (QUAINE, 1904) and by direct contact (WIDAL and JOLTRAIN; RUEDIGER; L. M. SMITH). Another very unusual mode of transmission was by way of the chin rest of a violin (HOPE).

The disease may sometimes be familial, usually because the members of a family are all exposed to the same source of infection (WIDAL and JOLTRAIN; CREGOR; NEVES; GARRETT and ROBBINS; SOARES et al.; GONZÁLEZ OCHOA, 1959; SILVA and GUIMARÃES).

Transmission through the placenta to the fetus has been shown in rats by DE BEURMANN, GOUGEROT and VAUCHER (1908g) and by FORNERO; but it has not been reported in man. DOMINICI and RUBENS DUVAL reported a case of a woman who had active lesions in the second half of her pregnancy and gave birth to normal offspring.

Carrier States and Infection via Gastrointestinal Tract: It has been shown that human beings may be carriers and harbor the fungus in the oropharynx after initial infection or after cure (DE BEURMANN and GOUGEROT, 1907a, e; MOUNT; OTTO-LENGHI) and that under certain circumstances it may invade the tissues and produce diesease. DE BEURMANN and GOUGEROT (1907d, p. 499) succeeded in infecting newborn guinea pigs by feeding the fungus in milk. DAVIS (1916) confirmed that the organism is able to pass through the wall of the gastrointestinal tract. EISEN-STADT reported a case of disseminated lesions in whom he suspected that the fungus had entered the body via the tonsils or pharynx. LOEWE had a case involving the cervical lymph nodes; he postulated that the infection may have been by way of the pharynx.

Contributing Factors: The prevalence of the fungus in nature and the fact that human beings may be carriers raises the question why only some of the contacts contract the disease. GOUGEROT (1911) felt that there were three factors which influence the virulence of the organism: (1) lowered resistance of the host usually due to some intercurrent infection, (2) increased virulence of the organism and (3) the development of a hypersensitivity to the toxins of the organism (DE BEURMANN and GOUGEROT, 1909d). With regard to the second factor, DE BEURMANN, GOUGEROT and VAUCHER (1908) have shown that the virulence of the human strain in rats has been increased by repeated passage through the animal. GOUGEROT (1911) postulated that in man the saprophyte may enter through the skin and continue its saprophytic existence on the mucous membranes until it becomes adapted to its environment and that it then becomes virulent for man.

Age Incidence

The disease is most common in young adults and in middle life. Table 1 shows the age incidence in 400 cases taken at random from the literature. The percentages in the younger age groups (0—10 and 11—20) are almost certainly unrealistically high because in case reports involving children the ages were always specified and were included in this count, whereas numerous cases, where the patients were simply referred to as adults, were omitted.

Table 1. *Age incidence based on 400 cases in which age was specified, taken at random*

Age, years	No. of cases	Percentage
0—10	83	21
11—20	78	19.5
21—30	38	9.5
31—40	57	14
41—50	61	15
51—60	43	11
61—70	33	8
71—80	7	2

The youngest case was that of a $2^1/_2$ month old baby in whom the lesion had been first noticed 24 h after birth (GOMEZ-OROZCO and ORTEGA) and the oldest was 76 years.

Sex Incidence

Of 400 cases taken at random from the literature, excluding the South African miners, there were 280 males (70%) and 120 females (30%), a ratio of slightly more than 3:1. If the South African miners had been included there would have been a much greater preponderance of males since there were approximately 3,000 cases, all male.

Incubation Period

HYDE and DAVIS stated that the lesion appears 6—12 days after the initial injury. DANGERFIELD and GEAR were of the opinion that it could take anything from 3 days to 3 weeks or even longer. SIMSON et al. infected human volunteers with spore suspensions; when the skin was previously scarified the lesion appeared

on the 14th day, but when the spores were applied to the unbroken skin it took
2 months before a lesion appeared. DE BEURMANN (1912) had one case in which the
incubation period was 3 months. According to HELM and BERMAN the incubation
period is usually 7—30 days but may be up to 6 months.

Anatomic Site of Primary Lesion

A review of 400 cases selected at random from the literature but excluding the
South African cases is summarized in Table 2.

Table 2. *Site of primary skin lesion based on
400 cases selected at random (excluding the
South African miners)*

Upper extremity	302	(75.5%)
Fingers, thumb, hand and wrist	241	
Forearm	47	
Elbow	6	
Upper arm	8	
Lower extremity	40	(10%)
Foot	4	
Ankle	2	
Leg	15	
Thigh	3	
Unspecified	16	
Head and neck	36	(9%)
Scalp	2	
Face	14	
Eyelids	15	
Neck	5	
Trunk	13	(3.25%)
Multiple primaries	9	(2.25%)

In the epidemic among the South African miners the organism was introduced
by contact with the fungus growing on the timber props. The miners habitually
wear heavy boots, trousers and a helmet. The amount of clothing worn above the
waist is variable, but the majority wear a sleeveless singlet or undershirt with
narrow shoulder straps. As a result the skin surface exposed to trauma was different from the usual and accounts for the complete absence of lesions on the feet, the

Table 3. *Site of primary skin lesion in 400
cases selected at random and 1,471 miners*

Upper extremity	63	%
Lower extremity	11	%
Head and neck		3.5%
Trunk	19	%
Multiple primaries		3.5%

scarcity of lesions on the scalp and the swimsuit area, and the greater frequency of
lesions on the trunk, which were mainly on the shoulders and scapular regions. If
the 1,471 miners reported by HELM and BERMAN are added to the 400 cases taken
at random from the rest of the world, there is a significant increase in the frequency
of lesions on the trunk with a diminution in those of the upper extremity, head
and neck. The distribution is summarized in Table 3.

It is of interest to note that SOLANO (1965) had 20 cases in children between the ages of 1 and 10 years, in all of whom the lesion was on the face; GOMEZ-OROZCO and ORTEGA, and LATAPÍ (1950) reported similar cases. MARIAT et al. are of the opinion that these facial lesions in infants are probably transmitted by insects.

Clinical Manifestations

GOUGEROT (1909) recognized the following clinical types:
1. Multiple disseminated subcutaneous gummatous
2. Multiple ulcerating gummatous
3. Localized lymphangitic
4. Dermal
5. Epidermal
6. Extracutaneous
7. Acute and subacute febrile
8. Carrier states.

Several different classifications of the clinical manifestations have been proposed (NORDEN, 1951; SINGER and MUNCIE; GONZÁLEZ OCHOA, 1953; MARIAT et al.; EVERETT; MIKKELSEN et al.; GONZÁLEZ OCHOA, 1965). Some of these classifications are based on the tissue involved, some on the route of dissemination and/or whether the lesions are primary or secondary. No one classification appears to be entirely satisfactory. The author suggests the following:

A. *Cutaneous*
  1. Epidermal
    a. primary
    b. secondary
  2. Dermal
    a. primary
    b. secondary
  3. Subcutaneous
    a. primary
    b. secondary
      i. lymphangitic (lymphogenous spread)
      ii. disseminated (hematogenous spread)
B. *Extracutaneous*
  1. Mucous membranes
  2. Musculoskeletal
  3. Visceral
  4. Central nervous system
  5. Organs of special senses
C. *Acute and subacute febrile*
D. *Sporotrichids and other allergic manifestations*
E. *Carrier states*

A. Cutaneous Sporotrichosis

1. Epidermal

DE BEURMANN and GOUGEROT (1912) described the following varieties:
Circinate
Vesicular
Vesiculopustular
Pustular and acneiform
Eczematous and pityriasiform
Pemphigoid

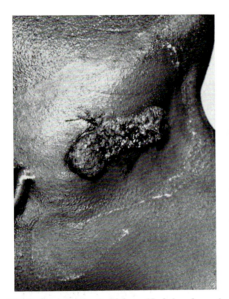

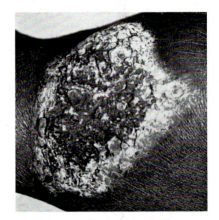

Fig. 3. Sporotrichosis of face. Nodular dermal lesion with areas of superficial ulceration

Fig. 4. Sporotrichosis of hand. Verrucous or papillomatous dermal lesion

du Toit described a flat scaly lesion which resembles ringworm. This may correspond to de Beurmann and Gougerot's pityriasiform type.

The epidermal lesions frequently surround ulcerated dermal lesions when they result from surface contact with infected serosanguinous discharge; rarely they may follow hematogenous dissemination or represent the initial primary infection in the "minimal" form of the disease reported from South America.

2. Dermal

These lesions may take any of the following forms:

Papule — a smooth, pink, raised papule often surrounded by other small discrete papules; sometimes several papules may coalesce. If untreated these lesions may become pustular and ulcerate.

Pustule — usually elevated, round or oval, often elongated in the line of a natural crease in the skin.

Furuncle — resembles a "boil" but lacking the acuteness of a pyogenic infection. A small scab appears in the center, which, when removed, reveals a crater-like sinus.

Flat plaque — usually oval, may be rough and covered with silvery scales or smooth and covered by atrophic-looking skin.

Nodule — at first covered by intact skin but may later ulcerate (Fig. 3). This type may be solitary or may consist of a group of nodules. They may be round, oval or elongated in a linear fashion.

Verrucous or papillomatous — round or oval, raised, hard, warty and scaling (Fig. 4).

Granulation tissue — a plaque-like area, varying in size and shape covered by exuberant granulation tissue (Fig. 5).

There are many intermediate types and combinations of types. The lesion may start as one type and change into another type; e.g. a papule may become a pustule and then ulcerate. It is of interest to note that four cases of onychomycosis

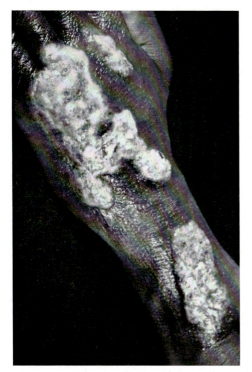

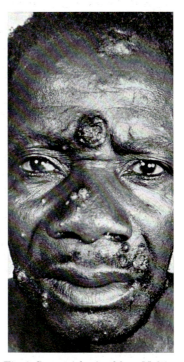

Fig. 5. Sporotrichosis of hand and arm. Granulation tissue type of dermal lesion

Fig. 6. Sporotrichosis of face. Multiple disseminated dermal lesions

or paronychia have been attributed to Sporotrichum infection (BOGGS and FRIED;
SARTORY et al., 1928; DO AMARAL; CONTI-DÍAZ).

HELM and BERMAN studied 2,825 cases in South Africa all of which were of the
dermal type, and found that with few exceptions the lesions were either papular,
pustular or ulcerated, flat plaques or verrucous. EVERETT, however, in reviewing
the American cases, found that the "chancre" was by far the most common. He
found only 17 primary cutaneous lesions which were "typical"; these included 7
pustular, 7 verrucous and 3 nodular varieties.

According to DU TOIT two factors govern the type of skin lesion which results
from an infection in any given case, viz.: the mode of infection and the area of skin
involved. Inoculation of the fungus via an abrasion results in the entire abraded
area being covered with fungating granulation tissue; when the infection enters
through a hair follicle the resultant lesion resembles a boil. He found that lesions
on the palm of the hand, where the skin is thick and resistant, are sometimes insignificant. On the lower leg, usually immediately above the top of the boot, they
take the form of superficial ulcers which have undermined edges or have a punched-out appearance. With few exceptions, the lesions he observed on the face were
of the verrucous or papillomatous variety, whereas other investigators have described facial lesions of all types (Fig. 6).

HELM and BERMAN are of the opinion that the appearance and course of the
lesion is dependent on the local resistance of the skin, the general resistance of the
patient and the depth of the infection. They confirmed this in part by experimental
inoculation of human volunteers, and found that subcutaneous inoculation is apt

to produce the pustular variety which is difficult to cure; that intradermal inoculation produces a more superficial and milder lesion; that scratch inoculation produces the papular type and is easier to cure, but that if left untreated for a sufficiently long period it becomes ulcerative. Evidence of natural resistance is borne out by the fact that in some cases attempts at producing an experimental infection failed. Also in some proven cases spontaneous cures were noted, especially in those with dry, flat plaques.

Others have reported similar spontaneous cures (D'Alessio et al.; Padilha Gonçalves, 1963 b). The present author is also of the opinion that the dry flat plaques and verrucous lesions occur in cases with some degree of immunity to the disease (Lurie, 1967). Carr et al. were impressed by the chronicity of their case of verrucous sporotrichosis; they expressed the opinion that this type of lesion probably represents a type analogous to the chronic, localized, cutaneous blastomycosis and that it may be the result of reinoculation or dissemination of the organism, rather than of primary inoculation.

The initial lesions appearing at the site of entry of the fungus are, with few exceptions, of the dermal type; if one lesion of this type is the only manifestation of the disease it is sometimes referred to as a "solitary" or "fixed" dermal lesion. However the initial lesion may be followed, after a varying interval, by lymphangitic spread and the appearance of additional lesions, in which case it is referred to as the "primary" lesion. A primary lesion of the nodular variety is frequently called a "sporotrichotic chancre". When secondary lesions appear along the course of the lymphatic vessels, the complex is commonly referred to as "localized lymphangitic sporotrichosis", presumably because it remains localized to one limb and there is no hematogenous dissemination. Deeply ulcerated lesions rarely persist as "fixed" lesions but usually result in rapid lymphangitic dissemination.

Localized Lymphangitic Sporotrichosis: This appears to be the most common clinical picture throughout the world. Both Foerster and Everett have stated that it is the most common type in the USA. du Toit, and Helm and Berman found it to be the most common in South Africa, as did Ramos E. Silva and Padilha Gonçalves, and Magalhães Pereira et al. (1964) in Brazil, Llerena in Salvador and González Ochoa (1965) in Mexico. In other countries too, although statistics are not available, this is suggested by the reports of fairly large series of cases, all of this type (Fukushiro et al. in Japan; Califano in Italy, etc.).

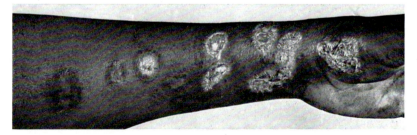

Fig. 7. Sporotrichosis. Localized lymphangitic type of hand and arm

Gómez Orozco and Ortega suggest that lymphangitic spread is uncommon in children. They reported 4 cases, Solano (1965) 20 cases and Gluckman 4 cases, all in children in whom the disease remained localized to the primary site of infection and no secondary lesions appeared. It would appear that lymphangitic spread is generally less common with lesions on the face (Candiota de Campos).

In the typical lymphangitic sporotrichosis the primary lesion is followed in a few days to several weeks by the appearance of secondary lesions along the course of the lymphatic vessels draining the area (Fig. 7). At first these take the form of small, hard, subcutaneous nodules freely movable over the underlying tissues and not attached to the skin. They gradually increase in size and later become attached to the deeper tissues and overlying skin. Then they soften in the center and superficially so that on palpation one feels a cup-shaped depression with marginal induration and eventually they ulcerate. Frequently there is an associated lymphangitis manifested by a palpable, painless, cord-like thickening of the lymph vessels (DE BEURMANN and GOUGEROT, 1907 b; HELM and BERMAN).

Lymph Node Involvement: In 1909 JOSSET-MOURE described a case showing lymphadenitis, but MARIE and GOUGEROT were the first to report a proved sporotrichotic lesion in a lymph node. A case of sporotrichotic osteitis of the tibia developed an inguinal adenitis; macroscopically the nodes were normal but on microscopic examination they showed the typical granulomata and the fungus was recovered on culture. DE BEURMANN, GOUGEROT and LAROCHE reported a case of fatal sporotrichosis with markedly enlarged preauricular and maxillary nodes.

SPOOR's case presented as a crop of boils over enlarged cervical nodes; WADE and MATHEW's case of a lesion in the mammary gland had enlarged axillary nodes and LIU reported a case of probable sporotrichosis with lymphadenopathy of the cervical, submaxillary, axillary and inguinal nodes.

With regard to the localized lymphangitic sporotrichosis, GOUGEROT (1913) stated hat there is usually no lymphadenopathy. CRUTCHFIELD reported two cases, one with cubital node and one with axillary node involvement. FOERSTER (1926) saw one case with the primary lesion on the hand and an enlarged epitrochlear node and one case with the primary on the forearm and enlarged axillary nodes. He stated that regional nodes may enlarge and become indurated and sometimes suppurate. DANGERFIELD and GEAR found that lymph nodes were enlarged in a few cases while DU TOIT reported that lymph nodes are practically never involved, the only exception to this rule being the epitrochlear node which is characteristically and frequently enlarged. HELM and BERMAN occasionally noted enlargement of the axillary or inguinal nodes but stated that it was difficult to assess whether this was due to sporotrichotic infection or to secondary bacterial infection. They confirmed du Toit's finding that with lesions on the hand or forearm the epitrochlear node is frequently considerably enlarged but never breaks down. MADDEN reported two cases in which both the epitrochlear and the axillary nodes were involved.

SINGER and MUNCIE stated that lymph nodes are infrequently involved and they reported a case of lymphangitic sporotrichosis spreading up the forearm and arm in whom the epitrochlear and the axillary nodes were not enlarged or tender. Most reports make no mention of lymph nodes while some specifically state that the nodes were not involved (MINTY et al.; MEAD and RIDLEY; CASTLETON and REES). It would appear, therefore, that lymph node involvement is uncommon, even in lymphangitic sporotrichosis.

3. Subcutaneous

The lesions which appear along the course of the lymphatic vessels following a primary dermal lesion start as subcutaneous nodules but eventually involve the overlying skin and ulcerate (Fig. 8). However the clinical category of subcutaneous sporotrichosis is usually confined to the cases with subcutaneous gummata resulting from hematogenous dissemination. There are two forms of these lesions, one in which the lesions rarely ulcerate and the other in which ulceration occurs early.

Non-Ulcerating Disseminated Gummatous Sporotrichosis: According to GOUGEROT (1909) this was the most common clinical picture of sporotrichosis in France. It is manifested by the insidious development of small, hard, elastic and painless subcutaneous nodules. There may be as few as 4 or 5 or as many as 100. There is no selective localization or systematic grouping. They may reach the size

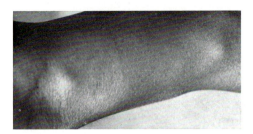

Fig. 8. Sporotrichosis of arm. Subcutaneous gummata

of a walnut, soften rapidly and within 3—6 weeks evolve into cold abscesses. The softening starts superficially and centrally so that on palpation one feels a soft central area, easily depressed and surrounded by an indurated wall. This "cup-shaped" depression was regarded by DE BEURMANN and GOUGEROT as constant and characteristic. GUILAINE, however, says that this is not always present. There is no associated inflammation, pain or systemic symptom. The abscesses remain quiescent, while new ones appear. They rarely ulcerate unless incised, when they discharge a thin serosanguinous material which later may become thick and purulent. The incision may close and the abscess reform, or it may develop into a "syphiloid" ulcer with persistent drainage and crusting over with a tendency to cicatrize and discharge through sinus tracts. The discharge may infect the surrounding skin resulting in dermal or epidermal lesions.

Multiple Ulcerating Gummatous Sporotrichosis: The lesions start as subcutaneous gummata, but ulcerate spontaneously within 2—3 weeks or after several months. The usual picture is that of an indurated, ulcerated lesion on the base of which one sees narrow, irregular openings of fistulous tracts with violaceous borders. The base of the ulcer is granular, bleeds easily and is usually covered with a crust. From the fistulae there is a scanty discharge of serous or serosanguinous material.

Frequently the lesions resemble tuberculosis with a cup-shaped depression and indurated periphery. Sometimes they resemble syphilis with large crateriform ulcers. Occasionally they resemble ecthyma with superficial and heavily crusted ulcers.

If they are not treated, involution of the lesions may take months or even years. The scars may be irregular, linear, or stellate with tongue-like tags or remaining fistulous walls, and surrounding pigmentation. Central keloidal masses may develop.

Rarely there may be an associated acute inflammatory reaction with erythema and edema. Generally the lesions are symptomless and the general health of the patient is unaffected. However, in long standing cases with multiple lesions, there may be steadily increasing debility, anemia and cachexia and some local disability. Subcutaneous gummata, non-ulcerated or ulcerated, are rarely associated with lymphadenopathy (DE BEURMANN, 1912; JAME).

Relative Frequency of Types of Cutaneous Sporotrichosis: The author reviewed 300 cases from the literature, selected at random, but excluding the South African miners. The distribution is shown in Table 4.

Table 4. *Relative frequency of types of Cutaneous Sporotrichosis in*
300 cases selected at random

Localized lymphangitic with primary dermal lesions . . .	86%
Fixed dermal lesions	9%
Disseminated subcutaneous	3%
Epidermal	2%

B. Extracutaneous Sporotrichosis

Sporotrichosis may involve any of the tissues or organs of the body. Usually these lesions result from hematogenous dissemination but in a significant number of cases the primary lesion cannot be found. DE BEURMANN and GOUGEROT (1907) postulate that in some instances the infection may be introduced through the gastro-intestinal tract. Pulmonary lesions may be the result of inhalation of spores.

1. Mucous Membranes

These include the nasopharynx, mouth, larynx, trachea, intestine and vagina. The infection may manifest itself as a rhinitis, pharyngitis, angina, stomatitis, glossitis, laryngitis, tracheitis, enteritis or vaginitis. The lesions may be erythematous, ulcerative, suppurative, vegetative or papillomatous. There is usually no evidence of membrane or pseudomembrane formation. However BANKS reported a case involving the fauces, palate and pharynx with a membrane resembling diphtheria. There may be accompanying lymphangitic gummatous chains and/or regional adenopathy. On healing, the mucous membranes remain soft and pliable with no resultant scarring or strictures.

The first case of a lesion in the oral mucosa was reported by DE BEURMANN and GOUGEROT in 1907a and since then there have been only 10 more cases. The pharynx and larynx are more frequently involved and the first example of this was reported by DE BEURMANN, BRODIER and GASTOU in 1907. LETULLE and DEBRÉ reported a case with lesions in the mouth, pharynx, larynx and trachea, and during the next 2 years 4 more cases were seen. In the 1920's there were 4 cases and since then another four. Lesions in the nasal cavity are rare; records of only 6 cases could be found (DANLOS and FLANDIN; S. COSTA; PAUTRIER and RICHOU; FOERSTER, 1924; ORTMEYER and HUMPHREYS; SCHMIDT and THEISSING). There have been only 3 cases of infection of the nasal sinuses (VON HAUFE; PASSOS; THEISSING and SCHMIDT). No more than 2 cases of involvement of the bowel could be found, viz. those of DE BEURMANN, GOUGEROT and VAUCHER (1909) and of BOGGS and FRIED. Vaginitis has not been recorded in human beings but DE BEURMANN, GOUGEROT and VAUCHER (1908f) produced this lesion in experimental animals.

2. Musculoskeletal System

The lesions in muscle may take the form of a diffuse or localized area of induration or of a gummatous lesion with destruction of tissue. The first lesions in muscle were reported by BRISSAUD and RATHERY and by DE BEURMANN and GOUGEROT in 1907c; during the next 4 years there were 7 more cases in France, but since that time there have been no further cases anywhere until LURIE reported one case in South Africa in 1963a.

Bone is the most common of the extracutaneous tissues to be involved in this disease. The lesions may take any of a variety of forms; there may be a small, solitary granuloma producing a focus of radiolucency (Fig. 9), a large gummatous lesion with much destruction of bone which may result in spontaneous fracture,

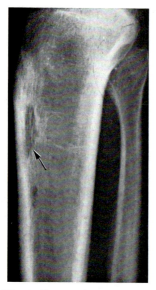

Fig. 9. Sporotrichosis of bone.
Osteolytic lesion in tibia

a type simulating a chronic pyogenic osteomyelitis, a diffuse hypertrophic osteosclerotic lesion or a periostitis.

The first case of sporotrichotic osteitis proved by culture was reported by Sicard et al. in 1908; the first osteomyelitis by Josset-Moure in 1908; the first granulomatous intra-osseous lesion by de Beurmann, Gougerot and Verne in 1909; the first hypertrophic osteitis by Marie and Gougerot in 1909 and the first periostitis by Fage in 1908. However there were several previous cases diagnosed by the association with cutaneous lesions but not proved by culture from the bone. Since then there have been many more cases, the last being reported by Wallk and Bernstein in 1964. The bones affected in order of frequency are as follows: tibia (19 cases), small bones of the hands and feet (8 cases), radius and ulna (5 cases), skull and facial bones (3 cases), ribs (2 cases), sternum, clavicle and spine (1 case each). In several instances the exact site was not stated.

Joint lesions may vary from a simple effusion to a chronic synovitis and a severe osteoarthritis with complete destruction of the joint. The first case of synovitis was reported by Hudelo et al. in 1908 and the first osteoarthritis by Moure in 1909. Since then there have been at least 20 more cases. The joints involved include the knee, elbow, wrist and sternoclavicular joint, the knee being the most frequent. The most recent case was reported by Riggs et al. in 1966 in the United States of America. Farha and Ford reported a case involving a synovial cyst of the knee. Gougerot and Lévy-Fraenkel reported a case of sporotrichotic tenosynovitis involving the flexor tendons of the hand; the only other similar case was that of Kedes et al. in 1964. Sartory et al. (1931) reported a case of an olecranon bursitis.

3. Visceral

a) Pulmonary

The only adequate description of a visceral lesion is that of the lung. This may take the form of diffuse fibrosis with or without granulomata and/or abscess-like cavities. The most detailed description of its gross and microscopic appearance is that of Forbus, in whose case the middle lobe of the right lung was consolidated and had a cartilagenous consistency. On section there was a mass of pigmented tissue which had a honeycomb-like structure with many small cavities traversed by bands of fibrous tissue. In addition there were scattered grey nodules with yellowish centers surrounded by semitranslucent connective tissue. Similar nodules but more heavily pigmented were seen throughout the lung. The left lung was also affected but the consolidation was confined to the upper part of the lower lobe and the lower part of the upper lobe. The walls of the cavities were quite clean and the cavities contained very small amounts of caseous necrotic material. The mediastinal lymph nodes were enlarged and firm and on section they showed hyaline strands of connective tissue and translucent nodules.

D. T. Smith (1945) reviewed the cases in the literature and found that in a few instances the lesion has simulated a pulmonary abscess. The most constant finding was enlargement of the mediastinal nodes, and the radiological findings consisted of conglomerations of linear fibrotic lesions.

SCOTT et al. had 2 cases: in one there was a 3 cm apical, thin-walled cavity containing a greyish-white exudate, and in the other lobes there were numerous greyish-white necrotic nodules. Their second case had a 3.5 cm cavity with a thick wall, lined by a greyish-white exudate and containing a yellow fluid.

The cases described by CRUTHIRDS and PATTERSON had a 2 cm subpleural, thin-walled cavity, lined by white necrotic tissue and communicating with a bronchus. In the neighbouring lung tissue there were several small fibrous and fibrocaseous nodules.

By 1912 DE BEURMANN and GOUGEROT had collected 6 case reports of pulmonary sporotrichosis from the literature, of which they accepted 4 on the basis of skin lesions proved by culture associated with a lesion in the lung and with the isolation of the *Sporotrichum* from the sputum. In the other 2 cases the fungus was isolated from the sputum but there were no physical signs in the lungs. Between 1912 and 1927 8 cases were reported. All the previous cases were reviewed by FORBUS who did not accept any of those approved by DE BEURMANN and GOUGEROT. He found sufficient justification for the diagnosis in only 4 cases, viz: those of LAURENT, DOMINGUEZ, WARFIELD, and NICAUD, and he added one of his own. Between 1927 and 1947 there were 7 more cases reported which were reviewed by D.T. SMITH (1947) who accepted only those of FORBUS and of MOORE and KILE. Since 1947 another 12 cases were reported. In 1962 RIDGEWAY et al. reviewed the literature since sporotrichosis was first described; they accepted a total of 12 cases only and added 2 of their own. Their basis for accepting the diagnosis was as follows: a pulmonary inflammatory lesion may safely be attributed to sporotrichosis if the fungus is repeatedly recovered on culture from the sputum and especially if no other etiological agent can be implicated. If the results of serological tests for sporotrichosis are positive and if there is a response to specific therapy, the diagnosis is established. In 1966 TREVATHAN and PHILLIPS considered their case to be the 16th on record, but it would appear that they had omitted the 2 cases reported by SCOTT et al. which would have raised the number to 18. The last, and therefore the 19th case, was that of CRUTHIRDS and PATTERSON in 1967.

b) Other Visceral Lesions

Only 2 cases of involvement of the gastrointestinal tract have been reported (BOGGS and FRIED; CORTELLA) and a similar number of renal lesions (ROCHARD et al.; MILHIT et al.). Although testicular lesions are the most common and characteristic lesions in experimental animals, they would appear to be rare in man, only 4 cases having been reported (BONNET, 1909; DE BEURMANN and GOUGEROT, 1909b; LAFFAILLE and PAVIE; KING). DE BEURMANN and GOUGEROT (1911b) mention 3 other cases but give no references and ARTHUR and ALBRITTAIN reported a case of disseminated sporotrichosis with involvement of the tunica vaginalis. Yet GUILAINE states that in disseminated gummatous sporotrichosis the fungus has a predilection for the eye and testis. GOUGEROT and BLUM reported a case with lesions in the parotid and submaxillary glands.

Probably the first case of widespread systemic involvement was that of WARFIELD in 1922. In 1934 PATSCHKOWSKI described a case with lesions in the thyroid, kidney, heart and larynx. Since then there have been only 4 more cases (CORTELLA; COLLINS; GERACI et al.; LURIE, 1963a).

4. Central Nervous System

There is hardly any information about the gross or microscopic appearance of sporotrichotic lesions in the central nervous system. From the evidence available it would appear that the lesion in the brain is like that of a localized granuloma or an abscess, and the meningeal lesion like that of any chronic meningitis.

The first but unproven case of meningitis was that of HYSLOP et al. in 1926, who found spores and mycelium in the cerebrospinal fluid; they were unable to grow the fungus or to infect animals. Further cases were reported by COLLINS, by GERACI et al. and by KLEIN et al. The two cases reported by AUFDERMAUR et al. and by FELLMAN were both caused by the so-called *S. Gougeroti*, which is no longer recognized as a Sporotrichum.

In the case reported by SHOEMAKER et al. the meninges at the base of the brain were thickened and opaque. On cutting the brain there was an area of hemorrhagic discoloration 1 cm posterior to the optic chiasma.

In the case of KLEIN et al. the cerebrospinal fluid showed glucose levels ranging between 12 and 40 mg/100 cc, protein between 164 and 326 mg/100 cc and cell counts between 130 and 240 WBC/cmm, at least 95% of which were lymphocytes.

5. Organs of Special Senses

Eye. BRANDT and BADER summarized the clinical manifestations of ocular sporotrichosis as follows:

1. Conjunctivitis and episcleritis with small yellow nodules, some ulcerating.

2. Dacryocanaliculitis with brown concretions. (They omitted to mention dacryocystitis which also has been reported.)

3. Corneal ulceration with confluent yellow nodules complicated by hypopyon.

4. Uveitis with nodular iritis, clouding of the vitreous and brown tumors in the retina.

5. Panophthalmitis. a. resulting from perforation following an exogenous infection; b. resulting from an endogenous spread from generalized sporotrichosis.

They did not include retrobulbar lesions in the orbit, which have also been reported (LURIE, 1963a). Involvement of the exterior of the eyelids is fairly common; in this presentation these have been included in the skin lesions.

The first case affecting the conjunctiva was presented in 1909 by MORAX and FAVA and reported independently; the first panophthalmitis was reported by DE BEURMANN and GOUGEROT in the same year (1909b), the first iritis by JEANSELME and POULARD in 1910, and the first dacryocystitis by MORAX in 1911. In 1947 GORDON reviewed the literature and found 34 cases of primary ocular sporotrichosis. Since then further cases have been reported by SUN KUEI-YÜ and CHÜ WEN-CHÜN (corneal) and ALVAREZ and LÓPEZ-VILLEGAS (conjunctival).

Middle Ear: The only case report of a lesion in the middle ear is that of DOMINGUEZ in 1914.

C. Acute and Subacute Febrile Sporotrichosis

Rarely the disease may start abruptly with fever and symptoms of an acute septicemia. Later multiple lesions, resembling acute coccal abscesses, appear anywhere on the body and develop rapidly, becoming adherent to the skin which appears red, edematous, painful and infiltrated like an erysipelas. They ulcerate in a few days and then slowly involute. Sometimes the disease is less acute with progressive asthenia, loss of weight, anemia and general debility associated with the development of gumma-like lesions anywhere on the body.

The first acute febrile case was reported by BRISSAUD and RATHERY in 1907, the second by BALZER and GALUP, and the third by BRODIER and FAGE. DE BEURMANN and GOUGEROT (1909a) reviewed these three cases and compared the clinical picture with that of a coccal infection. This type of sporotrichosis appears to be extremely rare. The case reported by HODARA and BEY, and that described by ANDERSON and SPECTOR as "rat-bite fever," probably fall into this category. CURCIO reported a case from Italy.

D. Sporotrichids and other Allergic Manifestations

The development of an allergy to the fungus may result in an -id eruption similar to the dermatophytids. HOPKINS and BENHAM ,who prefer to use the term sporotrichosides, are of the opinion that the epidermal lesions described by GOUGEROT belong in this category. However other observers have noted epidermal lesions which were either undoubtedly primary lesions, or due to surface contamination of the skin by discharge from ulcerated lesions, or to hematogenous dissemination of the organism. It is probably correct that the majority of the epidermal lesions do represent sporotrichids.

A few cases have been described in which a sporotrichotic infection has been accompanied by sarcoidosis. There have been many reports on the coexistence of Boeck's sarcoidosis and fungus infections. In some cases the sarcoidosis preceded the fungus infection but in others it was assumed to be a reaction to the mycosis. In the former category there have been many reports and the complicating mycoses include blastomycosis, cryptococcosis, histoplasmosis, coccidioidomycosis and nocardiosis (LEITHOLD et al.; HIATT and LIDE; PLUMMER et al.; HARRIS et al.); a case of sarcoidosis associated with an aspergillus infection was reported by HINSON et al. In the latter category, in which the sarcoidosis was considered to be a reaction to the fungus infection, both cryptococcosis and histoplasmosis have been incriminated (SHIELDS; REIMANN and PRICE; ISRAEL et al.; PINKERTON and IVERSON).

In 1963 LURIE reported the first case of disseminated systemic sporotrichosis in whom a sarcoid reaction appeared in lymph nodes and lung. In the same year MCFARLAND and GOODMAN reported a case in which disseminated sporotrichosis developed during the recovery phase of an illness thought to be sarcoidosis.

Those cases in whom the sarcoidosis preceded the fungus infection can be explained on the basis of lowered host resistance, impairment of the defense mechanism by the involvement of the reticulo-endothelial system or by steroid therapy, or merely coincidence. Cases in the second category, in which the sarcoid reaction followed the fungus infection, add support to the view that sarcoidosis is not a specific disease but that it represents a non-specific allergic reaction to a variety of stimuli, for example tuberculosis (SCADDING), beryllium (HARDY), pine pollen (CUMMINGS and HUDGINS) and nematodes (JAQUES).

A third type of allergic reaction to sporotrichosis has been reported by HELVE et al.; a case of primary ocular and mucosal sporotrichosis was followed by septicemia and visceral lesions. The histological features of these lesions were those of a necrotizing arteritis resembling periarteritis nodosa, and the authors suggest that this may represent a hypersensitivity affecting the vascular system rather than systemic spread. However in the present author's opinion the evidence presented as proof of sporotrichosis infection is not beyond doubt.

E. Carrier States

Pathogenic *Sporotrichum* has been isolated from otherwise healthy oral or pharyngeal mucosa and from the sputum of people with no evidence of lung disease. DE BEURMANN and GOUGEROT (1907a, 1908a) reported a case with ulcerated lesions in the buccopharynx who harbored the organism for a long time after the lesions were cured. In 1907e DE BEURMANN and GOUGEROT and again in 1911 GOUGEROT expressed the opinion that the organism may grow on the mucous membranes as a saprophyte without producing lesions. MOUNT had a similar case and confirmed their opinion. OTTOLENGHI isolated *Sporotrichum* species from the mouths of 10 out of 100 persons suffering from various pathological conditions and HOTCHKISS isolated the Sporotrichum from mucus obtained on bronchoscopy, but MAGALHÃES PEREIRA et al. (1964) were unable to culture the fungus from the oropharynx of 143 persons; some of these had been cured of the disease and others had no history of infection.

Relative Frequency of Clinical Types

Since sporotrichosis was first recognized there has been a remarkable change in the whole disease panorama. In the first 25 years there were numerous cases of disseminated gummatous and extracutaneous lesions reported, the large majority of them from France and neighbouring countries and only a few from the United

States. Subsequently these cases were seen less frequently in France, only two severe cases having been reported during the last decade, while during the same period the number increased in the USA, although never to as high a frequency as that in France at the beginning of the century. In the rest of the world cases with disseminated lesions have always been and continue to be exceedingly rare, even in South Africa and in South America where thousands of cases of sporotrichosis have occurred.

The change in the pattern of the disease is best exemplified by the bone lesions. Of 43 case reports reviewed by the author, 26 were seen between the years 1907 and 1913, most of them in France; during the next 20 years there were 5 cases and from 1934 to date there have been merely 12 cases, only one of which was in France. The first American case was described by CREGOR in 1922; since then very few cases have been reported from that country (MIKKELSEN et al., 2 cases; HANRAHAN and ERICKSON, 2 cases). In South Africa 3 cases have been seen (LURIE, 1963a).

Included in the first 100 cases from France and neighbouring countries there were 8 cases with disseminated gummatous lesions, 13 with bone lesions, 4 with arthritis, 8 with lesions in muscle, 1 with tenosynovitis, 3 with visceral involvement, 7 with lesions in the mouth, pharynx or larynx, 2 with testicular involvement, 1 with renal involvement and 1 with an ocular lesion. BÈZES stated that 20% of all cases had some bone involvement. By contrast, in the USA there were only 8 cases with disseminated gummatous lesions during the first 25 years, after which they increased in frequency in that country; at the same time the incidence decreased rapidly in France. In 1948 JAME quoted PAUTRIER as stating that gummatous lesions were frequently seen in France between 1908 and 1914 but since then they have been very rarely seen. This change in the distribution of the disease is summarized in Table 5.

Table 5. *Cases of disseminated gummatous and/or extracutaneous lesions reported*

	1903—1920	1921—1940	1941—1966
France	58	8	2
United States of America	5	10	24
South Africa	0	0	5
South America	0	0	7

It has been shown that there is no difference in the virulence for laboratory animals of the strains of *Sporotrichum* from different parts of the world, and that the fungus does not lose its virulence in the test tube even after many years. The change in pattern cannot be attributed to more rapid diagnosis and earlier treatment, for among the South African cases there were some who, on religious grounds, refused any treatment yet never developed hematogenous dissemination. That it is not due to improved therapy is evidenced by the fact that the treatment today is exactly the same as it was when the disease was first recognized.

The frequency of the different types of lesions in more recent times is shown in the following reviews. In 1963 EVERETT reviewed 117 cases in the USA and found the distribution to be:

Localized lymphangitic   80%
Cutaneous (fixed) 10%
Hematogenous 5%
Systemic 5%

These figures are probably subject to the same inaccuracies that any other review of the more recent literature would have, namely that the disease is now so well known that only unusual cases would be reported unless the disease was rare in the author's area.

Among the 117 cases reviewed by EVERETT he found 8 which were extra-cutaneous; mucous membranes 2, bones and joints 4 and pulmonary 2.

In Mexico GONZÁLEZ OCHOA (1965) found the distribution to be as follows:

Localized lymphangitic . . . 67%
Cutaneous (fixed) 32%
Disseminated gummatous . . 1%

He stated that systemic involvement was extremely rare.

Histopathology

The description which follows differs only in a few insignificant minutiae from the detailed description given by DE BEURMANN and GOUGEROT in 1906 and 1907d. The basic response of the tissues is the same whatever the type of lesion: primary or secondary, "chancre", dermal papule, subcutaneous gumma or visceral lesion. The majority of cases biopsied are those of fixed cutaneous lesions of fairly long duration, as once secondary nodules appear the diagnosis is usually obvious and biopsies are not taken. As most of the fixed lesions are variants of the nodular type this will be used as a prototype and its histology described in detail, followed by a few remarks about other types of lesions.

Nodular Dermal Lesion

Epidermis: There is usually little or no evidence of ulceration, the epidermis showing hyperkeratosis, parakeratosis, and irregular acanthosis which in many cases may reach the proportions of pseudo-epitheliomatous hyperplasia (Fig. 10) (HEKTOEN and PERKINS; HYDE and DAVIS; LEWIS and CUDMORE; MONTGOMERY and HOLMAN; GRAHAM; SKEER; PINKUS and GREKIN; COSTA and JUNQUIRA; MOORE and ACKERMAN; MINTY et al.; MEAD and RIDLEY; OKUDAIRA et al., 1959; MARIAT et al.; LURIE, 1963b; MORAES and MIRANDA). In the nodular-pustular lesions described by FUKUSHIRO et al. the epithelium is partially destroyed and flattened. Lesions referred to as "chancres" show on section areas of superficial ulceration alternating with non-ulcerated areas in which the epithelium may be either acanthotic or flattened. One of the most constant findings is the presence of intraepidermal micro-abscesses, even in the flattened epithelium (HEKTOEN and PERKINS; DE BEURMANN and GOUGEROT, 1907d; GRAHAM; MINTY et al.; LAVALLE et al.; MARIAT et al.; LURIE, 1963b; MORAES and MIRANDA; FUKUSHIRO et al.). These abscesses sometimes rupture into the dermis, resulting in the appearance of foreign-body giant cells in the immediate vicinity (LURIE, 1963b). Similar intra-epidermal micro-abscesses are seen in other fungal infections such as blastomycosis.

Dermis: There is a diffuse cellular infiltrate involving the entire thickness of the dermis. At the periphery of the lesion it consists of lymphocytes and plasma cells with a few large mononuclear cells. It is not sharply circumscribed but extends for some distance around the blood vessels which may show endarteritis (DE BEURMANN and GOUGEROT, 1907d; B. F. DAVIS, 1914; MARIAT et al.; LURIE, 1963b). In the central portion of the lesion there is an admixture of other inflammatory cells with the lymphocytes and plasma cells; hemosiderin-laden histiocytes are not uncommonly seen (DE BEURMANN and GOUGEROT, 1907d; LURIE, 1963b). Most reports mention the presence of eosinophils (BRISSAUD et al.; DE MASSARY et al.;

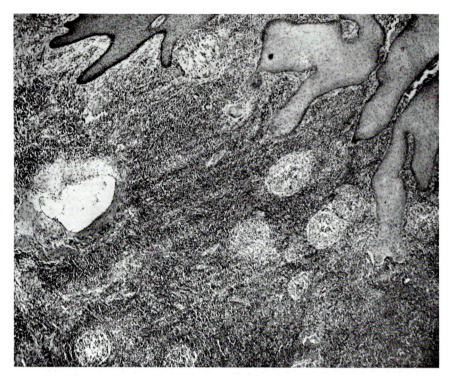

Fig. 10. Sporotrichosis. Section of dermal lesion showing pseudo-epitheliomatous hyperplasia of the epidermis, diffuse mononuclear cell infiltrate and granulomata in the dermis. H & E, × 35

HUDELO et al.; HAMBURGER; DU TOIT; MOORE and ACKERMAN; SIMSON et al.; PINKUS and GREKIN; SINGER and MUNCIE; MINTY et al.; OKUDAIRA et al., 1959; LAVALLE et al.; LURIE, 1963b). In the majority of cases they are fairly numerous but in some instances none were seen (LURIE, 1963b). Other authors make no mention of the presence or absence of eosinophils (MORAES and MIRANDA; FUKUSHIRO et al.). Some report the presence of mast cells (DE BEURMANN and GOUGEROT, 1907d; OKUDAIRA et al., 1959). DE BEURMANN and GOUGEROT (1907d) found numerous giant cells, frequently phagocytosing polymorphonuclear leucocytes and red cells. They also described the presence of irregular anastomosing aggregations of epithelioid cells, sometimes forming large sheets; among these cells there were fairly numerous giant cells, usually of the foreign body type. In LURIE's (1963b) cases the giant cells were situated mainly in the areas where intra-epidermal micro-abscesses had ruptured into the dermis. In some lesions LURIE (1963b) found poly-morphonuclear leucocytes dispersed among the mononuclear cells, but in most cases they are aggregated in clusters forming micro-abscesses varying in size from groups of about 10 cells to spheres several hundred microns in diameter (DE BEUR-MANN and GOUGEROT, 1906, 1907d; LAVALLE et al.; MARIAT et al.; LURIE, 1963b; MOREAS and MIRANDA; FUKUSHIRO et al.). In some of these abscesses the borders are indistinct and merge with the surrounding infiltrate. Usually, however, the borders are clearly demarcated and they are surrounded by a condensation of reti-culin fibers (LURIE, 1963b).

The most diagnostic histological feature is the presence of characteristic gra-nulomata (Fig. 10). These have been described by DE BEURMANN and GOU-

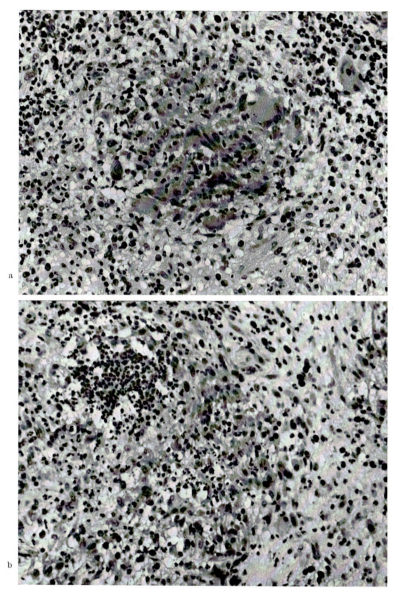

Fig. 11. Sporotrichosis. Section of dermal lesion showing development of granuloma; a. stage 1, an aggregation of histiocytic cells; b. stage 2, infiltration of neutrophil polymorphonuclear leucocytes in center of aggregation of histiocytes. H & E, × 220

GEROT (1906, 1907d), EISENSTAEDT, CREGOR, FOERSTER (1924), MONTGOMERY and HOLMAN, DU TOIT, MOORE and ACKERMAN, SIMSON et al., PINKUS and GREKIN, MINTY et al., MEAD and RIDLEY, LAVALLE et al., MARIAT et al., LURIE (1963b), MORAES and MIRANDA, and by FUKUSHIRO et al. Each granuloma commences as an aggregation of large histiocytes with homogenous eosinophilic cytoplasm. The number of histiocytes increases and the mass becomes rounded and circumscribed. The central area is then infiltrated by polymorphonuclear leucocytes, which are

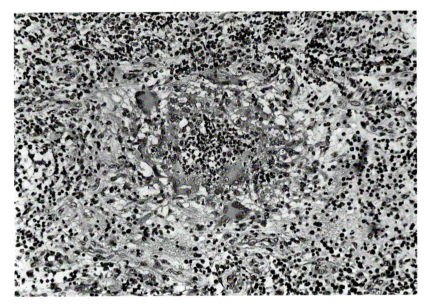

Fig. 12. Sporotrichosis. Section of dermal lesion showing fully developed granuloma (stage 3), consisting of central microabscess surrounded by a definite zone of histiocytes and multinucleated giant cells. H & E, × 160

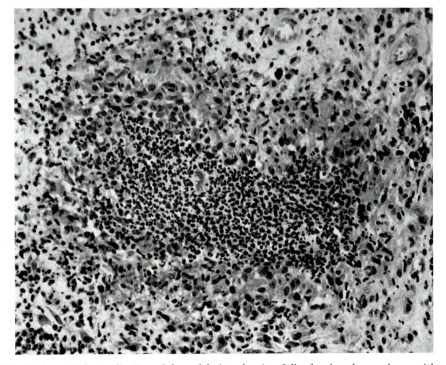

Fig. 13. Sporotrichosis. Section of dermal lesion showing fully developed granuloma with a central asteroid body. H & E, × 220

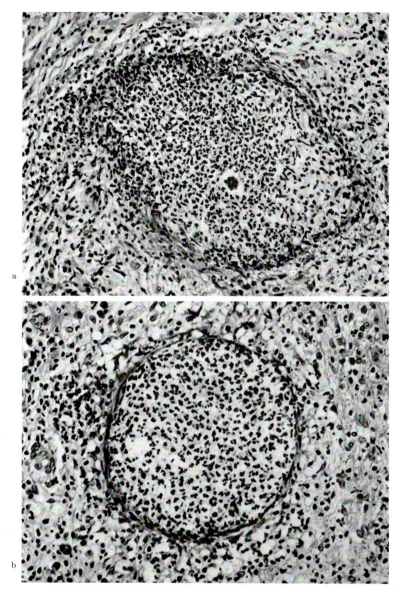

Fig. 14. Sporotrichosis. Section of dermal lesion showing development of microabscesses from granulomata. In (a) an asteroid body is visible. In (b) the zone of histiocytes is so compressed as to be almost unrecognizable. H & E, × 220

at first few in number but later increase to form a micro-abscess (Figs. 11—14). At the same time multinucleated giant cells appear at the periphery; these are formed either by fusion of histiocytes or by failure of the cytoplasm to divide after nuclear fission (LURIE, 1963b).

The fully developed granuloma has three distinct zones (Fig. 13) (MARIAT et al.; LURIE 1963b; MORAES and MIRANDA). According to LURIE (1963b), MORAES and MIRANDA and FUKUSHIRO et al. the central zone consists of polymorphonuclear leucocytes and is in fact a micro-abscess. DE BEURMANN and GOUGEROT (1906, 1907d) found an admixture with macrophages, while MARIAT et al. described in addition a variable number of histiocytes, lymphocytes and eosinophils. The middle zone is variously described as consisting of epithelioid cells (DE BEURMANN and GOUGEROT, 1906, 1907d; MARIAT et al.), epithelioid cells and giant cells (MORAES and MIRANDA), histiocytes and giant cells (LURIE, 1963b). The outer zone consists of plasma cells, lymphocytes and fibroblasts (MARIAT et al.), mononuclear cells (MORAES and MIRANDA) or lymphocytes and plasma cells only (LURIE, 1963b).

Further increase in size of the granuloma results in an enlargement of the micro-abscess and progressive compression and attenuation of the middle and outer zones (Fig. 14).

Many reports mention the presence of giant cells in the lesion but the large majority do not specify where they are located nor the type of giant cell (WALKER and RITCHIE; RUEDIGER; HAMBURGER; EISENSTAEDT; CREGOR; LEWIS and CUDMORE; MONTGOMERY and HOLMAN; GRAHAM; SIMSON et al.; MEAD and RIDLEY; FUKUSHIRO et al.). Some describe them as of the foreign body type (DU TOIT; COLLINS; MINTY et al.; LURIE, 1963b), while others call them Langhans type (HYDE and DAVIS; B. F. DAVIS, 1914; FOERSTER; COSTA and JUNQUEIRA; MOORE and ACKERMAN; SINGER and MUNCIE; LIU), and some authors report the presence of both types of giant cells (DE BEURMANN and GOUGEROT, 1907d; LAVALLE et al.; MARIAT et al.).

Generally there is no evidence of necrosis but some investigators report the presence of small foci of necrosis, or individual cell necrosis.

In addition to the typical granulomata described above, LURIE (1963b) and MORAES and MIRANDA noted the presence of tuberculoid granulomata and LURIE (1963b) also observed, in one case only, a foreign body granuloma consisting of an admixture of lymphocytes, plasma cells, histiocytes and foreign body giant cells.

There is a variable amount of fibrosis, depending on the duration of the lesion.

Other Dermal Lesions

The histopathological picture of other dermal lesions is essentially the same, varying mainly in the epidermal changes, the extent of the diffuse inflammatory cell infiltrate in the dermis, the number of granulomata, the number and size of the abscesses and the presence or absence of fibrosis.

The histological features of the *verrucous or papillomatous type* have been described by DE BEURMANN and GOUGEROT (1907d), SMITH and GARRATT, SINGER and MUNCIE, LAVALLE et al., and CARR et al. In these cases the epidermis shows papillomatosis and no evidence of ulceration, while the other features are essentially similar to those already described. The granulation tissue type of dermal lesion is, as the name implies, covered by exuberant granulation tissue. In the papular lesions the dermal infiltrate is less extensive and more superficial than in the nodular type and there is little or no fibrosis. In the pustular variety the micro-abscesses become confluent and form larger abscesses. (The process is similar to that described in detail under the gummatous lesion.)

Epidermal Lesions

No description of the histology of these lesions could be found in the literature reviewed.

Subcutaneous Gumma

In the non-ulcerated lesion the overlying epidermis and upper dermis show no significant changes. The lesion usually originates in the lower dermis at the

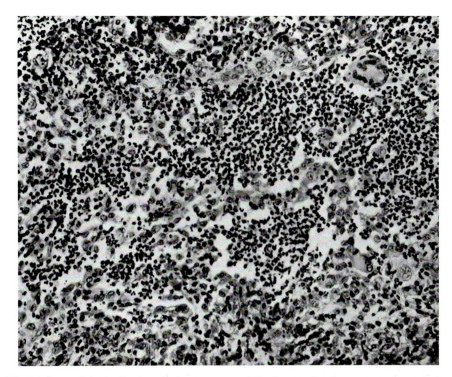

Fig. 15. Sporotrichosis. Section of subcutaneous nodule showing development of gumma by the breaking down and confluence of granulomata. H & E, × 220

junction with the subcutaneous tissue (LURIE, 1963b; FUKUSHIRO et al.). According to FUKUSHIRO et al. the initial reaction is primarily histiocytic and from this a granuloma develops. LURIE (1963b), however, found that the earliest lesion consists of a diffuse infiltration by lymphocytes and plasma cells, among which there is an admixture of a variable number of eosinophils, neutrophils, giant cells and histiocytes. Later, granulomata appear within the infiltrate, following the same pattern as that in the dermal lesions and having the same morphology. They continue to enlarge and eventually disintegrate. Adjacent granulomata become confluent, resulting in irregular, branching and anastomosing aggregations of polymorphonuclear leucocytes surrounded by large histiocytes (Fig. 15). Finally all the granulomata fuse into a single large granuloma or gumma, the characteristic morphology of which was originally described by DE BEURMANN and GOUGEROT in 1906, 1907d. The central area consists of numerous polymorphonuclear leucocytes only. The wall is made up of three zones: an inner zone of large histiocytes, an intermediate zone of large histiocytes and multinucleated giant cells of the foreign body type, and an outer zone of lymphocytes and plasma cells (Fig. 16). The features are therefore identical with those of the small granuloma in the nodular dermal lesion but on a greatly enlarged scale. Some of the reports mention the presence of central necrosis (DE BEURMANN and GOUGEROT, 1906, 1907d; RUEDIGER, FOERSTER, 1924, MONTGOMERY and HOLMAN, etc.). Most of these do not specify the type of necrosis; a few describe typical coagulative necrosis. DE BEURMANN and GOUGEROT state that it is not caseation, while R. D. BAKER (1947b) specifically states that caseation is a conspicuous feature. The entire lesion is usually

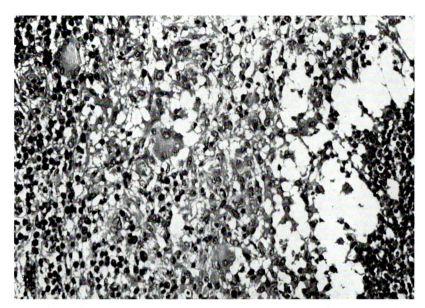

Fig. 16. Sporotrichosis. Section of wall of fully developed gumma showing: at right the central mass of polymorphonuclear leucocytes, in middle the zone of histiocytes, and at left lympho-cytes and plasma cells. H & E, × 240

fairly well circumscribed and surrounded by a variable amount of fibrous tissue which in older lesions may form a distinct capsule (DE BEURMANN and GOUGEROT, 1907 d).

LURIE (1963b) reported that in the early stages, when the small granulomata are appearing in the diffuse infiltrate, an occasional granuloma in some cases may be typically tuberculoid in nature.

Musculoskeletal Lesions

Granulomata indentical with those already described have been seen in bone (MARIE and GOUGEROT; LURIE, 1963a) and in muscle (LURIE, 1963a).

Pulmonary Sporotrichosis

The histopathology of the case described by FORBUS is as follows: the nodules seen in the lung on gross examination had a reticular structure. The spaces between the fine reticular septa were filled with large mononuclear cells which varied in shape and size, most being polygonal, some spherical and others spindle-shaped. In some areas there were scattered lymphocytes, plasma cells and eosinophils. Numerous giant cells were seen but their position was not constant. There was not true central caseation. The young nodules were highly vascular but the older ones became hyalinized and eventually ended up as scar tissue. The cavities within the scar tissue appeared to be the remains of bronchi.

The tissue reactions in the cases reported by SCOTT et al. and by CRUTHIRDS and PATTERSON were those of a non-specific inflammatory reaction, and the latter found a few ill-defined giant cells.

Central Nervous System

In the case reported by SHOEMAKER et al. the meninges were infiltrated by lymphocytes, plasma cells and large mononuclear cells, as were some of the Virchow-Robin spaces. In the glomus choroideum there was an infiltrate consisting of similar cells plus giant cells. In addition there was an area of necrosis bordered by palisading epithelioid cells, in the center of which there were some polymorphonuclear leucocytes, and cigar bodies seen with the PAS stain.

The case reported by COLLINS et al. had granulomata in the cerebral cortex, consisting of areas of necrosis infiltrated by macrophages, lymphocytes, polymorphonuclear leucocytes and occasional giant cells.

GERACI et al. found in their case a granuloma in the first sacral nerve and an infarct-like lesion in the brain.

Ocular Sporotrichosis

BRANDT and BADER described the histology of global sporotrichosis in great detail. The lesions are apparently identical with those already described. The early lesion consists of an infiltration by lymphocytes, plasma cells and a few granulocytes, and within this infiltrate granulomata appear; they commence as aggregations of histiocytes which change into epithelioid cells and giant cells of the foreign body type. The central area is then infiltrated by polymorphonuclear leucocytes and a micro-abscess is formed with non-caseous necrosis. Old lesions may become calcified. The authors found no fungal elements in the granulomata but they observed spores in preparations made from the vitreous humor.

Fungal Elements in Smears of Exudates and in Tissue Sections

At the beginning of the century several non-specific staining procedures were used to visualize the fungal elements. These were followed by the Gram's stain, the PAS and its modifications such as Gridley's and Hotchkiss-McManus, and then by the Gomori's silver impregnation. KUNZ, and KAPLAN and IVENS, utilized the fluorescent antibody technique in demonstrating spores in material from experimental animals infected with sporotrichosis, and in 1963 KAPLAN and GONZÁLEZ OCHOA, using this technique, found spores in exudates of 26 out of 27 cases proved by culture, and in 1 case out of 7 which were negative on culture but clinically resembled sporotrichosis. The value of this method was confirmed by GONZÁLEZ OCHOA (1964). LURIE (1963b) described a technique of incubating exudates at 37°C overnight and preparing smears the following day; the spores multiply rapidly so that clusters of 100 or more are readily seen. FETTER and TINDALL recommend preliminary diastase digestion of tissue sections before staining.

Smears of Exudates: In numerous cases the authors have failed to detect any fungal elements in smears prepared from exudates (GOLDBERG and PIJPER; CAMPBELL et al.; LEWIS and CUDMORE; GRAHAM; SMITH and GARRETT; BARRACK and POWELL; SINGER and MUNCIE; MIRANDA et al., 1955; BELLIBONI et al.; GLUCKMAN). Other reports indicate that spores are very scanty or rarely found (DE BEURMANN and GOUGEROT, 1907d; DU TOIT; SINGER and MUNCIE; LURIE, 1963b). DANGERFIELD and GEAR found that in exudates from primary skin lesions spores are seldom seen but that in the exudates from secondary lesions they were seen in almost every case. CRUTCHFIELD found numerous spores in his case, as did LURIE (1963b) in one case only of a large series. FUKUSHIRO et al. found numerous spores in preparations from 2 cases only in a series of 55 cases.

41*

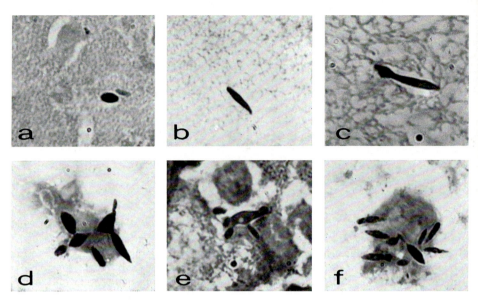

Fig. 17. Sporotrichosis. Fungal elements in pus: a. yeast-like body, b., c. and f. cigar bodies, d. and e. budding forms. Gram stain, × 1500

When fungal elements were detected most of them were described as round, oval or cigar-shaped bodies (Fig. 17). They have been described as yeast forms varying in size from that of nuclear debris to that of a red blood cell (Lawless), small, round yeast-like bodies (Ghose), oval bodies (Wade and Matthews; de Beurmann and Gougerot, 1906, 1907d), cigar-shaped bodies often surrounded by a clear halo resembling a capsule (Dangerfield and Gear), cigar-shaped bodies (du Toit), round and cigar-shaped bodies (Arêa Leão and Goto), yeast cells and spindle-shaped bodies, occasionally in chains (Liu), cigar bodies, round spores and budding yeast-like bodies (Fig. 17) (Lurie, 1963b), large round or oval spores attached to which were one or more cigar-shaped bodies resembling buds or short filaments suggesting germination (Lurie, 1963b), cigar-shaped bodies, single or budding, oval or elliptical, bacillary forms and globose structures (Kaplan and González Ochoa). Some reports merely mention the presence of spores without describing their shape (Crutchfield; Hope).

These spores are Gram positive (Hope; Dangerfield and Gear; du Toit; Liu; Lurie, 1963b). They may be intracellular or extracellular (Lawless; Ghose; Lurie, 1963b; Fukushiro et al.).

In only two reports were asteroid bodies found in direct smears (Borelli in 3 cases; Fukushiro et al. in 2 cases). In a few instances hyphae have been observed in smears of exudates. Wohl found elongated, sausage-like filamentous forms; along the sides of the filaments there were oval, refractile bodies. In a case of meningitis, Hyslop et al. observed spores and mycelium in the cerebrospinal fluid and Fukushiro et al. observed a long hypha in the exudate from one skin lesion.

In the Tissues: Most workers specifically state that no spores were seen in histological sections of sporotrichotic lesions (Schenck; Hektoen and Perkins; Hyde and Davis; Davis, 1914; Lawless; Hopkins and Benham; Campbell et al.; Lewis and Cudmore; Graham; Skeer; Smith and Garrett; Carr et al.). Some state that spores are difficult to find or are only occasionally seen (Walker and

RITCHIE; RUEDIGER). Others describe three main types of fungal elements as occurring in the tissues, viz. cigar bodies and their variants, asteroid bodies and hyphae.

Cigar Bodies and their Variants

The first observation of spores in tissue sections and in smears was made by DE BEURMANN and GOUGEROT in 1906 who described them as resembling cigars. Others have observed the typical cigar bodies (Fig. 18) (ALEIXO; AZULAY and MIRANDA; ARÊA LEÃO and GOTO; SIMSON et al.; LURIE, 1963b; CRUTHIRDS and PATTERSON). On the contrary, FUKUSHIRO et al. specifically state that a wide variety of shapes was seen but none of the spores observed were typically cigar-shaped.

These spores have been described as oval (DE BEURMANN and GOUGEROT, 1907d; DAVIS, 1913; SCOTT et al.), yeast-like (MEAD and RIDLEY), ovoid (MILLER), round (MORAES and MIRANDA), round or oval (FETTER; LURIE, 1963b), round or elongated (OKUDAIRA et al., 1959; CRUTHIRDS and PATTERSON), short rod-like blunt cells (MOORE and KILE), round, oval, spindle, semilunar or shrunken (FUKUSHIRO et al.), spherical, crescentic or comma-shaped (GONZÁLEZ OCHOA and SOTO PACHECO). Several reports refer to navicular cells; from their description and illustrations these appear to the author to be identical with the cigar bodies.

It is apparent, therefore, that these spores may vary enormously in shape; round, oval (or yeast-like), cigar-shaped (or navicular), elongated bodies with blunt ends, or spindle-shaped with sharply pointed ends. Some may become distorted or shrunken and appear as semilunar. In the author's opinion these are all variants of the same spore and represent the conidia of the yeast phase of the fungus. All of these variations have been observed in cultures. The small, round forms probably represent cigar bodies cut in cross section. Some of the round spores are larger than the usual and appear to develop thicker walls (double-contoured) and probably represent chlamydospores.

They may vary in size; according to DE BEURMANN and GOUGEROT (1906, 1907d) they measure 2—5 μ by 1—3 μ; OKUDAIRA et al. (1959) found that the smallest was 1 μ and the largest 10 μ. FUKUSHIRO et al. separate the round spores into three groups: (1) 5—7.9 μ, average 6.4 μ; (2) 3.1—4.5 μ, average 3 μ; (3) 2.1—2.9 μ, average 2.4 μ.

They are usually single but may occur in clumps or clusters (OKUDAIRA et al., 1959; FUKUSHIRO et al.). They may show budding (DAVIS, 1913; MEAD and RIDLEY; FETTER; CRUTHIRDS and PATTERSON). OKUDAIRA et al. (1959) observed 1—3 buds from a single spore, and FUKUSHIRO et al. saw 1—4 buds. The latter also observed short germ tubes emerging from the larger spores.

DE BEURMANN and GOUGEROT (1906, 1907a, d) stated that they are surrounded by an unstained, transparent zone. DANGERFIELD and GEAR confirmed that they were frequently surrounded by a clear halo resembling a capsule, and GONZÁLEZ OCHOA and SOTO PACHECO found an amoeba-shaped, eosinophilic halo. FUKUSHIRO et al. stated that there is a pseudocapsule, while both NORDEN (1951) and CRUTHIRDS and PATTERSON refer to a definite capsule. NEILL et al. claim to have demonstrated the presence of a capsule by the use of immune serum similar to the Quellung reaction of pneumococci. However KLIGMAN and BALDRIDGE were unable to detect a capsule in India ink preparations or by the use of immune serum even under the electron microscope; they have shown that the transparent halo is an artefact.

These spores may be intracellular (WALKER and RITCHIE; CRUTCHFIELD; WADE and MATTHEWS; COLLINS) or extracellular (MEAD and RIDLEY; MORAES and Miranda; Lurie, 1963b). Fukushiro et al. found intracellular spores in 12 out of 28 cases of lymphangitic sporotrichosis and in 12 out of 27 cases of localized or fixed sporotrichosis, but more commonly they were extracellular, in 26 out of 28 cases of the lymphangitic type and in 25 out of 27 localized lesions. de Beurmann and Gougerot (1906, 1907d), Okudaira et al. (1959), and Cruthirds and Patterson found intra- and extracellular spores in the same sections. Fukushiro et al. state that intracellular spores are never seen unaccompanied by extracellular forms. The intracellular spores are usually in giant cells (Okudaira et al., 1959; Fukushiro et al.), but are sometimes seen in macrophages, and in one pus smear small round bodies have been observed in polymorphonuclear leucocytes (Fukushiro et al.). Within the giant cells or macrophages they are usually single, but occasionally 2 and rarely numerous spores have been seen; Fukushiro et al. saw as many as 7 spores in one giant cell. The intracellular organisms may be round, oval, seldom semilunar or shrunken (Fukushiro et al.), round or elongated (Okudaira et al., 1959). They vary in size, the round forms from 2.1—6.8 μ with an average of 4.4 μ and the oval from 3.2—7.1 μ by 3.7—7.4 μ with an average of 4.6 μ by 5.6 μ (Fukushiro et al.). Occasionally intracellular budding forms with 1 or 2 buds were seen (Fukushiro et al.; Moraes and Miranda).

These cigar bodies and their variants are Gram positive when viable, PAS positive, and they stain well with the Gridley or Gomori stain. They are not seen in sections stained with H & E but are easily visualized with fluorescent antibody techniques.

In tissue sections these spores are found in the center of granulomata, in the micro-abscesses, or in association with small aggregations of polymorphonuclear leucocytes (Fukushiro et al.).

Most reports state that these spores are seldom seen in human tissues, and when present are usually very scanty (Davis, 1913; Simson et al.; Singer and Muncie; Lurie, 1963b). Fukushiro et al. in Japan have reported the largest series of cases in which these spores have been seen: in a total of 56 out of 69 biopsies from 55 cases; in 9 cases they were very numerous (7 to 12 per high power field).

The Asteroid Body

The first observation of stellate forms in human sporotrichotic lesions was by Splendore in 1908, who termed it asteroid formation. He isolated the fungus and called it *Sporotrichum asteroides*, Splendore 1908, and sent the cultures to de Beurmann and Gougerot for their opinion. They maintained that there was insufficient reason to regard it as a new species and renamed it *S. Beurmanni* var. *asteroides* (Splendore) de Beurmann and Gougerot (1911).

In the same year Greco described radiating forms in the tissues of man and rats from Uruguay and in 1909 Harter and Gruyer, in France, demonstrated radiate formation in experimental sporotrichosis in guinea pigs. In 1934 Bordes et al. published 4 cases of sporotrichosis in Uruguay, and in one of his own, Talice found radiate formation. Talice and Mackinnon reported that they had found radiate formation in pus from 6 out of 7 cases of sporotrichosis. Moore and Ackerman observed the asteroid form of Splendore in a gummatous lesion in Missouri, USA, which was the first asteroid body recorded in that country. Simson et al. reported that asteroid bodies were consistently found in South African cases. Lurie (1963b) confirmed their findings and observed these bodies in 39 out of 63 cases (61.9%). Pinkus and Grekin found that asteroid bodies were not uncommon in South America but were rare in the Northern Hemisphere; they could find no reports of their presence in European cases. Their frequency in South America was confirmed by Moraes and Miranda, who observed asteroid bodies in 10 out of 16 cases in Brazil. Fukushiro and Kagawa observed asteroid bodies in Japan; Fukushiro et al. found them in 37 out of 55 (67.3%) cases and mentioned that of 79 cases of sporotrichosis seen in Japan since the second World War, 8 had asteroid bodies. Mead and Ridley observed them in Australia. In all of the above reports, the

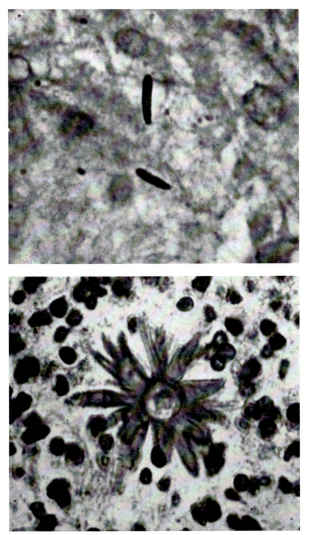

Fig. 18. Sporotrichosis. Fungal elements in tissue sections; (above) cigar bodies (PAS) and (below) an asteroid body (H&E), × 1500

asteroid bodies were seen in cutaneous lesions. There is only one report of their presence in an extracutaneous lesion, namely that of CRUTHIRDS and PATTERSON who observed these bodies in a pulmonary lesion.

Morphology of the Asteroid Body: At the outset it must be emphasized that the asteroid body should not be confused with the asteroid forms which were described originally by GOUGEROT (1912) in a strain of the fungus which he called *Sporothrix asteroides*. He found that, *in vivo* only, the fungus developed a central body with radially arranged elongated spores. DAVIS (1913) expressed the opinion that these were not distinctive forms and that they resembled the growth of *Actinomyces* in tissues.

As early as 1910 HYDE and DAVIS reported that in animal lesions it was common to see oblong bodies arranged radially in groups of 6 or 8 about a central spore, and at times there is present a delicate connecting pedicle. They stated that stellar forms may be seen in artificial cultures, and that these structures are produced by budding which may occur at any point on a spore. TAYLOR stated that the organism grows by elongation of the spore which usually divides into two. Buds push out from one or both of these new spores and grow rapidly, forming the mycelium which radiates from the center.

The true asteroid body consists of a central spore surrounded by a mass of eosinophilic material, typically stellate in shape (Fig. 18).

The Central Spore: This is typically a round thick-walled (double contoured) spore. Its diameter according to TALICE and MACKINNON varies from 5—8 μ with a mean of 7 μ; according to LURIE (1963b) 5—8 μ, with a mean of 7 μ; to MORAES and MIRANDA 5—6 μ; and to FUKUSHIRO et al. 1.8—7.9 μ, with an average of 4.7 μ. Sometimes they are oval or semilunar, the oval spores measuring 2.9—6.9 μ × 3.9—7.9 μ with an average of 4.3 × 5.2 μ (FUKUSHIRO et al.). LURIE (1963b) studied one unusual case of bone sporotrichosis in which giant forms were seen. They measured 14—22 μ with a mean of 17 μ. The author is of the opinion that although culture resulted in the growth of typical *Sporotrichum Schenckii*, the fungus represents a new species akin to the *Histoplasma duboisi*.

The spore contains some nuclear material which sometimes shows as an area of basophilic staining. Several authors have observed budding (PINKUS and GREKIN; MINTY et al.; LURIE, 1963b; MORAES and MIRANDA; FUKUSHIRO et al.). Sometimes the budding results in a chain of 3 or 4 spores (LURIE, 1963b; FUKU-SHIRO et al.) and the present author has observed a short fragment of a hypha in the center of an asteroid body.

SIMSON et al. traced the development of this spore from a cigar body through several cryptococcal stages. They concluded that it was not a degenerate form as it was capable of germinating on artificial media. PINKUS and GREKIN described it as a thick-walled small cyst. They quote GRUTZ' opinion that it resembled a chlamydospore which is quite readily found in old cultures of *Sporotrichum*. LURIE (1963b) is of the same opinion.

The Eosinophilic Material: This is extremely variable in size and shape. LURIE (1963b) found that the greatest diameter of the entire asteroid body varies from 7—25 μ, with a mean of 20 μ. MORAES and MIRANDA and FUKUSHIRO et al. measured the thickness of the eosinophilic material (length of the rays); the former found it to be 2—9 μ and the latter reported a maximum of 7 μ. The typical shape is that of a star with radially arranged spindle-shaped or elliptical projections, the tips of which may be sharply pointed or rounded. Many cases have been described in which the eosinophilic material consists only of a very thin uniform film on the surface of the spore, or a wider but uniform coating; it may be clumped and irregularly distributed, giving a tuberculated, nodular, or spiny appearance (TALICE and MACKINNON; SIMSON et al.; PINKUS and GREKIN; MINTY et al.; MEAD and RIDLEY; LURIE, 1963b; FUKUSHIRO et al.). It is homogenous and intensely eosinophilic. WEIDMAN found that the asteroid material associated with the *Aspergillus* stained greenish blue to purple with Gram's stain, a deep blue with Giemsa and black with Heidenhain's hematoxylin. MORAES and MIRANDA found it to be PAS negative, but both LURIE (1963b) and FUKUSHIRO et al. reported weakly positive staining with PAS. LURIE (1963b) was unable to stain this material with the Gridley stain or Gomori's silver impregnation. Histochemical reactions suggest the presence of a glycoprotein (LURIE, 1963b). SIMSON et al. found that in their experimental material the whole asteroid structure was very delicate and behaved like mucoid matter. Its form was easily disturbed and destroyed by manipulation. The projecting processes tended to stick together, forming a rolled up mass in prepared films of pus, and they appeared to be easily separated from the body of the crypto-coccus.

In the large majority of cases these asteroid bodies are extracellular but they have rarely been observed intracellularly within giant cells (TALICE and MACKIN-NON; LURIE, 1963b; YAMADA and WATANABE; FUKUSHIRO et al.). In tissue sections the asteroid bodies are found within the micro-abscesses and in the central poly-morphonuclear zone of the granulomata (Fig. 18). According to LURIE (1963b), MORAES and MIRANDA and FUKUSHIRO et al. this is invariably so but the author has since found an occasional one lying free in the tissues but always in association with a few polymorphonuclear leucocytes. There is usually only one asteroid body in each micro-abscess or granuloma. In the fully developed secondary nodule or gumma, LURIE (1963b) has found several asteroid bodies distributed irregularly in the pus. LURIE (1963b) in a series of 63 cases found asteroid bodies in 17 out of 32 (53.1%) of primary lesions and in 22 out of 31 (71.0%) secondary lesions. FUKU-SHIRO et al., however, found them more frequently in primary lesions, viz. in 34 out of 48 (70.8%) primary lesions and in 11 out of 21 (52.4%) secondary lesions.

Significance of the Asteroid Body: It was first thought that the formation of asteroid bodies in the tissues was a characteristic of the strain of *Sporotrichum*, be-cause of the marked frequency of their occurrence in South Africa and South America, as compared to their paucity in North America and Europe. MACKINNON (TALICE and MACKINNON), however, produced asteroid bodies in animals inoculated with European strains and SIMSON et al. found asteroid bodies in rats inoculated with cultures from North America. In contrast to this, MARIAT and DROUHET found a significant variation in the production of asteroid bodies in hamsters with different strains of *Sporotrichum*. MORAES and MIRANDA were of the opinion that the varia-tion bore no relationship to the strain of the fungus.

Some writers are of the opinion that there may be a relationship between the clinical manifestations and the presence of asteroid bodies. PINKUS and GREKIN noted that asteroid bodies were seen in two American cases which clinically appeared to be very mild and ran a protracted and bland course. FUKUSHIRO et al. found asteroid bodies in 20 out of 28 (71.4%) cases of lymphangitic sporotrichosis and in 17 out of 27 (63%) cases of localized sporotrichosis. LAVALLE et al. describe 3 cases of verrucous sporotrichosis in all of whom numerous asteroid bodies were found. They state that there may be an association of the clinical picture and the presence of these bodies, but that it may have been merely a coincidence. MORAES and MIRANDA found no relationship between the presence of asteroid bodies and the clinical form of the disease.

There has been much speculation about the nature of the eosinophilic material of the asteroid body. MOORE proposed the following theories:

1. The radiating material is an aborted product of the fungus.
2. It is living protoplasm capable of multiplying.
3. It is the result of a host-parasite relationship.
4. It is a protective mechanism set up by the fungus.
5. It is the result of an associated growth of certain bacteria.
6. It is an accompaniment of a reproductive process.
7. It results from the allergic state established by the organism in the tissue.
8. It may be similar to or related to leukotaxine.

SIMSON et al. thought that the formation of the eosinophilic material was a pro-tective mechanism. MORAES and MIRANDA were of the opinion that the eosinophilic material is not a cell membrane but they were unable to determine whether it is produced by the host or by the fungus. FUKUSHIRO et al. felt that it may be a defence mechanism of the fungus cells and that the eosinophilic rays develop as a result of the action of the tissue against the fungus.

Weidman found radiate formation around fungal elements, probably *Aspergillus*, in an infection in a capybara rodent. He identified it with similar structures seen around a *Cryptococcus neoformans* spore in the brain, around a spherule of *Coccidioides*, and with the material surounding an actinomycotic granule. He concluded that the encrustment is a measure of resistance against adverse environment or that it is an accompaniment of reproductive processes; it is produced by the fungus and not by the host. Moore and Ackerman stated that radiate formation is seen in actinomycosis, coccidioidal granuloma, aspergillosis, sporotrichosis, maduromycosis, paracoccidioidal granuloma, chromoblastomycosis and North American blastomycosis. In all these there is a granulomatous response of the tissue accompanied by a variable degree of suppuration. There is a marked inflammatory reaction with massing of leucocytes in close association with radiate forms.

Recently typical asteroid bodies were observed in a *Trichophyton rubrum* infection by Cooper and Mikhael and in a case of candidiasis by Berge and Kaplan.

In 1949 Negroni et al. found that primary inoculation of animals with *C. immitis* resulted in large spores with thin walls. On reinoculation, however, the spores showed thick walls and were surrounded by an areola of acidophilic radial formation. It is well known that intratesticular inoculation of rats produces numerous cigar bodies. However Negroni and Prado first sensitized guinea pigs and rats by giving 3 intramuscular injections of *Sporotrichum* suspension at 3-day intervals and then gave an intratesticular injection. This resulted in early formation of tuberculoid granulomata and in the simultaneous appearance of asteroid bodies. They believe that the asteroid bodies were an expression of the resistance of the host.

Mariat and Drouhet observed that in hamsters navicular spores transform directly to round forms. These then assume a double contour and resemble chlamydospores. They become coated with an eosinophilic material 1—2 μ thick, sometimes not covering the entire surface. This material increases in amount and projections of it radiate in all directions. The ends of the rays may be blunt or pointed. They concluded that the asteroid body is a result of a defence mechanism. The eosinophilic material is a mucoid substance secreted by the fungus or by the tissues of the host or by both.

The radial formation of eosinophilic material is seen not only in relationship to fungi. It also occurs around Bilharzia ova (Hoeppli phenomenon), microfilaria (Lurie, 1963b) and *Angiostrongyloides cantonensis*. Koppisch is of the opinion that the Hoeppli phenomenon represents a specific antigen-antibody reaction such as is seen when Schistosome eggs are placed in serum of infected persons (Oliver-González). Smith and von Lichtenberg have shown that an antigenic cystine- and cysteine-rich protein leaks through the shell of the ovum, evokes an immune response in the host and precipitates with a tryptophan-rich host globulin to produce the Hoeppli phenomenon. Thus the Hoeppli phenomenon is contingent upon a high degree of host sensitization.

Lurie (1963b) is of the opinion that the radial material in sporotrichosis is identical with the material at the periphery of the actinomycotic, nocardial and maduromycotic granules, around the hyphae in subcutaneous phycomycosis, around the spores of the other fungi mentioned previously, around Bilharzia ova, microfilaria and *Angiostrongyloides cantonensis*. In 1967 he postulated that the host is usually infected with conidia from the fungus growing on plants, moss, etc. These conidia appear in the tissues as cigar bodies or their variants. When resistance of the host is low, these cigar bodies multiply and are easily found in tissue sections and in smears of exudates. Magalhães Pereira et al. confirm that in cases with no immunity numerous yeast forms are found in the lesions. MARIAT et al. expressed the opinion that the cigar bodies and yeast-like forms are the multiplying forms, whereas the round are stable.

In rare instances fragments of hyphae enter the inoculation site. SIMSON et al. have shown that in experimental animals these hyphae disappear in 4 or 5 days. However, on occasion they appear to persist and even to grow in the tissues. When the host resistance is high the conidia, or cigar bodies, change into chlamydospores. As antibodies appear in the blood and react with the fungus, the asteroid eosinophilic material is deposited. NEGRONI and PRADO are also of the opinion that asteroid formation is an expression of host resistance.

Evidence in favor of this concept is provided by PINKUS and GREKIN's finding of asteroid bodies in two North American cases which clinically appeared to be very mild and ran a protracted and bland course. LURIE (1963a) reported that only 5 cases out of about 3,000 seen in South Africa showed systemic involvement. He feels that this may be due to some relative immunity of the local population, since animal experiments have shown no difference in the virulence of the fungal strains. In his opinion this may account for the prevalence of asteroid body formation. In 1967 he found a relationship between the amount of eosinophilic material around the fungal spore and the severity of the illness; the largest asteroid bodies were found in a solitary, dry, verrucous lesion which had been present for 1 year, and in a 7 month old recurrent lesion in a case which had been inadequately treated 10 years previously; asteroid bodies with moderate amounts of eosinophilic material were found in a 1 month old lesion in a garden worker in whom secondary nodules had appeared 2 weeks after the primary lesion; "asteroid bodies" with a minimal amount of eosinophilic material were found in a secondary nodule in a case in which the primary lesion could not be identified, but whose hands, face and neck were covered with innumerable secondary lesions and in whom a bone lesion was present; similar minimal "asteroid bodies" were observed in a case with wide-spread visceral involvement, in whom numerous cigar bodies were found in pus smears from lesions in a rib and from an abscess in the orbit.

MORAES and MIRANDA report an interesting case that failed to respond to several courses of treatment. Biopsy revealed granulation tissue but no microabscesses or spores. After treatment with potassium iodide, glucantime and sulfa drugs there was a marked improvement, and at this stage another biopsy showed the typical histology and asteroid bodies.

Evidence for the theory of relative immunity in a population is the fact that antibodies can be detected by means of skin tests with sporotrichin in patients who have been cured of the disease, as well as in people living in endemic areas who have no recollection of having had the disease (for details see under Skin Tests). However the state of affairs in Brazil appears to be contrary to this explanation on the basis of relative immunity. The skin test positivity rate in healthy adults is much higher there than elsewhere, and a "minimal" form of the disease is not uncommonly seen, yet since LUTZ and SPLENDORE first described the asteroid body in that country these spores were not seen there again until 1964.

Hyphal Forms

DAVIS (1913) and MOORE (1955) stated that hyphae have not been observed in living tissues. They have, however, been reported in a very few cases. As yet there is no explanation for their presence. The first report was by ADAMSON in 1911 who found, in sections of a skin nodule, pieces of mycelium, some jointed, some ending in a club-shaped spore; they occurred in areas where the infiltrate was sparsely cellular. McDONAGH confirmed their presence in other sections of a lesion he obtained from Adamson's case. Miller found similar branching mycelium in smears prepared from a lesion. Dohi et al. observed hyphae in one case in Japan. Hyslop et al. found foci of mycelium in the tissues in a case of meningitis and Forbus detected masses of mycelium within a cavity in a lung and embedded in the surrounding hyaline scar tissue. Wade and Matthews made KOH preparations of tissue from the edge of an ulcer and found dense clusters of fine filaments in the deeper layer of the skin. Okudaira et al. (1959) found a hyphal fragment 18 μ in length within a giant cell. Definite septate hyphae have been observed in tissue sections by Mount, Collins, Okudaira et al. (1959), Lurie (1963b), Fukushiro et al. in 2 cases, and Maberry et al.

Fungal Elements in the Circulating Blood

The *Sporotrichum* has been recovered from the blood stream in two of the early French cases (Widal and Weil; Landouzy), but no subsequent reports of positive blood cultures have been found.

Eosinophilia in the Circulating Blood

In addition to an infiltration of eosinophils in the tissues, some cases have had an eosinophilia in the circulating blood (Widal and Weil; Widal and Joltrain; Gaucher et al.; Brissaud et al.).

Serology

1. Complement Fixation Test

The first time this test was used in the diagnosis of sporotrichosis was in 1908 by Widal and Abrami and subsequently by several others (Adamson; Davis, 1914; Moore and Davis; Warfield; Lawless). Gougerot (1913) maintained that the test always gave a positive result but was not specific as sera from other mycoses also reacted. However negative reactions have been reported (Califano in 8 cases). du Toit found this test to be unreliable and of no practival value in the diagnosis of sporotrichosis. Padilha Gonçalves and Magalhães Pereira found only 60% positives in localized cases and, in another study, Magalhães Pereira et al. (1964) found 69% of these cases to be positive. Padilha Gonçalves (1962) stated that only some cases give positive reactions, that it may remain positive after cure and that positive reactions have been obtained in people without evidence of sporotrichosis. Magalhães Pereira et al. (1962, 1964) found 30% positive 1 month to 12 years after cure, and they obtained positive reactions in 24% of healthy people.

Norden found that autoclaved antigen gave no cross reactions with other fungi but that ground antigen, fresh antigen and methylated antigen gave variable cross reactions.

2. Agglutination Reaction

The first use of this test also was made by Widal and Abrami in 1908. Since then there have been many reports of positive agglutination tests in cases of sporotrichosis (Davis, 1914; Moore and Davis; Warfield; Wohl; Arěa-Leão and Goto, etc.). Magalhães Pereira et al. state that it is always positive in localized cases. The titers which have been obtained range from 1:10 (Wohl) to 1:1500 (de Beurmann, Gougerot and Vaucher, 1909d). Anderson and Spector found that the patient's serum agglutinated spores from the strain isolated from his own lesion to a titer of 1:2560 but those from an old culture to a titer of 1:640. Moore and Davis reported negative reactions with 1:20 dilutions of control serum. Widal et al. regarded 1:100 as a diagnostic titer. GOUGEROT (1913) reviewed 18 reports of agglutination tests and concluded that the titer may range from 1:200 to 1:500, the average being 1:400. The controls ranged from 1:10 to 1:80 and sera from patients with other fungal infections were rarely as high as 1:150. However FOERSTER (1924) states that normal human serum may agglutinate *Sporotrichum* spores to a titer of 1:40 to 1:150, or sometimes higher. DU TOIT, who obtained a titer of 1:600 in 100 cases of sporotrichosis, found that the controls were not significantly lower. D'IMEUX states that titers as high as 1:250 to 1:500 may be obtained in $^1/_4$ hour and that it may go up to 1:1500 to 1:4000 after a longer interval. NORDEN (1951) made a thorough study of the serology of sporotrichosis: his rabbit antiserum agglutinated suspensions of *Histoplasma capsulatum* to a titer of 1:80 and *Candida albicans* to a titer of 1:40, whereas against the homologous antigen it was 1:640. Antiblastomyces rabbit serum agglutinated the *Sporotrichum* antigen but the serum from a case of blastomycosis did not. However in a series of 11 human cases of sporotrichosis he found this test to be of limited value. ROTHE found that the serum of a case of actinomycosis agglutinated the *Sporotrichum* antigen.

DE BEURMANN, RAMOND, GOUGEROT and VAUCHER reported that their first case diagnosed in 1903 gave a negative reaction 5 years later and that 2 cases diagnosed 1 year previously were only weakly positive (1:80 and 1:60). GOUGEROT in 1913 stated that the reaction persists after cure but did not specify the length of time. CREGOR stated that this test has been found to be positive 1 year after cure and negative 3 years after cure. MAGALHÃES PEREIRA et al. (1962, 1964) found 90% positive 1 month to 12 years after cure and obtained positive reactions in 38% of healthy people.

3. Precipitin Reaction

This was first used by GONZÁLEZ OCHOA and SOTO FIGUERO in 1947 and then by NORDEN (1951). MAGALHÃES PEREIRA et al. (1964) state that it may be positive or negative in localized cases and negative in disseminated cases. More recently this test has been improved, some investigators using the agar precipitation technique (KADEN). However it is too early to evaluate the specificity and sensitivity of the latest modifications.

4. Hemagglutination Reaction

NORDEN (1951) found this to be unsatisfactory in sporotrichosis.

Dermal Reaction

Sporotrichin or Sporotrichosin Test

The first use of this test was made by BLOCH, followed by PAUTRIER and LUTEMBACHER and by LEBAIN and ST. GIRONS in 1909. MOORE and DAVIS also obtained dermal reactions and proved the specificity of the antigen by failing to elicit a reaction in a case of blastomycosis. Subsequently many reports of positive skin tests followed (DU TOIT; GELBER; SINGER and MUNCIE, etc.). DE BEURMANN and GOUGEROT (1909) and DU TOIT stated that a negative skin test practically excludes the diagnosis of sporotrichosis but that a positive reaction is not diagnostic as, according to the former, carriers may give positive reactions and, according to the latter, cross reactions may occur with other fungal infections. PADILHA GONÇALVES and PONTES DE CARVALHO noted strong reactions in all of 33 cases; MARTINS DE CASTRO obtained positive reactions in 64 out of 65 cases and MAGALHÃES PEREIRA et al. (1964) reported that 3 cases out of 67 gave negative reactions.

Gómez-Orozco and Ortega are of the opinion that the reaction is specific. However Ansel D'Imeux stated that the reaction is positive in 100% of cases of sporotrichosis but 50% of cases with other mycoses and 33% of cases with non-mycotic diseases also give positive reactions. González Ochoa and Soto Figueroa prepared an antigen from polysaccharides extracted from yeast phase growth and expressed the opinion that with this antigen the dermal reaction was not only consistently positive but it was also specific. However in disseminated sporotrichosis the reaction may be negative due to anergy (Padilha Gonçalves, 1962; Magalhães Pereira et al., 1964).

Padilha Gonçalves (1962) stated that the intradermal test is always positive in localized cutaneous cases and remains positive after cure of the disease. Martins de Castro and Belliboni found that the reaction was still positive up to 14 years after cure. It would appear that in fact it remains positive for life as Hektoen and Perkins' original case still has a positive reaction 65 years after his infection (McFarland).

González Ochoa (1965) stated that: when the polysaccharide antigen made from the mycelial phase was used, the reaction was positive only in the active phase and reverted to negative in 1—3 years; however when the antigen was made from yeast phase organisms it gave a positive reaction even in the absence of clinical symptoms, and this reaction may remain positive indefinitely. Magalhães Pereira et al. (1964), however, had one case which still gave a positive reaction with the polysaccharide antigen 12 years after cure, as did healthy individuals with no history of infection.

du Toit found that in a human volunteer a dermal reaction was discernible 5 days after experimental inoculation.

Immunity

There is evidence to suggest that some people are immune to infection or have a partial immunity. Simson et al. succeeded in infecting only 1 out of 10 human volunteers by applying a spore suspension to the intact skin. Helm and Berman reported that in some experimental cases neither injection nor scratch inoculation of a pathogenic culture has produced a progressive lesion in the human subject. Padilha Gonçalves (1962) reported that experimental inoculation of human volunteers failed to produce the disease in a few cases.

Spontaneous cures have been reported by Errecart, Mead and Ridley, Torrico and Romana, Crevasse and Ellner, Padilha Gonçalves, and Magalhaes Pereira et al. (1964). Helm and Berman noted such cures, particularly in those with the dry, flat plaque type of lesion. D'Alessio et al. mentioned an interesting case of a spontaneous cure in a 72 year old man who had worked at a tree nursery for 20 years.

Padilha Gonçalves (1962) reported that patients with sporotrichosis were successfully superinfected. The new lesions, however, showed a marked tendency to spontaneous regression. Magalhães Pereira et al. (1964) reinfected 3 cases; in one of these regression occurred, while in the others the lesions progressed and necessitated treatment.

Padilha Gonçalves (1962) and Magalhães Pereira et al. (1964) are of the opinion that when the portal of entry of the fungus is through the skin and the usual chancreform lesion is produced, there is time for antibodies to form, and immunity is developed sufficiently to prevent the disease from spreading. Under these circumstances fungal elements are difficult to find in the tissues. They suggest that the rare cases of disseminated sporotrichosis are due to the fungus' gain-ing entry into the body by inhalation or ingestion, and/or to the lack of immunity of the host, evidence for which is seen in a negative intradermal reaction (anergy). In the lesions of these cases fungal elements are numerous and easily found. LURIE (1967) is also of the opinion that the type of lesion and the number and type of spores observed are related to the presence or absence of immunity.

GARRETT and ROBBINS reported 8 cases among employees at a store in Mexico. Of these 8, only 1 showed the classical picture of a primary lesion and lymphangitic spread. The other 7 had small localized lesions resembling warts which in the ordinary course of events would not have been recognized as sporotrichosis in origin, unless this had been specifically sought. A "minimal" form of the disease is frequently seen in South America (RAMOS E. SILVA, 1945).

Subclinical Infections: There is strong evidence that subclinical infections with *Sporotrichum Schenckii* can occur and probably do so frequently, especially in people who are constantly exposed to the fungus. MAGALHÃES PEREIRA et al. (1962) after finding positive dermal reactions in 47 out of 49 cases, 1 month to 12 years after cure, concluded that the finding of a positive reaction in a healthy person was not a false positive but signified a previous infection. This explained the low incidence of "false" positive reactions in children.

WERNSDÖRFER et al. tested 55 residents of Germany, where sporotrichosis is not endemic, and found all to be negative; but in Brazil, where the disease is endemic, they found that 9 out 38 (23.8%) persons with no history of having had sporotrichosis gave positive reactions. NAVARRO DA SILVA et al. tested people in Portugal in areas free of sporotrichosis and in areas where the disease had been previously reported. They found no positive reactions in the former area but 2.5% of 39 persons tested in the latter area were positive. PADILHA GONÇALVES (1962) found positive reactions in 6% of Brazilian children, in 27% of a heterogeneous group of Brazilian adults and in 57% of persons working in a dermatological clinic in an endemic area. ROTBERG and ABRAMCZYK tested 59 boys in a boarding school in which 2 cases had been diagnosed; of these, 28.8% had positive dermal reactions. Of 19 of this group of boys who had often received scratches or bruises while playing in the woods, 63.1% reacted positively. SCHNEIDAU et al. tested 383 prison inmates and hospital patients with no history of sporotrichosis, in Louisiana, USA, and found 11.2% positive. However 32.3% of 34 employees at a plant nursery gave positive reactions. Of the employees who had worked there for more than 10 years, 58.3% were positive reactors.

MAGALHÃES PEREIRA et al. (1964) concluded that there was still some doubt about the presence of a natural immunity but that there was sufficient evidence to prove that subclinical infections impart a degree of immunity; that cases with localized lesions have a relatively high immunity, give a positive dermal reaction and are easily cured, while those with disseminated lesions have no immunity and may give negative dermal reactions.

Experimental Evidence of immunity is only suggestive and not at all conclusive. DE BEURMANN and GOUGEROT (1910) stated that it was possible to immunize animals. TAYLOR's experiment with rats suggested the possibility of producing immunity by injections of small doses of a culture of *Sporotrichum*. JESSNER also felt that in rats there was partial immunity to cutaneous infection. KESTEN and MARTINSTEIN found that previous subcutaneous inoculation in rats produced a shortening of the duration of survival of the organisms in the blood after intracardiac injection.

BENHAM and KESTEN inoculated a monkey by pricking its finger with an infected barberry thorn, producing a local lesion and lymphadenopathy. After 5 weeks the monkey was inoculated intravenously, producing numerous disseminated papular and nodular lesions. After these lesions had almost disappeared spontaneously they inoculated the animal intracardially, and this resulted in the appearance of only a few small papules. They were unable to recover the fungus from the lesions or from the blood. One month later they again inoculated intracardially and after 5 weeks there were no lesions but a generalized lymphadenopathy was present. The animal was sacrificed and no evidence of sporotrichosis was found.

Hasenclever and Mitchell were able to produce a slight protection in mice by immunization with formalin-killed suspensions of *S. Schenckii*. Sethi and Schwarz using subcutaneous immunization reduced the mortality rate in mice after intravenous challenge with the same strain. However, immunization failed to modify the pathology in the liver and spleen, although in some cases dissemination to the lungs was prevented.

Experimental Sporotrichosis in Laboratory Animals

Rats: The rat has always been considered to be the most susceptible of the laboratory animals and intraperitoneal inoculation of this animal is the recognized biological test for the presence of *S. Schenckii* (de Beurmann, Gougerot and Vaucher, 1908a, b, c).

de Beurmann, Gougerot and Vaucher (1908a, b) described the gross and microscopic appearance of the lesions in great detail. After intraperitoneal inoculation, swelling and induration of the testes appears in 10—15 days. After 20—25 days the scrotum is markedly swollen, red and tender and the skin ulcerates. The infection becomes generalized and the rat dies in 28—175 days after inoculation.

At autopsy the peritoneum is seen to be studded with discrete granulomata and abscesses. The entire genito-urinary tract is affected. The testes are adherent to the scrotum and they are covered by an inflammatory exudate in which there are numerous gray, translucent granulomata and white opaque abscesses. These may extend into the parenchyma of the testes and in severe cases the entire testes may be replaced by abscess cavities. The epididymis is generally spared.

Most reports confirm that intraperitoneal inoculation results in the development of nodules, tubercles or abscesses on the peritoneal surface (Hektoen and Perkins; Lutz and Splendore, 1908; Hyde and Davis; Taylor; Moore and Davis; Pijper and Pullinger; Lewis and Cudmore; du Toit; Simson et al.). The abscesses are said to contain a viscid, purulent, yellowish-grey material. Intraperitoneal or intratesticular inoculation also produces a severe orchitis (Figs. 19, 20, 21, 22) (Hektoen and Perkins; Lutz and Splendore, 1908; Hyde and Davis; Taylor; Moore and Davis; Pijper and Pullinger; Hopkins and Benham; Lewis and Cudmore; Graham; du Toit; Gelber; Panja et al.; Simson et al.; Mariat and Drouhet). Some investigators also found disseminated lesions: in liver and spleen (Hamburger; Hopkins and Benham; Simson et al.), in all organs (Kren and Schramek; Mariat and Drouhet), in bones (Moore and Davis; Benham and Kesten). de Beurmann, Gougerot and Vaucher (1909e) and Davis (1916) were able to infect rats by mouth by mixing the fungus in their food over a period of months. Lesions appeared in the omentum, mesentery and lymph nodes. On the other hand, Walker and Ritchie, and Campbell et al. failed to produce an infection in rats by intraperitoneal inoculation.

Mackinnon and Conti-Díaz showed that the atmospheric temperature affects the pathogenicity of the *Sporotrichum* in rats; those kept at a temperature of 5—20°C developed lesions in the bones of the paws and tail while those kept at 31°C did not.

The histological appearance of the rat lesions has been described by several workers. According to de Beurmann, Gougerot and Vaucher (1908a, b) the lesions consist of granulomata, abscesses, focal infiltrations with polymorphonuclear cells and macrophages, diffuse lymphoid infiltration, foci of necrosis with

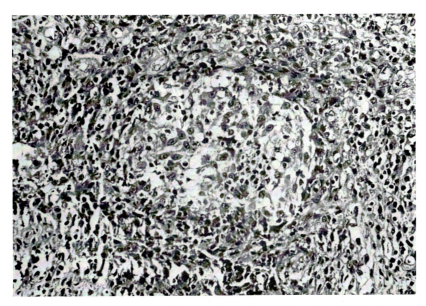

Fig. 19. Experimental sporotrichosis. Section of experimentally produced lesion in rat testis showing early granuloma. H & E, × 300

giant cells and areas of diffuse fibrosis. The granulomata may undergo central necrosis and become walled off by fibrous tissue or they may be infiltrated by polymorphonuclear cells and develop into abscesses. They may vary in size. The small ones resemble tuberculoid follicles with or without giant cells; the center is composed of eosinophilic epithelioid cells and multinucleated giant cells with central or peripheral nuclei, and the periphery is made up of a narrow zone of lymphocytes and is sharply demarcated (Fig. 19). The medium sized granuloma arises from the enlargement of a single small follicle or from the fusion of several follicles. Its center, which is at first epithelioid, later undergoes caseation necrosis. A few polymorphonuclear leucocytes may be seen in the interior of the granuloma and towards the edge vacuolated macrophages are moderately numerous. The periphery is indistinct and merges with the surrounding infiltrate (Fig. 20). The large granuloma shows central necrosis surrounded by a wall with threee zones: a zone of epithelioid cells, with or without giant cells, a zone of infiltration with lymphocytes and a zone of fibrous tissue at the periphery. These granulomata evolve into thick-walled fibrous cysts enclosing a mass of necrotic tissue, in which fungal spores are extremely numerous and often form a large confluent mass. Granulomata with central microabscesses are very rare, but when present, their middle and external zones have a tuberculoid structure (Fig. 21). Some of the granulomata become completely sclerosed.

HEKTOEN and PERKINS, and PIJPER and PULLINGER both described the lesions as cavities containing polymorphonuclear leucocytes and nuclear detritus enclosed by a wall of recent fibrous tissue. GRAHAM referred to them as acute purulent inflammation with abscess formation. CAMPBELL et al. described the cavities as containing only necrotic material and the walls as poorly vascularized granulation tissue, in the deeper layers of which there are several small round cells and occasional giant cells. TAYLOR described granulomata, usually with a central area of necrosis, surrounded by a zone of dense cellular infiltration, the predominant cell

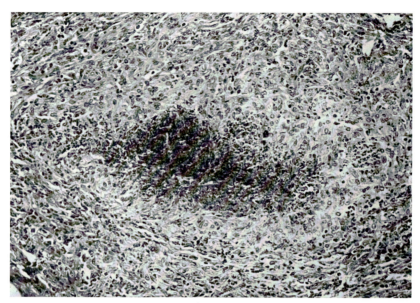

Fig. 20. Experimental sporotrichosis. Section of experimentally produced lesion in rat testis showing granuloma consisting of an area of central necrosis surrounded by histiocytic cells. H & E, × 200

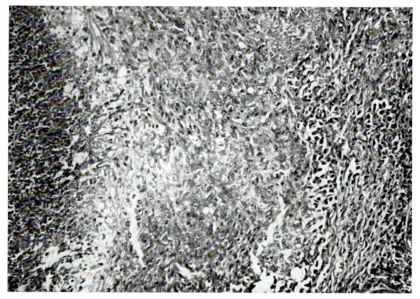

Fig. 21. Experimental sporotrichosis. Section of experimentally produced lesion in rat testis showing the wall of an abscess; at left necrotic debris, in the center a zone of histiocytic cells and fibroblasts, and at right fibrous tissue and mononuclear cell infiltrate. H & E, × 200

being the polymorphonuclear leucocyte. At the periphery there is an extensive area showing proliferation of connective tissue, congestion, hemorrhage and infiltration by histiocytes, small mononuclear cells, eosinophils and numerous giant cells. HAMBURGER found numerous eosinophils but no giant cells. SIMSON et al. described the lesions as being very similar to those in human cases, varying from acute necrotic lesions to typical granulomata with a central collection of pus surrounded by a zone of histiocytes and giant cells.

Hamsters: In the opinion of MARIAT and DROUHET the hamster is superior to the rat as a laboratory animal. In the rat subcutaneous gummata are rarely obtained, but in the hamster subcutaneous inoculation produces a disease similar to that in man, with gummatous lesions along the lymphatic vessels; in a few cases the disease becomes generalized. Intraperitoneal inoculation may produce either a generalized infection or a more chronic type with subcutaneous gummata, osteoarthritis of the paws or an orchitis.

The lesion in the paw rarely ulcerates. It consists of granulation tissue infiltrated by plasma cells and in it are aggregations of epithelioid cells with necrotic centers and micro-abscesses. Asteroid bodies are present in the centers of typical granulomata which have three distinct zones: a central zone of polymorphonuclear cells and necrotic cells, a middle zone of epithelioid cells and giant cells and a peripheral zone of plasma cells. The testes are swollen and suppuration extends through sinuses to the skin. The surface of the testes is covered with nodules which consist of abscesses with central necrosis teeming with fungal spores. MARIAT et al. and the present author (unpublished) confirmed the marked susceptibility of the hamster to experimental infection. Intraperitoneal inoculation produced a peritonitis, an orchitis, lesions in the spleen, liver, abdominal and thoracic lymph nodes.

Mice: The experiences of various investigators using this animal are extremely variable. Several have reported the development of a local lesion after subcutaneous inoculation (SCHENCK; HEKTOEN and PERKINS; FOULERTON; WALKER and RITCHIE; BAKER, 1942, 1947a), and in some instances dissemination has occurred with visceral involvement (SCHENCK: peritoneum, spleen, testis; FOULERTON: liver; BAKER, 1947a: bone, lymph nodes, viscera; OKUDAIRA et al.: generalized; SETHI and SCHWARZ: generalized).

Most workers have found that intraperitoneal inoculation produces a peritonitis but their reports of organ involvement differ (HEKTOEN and PERKINS: peritonitis only; FOULERTON: liver and spleen; BAKER, 1947a: liver and testis; PANJA et al.: testis; LIU: testis; MARIAT et al.: viscera and rarely testis). On the contrary, WALKER and RITCHIE, and MOORE and ACKERMAN failed to infect mice by the intraperitoneal route, but MOORE and ACKERMAN produced lesions in the testis by direct inoculation into that organ. HYDE and DAVIS successfully infected mice by scarification of the tail and SETHI et al. produced pulmonary lesions following intranasal infection. SETHI and SCHWARZ found that cortisone administration led to severe dissemination and early death.

Dogs: SCHENCK found that the dog has a natural immunity to sporotrichosis. Intravenous injection failed to produce an infection, but subcutaneous inoculation resulted in a local abscess which resolved spontaneously in 3—4 weeks. HEKTOEN and PERKINS confirmed these findings. However GOUGEROT and CARAVAN (1908d) produced lesions in the subcutaneous tissue, bone, peritoneum and liver; and KREN and SCHRAMEK found that nearly all the organs were affected. DE BEURMANN, GOUGEROT and VAUCHER (1909c) stated that the adult dog is resistant to infection but that the young animal is susceptible. In addition to the usual acute, subacute and chronic type of sporotrichosis, they reported in 1909c a chronic form with a slow evolution which responds readily to treatment. They produced a gummatous subcutaneous lesion which ran a benign course, but were unable to produce any visceral lesions. They stated that WIDAL had had the same experience with dogs.

42*

Cats: DE BEURMANN, GOUGEROT and VAUCHER (1909a, b) found that the adult cat is relatively resistant to infection. Inoculation may fail to produce a lesion or it may result only in a local lesion which is easily curable. However newborn and young cats are very susceptible; some die within 3—8 days, others run a more subacute course with multiple subcutaneous and visceral lesions.

Guinea Pigs: The susceptibility of guinea pigs to infection with the *Sporotrichum* is equivocal. SCHENCK failed to produce any lesions by subcutaneous or intraperitoneal injections. HEKTOEN and PERKINS also failed by intraperitoneal injections but were able to produce small abscesses by subcutaneous inoculation. FOULERTON produced lesions in the liver and spleen in 1 out of the 3 guinea pigs injected intraperitoneally. WALKER and RITCHIE, however, were unable to do so, but PINOY and MAGROU recommended direct inoculation of pus into guinea pigs as a diagnostic procedure. HAMBURGER succeeded in producing multiple abscesses in the peritoneum as well as in the liver and spleen. TAYLOR produced small abscesses in the peritoneum, a large abscess in the abdominal muscles and an orchitis. WARFIELD found multiple visceral lesions with a strain isolated from a case of pulmonary sporotrichosis. PANJA et al. reported a severe destructive orchitis and DE BLASIO succeeded in producing the disease in adult guinea pigs.

Rabbits: The rabbit appears to be the most resistent of all laboratory animals to infection. Intraperitoneal or intravenous inoculation fails to produce any lesions (SCHENCK; HEKTOEN and PERKINS; PAGE et al.; WALKER and RITCHIE). However DE BEURMANN, GOUGEROT and VAUCHER (1908c) produced lesions in the lungs, kidney, caecum and skin, and WARFIELD produced multiple visceral lesions with a strain isolated from a case of pulmonary sporotrichosis. PANJA et al. produced a severe destructive orchitis by intraperitoneal injection. BRAUDE et al. produced an acute febrile illness by intravenous inoculation of viable or killed spores.

Pigeons: Only one report could be found in which pigeons were inoculated, namely that of HEKTOEN and PERKINS, who failed to produce any lesions by subcutaneous inoculation.

Monkeys: Only three reports of the use of monkeys were found. HYDE and DAVIS inoculated a monkey subcutaneously, producing subcutaneous abscesses which healed spontaneously. HOPKINS and BENHAM produced a typical lymphangitic type of lesion. BENHAM and KESTEN infected a monkey by pricking its forefinger with a contaminated barberry thorn; this resulted in the development of a local papular lesion and a generalized lymphadenopathy which regressed spontaneously. The same animal was then inoculated intravenously resulting in disseminated papular and nodular lesions on the arms and face.

Fungal Elements in Tissue of Experimental Animals

Cigar Bodies and Their Variants (Fig. 22): Most investigators report that numerous spores were found, especially at the edge of the abscess in the necrotic tissue (SCHENCK; DE BEURMANN, GOUGEROT and VAUCHER, 1908 b; TAYLOR). They have been described as round, oval or clubshaped (SCHENCK), oval, oblong or lanceolate (HEKTOEN and PERKINS), oval, cylindrical or rod-shaped (FOULERTON), oblong, oval or pear-shaped (HYDE and DAVIS), oval (HAMBURGER), elongated or oval (DAVIS, 1913), cigar-shaped (TAYLOR; GELBER), fusiform or oval (BAKER, 1947a), first elongated or oval, later becoming spherical (SIMSON et al.), spindle-shaped (LIU), cigar-shaped and round (MARIAT et al.), cigar-shaped and ring forms (OKUDAIRA et al., 1961; SETHI and SCHWARZ). Three types of ring forms

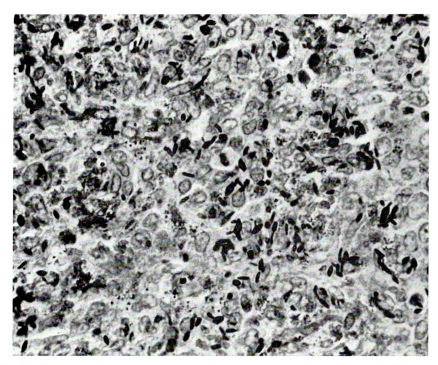

Fig. 22. Experimental sporotrichosis. Fungal elements in experimentally produced lesion in rat testis. PAS, × 550

were described by OKUDAIRA et al. (1961), viz: one that stains intensely and homogeneously with PAS, one with a prominent, darkly staining central mass, and one with a thin wall. Many authors, especially when writing in the Spanish language (e.g. MARIAT and DROUHET) refer to navicular or boat-shaped spores, which, from the description and illustrations, seem to be indistinguishable from cigar bodies.

The size of the spores in the various reports ranges between the extremes of $1—2 \mu \times 2—4 \mu$ (SCHENCK) and $1—3 \mu \times 10—12 \mu$ (HYDE and DAVIS). They have been reported as being usually extracellular (TAYLOR), usually intracellular (BAKER, 1947a), extra- or intracellular (SCHENCK; HAMBURGER). Budding has been observed (HYDE and DAVIS; DAVIS, 1913). Two reports mention that they may be arranged radially around a central spore (HYDE and DAVIS; DAVIS, 1913).

Asteroid Bodies: These have been seen in animal tissues on several occasions (GRECO, 1908; HARTER and GRUYER; TALICE and MACKINNON; SIMSON et al.; NEGRONI and PRADO). In the hamster asteroid bodies are apparently very numerous (MARIAT and DROUHET; MARIAT et al.).

Hyphae: WALKER and RITCHIE found a few short threads of mycelium in one animal. TAYLOR found mycelium in a preparation of pus from an abscess in a rat injected with a broth culture, but was unable to detect hyphae in sections. Indisputible hyphal filaments in the tissues were observed by CAMPBELL, OKUDAIRA et al. (1961), MARIAT et al., and SETHI et al. It is of interest to note that OKUDAIRA et al. (1961) were able to induce the development of hyphae in the tissues by the administration of Amphotericin B or Griseofulvin.

Therapy

Sporotrichosis was the first of the deep mycoses for which an effective drug therapy was found. The oral administration of *sodium or potassium iodide* was first used by the French, viz: DE BEURMANN, GOUGEROT and their colleagues, in 1903. It is still the treatment of choice for cutaneous sporotrichosis.

The largest experience in the use of this drug was that of HELM and BERMAN, who treated 2,829 cases in a period of about 3 years. They recommended that the patient be given 2 grams of *potassium iodide* 3 times a day for 2 days as a test for iodism, which usually would become apparent in this time. If there are only mild symptoms of iodism, the treatment is not interrupted as the symptoms usually disappear. If they are more severe, treatment is stopped for a period of 24—36 h and then started again. 130—200 g in 4—5 weeks is generally adequate for most cases. Some require less, others more, up to 520 g. If response is slow, the dose may be stepped up to 10 g per day. In the majority of cases cultures are negative after 26 g have been given, but treatment should be continued for several weeks after the lesions have healed to avoid the possibility of a recurrence.

Potassium iodide appears to act locally, as ROBINSON and ORBAN cured a case of extensive lymphangitic sporotrichosis by local applications twice daily. SHAFFER and ZACKHEIM employed iontophoresis. It would appear that this drug is most effective when given intravenously (M. SILVA) as this route of administration proved successful after oral administration failed (RAY and ROCKWOOD).

Other iodine compounds are also effective. BLAIR and YARIAN found no differences in the response in two cases, one treated with *potassium iodide* and the other with *sodium iodide*. LANE used *ethyl iodide* to cure a case who was resistant to *potassium iodide*. Others have supplemented the iodide therapy with superficial irradiation (HOLLAND and MAURIELLO; ROBINSON). Some cases have proved to be completely resistant to iodides, even to a dose of 17.5 g per day (LOEWE); for this and other reasons many different drugs have been tried.

Several cases have been cured with *Stilbamidine* (HARREL et al.; MIKKELSEN et al.). *Sulfonamides* have been equally successful (MARTINEZ NAVARRO; NOOJIN and CALLAWAY; ALGODOAL; BAKER and MALONE). One case has been cured with *Sulphone* orally and *zinc oxide* ointment locally (LEFROU). In Brazil several resistent cases have responded to *Glucantime* (*N-methylglucamine antimoniate*) given intramuscularly (BAPTISTA et al.; BELLIBONI and PATRICIO).

Some cases have been cured with *Griseofulvin* (GONZÁLEZ OCHOA, 1959; LOEWENTHAL; LATAPÍ et al.; LATAPÍ, 1960; BRAITMAN; LEAVELL). However WATT and LINTON and PADILHA GONÇALVES (1962) found this drug unsuccessful. GONZÁLEZ OCHOA (1965) treated 196 cases of which only 50% were cured and 25% were improved, and in 25% there was no effect. DE MARCO claims to have cured 2 cases with *Penicillin* but the case of SHAFFER and ZACKHEIM failed to respond to *Penicillin*. *Amphotericin B* is effective in sporotrichosis when given by mouth (NEWCOMER and HOMER) or parenterally (LONDOÑO; FINLAYSON et al.; KLEIN et al.; SEABURY and DASCOMB).

Radiotherapy alone was first used on cutaneous lesions by ATILLJ in 1925. Later it was used successfuly by others (NOGUER MORÉ and DAUSÁ). BURGEL and MEESSEN cured a case of sporotrichosis of the shoulder joint by immobilization and deep X-ray therapy only.

THOMAS et al. found that hyperthermia produced a dramatic improvement in the lesions which were rendered sterile, but they were forced to abandon the trial and had to resort to *potassium iodide* as the patient was uncooperative. However GALIANA and CONTI-DÍAZ successfully treated 9 cases with local heat and a rubifacient, and MACKINNON and CONTI-DÍAZ cured 1 case with hot, wet dressings only. TREJOS and RAMIREZ treated a woman with 300 lesions on the leg by immersing the limb in a waterbath at 45°C for 30 min 4 times a day for 8 weeks. She has remained cured for more than a year. HELM and BERMAN cured some cases by freezing the lesions with *ethyl chloride* spray. NIEMEYER stated that experience over 20 years has shown that freezing with carbon dioxide snow is the best basic therapy for both superficial and deep lesions; many cases respond to this treatment alone but some require, in addition, the use of *iodine, Streptomycin* or *Sulfone*.

Solitary lesions can be cured by surgical excision (ROBINSON and FROST) or by electrocoagulation (M. SILVA). For cavitary lesions of the lung a segmental resection or lobectomy has been found necessary and curative (CRUTHIRDS and PATTERSON).

SEZARY et al. used an autogenous vaccine in their case. MIRANDA et al. (1958), and PADILHA GONÇALVES (1962, 1963) cured cases by desensitization by intradermal injections of heat-killed suspensions of a yeast phase growth of *S. Schenckii*.

In conclusion, *potassium iodide* by mouth is the least expensive, simplest and usually the most effective therapy and is the treatment of choice in cutaneous cases. When iodides are contraindicated or are ineffective, one may use *Stilbamidine, sulfonamides, Glucantime, Sulfones* or possibly *Griseofulvin*.

In disseminated sporotrichosis, especially when there is visceral or brain involvement, *Amphotericin B* is advisable as its action would probably be more rapid.

Prognosis

Sporotrichosis is usually a slowly progressive, minor disease, having no effect on the general health of the patient. Most cases respond readily to the standard therapy of *potassium iodide* and there are no after-effects. Some cases undergo spontaneous cure. A few cases are more resistent to the usual therapy but generally respond to one of several other drugs.

A small percentage of cases have disseminated lesions and the viscera or brain may be involved; these cases are amenable to treatment with *Amphotericin B*. Some are curable surgically, for example pulmonary sporotrichosis. If the disease is diagnosed before extensive damage to the tissues occurs there are no after-effects. There have been only 3 deaths directly attributable to the disease (DE BEURMANN and GOUGEROT, 1912), all having occurred before the discovery of antibiotics.

References

ACEVES ORTEGA, R., AGUIRRE CASTILLO, R., SOSTO PERALTA, F.: Esporotricosis. Análisis de 70 casos estudiados en la Ciudad de Guadalajara. Bol. Derm. Méx. **1**, 5, 15 (1961). — ADAMSON, H.G.: A case of sporotrichosis. Brit. J. Derm. **23**, 239 (1911). — ALBORNOZ, J.E.: Primer caso de sporotricosis equina comprobada en el país. Rev. med. vet. (Bogotá) **14**, 88, 32 (1945). — ALEIXO, A.: Esporotrichose produzida por um esporotricho em forma de lêvedo. Brasil-méd. **35**, part 2, 383 (1921). — ALGODOAL, F.C.: Sobre um caso de esporotricose tratado pela sulfadiazina. Rev. clin. S. Paulo **18**, 1 (1945). — ALVARES, D., PRAZERES, C.: Un caso de sporotrichose humana. Med. contemp. **32**, 24, 187 (1914). — ALVAREZ, R.G., LÓPEZ-VILLEGAS, A.: Primary ocular sporotrichosis. Amer. J. Ophthal. **62**, 1, 150 (1966). — ALVAREZ PUEYO, J., DE ARMAS, V.: Esporotricosis mixta, tipo Schencki-Beurmanni (primera observación registrada en la casuística micológica). An. Inst. Llorente **1**, 25 (1943). — ANDERSON, N.P., SPECTOR, B.K.: Rat-bite fever associated with Sporothrix. J. infect. Dis. **50**, 344 (1932). — ANSEL D'IMEUX: Maladies infectieuses. Encyclopédie Médico-chirurgicale, Paris. Section 8124 A 10. pp. 1—4 (1949). — ARAVYSKY, A.H.: Personal communication (1966). — ARAVYSKY, A.H., ARIYEVICH, A.M.: In: Handbook on Dermato-Venereology, Vol. 2, Chapter 12. Leningrad: State Publishing House of Medical Literature (Medgiz.) 1961. — ARÊA LEÃO, A.E., GOTO, M.: Esporotrichose. Observação e estudo de um novo caso. Hospital (Rio de J.) **30**, 409 (1946). — ARMSTRONG, J.M.: A new case of sporotrichial infection. St. Paul med. J. **14**, 4, 218 (1912). —

Arndt, G.: Vorläufige Mitteilung über einen Fall von Sporotrichose der Haut. Berl. klin. Wschr. **46**, 2, 1966 (1909). — Arthur, G. W., Albrittain, J. W.: Disseminated cutaneous sporotrichosis with systemic involvement. Arch. Derm. **77**, 2, 187 (1958). — Atillj, S.: La Röntgen-terapia in un caso di sporotricosi. Arch. Radiol. (Napoli) **1**, 726 (1925). — Audebaud, G., Escudié, A., Courmes, E.: Les mycoses humaines en Guadeloupe. Premiers cas de chromo-blastomycose et de sporotrichose. Résultats d'une enquête histoplasminique. Bull. Soc. Path. exot. **57**, 5, 1012 (1964). — Aufdermaur, von M., Piller, M., Fischer, E.: Sporotrichose des Hirns. Schweiz. med. Wschr. **84**, 5, 167 (1954). — Azulay, R. D., Miranda, J. L.: Caso de esporotricose generalizada com presenca de cogumelos em corte histológico. An. bras. Derm. Sif. **30**, 3, 222 (1955). — Baker, K. C., Malone, J. T.: Sporotrichosis. Report of a case. Ariz. Med. **9**, 1, 28 (1952). — Baker, R. D.: Chronic progressive sporotrichosis in mice. Fed. Proc. **1**, 1, part 2, 173 (1942). ∼ Experimental sporotrichosis in mice. Amer. J. trop. Med. **27**, 6, 749 (1947a). ∼ Tissue changes in fungus disease. Arch. Path. **44**, 5, 459 (1947b). — Balabanoff, V. A.: Critical survey of medical mycological literature in Bulgaria for the period 1946—1961. Mycopathologia (Den Haag) **20**, 1—2, 157 (1963). — Baliña, P., Marcó del Pont: Dos casos del esporotricosis en Buenos Ayres. Argent. Med. **2**, 23 (1908). — Balzer, Galup: Trois nouveaux cas de sporotrichose en gommes disséminées. Bull. Soc. franç. Derm. Syph. **19**, 145 (1908). — Banks, H. S.: Sporotrichosis resembling diphtheria. Report of an unusual case. Lancet **251, II**, 270 (1946). — Baptista, L., Belliboni, N., Martins Castro, R.: Caso de esporotricose tratado pelo antimoniato de N-metilglucamina. Rev. paul. Med. **41**, 1, 24 (1952). — Barrack, B. B.: Mycotic granulomata in Australia. Med. J. Aust. **44**, 1, 7, 189 (1957). — Barrack, B. B., Powell, R. E.: Sporotrichosis. Med. J. Aust. **39**, 2, 18, 624 (1952). — Bauckus, H. H.: In discussion of case presented by Singer and Muncie. 1952. — Beatty, W.: A case of sporotrichosis. Brit. J. Derm. Syph. **29**, 270 (1917). — Beinhauer, L. G.: Sporotrichosis. Penn. med. J. **39**, 787 (1936). — Belliboni, N., Martins Castro, R., Prado Sampaio, S. de A., De Brito, T.: Esporotrichose. Contribuição ao seu estudo clinico, micológico immunológico e histopatológico. Brasil-méd. **4**, 441 (1961). — Belliboni, N., Patricio, L. D.: Tratamento da esporotricose pelo glucantime; considerações a respeito de 2 cases. Rev. Hosp. Clin. Fac. Med. S. Paulo **11**, 118 (1956). — Benham, R. W., Kesten, B.: Sporotrichosis. Its transmission to plants and animals. J. infect. Dis. **50**, 437 (1932). — Berge, T., Kaplan, W.: Systemic candidiasis with asteroid body formation. Sabouraudia **5**, 4, 310 (1967). — Bertin, Bruyant, L.: Sporotrichose gommeuse du bras par inoculation accidentelle de laboratoire. Presse méd. **18**, 355 (1910). — Bessiere, L.: Sporotrichose: 1 cas. Bull. Soc. franç. Mycol. Med. **5**, 13 (1963). — Bèzes, H.: Mycoses osseuses. Encyclopédie Médico-chirurgicale. Paris. Section Os-articulations. 14020 A 10, pp. 1—8 (1949). — Blair, J., Yarian, N. C.: Two cases of sporotrichosis infection due to a barberry. J. Amer. med. Ass. **91**, 2, 96 (1928). — Bloch, B.: Fall von ausgedehnter Sporotrichose. Gesellschaft, Basel, 6. Mai. Quoted by Gougerot 1912. ∼ Die Sporotrichose. Beiheft zu Med. Klin. Berlin **5**, 179 (1909). — Boeck, C.: (Two cases of sporotrichosis.) Forh. med. Selsk. Krist., pp. 150—152 (1914). Quoted by Norden 1951. — Boggs, T. R., Fried, H.: Sporothrix infection of the large intestine and finger nails. Bull. Johns Hopk. Hosp. **37**, 164 (1925). — Bolaños, E. L., Trejos, W. A.: Múltiples coincidencias en dos casos de esporotricosis facial. Rev. méd. C. Rica **5**, 105, 369 (1943). — Bonnet, L. M.: Orchite sporotrichosique. Lyon Méd. **112**, 1113 (1909). — Bordes, C., Berhouet, A., Errecart, L. M.: Cuatro casos de esporotricosis. Bol. Soc. méd-quir. Cent. Repúb. **7**, 17 (1934). — Borelli, D.: Esporotricosis. Tres casos con cuerpos asteroides. Bol. Venez. Lab. Clin. **3**, 51 (1958). Quoted by Moraes and Miranda. — Braitman, M.: Sporotrichosis treated with Griseofulvin and iodides. J. med. Soc. N. J. **61**, 6, 228 (1964). — Brandt, H. P., Bader, G.: Zur Klinik und pathologischen Anatomie der Augensporotrichose. Ber. dtsch. ophthal. Ges. **64**, 491 (1961). — Braude, A. I., McConnell, J., Douglas, H.: Fever from pathogenic fungi. J. clin. Invest. **39**, part 2, 1266 (1960). — Brayton, A. W.: On refractory subcutaneous abscesses caused by a fungus possibly related to the sporotricha. Indiana med. J. **18**, 272 (1899). — Bremener, M. M.: Sluchaĭ sporotrikhoza. (A case of sporotrichosis.) Med. Obozren. Moscow **79**, 3, 238 (1913). — Bridré, J., Nègre, L., Trouette, G.: Recherches sur la lymphangite epizootique en algérie. Ann. Inst. Pasteur **26**, 701 (1912). — Brissaud, Et., Joltrain, E., Weill, A.: Eosinophilie sanguine et locale dans les sporotrichoses humaines et expérimentales. C.R. Soc. Biol. (Paris) **66**, 305 (1909). — Brissaud, Rathery, F.: Un cas de sporotrichose intramusculaire. C.R. Cong. Franç. Med. Paris 315 (1908). — Brodier, L., Fage: Sporotrichose nodulaire disséminée à forme febrile; sporo-agglutination positive. Bull. Soc. Méd. Hôp. Paris 3 s **26**, 2 (1908). — Brodskyi, L. M., Mitzenmacher, M. A.: (A case of vegetating sporotrichosis.) Nov. khir. Arkh. **48**, 4, 341 (1941). Quoted by Aravysky. — Brooks, R. H.: Personal communication to D' Alessio et al. (1965). — Brown, R., Weintraub, D., Simpson, M. W.: Timber as a source of sporotrichosis infection. Sporotrichosis infection on mines of the Witwatersrand, pp. 5—28. Johannesburg: The Transvaal Chamber of Mines 1947. — Bürgel, E., Meessen, H.: Zur Diagnose und Therapie der Knochensporotrichose. Fortschr. Röntgenstr. **71**, 5, 832 (1949). — Burgess, J. F.: Sporotrichosis in man. Report of a case. Arch. Derm. Syph. (Chic.) **12**, 5, 642 (1925). — Burkholder,

P.R., MOYER, D.: Vitamin deficiencies of fifty yeasts and molds. Bull. Torrey Botan. Club 70, 4, 372 (1943). — CALERO, C.M., TAPIA, A.: Two cases of sporotrichosis in the Isthmus of Panama. Amer. J. trop. Med. Hyg. 11, 5. 676 (1962). — CALIFANO, A.: Relievi e considerazioni su otto casi di sporotricosi cutanea. G. ital. Derm. 106, 551 (1965). — CAMPANA, R.: La sporotricosi come malattia della pelle e nella patologia. Clin. Dermosif. Univ. di Roma 28, 3 (1910). ~ Ancora della sporotricosi. Clin. Dermosif. Univ. di Roma 28, 75 (1910). — CAMPANELLA, P.: Su di un caso di sporotricosi. Rif. med. 63, 29, 692 (1949). — CAMPBELL, C.H.: A case of sporotrichosis occurring in Papua. Med. J. Aust. 2, 1, 23 (1965). — CAMPBELL, H.S., FROST, K., PLUNKETT, O.A.: Sporotrichotic chancre. Arch. Derm. Syph. (Chic.) 28, 1, 61 (1933). — CANDIOTA DE CAMPOS, E.: Sôbre as lesões iniciais da esporotricose. Rev. med. Rio Grande do Sul 15, 85, 29 (1959). — CĂPUŞAN, I., SÍRBU, I., RADU, H., ROSENBERG, A.: Sporotricozǎ limfatica gomoasǎ, Derm.-vener. Halad. 6, 3, 219 (1961). — CAROUGEAU, F.: Sur une nouvelle mycose sous-cutanée des équidés. J. med. vet. Zootech. 60, 8, 75, 148 (1909a). ~ Premier cas africain de sporotrichose de DE BEURMANN; transmission de la sporotrichose du mulet à l'homme. Bull.Soc. Méd. Hop. Paris 3 s 28, 507 (1909b). — CARR, R.D., STORKAN, M.A., WILSON, J.W., SWATEK, F.E.: Extensive verrucous sporotrichosis of long duration. Report of a case resembling cutaneous blastomycosis. Arch. Derm. 89, 1, 184 (1964). — CARTER, R.M.: Sporotrichosis. Report of two cases. J. Amer. med. Ass. 86, 23, 1751 (1926). — CASTLETON, K.B., REES, V.L.: Sporotrichosis. Report of two cases from Utah. J. Amer. med. Ass. 148, 7, 541 (1952). — CASTRO: see MARTINS DE CASTRO. — CATANEI, A.: Recherches parasitologiques et expérimentales sur la sporotrichose, les blastomycoses et l'actinomycose, en Algérie. Arch. Inst. Pasteur Algér. 12, 351 (1934). — CIPOLLARO, A.C.: Presented for J.L. SINGER. Sporotrichosis, lymphangiectatic type. Arch. Derm. Syph. (Chic.) 68, 5, 598 (1953). — COLE, D.P., LOBITZ, W.C., JR.: Sporotrichosis in New Hampshire. New Engl. J. Med. 243, 4, 132 (1950). — COLLES, P.: Sporotrichose gommeuse disséminée chez un jeune chien. Bull. Soc. Sc. Vet. Lyon 37, 72 (1934). — COLLINS, W.T.: Disseminated ulcerating sporotrichosis with widespread visceral involvement. Report of a case. Arch. Derm. Syph. (Chic.) 56, 4, 523 (1947). — CONTI-DÍAZ, I.A.: Estudio micológico de 85 casos de onicopatías. An. Fac. Med. Montevideo 49, 5—6, 535 (1964). — COOKE, W.B., FOTER, M.J.: Fungi in used bedding materials. Appl. Microbiol. 6, 3, 169 (1958). — COOPER, J.L., MIKHAIL, G.R.: Trichophyton rubrum. Perifolliculitis on amputation stump. Arch. Derm. 94, 1, 56 (1966). — CORTELLA, E.: Un caso di sporotricosi. G. med. Alto Adige 9, 645 (1937). — COSTA, O.G.: Esporotricose no Brasil. Brasil-méd. 57, 34, 343 (1943). — COSTA, O., JUNQUEIRA, M.A.: Papular sporotrichosis. Arch. Derm. Syph. (Chic.) 51, 4, 261 (1945). — COSTA, S.: Chancre syphiloïde de la muqueuse nasale, lymphangite et adénites provoques par Sp. Beurmanni. C.R. Soc. Biol. (Paris) 71, 2, 35 (1911). — CREGOR, F.W.: Sporotrichosis. J. Amer. med. Ass. 79, 812 (1922). — CREVASSE, L., ELLNER, P.D.: An outbreak of sporotrichosis in Florida. J. Amer. med. Ass. 173, 1, 29 (1960). — CRUTCHFIELD, E.D.: Sporotrichosis. Arch. Derm. Syph. (Chic.) 7, 2, 226 (1923). — CRUTHIRDS, T.P., PATTERSON, D.O.: Primary pulmonary sporotrichosis. Amer. Rev. resp. Dis. 95, 5, 845 (1967). — CUMMINGS, M.M., HUDGINS, P.C.: Chemical constituents of pine pollen and their possible relationship to sarcoidosis. Amer. J. med. Sci. 236, 311 (1958). — CURCIO, A.: Sporotricosi setticemica a forma anemizzante con decorso febbrile. Policlinico, Sez. chir. 18, 203 (1911). — DABROWA, N., LANDAU, J.W., NEWCOMER, V.D., PLUNKETT, O.A.: A survey of tide-washed coastal areas of Southern California for fungi potentially pathogenic to man. Mycopathologia (Den Haag) 24, 2, 137 (1964). — D'ALESSIO, D.J., LEAVENS, L.J., STRUMPF, G.B., SMITH, C.D.: An outbreak of sporotrichosis in Vermont associated with sphagnum moss as the source of infection. New Engl. J. Med. 272, 20, 1054 (1965). — DANGERFIELD, L.F., GEAR, J.: Sporotrichosis among miners on the Witwatersrand gold mines. S. Afr. med. J. 15, 128 (1941). — DANLOS, FLANDIN, CH.: Sporotrichose cutanee simulant l'epithelioma ou la tuberculose papillomateuse; sporotrichose de la portion cartilagineuse de la cloison des fosses nasales. Bull. Soc. franç. Derm. Syph. 20, 251 (1909). — DAS GUPTA, S.N., SHOME, S.K., MAJUMDAR, S.S.: Medical mycology in India. Mycopathologia (Den Haag) 13, 4, 339 (1960). — DA SILVA, M.F.N.: see NAVARRO DA SILVA. — DAVIS, B.F.: Report of a case of sporotrichosis. J. Surg. Gynec. Obstet. 19, 490 (1914). — DAVIS, D.J.: The morphology of Sporothrix Schenckii in tissues and in artificial media. J. infect. Dis. 12, 453 (1913). ~ The formation of chlamydospores in Sporothrix Schenckii. J. infect. Dis. 15, 482 (1914). ~ The permeability of the gastro-intestinal wall to infection with Sporothrix. J. infect. Dis. 19, 688 (1916). — DAVIS, H.H., WORTHINGTON, W.E.: Equine sporotrichosis. J. Amer. vet. med. Ass. 145, 7, 692 (1964). — DE AGUIAR PUPO, J.: Frequencia da sporotrichose em S. Paulo. Ann. paul. Med. Cirurg. 8, 53 (1917). ~ Sporotrichoses no Brasil. Ann. paul. Med. Cirurg. 11, 200 (1920). — DE ALMEIDA, F., SAMPAIO, S.A.P., DA SILVA LACAZ, C., DE CASTRO FERNANDES, J.: Dados estatisticos sôbre a esporotricose: analise de 344 casos. An. bras. Derm. Sif. 30, 1, 9 (1955). — DEAN, K.F., HALEY, L.D.: A search for pathogenic fungi in Connecticut soils. Publ. Hlth Rep. (Wash.) 77, 1, 61 (1962). — DE BEURMANN, L.: On sporotrichosis. Brit. med. J. 2, 289 (1912). — DE BEURMANN, BRODIER, GASTAU: Sporotrichose gommeuse disséminée avec lçsions laryngées. Bull. Soc. Méd. Hôp. Paris 3 s 24, 1060 (1907). — DE BEURMANN,

L., Gougerot, H.: Les sporotrichoses hypodermiques. Ann. Derm. Syph. (Paris) 4 s 7, 837, 914, 993 (1906). ~ Sporotrichoses des muqueuses (sporotrichosides muqueuses ulcéreuses et saprophytisme du Sporotrichum Beurmanni sur les muqueuses). Bull. Soc. Méd. Hôp. Paris 3 s 24, 585 (1907a). ~ Treiziéme cas de sporotrichose. Sporotrichose localisée du bras. Lymphangite gommeuse ascendante. Bul. Soc. Méd. Hôp. Paris 3 s 24, 950 (1907b). ~ Associations morbides dans les sporotrichoses. IIe. Observation de sporotrichose: syphilis, tuberculose et sporotrichose. ii. Gomme de la cuisse droite. Bull. Soc. Méd. Hôp. Paris 3 s 24, 591 (1907c). ~ Sporotrichoses tuberculoïdes. Ann. Derm. Syph. (Paris) 4 s 8, 497, 603, 655 (1907d). ~ Saprophytisme du "Sporotrichum Beurmanni" dans le buccopharynx et dans le larynx. Bull. Soc. Méd. Hôp. Paris 3 s 24, 1069 (1907e). ~ Étiologie et pathogénie de la sporotrichose. Trib. Med. Paris 40, ns 44, 693 (1907f). ~ Diagnostic rétrospectif de la sporotrichose par la culture du Sporotrichum resté saprophyte dans le bucco-pharynx. Bull. Soc. Méd. Hôp. Paris 3 s 26, 77 (1908a). ~ Découverte du Sporotrichum Beurmanni dans la nature. Bull. Soc. Méd. Hôp. Paris 3 s 26, 733 (1908b). ~ Comparaison des sporotrichoses et des infections cocciennes. Sporotrichoses aiguës et subaiguës disséminées; Sporotrichomes à évolution phlegmasique. Ann. Derm. Syph. (Paris) 4 s 10, 81 (1909a). ~ Sporotrichose cachectisante mortelle. Bull. Soc. Méd. Hôp. Paris 3 s 27, 1046 (1909b). ~ Intra-dermoréaction sporotrichosique. Bull. Soc. Méd. Hôp. Paris 3 s 28, 141 (1909c). ~ L'état de "sensibilisation" des sporotrichosiques. Bull. Soc. Méd. Hôp. Paris 3 s 28, 397 (1909d). ~ Les Mycoses. Nouveau Traité de Médicine et de Thérapeutique. Edited by A. Gilbert and L. Troinot. Paris: J. B. Bailliere et Fils 1910. ~ Les Sporotrichum pathogènes. Classification botanique. Arch. Parasit. Paris 15, 5 (1911a). ~ État actuel de la question des Sporotrichoses. Les progrès accomplis: Les discussions botaniques. Intérêt pratique, pronostique, thérapeutique et économique. Intérêt doctrina des Sporotrichoses. Arch. Derm. Syph. (Leipzig) 110, 25 (1911b). ~ Les Sporotrichoses. Paris: Felix Alcan Edit. 1912. — de Beurmann, L., Gougeroth, H., Laroche: Sporotrichose faciale dermique et ganglionnaire. Gommules dermiques acnéiformes, lymphangite noueuse, adénites pré-auriculaire et angulo-maxillaire sporotrichosiques. Bull. Soc. Méd. Hôp. Paris 3 s 27, 782 (1909). — de Beurmann, L., Gougerot, H., Vaucher: Gomme sporotrichosique du chat. Bull. Soc. Méd. Hôp. Paris 3 s 24, 1071 (1907). ~ La sporotrichose du rat. Bull. Soc. Méd. Hôp. Paris 3 s 25, 718 (1908a). ~ La sporotrichose expérimentale du rat. Étude histologique de quelques localizations (1). Bull. Soc. Méd. Hôp. Paris 3 s 25, 800 (1908b). ~ Orchite sporotrichosique du rat. (Épreuve diagnostique). (2) Bull. Soc. Méd. Hôp. Paris 3 s 25, 837 (1908c). ~ Sporotrichose expérimentale généralisée du chien. Bull. Soc. Méd. Hôp. Paris 3 s 26, 9 (1908d). ~ Sporotrichose expérimentale du lapin. Caverne pulmonaire. Gomme rénale. Sporotrichome hypertrophique du caecum. Sporotrichose verruqueuse cutanée. Bull. Soc. Méd. Hôp. Paris 3 s 26, 61 (1908e). ~ Épididymite, orchite et vaginalite sporotrichosiques. Contribution à l'étude de sporotrichoses internes. Ann. Derm. Syph. (Paris) 4 s 9, 465 (1908f). ~ Hérédo-sporotrichose expérimentale. Bull. Soc. Méd. Hôp. Paris 3 s 26, 876 (1908g). ~ Sporotrichose expérimentale du chat. C.R. Soc. Biol. (Paris) 66, 338 (1909a). ~ Sporotrichoses cutanées du chat. C.R. Soc. Biol. (Paris) 66, 370 (1909b). ~ Sporotrichoses expérimentales; Sporotrichoses torpides chroniques; Sporotrichoses curables. C.R. Soc. Biol. (Paris) 66, 597 (1909c). ~ Sporotrichose osseuse et ostéo-articulaire. Rev. Chir. (Paris) 39, 661 (1909d). ~ Sporotrichose d'origine alimentaire. Porte d'entrée bucco-pharyngienne et gastro-intestinale du Sporotrichum Beurmanni. Bull. Soc. Méd. Hôp. Paris 3 s 27, 909 (1909e). — de Beurmann, L., Gougeroth, H., Verne: Ostéomyélite gommeuse sporotrichosique primitive. Abcès intra-osseux du tibia. Bull. Soc. Méd. Hôp. Paris 3 s 27, 1123 (1909). — de Beurmann, L., Ramond, L.: Abcès sous-cutanés multiples d'origine mycosique. Ann. Derm. Syph. (Paris) 4 s 4, 678 (1903). — de Beurmann, L., Ramond, L., Gougerot, H., Vaucher: Diagnostic rétrospectif de la sporo-agglutination. Bull. Soc. Méd. Hôp. Paris 3 s 26, 75 (1908). — de Beurmann, L., Saint-Girons, F.: Sporotrichose dermique ulcereuse localisée inoculée par une écharde d'epine-vinette. Bull. Soc. Méd. Hôp. Paris 3 s 28, 174 (1909). — de Blasio, R.: Transmissione dell'infezione sporotricosica alla cavia adulta. Rinasc. med. 12, 471 (1935). — Degos, R.: Personal communication (1967). — de Gregoriis, A.: Primeros casos de esporotrichosis observados in el norte de la República. An. Dep. Nac. Hig. B. Aires 26, 103 (1920). — del Guasta, F.: Sporotricosi cutanea a gomme ipodermiche (prima observazione in Provincia di Arrezzo). Arch. ital. Derm. 16, 193 (1940). — de Magalhaes, O.: Ensaios de micologia. Contribuičao ao conbecimento dos cogumelos patogênicos em Minas Gerais. Mem. Inst. Osw. Cruz 42, 1, 41 (1945). — de Marco, F.: Esporotricose e Penicilina. Arch. Biol. (S. Paulo) 29, 266, 55 (1945). — de Massary, Doury, Monier-Vinard: Gomme sporotrichosique du triceps brachial; ostéite astragaliene et ramollissement du sommet d'un poumon de nature indéterminée. Bull. Soc. Méd. Hôp. Paris 3 s 24, 1526 (1907). — de Montemayor, L.: Síntesis estadística y algunas conclusiones sobre 206 exámenes micológicos. Rev. med. vet. Parasit. 9, 1—4, 85 (1950). — de Montemayor, L., Heredia de Gamero, B.: Análisis de 6000 espécimenes micológicos Síntesis estadística — Comentarios. Mycopathologia (Den Haag) 18, 1—2, 1 (1962). — de Oyarzabal, E.: Sporotricosis gomose enfermedad de gran obuso. Act. Dermo-Syphilog. Madrid, Feb., March.

Quoted by DE BEURMANN and GOUGEROT 1912. — DE REZENDE, C.: Contribuição para o estudo da sporotrichose no Brasil. Brasil-méd. **32**, 33 (1918). — DESPOTOV, B., SHICK, G.: Treti sluchoĭ ot sporotrikhoza v stranata. (The third case of sporotrichosis in Bulgaria.) Derm.-Vener. (Sophia) **4**, 2, 130 (1965). — DEY, N.C.: Epidemiology and incidence of fungus diseases in India. Indian J. Derm. **8**, 1, 21 (1962). — DEY, N.C., SAIKIA, T., MAJUMDAR, C.T.: Sporotrichosis in Assam (India). Indian J. Derm. **3**, 3, 103 (1958). — DO AMARAL, Z.: Panaricio esporotrichosico. Rev. paul. Med. **8**, 372 (1936). — DOCKX, L.: Un cas de sporotrichose. Arch. belges Derm. **2**, 159 (1946). — DOHI, K., HASHIMOTO, T., TERAO, H.: (A case of sporotrichosis.) Jap. J. Derm. **20**, 741 (1920). — DOMINGUEZ, F.: A case of sporotrichosis with multiple localizations; importance of X-ray examination to determine the foci. Med. Rec. (N.Y.) **85**, 608 (1914). — DOMINICI, H., RUBENS DUVAL, H.: Sporotrichose de l'index; lymphangite sporotrichosique consécutive. Bull. Soc. Méd. Hôp. Paris 3 s **24**, 1055 (1907). — DROUHET, E., MARIAT, F.: La pyrimidine facteur de croissance pour les Sporotrichum. Ann. Inst. Pasteur **79**, 3, 306 (1950). — DU BOIS, C.: Sporotrichose généralisée à gommes disséminées multiples et non ouvertes. Rev. méd. Suisse rom. **32**, 757 (1912). — DUNN, Y.O.: Personal communication (1966). — DUQUE, M.: Surgical treatment of cutaneous sporotrichosis. Amer. J. Derm. **12**, 240 (1908). — DURIE, E.B., FREY, D., BECKE, R.F.A.: Sporotrichosis. Report of a case from Sydney, Australia. Aust. J. Derm. **6**, 1, 71 (1961). — DU TOIT, C.J.: Sporotrichosis on the Witwatersrand. Proc. Mine med. Offrs' Ass. **22**, 111 (1942). — *Editorial:* Sporotrichosis. Brit. med. J. **1969**, 779. — EISENSTAEDT, J.S.: Sporotrichosis resembling tuberculosis cutis. Report of a case. J. Amer. med. Ass. **71**, 726 (1918). — EL-MOFTY, A.M., NADA, M.: Sporotrichosis in Egypt. Brit. J. Derm. **77**, 7, 357 (1965). — EMMONS, C.W.: The isolation from soil of fungi which cause disease in man. Trans. N.Y. Acad. Sci. **14**, 1, 51 (1951). ~ The significance of saprophytism in the epidemiology of the mycoses. Trans. N.Y. Acad. Sci. **17**, 2, 157 (1954). — ERRECART, L.M.: Sobre veinticinco casos de esporotricosis en el Departamento de Flores. Arch. urug. Med. **28**, 3, 249 (1946). — ESCOMEL, E.: A propos de deux cas de sporotrichose pharyngée observés à Aréquipa (Perou). Arch. int. Laryng. **29**, 12 (1923). ~ Acerca de dos casos de esporotrichosis faringea en Aréquipa, Perú. Bol. Inst. Clin. quir. (B. Aires) **4**, 520 (1928). — EVERETT, M.A.: Atypical sporotrichosis. J. Okla. med. Ass. **56**, 10, 483 (1963). — FAGE, A.: Gomme sporotrichosique périostée avec périostose du tibia. Bull. Soc. Méd. Hôp. Paris 3 s **25**, 879 (1908). — FARHA, S.J., FORD, C.R.: An unusual sporotrichosis infection. Amer. Surg. **30**, 5, 335 (1964). — FAVA, A.: Un cas de sporotrichose conjunctivale et palpébrale primitives. Ann. Oculist. (Paris) **141**, 338 (1909). — FELLMAN, H.: Über einen Fall von Sporotrichose des Gehirns. Helv. med. Acta **20**, 4—5, 370 (1953). — FETTER, B.F.: Human cutaneous sporotrichosis due to Sporotrichum Schenckii; technique for demonstration of organisms in tissues. Arch. Path. **71**, 4, 416 (1961). — FETTER, B.F., TINDALL, J.P.: Cutaneous sporotrichosis. Clinical study of nine cases utilizing an improved technique for demonstration of organisms. Arch. Path. **78**, 6, 613 (1964). — FIELITZ, H.: Ueber eine Laboratoriumsinfektion mit dem Sporotrichum de Beurmanni. Zbl. Bakt., I. Abt. Orig. **55**, 361 (1910). — FINLAYSON, G.R., MIRANDA, J.L., MAILMAN, C.J., CALLAWAY, J.L.: Sporotrichosis treated with Amphotericin B. Nephrocalcinosis as a therapeutic complication. Arch. Derm. **89**, 5, 730 (1964). — FISCHER, J.B., MARKKANEN, M.V.: Sporotrichosis. Canad. med. Ass. J. **65**, 1, 49 (1951). — FLO, S.C., SMITH, P.E.: Sporotrichosis. Report of a case. New Engl. J. Med. **234**, 2, 50 (1946). — FOERSTER, H.R.: Sporotrichosis. Amer. J. med. Sci. **167**, 54 (1924). ~ Sporotrichosis. An occupational dermatosis. J. Amer. med. Ass. **87**, 20, 1605 (1926). — FONTOYNONT, M.: Sur quelques lésions mycosiques observées à Madagascar. Bull. Soc. Chirurgie Paris **48**, 439 (1922). — FONTOYNONT, M., CAROUGEAU, F.: Abcès sous-dermiques et gommes ulcérées produits par le Sporotrichum Carougeaui Langeron 1913, associé à la tuberculose chez un enfant Malgache. Bull. Soc. Path. exot. **15**, 444 (1922). — FORBUS, W.D.: Pulmonary sporotrichosis. Amer. Rev. Tuberc. **16**, 2, 599 (1927). — FORNERO, A.: L'anatomia patologica della sporotricosi geniale e la sporotricosi localizzata e generalizzata nei suoi rapporti col concepimento e colla transmissione materno e paterno fetale. Folia gynaec. (Pavia) **11**, 383 (1916). — FOULERTON, A.G.R.: On the morphology and pathogenic action of Sporothrix Schenckii. Trans. path. Soc. Lond. **52**, 259 (1901). — FRANÇOIS, J., DE VOS, E., HANSSENS, M., ELEWAUT-RIJSSELAERE, M.: Mycoses intra-oculaires. Ann. Oculist. (Paris) **195**, 97 (1962). — FUKUSHIRO, R., KAGAWA, S.: (Observations of eight cases of sporotrichosis.) Jap. J. Derm. **64**, 342 (1954). — FUKUSHIRO, VON R., KAGAWA, S., NISHIYAMA, S., TAKAHASHI, H., ISHIKAWA, H.: Die Pilzelemente im Gewebe der Hautsporotrichose des Menschen. Hautarzt **16**, 18 (1965). — GALIANA, J., CONTI-DÍAZ, I.A.: Healing effects of heat and a rubefaciant on nine cases of sporotrichosis. Sabouraudia **3**, 1, 64 (1963). — GARRETT, H.D., ROBBINS, J.B.: An unusual occurrence of sporotrichosis. Eight cases in one residence. Arch. Derm. **82**, 4, 570 (1960). — GASTINEAU, F.M., SPOLYAR, L.W., HAYNES, E.: Sporotrichosis. Report of six cases among florists. J. Amer. med. Ass. **117**, 13, 1074 (1941). — GAUCHER, LOUSTE, ABRAMI, GIROUX: Sporotrichose cutanée (gommeuse disséminée). Bull. Soc. franç. Derm. Syph. **19**, 283 (1908). — GAVIÑA ALVARADO, E.R., NEGRI, T., MOSTO, D.: Esporotricosis de pierna. Pren. méd. Argent. **25**, 1685 (1938). — GELBER, A.: Sporotrichosis. Report of a case and its occurrence in California. Arch. Derm. Syph. (Chic.) 54, 2, 208 (1946). — Geraci, J. E., Dry, T. J., Ulrich, J. A., Weed, L. A., MacCarty, C. S., Sayre, G. P.: Experiences with 2-Hydroxystilbamidine in systemic sporotrichosis. Report of a case. Arch. intern. Med. 96, 4, 478 (1955). — Ghose, L. M.: An unusual case of sporotrichosis. Indian med. Gaz. 67, 570 (1932). — Giroux, J. M., Perry, H. O.: Sporotrichosis. An important fungous disease in Minnesota. Minn. Med. 47, 2, 136 (1964). — Gluckman, I.: Sporotrichosis in children. S. Afr. med. J. 39, 991 (1965). — Goldberg, M., Pijper, A.: Sporotrichosis in a white man. J. med. Ass. S. Afr. 5, 140 (1931). — Gómez-Orozco, L., Ortega, H. G.: Esporotricosis facial en el niño. Reporte de cuatro casos. Bol. méd. Hosp. infant. (Méx.) 22, 331 (1965). — Gonçalves: see Padilha Gonçalves. — González Benavides, J.: La esporotricosis como enfermedad ocupacional en los trabajadores de alfarerias. Bol. Soc. cuba. Derm. Sif. 13, 3, 89 (1956). ~ Sporotrichose als Berufskrankheit in Töpfereibetrieben. Berufsdermatosen 7, 1, 22 (1959). — González Ochoa, A.: Sporotrichosis. Handbook of Tropical Dermatology and Medical Mycology. Vol. 2, p. 1332. Edited by Simons. Amsterdam: Elsevier Publishing Co. 1953. ~ Dos casos de esporotricosis curados con Griseofulvin. Rev. Inst. Salubr. Enferm. trop. (Méx.) 19, 2, 245 (1959). ~ El uso de anticuerpos fluorescentes en el estudio de algunas enfermedades infecciosas. ii. Diagnóstico rapido de la esporotricosis. Gac. méd. Méx. 94, 309 (1964). ~ Contribuciones recientes al conocimiento de la esporotricosis. Gac. méd. Méx. 95, 5, 463 (1965). — González Ochoa, A., González Mendoza, A.: La micología médica en México. Revisión de la bibliografía aparecida durante el período de 1946 a 1958. Mycopathologia (Den Haag) 13, 1, 48 (1960). — González Ochoa, A., Soto Figueroa, E.: Polisacáridos del Sporotrichum Schenckii. Datos immunológicos; Intradermo-reactión en el diagnóstico de la esporotricosis. Rev. Inst. Salubr. Enferm. trop. (Méx.) 8, 2, 143 (1947). — González Ochoa, A., Soto Pacheco, R.: Desarollo del Esporotrichum schencki en el pus obtenido de gomas esporotricósicas. Algunos datos sobre su ciclo evolutivo. Rev. Inst. Salubr. Enferm. trop. (Méx.) 11, 1, 3 (1950). — Gonzalo Calle, V., Angela Restrepo, M.: La esporotricosis. Antioquia Méd. 11, 444 (1961). — Gordon, D. M.: Ocular sporotrichosis. Report of a case. Arch. Ophthal. 37, 1, 56 (1947). — Gougerot, H.: Formes cliniques de la sporotrichose de de Beurmann. Gaz. Hôp. (Paris) 82, 537 (1909). ~ Les polymycoses: les cosensibilisations mycosiques (1). Progr. méd. (Paris) 47, 569 (1911). ~ Die Sporotrichosen. Die pathogenen Sporotrichen und die Sporotrichosen. In: Handbuch der pathogenen Mikroorganismen, pp. 211—266. Edited by W. Kolle and A. von Wassermann. Jena: Gustav Fischer 1912. ~ Importance prognostique et thérapeutique du diagnostic de sporotrichose. A propos d'un malade atteint d'ostéomyélite sporotrichosique primitive du tibia qui faillit être amputé et subit pendant deux ans sans succès le traitement mercuriel. Mouv. Med. Paris 1, 205 (1913). — Gougerot, H., Blanchetière, A.: Endotoxines, sporotrichosiques. 1. Action pathogène des corps microbiens tués et des corps résiduels. 11. Sporoéthérines, sporo-chloroformines. C.R. Soc. Biol. (Paris) (1) 67, 247, (11) 67, 352 (1909). — Gougerot, H., Blum, P.: Sporotrichose des ganglions parotidiens et sous-maxillaires simulant la tuberculose. Orthop. Tuberc. Chir. (Paris) 1, 415 (1914). — Gougerot, H., Caraven: Sporotrichose spontanée du chien. Gommes hypodermiques, péritonite granuleuse et gommes hépatiques. Presse méd. 16, 337 (1908). — Gougerot, H., Lévi-Frankel, G.: Synovite sporotrichosique. Rev. Chir. (Paris) 46, 11, 687 (1912). — Graham, P. V.: Solitary gummatous sporotrichosis of two years duration. Report of a case. Arch. Derm. Syph. (Chic.) 43, 5, 805 (1941). — Gray, A. M., Bamber, G. W.: Sporotrichosis. Proc. roy. Soc. Med. 25, 668 (1932). — Greco, N. V.: Sporotricosis linfangítica nodular vegetante, estudio experimental. Argent. med. 45, 699 (1907). ~ Biología del Sporotrichum Schenckii-Beurmanni. Etiología y patogenia de la esporotricosis. Rev. Dermat. Argent. 1, 78 (1908). — Greenburg, W.: Sporotrichosis. Report of a case in California. Arch. Derm. Syph. (Chic.) 36, 355 (1937). — Greig, D. M.: A case of sporotrichosis. Edinb. med. J. 18, 42 (1917). — Grütz, O.: Sporotrichosen und verwandte Krankheiten. In: J. Jadassohn, Handbuch der Haut- und Geschlechtskrankheiten, Vol. 11, pp. 751 and 753. Berlin: Springer 1928. — Guilaine, J.: Gommes sous-cutanées. Encyclopédie Médicochirurgicale. Section Dermatologie 12560 A 10., pp. 1—8 (1949). — Guilhon, J., Obry, J.: Sporotrichose cutaneo-muqueuse du chien. Bull. Acad. vét. Fr. 26, 6, 301 (1953). — Hamburger, W. W.: Sporotrichosis in man with a summary of the cases reported in the United States and a consideration of the clinical varieties and the important factors in the differential diagnosis. J. Amer. med. Ass. 59, 18, 1590 (1912). — Hanrahan, J. B., Erickson, E. R.: Sporotrichosis in Western Pennsylvania. Report of two cases. J. Amer. med. Ass. 197, 10, 814 (1966). — Harant, Nguyen-Duc, Huttel: Remarques sur la maladie des Cannes de Provence. Bull. Soc. Path. exot. 37, 7—8, 310 (1944). — Hardy, H. L.: Differential diagnosis between beryllium poisoning and sarcoidosis. Amer. Rev. Tuberc. 74, 885 (1956). — Harrell, E. R., Bocobo, F. C., Curtis, A. C.: Sporotrichosis successfully treated with Stilbamidine. Arch. intern. Med. 93, 1, 162 (1954). — Harris, T. R., Blumenfield, H. B., Cruthirds, T. P., McCall. C. B.: Coexisting sarcoidosis and cryptococcosis. Arch. intern. Med. 115, 6, 637 (1965). — Harsh. G. F., Allen, S. E.: A study of the fungus contaminants of the air of San Diego and vicinity. J. Allergy 16, 3, 125 (1945). — Harter, A., Gruyer: Formes actinomycosiques dans la sporotrichose expérimentale. C.R. Soc. Biol. (Paris) **66**, 399 (1909). — *Harvard African Expedition* (1926—1927): The African Republic of Liberia and the Belgian Congo. Vol. 1, chapter 23. Contributions from the Department of Tropical Medicine and Institute for Tropical Biology and Medicine. No. 5. Cambridge: Harvard University Press 1930. — HASENCLEVER, H. F., MITCHELL, W.: Attempts to immunize mice against sporotrichosis. J. invest. Derm. **33**, 3, 145 (1959). — HAWKS, G. H.: Sporotrichosis. Report of three cases from Toronto. Canad. med. Ass. J. **72**, 1, 28 (1955). — HAYES, W. N.: Sporotrichosis in employees of a tree nursery. GP (Kansas) **22**, 4, 114 (1960). — HECHT, H.: Ein Fall von Sporotrichosis. Arch. Derm. Syph. (Leipzig) **116**, 846 (1913). — HEKTOEN, L., PERKINS, C. F.: Refractory subcutaneous abscesses caused by Sporothrix Schenckii. A new pathogenic fungus. J. exp. Med. **5**, 77 (1900). — HELM, M.A.F., BERMAN, C.: The clinical, therapeutic and epidemiological features of the sporotrichosis infection on the mines. Sporotrichosis Infection on Mines of the Witwatersrand, pp. 59—67. Johannesburg: The Transvaal Chamber of Mines 1947. — HELVE, O., PÄTIÄTÄ, R., SAXÉN, E.: Sporothrichosis associated with vesicular lesions resembling periarteritis nodosa. Acta path. microbiol. scand. **28**, 1, 44 (1951). — HENRY: Un cas de sporotrichose en Guyane. Rev. méd. Hyg. Trop. (Paris) **8**, 37 (1911). — HIATT, J.S., JR., LIDE, T.N.: Blastomycosis complicating Boeck's sarcoid. Report of a case. N. Carolina med. J. **10**, 12, 650 (1949). — HIGUCHI, K., MINAMI, K., TOTOGAWA, Y., YOSHIZUMI, M., KODA, H.: (Application of fluorescent antibody technique for the identification of Sporotrichum schenckii.) Derm.-Urol. Fukuoka **27**, 5, 601 (1965). — HINSON, K.F.W., MOON, A.J., PLUMMER, N.S.: Broncho-pulmonary aspergillosis. Thorax **7**, 317 (1952). — HODARA, M., BEY, F.: (Trois cas de sporotrichose de de Beurmann.) Bull. med. Constantinople 13 December 1910, p. 97. Quoted by DE BEURMANN and GOUGEROT 1912. ~ Un cas de septicémie sporotrichosique (avec demonstrations des cultures et des pièces microscopiques à la Societé Imperiale de Medicine de Constantinople.) Arch. Derm. Syph. (Leipzig) **110**, 387 (1911). — HOEPPLI, R.: Histological observations in experimental Schistosomiasis Japonica. Chin. med. J. **46**, 1179 (1932). — HOLLAND, M.H., MAURIELLO, D.A.: Sporotrichosis. J. med. Soc. N.J. **46**, 9, 419 (1949). — HOPE, E.: Sporotrichosis among violinists. J. Lab. clin. Med. **22**, 7, 708 (1937). — HOPKINS, J.G., BENHAM, R.W.: Sporotrichosis in New York State. N.Y. med. J. **32**, 10, 595 (1932). — HOTCHKISS, M.: Studies on the mycological flora of the bronchi; 1. Sporotrichum isolated from mucus obtained on bronchoscopy. Bull. N.Y. med. Coll. Flower and Fifth Ave. Hosps. **4**, 128 (1941). — HUDELO, MONIER-VINARD (with BRAUN, MERLE): Deux cas de sporotrichose; localizations hypodermiques, intra-musculaires et probablement synoviales. Bull. Soc. Méd. Hôp. Paris 3 s **25**, 914 (1908). — HUGEL, G.: Ein Fall von Sporotrichose. Arch. Derm. Syph. (Leipzig) **102**, 95 (1910). — HUMPHREYS, F.A., HELMER, D.E.: Pulmonary sporotrichosis in a cattle beast. Canad. J. comp. Med. **7**, 7, 199 (1943). — HYDE, J.N., DAVIS, D.J.: Sporotrichosis in man. With incidental consideration of its relation to mycotic lymphangitis in horses. J. cutan. Dis. **28**, 7, 321 (1910). — HYSLOP, G.H., NEAL, J.B., KRAUS, W.M., HILLMAN, O.: A case of sporotrichosis meningitis. Amer. J. med. Sci. **172**, 726 (1926). — ISRAEL, H.L., DEAMATER, E., SONES, M., WILLIS, W.D., MIRMELSTEIN, A.: Chronic disseminated Histoplasmosis. An investigation of its relationship to sarcoidosis. Amer. J. Med. **12**, 252 (1952). — JADASSON: Ein Fall von Sporotrichosis de Beurmann. Cor. Bl. Schweiz. Ärzte (Basel) **39**, 735 (1909). — JAME, L.: Gommes. Encyclopédie Médico-chirurgicale, Paris. Section Dermatologie 12084. No. 14, p. 1 (1949). — JAQUES, W.E.: Relationship of Nematode larvae to generalized sarcoidosis. Report of case and review of literature. Arch. Path. **53**, 550 (1952). — JEANSELME, BURNIER, HOROWITZ: Trois cas de sporotrichose consécutifs à un traitement arsenical. Bull. Soc. franç. Derm. Syph. **35**, 7, 552 (1928a). — JEANSELME, E., CHEVALLIER, P.: Chancres sporotrichosiques des doigts produits par la morsure d'un rat inoculé de sporotrichose. Bull. Soc. Méd. Hôp. Paris 3 s **30**, 176 (1910). — JEANSELME, L., HUET, L., HOROWITZ: Quatre cas de gommes et ulcérations sporotrichosiques accidentelles, survenues à la suite d'intradermo-réactions. Bull. Soc. franç. Derm. Syph. **35**, 416 (1928b). — JEANSELME, POULARD: Sporotrichose de l'iris. Ann. Oculist. (Paris) **144**, 65 (1910). — JESSNER, M.: Experimentelle und histologische Studien über Rattensporotrichose. Klin. Wschr. **1**, 2, 2428 (1922). — JIMINEZ-RIVERO, M., BRICEÑO-IRAGORRI, L.: La esporotricosis y el primer caso de Rhinocladiosis schencki en Venezuela. Gac. méd. Caracas **43**, 225 (1936). — JONES, T.C., MAURER, F.D.: Sporotrichosis in horses. Bull. U.S. Army med. Dep. **1**, 74, 63 (1944). — JOSSET-MOURE: Sporotrichose du tibia ayant simulé une ostéomyélite chronique et necessité quatre interventions chirurgicales. Diagnostic par la sporo-agglutination et la réaction de fixation, Guérison. Bull. Soc. Méd. Hôp. Paris 3 s **26**, 738 (1908). ~ Adénite sporotrichosique. Bull. Soc. Méd. Hôp. Paris 3 s **27**, 133 (1909). — JUNG, VON H.D.: Zur Pilzflora in Ost-Mecklenburg. Mykosen **8**, 3, 101 (1965). — KADEN, R.: Präzipitation von Sporotrichon-Antiserum im Agarmedium. Z. Haut- u. Geschl.-Kr. **21**, 4, 87 (1956). — KAPLAN, W., GONZÁLEZ OCHOA, A.: Application of the fluorescent antibody technique to the rapid diagnosis of sporotrichosis. J. Lab. clin. Med. **62**, 5, 835 (1963). — KAPLAN, W., IVENS, M.S.: Fluorescent antibody staining of Sporotrichum Schenckii in cultures and clinical materials. J. invest. Derm. **35**, 3, 151 (1960). — KEDES, L.H., SIEMIENSKI, J., BRAUDE, A.I.: The syndrome of the alcoholic rose gardener; sporotrichosis of the radial tendon sheath. Report of a case cured with Amphotericin B. Ann. intern. Med. **61**, 6, 1139 (1964). — KEHRER, J. K. W., Een geval van sporotrichose. Ned. T. geneesk. (Amst.) **61**, 2, 386 (1917). — KESTEN, B., ASHFORD, B. K., BENHAM, R. W., EMMONS, C. W., MOSS, M. C.: Fungus infections of the skin and its appendages occurring in Porto Rico. A clinical and mycological study. Arch. Derm. Syph. (Chic.) **25**, 6, 1046 (1932). — KESTEN, B., MARTENSTEIN, H.: Experimental sporotrichosis; cutaneous and intracardial inoculation. A preliminary report. Arch. Derm. Syph. (Chic.) **20**, 441 (1929). — KING, H.: Sporotrichosis with report of an unusual case. Sth. med. J. (Bgham, Ala.) **20**, 541 (1927). — KLEIN, R. C., IVENS, M. S., SEABURY, J. H., DASCOMB, H. E.: Meningitis due to Sporotrichum Schenckii. Arch. intern. Med. **118**, 145 (1966). — KLIGMAN, A. M., BALDRIDGE, G. D.: Morphology of Sporotrichum Schenckii and Histoplasma capsulatum in tissue. Arch. Path. **51**, 6, 567 (1951). — KOBAYASI, T.: Über einen typischen Fall von Sporotrichose. Jap. J. Derm. Urol. **36**, 114 (1934). — KOPPISCH, E.: Studies on Schistosomiasis Mansoni in Puerto Rico; vi. Morbid anatomy of the disease as found in Puerto Ricans. Puerto Rico J. publ. Hlth **16**, 395 (1941). — KREN, O., SCHRAMEK, M.: Ueber Sporotrichose. Wien. klin. Wschr. **22**, 1519 (1909). — KUNZ, C.: Fluorescenz-serologische Untersuchungen an einem pathogenen Pilzstamm (Sporotrichum Schenckii). Arch. klin. exp. Derm. **209**, 2, 200 (1959). — LAFFAILLE, A., PAVIE, P.: Un cas d'épididymite sporotrichosique. Ann. Anat. path. **7**, 373 (1930). — LANDOUZY, L.: Sporotrichose hypodermique gommeuse, ulcéreuse, disséminée (sporotrichose de de Beurmann). Presse méd. **17**, 785 (1909). — LANE, C. G.: Sporotrichosis. Arch. Derm. Syph. (Chic.) **40**, 102 (1939). — LATAPÍ, F.: Esporotricosis facial infantil, nota clinica. Pren. med. Mex. **15**, 259 (1950). ~ Griseofulvin in the treatment of some deep mycoses. Arch. Derm. **81**, 5, 841 (1960). ~ La sporotrichose au Mexique. Laval Méd. **34**, part 2, 6, 732 (1963). — LATAPÍ, F., LAVALLE, P., NOVALES, J., ORTIZ, Y.: Griseofulvina en micosis cutáneas profundas. Nota preliminar sobre resultados terapéuticos en un caso de micetoma por N. brasiliensis y en uno de esporotricosis por S. Schenckii. Dermatologia (Napoli) **3**, 1, 34 (1959). — LAURENT, C.: Sporotrichose osseuses et sporotrichose pulmonaires simulant la tuberculose. Presse méd. **21**, 793 (1913). — LAVALLE, P., NOVALES, J.: Esporotricosis localizada al dorso con lesión vegetante y presencia de "cuerpos asteroides" en los cortes. Ses. Clin. Soc. Derm. Quoted by LAVALLE, NOVALES and MARIAT (1958). — LAVALLE, P., NOVALES, J., MARIAT, F.: Esporotricosis. Nuevas observaciones clínicas, histopatológicas y micológicas. Mem. Congr. Mex. Derm. **1**, 276 (1961). — LAWLESS, T. K.: The diagnosis of sporotrichosis. Arch. Derm. Syph. (Chic.) **22**, 3, 381 (1930). — LEAO: see AREA LEAO. — LEARMONTH, G. E.: Observations on a Sporothrix bearing some resemblance to Sporothrix Beurmanni. Canad. med. Ass. J. **5**, 32 (1915). — LEAVELL, U. W., JR.: A case of sporotrichosis cleared when given Griseofulvin. J. Ky med. Ass. **63**, 415 passim. (1965). — LEBAR, SAINT-GIRONS: Sporotrichose de de Beurmann. Ulcération cutanée de l'avant bras avec ostéite du cubitus. Séro-diagnostic et intradermo-réaction positifs. Bull. Soc. Méd. Hôp. Paris 3 s **28**, 168 (1909). — LEFROU, G.: Action curative des sulfones dans un cas de sporotrichose. Bull. Soc. Path. exot. **43**, 9—10, 536 (1950). — LEHMANN, C. F., PIPKIN, J. L.: Sporotrichosis. Arch. Derm. Syph. (Chic.) **31**, 589 (1935). — LEITE: see SALAZAR LEITE. — LEITHOLD, S. L., REEDER, P. S., BAKER, L. A.: Cryptococcal infection treated with 2-Hydroxystilbamidine in a patient with Boeck's sarcoid. Arch. intern. Med. **99**, 5, 736 (1957). — LERAT: Un cas de sporotrichose tuberculoïde. Presse méd. (Belge) **61**, 525 (1909). — LETULLE, M., DEBRÉ, R.: Sporotrichose de la peau, de la bouche, du pharynx, du larynx et de la trachée. Bull. Soc. Méd. Hôp. Paris 3 s **25**, 379 (1908). — LEWIS, G. M., CUDMORE, J. H.: Sporotrichosis. Report of a case originating in New York. Ann. intern. Med. **7**, 2, 991 (1934). — LINDENBERG, A.: Dermatomycoses brasileiras. Rev. med. cirurg. S. Paulo **12**, 313 (1909). — LIU, C. L.: Sporotrichosis. Report of a case. Chin. med. J. **73**, 4, 330 (1955). — LLERENA, J.: La esporotricosis en El Salvador. Trab. xvi Congr. Med. Nac. Salvador (1964). — LOEWE, G. M.: Sporotrichosis of the cervical area. J. Amer. med. Ass. **107**, 13, 1040 (1936). — LOEWENTHAL, L. J. A.: Sporotrichosis treated with Griseofulvin. Med. Proc. **5**, 26, 563 (1959). — LONDERO, A. T., DE CASTRO, R. M., FISCHMAN, O.: Two cases of sporotrichosis in dogs in Brazil. Sabouraudia **3**, 4, 273 (1964). — LONDERO, A. T., FISCHMAN, O., RAMOS, C. D.: A esporotricose no Rio Grande do Sul. (Observaçóes no interior dêsse Estado.) Hospital (Rio de J.) **63**, 6, 1441 (1963). — LONDOÑO, F.: Apuntes sobre esporotricosis. A propósito de un caso tratado con Anfotericin B. Rev. Fac. Med. (Bogotá) **28**, 1—3, 23 (1960). — LÜ, YAU-CHIN: Sporotrichosis. Report of five cases. J. Formosan med. Ass. **58**, 5, 245 (1959). — LUDWIG, J. S.: Sporotrichosis. Report of an unusual case. Penn. med. J. **59**, 5, 576 (1956). — LURIE, H. I.: Pathogenic sporotricha; their carbohydrate reactions. Mycologia **42**, 5, 624 (1950). ~ Sporotrichon species; their nitrogen metabolism. Mycologia **43**, 2, 117 (1951). ~ Five unusual cases of sporotrichosis from South Africa showing lesions in muscles, bones and viscera. Brit. J. Surg. **50**, 224, 585 (1963a). ~ Histopathology of sporotrichosis. Notes on the nature of the asteroid body. Arch. Path. **75**, 4, 421 (1963b). ~ Sporotrichosis. The significance of variations in morphology of spores in the tissues. Med. Coll. Va. Quart. **3**, 1, 13 (1967). — LUTZ, A., SPLENDORE, A.: Sopra una micosi osservata in uomini e topi (Mus decumanus). Contribuzione alla conoscenza delle cosi dette Sporotricosi. Ann. Igiene Sper. n. s. 17, 581 (1907a). ~ Über eine bei Menschen und Ratten beobachtete Mykose. Ein Beitrag zur Kenntnis der sogenannten Sporotrichosen. Zbl. Bakt., I. Abt. Orig. 45, 7, 631 (1907b); 46, 1, 21 (1908); 46, 2, 97 (1908). ~ Sóbre uma micose observada em homens e ratos. Contribuição para o conhecimento das assim chamadas esporotricoses. Rev. med. cirurg. S. Paulo 10, 433 (1907c). — LYONS, R.E.: Sporotrichosis; a case occurring in a brickyard worker. Arch. Derm. 86, 5, 634 (1962). — McDONAGH, J.E.R., see ADAMSON, H.G.: A case of sporotrichosis. Proc. roy. Soc. Med. 4, part 1. Dermatological Section, pp. 113—121 (1911). — McFARLAND, R.B.: Sporotrichosis revisited. 65 year follow-up of the second reported case. Ann. intern. Med. 65, 2, 363 (1966). — McFARLAND, R.B., GOODMAN, S.B.: Sporotrichosis and sarcoidosis. Report of a case with comment upon possible relationships between sarcoidosis and fungus infections. Arch. intern. Med. 112, 5, 760 (1963). — MABERRY, J.D., MULLINS, J.F., STONE, O.J.: Sporotrichosis with demonstration of hyphae in human tissue. Arch. Derm. 93, 1, 65 (1966). — MACKINNON, J.E.: Resumen sobre 46 observaciones de esporotricosis realizadas en el Uruguay. An. Inst. Hig. Montevideo 2, 1, 44 (1949a). ~ Estadística sobre 1000 casos de micosis cutáneas en el Uruguay y determinación de las especies causantes. An. Inst. Hig. Montevideo 3, 83 (1949b). ~ Las condiciones meteorológicas causa determinante de la frequencia de la esporotricoses. An. Inst. Hig. Montevideo 2, 1, 50 (1949c). ~ The dependance on the weather of the incidence of sporotrichosis. Mycopathologia (Den Haag) 4, 4, 367 (1949d). — MACKINNON. J.E., CONTI-DÍAZ, I.A.: The effect of temperature on sporotrichosis. Sabouraudia 2, 2, 56 (1962). — MADDEN, J.F.: Sporotrichosis in Minnesota. Minn. Med. 30, 8, 854 (1947). — MAGALHÃES PEREIRA, A., PADILHA GONÇALVES, A., LACAZ, C.S., FAVA NETTO, C., MARTINS DE CASTRO, R.: Immunologia da esporotricose. i. A prova da esporotriquina após a cura da esporotricose. ii. A prova da esporotriquina em Crianças sem esporotricose. Rev. Inst. Med. trop. S. Paulo 4, 6, 383, 386 (1962). ~ Estudos sôbre a imunopatologia da esporotricose. An. bras. Derm. Sif. 39, 1, 34 (1964). — MARIAT, F., DROUHET, E.: Sporotrichose expérimentale du hamster. Observation de formes astéroides de Sporotrichum. Ann. Inst. Pasteur 86, 4, 485 (1954). — MARIAT, F., LAVALLE, P., DESTOMBES, P.: Recherches sur la sporotrichose. Etude mycologique et pouvoir pathogène de souches mexicaines de Sporotrichum schenckii. Sabouraudia 2, 2, 60 (1962). — MARIE, P., GOUGEROT, H.: Sporotrichose de de Beurmann. Ostéite sporotrichosique hypertrophiante primitive du tibia, compliquée du lymphangite gommeuse ulcéreuse ascendante et d'adénite inguinale sporotrichosiques. Bull. Soc. Méd. Hôp. Paris 3 s 27, 994 (1909). — MARROQUIN: see SANCHEZ MARROQUIN. — MARTINEZ NAVARRO, A.: Un caso de esporotricosis tratado con la sulfonamida de Damagk; nota clínica. Actas Dermosif. 32, 271 (1940). — MARTINS DE CASTRO, R.: Prova da esporotriquina. Contribuição para o seu estudo. Rev. Inst. A. Lutz (S. Paulo) 20, 5, 5 (1960). — MARTINS CASTRO, VON R., BELLIBONI, N.: Über Sporotrichintest bei Patienten mit geheilter Sporotrichose. Mykosen 5, 1, 24 (1962). — MASON, L.M., McCORMICK, W.C., GLOSSON, J.R.: Cutaneous sporotrichosis. Report of two cases. J. Indiana med. Ass. 44, 1, 31 (1951). — MATRUCHOT, L.: Sur un nouveau groupe de champignons pathogènes, agents des sporotrichoses. C.R. Acad. Sci. (Paris) 150, 9, 543 (1910). — MATRUCHOT, L., RAYMOND: Un type nouveau de champignon pathogène chez l'homme. C.R. Soc. Biol. (Paris) 59, 379 (1905). — MAY, J.: Dos casos de esporotricosis. Arch. urug. Med. 4, 127 (1934). — MEAD, M., RIDLEY, M.F.: Sporotrichosis and chromoblastomycosis in Queensland. Med. J. Aust. 44, 1, 7, 192 (1957). — MENOCAL, R.: Tres casos de esporotricosis. Rev. méd. Cuba. 19, 264 (1911). — MERKLEN, F.P., RIVALIER, E., MOLINE, R., MERCIER, J.N.: Un cas de sporotrichose cutanée. Bull. Soc. franç. Derm. Syph. 63, 4, 425 (1956). — MESCHTSCHERSKI, G.I.: La sporotrichose nouvelle forme de mycose cutanée. Med. Revue (Med. Obosteniye) 70, 16, 437 (1908). — MEYER, K.F.: The relation of animal to human sporotrichosis (studies on American sporotrichosis iii). J. Amer. med. Ass. 65, 7, 579 (1915). — MEYER, K.F., AIRD, J.A.: Various sporotricha differentiated by the fermentation of carbohydrates (studies on American sporotrichosis i.). J. infect. Dis. 16, 399 (1915). — MIKKELSEN, W.M., BRANDT, R.L.: HARRELL, E.R.: Sporotrichosis. A report of 12 cases including two with skeletal involvement. Ann. intern. Med. 47, 3, 435 (1957). — MILHIT, J., MARTIN, A., DELON, J.: Un cas de sporotrichose rénale. Bull. Soc. Pédiat. Paris 33, 592 (1935). — MILLER, M.B.: Sporotrichosis. Ann. Surg. 58, 540 (1913). — MINTY, C.C.J., MEAD, M., McCAFFREY, M.F.: Sporotrichosis. A case report from Queensland. Med. J. Aust. 43, 1, 18, 704 (1956). — MIRANDA, R.N., CUNHA, C., PINHO, A., SCHWEIDSON, J.: A esporotricose. Rev. méd. Paraná 24, 1—2, 23 (1955). — MIRANDA, R.N., CUNHA, C., SCHWEIDSON, J.: Tratamento da esporotricose pela esporotriquina. Hospital (Rio de J.) 54, 2, 257 (1958). — MONTGOMERY, H., HOLMAN, J.C.: Pseudo-epitheliomatous hyperplasia in a case of sporotrichosis. Mayo clin. Proc. 13, 30, 465 (1938). — MONTPELLIER, J., CATANEI, A., LE FRANC, R.: Un nouveau cas de sporotrichose humaine observé en Algérie. Bull. Soc. Path. exot. 25, 297 (1932). — MOORE, M.: Radiate formation on pathogenic fungi in human tissues. Arch. Path. 42, 2, 113 (1946). ~ Morphologic variation in tissue of the organisms of blastomycosis and of histoplasmosis. Amer. J. Path. 31, 6, 1049 (1955). — MOORE, M., ACKERMAN, L.V.: Sporotrichosis with radiate formation in tissue. Report of a case. Arch. Derm. Syph. (Chic.) 53, 3, 253

(1946). — MOORE, J.J., DAVIS, D.J.: Sporotrichosis, following mouse bite, with certain immunologic data. J. infect. Dis. 23, 252 (1918). — MOORE, M., KILE, R.L.: Generalized, subcutaneous, gummatous, ulcerating sporotrichosis. Report of a case with a study of the etiologic agent. Arch. Derm. Syph. (Chic.) 31, 672 (1935). — MOORE, M., MANTING, G.: Sporotrichosis following a mosquito bite; description of lesions in a girl of Indian and French descent. Arch. Derm. Syph. (Chic.) 48, 5, 525 (1943). — MORAES, M.A.P., MIRANDA, E.V.: Sōbre a presenca de formações radiadas (asteroides) na esporotricose. Rev. Inst. Med. trop. S. Paulo 6, 1, 5 (1964). — MORALES, R.: Un cas de lymphangite sporotrichosique au Guatemala. Ann. Parasit. hum. comp. 9, 366 (1931). — MORAX, V.: La sporotrichose de l'appareil visuel. Ann. Oculist. (Paris) 141, 321 (1909); Bull. Soc. Ophtal. Fr. 26, 240 (1909). ~ Sporotrichose primitive du sac lacrymal. Ann. Oculist. (Paris) 145, 49 (1911). — MORAX, V., FAVA, A.: Sporotrichose de la conjunctive. Bull. Soc. Ophtal. Fr. 6 avril, 1909. Quoted by DE BEURMANN and GOUGEROT 1912. — MOUNT, L.B.: Sporotrichosis. With a report of a rather unusual case. Arch. Derm. Syph. (Chic.) 25, 1, 528 (1932). — MOURE, M.P.: Arthrite sporotrichosique du genou. Bull. Soc. Méd. Hôp. Paris 3 s 28, 948 (1909). — MUMFORD, E.P.: Human mycoses in the Near and Middle East. J. trop. Med. Hyg. 67, 2, 35 (1964). — MUMFORD, E.P., MOHR, J.L.: Manual on the distribution of communicable diseases and their vectors in the tropics: Pacific Islands section, Part 1. Amer. J. trop. Med. 24, 3 (suppl.), 1 (1944). — NAVARRO, A. MARTINEZ: see MARTINEZ NAVARRO. — NAVARRO DA SILVA, M.F., NEVES, H., PEREIRA, A., GONÇALVES, A.P., LACAZ, C.S., FAVA NETTO, C., CASTRO, R.M.: Imunologia da esporotricose. iii. A prova da esporotriquina em Portugal, em pessoas sem esporotricose. Rev. Inst. Med. trop. S. Paulo 5, 1, 12 (1963). — NEGRONI, P., PRADO, J.M.: Alergia e immunidad en la esporotricosis experimental. An. Soc. Cient. Argent. 151, 1, 32 (1951). — NEGRONI, P., VIVOLI, D., BONFIGLIOLI, H.: Estudios sobre el Coccidioides immitis Rixford et Gilchrist; reacciones immunoalérgicas en la infeccion experimental del cobayo. Rev. Inst. bact. Malbrán 14, 273 (1949). — NEILL, J.M., CASTILLO, C.G., SMITH, R.H., KAPROS, C.E.: Capsular reactions and soluble antigens of Torula histolytica and of Sporotrichum schenckii. J. exp. Med. 89, 1, 93 (1949). — NETHERTON, E.W., CURTIS, G.H.: Sporotrichosis (Lymphangitic type with primary lesion on the finger). Arch. Derm. Syph. (Chic.) 40, 453 (1939). — NEVES, A.: Contribuição ao estudo da esporotrichose familiar. Brasil-méd. 43, 92 (1929). — NEVES, H., NAVARRO DA SILVA, M.F.: A esporotricose em Portugal. J. med. Porto. 49, 1035, 671 (1962). — NEWCOMER, V.D., HOMER, R.S.: Localized lymphangitic sporotrichosis treated with oral Amphotericin A and B. Arch. Derm. 81, 472 (1960). — NICAUD, P.: Les mycoses pulmonaires. Presse méd. 34, 97, 1521 (1926). — NIEMEYER, A.: Tratamento da esporotrichose pela neve carbônica. Rev. med. Rio Grande do Sul 10, 56, 66 (1953). — NOGUER MORÉ, S., DAUSÁ, J.: La esporotricosis dermato-micosis frequente en Cataluña. Nuevo tratamiento por la radioterapia. Ars. med. (Barcelona) 10, 65 (1934). — NOOJIN, R.O., CALLAWAY, J.L.: Effectiveness in vitro of sulfonamide on Sporotrichum schenckii. Report of 5 cases of sporotrichosis in North Carolina. Arch. Derm. Syph. (Chic.) 49, 5, 305 (1944). — NORDBRING, B.: Studies on growth factors for Sporotrichum schenckii. Physiol. Pl. 5, 1 (1952). — NORDÉN, A.: Sporotrichosis. Clinical and laboratory features and a serologic study in experimental animals and humans. Acta path. microbiol. scand., 89, 119 pages (1951). ~ Interna svampojukdomar (systemic mycoses). Nord. Med. 47, 9, 271 (1952). — O'DONNELL, J.M.: A case of sporotrichosis. Med. J. Aust. 49, 1, 14, 517 (1962). — OKUDAIRA, M., ARAKI, T.O., ARAKI, T., FUKUSHIRO, R.: Sporotrichosis with hyphal elements in tissues. Report of a biopsy case. Trans. Soc. path. Jap. 48, 254 (1959). — OKUDAIRA, M., TSUBURA, E., SCHWARZ, J.: A histopathological study of experimental murine sporotrichosis. Mycopathologia (Den Haag) 14, 4, 284 (1961). — OLIVER-GONZÁLEZ, J.: Anti-egg precipitins in serum of humans infected with Schistosoma Mansoni. J. infect. Dis. 95, 86 (1954). — OLSON, G.M.: A case of sporotrichosis in North Dakota; probable infection from gophers. J. Amer. med. Ass. 59, 12, 941 (1912). — ORTMEYER, M., HUMPHREYS, E.M.: Intranasal granuloma of the sporothrix type producing marked nasal deformity. Ann. Surg. 113, 118 (1941). — OTTOLENGHI, R.: The mycotic flora of the oral cavity in normal and pathological conditions. Dent. Items. 66, 2, 134 (1944). — PADILHA GONÇALVES, A.: Tratamento da esporotricose. Brasil-méd. 76, 5—6, 144 (1962). ~ Tratamento da esporotricose pela esporotriquina. An. bras. Derm. Sif. 38, 85 (1963a). ~ Immunologic aspects of sporotrichosis. Proc. XII Int. Derm. Congr. (1962), Vol. 1, 511 (1963b). — PADILHA GONÇALVES, A., MAGALHÃES PEREIRA, A.: Contribuição para o estudo immunológico da esporotrichose. XIII Reuniao An. Derm. Brasil, Fortaleza (Ceará) 1961. Quoted by MAGALHÃES PEREIRA et al. 1964. — PADILHA GONÇALVES, A., PERYASSU, D.: A esporotricose no Rio de Janeiro (1936—1953). Hospital (Rio de J.) 46, 1, 1 (1954). — PADILHA GONÇALVES, A., PONTES DE CARVALHO, L.: Apreciação do teste intradermico com a esporotriquina. An. bras. Derm. Sif. 29, 2, 103 (1954). — PAGE, C.G., FROTHINGHAM, L., PAIGE, J.B.: Sporothrix and epizootic lymphangitis. J. med. Res. 23, 137 (1910). — PANJA, D., DEY, N.C., GHOSH, L.M.: Sporotrichosis of the skin in India. (A new species described.) Indian med. Gaz. 82, 4, 200 (1947). — PARDO-CASTELLO, V., TRESPALACIOS, F.: Superficial and deep mycoses in Cuba. A report based on 1,174 cases. Sth. med. J. (Bgham,

Ala.) **52**, 1, 7 (1959). — PASSOS, P.: Sinusite maxilar-sporotricose. Rev. bras. Oto-rino-laring. **11**, 167 (1943). — PATSCHKOWSKI: Beitrag zur Klinik der Sporotrichose. Münch. med. Wschr. **81**, 938 (1934). — PAUTRIER, L. M., LUTEMBACHER: Premier cas de sporotrichose diagnostiqué par une sub-cuti-réaction positive. Bull. Soc. Méd. Hôp. Paris 3 s **28**, 137 (1909). — PAUTRIER, L. M., RICHOU: Sporotrichose du nez; lésions multiples osseuses, endonasales et cutanées, simulant les accidents syphilitiques tertiares et la tuberculose verruqueuse. Bull. Oto-rhino-laryngol. (Paris) **15**, 54 (1912). — PEÑA, C. E.: Deep mycotic infections in Colombia. A clinicopathologic study of 162 cases. Amer. J. clin. Path. **47**, 4, 505 (1967). — PEPPLER, H.J., TWIEHAUS, M.J.: Equine sporotrichosis. Trans. Kansas Acad. Sci. **45**, 40 (1942). — PEREIRA: see MAGALHÃES PEREIRA. — PERKEL, I. D.: (Sporotrichosis; Beurmann's disease; different forms of sporotrichosis and their diagnosis, differentiation from syphilis and tuberculosis; case of gummatous verrucous sporotrichosis in a syphilitic). Vrach Gaz. S. Petersb. **17**, 985, 1005 (1910). — PESHKOVSKI, N. YA.: (Sporotrichosis). Sib. Vrach. Gaz. **3**, 461; **4**, 473 (1910). — PESTANA, M., GAUCHE, F., MOSTACCI, R.: Esporotricosis linfangítica. Sem. méd. (B. Aires) **2**, 1502 (1938). — PEYRI, T.: Quoted by DE BEURMANN 1912. — PIJPER, A., PULLINGER, D.: An outbreak of sporotrichosis among South African native miners. Lancet **II**, 914 (1927). — PINKERTON, H., IVERSON, L.: Histoplasmosis. Three fatal cases with disseminated sarcoid-like lesions. Arch. intern. Med. **90**, 4, 456 (1952). — PINKUS, H., GREKIN, J. N.: Sporotrichosis with asteroid tissue forms. Report of a case. Arch. Derm. Syph. (Chic.) **61**, 5, 813 (1950). — PINOY, E., MAGROU, J.: Sur une méthode de diagnostic possible de la sporotrichose par inoculation directe de pus au cobaye. C.R. Soc. Biol. (Paris) **71**, 387 (1911). — PIRATININGA, S. N.: Esporotricose em muar. Rev. Fac. Med. vet. (S. Paulo) **2**, 3, 219 (1943). — PLUMMER, N.S., SYMMERS, W. ST. C., WINNER, H. I.: Sarcoidosis in identical twins with torulosis as a complication in one case. Brit. med. J. **2**, 599 (1957). — POSADA BERRIO, L.: Nueva enfermedad. Esporotricosis o enfermedad de de Beurmann y Gougerot. An. Acad. méd. Medellin. **2**, 35 (1910). Quoted by DE BEURMANN and GOUGEROT 1912. — POSADA TRUJILLO, J., et al.: Esporotricosis epidérmica. Antioquia Méd. **12**, 485 (1962). — PRINGUALT, E., VIGNE, P.: Note sur un cas de sporotrichose naturelle du rat. Bull. Soc. franç. Derm. Syph. **28**, 342 (1921). — QUAINE, E. P.: Report of six cases of tubercular ulcers and tubercular lymphangitis of the upper extremity. St. Paul med. J. **6**, 8, 615 (1904). ~ In discussion of case presented by RUEDIGER and MILLER (1911). — QUIROGA, R.: Esporotricosis por Rhinocladium Beurmanni. Bol. Inst. Clin. quir. (B. Aires) **4**, 1, 523 (1928). — RAMOS E SILVA, J.: Formas minimais da esporotricose: seu interêsse clinico. Hospital (Rio de J.) **28**, 925 (1945). ~ La sporotrichose au Brésil. Laval Méd. **34**, part 2, 6, 739 (1963). — RAMOS E SILVA, J., PADILHA GONÇALVES, A.: Sôbre as formas clinicas da esporotricose. Hospital (Rio de J.) **45**, 2, 155 (1964). — RAPPAPORT, M.A., MEKLER, I.S.: (A case of sporotrichosis caused by the fungus Sporotrichum Beurmanni.) Vrach. Delo. **12**, 1315 (1958). — RAY, L.F., ROCKWOOD, E.M.: Sporotrichosis. Report of a case in which it was resistant to treatment. Arch. Derm. Syph. (Chic.) **46**, 2, 211 (1942). — REIMANN, H.A., PRICE, A.H.: Histoplasmosis resembling sarcoidosis. Trans. Ass. Amer. Phycns **62**, 112 (1949). — RICHARDS, M.: A census of mould spores in the air over Britain in 1952. Trans. Brit. Mycol. Soc. **39**, 4, 431 (1956). — RICHTER, R., ERBAKAN, N.: Der heutige Stand der medizinischen Mykologie in der Türkei. Mycopathologia (Den Haag) **10**, 1, 41 (1958). — RIDDELL, R.W.: Survey of fungus diseases in Britain. Brit. med. Bull. Part 1, **7**, 3, 197 (1951). — RIDGEWAY, N.A., WHITCOMB, F.C., ERICKSON, E.E., LAW, S.W.: Primary pulmonary sporotrichosis. Report of two cases. Amer. J. Med. **32**, 1, 153 (1962). — RIGGS, S., MOORE, A.J., GYORKEY, F.: Articular sporotrichosis. Arch. intern. Med. **118**, 584 (1966). — RIORDAN, T.J.: Sporotrichosis. Arch. Derm. Syph. (Chic.) **60**, 5, 979 (1949). — RISPAL, DALOUS: Deux cas de sporotrichose. An. Derm. Syph. Paris 4 s **10**, 689 (1909). — RITCHIE, H.: In discussion of case presented by RUEDIGER and MILLER 1911. — ROBINSON, H.M.: Industrial sporotrichosis. Sth. med. J. (Bgham, Ala.) **42**, 4, 343 (1949). — ROBINSON, F.W., FROST, T.T.: Cutaneous sporotrichosis treated surgically. Plast. reconstr. Surg. **32**, 657 (1963). — ROBINSON, C.F., ORBAN, T.D.: A case of regional lymphatic sporotrichosis. Aust. J. Derm. **1**, 2, 142 (1951). — ROBINSON, E.M., PARKIN, B.S.: A case of sporotrichosis in the horse. Jl. S. Afr. vet. med. Ass. **1**, 3, 17 (1929). — ROCHARD, DUVAL, R., BODOLEC: Pyélonéphrite sporotrichosique. Gaz. Hôp. (Paris) **82**, 1147 (1909). — ROGERS, A.L., BENEKE, E.S.: Human pathogenic fungi recovered from Brazilian soil. Mycopathologia (Den Haag) **22**, 1, 15 (1964). — ROMAÑA, C., UGHETTI, R.: Sôbre un caso de esporotrichosis. An. Inst. Med. region. (Tucumán) **1**, 2, 185 (1945). — ROTBERG, A., ABRAMCZYK, J.: Estudo sôbre alergia nas micoses. i. Pesquisa epidemiológica com esporotriquinas favoravel à hipótese da esporotricose-infecção. Rev. Fac. Med. (Ceará) **3**, 1, 95 (1963). — ROTBERG, A., DEFINA, A.F., PEREIRA, C.A.: Dados sôbre a freqüência das micoses profundas em especial da esporotricose, na clinica dermatológica da Escola Paulista de Medicina (1951—1960). Rev. Fac. Med. (Ceará) **3**, 1, 84 (1963).— ROTHE, L.: Ueber die Agglutination des Sporotrichon de Beurmann durch Serum von Aktinomykosekranken. Dtsch. med. Wschr. **36**, 1, 30 (1910). — ROUSLACROIX: Dog bite. Quoted by DE BEURMANN and GOUGEROT, p. 278 (1912). ~ Parrot bite. Quoted by DE BEURMANN and GOUGEROT in 'Les Sporotrichose des Animaux'. Rev. Gen.

Med. Vet. **30**, 557 (1913). — Ruediger, G. F.: Sporotrichosis in the United States. J. infect. Dis. **11**, 2, 193 (1912). — Ruediger, G. F., Miller, H. W.: Sporotrichosis in North Dakota. Report of a case. J. Minn. St. med. Ass. **31**, 507 (1911). — Rugiero, H. R., González Camba-ceres, C. E., Yerga, M., Maglio, F.: Esporotricosis por mordedura de rata. Primer caso en la República Argentina. Rev. Asoc. méd. Argent. **75**, 9, 491 (1961). — Salazar Leite, A., Bastos da Luz, J.: Contribuição para o estudo das esporotricoses na provincia ultramarina de Moçambique. An. Inst. Med. trop. (Lisbon) **3**, 187 (1946). — Saliba, A. M., Soerensen, B., Marcon des Veiga, J. S.: Esporotricose em muar. Biológico **29**, 10, 209 (1963). — Salvin, S. B.: Endotoxin in pathogenic fungi. J. Immunol. **69**, 1, 89 (1952). — Sampaio, S. A. P., da Silva Lacaz, C.: Klinische und statistische Untersuchungen über Sporotrichose in São Paulo (Brasilien). Hautarzt **10**, 11, 490 (1959). — Sanchez Marroquin, A., Ma de los Angeles González: Estudio micológico de 16 casos de esporotricosis en la ciudad de México. An. Esc. Nac. Cienc. Biol. (Mexico) **4**, 1, 19 (1945). — Sartory, A.: Présence du Sporotrichum Beurmanni sur un épi de bié. C.R. Soc. Biol. (Paris) **78**, 740 (1915). — Sartory, A., Sartory, R., Meyer, J.: Sur un cas d'onychomycose produit par le Sporotrichum Beurmanni de Beurmann et Ramond. Bull. Acad. Méd. (Paris) **99**, 386 (1928). — Sartory, A., Sartory, R., Meyer, J., Hufschmitt: Un cas de bursite olécranienne sporotrichosique. Strasbourg Méd. **91**, 293 (1931). — Scadding, J.G.: Mycobacterium tuberculosis in the etiology of sarcoidosis. Brit. med. J. 5213, 2, 1617 (1960). — Schenck, B. R.: On refractory subcutaneous abscesses caused by a fungus possibly related to the Sporotricha. Bull. Johns Hopk. Hosp. **9**, 286 (1898). — Schmidt, W., Theissing, G.: Zur Kasuistik der Haut- und Schleimhautsporotrichose. Derm. Wschr. **135**, 22, 545 (1957). — Schneidau, J. D., Lamar, L. M., Hairston, M. A.: Cutaneous hypersensitivity to Sporotrichin in Louisiana. J. Amer. med. Ass. **188**, 4, 371 (1964). — Scott, S. M., Peasley, E. D., Crymes, T. P.: Pulmonary sporotrichosis. Report of two cases with cavitation. New Engl. J. Med. **265**, 10, 453 (1961). — Seabury, J. H., Dascomb, H. E.: Results of the treatment of systemic mycoses. J. Amer. med. Ass. **188**, 6, 509 (1964). — Segrè, G.: Su di un caso di sporotricosi cutanea. G. ital. Mal. vener. **55**, 893 (1914). — Sequin: (Sur un cas de mycose généralisée.) Bull. Soc. Med. Chirurg. Indo China **1**, 9, 462 (1910). Quoted by de Beurmann and Gougerot 1912. — Sethi, K. K., Kneipp, V. L., Schwarz, J.: Pulmonary sporotrichosis in mice following intranasal infection. Amer. Rev. resp. Dis. **93**, 463 (1966). — Sethi, K. K., Schwarz, J.: Experimental cutaneous sporotrichosis. Mykosen **8**, 4, 128 (1965). — Sézary, A., Combe, E., Benoist, F.: Sporotrichose cutanée traitée par un auto-vaccin. Contribution à l'étude du mode d'action de la vaccinothérapie. Bull. Soc. Méd. Hôp. Paris 3 s **51**, 619 (1927). — Shaffer, L. W., Zackheim, H. S.: Sporotrichosis. Report of a case in which treatment with iontophoresis was successful. Arch. Derm. Syph. (Chic.) **56**, 2, 244 (1947). — Sherwell, S.: In discussion of case presented by G. M. Turrell. Long Isl. med. J. **5**, 484 (1911). — Shields, Lee H.: Disseminated cryptococcosis producing a sarcoid type reaction. The report of a case treated with Amphotericin B. Arch. intern. Med. **104**, 5, 763 (1959). — Shoemaker, E. H., Bennett, H. D., Fields, W. S., Whitcomb, F. C., Halpert, B.: Leptomeningitis due to Sporotrichum schenckii. Arch. Path. **64**, 222 (1957). — Shrank, A. B., Harman, R. R. M.: The incidence of skin diseases in a Nigerian teaching hospital dermatological clinic. Brit. J. Derm. **78**, 4, 235 (1966). — Sicard, Bith, Gougerot: Sporotrichose osseuse du tibia (présentation de malade). Bull. Soc. Méd. Hôp. Paris 3 s **25**, 877 (1908). — Silva, M.: Sporotrichosis in Colombia. Arch. Derm. Syph. (Chic.) **65**, 3, 355 (1952). — Silva, Y. P., Guimarães, N. A.: Esporotricose familiar epidêmica. Hospital (Rio de J.) **66**, 3, 573 (1964). — Silva-Correa, M. R.: Dos casos de esporotricosis en Cerro Largo. Arch. urug. Med.-Cir. **13**, 697 (1938). — Silverie, C. R., Ravisse, P.: Premiers cas de sporotrichose observés en Guyane Française. Bull. Soc. Path. exot. **55**, 5, 756 (1962). — Simson, F. W., Helm, M. A. F., Bowen, J. W., Brandt, F. A.: The pathology of sporotrichosis in man and experimental animals. Sporotrichosis infection on Mines of the Witwatersrand, pp. 34—48. Johannesburg: The Transvaal Chamber of Mines 1947. — Singer, J. I., Muncie, J. E.: Sporotrichosis. Etiologic considerations and report of additional cases from New York: N.Y. med. J. **52**, 17, 2147 (1952). — Skeer, J.: Sporotrichosis. Report of a case of localized lymphatic type originating in New York city. Med. Tms (N.Y.) **71**, 1, 7 (1943). — Slamjer: Quoted by de Beurmann 1912. — Smith, D. T.: Pulmonary mycoses. Clinics **4**, 4, 994—1034 (1945). ~ Fungus diseases of the lungs. Springfield, Ill.: Charles C. Thomas 1947. — Smith, L. M.: Sporotrichosis. Report of four clinically atypical cases. Sth. med. J. (Bgham, Ala.) **38**, 8, 505 (1945). — Smith, L.H., Garrett, H. D.: Verrucous sporotrichosis. Arch. Derm. Syph. (Chic.) **56**, 4, 532 (1947). — Smith, J. H., von Lichtenberg, F.: The Hoeppli phenomenon in schistosomiasis. ii. Histochemistry. Amer. J. Path. **50**, 6, 993 (1967). — Soares, J. A., de Oliveira Ribeiro, D., da Silva Lacaz, C.: Esporotricose familiar. An. bras. Derm. Sif. **27**, 1, 5 (1952). — Solano, E. A.: Dermatomicosis. Rev. méd. C. Rica **18**, 325 ,229 (1961). ~ Esporotricosis en niños. Rev. méd. C. Rica **22**, 211 (1965). — Souza, J.J.: Esporotricose em cão. VII Congr. Brasil Vet. (Recife) 1957. Quoted by Londero et al. 1964. — Splendore, A.: Sobre a cultura de uma nova especie de cogumelo patogénica do homen (Sporotrichum Splendore) ou "Sporotrichum asteroides" n. sp. Rev. Soc.

Cient. S. Paulo **3**, 62 (1908). — Spoor, A. A.: Sporotrichosis. Report of a case. J. Amer. med. Ass. **68**, 21, 1548 (1917). — Stancanelli, P.: Sulla sporotricosi cutanea: O Malattia di de Beurmann e Gougerot. G. intern. Sci. Med. **31**, 933 (1909). — Stein, R.: Die Sporotrichosis de Beurmann und ihre Differentialdiagnose gegen Syphilis und Tuberkulose. Arch. Derm. Syph. (Leipzig) **98**, 1, 3 (1909). — Stickney, V. H.: In discussion of case presented by Ruediger and Miller (1911).. — Stout: A case for diagnosis. J. cutan. Dis. **27**, 131 (1909).— Sun Kuei-Yü, Chü Wen-Chün: Corneal sporotrichosis. A case report. Chin. med. J. **85**, 1, 44 (1966). — Sutton, R. L.: Sporotrichosis in America. J. Amer. med. Ass. **55**, 2213 (1910). ~ Sporotrichosis in the Mississippi Basin. J. Amer. med. Ass. **63**, 14, 1153 (1914). — Takahashi, Y.: A critical survey of medical mycology for the years 1946—1956 in Japan. Mycopathologia (Den Haag) **19**, 1—2, 105 (1963). — Talice, R. V.: Deux case de sporotrichose produits par le Sporotrichum asteroides de Splendore. Ann. Parasit. hum. comp. **13**, 576 (1935). — Talice, R. V., Mackinnon, J. E.: The asteroides form of Splendore in spontaneous and experimental sporotrichosis. Proc. Third Int. Congr. Microbiol. New York (1939), pp. 510—511 (1940). — Taylor, K.: Sporotrichum schenckii. J. Amer. med. Ass. **60**, 15, 1142 (1913). — ten Brink, K. B. M.: Sporotrichose. Geneesk. T. Ned.-Ind. **56**, 178 (1916). ~ Sporotrichose in Nederlandsch-Indië. Ned. T. Geneesk **62**, 1, 5 (1918). — Theissing, G., Schmidt, W.: Über das seltene Krankheitsbild der Sporotrichose im Nebenhöhlen- und Mundbereich mit Hautbeteiligung. Z. Laryng. Rhinol. **36**, 3, 141 (1957).— Thomas, C. C., Pierce, H. E., Jr., Labiner, G. W.: Sporotrichosis responding to fever therapy. J. Amer. med. Ass. **147**, 14, 1342 (1951). — Thorold, P. W.: Equine sporotrichosis. J. S. Afr. vet. med. Ass. **22**, 2, 81 (1951). — Torrico,, R. A., Romaña, C.: Caso de cura espontánea de una infección esporotricósica. An. Inst. Med. region. (Tucumán) **5**, 1, 59 (1959). — *Transvaal, Orange Free State Chamber of Mines:* Third annual research review, p. 55 (1965). — Trejos, A., Ramirez, O.: Local heat in the treatment of sporotrichosis. Mycopathologia (Den Haag) **30**, 1, 47 (1966). — Trevathan, R. D., Phillips, S.: Primary pulmonary sporotrichosis. Case report. J. Amer. med. Ass. **195**, 11, 965 (1966). — Tyau, E. S.: Human sporotrichosis with report of a case. China med. J. **30**, 233 (1916). — van Dijk, E., der Kinderin, P. J.: Sporotrichose. Ned. T. Geneesk **102**, 40, 1959 (1958). — Vignolo Lutati, C.: Sopra un caso di sporotrichosi. Gazz. med. Ital. **62**, 91, 101; G. ital. Mal. vener. **52**, 23 (1910). — von Haufe, F., Osswald, M.: Atypischer Verlauf einer Sinusitis maxillaris durch Sporotrichon Schenckii. Z. ärztl. Fortbild. **57**, 79 (1963). — von Ofenheim, E.: Sporotrichosis. Lancet **I**, 659 (1911). — Voss, J. A.: Et tilfelle av sporotrichosis pulmonum. Norsk Mag. Laegevidensk. **96**, 14 (1935). Quoted by Norden 1951. — Wade, J. L., Matthews, A. R. K.: Bilateral sporotrichosis of the breast. Report of a case. Arch. intern. Med. **61**, 916 (1938). — Walker, N., Ritchie, J.: Remarks on a case of sporotrichosis. Brit. med. J. **2**, 1 (1911). — Wallk, S., Bernstein, G.: Systemic sporotrichosis with bony involvement. Arch. Derm. **90**, 3, 355 (1964). — Warfield, L. M.: Report of a case of disseminated gummatous sporotrichosis with lung metastasis. Amer. J. med. Sci. **164**, 72 (1922). — Watt, D. L., Linton, W. T. R.: Sporotrichosis treated by Griseofulvin — a failure. Canad. med. Ass. J. **83**, 21, 1103 (1960). — Weidman, F. D.: Radiate formation due to a Hyphomycete (Aspergillus?). Arch. Path. **13**, 725 (1932). — Wendt, D. O.: Sporotrichosis in a jack. Vet. Med. **36**, 321 (1941). — Wernsdörfer, R., Magalhães Pereira, A., Padilha Gonçalves, A., Silva Lacaz, C., Fava Netto, C., Martins Castro, R., de Brito, A.: Immunologia da esporotricose iv. A prova da esporotriquina na Alemanha e no Brasil, em pessoas sem esporotricose. Rev. Inst. Med. trop. S. Paulo **5**, 5, 217 (1963). — Widal, F., Abrami, P.: Sérodiagnostic de la sporotrichose par la sporoagglutination. La coagglutination mycosique et son application au diagnostic de l'actinomycose. La réaction de fixation. Bull. Soc. Méd. Hôp. Paris 3 s **25**, 947 (1908). — Widal, F., Joltrain, E.: Sporotrichose chez deux membres d'une même famille. Diagnostic immédiat chez l'un d'eux et rétrospectif chez l'autre par la sporoagglutination et la réaction de fixation. Bull. Soc. Méd. Hôp. Paris 3 s **26**, 647 (1908). — Widal, F., Joltrain, E., Brissaud, E., Weill, A.: Séro-diagnostic mycosique. Applications au diagnostic de la sporotrichose et de l'actinomycose. Les coagglutinations et cofixations mycosiques. Ann. Inst. Pasteur **24**, 1 (1910). — Widal, F., Weill, A.: Sporotrichose gommeuse disséminée à noyaux très confluents. Gommes dermiques peur la plupart; gommes hypodermiques et intra-musculaires; gomme sous-periostée tibiale. Présence du parasite dans le sang. Bull. Soc. Méd. Hôp. Paris 3 s **25**, 944 (1908). — Widirøe, S.: Ein Fall von Sporotrichosis. Nord. med. Ark. 3f 12, Afd. 1, n 3, No. 6, 4 pages (1912). — Wilder, W. H., McCullough, C. P.: Sporotrichosis of the eye. J. Amer. med. Ass. **62**, 1156 (1914). — Wohl, M. G.: Fungous diseases of man in the state of Nebraska. Sporotrichosis; Blastomycosis; Actinomycosis. J. Amer. med. Ass. **81**, 8, 647 (1923). — Wolff, A.: Ein Fall von Sporotrichose. Arch. Derm. Syph. (Leipzig) **102**, 1, 95 (1910). — Wyse-Lauzun: Quoted by de Beurmann 1912. — Yamada, M., Watanabe, S.: (Supplementary report on sporotrichosis; the asteroid body in giant cells found in a case.) Acta Derm. (Kyoto) **59**, 185 (1964). — Zeleneff, I. F.: (The problem of sporotrichosis.) Russk. Zh. Kozhn. Vener. Bolěz. **16**, 177 (1908). — Ziprkowski, L., Altman, G., Krakowski, A.: (Sporotrichosis.) Harefuah **60**, 8, 252 (1961).

Rhinosporidiosis

L. N. MOHAPATRA, New Delhi, India

With 9 Figures

Definition

Rhinosporidiosis is a chronic fungous infection produced by *Rhinosporidium seeberi* usually involving the nasal mucosa and resulting in a polypoid growth (Figs. 1, 3). It may also involve the conjunctiva, skin (Fig. 2) and other parts of the body.

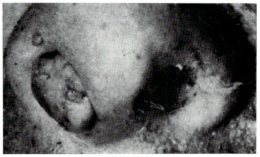

Fig. 1. Rhinosporidiosis. A protruding polypoid growth in the right nostril. Note the sporangia visible as white dots on the surface. (Through the courtesy of Dr. S. N. JAIN, KAKINADA, A. P., India)

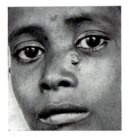

Fig. 2. Rhinosporidiosis. A small nodule on the skin below the inner canthus of the eye. Proved by biopsy. (Through the courtesy of Dr. S. N. JAIN)

Geographic Distribution

Though about 90% of the reported cases are from India and Ceylon (KARUNA-RATNE, 1964), the disease occurs in all the countries of the world except Australia and New Zealand. The first two cases were seen by MALBRAN (1892) and GUILLERMO SEEBER (1900) in Argentina. O'KINEALY (1903) reported the first case from India in a person who had worked in a store where hides were sold.

Subsequently, cases were reported from Africa (Belgian Congo, Liberia, Madagaskar, Natal, Rhodesia, South Africa and Uganda), Cuba, England and Scotland, Indonesia, Iran,

Italy, Malay, Mexico, the Philippines, Russia, South America (Argentina, Boliva, Brazil, Colombia, Ecuador, Paraguay), Thailand, Turkey, United States and Vietnam. The disease is also found in animals including horse, cattle, buffalo, mule and dog (AYYER, 1927, 1932; MAYER and DIAZ, 1954; RAO, 1938; SAHAI, 1938).

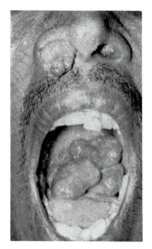

Fig. 3. Rhinosporidiosis. Polypoid growth blocking the right nostril and several fleshy masses in the oral cavity. Proved by biopsy. (Through the courtesy of Dr. S. KAMESWARAN, Madurai Medical College, Madras, India)

Epidemiology

Rhinosporidiosis is seen more often in the younger age group (20—30 years) but it can occur at any age. The largest number of cases reported in India and Ceylon (the two countries with the highest incidence of this disease in the world) are in the age group of 15—39 years (KARUNARATNE, 1964). In a recent report from BHILAI, an endemic focus in Madhya Pradesh, India, 123 cases have been recorded from the main hospital during the past eight years (1960–1968) and the largest number (76) were in the age group of 13—30 years (KULKARNI, 1968, personal communication).

Males suffer from it more often than females (3:1). This probably reflects the increased exposure to the infection in males.

There is no significant difference in susceptibility of different *races* or communities to the infection, but persons of the working class who are much exposed to water in tanks and pools in the endemic areas suffer most (ANDLEIGH, 1952; KARUNARATNE, 1964; MANDLIK, 1937; NORONHA, 1933; REDDY and LAKSHMINARAYANA, 1962). The infection is believed to be exogenous in origin and the fungus to come from its natural habitat in water or water vegetation (CHERIAN and SATYANARAYANA, 1949; JAIN, 1967; RAJAM et al., 1955). The disease is not contagious and spread of infection from person to person is not known. Spread of infection from husband to wife in a single instance (with lesions in the genitalia) is suspected by SYMMERS (personal communication).

The lesions are chronic in nature and may be present for as long as 20—30 years before the patient seeks medical advice. Failure to grow the aetiologic agent *in vitro* and *in vivo* and lack of knowledge about its free-living saprophytic stage are responsible for the ignorance of the life cycle of this parasite (DATTA, 1965; GUPTA, 1959; REDDY and LAKSHMINARAYANA, 1962).

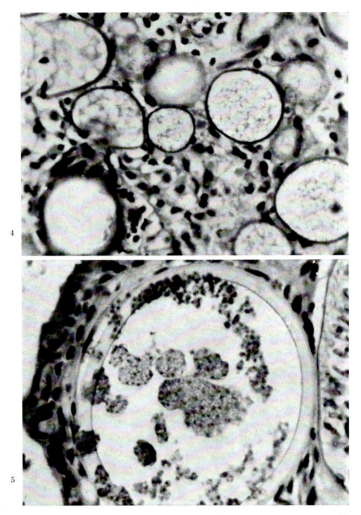

Fig. 4. *Rhinosporidium seeberi*. Developing sporangia of various sizes (H & E, ×450)

Fig. 5. *Rhinosporidium seeberi*. A thick-walled sporangium with granular material within (H & E, ×450)

Etiologic Agent

The causative agent is seen in the infected tissue in abundance in the form of spores and sporangia containing them (ASHWORTH, 1923) (Figs. 4—9). The sporangia vary in size and maturity, the small young ones with a well defined wall are almost empty of contents. As the parasite grows in age and increases in size to about 50 μ the cytoplasm gets filled with granules and globules. Successive nuclear division goes on and the parasite increases in sizes gradually with a cellulose material deposited in the wall. In a fully matured sporangium measuring up to 250—300 μ there are 15,000—20,000 young spores. These escape through the pore, a thin area on the wall without the thick cellulose deposit. These spores vary in size, the matured ones measuring 8—9 μ in diameter, and contain a

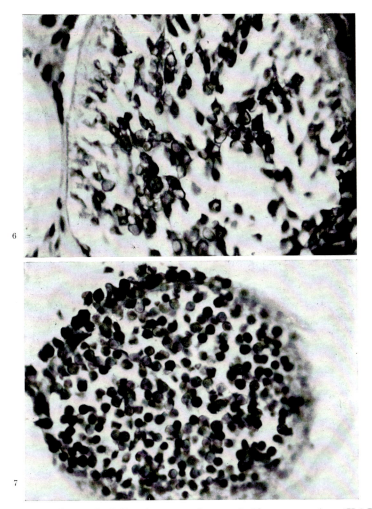

Fig. 6. *Rhinosporidium seeberi*. Development of spores inside a sporangium (H & E, ×450)

Fig. 7. *Rhinosporidium seeberi*. Showing mature spores (H & E, ×450)

number of highly refringent granules. In a mature sporangium both young and mature spores are seen, the former often concentrated in the center (Figs. 4—8). The rupture of the sporangium results in escape of the spores into the tissue with spread of infection to fresh areas and perpetuation of this process. Histochemical reactions together with colloidal iron reaction, enzyme digestion studies and reactions that modify carbohydrate groups, show that the sporangial wall and spore wall are rich in mucopolysaccharides. The spores possess periodic-acid Schiff (PAS) reactivity. Histochemical reactions with mercury bromophenol blue, potassium ferrocyanide-ferric chloride and tannic acid-ferric chloride indicate the presence of protein in the spores (NARAYANA RAO, 1966).

SEEBER considered this parasite to be a protozoon of the sporozoon group but ASHWORTH (1923) placed it in the group of *lower fungi* (phycomycete) closely related to the chytridiales. The composition of the wall of the sporangium, develop-

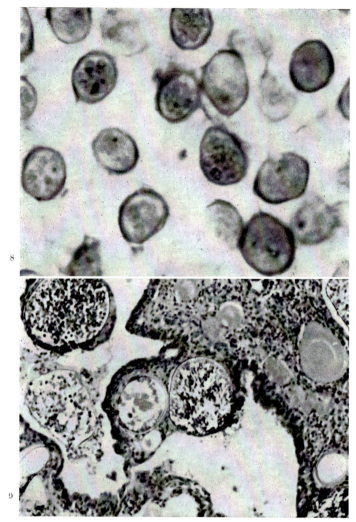

Fig. 8. *Rhinosporidium seeberi*. Mature spores showing karyosome and several globular bodies within (H & E, ×2000)

Fig. 9. *Rhinosporidium seeberi*. Tissue containing sporangia of various size and of varying degrees of maturity. Note the "round cell" chronic cellular infiltrate and the covering stratified columnar epithelium (H & E, ×100)

ment of a definite pore in it, presence of a mucoid substance between the spores and repeated nuclear division prior to formation of spores support the above view.

Attempts to grow this fungus *in vitro* and to infect animals with tissue removed from lesions teeming with spores have been unsuccessful (Dhayagude, 1941; Gupta, 1959; Rajam et al., 1955; Rao, 1938; Reddy and Lakshminarayana, 1962; Satyanarayana, 1960).

Pathologic Anatomy

Though gross appearance of the lesion does not prove the nature of the infection, microscopic examination of the H & E stained section reveals the diagnosis readily. The lesion usually involving the nasal mucosa is seen as a polypoid mass (GRAHAM, 1932; HABIBI, 1944; JAIN, 1967; KARUNARATNE, 1964; O'KINEALY, 1903; PURANDARE and DEORAS, 1935; SHARMA, JUNARKAR and AGARWAL, 1962; SATYANARAYANA, 1960; TIRUMURTHI, 1924) (Figs. 1, 3). The stroma is dense with a chronic inflammatory reaction with neutrophils, plasma cells and lymphocytes and occasional giant cells of the foreign body type (Figs. 4, 9). The presence of numerous well circumscribed globular structures varying in size from 10—250 μ in the stroma covered by hyperplastic squamous or columnar epithelium is the diagnostic feature (Figs. 4, 9). These sporangia are of varying size and age with thick chitinous wall (Fig. 5) and contain immature and mature spores. The latter are larger than erythrocytes and contain a karyosome and several globular eosinophilic bodies (Fig. 8). The epithelium (squamous or columnar) covering the polypoid growth shows considerable hyperplasia.

Clinical Features

The commonest site of rhinosporidiosis in man is the *nose*. It is affected in 70% of the cases (KARUNARATNE, 1964) and the lesions are most frequently in the septum, inferior turbinate or in the floor of the nose. Multiple lesions are not rare. Commonly only one nostril is affected but bilateral infection is occasionally seen. The patient usually has a sessile or pedunculated growth in the nose (the commonest site of infection) which is vascular, friable and sometimes ulcerated (Fig. 1). In cases of long duration the lesions spread and may extend beyond the mucocutaneous border. These lesions in the nose may protrude through the nostril as a polyp and produce discomfort as they increase in size (PEÑA, 1967; SATYANARAYANA, 1960).

Next to the nose is the *eye* in order of frequency of involvement, the lesion being mostly confined to the palpebral conjunctiva (SENGUPTA, MITRA and SARKAR, 1958). Lesions in the conjunctiva are more conspicuous and produce lacrimation and photophobia. These may spread to and cause eversion of the lid. The lesion is usually small and because of its situation medical advice is sought early (DARBARI and SRIVASTAVA, 1961; HAFEEZ and TANDON, 1965; SOOD and NARAYANA RAO, 1967; SRINIVASA RAO, 1962; WRIGHT, 1922). Infection of the lacrymal sac presents as a swelling which may suppurate and cause ulceration of the overlying skin. WRIGHT (1922) reported the first case and SATYANARAYANA (1960) saw three cases in his series.

Several cases of *skin* infection are reported. The lesion in the nasal mucous membrane may also involve the skin at the nasal orifice (ALLEN and DAVE, 1936; HABIBI, 1944). DHAYAGUDE (1941) reported a case of multiple nodular lesions in the skin and subcutaneous tissue without infection of the nose.

The case reported by AGGARWAL et al. (1959) as generalised rhinosporidiosis with visceral involvement had multiple nodules over the chest, back, lower extremities and scalp without any lesion in the nasal cavity. Solitary skin lesions have been reported by PURANDARE and DEORAS (1953), CHERIAN and SATYANARAYANA (1949) and REDDY (1954). The skin lesion starts as a painless nodule which becomes warty. Some of them ulcerate and are secondarily infected (Fig. 2).

Lesions in rare sites like the oral cavity (Fig. 3), the ear, the male and female genitalia and the rectum have been recorded (DHAYAGUDE, 1941; INGRAM, 1910; MAHADEVAN, 1952; SYMMERS, 1961; THOMAS, GOPINATH and BETTS, 1956).

Infection of nasopharynx, epiglottis, uvula, palate, tonsils, larynx and trachea has been reported by SATYANARAYANA (1960) in a series of 255 cases. Lesions in the lower respiratory tract are very rare. Unusual extranasal lesions in a Hindu male farmer with involvement of paranasal sinuses is reported by GUPTA (1966). A parotid salivary cyst due to this infection has been reported by MAHADEVAN (1952).

BEATTIE (1906) reported a case of an aural polyp.

The first case of infection of the glans penis with papillomatous growth was reported by Ingram (1910). Dhayagude (1941) described a case of urethral involvement with a pedunculated growth. Infection of the vulva (Borzone et al., 1951) and that of vagina (Karunaratne, 1936) are known to occur.

The infection is most commonly localized in a single organ such as in the nose or eye, but two cases with *disseminated lesions* seen in several organs were described by Agarwal et al. (1959) and Rajam et al. (1955). In the former case the diagnosis during life was established by examination of the biopsy specimens from the palate and right leg. After death lesions in the skin, eye, palate, tongue, larynx and lungs were histologically positive for rhinosporidiosis. In the second case the diagnosis of hematogenous spread of the infection from the primary lesion in the nose was suspected during life by demonstration of the parasite in the blood and confirmed by finding the organism in many viscera after death. Dhayagude's (1941) case was rare and unusual in that though multiple subcutaneous localizations of the lesions could have occured through hematogenous spread of the infection, adequate proof of the same is lacking.

Bony lesions are almost unknown except for the cases reported by Nguyen-Van-Ai et al. (1958) and Atav et al. (1955).

Diagnosis

Examination of the surface of the polypoid growth shows small white dots which contain the sporangia of varying size (Figs. 1, 3). The mucoid exudate on the surface of these lesions may show the presence of spores discharged from the sporangia.

Examination of the H & E stained slide of the biopsy taken from the lesion readily reveals the histologic diagnosis (Fig. 9).

Neither culture of the fungus nor animal inoculation with the clinical material is successful. No immunologic test is designed for diagnosis of a case (Emmons et al., 1964).

Prognosis

Unless surgically removed the growth in the nose increases in size and frequently ulcerates with secondary bacterial infection. The disease being strictly localized to the affected site, the prognosis is good after complete excision of the diseased tissue (Conant et al., 1954).

Occasionally there is recurrence presumably due to some infected tissue being left at the site during surgical excision. Only in a very few cases have disseminated visceral lesions with fatal result been reported (Rajam et al., 1955; Agarwal et al., 1959).

Treatment

Several chemotherapeutic agents like trivalent and pentavalent antimony preparations have been tried without much success (Allen and Dave, 1936). Careful dissection and complete removal of the lesion are the only sure ways to get rid of this infection. In advanced cases extensive surgical excision may be supplemented by cauterization to prevent recurrence (Kameswaran, 1966).

References

Agarwal, S., Sharma, K.D., Srivastava, J.B.: Generalized rhinosporidiosis with visceral involvement (Report of a case) A.M.A. Arch. Dermatol. **80**, 22 (1959). — Allen, F.R.W.K., Dave, M.L.: The treatment of rhinosporidiosis in man based on a study of 60 cases. Indian med. Gaz. **71**, 376 (1936). — Andleigh, H.S.: Rhinosporidiosis in Rajasthan. Indian J. med. Sci. **6**, 16 (1952). — Ashworth, J.H.: Transactions of the Royal Society, Edinburgh

53, 301 (1923). Quoted by KARUNARATNE (1964). — ATAV, N., GOKSAN, T., URAL, A. (1953). Quoted by KARUNARATNE (1964). — AYYER, V.K.: Rhinosporidiosis in cattle, case recorded in bullock; Transactions of VII Congress. Far East. Ass. Trop. Med. **3**, 658 (1927). ~ Rhinosporidiosis in equines. Indian J. vet. Sci. **2**, 49 (1932). — BEATTIE, J.M.: A sporozoon in aural polyp. Brit. med. J. **2**, 1402 (1906). — BORZONE, R.A., LAPIEZA CABRAL, P.: (1951). Quoted by KARUNARATNE (1964). — CHERIAN, P.V., SATYANARAYANA, C.: Rhinosporidiosis. Indian J. Otolaryng. **1**, 15 (1949). — CONANT, N.F., SMITH, D.T., BAKER, R.D., CALLAWAY, J.L., MARTIN, D.S.: Manual of Clinical Mycology, pp. 456, figures 201. Philadelphia and London: Saunders Company 1954. — DARBARI, B.S., SRIVASTAVA, S.P.: Rhinosporidiosis of conjunctiva. J. All-India ophthal. Soc. **9**, 39 (1961). — DATTA, S.: *Rhinosporidium seeberi* — its cultivation and identity. Indian J. vet. Sci. **35**, 1 (1965). — DHAYAGUDE, R.G.: Unusual rhinosporidiosis infection in man. Indian med. Gaz. **76**, 513 (1941). — EMMONS, C.W., BINFORD, C.H., UTZ, J.P.: Medical Mycology, pp. 380. Philadelphia: Lea & Febiger 1964. — GRAHAM, G.S.: *Rhinosporidium seeberi* in nasal polyp, 4th North American case. Amer. J. clin. Path. **2**, 73 (1932). — GUPTA, I.M.: An attempt to grow *Rhinosporidium seeberi*. Indian J. Path. Bact. **2**, 76 (1959). — GUPTA, O.P.: Unusual extranasal manifestations of rhinosporidiosis. Laryngoscope (St. Louis) **76**, 1842 (1966). — HABIBI, M.: 1944. Quoted by KARUNARATNE (1964). — HAFEEZ, M.A., TANDON, P.L.: Rhinosporidiosis of conjunctiva J. All-India ophthal. Soc. **13**, 114 (1965). — INGRAM, A.C.: *Rhinosporidium kinealyi* in unusual situations. Lancet **2**, 716 (1910). — JAIN, S.N.: Etiology and incidence of rhinosporidiosis. Indian J. Otolaryng. **19**, 1 (1967). — KAMESWARAN, S.: Surgery in rhinosporidiosis. Experience with 293 Cases. Int. J. Surg. **46**, 602 (1966). — KARUNARATNE, W.A.E.: The pathology of rhinosporidiosis. J. Path. Bact. **42**, 193 (1936). ~ Rhinosporidiosis in man, pp. 146. University of London: The Athlone Press 1964. — MAHADEVAN, R.: A rare case of parotid salivany cyst due to rhinosporidiosis. Indian J. Surg. **14**, 271 (1952). — MALBRAN, 1892. Quoted by KARUNARATNE (1964). — MANDLIK, G.S.: A record of rhinosporidial polyp, with some observations on the mode of infection. Indian med. Gaz. **72**, 143 (1937). — MAYER, H.F., DIAZ, B.E. (1954). Quoted by KARUNARATNE (1964). — NARAYANA RAO, S.: *Rhinosporidium seeberi* — A histochemical Study. Indian J. exp. Biol. **4**, 10 (1966). — NGUYEN-VAN-AI, PHAN-NGOC-DUONG, NGUYEN-TRI-LOC (1958). Quoted by KARUNARATNE (1964). — NORONHA, A.J.: A preliminary note on the prevalence of rhinosporidiosis among sand workers in Poona. J. trop. Med. Hyg. **36**, 115 (1933). — O'KINEALY, F.: Localized sporopermiosis of the mucosa of the septum nasi. Proc. laryng Soc. Lond. **10**, 109 (1903). — PEÑA, CARLOS E.: Deep mycotic infections in Colombia (A clinico-pathological study of 162 cases). Amer. J. clin. Path. **47**, 505 (1967). — PURANDARE, N.M., DEORAS, S.M.: Rhinosporidiosis in Bombay. Indian J. med. Sci. **7**, 103 (1935). — RAJAM, R.V., VISWANATHAN, G.C., RAO, A.R., RANGIAH, P.N., ANGULI, C.V.: Rhinosporidiosis, a study with report of a fatal case of systemic dissemination. Indian J. Surg. **17**, 269 (1955). — RAO, M.A.N.: Rhinosporidiosis in bovines in the Madras presidency, with a discussion on probable modes of infection. Indian J. vet. Sci. **8**, 187 (1938). — REDDY, D.B.: Rhinosporidiosis (a review based on the study of 156 biopsies). Antiseptic **51**, 702 (1954). — REDDY, D.G., LAKSHMINARAYANA, C.S.: Investigation into transmission, growth and serology in rhinosporidiosis. Indian J. med. Res. **50**, 363 (1962). — SAHAI, L.: Rhinosporidiosis in equines. Indian J. vet. Sci. **8**, 221 (1938). — SATYANARAYANA, C.: Rhinosporidiosis with a record of 255 cases. Acta olotaryng. (Stockh.) **51**, 348 (1960). — SEEBER, G.R. (1900). Quoted by KARUNARATNE (1964). — SENGUPTA, M., MITRA, B.K., SARKAR, P.K.: Rhinosporidiosis of the conjunctiva. J. All-India ophthal. Soc. **6**, 39 (1958). — SHARMA, K.D., JUNARKAR, R.V., AGARWAL, S.: Rhinosporidiosis. J. Indian med. Ass. **38**, 640 (1962). — SOOD, N.N., NARAYANA RAO, S.: Rhinosporidium granuloma of the conjunctiva. Brit. J. Ophthal. **51**, 61 (1967). — SRINIVASA RAO, P.N.: Rhinosporidiosis of conjunctiva. J. Indian med. Ass. **39**, 601 (1962). — SYMMERS, W.St.C.: Symposium on fungus diseases; further cases of exotic mycoses seen in Britain — histoplasmosis, chromoblastomycosis, rhinosporidiosis and phycomycosis. Trans. roy. Soc. trop. Med. Hyg. **55**, 201 (1961). — THOMAS, T., GOPINATH, N., BETTS, R.H.: Rhinosporidiosis of the bronchus. Brit. J. Surg. **44**, 316 (1956). — TIRUMURTHI, T.S.: *Rhinosporidium seeberi* (KINEALYI) in a Malabar woman. Lancet **1**, 802 (1924). — WRIGHT, R.E.: *Rhinosporidium Kinealyi* of the conjunctiva. Indian med. Gaz. **57**, 81 (1922).

Subcutaneous Phycomycosis and Rhino-Entomophthoromycosis

BETTY M. CLARK and GEORGE M. EDINGTON, Ibadan, Nigeria

With 3 Figures

Entomophthoromycosis describes infection caused by fungi belonging to the order Entomophthorales and includes subcutaneous phycomycosis (JOE et al., 1956) and a condition previously described as rhinophycomycosis (MARTINSON, 1963) but now termed rhinophycomycosis entemophthorae (MARTINSON and CLARK, 1967) or rhino-entomophthoromycosis (CLARK, 1967) in order to distinguish it from rhinomucormycosis (rhinophycomycosis) (DWYER and CHANGUS, 1968). Rhinomucormycosis is described in the chapter on mucormycosis by BAKER.

The histopathology of subcutaneous phycomycosis and rhino-entomophthoromycosis is essentially similar and is dealt with in detail when the pathology of subcutaneous phycomycosis is considered. Rhino-entomophthoromycosis is however a separate entity both clinically and mycologically and attention is given to the distinguishing features when the condition is described.

Subcutaneous Phycomycosis

Subcutaneous phycomycosis is characterized by a firm progressive swelling of the subcutaneous tissues. It is caused by *Basidiobolus haptosporus* DRECHSLER, 1947 and 1956.

Historical: The condition was first described in Indonesia in 1956 by JOE et al. Since then the disease has been reported from other parts of the world.

Epidemiology: Although originally described in Indonesia the great majority of the cases have been described in Africa from the following countries:

Uganda (JELLIFFE et al., 1961; BURKITT et al., 1964:) Sudan (LYNCH and HUSBAND, 1962): Nigeria (ELEBUTE and OKUBADEJO, 1962; HARMAN et al., 1964): Senegal (BASSET et al., 1963): Ivory Coast (ANGATE et al., 1963; VILLASCO et al., 1966): Cameroons (GAMET and BROTTES, 1963): Ghana (BURKITT et al., 1964): Kenya (NEVILLE and MILLER, 1964): Upper Volta (LASCH et al., 1965).

Cases have also been reported from India (MUKERJI et al., 1962; KLOKKE et al., 1966; GRUEBER, 1966): England (SYMMERS, 1964): Burma (STOCKDALE, 1964) and Iraq (RIDLEY and WISE, 1965).

The condition is predominantly a disease of *childhood* and *adolescence* but adults are occasionally affected. *Boys* are more often affected than girls. *B. haptosporus* is a common saprophyte of soil and decaying vegetation. It was first isolated by DRECHSLER (1947) from leaf mould from woods in Wisconsin, USA. It has also been isolated from soil and from the intestinal tract of frogs, toads, gekkoes, chameleons and lizards. The infection is most frequently seen in the tropics, the case reported from England being an exception. Minor trauma is probably the portal of entry and this is borne out by the limbs and buttocks being the most common sites of the subcutaneous swellings. The possibility of insect vectors has been considered (BAKER et al., 1962) but as yet the fungus has not been isolated from insects investigated.

Clinical Features: The lesions present as firm, moveable, well defined sub-cutaneous swellings (Fig. 1). Satellite small nodules may be palpable at the advancing edge. The skin over the lesion is usually intact but ulceration occasionally occurs. There is usually no pain, tenderness or constitutional upset but occasionally patients present with lesions which are hot tender and painful. Involvement of deeper tissues and the viscera may occur either by direct spread or in rare cases by haematogenous dissemination (RIDLEY and WISE, 1965). The condition may be

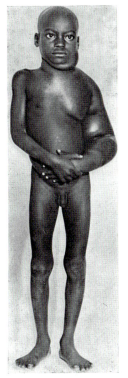
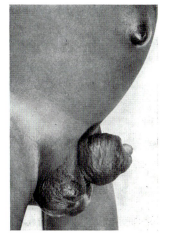

Fig. 1   Fig. 2

Fig. 1. Subcutaneous phycomycosis in an East African Child. (From JELLIFFE, BURKITT, O'CONNER and BEAVER, T. Pediat. **59**, 124, 1961, with permission)

Fig. 2. Subcutaneous phycomycosis of the scrotum and penis. (From EDINGTON, G.M. Trans. roy. Soc. trop. Med. Hyg. **58**, 242, 1964, with permission)

benign and self limiting (JOE and ENG, 1960; JELLIFFE et al., 1962) or may end fatally. We have seen one male child dying from the effects of infiltration of tissues of the penis, perineum, pelvic organs and large bowel (Fig. 2) (EDINGTON, 1964) and another from massive infiltration of the tissues of the neck and mediastinum.

Pathology: The subcutaneous, fatty tissue and dermis are mainly affected. Macroscopically the lesion is firm, creamy white in colour and tough on section. Yellowish areas of necrosis are present. A wide variety of histopathological changes may be seen in the one patient probably depending upon the duration of

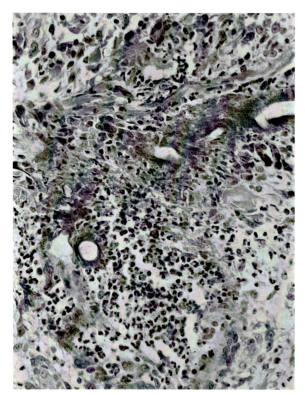

Fig. 3. Subcutaneous phycomycosis. Photomicrograph of slide from case shown in Fig. 2. The broad hyphae, cut lengthwise and crosswise, are surrounded by eosin-staining hyaline material and lie in microabscesses or directly in fibroblastic scar tissue which contains eosinophils. Giant cells may also participate in the response. H & E, ×370

the infection and the immunological response of the host (Burkitt et al., 1964) and they can be classed as acute, subacute, and chronic.

The characteristic and *diagnostic* acute lesion is the *eosinophilic microabscess* containing fungal elements at its centre, the predominant cell being the eosinophil polymorphonuclear leucocyte. The striking feature is the cuff of granular intensely eosinophilic material, a few microns in diameter surrounding the fungus (Fig. 3). These lesions are most frequently seen at the advancing edge of the tumor. The fungi stain poorly with routine H & E stains and, as the cytoplasm is often absent, may appear as circular, oval or longitudinal spaces surrounded by a slightly refractile envelope at the centre of the eosinophilic material (Fig. 3). The hyphae stain well with methenamine silver, are thin walled and vary from 5—15 μ in width. Branching forms are present but only occasionally are septa noted. They are usually discrete in the tissues. The circumfungal eosinophilic precipitation which is common to subcutaneous phycomycosis and rhino-entomophthoromycosis gives the staining reactions of fibrin and is thought to indicate an immunological reaction to the fungus in the tissues of the host. This eosinophilic reaction is evoked by a number of fungi and parasites.

Burkitt et al. (1964) noted the similarity of this material to that surrounding the asteroids of sporotrichosis, grains of actinomycosis and the nocardial type of Madura foot. We have noted the similarity to the reaction seen surrounding ova in the acute stages of schistosomiasis

(HOEPPLI, 1932) and other tissue parasites. SMITH and VON LICHTENBERG (1967) have confirmed the immunological relationship of this precipitation to the ova of schistosomiasis by fluorescent antibody techniques and have described its histochemical characteristics. WILLIAMS (1968) has shown that the eosinophilic deposits in subcutaneous phycomycosis and rhino-entomophthoromycosis are identical histochemically but differ somewhat from the precipitate found in the HOEPPLI phenomenon in schistosomiasis.

The *eosinophilic precipitate* is not seen in all lesions. In the subacute stage there may be palisading of epithelioid cells round the hyphae with plasma cells, lymphocytes, and giant cells of the foreign body or Langhans type at the periphery. Masses of disintegrating "fibrinoid" material may be seen with a variable infiltration of eosinophils, histiocytes, plasma and giant cells. The eosinophilic material may be seen within giant cells frequently accompanied by hyphal remnants. Areas of necrosis with microabscesses devoid of fungal elements may be present. Extensive fibrosis with a variable cellular infiltration exemplifies the chronic stages of the disease and is most commonly found centrally and distally in the lesion. Intense plasma cell and lymphocytic infiltration with prominent Russell bodies are inconstant findings. In contrast to mucormycosis the vessel walls are rarely invaded by hyphae and invasion has only been described in two cases (LYNCH and HUSBAND, 1962; SYMMERS, 1962). Vascular proliferation with haemosiderin deposition however, may be a feature and obliterative endarteritis occurs in the more chronic areas of the lesion.

Mycology: Subcutaneous phycomycosis was originally considered to be caused by *Basidiobolus ranarum* Eidam 1886 (JOE et al., 1956). It has since been established that the species which causes disease in man does not produce the rough-walled zygospores characteristic of *B. ranarum* (DRECHSLER, 1958) but the exact taxonomic position of the pathogen is still controversial. It has been classified as *B. meristosporus* DRECHSLER (1955) by GREER and FRIEDMAN (1966) and as *B. haptosporus* DRECHSLER (1947, 1956) by SRINIVASAN and THIRUMALACHER (1964 and 1967). The latter consider *B. haptosporus* and *B. meristosporus* to be one species.

The fungus grows readily at room temperature and at 37°C. on Sabouraud's dextrose agar. The colonies which are at first flat waxy and yellowish grey in colour soon become heaped up and folded with radial furrows. The surface of the colony may become covered with a fine white down of aerial hyphae and conidia or may remain waxy, gradually becoming grey brown with age. Satellite colonies are frequently seen.

Asexual sporulation occurs by means of globose conidia, adhesive conidia and sporangiospores arising from these. Sexual reproduction results in the formation of smooth walled zygospores from the union of adjacent hyphal cells. A detailed morphological description of a strain isolated from an Indonesian patient has been given by DRECHSLER (1958). It should be noted that the fungus soon dies off in tissue kept in a refrigerator (BURKITT et al., 1964).

Diagnosis: The histopathology in biopsies taken from the edge of the lesion is, in our experience, diagnostic of either subcutaneous phycomycosis or rhino-entomophthoromycosis. Culture is necessary to differentiate the two conditions.

Rhino-Entomophthoromycosis

Synonyms: Rhinophycomycosis: Rhinophycomycosis entomophthorae.

Rhino-entomophthoromycosis is caused by the fungus *Delacroixia coronata* (Costantin) SACCARDO and SYDOW (1899) and is characterized by nasal obstruction and swelling of the tissues of the nose, cheek and upper lip.

Historical: The disease was first reported as a chronic granulomatous condition affecting the skin and mucous membranes of the nostrils and the lips of horses (Emmons and Bridges, 1961; Bridges et al., 1962).

Martinson (1963) in Nigeria described three cases of a disease in man involving the upper respiratory tract and face. The histological features of this condition were indistinguishable from those of subcutaneous phycomycosis but because of the peculiar anatomical distribution of the lesions he called the disease rhinophycomycosis. He also postulated that the aetiological agent might belong to a species or genus different from that responsible for subcutaneous phycomycosis. This was confirmed by Bras et al. (1965) who reported the first proven case of infection with D. coronata in man.

In 1956 Ash and Raum described a case of "Mucormycosis" of the nose with clinical and histological features identical to that of rhino-entomophthoromycosis. Since then there have been several reports in the literature of cases of "subcutaneous phycomycosis" affecting the nose in which the diagnosis was based on the histological findings (Blaché et al., 1961; Straatsma et al., 1962; Basset et al., 1963; Harman et al., 1964; Peloux and Foucard, 1964 anol Klokke et al., 1966). Mycological investigations of these patients would probably have shown that their disease was caused by D. coronata.

Epidemiology: In contrast to subcutaneous phycomycosis the patients are usually *adults* between the ages of 20 and 40 years. Males are affected more often than females. The majority of cases have been reported from areas of tropical rain forest; agricultural and other outdoor workers are the most frequently affected.

D. coronata occurs in decaying vegetation and soil. The fungus causes disease in insects (Kevorkian, 1937) but unlike B. haptosporus it has never been isolated from the gastro-intestinal tract of reptiles. Infection probably occurs by implantation of inhaled spores into the nasal mucosa through minor trauma or insect bites.

Proven cases of infection with D. coronata have been reported from the Cayman Islands (Bras et al., 1965): Congo (Kinshasha) (Renoirte et al., 1965): Brazil (Andrade et al., 1967): Columbia (Restrepo, M., et al., 1967) and Nigeria (Martinson and Clark, 1967). Probable cases, lacking mycological confirmation have been reported from the Cameroons (Blaché et al., 1961): Senegal (Basset et al., 1963): Central Africa (Peloux and Foucard, 1964) and India (Klokke et al., 1966). The origin of the case reported by Ash and Raum (1956) is unknown and that of Straatsma et al. (1962) is uncertain but may have been Puerto Rico (Zimmerman, 1966).

Clinical Features: Nasal obstruction due to polypoid tumours of the mucosa is the earliest clinical finding; the paranasal sinuses and the dorsum of the nose are frequently involved. In more advanced cases the lesions may have spread to the cheek, upper lip, palate and pharynx. In contrast to subcutaneous phycomycosis the early facial lesions are not attached to the skin and are not moveable over deeper structures.

Pathology: The respiratory epithelium may show transitional or squamous metaplasia but ulceration is uncommon; subepithelial tissue and muscle are affected. Otherwise the macroscopic and microscopic pathology is identical to that described previously in subcutaneous phycomycosis.

Mycology: *Delacroixia coronata* (Constantin) Saccardo and Sydow 1899. Synonym: *Boudierella coronata* Costantin 1897: *Conidiobolus villosus* Martin 1925; *Entomophthora coronata* (Costantin) Kevorkian 1937; *Conidiobolus coronatus* (Costantin) Srinivasan and Thirumalacher 1964.

Couch (1939) and more recently Kjoller (1967) revived the genus Delacroixia for fungi with asexual reproduction similar to that of the genus Conidiobolus but for which no perfect state was known.

Delacroixia coronata grows readily on Sabourand's dextrose agar at $25°—30°$C. The young colony is similar in appearance to that of *B. haptosporus (vide supra)* but within 2—3 days the surface soon becomes white and powdery due to the production of numerous propulsive globose conidia, $10—20$ μ in diameter. When cultures are grown in petridishes the conidia form a thick mat in the inverted lid.

Conidia which fall on to the agar surface give rise to numerous satellite colonies which soon coalesce. Those that fall on to the glass may give rise to secondary globose conidia, multiple secondary microconidia or give villous appendages.

Diagnosis: The characteristic clinical features combined with a histopathological picture identical with that of subcutaneous phycomycosis are highly suggestive of rhino-entomophthoromycosis, but culture of the fungus is the only definitive method of diagnosis.

References

ANDRADE, Z. A., PAULA, L. A., SHERLOCK, I. A., CHEEVER, A. W.: Nasal granuloma caused by *Entomophthora coronata*. Amer. J. trop. Med. Hyg. **16**, 31 (1967). — ANGATE, Y., OUEDRAOGO, H., DIARRA, S., CAMAIN, R.: Sur un cars de Phycomycase en cote d'Ivoire. Bull. Soc. Path. exot. **56**, 112 (1963). — ASH, J. E., RAUM, M.: In: An Atlas of Otolaryngic Pathology, p. 179. Washington, D.C.: A.F.I.P. 1956. — BAKER, R. D., SEABURY, J. H., SCHNEIDEN, J. D.: Subcutaneous and cutaneous mucormycosis and subcutaneous phycomycosis. Lab. Invest. **11**, 1091 (1962). — BASSET, A., CAMAIN, R., LARIVIERE, M.: Trois cas Senegalais de phycomycose. Bull. Soc. Path. exot. **56**, 108 (1963). — BLACHÉ, R., DESTOMBES, P., NAZIMOFF, O.: Nouvelles mycoses sous-cutanees au Sud-Cameroun. Bull. Soc. Path. exot. **54**, 56 (1961). — BRAS, G., GORDON, G.G., EMMONS, C.W., PRENDERGAST, K.M., SUGAR, M.: A case of phycomycosis observed in Jamaica, infection with *Entomophthora coronata*. Amer. J. trop. Med. Hyg. **14**, 141 (1965). — BRIDGES, C. H., ROMANE, W. M., EMMONS, C.W.: Phycomycosis of horses caused by Entomophthora coronata. J. Amer. vet. med. Ass. **140**, 673 (1962). — BURKITT, D. P., WILSON, A. M. M., JELLIFFE, D. B.: Subcutaneous phycomycosis: A review of 31 cases seen in Uganda. Brit. med. J. i, 1669 (1964). — CLARK, B. M.: The epidemiology of phycomycosis. In: The Systemic Mycoses. Ciba Foundation. Ed. by A. E. W. WOLSTENHOLME and R. PORTER. London: J. A. Churchill, Ltd. 1968. — COUCH, J. N.: A new conidiobolus with sexual reproduction. Amer. J. Botany **26**, 119 (1939). — DRECHSLER, C.: A Basidiobolus producing elongated secondary conidia with adhesive breaks. Bull. Torrey botan. Club **74**, 403 (1947). — DRECHSLER, C.: Formation of sporangia from conidia and hyphal segments in an Indonesian Basidiobolus. Amer. J. Botany **45**, 632 (1958). — DWYER, G.K., CHANGUS, G.W.: Rhinomucormycosis resulting in fatal cerebral mucormycosis. Arch. Otolaryng. **67**, 619 (1958). — EDINGTON, G.M.: Phycomycosis in Ibadan, Western Nigeria. Two post mortem reports. Trans. roy. Soc. trop. Med. Hyg. **58**, 242 (1964). — ELEBUTE, E.A., OKUBADEJO, O.A.: Subcutaneous phycomycosis in West Africa. W. Afr. med. J. **11**, 217 (1962). — EMMONS, C.W., BRIDGES, C. H.: *Entomophthora coronata*, the etiologic agent of a phycomycosis of horses. Mycologia **53**, 307 (1961). — GAMET, A., BROTTES, H.: Processus pseudo-tumoral du a un phycomycete *Basidiobolus ranarum*. Bull. Soc. Path. exot. **56**, 285 (1963). — GREER, D.L., FRIEDMAN, L.: Studies on the genus Basidiobolus with reclassification of the species pathogenic for man. Sabouraudia **4**, 231 (1966). — GRUEBER, H. L. E.: Subcutaneous phycomycosis in India. J. Christ. med. Ass. India **41**, 284 (1966). — HARMAN, R. R. M., JACKSON, H., WILLIS, A. J. P.: Subcutaneous Phycomycosis in Nigeria. Brit. J. Derm. **76**, 408 (1964). — HOEPPLI, R.: Histological observations in experimental schistosomiasis japonica. Chir. med. J. **46**, 1179 (1932). — JELLIFFE, D.B., BURKITT, D., O'CONNOR, G.T., BEAVER, P.C.: Subcutaneous phycomycosis in an East African child. J. Pediat. **59**, 124 (1961). — JELLIFFE, D.B., WILSON, A.M.M., BURKITT, D.: Subcutaneous phycomycosis — response to oral iodide therapy. J. Pediat. **61**, 448 (1962). — JOE, L.K., ENG., N.I.T., POHAN, A., MEULEN, H. VAN DER, EMMONS, C.W.: Basidiobolus ranarum as a cause of subcutaneous mycosis in Indonesia. Arch. Derm. **74**, 378 (1956). — JOE, L.K., ENG, N.I.T.: Subcutaneous phycomycosis a new disease found in Indonesia. Ann. N.Y. Acad. Sci. **89**, 4 (1960). — KEVORKIAN, A.G.: Studies in the Entomophthoraceae. I. Observations on the genus *Conidiobolus*. J. Agric. Univ. Puerto Rico **21**, 191 (1937). — KJOLLER, A.: Microfungi isolated from tropical soils with notes on *Trichoderma viride* and *Delacroixia coronata*. Saertryk af Botanisk Tidsskrift **62**, 323 (1967). — KLOKKE, A.H., JOB, C.K., WARLOW, P.F.M.: Subcutaneous phycomycosis in India. Report of four patients with a review of the disease. Trop. geogr. Med. **18**, 20 (1966). — LASCH, E.E., LUONG, N'G.T., ROMANI, J.: A propos d'un cas de phycomycose en Republique de Haute-Volta. Med. Trop. **25**, 642 (1965). — LYNCH, J.B., HUSBAND, A.D.: Subcutaneous phycomycosis. J. clin. Path. **15**, 126 (1962). — MARTINSON, F.D.: Rhinophycomycosis. J. Laryng **77**, 691 (1963). — MARTINSON, F.D., CLARK, B.M.: Rhinophycomycosis entomophthorae in Nigeria. Amer. J. trop. Med. Hyg. **16**, 40 (1967). — MUKERJI, S., GORE, S.B., MANSUKHANI, S.H., KINI, V.M.: Subcutaneous phycomycosis. Indian J. Child Hlth. **11**, 502 (1962). — NEVILLE, G., MILLER, R.: (1962). Quoted by BURKITT et al. (1964). — PELOUX, Y., FOUCARD, H.: La phycomycose. Méd. trop. **24**, 447 (1964). — Renoirte, R., Vandepitte, J., Gatti, F., Werth, R.: Phycomycose nasofaciale (rhinophycomycose) due a *Entomophthora coronata*. Bull. Soc. Path. exot. **58**, 847 (1965). — Restrepo, M.A., Greer, D.L., Robledo, V.M., Diaz, G.C., Lopez, M.R., Bravo, R.C.: Subcutaneous phycomycosis: report of the first case observed in Columbia, South America. Amer. J. trop. Med. Hyg. **16**, 34 (1967). — Ridley, D.S., Wise, M.: Unusual disseminated infection with a phycomecete. J. Path. Bact. **90**, 675 (1965). — Smith, J.H., von Lichtenberg, F.: The Hoeppli phenomenon in schistosomiasis. Amer. J. Path. **50**, 993 (1967). — Srinivasan, M.C., Thirumalacher, M.J.: Basidiobolus species pathogenic for man. Sabouraudia **4**, 32 (1964). ~ Studies on Basidiobolus species from India with discussion on some of the characters used in the speciation of the genus. Mycopathologia (Den Haag) **33**, 56 (1967). — Symmers, W.St.C.: Histopathologic aspects of the pathogenesis of some opportunistic fungal infections, as exemplified in the pathology of aspergillosis and the phycomycetosis. Lab. Invest. **11**, 1073 (1962). ~ Symmers, W.St.C.: The occurrence of deep seated fungal infections in general hospital practice in Britain today. Proc. roy. Soc. Med. **57**, 405 (1964). — Stockdale, P.M.: (1964). Quoted by Clark (1967). — Straatsma, B.R., Zimmerman, L.E., Gass, J.D.M.: Phycomycosis. A clinicopathologic study of fifty-one cases. Lab. Invest. **11**, 963 (1962). — Villasco, J., Camain, R., Mazere, J., Orio, J., Segretain, G.: Description d'un deuxieme cas de phycomycose en cote d'Ivoire avec isolement de la souche. Bull. Soc. Path. exot. **59**, 781 (1966). — Williams, A.O., Nwabuebo, I.O.E., Ajumobi, A.: Pathology of phycomycosis due to Entomophthora and Basidiobolus species. (In press) (1968). — Zimmerman, L.E.: (1966). Quoted by Clark (1967).

Chromoblastomycosis[1]
Chromomycosis

RODOLFO CÉSPEDES F., San José, Costa Rica

With 4 Figures

Definition: Chromoblastomycosis is a chronic cutaneous mycosis, usually without tendency to generalization or deep invasion. It occurs most frequently on a lower extremity of an adult male and forms verrucous nodules.

The disease is called chromoblastomycosis because of the resemblance of the lesions to those of blastomycosis. Since the fungus does not multiply in the tissues by budding but by the formation of internal septa, some students of the disease prefer the term chromomycosis, but this has not been widely accepted. Unfortunately, chromomycosis implies that the disease is pigmented, whereas only the causative organism is pigmented.

Geographical Distribution and Incidence

The disease has been reported from all the continents, but most cases have been seen in the tropical regions of America and Africa. Cases reported from North America have been few.

In 1954 there were 21 cases reported from the United States, 9 of which were from Louisiana (GARDNER et al., 1964; HOWLES et al., 1954; MOORE et al., 1943; ROMERO and TREJOS, 1953). In Europe, cases have been reported only in the eastern regions (U.S.S.R. and Finland). A few cases have been seen in Australia, Asia and Japan (SASANO et al., 1961). Until 1964, only 3 cases of chromoblastomycosis had been reported in India (KLOKKE, 1964). In Costa Rica, a tropical country of 1,400,000 inhabitants, 140 cases had been diagnosed as of May, 1966, and 14 new cases per year were diagnosed from 1961—1966. In Madagascar, 129 cases have been studied in 4 years (BRYGOO and SEGRETAIN, 1960). In Colombia, Duque has collected 59 cases and observes about 8 new cases every year.

A survey of pathology laboratories in Latin America gives an idea of the number of cases diagnosed by histological examination each year: Buenos Aires, Argentina, 0; La Plata, Argentina, 0; Santos, Brazil, 1; Manaos (Amazonas), Brazil, 1; Recife, Pernambuco, Brazil, 1; Medellín, Colombia, 8; San José, Costa Rica, 14; Santiago, Chile, 0; Concepción, Chile, 0; Quito, Ecuador, 0; San Salvador, El Salvador, 2; Tegucigalpa, Honduras, 1; Chihuahua, México, 0; Monterrey, México, 1; Yucatán, México, 5; Durango, México, 2; México, D.F., México, 1; León, Nicaragua, 1; Panamá, Panamá, 6; Asunción, Paraguay, 3; Ica, Perú, 0; San Juan, Puerto Rico, 1; Aquadilla, Puerto Rico, 2; Valera, Venezuela, 0.

Since chromoblastomycosis is also diagnosed clinically without histological examination, the number of cases must be larger than that indicated in the above inquiry. On the other hand, in a few cases the diagnosis is not suspected clinically and the etiology of the lesion is a surprising finding on histological examination (KEMPSON and STERNBERG, 1963). The reported incidence of the disease will probably increase when the agricultural, developing countries have more and better laboratories for diagnosis, but it is apparent that countries of temperate climates have few cases.

1 Doctors JORGE SALAS, JORGE PIZA, SAEED MEKBEL and PEDRO MORERA, and Mrs. CECILIA CHACÓN, assisted in the preparation of the manuscript. The members of the Sociedad Latino Americana de Anatomía Patológica contributed by answering the questionnaire of the survey.

Epidemiology: The condition is usually seen in *adults* and only exceptionally in children. There is no racial predilection, since the disease has been seen in caucasians, orientals, Negroes and even American Indians. All authors agree that chromoblastomycosis is much more frequent in males than in females. In our case material the rate is 10 to 1. Predilection for the male sex is explained by the fact that men do more agricultural work than women and are more exposed to trauma and contamination. Most patients are field and forest workers. There is usually no history of a definite incident that initiated the disease. A few patients tell of antecedent injury with wood or thorns at farm work. Later they notice the appearance of an erythematous papule which then begins to enlarge and fungate. Fungi morphologically and serologically identical with *Phialophora verrucosa* have been isolated from wood pulp (Conant et al., 1954).

Chromoblastomycosis as a spontaneous disease has not been reported in animals. Experimentally, it can be induced in rabbits, mice and cold-blooded animals (Binford et al., 1952; Trejos, 1963).

Several different species of fungi have been implicated in this disease. It is probable that climatic conditions have something to do with the species of fungus that predominates in a given area. In Madagascar (Brygoo and Segretain, 1960) it was established that cases of chromoblastomycosis from an area with little rain (500—600 mm per year) are caused by *Cladosporium carrionii*, while cases from rainy areas (2,200—3,000 mm per year) are caused by *Fonsecaea pedrosoi*. The fungi live in wood or soil, and on passing to the human host probably undergo a process of adaptation for which some species must have a better potential. It is possible that the climatic characteristics of certain geographical regions foster the emergence of certain pathogenic species.

It has been shown (Binford et al., 1952) that *Cladosporium trichoides* inoculated into mice and rabbits by the intravenous route, causes fatal cerebral lesions. Intracutaneous inoculation of rats and mice, which are the most susceptible animals, does not produce chronic verrucous or papillomatous lesions, but abscesses that later rupture and heal spontaneously (Laskowski, 1960). With *H. pedrosoi* it has been possible to cause systemic infections. So, in chromoblastomycosis, as in other diseases, the species of fungus, the host route of inoculation, occupation, age and sex, are factors that determine the disease process.

Mycology: Chromoblastomycosis is caused by several pigmented fungi, all of which produce similar lesions in the human skin, so that it is not possible to identify the species by their appearance in tissues. There are five species that are pathogenic for man: 1. *Phialophora verrucosa*; 2. *Fonsecaea (Hormodendrum) pedrosoi*; 3. *Fonsecaea (Hormodendrum) compactum*; 4. *Fonsecaea (Hormodendrum) dermatitidis* and 5. *Cladosporium carrionii*. The etiological agents of chromoblastomycosis grow at room temperature on Sabouraud's medium. Colonies grow slowly and have a dark color, varying from gray to olive to black, with a velvety appearance. There are variants according to the species (Laboratory Procedures in Clinical Mycology 1964).

Carrion stated that the species which most frequently produces lesions of chromoblastomycosis is *Fonsecaea (Hormodendrum) pedrosoi*, but in the light of recent investigation (Brygoo and Segretain, 1960), especially in geographical pathology, this may have to be changed. In the opinion of Duque the classification of the species of fungi that cause chromoblastomycosis should be submitted to revision.

Mycological Diagnosis: A simple preparation of scrapings from the lesion in 10% KOH with warming on a glass slide, without the addition of any stain,

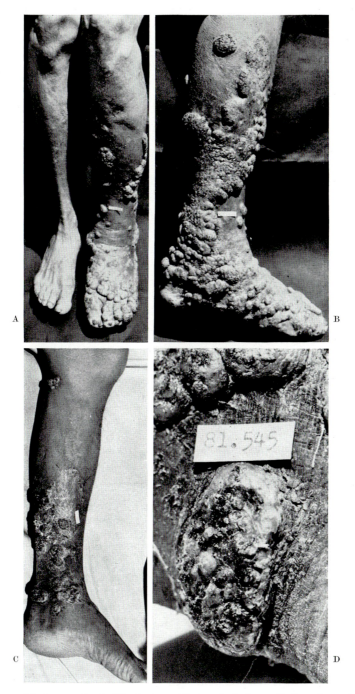

Fig. 1. Chromoblastomycosis. A. The lesions affect a single lower limb and consist of con-fluent, verrucous nodules. Note the edema of the skin between the nodules. B. Detail of A to show "mossy skin". C. A lesion of the lower half of the leg, with a metastasis to the inner aspect of the knee. D. A well circumscribed cauliflower lesion of the patient in A and B

suffices for diagnosis. Dark brown, spherical bodies with thick walls (Fig. 2 B) and often with septa are easily seen. Sometimes the fungus cell gives origin to germinative tubules of thick and septated mycelia (Fig. 2A). The dark brown, spherical bodies, measuring from 7 to 10 microns approximately, are also easily recognized in histological sections with any stain, and even without staining. The organisms are either in microabscesses or in giant cells (Fig. 4D and E). It is helpful to add penicillin and streptomycin to the media to suppress bacterial growth when culturing material from lesions.

For species identification, it is necessary to use meticulous cultural procedures with special media at room temperature, and also slide cultures that allow observation of the type of sporulation. There are four types of sporulation: phialophora, hormodendrum, cladosporium and acrotheca (Fig. 2C, D, E, F, G). All four types can be found in a single species! The work of typing takes weeks. Physiological characteristics are used to complete species identification.

Serological methods have no important practical application, but it is possible to demonstrate the existence of antibodies (EMMONS et al., 1963; FRENCH and RUSSELL, 1953; GAMET and BROTTES, 1963; GARDNER et al., 1964; HOWLES et al., 1954; KEMPSON and STERNBERG, 1963; KOKKE, 1964; Laboratory Procedures in Clinical Mycology, 1964; LASKOWSKI, 1960). Experimental inoculation of rats, rabbits and cold-blooded animals is not used in clinical practice for mycological diagnosis.

Pathogenesis: A history of local trauma is present in only a small number of cases of chromoblastomycosis. Most patients do not seek medical care until the lesion has been present for many years and they do not recall a history of trauma. The disease spreads locally over a period of several years. Sometimes satellite lesions appear, with unaffected skin surrounding the original lesion. These satellites are probably the result of lymphatic spread. No regional lymph node involvement has been reported except in cases with superimposed bacterial infection. On the other hand, there have been reports of lymph node involvement by chromoblastomycosis, without skin lesions (TSAI et al., 1966). The process rarely invades the subcutaneous tissue, a fact which allows plastic surgeons to resect the lesion entirely (Fig. 4A, B). Usually extensive lesions are found in only one lower limb (Fig. 1A). It is infrequent that other cutaneous regions are affected. The incubation period in man is difficult to establish, for a history of antecedent trauma seldom exists. TREJOS (personal communication) reported a case of autoinoculation. The lesions appeared a few days later, and, at the time of resection several weeks later, measured 11 mm in diameter and 2 mm in depth. Microscopically there were already typical microabscesses and fungal cells. We have also seen metastatic lesions appear 15—20 cm from the primary site, 90 days after surgical resection of chromoblastomycosis (Fig. 1C). These attained a diameter of 35 mm over a period of 5 months.

The disease sometimes takes 15—20 years completely to involve a limb. That it eventually involves an entire limb suggests that the microorganisms do not provoke antibody formation in sufficient amount as to limit the spread of the infection. The fact that the disease does not involve the viscera is in favor of a low virulence of the causative organism. Most cases reported as cerebral abscesses, or hepatic granulomas of chromoblastomycotic origin, are probably examples of cladosporiosis (BINFORD et al., 1952; RILEY and MANN, 1960; SASANO et al., 1961; SUGAWARA et al., 1964; WATSON, 1962). Rarely, chromoblastomycosis is associated with a deep mycosis; SAENZ and MORERA reported a case of South American blastomycosis with pulmonary involvement in a patient who had chromoblastomycosis of a lower extremity for over 30 years. The blastomycosis was cured by medical treatment, whereas the chromoblastomycosis progressed to the point of

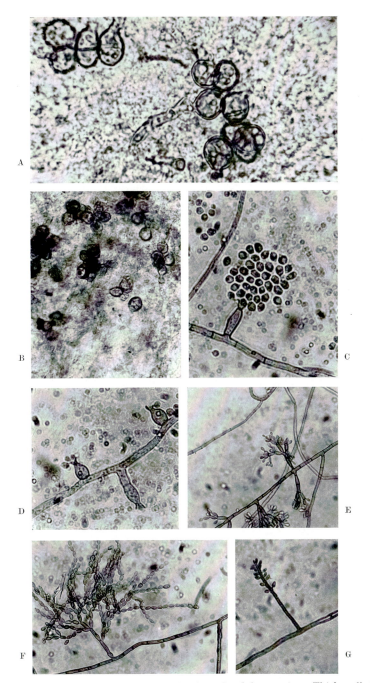

Fig. 2. Chromoblastomycosis. A. Direct examination of nodule scrapings. Thick walled fungus cells. Septate cells are seen in the upper left corner. A hypha is growing from one of the fungus cells. B. Same specimen as in A, seen under lower power; clusters of dark fungus cells. C. "Slide culture". Mature phialide of *Phialophora verrucosa*. D. Young phialides. E. Hormo-dendrum type of sporulation. F. Cladosporium type of sporulation. G. Acrotheca type of sporulation

making amputation necessary. Recurrence of the lesion appeared in the stump several months later.

No cases of *transmission* of the disease from man to man are known, nor are there reported cases of spontaneous infection in animals.

As stated before, antibodies may be detected in the serum of chromoblasto-mycosis patients, by means of a complement fixation test (LASKOWSKI, 1960). In clinical practice, no skin reaction is used for the diagnosis of the disease.

Gross and Microscopic Appearances: The basic lesion is a warty, discrete, firm nodule (Fig. 1D). It may be single or multiple, sometimes coalescing to give the appearance of "a mossy skin" (Fig. 1B). The skin surface may or may not be ulcerated and may be keratinized. The intervening skin may be edematous (Fig. 1A) or atrophic; usually it is hard and cyanotic. The early single lesion looks much like that of cutaneous leishmaniasis or chronic sporotrichosis (Fig. 3A). If there is superimposed bacterial infection, the surface of the lesion is wet with serosanguineous or purulent, foul-smelling exudate.

If resection is performed and the defect covered with a skin graft, the lesion often recurs in the grafted skin in the following months. This recurrence does not preclude a new resection, followed by another skin graft.

The low power microscopic appearance shows marked papillomatosis, hyper-keratosis and acanthosis (Fig. 4C). There is a granulomatous infiltrate- both in the upper and lower dermis, but the hypodermis is spared (Fig. 4B). This allows for radical surgery. The edges of the lesion are sharply defined (Fig. 4A, B). The dermal granulomas may resemble tubercles, with clusters of epithelioid cells surrounding brown fungus cells, single or multiple (Fig. 4E). Septa within the fungus spherules are not always seen in histologic sections; sometimes only peri-pheral portions of the fungus cells are visible; but the brown color facilitates their identification. Microabscesses are also seen, and consist of masses of polymorpho-nuclear leukocytes surrounded by histiocytes or epidermal epithelial cells. Within these abscesses one may see the chromoblastomycotic spherules (Fig. 4D). Among the tubercles and microabscesses there is a pleomorphic infiltrate composed of lymphocytes and plasma cells, less than in leishmaniasis, some eosinophils, multinucleated giant cells, either of LANGHANS or foreign-body type, and a slight fibroblastic proliferation. Fungus cells are often seen within the giant cells. Chromoblastomycosis does not usually tend to spontaneous healing, and may show slight fibrosis and a scant blood vessel proliferation. Although the usual picture is that of epidermal hyperplasia, atrophic areas are seen. One may observe hyphae and germinal tubes within the debris of the horny layer.

Differential Diagnosis: Grossly, chromoblastomycosis appears as a verrucal dermatitis which may be confused with leishmaniasis, chronic forms of sporo-trichosis, North American and South American blastomycosis; less frequently, it may have to be distinguished from yaws, syphilis, leprosy and tuberculosis. The differential diagnosis cannot be made grossly. It requires biopsy and culture. When fungus cells are present, the microscopic diagnosis is easily made although chromoblastomycosis and leishmaniasis sometimes occur together (MEDINA and BORELLI, 1958).

Keloidal blastomycosis (Lobo's disease) may be easily ruled out because of the absence of epithelial hyperplasia and the presence of marked fibrous proliferation, as well as abundant non-pigmented organisms. In leishmaniasis, epithelial hyper-plasia is less severe than in chromoblastomycosis; the granulomas show histio-cytes and plasma cells, but there are no abscesses. If no parasites are seen and the microscopic picture is not diagnostic, the formalin-picrofuchsin stain of GALLEGO may be helpful in the search for organisms of leishmaniasis.

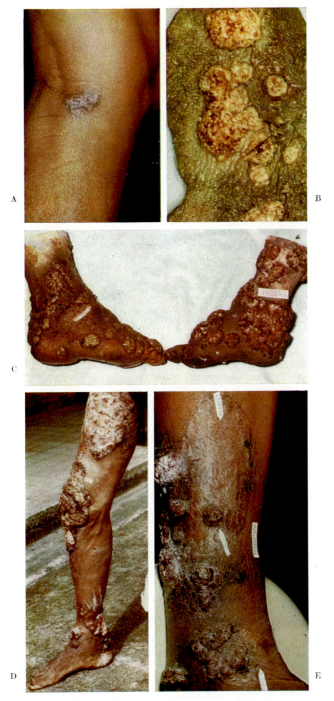

Fig. 3. Chromoblastomycosis. A. Young lesion (90 days), quite similar to those of leishmaniasis and sporotrichosis. B. Resected verrucous nodules. C. Two amputated feet. D. Widespread lesions involving the entire lower extremity. E. Recurrence after resection; the arrows point to the skin grafts and the new lesions

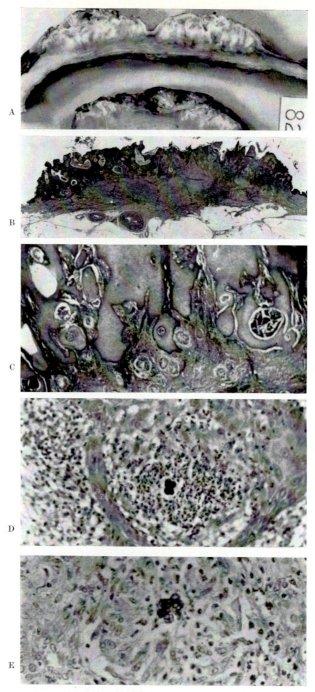

Fig. 4. Chromoblastomycosis. A. Section through verrucous nodules. Note the well-defined demarcation. B. Same specimen as in A; section stained with H & E (2×). The inflammatory infiltrate does not extend into the subcutaneous tissue. The nodule is sharply limited. C. Low-power microscopic field showing hyperkeratosis, ancanthosis, papillomatosis, and abscesses, both "intraepidermal" and dermal. D. Microabscess surrounded by epidermis and containing spherules of chromoblastomycosis. E. Tubercle made up of epitheloid cells showing central fungus cells, one of which is septate

The most difficult differential diagnosis is between chromoblastomycosis and sporotrichosis when no microorganisms are seen in the sections. It must be borne in mind that the predominant cell in *sporotrichosis* is the *neutrophil*, and eosinophils are absent. In *chromoblastomycosis*, on the other hand, microabscesses are surrounded by *histiocytes*, and there are eosinophils. These criteria are not enough to establish a diagnosis with certainty. Better results are obtained by multiple sectioning in search of the causative agent, and also the periodic acid-Schiff stain, which may bring out the microorganism in cases of sporotrichosis. Direct examination and culture may also be of great help. South American and North American blastomycosis show characteristic blastospores which are easily seen with special stains.

The tuberculoid form of leprosy may be confused with chromoblastomycosis; however, there is neither epithelial hyperplasia nor papillomatosis, nor microabscesses, but there are tubercles, or granulomas (ASH and SPITZ, 1945; BAKER, 1966; FRENCH and RUSSEL, 1953; GAMET and BROTTES, 1963; THYS, 1964). Syphilis has a characteristic microscopic picture and no tendency to abscess formation.

Lastly, there remains the problem of cutaneous granulomas without demonstrable etiologic agents. This cannot be solved by the pathologist. Sometimes immunologic methods are of value.

Clinical Picture: In the tropics, the patient usually seeks medical care only after many years of evolution of the disease that began as a papule, then became a wart and spread slowly, in spite of treatment with ointments and electrofulguration. Finally, the patient requests an amputation, not because of the pain or itching, but because of the repugnant appearance of the lesion, which he considers depressing and incurable (Fig. 3 C). When the disease is widespread, and there is involvement of a whole limb, nothing can be done. If it affects a foot, no shoe can be worn.

Clinical Case: A farmer, aged 74 years, had had chromoblastomycosis of his left foot and the lower third of his left leg for 5 years. The lesions were completely resected in December, 1965. Skin grafts measuring 15 by 17 cm were applied to the foot and medial aspect of the leg (Fig. 3 E). Three months later there was recurrence of the mycosis in the lower third of the leg, with progressive invasion of the grafts; a month later a metastatic lesion appeared on the medial aspect of the knee (Fig. 1 C). Photographs 1 C and 3 E were taken in August, 1966, eight months after the operation. The lesions were again completely excised, including subcutaneous tissues (Fig. 3 B and Fig. 4A, B).

A new skin graft was performed. No recurrence had occured after 4 years.

Prognosis: The disease does not heal spontaneously, and evolves slowly over a period of 15—20 years. It does not kill or spread to internal organs. If diagnosed in time, radical resection down to hypodermis may be curative. Resections not sufficiently deep are commonly followed by recurrences. No satisfactory drug therapy is available.

References

AKÜN, R.: Eine chromoblastomykoseähnliche Pilzkrankheit beim Pferde. Zbl. Path. **90**, 294 (1953). — ASH, SPITZ: Pathology of Tropical Diseases, an Atlas. Philadelphia: W. B. Saunders Co. 1945. — AUDEBAU, G., ESCUDIÉ, A., COURMES, E.: Les Mycoses Humaines en Guadeloupe. Premiers cas de chromoblastomycose et de sporotrichose. Résultats d'une enquete histoplasminique. Bull. Soc. Path. exot. **57**, 1012 (1964). — BAKER, R. D.: Fungus Infections. In: ANDERSON's Pathology, Fifth ed. St. Louis: C. V. Mosby Co. 1966. — BINFORD, C. H., THOMPSON, R. K., GORHAM, M. E., EMMONS, C. W.: Mycotic brain abscess due to *Cladosporium trichoides*, a new species. Amer. J. clin. Path. **22**, 535 (1952). — BRYGOO, E. R., SEGRETAIN, G.: Étude clinique epidemiologique et mycologique de la chromoblastomycose a Madagascar. Bull. Soc. Path. exot. **53**, 443 (1960). — CARRION, A. L.: The specific fungi of chromoblastomycosis. Puerto Rico J. publ. Hlth **15**, 340 (1940). — CONANT, N. F., SMITH, D. T., BAKER,

R.D., Callaway, J.L., Martin, D.S.: Manual of Clinical Mycology, Second ed. Philadelphia and London: W.B. Saunders Co. 1954. — Duque, O.: Cromoblastomicosis. Revisión general y estudio de la enfermedad en Colombia. Antioquía méd. 11, 499 (1961). — Emmons, C.W., Binford, C.H., Utz, J.P.: Medical Mycology. Philadelphia: Lea & Febiger 1963. — French, A.J., Russell, S.R.: Chromoblastomycosis. Report of a case recognized in Michigan, apparently contracted in South Carolina. A.M.A. Arch. Derm. Syph. 67, 129 (1953). — Gamet, A., Brottes, M.: Les chromoblastomycoses au Cameron. Bull. Soc. Path. exot. 56, 117 (1963). — Gardner, J.T., Pace, B.F., Freeman, R.G., et al.: Chromoblastomycosis in Texas. Report of four cases. Tex. St. J. Med. 60, 913 (1964). — Howles, J.K., Kennedy, C.B., Garvin, E., Brueck, J.W., Buddingh, G.J.: Chromoblastomycosis: Report of nine cases from a single area in Louisiana. A.M.A. Arch. Derm. Syph. 69, 83 (1954). — Kempson, R.L., Sternberg, W.H.: Chronic subcutaneous abscesses caused by pigmented fungi, a lesion distinguishable from cutaneous chromoblastomycosis. Amer. J. clin. Path. 39, 598 (1963). — Klokke, A.H.: Chromomycosis. J. Indian med. Ass. 43, 340 (1964). — Laboratory Procedures in Clinical Mycology. Dept. of the U.S. Army Technical Manual, Feb., 1964. — Laskowski, L.F., Jr.: Chromomycosis (chromoblastomycosis, dermatitis verrucosa). Basic techniques and newer concepts in clinical diagnostic medical mycology. Catholic Hospital Association, St. Louis, Mo., 153—157, Oct., 1960. — Martin, D.S., Baker, R.D., Conant, N.F.: Case of verrucous dermatitis caused by *Hormodendrum pedrosoi* (chromoblastomycosis) in North Carolina. Amer. J. trop. Med. 16, 593 (1936). — Medina, Rafael, Borelli, Dante: Leishmaniasis tegumentaria asociada a cromomicosis. Acta méd. Venez. 6, 202 (1958). — Moore, M., Cooper, Z.K., Weiss, R.S.: Chromomycosis (chromoblastomycosis), report of two cases. J. Amer. med. Ass. 122, 1237 (1943). — Moss, E.S., McQuown, A.L.: Atlas of Medical Mycology. Baltimore: Williams & Wilkins Co. 1960. — Niño, F.L.: Lecciones de Micología y Micopatología Médica. Cajica, Buenos Aires, 1959. — Romero, A., Trejos, A.: La cromoblastomicosis en Costa Rica. Rev. Biol. trop. (S. José) 1, 95 (1953). — Riley, O., Mann, S.H.: Brain abscess caused by *Cladosporium trichoides*. Amer. J. clin. Path. 33, 525 (1960). — Sáenz, L., Morera, P.: Sobre un caso de blastomicosis suramericana asociada a cromomicosis. Acta méd. costarric. 6, 55 (1963). — Salomon, L.M., Berman, H.: Amphotericin B and electrodesiccation for chromoblastomycosis. Arch. Derm. 87, 492 (1963). — Sasano. N., Okamoto, T., Takahashi, T., Suzuki, S.: An autopsy case of primary chromoblastomycosis arising from the internal organs. Dark-brown granulomas in the liver and the brain without skin symptoms, observed in a smoking child 3 years old. Tohoku J. exp. Med. 73, 180 (1961). — Simpson, F.W., Harington, C., Barnetson, E.J.: Chromoblastomycosis: A report of six cases. J. Path. Bact. 55, 191 (1943). — Solano, E.: Cromomicosis. Acta méd. costarric. 9, 77 (1966). — Sugawara, M., Sobajima, Y., Tamura, H.: A case of generalized chromoblastomycosis. Acta path. jap. 14, 239 (1964). — Thys, A.: Personal observation on the histopathology of Congolese mycoses. Ann. Soc. belge Méd. trop. 44, 887 (1964). — Trejos, A.: *Cladosporium carrionii* n. sp. and the problem of Cladosporia isolated from chromoblastomycosis. Rev. Biol. trop. 2, 75 (1954). ~ Cromoblastomicosis experimental en Bufo marinus. Rev. Biol. trop. 1, 39 (1963). ~ Communicación personal. — Tsai, C.Y., Lu, C., Wang, L.T., Hsu, T.L., Sung, J.L.: Systemic Chromoblastomycosis due to *Hormodendrum dermatitidis* (Kano) Conant. Report of the first case in Taiwan. Amer. J. clin. Path. 46, 99 (1966). — Watson, K.C.: Cerebral chromoblastomycosis. J. Path. Bact. 84, 233 (1962). — Zapater, R.C.: Atlas de diagnóstico micológico (aplicación del Laboratorio) VI + 251. Buenos Aires: El Ateneo 1962.

Cladosporiosis of the Central Nervous Tissue

Oscar Duque, Medellín, Colombia

With 17 Figures

Definition: Cladosporiosis may be defined as infection of the central nervous system and meninges by *Cladosporia*, and the fungi causing chromoblastomycosis (*Cladosporium, Hormodendrum, Phialophora, Fonsecaea*).

Historical: In 1911 Guido Banti presented to the Academia Medico Fisico Fiorentina the case of a woman who died with symptoms of brain tumor. The autopsy disclosed multiple nodular dark brown areas in the cerebrum and cerebellum formed by granulomatous inflammation with necrosis. In these lesions brown septate hyphae and spherical forms of a fungus were found. Cultures of this microorganism were studied by Saccardo who published its description and biological characteristics in 1912 with the name of *Torula bantiana*. It produced brain lesions when inoculated into rabbits. The observations of Banti and Saccardo remained largely ignored until Borelli (1960), and Stigliani called attention to it. In 1952 Binford and associates described the case of a man who suffered from headache and drowsiness. An abscess was found in the left frontal lobe of his brain which again consisted of a granulomatous inflammation with necrosis and purulent material from which a fungus was grown. This was studied by Emmons (in Binford et al.) who noted that by its morphology and brown pigment it should be classified with *Cladosporia*. He named it *Cladosporium trichoides* "signifying its hyphal growth in human brain tissue". There can be little doubt today that both the cases of Banti and Binford were caused by the same fungus. The figures of *T. bantiana*, published by Saccardo, are very similar to those of *Cl. trichoides*; both are highly pathogenic for laboratory animals, and both grew well at 37 °C, unlike other species of saprophtic *Cladosporia* which are not thermophilic. Emmons has pointed out that the spore size of *Torula bantiana*, as registered by Saccardo, is larger than that of *Cladosporium trichoides*; however, one wonders if the difference could not be within the limits of strain variation. Borelli (1960) proposed a new combination to designate the species: *Cladosporium bantianum* (Saccardo, 1912; Borelli, 1960). Both names will be used here to avoid the question of priority which will have to be solved by the proper authorities.

A total of 31 acceptable cases of cladosporiosis has been reported (see Table 1). Fourteen of the cases were caused by *C. trichoides* making this species the most important agent of cladosporiosis (Banti, Binford, King, McGill, Dereymäker, Watson, Watson and Lines, Garcin (1957), Riley, Barnola, Duque, Coudert, Chevrel, Dastur). Two cases were caused by *Hormodendrum pedrosoi* (Fukushiro, Lucasse); the fungus isolated from the case of Lucasse was studied by Vanbreuseghem who described it as *C. trichoides* but commented that it produced the acrotheca type of sporulation. Borelli (1956) re-examined this fungus and concluded that it was *H. pedrosoi*. The cases of Shimazono, and Tsai were due to *Hormodendrum dermatitidis*. *Cladosporium gougeroti* was the causative agent in the case of Aufdermaur. In the other 12 cases the fungus was not isolated but diagnosis was established by the morphology and characteristic brown color of the fungi in tissue sections (Bonne, two Indonesian cases; Garcin, 1949; Franca-Netto, Bobra, Manson, Symmers, Horn, Sasano, Duque, Warot, Bagchi). The case of Wybel, cited by some authors, is doubtful as no mention is made of the fungus being pigmented.

Table 1. *Reported cases of cladosporiosis*

Case No. Age, Sex	Chief Manifestations	Associated Conditions	Outcome and Duration	Post Mortem Findings			Organism Responsible
				Central Nervous System	Meningitis	Other Organs	
Case 1 43, F	Symptoms of brain tumor. Mental deterioration. Vomiting, headache, coma	Patient was deaf	Death 6 months after onset	Multiple, melanoma-like granulomas; brain and cerebellum		Nothing of note	*Torula bantiana*
Case 2 23, F	Fever, paralysis of left arm and leg, and R. sixth and seventh cranial nerves		Death a few weeks after onset of symptoms	Meningeal and pontine granulomas	Nodular	Nothing of note	Not isolated
Case 3 20, M	Cachexia; right hemiplegia; papilloedema	Scabies; decubitus ulcer	Death 1 month after admission	Hemorrhagic left frontal granuloma	?	Nothing of note	Not isolated
Case 4 37, M	Fever, headache; R. hemiplegia, papilloedema, leucocytosis, cachexia		Death 8.5 mos. after onset of symptoms	Ependymitis. Discrete lesions in left frontal lobe. Hydrocephalus	Nodular thickening of basal meninges	Not examined	Not isolated
Case 5 22, M	Headache, drowsiness, fever, leucocytosis		Free from symptoms 2 years after operation	3 cm left frontal abscess shelled out	No		*Cl. trichoides*
Case 6 47, M	One month history of headache, fever, dysarthria; R. hemiplegia, convulsions	Arteriosclerosis, hypertension. Left otorrhea	Death about 3 months after first symptoms	Large left frontal lobe abscess and multiple secondary abscesses	?	Arteriosclerosis	*Cl. trichoides*
Case 7 34, M	Fever, headache, convulsions, diplopia, meningism, paresis		Death 1 year after onset of symptoms		Chronic sclerosing	Old rheumatic mitral valve disease	Not isolated
Case 8 42, M	3 mos. history of headache, tiredness, disorientation; ataxia, meningism		Death 4 months after onset of symptoms	Small abscesses in brain	Basal meningitis	Hyphae in lungs (contaminant?)	*Cl. gougeroti*
Case 9 10, M	4 mos. history of fever, anemia, convulsions, papilloedema	Filariasis	Death 9 months after first symptoms	Ependymitis and small brain abscesses	Basal meningitis	Nothing of note	*H. pedrosoi* (BORELLI, 1956)
Case 10 27, F	4 mos. history of vomiting, headache, meningism, fever, R. hemiplegia		Death about 10 mos. after onset of symptoms	2 chronic left lobe abscesses. Two secondary abscesses		No autopsy	*Cl. trichoides*
Case 11 32, M	5 mos. history of headache, vomiting, papilloedema, ataxia, failing sight		Death 7 months after onset of symptoms	Fibrino purulent basal meningitis (operation)		No autopsy	*Cl. trichoides*

Case	Symptoms / History	Predisposing conditions	Course	Brain lesion	Post surgical infection of meninges	Other findings	Organism
Case 12 37, F	One mos. history of R. hemiplegia; Jacksonian epilepsy	Old laceration of scalp syphilis, skin abscess	Death 7.5 months after first symptoms	Left parietal abscess (removed), Large secondary abscess		Lung infarct	Cl. trichoides
Case 13 8, F	6 mos. history of chromoblasto-mycosis of the face; then headache, fever, paralysis of increasing severity	chromoblasto-mycosis of skin of face	Death 12 mos. after appearance of skin lesions	Multiple dark green granulomas in brain, cerebellum, pons	Nodular meningitis. Arteritis	Autopsy confined to CNS	H. pedrosoi
Case 14 30, M	Fever, headache, meningism, mental deterioration		Death about 24 days	2 cm encysted abscess in right frontal lobe	No	Horseshoe kidney	"Hormodendr." probably Cl. trichoides
Case 15 3, M	Fever; R. hemiplegia; swollen abdomena, leucocytosis	Neglected, smoking, allotriophagic child	Death 1 month after onset of symptoms	Multiple disseminated dark brown nodules	Nodular basal meningitis	Dark brown nodules in liver, kidney and lymph nodes	Not isolated
Case 16 57, M	10 mos. history of mental deterioration. Hemiplegic strokes; papilloedema	Hypertension	Sudden death 10 mos. after onset of symptoms	3 cm left parieto-occipital abscess with extension to chiasm	?	Arteriosclerosis and hypertension	Not isolated
Case 17 44, M	2 weeks history of weakness of l. limbs, then l. hemiplegia, meningism		Death 6 weeks after first symptoms	Large right occipital, left frontal and temporal abscesses	No	Pulmonary emphysema. Bantu siderosis	Not isolated
Case 18 22, F	1 month history of fever, loss of weight associated with polyarteritis. Left hemiplegia following cortisone therapy	Polyarteritis nodosa, cortisone treatment	Death about 5 mos. after first symptoms	Right fronto-parietal abscess (infected infarct ?)	No	Healed and healing lesions of arteritis nodosa	Not isolated
Case 19 68, F	Fever, opisthotonus, coma	Mild diabetes. Neurogenic hyper-natremia	Death within 3 mos. after onset of symptoms	Multiple nodular granulomatous lesions	No	Left fibrinous exudate with hyphae	Not isolated
Case 20 24, M	3 episodes of seizures; cough, fever, headache, vomiting	Dental caries. Scarred right ear drum	Well 3 mos. after operation	Small purulent mass in right frontal lobe	No		Cl. trichoides
Case 21 23, F	3 months history of headache. Left hemiplegia		Progressive worsening sudden death	Gray black area surrounding abscess cavity of 5 cm r. fronto parietal	No	Small mycotic abscess in right lung	Cl. trichoides (brain and lung)

Reported cases by:

1 = BANTI (1911); 2 = BONNE et al. (1948); 3 = BONNE et al. (1948); 4 = GARCIN et al. (1949); 5 = BINFORD et al. (1952); 6 = KING and COLLETE (1952); 7 = FRANCA NETTO et al. (1953); 8 = AUFDERMAUR et al. (1954); 9 = LUCASSE et al. (1954); 10 = SEGRETAIN (1955) and GARCIN (1957); 11 = DEREYMAKER and DE SOMER (1955); 12 = MCGILL and BRUECK (1956); 13 = NISHI (1956), OKUDAIRA (1956) and FUKUSHIRO (1957); 14 = WATSON and LINES (1957); 15 = SASANO et al. (1958, 1961); 16 = BOBBA (1958); 17 = MANSON (1958); 18 = SYMMERS (1960); 19 = HORN et al. (1960); 20 = RILEY and MANN (1960); 21 = BARNOLA and ANGULO (1961)

Table 1 (continued)

Case No. Age, Sex	Chief Manifestations	Associated Conditions	Outcome and Duration	Post Mortem Findings			Organism Responsible
				Central Nervous System	Meningitis	Other Organs	
Case 22 22, M	Headache, fever, vomiting 20 day, then vertigo, staggering gait, anisocoria	"sore throat"	Discharged 1 month after operation	Abscess in left parietal lobe	No		Cl. trichoides
Case 23 29, M	Laceration of face and scalp 9 mos. prior to admission. Headache, vomiting, ataxia, dysarthria, meningism, papilloedema		Death 9 mos. after accidental laceration of scalp	Granular ependymitis Hydrocephalus	Basal granular meningitis	Autopsy confined to CNS	Not isolated
Case 24 40, M	2 episodes of epileptic seizures. Paresis of left face and limbs; vomiting, meningism	Sarcoidosis	Death 3 mos. after first symptoms	3 black nodules in right frontal lobe resected surgically		No autopsy	Not isolated
Case 25 25, M	15 days history of facial paralysis, dysarthria; then aphasia, R. hemiplegia		Death 3 weeks after onset; 5 days after operation	3 cm abscess in left frontal lobe		No autopsy	Cl. trichoides
Case 26 54, M	2 months history of fever, headache, paresis, vomiting, convulsions, papilloedema		Death 10 mos. after first symptoms	Mass in right parietal area with multiple abscesses; resected			Not isolated
Case 27 18, M	18 months history of headache, impaired vision, dizziness, meningism, papilloedema	Right middle ear infection, 3 years prior to admission	Discharged in good condition after operation. No follow up	Large abscess in right temporo-occipital area			Cl. trichoides
Case 28 12, M	Syndrome of intracraneal hypertension		Well 10 mos. after operation	Multiple abscesses in left temporal lobe	No		Cl. trichoides
Case 29 30, F	Headache, vomiting, facial paralysis, confusion, nystagmus, left hemiplegia		Death about 3 mos. after operation	Multiple disseminated abscesses	Nodular basal meningitis	Slight fibrosis of pancreas	H. dermatitidis
Case 30 19, F	Weakness of right leg. Epileptic seizures; pyramidal signs; involvement of cranial nerves	Jaundice and lymph node enlargement 3 years prior to admission	Death 7 mos. after onset of neurological symptoms	Large greenish nodule in left frontal lobe. Multiple disseminated nodules	Basal and spinal	Mycotic granulomas in liver, kidney pancreas, lymph n.	H. dermatitidis
Case 31 24, M	Paresthesia, headache, vomiting, hemiparesis, convulsions, leucocytosis	Scaly skin eruption from which "Cladosporium sp." was recovered	Death about 8 mos. after first symptoms	3 encapsulated purulent nodules in left fronto-parietal region		No autopsy	Cl. trichoides (brain), Cladosporium sp. (skin)

Reported cases by:

22 = Duque (1961); 23 = Duque (1961); 24 = Warot et al. (1961); 25 = Chevrel et al. (1962); 26 = Bagchi et al. (1962); 27 = Watson (1962); 28 = Coudert et al. (1962); 29 = Shimazono et al. (1963); 30 = Tsai et al. (1966); 31 = Dastur et al. (1966).

Epidemiology: Cases of cladosporiosis have been reported from Europe, North and South America, Africa, India, Indonesia, Japan and Taiwan. Both sexes are about equally affected. The disease occurred in a Japanese smoking child of 3 years (SASANO), and in an 8 year old Japanese girl (FUKUSHIRO), but most of the cases were in adults. White, negro, oriental and mixed races are susceptible.

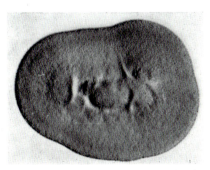

Fig. 1. *Cladosporium trichoides* (bantianum). Three weeks old culture in Sabouraud's glucose agar at room temperature

Mycology: *Cladosporium trichoides* grows well in Sabouraud's glucose agar at room temperature producing black-grey to olive-brown velvety colonies that may reach 4 cm in diameter after a month in a plate culture; folds may be present in older colonies (Fig. 1). Unlike other *Cladosporia*, *C. bantianum* grows well at 37°C and has no proteolytic action on Loeffler's medium. In culture, hyphae are brown, septate, 1—2 μ in diameter, smooth and doubly walled. Conidiophores

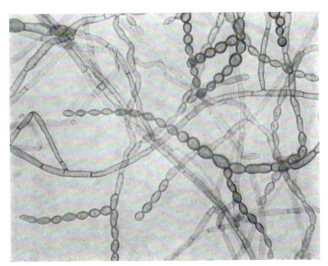

Fig. 2. *Cladosporium trichoides*, slide culture

vary in length, straight or shield shaped, bearing one or several long, branched chains of elliptical or fusiform conidia 2—4 μ in diameter, 5—20 μ in height; younger conidia are produced at the ends of chains, basal conidia may be septate (Figs. 2 and 3). In pus from the lesions, the fungus appears as olive green to brown septate branched hyphae with bulbous extremities (Fig. 4). In tissues the hyphal phase is abundant (Fig. 5), but vesicular and large spherical forms, like the "sclerotic cells" of chromoblastomycosis of the skin may be also observed (Fig. 6).

C.trichoides is highly pathogenic for mice, rats, guinea pigs, and rabbits when inoculated into these animals from cultures by intracerebral or intravenous routes. It kills mice within 5—25 days, growing so abundantly in the brain that the

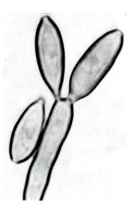

Fig. 3. *C.trichoides*, slide culture. Conidiophore with two terminal conidia. ×2500

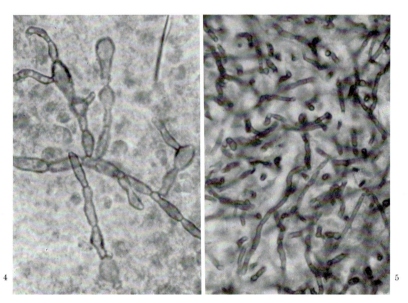

Fig. 4. Septated, branched hyphae with bulbous extremities of *C.trichoides* as observed in pus from a brain abscess. Unstained preparation. ×600

Fig. 5. Abundant hyphal growth of *C.trichoides* in brain lesion. H & E, ×600

lesions present a characteristic black greenish color (Fig. 7). Direct inoculations into animals of material from the human brain lesions is less successful. The fungus is distinctly neurotropic; when inoculated intravenously the main lesions are always in the brain although limited growth may be observed in other organs. Intraperitoneal inoculations in new born mice (DUQUE, 1961, 1963) produce small

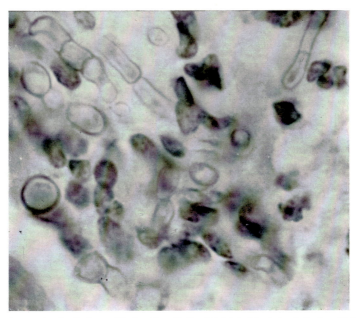

Fig. 6. Hyphae and spheric forms ("sclerotic cells") of *C. trichoides* in brain lesion. H & E, ×1250

granulomatous nodules in the serosa and severe lesions in the brain. Because of the close morphological similarity between *C. trichoides* and one of the etiological agents of chromoblastomycosis, *Cladosporium carionii*, the question arose as to whether or not other dematiaceous fungi could cause brain lesions also. In 1958 Iwata reported that the fungus isolated from the case of Fukushiro, an 8 year old Japanese girl with chromoblastomycotic lesions of the skin of the face and metastatic lesions in the brain, was *Hormodendrum pedrosoi*. Then, Duque, and Felger demonstrated experimentally that *H. pedrosoi*, *H. compactum*, *Phialophora verrucosa*, and *H. carrionii* produce brain lesions when inoculated intracerebrally or intravenously in new born or cortisone treated mice. The neurotropism of these fungi and the severity of the brain lesions that they produce varied from very intense with *H. pedrosoi* to mild and limited with *C. carrionii*, but, unlike *C. bantianum*, these microorganisms did not reach the brain when inoculated intra-peritoneally. The case of Aufdermaur caused by *Cladosporium gougeroti*, and those of Shimazono, and Tsai due to *Hormodendrum dermatitidis* enlarged the number of dematiaceous fungi causing chromoblastomycosis that may also infect the central nervous system.

Cladosporium trichoides cannot be differentiated in tissue sections from *H. pedrosoi* or the other fungi of chromoblastomycosis. All of these microorganisms produce pigmented hyphae and spherical forms in the lesions. They are Schiff positive and stain black with Grocott's methenamine silver stain, but these special stains offer little advantage as the fungi are readily demonstrable in unstained or in ordinary H & E preparations because of their brown color. Cultures are necessary to establish the identity of the species in this group of fungi. Studies of *C. trichoides* and *C. carrionii* with immuno-fluorescence methods by Al Doory showed that both fungi react with a number of dematiaceous species in addition to the homologous organism, but selective dilution and absorption resulted in conjugates specific for each of the two species.

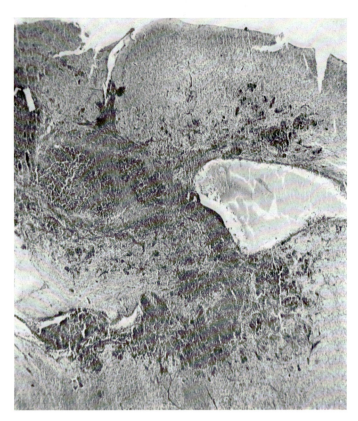

Fig. 7. Brain lesions produced by intracerebral inoculation of *C.trichoides* in a new born mouse. H & E, ×20

Pathogenesis: The portal of entry of *Cladosporium trichoides* is unknown. Direct inoculation was suspected in the cases of McGill and Duque, which had sustained trauma to the face and scalp. In three cases (King, Riley, Watson) there was inflammation or healed lesions of one of the ears, and Banti's patient was deaf. King isolated *C.bantianum* from the inner ear of his case, but whether the infection of the ear was primary or secondary to the brain lesion in these cases cannot be determined. There is some evidence that, as in other systemic mycoses, the portal of entry may be respiratory; *Cladosporium trichoides* was recovered from lung lesions in the case of Jaffe and Barnola (reported by Barnola). Hyphae were seen in lung lesions by Horn, and in the lungs and other organs by Sasano, but no cultures were made in these last two cases. Hyphae were also seen in the lung of the case of Aufdermaur due to *C.gougeroti*. The work of Fernandez-Baquero has thrown new light on the role of the respiratory tract in chromoblastomycosis. He isolated *Hormodendrum pedrosoi* from the bronchial washings of 4 patients with cutaneous chromoblastomycosis; the identity of the fungus was established by its cultural characteristics and by inoculation into 6 men who developed typical lesions at the sites of injection. Furthermore, as more cases of disseminated chromoblastomycosis are reported (Sugawara, Azulay) it is becoming increasingly evident that hematogenous dissemination of its etiological agents may be a feature of the disease. The close biological similarity between

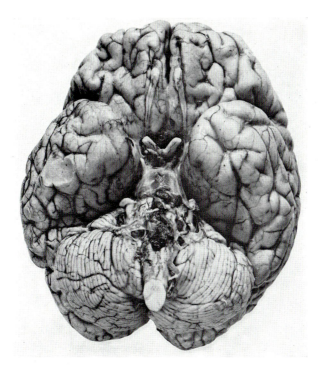

Fig. 8. Meningitis due to *Hormodendrum dermatitidis* (case of Shimazono et al.). Black nodules scattered on the basal surface of the brain and brain stem

C.bantianum and the species causing chromoblastomycosis is emphasized by the fact that in the case of Dastur (studied also by Desai), *C.trichoides* infection of the brain was associated with a scaly, olivaceous dermatitis and a subcutaneous abscess; in these skin lesions brown septate hyphae were found. Emmons (1963) mentions that this fungus was identified in a lesion of the skin of the abdomen in a patient that had no signs of cerebral mycosis. These facts lead one to to suppose that *C.trichoides*, and the fungi of chromoblastomycosis, may reach the brain by hematogenous dissemination from an infected wound, or from the respiratory tract. The presence of arteritis in some of the reported cases of cladosporiosis lends weight to this hypothesis.

C.trichoides (bantianum) does not seem to be a merely opportunistic agent of disease like certain fungi that invade only the debilitated individual. In most of the cases of cladosporiosis the patients were in good health until the onset of cerebral symptoms. Exceptions are the case of Horn which occured in a diabetic, and the patient of Symmers who had been receiving high doses of corticoesteroids for polyarteritis nodosa. Hypertension was present in the cases of King, and of Bobra. No relation with a particular occupation has been reported.

Pathologic Anatomy: The gross and microscopic appearances of the *central* nervous system lesions caused by *C.trichoides*, *C.gougeroti*, *H.pedrosoi*, and *H.dermatitidis* are entirely similar. Two main forms of cladosporiosis have been described, meningeal and cerebral, but lesions in both meninges and brain may be frequently seen. Meningitis has always been basal (Dereymaker, Lucasse, Tsai, Aufdermaur, Bonne, Garcin, 1949; Duque, 1961; Shimazono), consisting of fibrous thickening with or without granules or small nodules; when

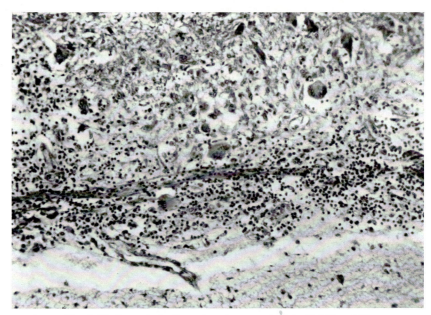

Fig. 9. Cladosporiosis. Granulomatous meningitis. H & E, ×120

these were present they were described as grey, green, or black-red in color (Fig. 8). The lesions may extend around the brain stem and even down to the cervical spinal cord, and it may be accompanied by fibrinopurulent exudate. Involvement of the ependyma is frequent in these cases, presenting as small disseminated granules on the walls of the ventricles. Choroid plexus may also be affected, and hydrocephalus was described in the cases of Garcin, and of Duque. Microscopically the lesion consists of a granulomatous inflammation with abundant giant cells of the foreign body and Langhans types, and an admixture of polymorphonuclear leucocytes and lymphocytes (Fig. 9). Microabscesses are frequently present; the degree of fibrosis is variable, probably in accord with the virulence and duration of the process. Superficial involvement of the nervous tissue is always present either as small granulomas and abscesses, or in the form of non specific inflammatory reaction. Coexistence of meningitis and deep cerebral lesions were found by Tsai, Aufdermaur, Garcin, and Shimazono. Severe arteritis and partial destruction of the roots of cranial nerves by the inflammatory process may be found. In these lesions the fungus grows mainly in the form of hyphae but spherical forms are also present.

In the cerebral form of the disease the brain is mainly affected, but cerebellum and brain stem may also be involved. The lesion occurs slightly more frequently on the left than on the right side, and it may be single or multiple, varying in size from a few milimeters to 5 cm in diameter. It appears as a firm pigmented nodule, sometimes with a necrotic or purulent center, or as a poorly limited necrotic or abscessed area surrounded by an irregular area of pigmented granulation tissue (Figs. 10 and 11); a true capsule is rarely found. Pigmentation is due in part to the pigment of the fungus itself; it has been described as brown, greenish, grey, or black-red but it may be so intense as to be taken for metastasis of a melanoma (Banti, Warot). Microscopic structure of the lesion is that of a granuloma with abundant giant cells, polynuclear and eosinophil leucocytes, and lymphocytes.

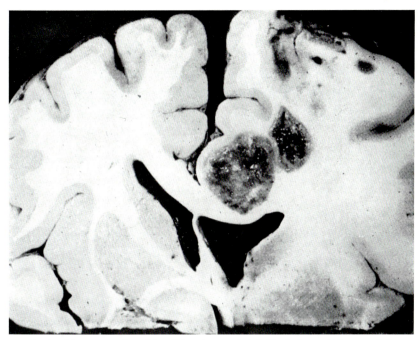

Fig. 10. Cerebral lesions produced by *C.bantianum (trichoides)*. Case of KING and COLLETTE.
Multiple abscesses and distortion of ventricular system

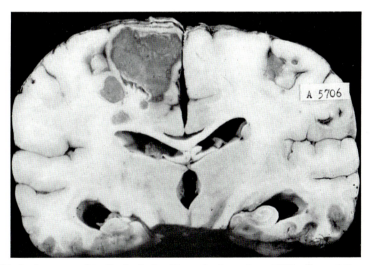

Fig. 11. Lesions caused in the brain by *Hormodendrum dermatitidis*. Case of TSAI et al.

Tubercle formation is uncommon but microabscesses and areas of necrosis are
found scattered in the granulomatous tissue (Fig. 12). Proliferation of glia cells and
areas of scar tissue are found in older lesions (Fig. 13). Condensation of glia and
collagen towards the periphery may give the appearance of a true capsule but this
usually fails to confine the growth of the fungus. Occasionally the core of the

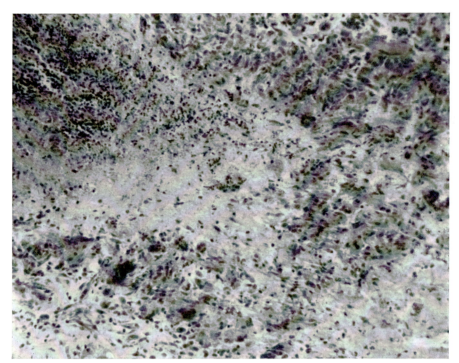

Fig. 12. Cerebral lesions of *C.trichoides*. Purulent exudate (upper left) is confined by necrotic tissue (center left); this area is surrounded by granulomatous inflammation with many giant cells. H & E, ×150

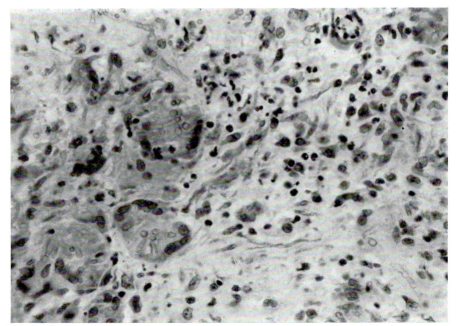

Fig. 13. Cerebral cladosporiosis. Granulomatous inflammation, fibrosis and gliosis are seen in the periphery of older lesions. Note hyphae within giant cells and free in the tissue. H & E, ×450

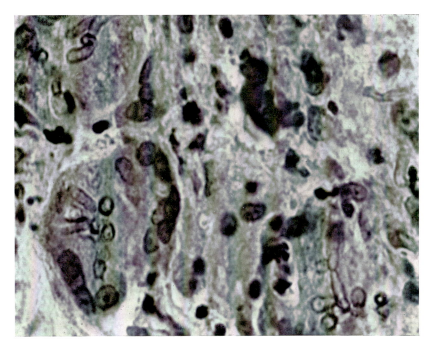

Fig. 14. Detail of Fig. 13 showing the fungus within giant cells. H & E, ×1250

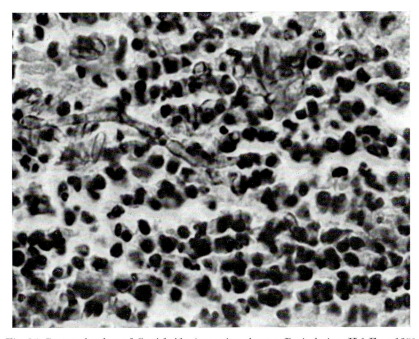

Fig. 15. Septate hyphae of *C. trichoides* in a microabscess. Brain lesion. H & E, ×1250

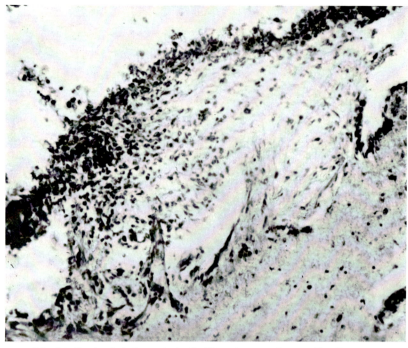

Fig. 16. Cerebral cladosporiosis. Proliferative ependimitis. H & E. ×200

lesion is surrounded by necrotic brain tissue permitting the surgeon to "shell-out" the granuloma as in the cases of BINFORD, and KING and COLLETTE. Hyphae are abundant in the lesions; they are seen within the giant cells (Fig. 14), or free in the tissue (Fig. 15), clearly septate, pigmented, measuring about 4 μ in diameter. Branching is rarely seen in tissue sections but it is easily demonstrable in fresh preparations. The large spheric elements ("sclerotic cells", "chlamydospores") are usually less numerous, although they were predominant in the case of FRANCA-NETTO. Granulomatous and proliferative inflammation of the ependyma and choroid plexus is found frequently, accompanying the cerebral lesion (Figs. 16 and 17).

Clinical Picture: The disease may have a sudden onset and a rapid course of less than a month. More commonly, symptoms appear gradually and the process extends for a period of from several months to two years. Symptoms are those of intracranial hypertension, space occupying lesion, and meningismus. Irregular fever is common; headache is mentioned in the majority of the cases, sometimes accompanied by nausea, vomiting and vertigo. Paralysis of the face and extremities develops in most cases, preceded by a period of sudden or gradual paresis. Papillary edema has been mentioned in 9 patients, and loss of weight in 12. In one third of the cases there have been convulsions. The symptoms of meningitis are frequently obscured by signs of cranial nerve involvement. In 14 cases the cerebrospinal fluid was examined; it was normal in 5. In the rest it was described as turbid, pressure variable, proteins generally increased, but data on sugar and chloride was inconsistent. Cells were generally increased, up to 4,450 per cmm, mostly polymorphonuclear leucocytes. The fungus has never been seen in the spinal fluid and its inoculation has been negative. In only one instance (case of

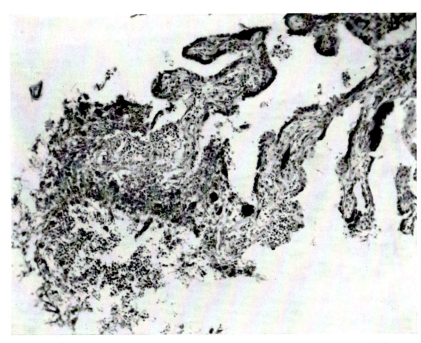

Fig. 17. Section of choroid plexus revealing involvement with granulomatous inflammation. Case of meningo-encephalitis caused by *C. trichoides*. H & E, × 200

DASTUR, studied by DESAI) has the fungus been isolated from the cerebrospinal fluid. Leucocytosis of the peripheral blood is frequently observed, with counts as high as 21 400 per cmm, with an increased number of neutrophils. Ventriculograms and carotid angiography appear to be most succesful diagnostic procedures.

It is clear from this brief description that cladosporiosis has no specific diagnostic features that permit it to be separated from other cases of brain abscess or meningitis of different etiology. Cladosporiosis is a serious disease, 25 of the cases having ended in death. The patient of BINFORD was seen again two years after operation, free from symptoms, and this is the only case that could be considered as cured. COUDERT's patient was well 10 months after operation, and in three other cases the patients were discharged in good condition but were not seen again. No effective therapy is available; penicillin, wide spectrum antibiotics, mycostatin, amphotericin B, izoniazide, chloramphenicol, cortisone, and potassium iodide have been tried without succes.

Summary of Illustrative Cases

Case of KING and COLLETTE *(Cladosporium trichoides)*

A 47-year-old white laborer was admitted with severe headaches. A short time after the onset of purulent drainage from the left ear the patient experienced headaches in the occipital and parietal regions. It was then noted that his speech was becoming inarticulate. A month after the onset of symptoms, weakness of the right extremities developed. Physical examination disclosed arteriosclerosis and a blood pressure of 156/100; dulled mental state and a motor speech aphasia were noted. There was also moderately severe right hemiparesis with Babinsky response. Laboratory studies were within normal limits. A left carotid angiogram showed an avascular area in the left frontal lobe. Puncture of the right ventricle yielded 25 ccm of clear fluid; only a few drops of fluid could be obtained from the left ventricle. Roentgenograms disclosed a mass in the frontal lobe near the midline.

A left frontal flap was reflected. The brain was not under tension. A firm mass was palpated subcortically near the midline about halfway between the tip of the frontal lobe and the Rolandic fissure. Needle aspiration of the mass produced a thick green pus. The abscess was shelled out in toto. After the operation speech became spontaneous and more articulate. There was no actual paralysis but the patient was unable to perform isolated movements of the right arm or leg. By the time of discharge the patient was sitting in a chair but could not walk. The specimen removed at operation was 3.5 cm in diameter and contained a light green pus from which a fungus was grown. The wall of the abscess was 3 cm in thickness. Microscopic examination showed a marked glial reaction with a rich round cell and some polymorphonuclear infiltration. Three weeks later the patient was readmitted because of convulsions; he was drowsy and could not talk. The right hemiplegia was now profound, the neck was stiff; early papilledema was present. Leucocyte count was 13,800 with a differential count of 82% polymorphonuclears. Spinal fluid contained 6 cells per cmm, 60 mg protein and 102 mg of sugar. Bacteriological cultures remained sterile. Ventriculogram demonstrated a mass in the posterior part of the left frontal lobe. About 20 ccm of a thick gelatinous green material was aspirated. The patient's course was one of steady decline. The temperature fluctuated from 98°—102°F. The patient expired two weeks after his second admission. Penicillin and potassium iodide were given without any noticeable effect. Postmortem findings included marked arteriosclerotic cardiovascular disease. In the brain a large hemorrhagic area was present at the site of enucleation of the original abscess; multiple daughter abscesses were also found in the surrounding white matter (Fig. 10), with little capsule formation. The walls of the ventricle were lined by a thin layer of pus and the choroid plexus on the left was swollen and edematous. The middle ears and paranasal sinuses were opened but no evidence of infection was found. Microscopically, besides a moderate glial reaction, there was a mild infiltration by round cells, and many giant cells were noted. Hyphae were present in the lesion and surrounding brain tissue. The fungus was studied by Dr. C.W. Emmons who concluded that it was *Cladosporium trichoides*. This fungus was grown also in cultures taken from the left petrous bone, but it might have been contaminated by the removal of the brain.

Case of Fukushiro et al. *(Hormodendrum pedrosoi)*

An 8-year-old Japanese girl consulted for verrucous lesions of the skin of the nose and right cheek of a year's duration. Previously she had suffered from tinea corporis caused by *Trichophyton ferrugineum*. She was in good physical condition. Tuberculin, trichophytin, and sporotrichin tests were negative, but she reacted with chromoblastomycetin antigen. Biopsy of the skin lesions revealed typical changes of chromoblastomycosis. *Hormodendrum pedrosoi* grew in cultures taken from these lesions. Three months after her first visit the girl developed neurological symptoms consisting of headaches, fever, nausea, and facial paresis that progressed to left facial paralysis and, two months later, to paralysis of the four extremities, accompanied by dysphasia. Leucocyte count was 12,000, sedimentation rate 65 mm, spinal fluid clear with pressure of 20 mm, Pandy test positive, and 10 cells per cmm; cultures of the fluid were negative. The patient's condition worsened steadily and she died of respiratory paralysis 9 months after the onset of neurological symptoms. Chlorophenol and sulphanil-amide were administered without improvement. At autopsy multiple "black-green granulo-matous tumors" were found in the basal meninges, cerebral hemispheres, cerebellum and pons. The larger one of the nodules, about 4 cm in diameter, was found in the left internal capsule. *Hormodendrum pedrosoi* pathogenic for mice was recovered from these lesions. Microscopically the lesions consisted of a granulomatous inflammation with many giant cells and polymorphonuclear leucocytes, and necrosis. Brown hyphae and spheric forms of the fungus were abundant in the lesions.

Case of Tsai et al. *(Hormodendrum dermatitidis)*

A 19-year-old female student from Taiwan became icteric in September 1961; jaundice fluctuated thereafter, and in March 1963 several swellings in her neck were observed. Strepto-mycin was given without benefit. Five months later, soreness and numbness developed in her right leg. On admission she exhibited mild jaundice; lymph nodes were palpated in the right side of her neck, and there was hepato-splenomegaly. White cell count 8,450 with 10% eosinophils. Liver tests revealed moderately altered hepatic function. Tuberculin was weakly positive; sedimentation rate was 120 mm. Lumbar puncture yielded clear fluid with a pressure of 120 mm, 23 cells predominantly lymphocytes, total protein 20 mg, sugar 60 mg, chloride 123 mEq. Cholecystography failed to visualize the gall bladder or bile ducts. Weakness of her right leg became progressive and Jacksonian seizures of the right hand developed. A lymph node biopsy revealed granulomatous inflammation with brown hyphae in the giant cells. *Hormodendrum dermatitidis* was obtained from a lymph node culture. Amphotericin B therapy was begun but because of severe side effects prednisolone was administered. In spite of treatment her general condition deteriorated progressively. Anemia increased, serum bilirubin rose to 11 mg and a high fever developed. In November she complained of abdominal pains, and this was followed by signs of acute peritonitis which became localized with abscess formation. Fungus was not seen in this abscess. A needle biopsy of the liver disclosed a few granulomatous lesions with multiple pigmented hyphae. In addition to the Jacksonian seizures and bilateral pyramidal signs, symptoms of involvement of cranial nerves appeared. An E.E.G. revealed generalized cortical abnormalities and severe involvement of the left central and parietal portions. She became comatose and died in April 1964. Iodide and Mycostatin therapy did not alter the course of the disease. Autopsy: no lesions were found in the lungs; fibrinopurulent exudate and adhesions were found between the peritoneum and the abdominal viscera, without perforation of hollow organs. The liver was cirrhotic, with white scarred patches, and intrahepatic pigment stones were found. Marked fibrosis and miliary brown spots were seen in the intrapancreatic portion of the common bile duct. Almost all the lymph nodes of the body presented yellow brown nodules. Over the leptomeninges of the spinal cord, brain stem and hypothalamic portions there were numerous raised black or red-black patches measuring up to 1 cm in diameter. Multiple green yellow nodular lesions were found in the cerebrum (Fig. 11), and cerebellum. The largest of these lesions, 7 cm in diameter, was found near the superior frontal pre- and post central gyri of the left hemisphere. Microscopically, the lymph node lesions consisted of granulomas with yellow brown hyphae and round structures of the fungus; this was found also in the lesions around the bile duct. Histologic changes in the brain consisted of conglomerate granulomas with or without fibrous capsule, and necrotic areas. Real abscesses were seen in a few daughter nodules adjacent to the large lesion in the mid brain; pigmented hyphae and some round bodies were found in these lesions. The ependyma of the fourth ventricle was covered by a thick layer of granulomatous tissue. The exuberant growth of the fungus in the meningeal lesions resembled a pure culture of the organism. Granulomatous angiitis in vessels invaded by the fungus was observed. *Hormodendrum dermatitidis* was grown from the various lesions. It produced abscesses in the brain, liver and spleen of mice inoculated intravenously.

Acknowledgements: The author wishes to express his appreciation to the Williams and Wilkins Company, of Baltimore, publishers of the American Journal of Clinical Pathology for their kind permission to use the pictures in the papers by Dr. TSAI, and by the author, for illustrations N° 2, 3, 4, 9, 11, 13, 16, and 17. The Editors of the Johns Hopkins Medical Journal graciously granted their permission to the author to use one of the brain photographs of Dr. King's paper for illustration N° 10. — Professor R. FUKUSHIRO and Dr. Y. SHIMAZONO, of Kanazawa University, provided the author with the beautiful photograph of the brain for illustration N° 8. Dr. A.B. KING, of Sayre, Pennsylvania, kindly allowed the author to use the picture for illustration N° 10. Dr. C.Y. TSAI, of the National Taiwan University graciously furnished the author with the potograph for illustration N° 11. To all these distinguished colleagues the author is deeply indebted.

References

AL DOORY, Y., GORDON, M.A.: Application of fluorescent antibody procedures to the study of pathogenic dematiaceous fungi. J. Bact. **86**, 332 (1963). — AUFDERMAUR, M., PILLER, M., FISCHER, E.: Sporotrichose des Hirns. Schweiz. med. schr. **84**, 167 (1954). — AZULAY, R.D., SERRUYA, J.: Hematogenous dissemination in chromoblastomycosis. Arch. Derm. **95**, 57 (1967). — BAGCHI, A., AIKAT, B.K., BARUA, D.: Granulomatous lesion of the brain produced by *Cladosporium trichoides*. J. Indian med. Ass. **38**, 602 (1962). — BARNOLA, J., ANGULO, A.: Cladosporiosis profunda. Mycopathologia (Den Haag) **15**, 422 (1961). — BINFORD, C.H., THOMPSON, R.K., GORHAM, M.E., EMMONS, C.W.: Mycotic brain abscess due to *Cladosporium trichoides*, a new species. With mycologic report by C.W. EMMONS. Amer. J. clin. Path. **22**, 535 (1952). — BOBRA, S.T.: Mycotic abscess of the brain probably due to *Cladosporium trichoides*. Report of the fifth case. Canad. med. Ass. J. **79**, 657 (1958). — BONNE, C., BROS, G., VER HAART, W.J.C.: Localized lesions of the meninges and the brain caused by a brown fungus with septate hyphae of unknown nature. Med. Maandbl. (Batavia) **1**, 465 (1948). — BORELLI, D.: Cladosporiosis profunda. Revisión de una cepa. Bol. venez. Lab. Clin. **1**, 29 (1948). ~ *Torula bantiana*, agente di un granuloma cerebrale. Riv. Anat. pat. **17**, 615 (1960). — CHEVREL, M.L., JAVALET, A., DOBY, J.M., DOBY-DUBOIS, M., LOUVET, M.: A propos d'une observation de cladosporiosis cérébrale. Ann. Anat. path. **7**, 607 (1962). [This same case was also studied by DOBY-DUBOIS, M. et al.: Ann. Parasit. hum. comp. **37**, 644 (1962)]. — COUDERT, J., ALLEGRE, G., TOMASSI, M., BATTESTI, M.R.: Un cas lyonnais de mycose cérébrale due á *Cladosporium trichoides* (EMMONS, 1952). Etude anatomo-clinique et mycologique. Rev. lyon. Méd. **11**, 847 (1962). [This case was also studied by TOMMASI, M. et al.: Arch. Anat. path. **12**, 48 (1964)].— DASTUR, H.M., CHAUKAR, A.P., REBELLO, M.D.: Cerebral chromoblastomycosis due to *Cladosporium trichoides* (bantianum). I. A review and case report. Neurology (Bombay) **14**, 1 (1966) (See Desai). — Desai, S.C., Bhatikar, M.L., Mehta, R.S.: Cerebral chromoblastomycosis due to *Cladosporium trichoides* (bantianum). II. Mycopathologic investigation of brain abscess and skin involvement. Neurology (Bombay) **14**, 6 (1966). — Dereymaeker, A., De Somer, P.: Arachnoidite fibrinopurulente cérebelocervical due á une moisissure (*Cladosporium*). Acta neurol. belg. **55**, 629 (1955). — Doby-Dubois, M., Chevrel, M.L., Doby, J.M., Robert, Y.: Abcès mycosique cérébral humain par *Cladosporium trichoides*. Ann. Parasit. hum. comp. **37**, 644 (1962). — Duque, O.: Cladosporiosis cerebral experimental. Rev. lat.-amer. Anat. pat. **7**, 101 (1963). ~ Meningoencephalitis and brain abscess caused by *Cladosporium* and *Fonsecaea*. Review of the literature, report of two cases, and experimental studies. Amer. J. clin. Path. **36**, 505 (1961). — Emmons, C.W., Binford, C.H., Utz, J.P.: Medical Mycology. Chapter 27, Cladosporiosis, pp. 330 to 338. Philadelphia: Lea & Febiger 1963. — Felger, C.E., Friedman, L.: Experimental cerebral chromoblastomycosis. J. infect. Dis. **111**, 1 (1962). — Fernández-Baquero, G., Reaud, B.: Cultivo del *Hormodendrum pedrosoi* del material obtenido por lavado bronquial en cuatro enfermos de cromoblastomicosis. Bol. Soc. Cuba. Derm. Sif. **17**, 99 (1960). — Fernández-Baquero, G., Barquin-Lopez, P., Reaud-Lescay, B.: Cromoblastomicosis experimental. Bol. Soc. cuba. Derm. Sif. **18**, 19 (1961). — Franca-Netto, A.S., De Britto, T., De Almeida, F.P.: Cromomicose do sistema nervoso. Etudo anatomoclinico de um caso. Arch. Neuropsiquiat. (S.Paulo) **11**, 265 (1953).— Fukushiro, R., Kagawa, S., Nishiyama, S., Takahashi, H.: Un cas de chromoblastomycose cutanée avec métastase cérébrale mortelle. Presse méd. **65**, 2142 (1957). [This same case was reported by several Japanese authors: Nagahata, M.: Pediatr. Univ. (Tokyo) **2**, 75 (1958). Nishi, M.: Trans. Soc. path. jap. **45**, 566 (1956). Okudaira, M.: Acta path. jap. **6**, 207 (1956)]. — Garcin, R., Martin, R., Bertrand, I., Gruner, J., Tourneur, R.: Mycose méningo-épendymaire. Etude anatomo-clinique. Presse méd. **57**, 1201 (1949). — Garcin, R., Martin, R., Maningand, G., Bertrand, I., Godlewski, S., Sureau, B.: Mycose cérébrale á *Cladosporium trichoides*. Sem. Hôp. Paris **33**, 2282 (1957). [The fungus from this case was studied also by Segretain, G. et al.: Ann. Inst. Pasteur **89**, 465 (1955)]. — Horn, I.H., Wilansky, D.L., Harland, W.A., Blank, F.: Neurogenic hypernatremia with mycotic brain granuloma due to *Cladosporium trichoides*. Canad. med. Ass. J. **83**, 1314 (1960). — Iwata, K., Wada, T.: Mycological studies on the strains isolated from a case of chromoblastomycosis with metastasis in central nervous system. Jap. J. Microbiol. **1**, 355 (1957). — King, A.B., Collette, F.S.: Brain abscess due to *C.trichoides*. Report of the second case due to this organism. Bull. Johns Hopk. Hosp. **91**, 298 (1952). — Lucasse, C., Chardome, J., Magis, P.: Mycose cerebrale par *Cladosporium trichoides* chez un indigène de Conge Belge, et note mycologique sur *Cladosporium trichoides* Emmons (1952), par R. Vanbreuseghem. Ann. Soc. belge Méd. trop. **34**, 475 (1954). — Manson, M.D.E.: Chromoblastomycotic brain abscess in a South African Bantu. Report of a case. S. Afr. J. Lab. clin. Med. **4**, 283 (1958). — McGill, H.C., Brueck, J.W.: Brain abscess due to *Hormodendrum* species. Arch. Path. **62**, 303 (1956). — Riley, O., Mann, S.H.: Brain abscess caused by *C.trichoides*. Review of 3 cases and report of fourth case. Amer. J. clin. Path. **33**, 525 (1960). — Saccardo, P.A.: Torula fungine bantiana. Ann. Mycol. **10**, 320 (1912) (reproduced in Stigliani, q.v.). — Sasano, N., Okamoto, T., Takahashi, T., Suzuki, S.: An autopsy case of primary chromoblastomycosis arising from the internal organs. Dark brown granulomas in the liver and the brain without skin symptoms, observed in a smoking child 3 years old. Tohoku J. exp. Med. **73**, 180 (1961). [Published originally in Japanese: Trans. Soc. path. jap. **47**, 400 (1958)]. — Segretain, G., Mariat, F., Drouhet, E.: Sur *Cladosporium trichoides* isolé d'une mycose cérébrale. Ann. Inst. Pasteur **89**, 465 (1955). — Shimazono, Y., Isaki, K., Torii, H., Otsuka, R., Fukushiro, R.: Brain abscess due to *Hormodendrum dermatitidis* (Kano) Conant 1953. Report of a case and review of the literature. Folia psychiat. neurol. jap. **17**, 80 (1963). [This case was reported also by Fukushiro, R.: Saishin Igaku **16**, 580 (1961)]. — Stigliani, R.: Particolaritá istologiche della torulose encefalica nei preparati originali Bantiana della prima osservazione conosciuta. Arch. De Vecchi Anat. pat. **36**, 329 (1961). — Sugawara, M., Sobajima, Y., Tamura, H.: A case of generalized chromoblastomycosis. Acta Path. jap. **14**, 239 (1964). — Symmers, W.St.C.: A case of cerebral chromoblastomycosis (Cladosporiosis) occurring in Britain as a complication of polyarteritis treated with cortisone. Brain **83**, 37 (1960). — Tsai, C.Y., Lü, Y,C., Wang, L.T., Hsu, T.L., Sung, J.L.: Systemic chromoblastomycosis due to *Hormodendrum dermatitidis* (Kano) Conant. Amer. J. clin. Path. **46**, 103 (1966). — Warot, P., Galibert, P., Meignie, S., Delandtsheer, J.M., Petit, H.: Mycose cérébrale á symptomatologie tumorale (*Cladosporium trichoides* probable). Rev. neurol. **105**, 489 (1961). — Watson, K.C., Lines, G.M.: Brain abscess due to the fungus *Hormodendrum*. S. Afr. med. J. **31**, 1081 (1957). — Watson, K.C.: Cerebral chromoblastomycosis. J. Path. Bact. **84**, 233 (1962). — Wybel, R.E.: Mycosis of cervical cord following intrathecal penicillin therapy. Report of a case simulating cord tumor. Arch. Path. **53**, 167 (1953).

Subcutaneous Abscesses due to Brown Fungi

HERBERT ICHINOSE, New Orleans/Louisiana USA

With 19 Figures

Introduction

The subcutaneous abscesses described in this chapter are apparently caused by members of the same general group of organisms that also give rise to chromo-blastomycosis. However, the two diseases show distinct differences in clinical manifestations and biologic course. In addition, the organisms in the lesions of chromoblastomycosis are almost exclusively yeast forms in contrast to the organisms in the subcutaneous abscess which characteristically exhibit dimorphism.

Definition of the Disease

The chronic subcutaneous abscesses caused by pigmented fungi are solitary lesions covered by normal epidermis. The lesions are often misdiagnosed clinically and the causative organisms have rarely been cultured. The infection remains localized and the lesions are readily cured in most instances by surgical excision. The patients frequently have unrelated serious diseases.

Cases of Subcutaneous Abscesses

The following is a listing of reported cases of such subcutaneous abscesses from 1908 to the present in literature available to the author:

YOUNG, J.M. and ULRICH, E., Memphis, Tenn./USA (1953) . . . . 1 case
MEAD, M. and RIDLEY, M.F., Brisbane, Australia (1957) . . . . 1 case
NITYANANDA, K., Colombo, Ceylon (1962) . . . . 1 case
MARIAT, F., et al., Paris, France (1967) . . . . 1 case
KEMPSON, R.L. and STERNBERG, W.H., New Orleans, La./USA (1963) . . . . 7 cases

Two other cases (DUKE nos. 2492 and 3326) included in an antigenic study by NIELSEN and CONANT have not been reported in detail. Five additional cases have been made available to the author by several pathologists including Dr. R.J. REED, Dr. F. HARRIS, and Dr. W.H. STERNBERG. The pathologic and clinical data to be presented have been derived largely from these 5 cases (ICHINOSE, unpublished data) and a restudy of the 7 cases reported by KEMPSON and STERNBERG.

Mycology

Organisms from the lesions have rarely been cultured. In two instances, the organisms were identified as *Hormiscium dermatitidis* (NIELSEN and CONANT; SCHNEIDAU). The preliminary report on organisms from another lesion was *Cladosporium sp.* (SAMUELS, personal communication.) In two other cases, the organisms were classified as *Sporotrichum gougerotii* by YOUNG and ULRICH and *Phialophora gougerotii* by MARIAT et al. The latter authors consider their isolate identical to that reported by YOUNG and ULRICH. They also refer to BORRELLI's opinion that this organism is synonymous with *H.dermatitidis*. It should also be that CARRION and SILVA studied the organisms from the lesion reported by and ULRICH as well as organisms from two other sources and reclassified trichum gougerotii as *Cladosporium gougerotti*. These opinions indicate that the lesions are caused by closely related fungi. Because of the small number of lesions from which organisms have been cultured, it is premature to assume that similar lesions might not be caused by other organisms.

Clinical

The patients were adults usually in their fifth or sixth decade. About half of the patients had some serious systemic disease unrelated to the fungal infection. Three patients had mild diabetes mellitus and two of these had severe hypertension and congestive heart failure. The third patient had severe cerebral atherosclerosis, three cerebral vascular accidents, and atherosclerosis obliterans of the legs. A fourth patient had minor infections of axillary sweat glands and a strong family history of diabetes mellitus. Another patient had dysglobulinemia, long standing lymphadenopathy, and serous cavity effusions. The patient reported by Young and Ulrich was being treated for pulmonary tuberculosis. Similarly, the patient described by Mariat et al. suffered from bilharziasis and the fungus disease was thought to be an example of an "opportunistic" infection. In this regard, the statement by Kempson and Sternberg is appropriate: "Although the series of cases complaine is too small for definite conclusions, it seems that subcutaneous chromoblastomycosis infections may tend to occur in patients with metabolic and debilitating diseases."

No important symptoms were attributed to these infections. The patients frequently regarded the lesions as small calluses and brought them to the attention of the physician for cosmetic reasons.

The subcutaneous abscesses probably developed from inconspicuous puncture wounds made by contaminated plant material. Wood splinters were present in three of the lesions and a fourth contained what appeared to be a portion of a thorn. The rapid healing which is characteristic of small skin punctures, in all likelihood, accounts for the normal epidermis overlying the lesions. Several of the patients lived in rural areas and engaged in agricultural work. Another patient raised flowers including roses as an avocation. The onset and duration of the lesions could rarely be accurately stated by the patients. The shortest reported duration was four days and the longest was two years.

On physical examination the lesions were situated in the distal parts of the upper extremities including the volar surfaces of the fingers and palm, the dorsum of the hand, the wrist and the forearm. Less commonly, the lesions were on the lower extremity, e.g., dorsum of the foot (Nityananda), the ankle, the leg near the lateral malleolus and the knee. The lesions were discrete solitary masses clinically situated in the subcutis. The overlying epidermis was normal in all instances, and no ulceration or sinus tracts were observed. An exception to this generalization was a sinus tract that developed between the lesion and the skin surface after the lesion had been aspirated for the second time (Young and Ulrich). The lesions were less than 2 cm in diameter. They frequently exhibited a soft fluctuant consistency and, therefore, were commonly misdiagnosed as sebaceous cysts or lipomas. When located near joints, the possibility of Baker's cyst or ganglion was occasionally considered. Sometimes, the lesions were firm giving some basis for a tentative diagnosis of giant cell tumor of tendon sheath. When a history of previous trauma to the area of the lesion could be elicited, the possibility of foreign body granuloma was also considered.

Gross Pathology

The typical specimen was a solitary cystic lesion surrounded by capsule to which subcutaneous adipose tissue was adherent (Fig. 1).

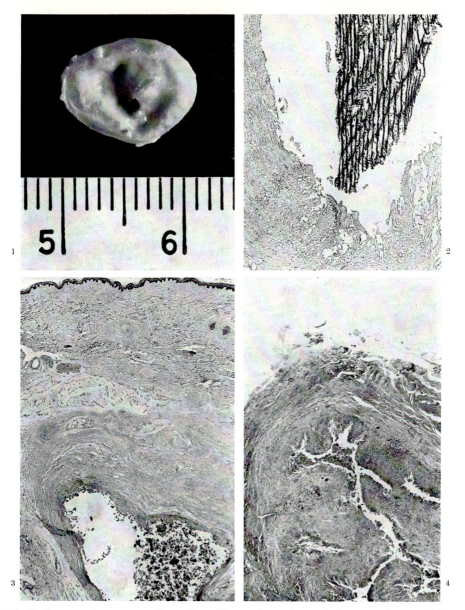

Fig. 1. Gross specimen, cut section surface: The specimen shows an abscess cavity containing whitish purulent exudate and showing a darker appearing granulation tissue lining. The lining is indistinct on the right side of the lesion. An intact fibrous capsule is present. The black circular body in the interior of the abscess cavity is a cut section of a sliver of plant material. Formalin fixed, ×4 approximately

Fig. 2. Foreign body: A foreign body is present in the abscess cavity and shows histologic features of plant tissue. Gridley stain, ×105

Fig. 3. Subcutaneous abscess, fluctuant stage: The lesion is situated in the subcutaneous tissue of the skin and the overlying epidermis and dermis are normal. A fibrous capsule is present around the abscess. (Refer to Acknowledgements.) H & E, ×8

Fig. 4. Subcutaneous abscess, stellate abscess stage: The lesion shows a stellate outline of the cavity with a festooned margin. Purulent exudate is present in the lumen. An intact fibrous capsule is present. H & E, ×15

cavity measured approximately 1 cm in diameter, was filled with viscid yellow exudate or cheesy material, and was lined by firm yellowish tan tissue. Rarely, the lining also showed granular areas of blackish discoloration probably representing colonies of organisms. Three lesions contained a sliver of foreign material believed to be a small wood splinter (Figs. 1 and 2) and one contained a foreign body that resembled a thorn. Less commonly, the lesion failed to show a cavity. In these instances, the nodule was made up of firm yellowish tan tissue contained within a fibrous capsule. When the overlying epidermis was also received, it showed no abnormalities.

Histopathology

The chronic abscess was characteristically located in the deeper dermis and adjacent subcutis. *Histologically*, the lesions showed three apparent stages of development: (1) tuberculoid phase, (2) stellate abscess, (3) fluctuant abscess. The combination of the fluctuant (Fig. 3) and stellate abscesses (Fig. 4) were typically found in most lesions although all three stages were observed in one of the lesions. In the tuberculoid stage, clusters of tubercles formed the main nodule (Fig. 8). The tubercles contained abundant organisms and were composed predominantly of epithelioid cells and foreign body giant cells. Small foci of coagulation and fibrinoid necrosis of epithelioid cells were present and were associated with a chronic and acute cellular reaction. As these foci of necrosis apparently increased in number and coalesced, a stellate abscess developed. The festooned outline of the lesion was still composed predominantly of epithelioid cells. The giant cells and occasional microabscesses were nearly always seen in that portion of the granulation tissue bordering the necrotic debris. This border showed sporadic fibrinoid and coagulation necrosis (Fig. 5). In this granulation tissue, capillaries showing prominent endothelial cells coursed toward the necrotic center. Occasional xanthoma cells were present and some lesions showed hyalinization of the granulation tissue (Fig. 6). With apparent progressive necrosis of granulation tissue, there was a loss of the stellate outline resulting in a more nearly spherical fluctuant abscess. Epithelioid cells continued to form a complete inner lining of the cavity which was considerably attenuated. The exudate filling the abscess cavity was composed predominantly of degenerating neutrophils. Occasional giant cells

---

Fig. 5. Abscess wall: The lining of the abscess is formed by granulation tissue rich in epithelioid cells and giant cells. A small microabscess is present near the upper part of the left margin of the picture. Fibrinoid necrosis of portions of the granulation tissue are present in the center and the left upper corner of the picture. Inflammatory cells, predominantly neutrophils, fill the abscess cavity and show varying stages of degeneration. The fibrous capsule is intact and exhibits mild chronic inflammation. H & E, ×105

Fig. 6. Abscess wall: The granulation tissue lining shows hyalinization of the luminal edge in occasional lesions. A group of xanthoma cells are present in the lower right corner of the picture. A paucity of neutrophils and predominance of lymphocytes and other chronic inflammatory cells are noted. This particular lesion contained only a small number of organisms. H & E, ×360

Fig. 7. Unstained section: The organism has an olive-brown color and is readily detected without staining. The aberrant hypha shows a "rounding out" of the second segment from the left. The fourth segment exhibits a similar change. These alterations are interpreted as stages in transformation to chlamydospores. Unstained, ×875

Fig. 8. Subcutaneous abscess, tuberculoid stage: The nodular lesion is formed by a conglomeration of tubercules best demonstrated in the lower portion of the picture. It is contained within a fibrous capsule. Large numbers of organisms are present and appear as black dots of various sizes. The arrow is directed at one of the larger groups of organisms. PAS, ×83

contained phagocytized foreign matter that resembled non-viable plant material. The chronic cellular infiltrate of leucocytes was predominantly composed of mature lymphocytes. Occasional aggregates of eosinophils were also present when the lymphocytic infiltrate was heavy. Only a few plasma cells were present. A dense collagenous capsule surrounded the lesion in all three developmental stages. No organisms were present in this fibrous capsule. In the tissue situated just exterior to the fibrous capsule, chronic inflammatory cellular reaction was present around blood vessels and was most prominent in the region deep to the lesion.

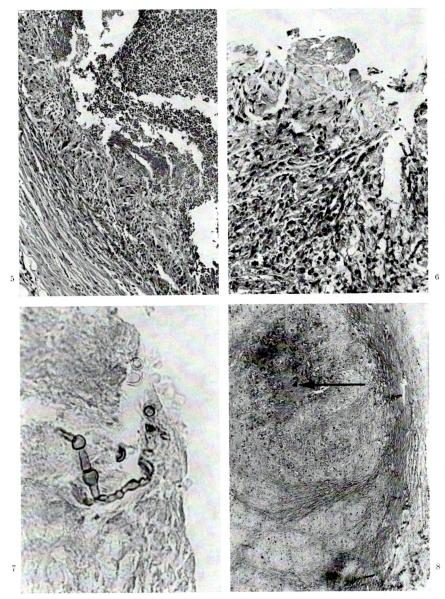

Figs. 5—8

46*

Organisms in Tissue

Terminology: Since the tissue phase of these organisms has not been previously described in detail, appropriate terminology has not as yet been firmly established. Therefore, in the following description the application of certain terms is arbitrary and, likewise, somewhat conjectural. The terminology employed by others in describing the tissue phase of the pigmented fungi is used whenever it appears appropriate.

By definition, a "blastospore" is a "spore that arises by budding" (Snell and Dick). Since terminal bud-fission was frequently observed at the ends of chains of organisms, the use of the term, blastospore chains, was adapted to describe this pattern of growth. The term is used in cognizance of the nearly identical sequential process of budding with the youngest cell at the apex in the Homodendrum type conidia of *H.pedrosoi* and *P.gougerotii* in culture. However, in these chains the oldest spore is attached to a conidiophore and, therefore, can be classically distinguished from the blastospore chain. In a larger sense, even the conidial chains of these two organisms might be considered a form of blastosporulation since they share phenomenon of terminal spore formation with blastospore chains.

Fig. 9. A cluster of chlamydospores is present within a degenerating giant cell. Two spores in the upper left portion of the cluster are budding. These organisms and those in Fig. 10 were present in the exudate of a fluctuant portion of the abscess. PAS, ×835

Fig. 10. A group of organisms has formed branching chains. Most of the organisms have thick dark staining walls and are interpreted as chlamydospores having developed from blasto-spores. The chain forming the left upper extremity of this group of organisms shows branching near its apex and terminal bud formation. The cells from which these buds have arisen show thin walls and are smaller in size than the chlamydospore to which the cells are attached. Septation is present in the right extremity of this group of organisms. PAS, ×835

Fig. 11. A short chain of organisms is present and includes a chlamydospore (sclerotic cell). The three cells attached to the inferior aspect of the chlamydospore are smaller in size and are believed to be blastospores. PAS, ×835

Fig. 12. Three spores forming a chain are separated by thick transverse disjunctors. The largest cell (sclerotic cell) is probably the oldest and exhibits a thickened wall. It has a dis-junctor in its upper extremity and probably broke off from a larger chain. The lower two cells are blastospores and the most inferior cell has probably been formed most recently. PAS, ×835

Fig. 13. A tubular type disjunctor separates the lowest cell from the cell situated in the middle of the chain. PAS, ×835

Fig. 14. An inverted L shaped structure is interpreted as a group of non-viable, degenerating organisms. Apparent shrinkage and distortion of overall shape are exhibited. The overall size is comparable to the organisms in Figs. 11, 12, and 13. Gridley, ×840

Fig. 15. A branching filament is partly enveloped by a coating with proteinaceous protuber-ances forming an asteroid body. The left upper extremity consists of three spores, the largest being a chlamydospore. The latter appears to have originated from a hypha and subsequently given rise to a short blastospore chain. Gridley, ×840

Fig. 16. A growth tube has developed from a large chlamydospore. The latter is attached by a tubular structure to two other spores. PAS, ×1410

Fig. 17. A chain of spores shows the member on the left extremity having formed a filament. Septation is present in the third and fourth cells from the right. The left portion of the picture was photographed at a different level of focus from the right part. PAS, ×1410

Fig. 18. Two hyphae have germinated from a fairly large chlamydospore. This particular germinating pattern has been frequently observed in epidermal scales and exudate from verrucous lesions of chromoblastomycosis. PAS, ×835

Fig. 19. Abundant hyphae are present. Several of these are extracellular in location. Aberrant filaments are more plentiful than "classic" hyphae. Some of the hyphae are believed to have formed after the specimen had been removed from the patient. PAS, ×692

TUBAKI employs the term, blastospore, for the conidia of Homodendrum type in a recent treatise. He is of the opinion that the use of the term in this sense has been accepted by many workers.

Description: The pigmented fungal organisms in our material showed considerable morphological variation. In unstained sections (Fig. 7) as well as in

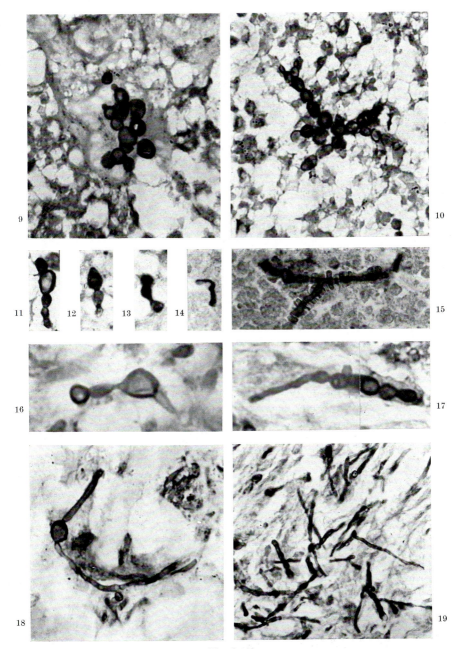

Figs. 9—19

sections stained with hematoxylin and eosin, the organisms exhibited an olive-brown color. With the PAS stain, the organisms were stained purple pink, and with Gridley stain, the organisms appeared dark purple. The Gomori methanamine silver stain was also employed to some advantage. Since organisms were plentiful (Fig. 8), more than 100 organisms and groups of organisms were available for study in all except two lesions. In the latter, only a few sparse organisms could be found even on careful study of all the available sections. Though the organisms were generally plentiful, the massive growths forming dense "mulberry clusters" in histologic sections of chorioallantoic membrane studied by Moore and the "black granules" found in a mycetoma-like lesion of the hand by Lewis et al. were not present in the subcutaneous abscess.

Chlamydospores, synonymous with sclerotic cells[1], were present in all instances and showed characteristic thickened walls and occasional septation. They were frequently grouped in conglomerate aggregations in giant cells. Some of the cells of a sclerotic cell aggregate occasionally gave rise to small buds (Fig. 9). More frequently, the sclerotic cells were attached to a chain of fairly uniform sized spherical fungal cells believed to be chains of blastospores. The chains occasionally were branched and propagated by sequential budding occurring at the ends of the chain (Fig. 10). Organisms propagating by budding have been previously observed in tissue sections of the subcutaneous abscess (Young and Ulrich). The branching chains of blastospores are identical to those described in culture (Carrion, 1950b). The spores which appeared to have been formed more recently were smaller in size in contrast to the older cells which were of the same size or larger than the parent cell (Figs. 10, 11, 12). Thick disjunctors were present, and structures interpreted as tubular disjunctors were also observed on rare occasion (Figs. 12, 13). Sclerotic cells and blastospore chains were the prevalent forms and were present in all lesions. Some of the blastospores in a chain had thickened cell walls and probably represent conversion to chlamydospores. Growth tubes and hyphae arose from chains as well as from isolated chlamydospores (Figs. 16, 17, 18). Such examples of germination are identical to those noted in epidermal scales and exudate of chromoblastomycosis lesions (Carrion, 1950a; Merrin; Da Fonseca). In the rare lesions containing abundant hyphae, the hyphae were commonly found in extracellular sites in the granulation tissue of the abscess wall (Fig. 19). This observation, as well as the finding of significant numbers of chlamydospores with growth tubes, suggests that at least some of the hyphae might have been formed after the lesions had been surgically excised. The hyphae were segmented, had fairly uniform width, and showed occasional branching, usually at acute angles. There were some fungal cells which appeared to be aberrant hyphae with segments showing variable dimensions and tapering at points of junction (Figs. 7, 19). These aberrant hyphae were usually more abundant than the "classic" hyphae and were found predominantly in giant cells as were most of the sclerotic bodies and blastospore chains. Organisms were also present in the exudate filling the abscess cavities and were usually widely distributed. They frequently exhibited degenerative changes consisting of distortion, shrinkage, and loss of some of their chromatic characteristics (Fig. 14). In the hematoxylin and eosin preparations, the organisms stained dark purple, and in unstained sections they showed a loss of their natural olive-brown color. Other organisms in the exudate retained normal morphologic features and occasionally exhibited acidophilic encrustations enveloping their exterior surfaces representing one type of asteroid formation (Fig. 15).

1 These two terms are employed in the sense used by Carrion (1950a) with the realization that both are not consistent with classic terminology.

Summary and Comment

Chlamydospores (sclerotic cells) divided by septation as well as gave rise to chains of blastospores. Of these two methods of multiplication, blastosporulation was more frequently observed. Some of these spores showed conversion back to chlamydospores. Some of the aberrant hyphal forms may represent a similar adaptive phenomenon. In this regard, SILVA has demonstrated the development of chlamydospores from "rounded out" and thick-walled hyphal segments as well as from occasional conidia in organisms growing *in vitro* and *in vivo*. The chlamydospores and blastospore chains were the prevalent fungal cells and probably represent the most favorable adaptation to the adverse environment created by the host tissue reaction. Degenerating organisms were present in the exudate filling the abscess cavities. Single chlamydospores as well as those situated in blastospore chains gave rise to hyphae. At least some of the hyphae may have formed after the lesions had been surgically removed. This opinion is partly supported by the observation that exposure to light favored abundant hyphal growth of *C. mansonii* in contrast to the near absence of these structures when cultures were incubated in the dark (SUSSMAN et al.). In addition, the continued growth of the organisms in tissue in spite of the specimens having been fixed in formalin might be considered on the basis of WEIDMAN and ROSENTHAL's findings. These workers added 10% formaldehyde to a dextrose bouillon culture of *F. pedrosoi* and observed continued growth of the colonies after several months. Under these conditions it is interesting that they found that the organisms were converted from yeast forms to straight hyphae, and conidia were absent.

Differential Diagnosis: Clinically, the fungus lesion most closely mimicking the subcutaneous abscess caused by the brown fungi is the rare case of subcutaneous nocardiosis (THORLAKSON and RUSNAK). The lesions are not attached to the normal overlying epidermis, may be solitary, and are associated with a history of trauma. The clinical features of the lesion may remain unchanged for long periods of time. Similarly, one of the rare instances of localized cutaneous histoplasmosis appeared as a painless nodule after having been previously incised. The lesion became ulcerated a little over 18 months later (SYMMERS, 1956). In disseminated chromoblastomycosis, rare skin lesions are subcutaneous abscesses. Some of these lesions are believed to be metastatic in origin. However, the possibility that these lesions may also have arisen from primary innoculations cannot be excluded.

In the early stages of their development, several different fungal diseases may show a close clinical resemblance to the subcutaneous abscesses caused by the brown fungi. The subcutaneous phycomycosis lesions of Indonesia (JOE and ENG) and parts of Africa as well as the early lesions of primary cutaneous coccidioidomycosis (LEVAN and HUNTINGTON), sporotrichosis, chromoblastomycosis, mycetoma pedia and manus fail to show ulceration and may present as solitary asymptomatic nodules initially. Also, the history of skin trauma may be obtained with some regularity in these other infections. Atypical acid-fast organism infections may occasionally present in an identical manner (BROCK et al.).

Treatment and Prognosis: The lesions were readily dissected and removed surgically under local anesthesia. However, in two instances the cavity ruptured during the procedure resulting in the spillage of the abscess contents into the surgical wound. It is noteworthy that, in these two instances as well as in all the remaining cases, no recurrences were noted during follow-up periods ranging up to nine years (KEMPSON and STERNBERG; ICHINOSE). The patients also failed to show clinical indications of systemic spread of the infection. This lack of local or systemic spread was further confirmed at autopsy in the patient who died with dysglobulinemia. Another patient died seven years after removal of the lesion. This patient died after a series of cerebral vascular accidents documented by carotid angiograms. No autopsy was performed but clinical evidence of disseminated fungus infection was absent.

The patients have a good prognosis in regard to the mycotic infection since it is localized and the contents of the abscess cavity apparently have a poor potential for infectivity. The latter observation suggests that the luminal contents containing degenerating organisms might be less likely to yield a positive culture than the tannish granulation tissue lining of the cavity. This may be especially applicable to lesions containing few organisms.

General Comment: The clinical manifestations of chromoblastomycosis include a variety of cutaneous lesions classified by Pardo-Castello et al. into five different groups: Verrucous, tuberculoid, syphiloid, psoriasiform, cicatricial and elephantiasic lesions. This listing does not include the lesion presenting as a solitary subcutaneous abscess covered by normal epidermis. No lesion of this character is described in several more recent studies including a report of 129 cases of chromoblastomycosis by Brygoo and Segretain. The indolent progressive course of chromoblastomycotic lesions differs also from the nearly static and quiescent behavior of the subcutaneous abscesses. For these reasons, the separation of the subcutaneous abscess caused by pigmented fungi from the general category of chromoblastomycosis made by Kempson and Sternberg as well as by Baker appears to be warranted.

In rare instances subcutaneous abscesses are seen in patients with disseminated chromoblastomycosis. These lesions are believed to be metastatic, and although they exhibit the same histopathologic changes as the subcutaneous abscess we have seen, they are associated with widespread lesions typical of ordinary chromoblastomycosis (Azulay and Serruya). Two of these lesions described by Carrion and Koppisch were present in subcutaneous tissue and a third lesion was found in the deep fascia of the right thigh. The possibility that at least some of these lesions are due to primary innoculations has not been excluded. However, further support for some of these lesions being metastatic is found in a report by Kakoti and Dey. Their patient developed extensive lesions of the labia majora and lymph nodes of both inguinal regions. The nodes were necrotic and apparently resembled tuberculous lesions grossly. The same organisms were isolated from the vulvar lesions as well as from the nodes. Tissue sections and smears of the nodes also showed these organisms. The massive deep abscesses also found in rare patients with chromoblastomycosis should likewise be set apart from the subcutaneous abscesses. Pedroso and Gomes found bacteria as well as fungi in such a lesion from the neck which measured 6×2 cm.

The medical significance of the subcutaneous abscess has not been determined with certainty because of the small number of cases studied up to the present time. As far as is known, the infection remains localized and is innocuous. This is somewhat surprising in view of the presence of unrelated serious diseases in many of these patients. One explanation for this limited infection is that the organisms may have such low virulence that they are unable to take further advantage of the lowered host resistance after having established the initial lesion. The observation that the abscess contents may be spilled into the surgical wound during attempts at excision without initiating a recurrence is somewhat in favor of this explanation. Indeed it is possible that some of these lesions sterilize themselves as is suggested by the extremely small number of fungi in two lesions and the presence of degenerating organisms in many lesions. On the other hand, pigmented fungus infections may be quite aggressive in certain instances. Fuku-

SHIRO et al. presented the case of an 8 year old child who developed lesions of the right cheek and ala nasi due to *H. pedrosoi*. Several months later the child died of brain abscesses caused by the same organism. At least 13 brain lesions were present and were believed to have been metastatic from the sores on the face. Although this is an isolated case, its validity and significance are difficult to ignore. A second observation of some pertinence is found in the experiences with experimental induction of subcutaneous abscesses in mice and rats using chromoblastomycosis organisms. The abscesses usually rupture and heal spontaneously (CONANT et al.). By contrast, the subcutaneous abscesses produced by IWATA and WADA penetrated the thoracic wall and extended into the lungs of mice. The organisms had been obtained from FUKUSHIRO et al. 's case. These workers had added a small amount of carboxy-methyl cellulose to the usually employed saline suspension of cultured organisms. The cellulose polymer may have been the critical factor responsible for the aggressive behavior of the lesions. On rare occasion, an intracutaneous innoculation in the mouse has apparently given rise to a brain lesion (WATSON).

The wide variety of organisms found in the subcutaneous abscess provides a bountiful opportunity to study the tissue phase of these fungi. Organisms showing authentic budding are found with regularity, a phenomenon not observed in the lesions of chromoblastomycosis. The blastospore chains studied by RAJAM et al. appear to be an exception. The conversion of blastospores to chlamydospores, likewise, seems to occur frequently. In addition, the germination of the spores as documented by the formation of growth tubes can be observed. Although both yeast and mycelia are characteristically present in the subcutaneous abscess, this dimorphism is not limited to that particular lesion. Dimorphism is also characteristic for organisms in lesions of cladosporiosis, the infection of brain and meninges by chromoblastomycosis organisms (SYMMERS, 1960). It is not known what factors are directly responsible for the development of two growth forms of the same organism in these diseases.

Acknowledgements: The author acknowledges the interest and inspiration of Drs. R.J. REED, CHARLES E. DUNLAP, and W.H. STERNBERG. Dr. STERNBERG also provided one of the figures and pathologic material on seven of the cases, two of which were originally contributed by Dr. FRIEDRICHS HARRIS. Dr. J.T. McQUITTY provided clinical follow-up on one case. Drs. LORRAINE FRIEDMAN and JOHN D. SCHNEIDAU, JR. (Tulane Department of Microbiology, Mycology Section) as well as Drs. EMMA MOSS and MARION HOOD (Charity Hospital, New Orleans, Louisiana) gave assistance in evaluation of fungi in tissue; each has some reservations about the terminology employed and, since they do not all agree, the responsibility becomes solely that of the author. Dr. RENÉE CORNILLE translated two of the French articles. Mr. RAYMOND JOHNSON made the photographs. Figure C is used with the permission of the Williams and Wilkins Co., Baltimore, Maryland and Drs. R.L. KEMPSON and W.H. STERNBERG. It is a reproduction of Fig. 1, page 599, American Journal of Clinical Pathology, Vol. 39, No. 6, 1963.

References

AZULAY, R.D., SERRUYA, J.: Hematogenous dissemination in chromoblastomycosis; report of a generalized case. Arch. Derm. **95**, 57 (1967). — BAKER, R.D., in ANDERSON, W.A.D., ed.: Pathology, ed. 5, Saint Louis, C.V. Mosby Co., 1966, Chapter 12, Fungus Infections, p. 310. — BROCK, J.M., KENNEDY, C.B., CLARK, W.G.: Cutaneous infection with atypical mycobacterium; report of a case. Arch. Derm. **82**, 918 (1960). — BRYGOO, E.R., SEGRETAIN, G.: Etude clinique épidémiologique et mycologique de la chromoblastomycose à Madagascar. Bull. Soc. Path. exot. **53**, 443 (1960). — CARRION, A.L.: Chromoblastomycosis. Ann. N.Y. Acad. Sci **50**, 1255 (1950a). ~ Yeastlike dematiaceous fungi infecting the human skin; special reference to so-called *Hormiscium dermatitidis*. Arch. Derm. Syph. (Chic.) **61**, 996 (1950b). — CARRION, A.L., KOPPISCH, E.: Observations on dermatomycosis in Puerto Rico; report on a case of chromoblastomycosis. Puerto Rico J. publ. Hlth. **9**, 169 (1933). — CARRION, A., SILVA, M.: Sporotrichosis; special reference: a revision of so-called *Sporotrichum gougerotti*. Arch. Derm. **72**, 523 (1955). — CONANT, N.F., SMITH, D.T., BAKER, R.D., CALLAWAY, J.L.,

Martin, D.C.: Manuel of Clinical Mycology, ed. 2, p. 278. Philadelphia: W.B. Saunders Co. 1954. — DaFonseca, O.: Sur l'état actuel de la question des chromoblastomycoses. Presse méd. **48**, 133 (1940). — Fukushiro, R., Kagawa, S., Nishiyama, S., Takahashi, H.: Un cas de chromoblastomycose cutanée avec métastase cérébrale mortele. Presse méd. **65**, 2142 (1957). — Ichinose, H.: Unpublished data. — Iwata, K., Wada, T.: Mycological studies on the strains isolated from a case of chromoblastomycosis with a metastasis in the central nervous system. Jap. J. Microbiol. **1**, 355 (1957). — Joe, L.K., Eng, N.T.: Subcutaneous phycomycosis: a new disease found in Indonesia. Ann. N.Y. Acad. Sci. **89**, 4 (1960). — Kakoti, L.M., Dey, N.C.: Chromoblastomycosis in India. J. Indian med. Ass. **28**, 351 (1957). — Kempson, R.L., Sternberg, W.H.: Chronic subcutaneous abscesses caused by pigmented fungi, a lesion distinguishable from cutaneous chromoblastomycosis. Amer. J. clin. Path. **39**, 598 (1963). — Levan, N.E., Huntington, R.W., Jr: Primary cutaneous coccidioido-mycosis in agricultural workers. Arch Derm. **92**, 215 (1965). — Lewis, G.M., Hopper, M.E., Sachs, W., Cormia, F.E., Potelunas, C.B.: Mycetoma-like chromoblastomycosis affecting the hand; further findings and comparative mycologic studies. J. invest. Derm. **10**, 155 (1948). — Mariat, F., Segretain, G., Destombes, P., Darrasse, H.: Kyste sous-cutane mycosique (Phaeo-sporotrichose) à *Phialophora gougerotii* (Matruchot, 1910) Borelli, 1955, observeé au Sénégal. Sabouraudia **5**, 209 (1967). — Mead, M., Ridley, M.F.: Sporotrichosis and chromoblastomycosis in Queensland. Med. J. Aust. **1**, 192 (1957). — Merrin, J.A.: Weitere Beobachtungen über den Erreger der europäischen Chromoblastomycosis. Arch. Derm. Syph. (Chic.) **166**, 722 (1932). — Moore, M.: The virulence of strains of *Phialophora verrucosa* determined by innoculating chorio-allantoic membranes of chick embryos. J. invest. Derm. **5**, 411 (1942). — Nielson, H.S., Jr., Conant, N.F.: Practical evaluation of antigenic relationships of yeastlike dematiaceous fungi. Sabouraudia **5**, 283 (1967). — Nityananda, K.: Chromoblastomycosis in Ceylon. Derm. Trop. **1**, 184 (1962). — Pardo-Castello, V., Leon, E.R., Trespalacios, F.: Chromoblastomycosis in Cuba. Arch. Derm. Syph. (Chic.) **45**, 19 (1942). — Pedroso, A., Gomes, J.M.: Four cases of dermatitis verrucosa produced by *Phialophora verrucosa*. Ann. paulist. de med. e. cir. **9**, 53 (March), 1920, as cited by F.D. Weidman and L.H. Rosenthal. Reference 21. — Rajam, R.V., Kandhari, K.C., Thirumalachar, M.J.: Chromoblastomycosis caused by a rare yeast like dematiaceous fungus. Mycopathologia (Den Haag) **9**, 5 (1958). — Samuels, M.S.: Personal communication, Feb. 1968. — Schneidau, J.D., Jr.: Personal communication, Feb. 1968. — Silva, M.: The parasitic phase of the fungi of chromoblastomycosis: development of sclerotic cells *in vitro* and *in vivo*. Mycologia **49**, 318 (1957). — Snell, W.H., Dick, E.A.: A Glossary of Mycology, p. 20. Cambridge: Harvard University Press 1957. — Sussman, A.S., Lingappa, Y., Bernstein, I.A.: Effect of light and media upon growth and melanin formation in *Cladosporium mansoni*. Mycopathologia (Den Haag) **20**, 307 (1963). — Symmers, W.St.C.: Localized cutaneous histoplasmosis. Brit. med. J. **2**, 790 (1956). ~ A case of cerebral chromoblastomycosis (cladosporiosis) occurring in Britain as a complication of polyarteritis treated with cortisone. Brain **83**, 37 (1960). — Throlakson, R.H., Rusnak, C.H.: Subcutaneous nocardiosis. Canad. med. Ass. J. **95**, 224 (1966). — Tubaki, K.: Sporulating Structures in Fungi Imperfecti. In: G.C. Ainsworth, and A.S. Sussman, eds.: The Fungi; An Advanced Treatise. New York and London: Academic Press 1966. Vol. II, The Fungal Organism, Chapter 4, p. 116. — Watson, K.C.: Cerebral chromoblastomycosis. J. Path. Bact. **84**, 233 (1962). — Weidman, F.D., Rosenthal, L.H.: Chromoblastomycosis: a new and important blastomycosis in North America; report of a case in Philadelphia. Arch. Derm. Syph. (Chic.) **43**, 62 (1941). — Young, J.M., Ulrich, E.: Sporotrichosis produced by *Sporotrichum gougerotii*; report of a case and review of the literature. Arch. Derm. **67**, 44 (1953).

Candidosis

H. I. WINNER, London, Great Britain

With 33 Figures

1. General

The intense interest in this subject in recent years is reflected in the great volume of published literature on all its aspects, especially the clinical and experimental. (WINNER and HURLEY, 1964).

a) Definition

Candidosis (candidiasis, moniliasis) is disease due to infection by *Candida albicans* and other species of candida.

The commonest variety of the disease is "thrush" or infection of the mucous membrane of the oral cavity or the vagina. Less commonly, however, the skin and any visceral organ may be affected.

b) Epidemiology

Systematic studies on the epidemiology of the disease are scanty. Superficial infection is contracted as a result of direct contact with infected persons. There is some evidence (CLAYTON and NOBLE, 1966) that airborne contamination may also occur. Infection of the gut frequently follows the ingestion of infected saliva. Systemic disease, due to bloodstream contamination, may arise by invasion of the tissues from superficial infection, or by direct implantation of the organism into the bloodstream during parenteral therapy or surgical operation.

c) Incidence and Predisposing Factors

Oral thrush is common in infants and children; it also frequently occurs in adults.

Vaginal thrush occurs in women of all ages, but particularly in the child bearing age and in pregnancy.

All types of the disease occur more commonly in the following conditions:

1. Physiological: Pregnancy, Early infancy
2. Traumatic: Maceration of skin, Allergic conditions of the skin, Chemical damage to mucous membranes
3. Endocrine disorders: Diabetes mellitus, Hypothyroidism, Hypoparathyroidism, Hypoadrenalism
4. Malnutrition and malabsorption syndrome.
5. Malignant disease, especially leukaemias.
6. Agranulocytosis and aplastic anaemia.
7. Post-operative states.
8. Antibacterial antibiotic therapy.
9. Therapy by immunosuppressive drugs.

2. Mycology

Candida albicans is a yeast-like fungus which exists in three morphological forms: yeast cells or blastospores, mycelium or pseudomycelium, and chlamydospores. For the purpose of this article, mycelium and pseudomycelium are regarded as identical.

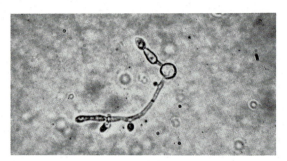

Fig. 1. *C.albicans* mycelium, chlamydospore, and blastospores. Unstained preparation after 24 h incubation on corn-meal agar at room temperature (×360). (From Winner and Hurley, 1964; Fig. 5, p. 24)

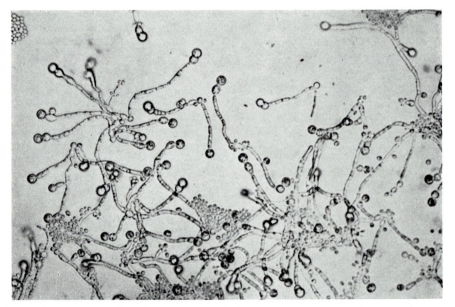

Fig. 2. *C.albicans* mycelium, blastospores, and chlamydospores. Unstained preparation after 24 h incubation on "Oxoid" corn-meal agar at 26°C (×480). (From Winner and Hurley, 1964; Fig. 6, p. 25)

Yeast cells and mycelium are the forms found in lesions in human cases. There is controversy about whether the yeast or the mycelium is the invasive form, or whether both may be invasive; the evidence is inconclusive. Chlamydospores are thick-walled, spherical, refractile structures found on artificial culture in poor media; their significance and function are unknown (Figs. 1, 2, 3).

Approximately 25% of cases of candidosis are due to species other than *C.albicans*. The most important are *C.stellatoidea*, *C.tropicalis*, *C.parapsilosis*,

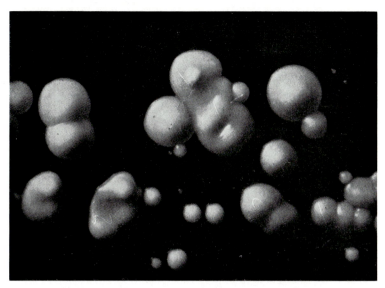

Fig. 3. Colonial appearance of *C.albicans* after 24 h incubation on peptone maltose agar at 37°C (×6). Note creamy consistency of colonies. (From WINNER and HURLEY, 1964; Fig. 10, p. 41)

C.pseudotropicalis, C.guilliermondii, and *C.krusei.* The species are all about the same size; they differ somewhat in morphology, in biochemical characteristics and in antigenic structure. The clinical pictures and pathology of the diseases they cause are broadly similar and for convenience may be considered together.

3. Diagnosis of Candida Infections

a) Identification from Clinical Specimens

From superficial lesions smears from swabs or loops of exudate should be examined microscopically both fresh and after gram staining. Direct cultures should be made on to Sabouraud's or other suitable media. On Sabouraud's agar all types of candida show a growth within 24 h after incubation at 37°C. The species may be identified by further cultural, biochemical and serological tests.

Portions of tissues suspected of infection by candidas should whenever possible be cultured in the fresh state before fixation. It is impossible to identify a candida with certainty, or even to assign an evident fungus to the candida genus, unless cultures are made from the material. In the absence of a culture, the morphological appearances of the genus are not sufficiently characteristic to enable more than a presumptive identification to be made from the examination of stained sections.

On the other hand, experienced histologists can identify certain features of the candida genus as seen in stained sections of histological tissues which enable them to name the genus, if not the species, with a fair degree of confidence.

C.albicans may be seen in tissue sections either in the mycelial or blastospore form; usually, but not always, both are present. When this is so, identification of the genus candida may be inferred since the dimorphic appearance is characteristic. However, the possibility of a dual infection must be borne in mind. Further difficulties arise when either the blastospore or the mycelial form is present by

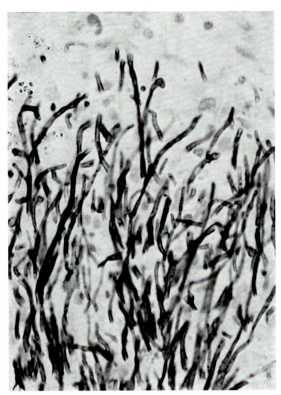

Fig. 4. *C. albicans* in the margin of a liver abscess in a case of septicaemic candidosis. Close-set, septate, rather narrow and angular hyphae; branching at various angles (Hexamine silver, ×930)

Table 1

Septa	Candida +	Aspergillus +	Mucor —
Section	Circular varying calibre	Circular, uniform calibre	Flat
Thickness	Varying; numerous constrictions	Uniform	Great variation mainly very broad. Numerous constrictions
Folds	Few	Few	Many, may give appearance of septa
Angle of branching	Various	Dichotomous	Mainly perpendicular

itself, and in such circumstances anything more than a tentative diagnosis is usually impossible in the absence of cultural confirmation.

Blastospores of *C. albicans* are spherical or slightly ovoid; all other candida species are more oval or elongated than *C. albicans*. The amount of tissue reaction is variable, and there may be none.

The candidas do not stain sharply with haemotoyxlin and eosin, but they can easily be stained by the modified periodic-acid-Schiff reaction and by silver impregnation methods such as Grocott's methenamine-silver technique. They are strongly gram positive.

Differentiation from *Cryptococcus neoformans* may be made by the absence of a capsule and the presence of filaments.

The mycelium of candida is usually uniform in thickness, with little branching; straight filaments are characteristic. Filaments of candida may be differentiated from those of mucor by the features shown in Table 1 (SYMMERS, 1964) (Fig. 4).

b) Serological Diagnosis

In cases of suspected deep-seated candidosis, in which it has not proved practicable to culture the organism from the lesion, attempts have been made to assist the diagnosis by the detection of antibodies in the patient's serum. Care is needed in the interpretation of serological tests, since the occurrence of candida antibodies is widespread throughout the human population even in the absence of clinical infection (WINNER, 1955).

On the other hand, a persistently high titre is undoubtedly supporting evidence of a candida infection. Various techniques have been tried, of which the most commonly used has been the agglutination reaction using killed whole candida cells as the antigen. Complement fixation and precipitin reactions have also been used, but are technically more exacting and the formulation of standard antigens is a difficulty. Moreover the results are less easy to control by comparison with "control" subjects who show no manifestations of infection.

At present much research is in progress on the elucidation of the antigenic structure of the candidas, the preparation of standardised antigens, and the significance of different types of antibody in infected subjects. This should lead to an increase in the value of serological methods of diagnosis.

c) Other Methods of Diagnosis

Skin tests: Dermal hypersensitivity to *C. albicans* was reported by RAMEL (1925) and by RAVAUT and RABEAU (1929), who showed that normal people would give positive skin reactions to extracts of candida. Since then, there have been many attempts to assess the significance of such reactions, and particularly to use them as a means of detecting latent infection. However, too many normal subjects have shown positive reactions (SCLAFER and FLAVIN, 1954; SCLAFER, 1957). LEWIS et al. (1937), showed that 43% of patients with candidosis gave negative skin reactions, and 46% without the disease gave positive reactions.

These results indicated that the test was useless as a means of diagnosis of infections. The possibility that they might be due to unsuitable antigenic preparations was propounded by AKIBA et al. (1957). They recommended the use of purified antigens. On the other hand, in the absence of exact chemical definition of the antigens, it is difficult to see how purified antigens can be obtained. MAIBACH and KLIGMAN (1962) concluded that the development of skin allergy in dermal candidosis was too inconstant to be of value in diagnosis. Moreover, skin reactions are not specific; patients infected with other fungi may cross-react to extracts of candida.

To summarise, it is doubtful whether tests for hypersensitivity have any place today in the diagnosis of deep-seated infection.

Radiology: Radiology has been tried as an ancillary method of diagnosis in suspected disease of the chest and the gastrointestinal tract. So far as chest radiology is concerned, there is no means of differentiating radiologically between infections with candida and those by other micro-organisms. Some authors have claimed (Marsh, 1959; Kaufman et al. ,1960) that the radiological appearances in candidosis of the oesophagus are sufficiently characteristic to warrant a confident diagnosis. It seems, however, that radiology, no matter how well performed, must still be confirmed by the isolation of the organisms from the lesions.

4. Pathogenesis of Candida Infections

It has repeatedly been observed that candida infections, both superficial and deep-seated, are particularly liable to occur in patients whose immune mechanisms are disturbed for any reason, or whose microbial flora has been assaulted by antimicrobial therapy. A list of the predisposing clinical conditions associated with candidosis is given earlier in this chapter. Such a list, however, cannot be exhaustive. Indeed, the first manifestation of one of the disorders listed may be the clinical appearance of a candida infection. The diagnosis of such an infection is therefore an indication for a searching clinical examination, including all ancillary tests. As Wilson (1962) points out, C.albicans is a better clinician and more able to detect patients with immunological abnormalities than are human physicians. In adults hitherto regarded as previously normal, the appearance of even a superficial candida infection is a manifestation of either some local damage at the site of the infection or of some systemic disorder. The only exceptions are the appearance of vaginal thrush in non-pregnant women, or candidosis anywhere in the body in pregnant women. Early infancy, that is to say, the first few weeks of extrauterine life, is another state in which immunity patterns are too immature to withstand tissue invasion by this organism, and there is no need to look for any predisposing cause of candidosis in a small infant.

In all other cases, the normal immune mechanisms of the individual are sufficient to withstand tissue invasion by candida. Such invasion only occurs in the breakdown of immune mechanisms, either locally or generally, and the appearance of a candida lesion is a clear indication for a search for such a breakdown.

5. Clinical Features and Pathology of Candida Infections

The commonest form of candidosis is thrush of the oral or vaginal mucous membranes. A more generalised infection, affecting surface areas in many parts of the body, is occasionally seen. Thus the skin and nails may be affected as well as the mucous membranes. Generalised candidosis, as this superficial disease is called, is usually associated with one of the predisposing conditions to which we have referred, and more specifically, may be part of a generalised endocrine deficiency syndrome sometimes called the *endocrine candidosis syndrome* (see later). Candida granuloma ("monilial granuloma") is a variety of superficial generalised candidosis.

Generalised candidosis is usually superficial. However, it may also be associated with the presence of the organisms in the bloodstream, and may therefore be a manifestation of septicaemic candidosis. The latter, as would be expected, is a much more serious and frequently fatal condition. The organism may set up metastatic lesions in almost any organ of the body, most commonly the kidneys. The heart valves may be affected in patients with pre-existing valvular lesions.

a) Infections of the Mouth

The commonest clinical manifestation of *C.albicans* infection is oral thrush, which occurs frequently in infants and in debilitated adults.

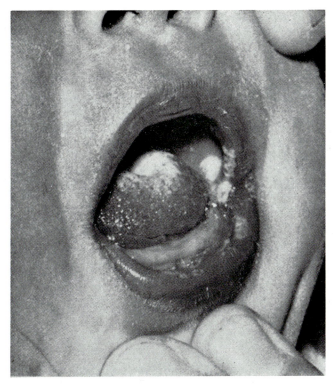

Fig. 5. Oral thrush in a child of eight days (From WINNER and HURLEY, 1964; Fig. 18, p. 95)

Clinical features: The disease first appears in the form of small white patches on the lining of the gums, the side of the tongue, the buccal mucosa, and the mucosa of the throat. The lesions coalesce and form pearly-white elevated patches which look like curdled milk, but, unlike these, can be removed only with difficulty. They are painless with no swelling, and they may heal within a few days of starting treatment. Occasionally erosion and ulceration may occur with necrosis and granuloma formation (Fig. 5).

Pathology: In oral thrush, the essential lesion is oedema of the infected mucous membrane. An oedematous plaque forms from the desquamating epithelial cells. This forms a pseudomembrane which consists of shed desquamating epithelium mixed with keratin, fibrin, necrotic tissue, food debris, leucocytes and bacteria, all matted together and anchored down to the living epithelium by the fungal hyphae. There may be little or no tissue response (LEHNER, 1966) (Fig. 6).

Candida leukoplakia. Some cases of oral leukoplakia are associated with, if not due to, candida infection (CAWSON and LEHNER, 1968). Clinically this may be indistinguishable from other forms of leukoplakia, though candida may readily be detected in smears of the exudate and in biopsy sections. Cases infected with candida also show a raised antibody titre to this organism. While some cases have responded to local antimycotic therapy, however, it is also possible that the changes initiated in the mucosa by candida infection may in some cases be progressive and irreversible, even after the infection has been removed (Fig. 7 and 8).

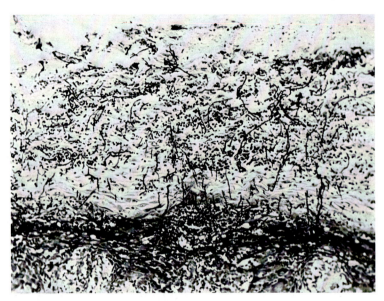

Fig. 6. Oral thrush. Loosely knit oedematous plaque of desquamating epithelial cells invaded by hyphae and infiltrated by inflammatory cells (PAS, ×120)

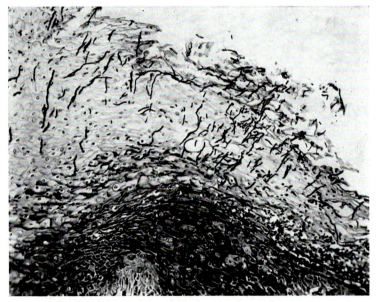

Fig. 7. Candida leukoplakia. Hyphae invading the parakeratotic zone. Oedema and inflammatory cells at the junction of the parakeratotic zone and the stratum spinosum (PAS, ×120)

The histological picture shows a marked parakeratosis, with hyphal invasion. There is an inflammatory reaction along the junction of the parakeratotic zone with the stratum spinosum. Some degree of acanthosis is present. Chronic inflammatory changes are also found in the corium.

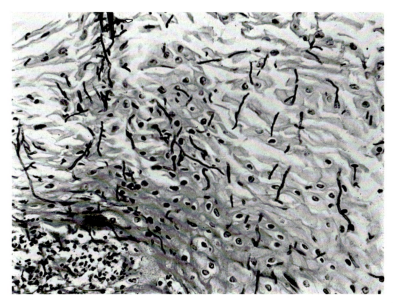

Fig. 8. Candida leukoplakia. Higher power from same lesions as Fig. 7, to show details of plaque (PAS, ×120)

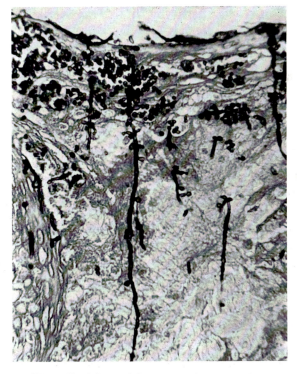

Fig. 9. Candidosis of the tongue (Grocott, ×390)

Lehner (1966) and Cawson (1966) have described the changes associated with other clinical varieties of oral candidosis. Acute atrophic candidosis is often associated with antibiotic therapy ("antibiotic sensitive tongue"). In this condition the pseudomembrane may be shed, leaving an intensely painful atrophic red mucosa. Denture stomatitis is frequently associated with candida infection; in fact, Cawson asserts that this is the commonest form of oral candidosis. It is characterised by erythema and oedema of the upper-denture bearing part of the mucosa, which becomes bright red and may be sharply differentiated from the surrounding mucosa at the margins of the denture (Fig. 9).

b) Skin

Maceration: The most important predisposing factor in candidosis of the skin is *maceration*, or damage by moisture. Those whose occupation involves frequent immersion of the hands in water are particularly liable to candidosis of the hands. Such occupational groups include housewives in whom candidosis of the fingers and chronic paronychia are common. Fishmongers, shoemakers, chefs and barmen are other groups subject to this occupational disease.

Another source of the damaging moisture is perspiration which is unable to evaporate freely, as in intertriginous lesions anywhere in the body. These are liable to infection by candida and other microbes. Soldiers are subject to candidosis of the feet.

In *infants*, the diaper region may be kept wet by the infants' excreta. Diaper rashes due to candida infection are common. They have been described by Bound (1956). The buttocks and inner thighs are most commonly involved, but the genitalia and lower abdomen may also be affected. At first the lesions consist of dull red areas which tend to coalesce. Flat vesicles soon form, after which desquamation occurs. Bound considers that the rash may easily be distinguished from two other common napkin rashes, namely, excoriated buttocks and ammonia dermatitis. Another type of illness was described by Robinson (1957). This is a sudden flare up of acute dermatitis in cases of infantile eczema.

Perlèche is a form of maceration of the corners of the mouth first described by Lemaistre (1886) among inhabitants of the Limousin district who moistened their lips with their tongue after sipping wine.

Candida invasion of intertriginous skin may occur in the axillae, the submammary regions, the umbilicus, the webs of the fingers and toes, the limb flexures, and the vulval area.

Candidosis may also occur in the *external ear* (La Touche, 1966).

Candida Granuloma: A well defined and serious skin infection in older children is *candida granuloma* (monilial granuloma). This takes the form of superficial inflammation with hyperkeratosis which may be very marked, giving rise to crust formation and sometimes to the formation of horns.

In the case described by Hauser and Rothman (1950) the patient was a well-developed and well-nourished boy of seven. Apparently there were no predisposing factors. Multiple horns developed on the skin, biopsy of which showed hyperkeratosis and acanthosis. The corium was filled with a dense infiltration of lymphocytes, plasma cells, polymorphs, and foreign body giant cells. The infiltrate extended downwards to the subcutis and was perifollicular and periglandular in some areas. Filaments thought to be hyphae were seen in the stratum corneum. Some years after this case report, Rothman (1959) further reported that the patient had suddenly developed diabetic coma and that he later died of diabetes.

In their comments on this and other reported cases, Hauser and Rothman considered that there might be a constitutional defect in defence mechanisms. They showed that the organisms which cause candida granuloma were not more pathogenic than other strains of candida and they noted, as additional evidence of subnormal resistance, the early age of death in patients with candida granuloma. NITYANANDA (1959) pointed out the early age of onset of the disease. On the other hand, several cases have been described in adults (ROCKWOOD and GREENWOOD, 1934; DANBOLT, 1940; CARSLAW et al., 1966).

Skin Allergy: Next to maceration, the most important predisposing cause of candidosis of the skin is allergy. OWEN et al. (1939) showed that spontaneous skin infections by *C.albicans* might lead to the development of "id" reactions, which could be acute or chronic. Invasion by candida has also often been noted in skin affected by allergy due to other causes.

c) Lungs

The frequency with which *C.albicans* can be cultured from the sputum, in apparent cases of acute and chronic chest infection, has led to much discussion on its possible pathogenic role in the lungs.

The mere fact of isolating *C.albicans* from the sputum is no indication of its possible pathogenic role in the chest. *C.albicans* is often present in the mouths of healthy people and it can appear in their sputum by contamination from the mouth. Moreover, unless the sputum specimen is fresh when cultured, and unless it is collected into a sterile container, the possibility of aerial contamination exists.

As it occurs so often in the mouths of healthy people, *C.albicans* will obviously be found no less frequently in the sputum of those with lung disease, and the numerous sanatorium and hospital surveys confirm this. Moreover, its occurrence, here as elsewhere in the body, is increased in patients on antibiotic therapy.

For there to be a reasonable assurance that organisms recovered from the *sputum* have come from the lungs, the following criteria should be fulfilled.

1. The specimen should be collected into a sterile container.

2. The specimen must either be refrigerated until it is cultured, or it must be cultured soon after collection — within an hour or two. ORIE (1946) recommended that it be washed.

3. Either the organisms should be grown frequently or invariably from the sputum and not from the mouth or throat or postnasal swabs, or they should be grown from a bronchial cast, plug or membrane from a bronchiectatic cavity or pulmonary abscess.

Any patients may harbour the organism in their mouths or throats whether or not they are suspected cases of pulmonary candidosis. Unless the above criteria are fulfilled, therefore, the presence of the organism in the sputum of such patients should be discounted, so far as the diagnosis of pulmonary candidosis is concerned. It is from such patients that a bronchial aspiration specimen may reasonably be demanded in order to confirm that the *C.albicans* has truly come from their lungs. It is not sufficient to cleanse the mouth.

There are, of course, many cases in which *C.albicans* is one of several types of fungus which are apparently playing a saprophytic role in the lung. Such cases are those of cavitation or bronchiectasis, where there is likely to be much stagnant organic material on which yeasts and other fungi may thrive. The bizarre name of "pulmonary intercavitary fungus ball" was given to this condition, in which *C.albicans* is rarely, if ever, the only fungus present (WIESE and BIXBY, 1941; GELLI, 1954).

No aspect of the pathogenicity of *C.albicans* has given rise to more controversy than the part it plays in lung disease. Apparent cases of pulmonary candidosis have been reported from most parts of the world. However, many experienced workers in this field have been inclined to decry the importance of *C.albicans* as a pulmonary pathogen, and indeed to deny it can ever cause primary lung disease. SHREWSBURY (1936) considered that the organism could not cause pneumonia, and that the extent of lung pathology produced by this yeast was secondary thrush of the bronchi. His view was endorsed by RIDDELL and CLAYTON (1958). Similar views have also been expressed by ROBERTSON (1945), FRISK (1952, and ORIE (1952).

This standpoint does not, of course, dispose of the importance of *C.albicans* as a lung pathogen. It is often difficult, and it may be impossible, to determine in any particular case whether the role of *C.albicans* in the lungs is that of a primary or a secondary invader. Moreover, this point, though important, does not seem to be crucial (OBLATH et al., 1951). The important question is not whether the role of *C.albicans* is primary or secondary, but whether it causes disease in the lungs at all. If it only does so as a secondary invader, it resembles several pathogenic bacteria in this respect, for Friedlander's bacillus and *Haemophilus influenzae* are often secondary invaders. This fact does not diminish their potential danger as pathogens.

If *C.albicans* can cause lung disease, this role is by no means incompatible with Shrewsbury's view, endorsed by RIDDELL and his colleagues, that the organism causes secondary thrush of the bronchi. It may, in such circumstances give rise to chronic bronchitis and hence pave the way for bacterial invasion of the lungs. It may give rise to allergic symptoms resembling asthma. It may cause bronchial obstruction leading to pulmonary collapse and its sequelae. It may cause mycomas in lungs affected by pulmonary tuberculosis (SCHULTE, 1957). If the organism fulfils any of these roles, whether as a primary or as a secondary invader, it is a lung pathogen. Moreover, in a small number of cases, of which that reported by SMITH and ARMEN (1955) is the most convincing, the organism has been shown to cause pneumonia, contrary to the view of SHREWSBURY and others.

The controversy surrounding this subject appears to be due to the chronic nature of the disease, and to the facts that histopathological studies are made late in the course of the illness, or post-mortem, if they are made at all, and that there is no clear-cut association of a particular clinical and a particular pathological picture at all stages of the disease. If pneumonia occurs, it occurs at a stage at which the patient does not die, rarely has a lung resected, and hence is unable to present a specimen for histological study. Inferences as to the possible role of *C.albicans* in causing pulmonary consolidation, the chief matter in dispute, have, therefore, had to be made retrospectively. None the less, they have been made, and with justifiable confidence.

Diagnostic Criteria: Neither the clinical features, or serological or radiological evidence are more than adjuvants in the diagnosis of pulmonary candidosis. For the reasons already given, cultural evidence too, is suspect, though clearly negative culture rules out the possibility of pulmonary candidosis. In the opinion of the present writer, the following are the necessary criteria for the diagnosis of primary pulmonary candidosis:

1. *C.albicans* is obtained consistently and in large amounts from the sputum or bronchoscopic swabbings.
2. *M.tuberculosis* is not found.
3. No other cause of disease is found.
4. Candida is demonstrated in histological sections of the lungs obtained from operation specimens, biopsy, or necropsy.

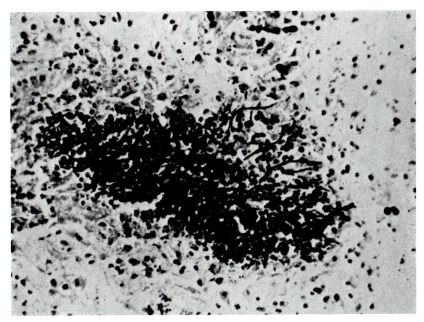

Fig. 10. Candidosis of the lung in a fatal case of septicaemic candidosis (PASH, ×107). (From the same case as Figs. 17, 23 and 33; from WINNER and HURLEY, 1964; Fig. 19, p. 110)

Using these admittedly exacting criteria, a number of convincing cases have been reported. (HURWITZ and YESNER, 1948; SMITH and ARMEN, 1955; OBLATH et al., 1951; FALKMER and WISING, 1955).

In addition to the above cases where candida has caused disease of the lung by direct invasion, candida may also be a cause of asthma. Moreover, it is a common cause of "secondary thrush of the bronchi" (SHREWSBURY, 1936).

In cases of septicaemic candidosis, *C.albicans* may invade the lungs as it does other organs (Fig. 10).

d) Gut

Candida infection of the oesophagus, stomach, and small or large intestines may occur as part of systemic candidosis, or in association with the predisposing conditions already mentioned, especially agranulocytosis, aplastic anaemia, and leukaemia.

Macroscopically the changes associated with candidosis of the alimentary tract are of two types. The mucous membrane may be covered by a thick, shaggy, cream-coloured confluent membrane for much of its length; for example, the whole of the oesophagus may be so covered. This membrane strips easily, revealing greyish-brown plaques of confluent ulceration. The second type of change consists of more localised, discrete and scattered multiple lesions, which may be few or many and may occur in any part of the gut. These are greyish-brown raised plaques or areas of shallow ulceration, and may be covered by a rough friable brown exudate. Mycotic lesions of the second type may be small and may be overlooked at necropsy unless the gut is carefully examined.

The histology of the mycotic lesions of the bowel was described by BEEMER et al. (1954) and by LANNIGAN and MEYNELL (1959). Both mycelium and yeast forms of candida were present, the latter predominating in the case of BEEMER

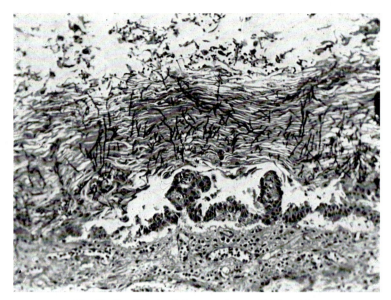

Fig. 11. Candidosis of the oesophagus (PAS, ×120)

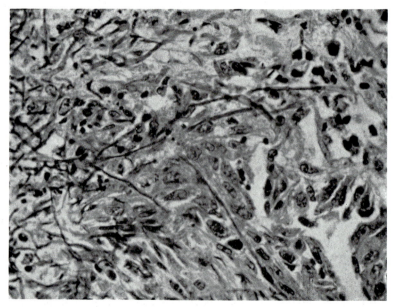

Fig. 12. Proliferating mycelium in the wall of the oesophagus. From a fatal case of disseminated candidosis in a child of 6 treated for acute leukaemia (PAS, ×450). (From WINNER and HURLEY, 1964; Fig. 21, p. 129)

et al. These authors noted a cellular reaction consisting of round cells and neutrophils, with some fibroblastic proliferation. LANNIGAN and MEYNELL reported a reaction which was predominantly lymphocytic and mononuclear, with variable numbers of plasma cells (Figs. 11, 12, 13).

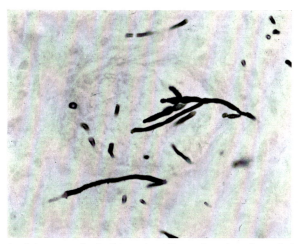

Fig. 13. Candidosis of the stomach. *C. albicans* invading a thrombosed venule in the submucosa in the vicinity of an ulcerating carcinoma, the surface of which was covered with the fungus (Hexamine silver, ×600)

e) Vagina

Candida albicans is now the commonest cause of vaginal discharge. However, in vaginal thrush there may be vulvitis with little or no discharge. The vulva is slightly swollen and tender, reddish blue or intensely red, sometimes with a grey surface. The epithelium may be injured from scratching. The area feels warm both subjectively and to the touch. Small whitish areas ("thrush spots") of caseous material may be observed, giving a granular appearance. The discharge may be thin and yellow, often with white flakes.

The diagnosis is readily confirmed by the microscopic examination and culture of smears of the discharge.

f) Candidosis and Endocrine Disorders

There is a well marked association between candidosis of the skin or mucous membranes and various endocrine disorders. This is most marked in the case of diabetes mellitus, and in many patients the first manifestation of this disease has been the appearance of a superficial candida infection. Other cases of candida infection have been reported in association with hypoadrenalism, hypopara-thyroidism, and hypothyroidism. Sometimes two or more of these disorders have been combined in the same patient who is usually a child. The association has been so well marked as to be given the title *"Candida endocrine syndrome"* (WHIT-AKER et al., 1956; LEHNER, 1966).

It is probable that the precipitating cause for the attack by candida on the host is different in different conditions. In the case of diabetes mellitus, an obvious factor might appear to be the abnormally high glucose content of the blood and tissues, which would be expected to favour the growth of candida. Probably this explanation is too facile; certainly it is now well recognised that changes in carbohydrate metabolism may precede by several years the development of clinical diabetes, and in this pre-diabetic period a candida infection may give warning of the impending disease (WILSON and PLUNKETT, 1965).

In other endocrine disorders it is no easier to find an explanation for the candida infection. Presumably there is some widespread disruption of the immunity mechanisms of the host. LEHNER (1966) suggests that auto-immunity may be a factor, but the rather scanty evidence is indirect.

g) Systemic (Septicaemic) Candidosis

Various terms have been given to this disease, such as acute disseminated (septicaemic) candidosis. There are numerous recent reviews and reports (WINNER and HURLEY, 1964; SYMMERS, 1966).

Diagnosis: One of the reasons for the increasing numbers of cases diagnosed is the increasing importance attached to the isolation of a candida. All too often in the past, if a candida was isolated from a necropsy lesion or from the bloodstream, it was regarded as a contaminant. This belief was undoubtedly mistaken in many cases, and has resulted in many instances of candida septicaemia being missed. It cannot be too strongly emphasized that the isolation of a candida from a lesion, whether during life or at necropsy, must not be regarded as an insignificant finding and full weight must be given to the presence of the organism.

Clinical varieties: SYMMERS (1964) has made a useful subdivision of the cases as follows:

1. Septicaemic candidosis occurring without recognised predisposing factors.

2. Septicaemic candidosis resulting from direct inoculation of the fungus into the body.

3. Septicaemic candidosis occurring as a complication of other diseases or of their treatment.

So far as the first category is concerned, the history of many of the cases described suggests that the underlying predisposing cause was missed. There seems no reason to suppose that candida septicaemia is an exception to what has already been propounded, that the disease does not occur in people hitherto well except in conditions of "physiological unorthodoxy", such as early infancy and pregnancy.

The direct inoculation of the fungus into the bloodstream is a curiously frequent precipitating cause of the disease. This has been known to follow injections of various kinds, including therapeutic substances and narcotic drugs; several cases have followed open-heart surgery (see later).

A large number of cases have been described of septicaemic candidosis arising as a complication of other diseases or of their treatment.

The disease has been described in both adults and children. It is associated with the predisposing causes already listed on page 731. Since such conditions are likely to be present in almost any group of hospital patients, the possibility of such patients developing septicaemic candidosis must always be borne in mind, especially during intense antibacterial or immunosuppressive therapy.

Portal of Entry: As has been stated, the portal of entry of the fungus may well be intravenous, when therapy has been given by this route. In other cases, it seems likely that the organism invades from the alimentary tract, where it is often present as a commensal. Mycotic ulcers of the gut may be small and may be overlooked at necropsy unless carefully sought (LUDLAM and HENDERSON, 1942). This may account for the apparently low incidence of alimentary tract lesions in the cases reviewed above.

Other cases are apparently secondary to superficial candidosis. In some patients who have developed systemic candidosis the portal of entry is obscure. Possibly the organism has entered the bloodstream by direct invasion through the wall of a blood vessel, a hypothesis which may be supported by the appearance of histological sections of the tissues of infected patients and experimentally infected animals.

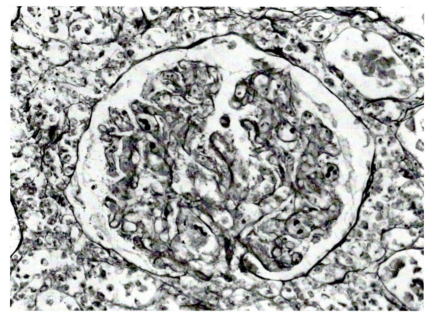

Fig. 14. Renal candidosis, showing yeasts in glomerulus (Hexamine silver, ×310)

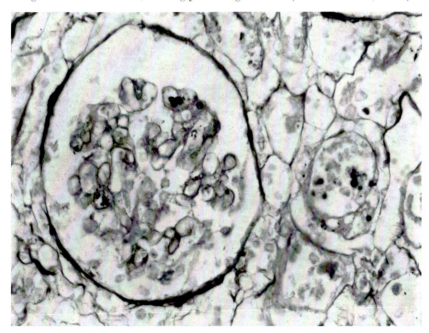

Fig. 15. Renal candidosis. Several fungal cells in a glomerulus and in a nearby dilated capillary (Hexamine silver, ×400)

Pathology: The general picture is that of an acute severe widespread mycotic infection. The organ most frequently involved is the kidney, which shows numerous areas consisting of fungus in both the mycelial and the yeast-like phase, and

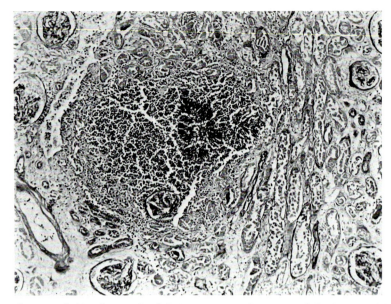

Fig. 16. Acute nephritic abscess. Candida is present in the centre of the lesion (PAS, ×65)

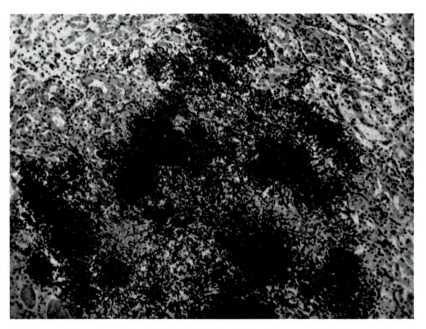

Fig. 17. Areas of fungal proliferation in the kidney. Note absence of cellular reaction. From the same case as Figs. 10, 23 and 33 (PAS, ×86). (From WINNER and HURLEY, 1964; Fig. 27, p. 148)

inflammatory cells. Some of the lesions are large enough to be seen with the naked eye. The lesions are usually confined to the cortex, but proliferating fungi may also occasionally be seen in the medulla. In some cases there is a marked poly-

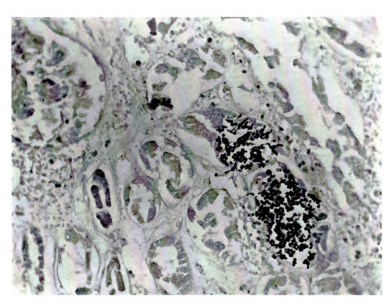

Fig. 18. Candida in kidney lesion (Gram stain, ×220)

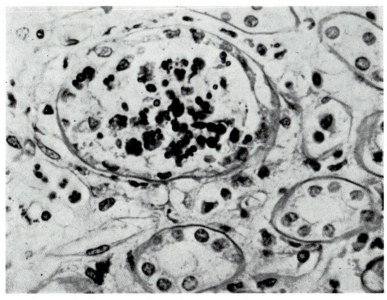

Fig. 19. Budding yeasts and cellular debris in a renal tubule. From a fatal case of disseminated candidosis in a woman of 50 (PASH, × 550). (From WINNER and HURLEY, 1964; Fig. 25, p. 146)

morphonuclear reaction to the fungus and the lesions are mycotic abscesses; in others, cellular reaction is minimal or absent (LEHNER, 1964) (Figs. 14—22).

Sometimes the fungus provokes a basal meningitis, in which small nodules, often less than 1 mm in diameter, are to be found close to blood vessels. The inflammatory exudate consists largely of lymphocytes and plasma cells, though a

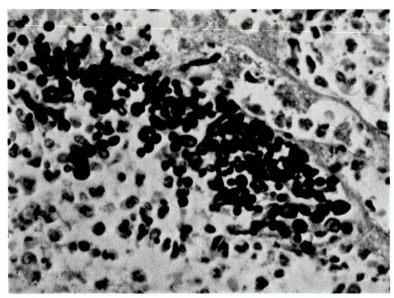

Fig. 20. Budding yeasts in renal tubule. From the same case as Fig. 19 (PASH, ×650). (From Winner and Hurley, 1964; Fig. 26, p. 147)

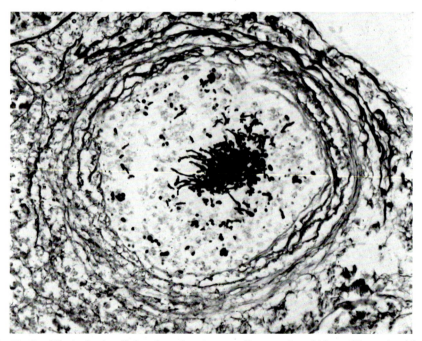

Fig. 21. Candida in fresh cellular thrombus in a small artery in a kidney (Hexamine silver, ×250)

few polymorphonuclear leucocytes may be present. The brain occasionally shows minute abscesses and granulomata, which may contain multinucleate giant cells (Fetter et al., 1967).

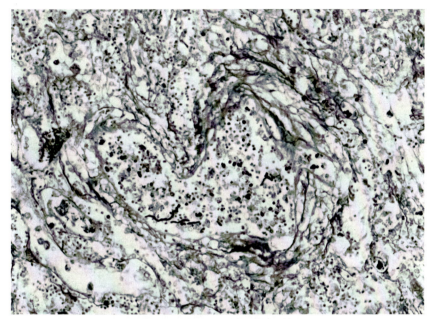

Fig. 22. Candida in a kidney venule (Hexamine silver, ×210)

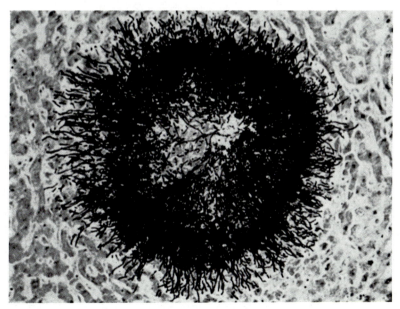

Fig. 23. Colony of Candida in the liver. There is no tissue reaction. From the same case as Figs. 10, 17 and 33 (PASH, ×130). (From WINNER and HURLEY, 1964; Fig. 28, p. 149)

Other organs which may be involved are the liver, lungs, blood vessels, spleen, thyroid, bone marrow, retina, skeletal muscles, and urinary bladder. These lesions do not show any particular features other than those which have already been described. Some of them are illustrated here (Figs. 23—28).

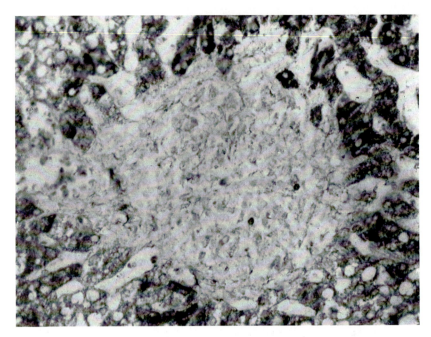

Fig. 24. Candidosis of the liver: A small focus of necrosis containing two candida cells in the liver of a patient with septicaemic candidosis (Hexamine silver, ×300)

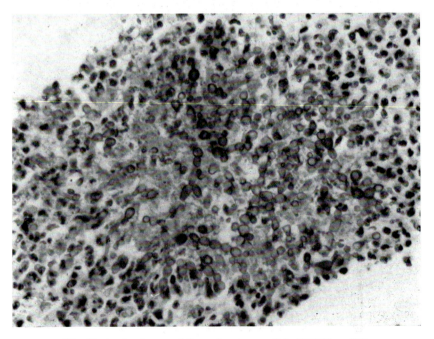

Fig. 25. Acute abscess of liver, showing candida (PASH, ×480)

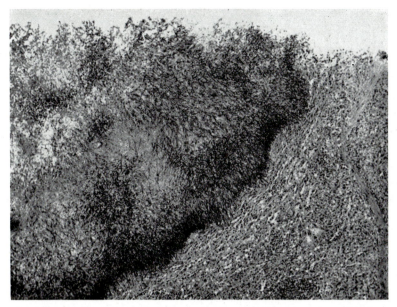

Fig. 26. Candida abscess of the spleen. From a fatal case of disseminated candidosis in a child of 6 treated for acute leukaemia (PASH, ×50). (From WINNER and HURLEY, 1964; Fig. 29, p. 150)

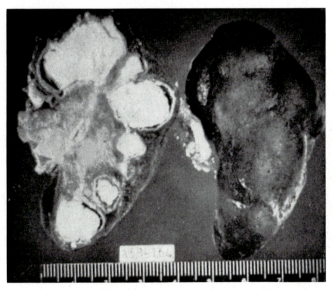

Fig. 27. Multiple infarcts in the kidney by emboli from candida vulvitis (From UTZ, WINNER and HURLEY, 1966; Fig. 5, p. 227)

h) Candida Endocarditis

This is a variant of acute disseminated (septicaemic) candidosis, with involvement of one or more heart valves as the predominant pathological feature. Predisposing factors are pre-existing disease of the heart valves, and more than

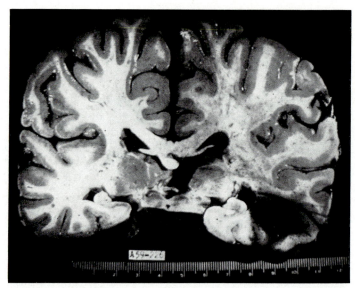

Fig. 28. Infarct of left cerebellum by embolus from candida valvulitis. (From Utz, ed. Winner and Hurley, 1966; Fig. 6, p. 227)

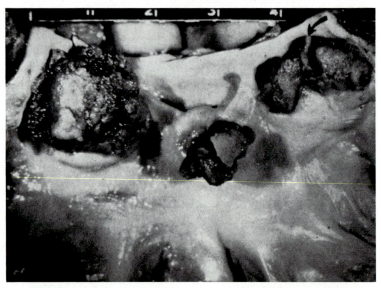

Fig. 29. Candida endocarditis of the aortic valve, viewed with heart opened. The arrow indicates the coronary ostium. (From Utz, ed. Winner and Hurley, 1966; Fig. 3, p. 226)

half the cases have a previous history of rheumatic heart disease; other cases have congenital lesions (Pearl and Sidransky, 1960; Andriole et al., 1962; Kaplan and Levin, 1967). The disease is always blood-born. In some cases it is iatrogenic, or self-inflicted, in that the infection may get into the bloodstream from intravenous therapy. Some of the self-inflicted cases have occured in "main-line" drug addicts, who may give themselves "shots" of drugs which are infected with candida (Wilson, 1961).

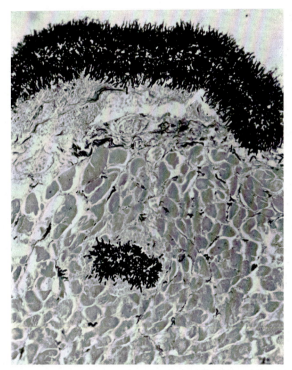

Fig. 30. Gross candida invasion of the pericardium and endocardium (Hexamine silver, ×120)

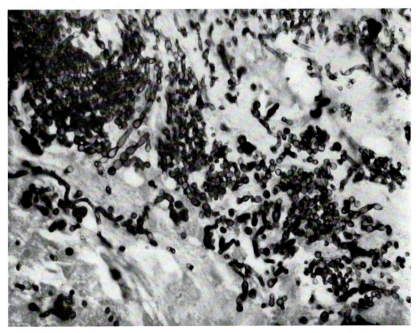

Fig. 31. *C.albicans* vegetation on mitral valve and invading the fibrotic tissue of the cusp
(PASH, ×400)

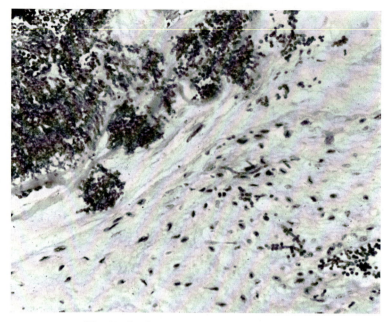

Fig. 32. Candida endocarditis (PASH, ×200)

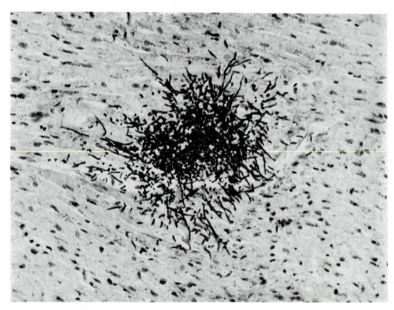

Fig. 33. Colony of *C. albicans* in the myocardium. From the same case as Figs. 10, 17 and 23 (PASH, ×160). (From WINNER and HURLEY, 1964; Fig. 32, p. 166)

Other cases have followed open-heart surgery for congenital or acquired valvular disease (ANDRIOLE et al., 1962; JAMSHIDI et al., 1963; CLIMIE and RACHMANINOFF, 1965) (Figs. 29—33).

Clinical Manifestations: The clinical manifestations of candida endocarditis are those of any infective endocarditis, together with those of a deep mycotic infection. Usually there has been some preceding systemic disorder, most commonly rheumatic heart disease. Special predisposing factors are those of other deep mycoses, that is to say, debilitating disease such as diabetes mellitus, antibiotic therapy or steroid therapy. The commonest clinical features are fever; abdominal pain; nausea and vomiting; heart failure, occurring in patients with recent or old cardiac murmurs; splenic or hepatic enlargement; and embolic manifestations. Embolism to the large arteries has been reported in one-third of the cases reviewed by ANDRIOLE et al. (1962).

Pathology: Necropsy or operation specimens of the heart valves show the presence of large friable vegetations. They are usually larger than those seen in bacterial endocarditis, which may, of course, precede mycotic infection. The incidence of infection on the various heart valves does not appear to differ from that in bacterial endocarditis.

Sections of the valves show filamentous and yeast forms of candida, as illustrated. Candida lesions may also be seen on the myocardium and pericardium.

i) Candidosis of the Urinary Tract

Candidosis of the urinary tract is a variety of the septicaemic disease (WINNER and HURLEY, 1964). It is clear both from experimental studies and from examination of cases of systemic infection that candida has a predilection for the kidney. It can apparently multiply in the parenchyma of that organ, probably more rapidly than in any other part of the body. The carriage of viable candida into the kidney by the bloodstream may therefore be sufficient in itself to initiate a candida lesion. It is not known whether pre-existing kidney disease is necessary for the successful establishment of candida; the large size of the organism may well produce blockage of the renal arterioles and hence bring about an embolic lesion which could favour the further multiplication of candida. Experimental studies give some colour to this idea (MACKINNON, 1936; EVANS and WINNER, 1954).

Unlike cases of candida septicaemia, which always occur in patients who are known to be suffering from some other constitutional disorder, candida infection of the urinary tract has been reported as a primary disease in those hitherto thought to be healthy (ALBERS, 1953; GUZE and HALEY, 1958; WINNER and HURLEY, 1964). This observation, of course, does not rule out the possibility, or, in the present author's view, the probability that the affected patients have been subject to some undetected disorder which has enabled the candida to change from a commensal to an invasive prasite.

Diagnosis: It appears to be a melancholy fact that many cases of candidosis of the urinary tract have been missed because the finding of *C. albicans* in urine specimens has been disregarded as insignificant. When searching for the cause of an apparent clinical urinary infection, clinicians (and pathologists) have perhaps been excessively obsessed by the overwhelming importance of coliform bacilli, faecal streptococci, and tubercle bacilli. Another factor is the unhygienic and septic conditions under which urine specimens are collected, which obviously may favour aerial contamination. A combination of these two factors has led to a situation in which any yeasts found in urine specimens are throught to be of no account.

This is far from the case, as the recent emergence of urinary candidosis as a clinical entity has shown. In all cases of suspected urinary infection, where no other microbiological cause has been demonstrated, a candida or other yeast isolated from the urine must be regarded as being the cause until this is proved otherwise.

Experimental studies have confirmed that candida in the bloodstream of animals can produce a chronic pyelonephritis (Hurley and Winner, 1963).

Thrush of the urinary bladder: This has been reported as a cause of acute cystitis (Moulder, 1946; Snyder, 1948; Sauer and Metzner, 1948). A distinct variety of this disease has been the appearance of candida in "fungus ball of the bladder" (Chisholm and Hutch, 1961).

6. Experimental Aspects of Candida Infections

Experimental aspects of candida infections have attracted many workers. The reasons for this are not hard to seek; the organism is accessible and easily handled, and it is not difficult to manipulate the host in such a way to as produce variations in immunity which might be expected to favour the onset of the disease.

In these days of antibiotics and immunosuppressive therapy it is obviously important to achieve a better understanding of the mechanisms whereby an "opportunistic" pathogen such as candida may cause disease; for this reason, experimental studies of candidosis have an importance far beyond the boundaries of the subject itself.

The earliest such studies, dating back well over a hundred years, were attempts to produce disease of the mucous membranes in animals and humans. These experiments led to attempts to reproduce systemic candidosis. Workers as early as the end of the 19th century reported that the organ most affected in systemic candidosis was the kidney. The experimental disease produced in laboratory animals by the intravenous injection of *C.albicans* has been described in great detail by several groups of workers. A comprehensive bibliography is to be found in the monograph by Winner and Hurley (1964).

At the time of writing, the main lines of research on candida infection in various centres may be summarised as follows:

1. Studies of variations in the parasite — differences in the pathogenicity of different species of candida, and of different strains of single species. (Hurley, 1967).

The different species of candida may now be placed in a descending order of pathogenicity, as follows: *C.albicans*, *C.stellatoidea*, *C.tropicalis*, *C.parapsilosis*, *C.pseudotropicalis*, *C.guilliermondii*, and *C.krusei*. An elegant demonstration of the differential pathogenicity of different species of candida is that of Stanley and Hurley (1967).

At the time of writing it is still doubtful whether the different strains of a particular candida species show different pathogenicity .Current studies of *Candida albicans* Types A and B, however, suggest that Type A is more pathogenic than Type B.

2. Studies of variations in the host:

(a) *Modification of host resistance* by external factors such as irradiation, toxic poisoning, surgical operations, damage to skin and mucous membranes, immunosuppressive and antibacterial therapy. The object of this work is to reproduce in the host conditions similar to those in which clinical candidosis may occur. A recent review with additional information is that of Hurley (1966).

(b) Study of *individual host factors* such as the effect of phagocytes and of antibodies on the candida cell. (Louria and Brayton, 1964) (1 and 2).

3. Studies of possible *pathogenic mechanisms*, such as the production of toxins by candida. (Winner and Hurley, 1964).

4. Detailed study of the *candida cell*, both intact and altered by disruption or exposure to antifungal antibiotics.

(a) Metabolism.

(b) Antigenic analysis (STALLYBRASS, 1964, 1965).

(c) Ultrastructure studies.

5. Experimental studies of mechanisms of immunity and allergy.

Work on some of these latter aspects is in progress at the time of writing, and it is premature to give references to these.

Acknowledgments for Illustrations: The author acknowledges with thanks the provision of Figs. 4, 13, 14, 15, 21, 22, 24, 25, 31 and 32 by Professor W. ST. C. SYMMERS; Figs. 6, 7, 8, 9, and 11 by Professor R. A. CAWSON; Figs. 16, 18, and 30 by Dr. T. LEHNER; Figs. 27, 28 and 29 by Dr. J. P. UTZ; Fig. 2 by Dr. D. W. R. MACKENZIE. Figs. 1, 2, 3, 5, 10, 12, 17, 19, 20, 23, 26, and 33 are reproduced from "Candida albicans" by H. I. WINNER and R. HURLEY (Churchill, London, 1964), by permission of the publishers. Figs. 28 and 29 are reproduced from "Symposium on Candida Infections", edited by H. I. WINNER and R. HURLEY (Livingstone, Edinburgh, 1966), by permission of the publishers. Fig. 27 is reproduced from the American Journal of Medicine, by permission of the publishers.

References

AKIBA, T., IWATA, K., INOUYE, S.: Studies on the serologic diagnosis of deep-seated Candidiasis. Jap. J. Microbiol. **1**, 11 (1957). — ALBERS, D. D.: Monilial infection of (the) kidney (s): case reports. J. Urol. (Baltimore) **69**, 32 (1953). — AMON, H., SCHREYER, W.: Sepsis mycotica (Candidiasis) mit disseminierter Thrombarteriitis. Frankf. Z. Path. **71**, 370 (1961). — ANDRIOLE, V. T., KRAVETZ, H. M., ROBERTS, W. C., UTZ, J. P.: Candida endocarditis: Clinical and pathologic studies. Amer. J. Med. **32**, 251 (1962). — BEEMER, A. M., PRYCE, D. M., RIDDELL, R. W.: *Candida albicans* infection of the gut. J. Path. Bact. **68**, 359 (1954). — BEUTHE, D.: Candida-Sepsis. Wiss. Z. Univ. Jena, Math.-nat. Reihe 4, S. 199 (1955). ~ Candidasepsis. Zbl. allg. Path. path. Anat. **93**, 241 (1955). — BICHEL, J. STENDERUP, A.: Investigaciones experimentales acerca del efecto de la monilia (Candida albicans) sobre la linfopoyesis del raton. Folia clin. int. (Barcelona) **5**, 273 (1955). — BOUND, J. P.: Thrush napkin rashes. Brit. med. J. **1**, 782 (1956). — CAPLAN, H.: Monilial (Candida) endocarditis following treatment with antibiotics. Lancet **II**, 957 (1955). — CARSLAW, R. W., RICHARDSON, Anne, CAMERON, J. A.: Monilial granuloma in an adult, successfully treated with amphotericin B. Brit. J. Derm. **78**, 242 (1966). — CAWSON, R. A.: Chronic Oral Candidosis, denture stomatitis, and chronic hyperplastic candidosis. In: *"Symposium on Candida infections"*, edited by H. I. WINNER and R. HURLEY, Livingstone, Edinburgh, pp. 138—153 (1966). — CAWSON, R. A., LEHNER, T.: Chronic hyperplastic candidiasis — Candidal leukoplakia. Brit. J. Derm. **80**, 9 (1968). — CHISHOLM, E. R., HUTCH, J. A.: Fungus ball *(Candida albicans)* formation in the bladder. J. Urol. (Baltimore) **86**, 559 (1961). — CLAYTON, YVONNE M., NOBLE, W. C.: Observations on the epidemiology of *Candida albicans*. J. clin. Path. **19**, 76 (1966). — CLIMIE, A. R. W., RACHMANINOFF, N.: Fungal (Candida) Endocarditis following open-heart surgery. J. thorac. cardiovasc. Surg. **50**, 431 (1965). — DANBOLT, N.: Deep cutaneous moniliasis, a fatal case of a peculiar type. Acta derm.-venereol. (Stockh.) **21**, 98 (1940). — DEBRÉ, R., MOZZICONACCI, P., DROUHET, E., DROUHET, V., HOPPELER, A., GRUMBACH, R., HABIB, R.: Les infections a Candida chez le nourrisson. Ann. paediat. (Basel) **184**, 129 (1955). — DUBOIS-FERRIÈRE, H., FEUARDENT, R., GOLDSCHLAG, H., BURSTEIN, L., BOUVIER, C., BÖHNI, H.: Septicémies à muguet (candida albicans) favorisées par les antibiotiques et la cortisone au cours d'hémopathies malignes. Helv. med. Acta **22**, 477 (1955). — EVANS, W. E. D., WINNER, H. I.: The histogenesis of the lesions in experimental moniliasis in rabbits. J. Path. Bact. **67**, 531 (1954). — FALKMER, S., WISING, P. J.: Fatal bronchopulmonary moniliasis. Acta med. scand. **151**, 117 (1955). — FETTER, B. F., KLINTWORTH, G. K., HENDRY, W. S.: *Mycoses of the Central Nervous System.* Baltimore: Williams & Wilkins Co. 1967. — FRISK, A.: Lungcandidos (monilos) och antibioticabehandlung. Svenska Läk.-Tidn. **49**, 1493 (1952). — GAVALLÉR, BELA DE: Contribucion a la patogenicidad de las monilias en recién nacidos a base de los hallazgos anátomo-pathológicos. Rev. sudamer. Morf. **10**, 117 (1952). — GELLI, G.: Micosi (candidosi) polmonare in forma cavitaria; (particolare riferimento al trattamento chirurgico). Riv. Clin. pediat. **54**, 155 (1954). — GERLÓCZY, F., SCHMIDT, K., SCHOLZ, M.: Beiträge zur Frage der Moniliasis im Säuglingsalter. Ann. paediat. (Basel) **187**, 119 (1956). — GIESSLER, G., GULOTTA, F.: Moniliasis des Zentralnervensystems. Zbl. allg. Path. path. Anat. **105**, 433 (1964). — GUZE, L. B., HALEY, L. D.: Fungus infections of the urinary tract. Yale J. Biol. Med. **30**, 292 (1958). — HAUSER, F. V., ROTHMAN, S.: Monilial granuloma: report of a case and review of the literature. Arch. Derm. Syph. (Chic.) **61**, 297 (1950). — Hoffmann, D. H.: Die experimentelle endogene Entzündung des Augeninneren durch Candida albicans. Ophthalmoskopische, histologische und mikrobiologische Studien zum Ablauf der Infektion beim Kaninchen. Ophthalmologica (Basel) Vol. 151 Suppl. Basel: S. Karger 1966. — Hoffmeister, W., Dickgiesser, F., Götting, H.: Tierexperimentelle und serologische Untersuchungen zur Diagnostik und Therapie der Infektion mit Candida albicans. Dtsch. Arch. klin. Med. **198**, 499 (1951). — Hurley, R.: Experimental infection with *Candida albicans* in modified hosts. J. Path. Bact. **92**, 57 (1966). — Hurley, R.: The Pathogenic Candida species: A Review. Rev. med. vet. Mycot. **6**, 159 (1967). — Hurley, R., Winner, H. I.: The pathogenicity of Candida tropicalis. J. Path. Bact. **84**, 33 (1962). — Hurley, R., Winner, H. I.: Experimental renal moniliasis in the mouse. J. Path. Bact. **86**, 75 (1963). ~ Pathogenicity in the genus Candida. Mycopathologia (Den Haag) **24**, 337 (1964). — Hurwitz, A., Yesner, R.: A report of a case of localized bronchopulmonary moniliasis successfully treated by surgery. J. thorac. Surg. **17**, 26 (1948). — Jamshidi, A., Pope, R. H., Friedman, N. H.: Fungal Endocarditis Complicating Cardiac Surgery. Arch. intern. Med. **112**, 370 (1963). — Kärcher, K. H.: Experimentelle Untersuchungen zur Pathogenität und biologischen Wirkung der Candida albicans an Mensch und Tier. Arch. klin. exp. Derm. **202**, 424 (1956). ~ Die Candidamykose (Candidosis, Candidiasis Moniliasis, Oidiomykosis), aus Pilzkrankheiten der Haut durch Hefen, Schimmel, Actinomyceten, Handbuch der Haut- und Geschlechtskrankheiten von J. Jadassohn, Ergänzungswerk Bd. IV/4, S. 1—74. Berlin-Göttingen-Heidelberg: Springer 1963. — Kaplan, B., Levin, S. E.: Candida Endocarditis Complicating Congenital Heart Disease: A case report. Med. Proc. **13**, 614 (1967). — Kaufman, S. A., Scheff, S., Levene, G.: Esophageal moniliasis. Radiology **75**, 726 (1960). — Khmelnitsky, O. K.: Pathologico-anatomical changes in visceral candidiasis. Arkh. Pat. (Mosk.) **24**, 20 (1962). — Lannigan, R., Meynell, M. J.: Moniliasis in acute leukaemia. J. clin. Path. **12**, 157 (1959). — La Touche, C. J.: Candida in Chronic Ear Infections. In: *"Symposium on Candida infections"*, edited by H. I. Winner and R. Hurley, Livingstone, Edinburgh, pp. 154—160 (1966). — Lehner, T.: Systemic Candidiasis and Renal Involvement. Lancet I, 1414 (1964). ~ Immunofluorescent investigation of Candida albicans antibodies in human saliva. Arch. oral Biol. **10**, 975 (1965). ~ Classification and Clinico-Pathological Features of Candida Infections in the Mouth. In: *"Symposium on Candida Infections"*, edited by H. I. Winner and R. Hurley, Livingstone, Edinburgh, pp. 119—137 (1966). — Lemaistre, J.: Etude sur l'air de la ville de Limoges: de la perlèche: du Streptococcus plicatilis. J. Soc. Méd. Pharm. Haute-Vienne **10**, 41 (1886). — Lewis, G. M., Hopper, M. E., Montgomery, R. M.: Infections of the skin due to Monilial albicans. I. Diagnostic value of intradermal testing with a commercial extract of Monilial albicans. N.Y. St. J. Med. **37**, 878 (1937). — Louria, D. B., Brayton, R. G.: A substance in blood lethal for *Candida albicans*. Nature (Lond.) **201**, 309 (1964). ~ Behaviour of Candida cells within leukocytes. Rev. med. vet. Mycol. **66**, 956 (1964). — Ludlam, G. B., Henderson, J. L.: Neonatal thrush in a maternity hospital. Lancet **1942**, I, 64. — Mackinnon, J. E.: Caracteres y grado de la virulencia experimental de las Torulopsidáceas de la subfamilia micotorulaceas (monilias). An. Fac. Med. Montevideo **21**, 320 (1936). — Maibach, H. I., Kligman, A. M.: The biology of experimental human cutaneous moniliasis (*Candida albicans*), Arch. Derm. **85**, 233 (1962). — Mankowski, Z. T.: Occurrence of malignancy, collagen diseases and Myasthenia gravis in the course of experimental infections with Candida albicans. Mycopathologia (Den Haag) **19**, 1 (1962). — Marsh, A. P.: Oesophageal moniliasis. Amer. J. Roentgenol. **82**, 1063 (1959). — Masshoff, W., Adam, W.: Histomorphologie der experimentellen Candida-Infektion. Arch. klin. exp. Derm. **204**, 416 (1957). — Miyake, M., Okudaira, Akiba, T., Inoue, S.: An immuno-pathologic study on deep seated candidiasis, especially on the precipitin reaction using the infected tissue extract as antigen. Acta path. jap. **10**, 25 (1960). — Moulder, M. K.: Thrush of the urinary bladder: case report. J. Urol. (Baltimore) **56**, 420 (1946). — Nezelof, C., Sarrut, S.: Infections mortelles à candida chez le nouveau-né et le nourrisson. Six observations anatomohistologiques. Ann. Pédiat. **1957**, 531. — Nilsby, I., Norden, A.: Studies of the occurrence of Candida albicans. Acta med. scand. **133**, 347 (1949). — Nityananda, K.: Monilial Granuloma. Brit. med. J. **1**, 690 (1959). — Oblath, R. W., Donath, D. H., Johnstone, N. G., Kerr, W. J.: Pulmonary moniliasis. Ann. intern. Med. **35**, 97 (1951). — Orie, N. G. M.: De aanwezigheid en de betekenis van gisten in de luchtwegen. Thesis. Utrecht 1946. ~ Candida (Monilia) infection of the respiratory tract. Dis. Chest. **22**, 107 (1952). — Owen, C. R., Anderson, M. B., Henrici, A. T.: Allergy in Monilia and yeast infections. Mycopathologia (Den Haag) **1**, 10 (1939). — Pearl, M. A., Sidransky, H.: Candida endocarditis: two new cases with a review of 12 previously reported cases. Amer. Heart J. **60**, 345 (1960). — Ramel, E.: Beitrag zur Kenntnis der Hautblastomykose mit besonderer Berücksichtigung der Allergieerscheinungen. Arch. Derm. Syph. (Berl.) **148**, 218 (1925). — Ravaut, P., Rabeau, H.: Parakeratoses eczematiformes provoquees par des injections intradermiques de levurine. Presse méd. **37**, 372 (1929). — Rey, J.C., Natin, I.: Moniliasis pulmonar. Pren. méd. argent. **1953**, 2306. — RIDDELL, R.W., CLAYTON, Y.M.: Pulmonary mycoses occurring in Britain. Brit. J. Tuberc. **52**, 34 (1958). — ROBERTSON, R.F.: Pulmonary moniliasis. Edinb. med. J. **55**, 274 (1945). — ROBINSON, R.C.V.: Cutaneous moniliasis in infants. J. Pediat. **50**, 721 (1957). — ROCKWOOD, E.M., GREENWOOD, A.M.: Monilial infection of the skin: report of a fatal case. Arch. Derm. Syph. (*Chic.*) **29**, 574 (1934). — ROTHMAN, S.: Some unusual forms of cutaneous moniliasis. Arch. Derm. **79**, 598 (1959). — RUHRMANN, G., ADAM, W.: Tödliche pulmonale Moniliasis eines Säuglings. Virchows Arch. path. Anat. **327**, 273 (1955). — SAUER, H.R., METZNER, W.R.T.: Thrush infection of the urinary bladder. J. Urol. (Baltimore) **59**, 38 (1948). — SCHABERG, A., HILDES, J.A., WILT, J.C.: Disseminated candidiasis. Arch. intern. Med. **95**, 112 (1955). — SCHULTE, H.W.: Die lokalisierte Candidamykose in Kombination mit der Lungentuberkulose. Tuberk.-Arzt **11**, 751 (1957). — SCLAFER, J.: L'allergie à Candida albicans (clinique; diagnostique; traitement). Sem. Hôp. (Paris) **33**, 1330 (1957). — SCLAFER, J., FLAVIAN, N.: Étude de l'allergie cutanée a Candida albicans chez les enfants. Sem. Hôp. (Paris) **30**, 1557 (1954). — SHREWSBURY, J.F.D.: Secondary thrush of the bronchi. Quart. J. Med. **5**, 375 (1936). — SKOBEL, P., JORKE, D., SCHABINSKI, G.: Akute, generalisierte Mykose. Sepsis durch Candida pseudotropicalis. Münch. med. Wschr. 194 (1955). — SMITH, G.M., ARMEN, R.M.: Pulmonary moniliasis treated by brilliant green aerosol: report of a case. Ann. intern. Med. **43**, 1302 (1955). — SNYDER, O.C.: Thrush of urinary bladder; case report. Urol. cutan. Rev. **52**, 80 (1948). — SOLOV, K.A.: Candida pneumopathies in neonates (Candidaerkrankungen der Lungen bei Neugeborenen). Arkh. Pat. (Mosk.) **26**, Nr. 1, S. 60—63 mit engl. Zusammenfassung (1964). — STALLYBRASS, F.C.: Candida precipitins. J. Path. Bact. **87**, 89 (1964). ~ Serotypes of Candida albicans. Nature (Lond.) **207**, 220 (1965). — STANLEY, VALERIE C., HURLEY, ROSALINDE: Growth of Candida species in culture of mouse epithelial cells. J. Path. Bact. **94**, 301 (1967). — STIEFEL, E., ANDRÉU URRA, J., LAZÁRO, J.: A propósito de la candidasis pulmonar, antigua moniliasis. Rev. esp. Tuberc. **22**, 225 (1953). — SYMMERS, W.ST.C.: The tissue reactions in deepseated fungal infection. The role of histological examination in mycological diagnosis. Ann. Soc. belge Méd. trop. **44**, 869 (1964). ~ Septicaemic candidosis. In: "Symposium on Candida infections", edited by H.I. WINNER and R. HURLEY, Livingstone, Edinburgh, pp. 196—212 (1966). — THJÖTTA, TH., AMLIE, R.: Three cases of infection with Monilia (Castellania) tropicalis Castellani. Acta path. microbiol. **24**, 161 (1947). — TOBLER, R., COTTIER, H.: Familiäre Lymphopenie mit Agammaglobulinämie und schwerer Moniliasis. Die "essentielle Lymphocytophthise" als besondere Form der frühkindlichen Agammaglobulinämie. Helv. paediat. Acta **13**, 313 (1958). — VIALATTE, J., SATGE, P., DROUHET, E., WOLF: La forme granulomateuse de la moniliase cutanée. Arch. franç. Pédiat. **19**, 37 (1962). — WHITAKER, J., LANDING, B.H., ESSELBORN, V.M., WILLIAMS, R.R.: The syndrome of familial juvenile hypoadrenocorticism, hypoparathyroidism and superficial moniliasis. J. clin. Endocr. **16**, 1374 (1956). — WIESE, E.R., BIXBY, E.W.: Bronchiectasis associated with monilia simulating pulmonary tuberculosis. Clinical Pathologic study. J. Lab. clin. Med. **26**, 624 (1941).—WILSON, J.W.: Abstract of discussion of "The biology of experimental human cutaneous moniliasis (*Candida albicans*)" (MAIBACH and KLIGMAN). Arch. Derm. **85**, 254 (1962). — WILSON, J.W., PLUNKETT, O.A.: The Fungous Diseases of Man, p. 175. University of California Press Berkeley: 1965. — WILSON, R.M.: Candidal endocarditis. J. Amer. med. Ass. **177**, 332 (1961). — WINNER, H.I.: A study of *Candida albicans* agglutinins in human sera. J. Hyg. (Lond.) **53**, 509 (1955). ~ Experimental moniliasis in the guinea-pig. J. Path. Bact. **79**, 420 (1960). — WINNER, H.I., HURLEY, ROSALINDE: *Candida albicans*. London: J. & A. Churchill (1964). — WINNER, H.I., HURLEY, R.: Symposium on Candida infections, pp. 226—227. Edinburgh: E & S Livingstone, Ltd. (1966).

Aspergillosis

CARLOS E. PEÑA, Washington/D.C., USA

With 35 Figures

Introduction

Aspergillus, a ubiquitous fungus with thin branching hyphae and stout sporulating fruiting heads, may sometimes mount the horse of opportunism to become a dangerous pathogen.

The genus includes 150 recognized species and varieties, of which only a relatively small number are pathogenic. The fungus has the ability to colonize living and dead matter, enjoys a worldwide distribution and possesses a wide spectrum of pathogenicity for man and for animals. In man the infections most often involve the lungs, but can also affect almost any organ of the body. In the veterinary field the fungus' importance stems from its ability to produce abortion in mares, cattle and sheep, to colonize the respiratory tract of birds, and to attack insects. In industry, where its fermentative properties can be utilized, workers are oftentimes exposed to heavy concentrations of air-borne spores.

Definition

Aspergillosis can be broadly defined as any infection or colonization of tissues or cavities by fungi of the genus *Aspergillus*. This includes proliferation in normal or dilated bronchi or caverns, a necrotizing or granulomatous pneumonitis sometimes with hematogenous dissemination, endocarditis, sinusitis, infections of the tegument and certain cases of mycetoma pedis. In addition the spores of the fungus may act in man as an allergen that when inhaled produces a hypersensitivity reaction similar to bronchial asthma.

History

Aspergillus, like many other mycological terms, was coined by MICHELI, a botanist from Florence, in the descriptivist atmosphere of the 18th century. According to him the fungus was thus called because of the similarity of its fruiting heads and the "aspergillum" (from *aspergere*, to sprinkle), a perforated globe used to sprinkle holy water in religious ceremonies. In his treatise "Nova Plantarum Genera", published in 1729, MICHELI listed nine different species, separated mainly on the basis of the characteristics of the fruiting heads, which he proceeded to identify with Latin sentences. This use of sentences to characterize the species is hardly surprising, since the system of binomial nomenclature, devised by LINNAEUS, did not appear until 1753.

Subsequently LINK (1809) described several species of the fungus from decaying vegetation, including *A. flavus*, *A. candidus* and *A. glaucus*. Recognition of the role of *Aspergillus* as an agent of disease waited more than 100 years after its first description, when Pasteur, Koch and others showed that many diseases were caused by microorganisms. In the case of *Aspergillus* this knowledge first came from observations in animals.

The earlier communications of the fungus infections which were probably aspergillosis, were those of MAYER (1815), who found a mold in the lungs of a jay (*Corvus glandarius*), and JÄGER (1816), who observed a similar condition in the lungs of two swans. However, they did not classify the fungus any further. DESLONGCHAMP (1841) also reported on a "mold developed during life" in the air pockets of a duck (*Anas mollissima*), but like his predecessors, did not give a precise classification of the fungus. The first definite account of an *Aspergillus* infection in an animal was that of RAYER and MONTAGNE (1842), who identified *A.candidus* in the air pockets of a tuberculous bullfinch (*Pyrrhula vulgaris*).

All too often HUGHES BENNETT of Edinburgh (1844) has been credited with the first description of a human case of the disease. However, according to the pictures and the description given, the fungus was probably not an *Aspergillus*.

The first human case in which *Aspergillus* seems to have been identified was that of SLUYTER (1847). The patient was a woman who died of a pulmonary disease. In a cavern of one of the lungs, BAUM, LITZMANN and EICHSTEDT found a black mycelial mass. The authors thought that the fungus was a MUCOR, but VIRCHOW believed that it was actually an *Aspergillus*. ROBIN (1853) reviewed the literature and reported *Aspergillus nigrescens* in the air pockets of a pheasant that died of tuberculosis.

VIRCHOW (1856) described four cases of bronchial and pulmonary aspergillosis in patients who died respectively of dysentery, pulmonary inflammation with emphysema, gastric carcinoma and pneumonia. The same year Friedreich in Würzburg recorded a case of "pneumomycosis aspergillina" characterized by the presence of the fungus in a tuberculous cavity. CRAMER in 1859 isolated *A.niger* from ear infections that he reported under the name of "*Sterigmatocystis antacustica*". FRESENIUS described in 1863 *A.fumigatus*, encountered in the respiratory tract of a bustard (*Otis tarda*) from the Frankfurt Zoological Park. WREDEN reported in 1867 two new types, *A.flavescens* and *A.nigricans*, isolated from human ear infections, which he considered to be varieties of *A.glaucus*. Other cases of human pulmonary infections were described by COHNHEIM (1865), FÜRBRINGER (1876) and LICHTHEIM (1882).

Towards the end of the 19th century came the discovery that many microbiological diseases occurring in man could be reproduced in experimental animals. *Aspergillus* was then used as a pioneer tool by GRAWITZ (1880) who produced lesions in the brains of rabbits and dogs by the injection of the fungus into the carotid artery.

The first cases of *Aspergillus* infections observed on this side of the Atlantic were reported by CHARLES BURNETT of Philadelphia, who studied a number of patients with otomycosis (1874, 1879, 1889). OSLER (1887) also recorded the case of a woman who expectorated bodies consisting almost completely of aspergillar hyphae.

During the same period SIEBENMANN (1889) published in Germany his comprehensive monograph on human ear infections, and WHEATON (1890) observed the first case ever published in Britain. SCHUBERT (1885) and MACKENZIE (1893) recorded cases of nasal and maxillary sinus infections.

At the same time French physicians started to show interest in the study of aspergillosis. In 1890 DIEULAFOY et al. first observed the disease in pigeon-crammers ("gaveurs de pigeons"). The duty of a "gaveur" consisted of chewing wet grain which they then fed to the animals, mouth to beak. The authors called the condition "pseudotuberculose mycosique" and described quite adequately its clinical picture, as well as the histopathology of the lesions in birds. Furthermore, they reproduced it experimentally and identified *A.fumigatus* as the etiologic agent. GAUCHER and SERGENT (1894) also observed a case of this condition in a pigeon-crammer. RÉNON's series of studies published in 1893, 1895 and 1897 examined the subject on a wider perspective. In his last study the author discussed four previously published instances of pulmonary aspergillosis in pigeon-crammers (DIEULAFOY et al., 1890; POTAIN and RÉNON, RÉNON, 1893; GAUCHER and SERGENT, 1894). In addition he commented on two cases, husband and wife, that he had observed beforehand (1895), in "peigneurs de cheveux" (hair-combers), who used rye flour for cleaning hair which was used in the manufacturing of wigs. The author also distinguished between primary and secondary disease according to the absence or presence of a pre-existing condition, and was able to compile 68 references on human aspergillosis.

English physicians were also active in this field as exemplified by the 2 cases reported by BOYCE (1893), and by ARKLE and HINDS (1895—1896).

OPPE (1897) recorded in Germany the first case of cerebral involvement, due to intracranial extension of a sphenoid sinusitis. LANGERON (1922) isolated a fungus, apparently *A.terreus*, from a case of otomycosis, which he called *Sterigmatocystis hortai*. Two Portuguese physicians, EGAS MONIZ and LOFF (1931) observed a case of cerebral aspergillosis in a patient from Lisbon.

The most recently described form of aspergillosis, and perhaps the most characteristic, was observed by DÉVÉ (1938). This French physician described the clinical and radiologic, as well as the anatomic features of the entity, which he called intrabronchiectatic megamycetoma.

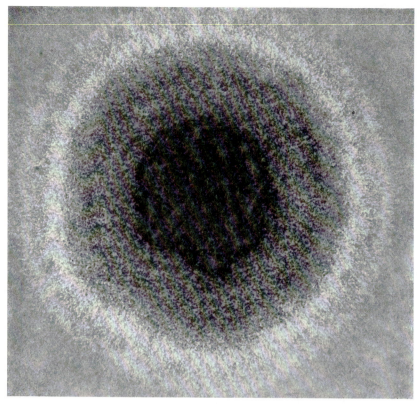

Fig. 1. Culture of *A.flavus* on Sabouraud's medium. Pigmentation proceeds centrifugally in the wake of the mycelial growth

Aspergillus restrictus has been the latest species found to be pathogenic for man and animals (MARSALEK et al., 1960).

The study of toxic metabolites of the *Aspergilli* has become quite important in recent years. Early studies in this field were carried out by CENI and BESTA in Italy (1902), by BODIN and GAUTIER in France (1906), and by HENRICI in the United States (1939). These investigations recently culminated in Britain with the discovery of aflatoxins, following outbreaks in 1960 and 1961 of an unknown "X" disease in poults, swine and cattle.

Mycology

RAPER and FENNELL (1965) recognize 150 species and varieties of *Aspergilli*, that are classified into 18 groups. In human infections of the lung and other viscera the species most frequently encountered is by far *A.fumigatus*, followed by *A.flavus*, *A.niger*, *A.terreus* and *A.versicolor*. In ear and skin infections the most frequent species is *A.niger*.

Direct examination and cultures are the techniques most frequently used in the diagnosis of the disease. Animal inoculations are generally not helpful.

Direct Examination: The suspected fluid (sputum) is placed on a slide and pressed under a coverslip. The use of sodium hydroxide improves the quality of

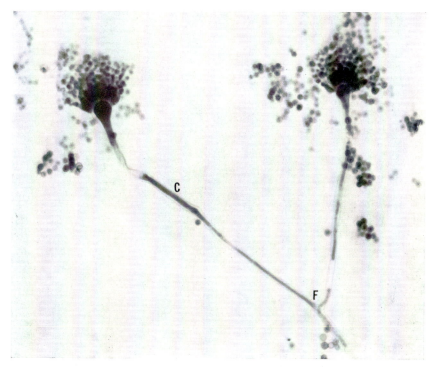

Fig. 2. Foot cell (F), conidiophores (C), and fruiting heads of *A. fumigatus*. Slide culture, lactophenol cotton blue stain. × 450

the preparation. Branching hyphae or fragments, greenish spores (3—5 μ in diameter) and fruiting heads may be seen.

Culture: The material to be examined may be inoculated on Sabouraud's glucose — agar slants with chloramphenicol and kept at temperatures ranging from normal room temperature to 45°C. The fungus grows in 2—5 days, appearing first as white filamentous colonies, that become bluish green or black, according to the species, due to the appearance of fruiting heads and spores (Fig. 1).

Small fragments of mycelium or slide cultures may be stained for microscopic examination with lactophenol cotton blue. The hyphae are seen as very long, gently curving structures, measuring approximately 10 μ in diameter, stained blue and covered by an unstained, somewhat refractile membrane. The septa are sharp and regularly spaced. Successive dichotomous branching is apparent, the branches originating at an angle of 45°. Conidiophores branch off at an angle close to 90°, from hyphae called "foot" cells. The identification of foot-cells is strong evidence that the fungus is an *Aspergillus*.

The fruiting heads are supported by a hypha (conidiophore) that widens progressively towards its distal end, where there is a spherical swelling (the vesicle) (Figs. 2, 3). No line of demarcation separates the vesicle from the conidiophore.

According to the species, the vesicle is surrounded by one or two rows of flask-like projections, the primary and secondary sterigmata to which chains of spores are attached. Brownish-green pigmentation is present in the elements of the fruiting head.

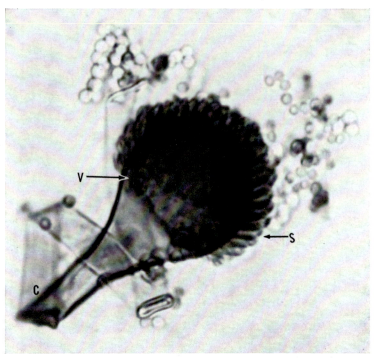

Fig. 3. Fruiting head of *A.fumigatus*. The conidiophore (C), the vesicle (V), a row of sterigmata (S), and a number of spores are seen. Unstained preparation. Approx. × 1200. (Courtesy of Dr. J.C. Sieracki, Pittsburgh, Pa.)

Species differences are related to the manner of implantation of the conidia (radial, columnar), to the shape of the vesicle, to the number of rows of sterigmata, to the shape of the conidia (globose, elliptical) and to the pigmentation of the head.

Further details may be found in manuals and textbooks (RAPER and FENNELL, 1965, or its preceding editions, THOM and RAPER, 1945; THOM and CHURCH, 1926).

Incidence and Epidemiology

Aspergillosis is worldwide in distribution and has been reported from all continents. It is stated that warm, humid climates are favorable for the growth of the fungus, but perhaps with the exception of otomycosis, there does not seem to be any evidence that the disease is more frequent in such regions. Its overall incidence is difficult to ascertain. HEFFERNAN et al. (1966) found aspergillosis in 0.7% of all the autopsies performed in the Johns Hopkins Hospital in the year 1963. CARBONE et al. (1964) reported an incidence of 1.7% in patients dying with *cancer* and of 5.8% in those dying with acute *leukemia*.

No important difference can be detected as to sex and race. However, some localizations are more frequent in men (bronchial aspergilloma) and others in women (infections of the paranasal sinuses). The condition is less frequently reported in children than in adults, although in the young it disseminates more frequently and runs a faster course.

An ever growing body of evidence indicates that in recent years there has been a progressive increase in the incidence of aspergillosis (KEYE and MAGEE, 1956;

TORACK, 1957; SIDRANSKY and PEARL, 1961; BAKER, 1962a; WAHNER et al., 1963; GRUHN and SANSON, 1963; CARBONE et al., 1964; HUTTER et al., 1962; 1964; HEFFERNAN et al., 1966). This higher frequency has been ascribed to the use of new drugs that may prolong the life of patients with low organic resistance, such as antibiotics, or that may themselves affect the individual's organic defenses such as steroids and cytotoxic drugs. Although dissenting opinions still persist (MACARTNEY, 1964) it is evident that the data gathered through the analysis of cases in humans, as well as through experimental observation show that certain chemotherapeutic agents have played an important role in such a rise.

Sources of Infection: *Aspergillus* is found widely distributed in nature and grows in a large number of natural substrates. RÉNON (1895, 1897) reported its isolation from the grain and flour used respectively by pigeon-crammers and hair cleaners. EMMONS (1960, 1962) has reported the occurrence of *Aspergillus fumigatus* in piles of vegetable compost during early stages of decomposition. When this material is exposed to rain, the subsequent microbial fermentation produces a rise in the temperature that supports the growth of the fungus. Contaminated hay and straw are a very important source of pathogenic *Aspergilli*. By means of quantitative methods, GREGORY and BUNCE (1960) were able to show that *A. fumigatus* was one of the main fungi in hay baled with a moisture content of 42%, and that *A. glaucus* was predominant at about 28% of moisture content. Furthermore GREGORY and LACEY (1963) demonstrated that, at a constant wind speed, an obviously moldy hay released 1000 times as many spores as a well preserved hay, and that the number of spores released at a given time increased at higher wind speeds. Other materials that may harbor the fungus are soil (SCHMIDT et al., 1962), household dust (SWAEBLY et al., 1952), bagasse used for litter (HUTSON, 1966), rye flour (WEINER, 1960), oilcake stored in a barn (STRELLING et al., 1966), feed pellets (FORGACS et al., 1954), groundnuts (SARGEANT et al., 1961), hop manure (HINSON et al., 1952), corn, and bark of various tropical fruits (LARA, 1928).

The air-borne spores of *Aspergillus* can readily be isolated by exposing culture plates to the air.

In addition the use of samplers or spore traps allows a quantitative determination that can be expressed as number of colonies obtained per unit volume of air. Isolation of the fungus by air sampling has been carried out in various countries which include France (VALLERY-RADOT et al., 1950), United States (BRUSKIN, 1953), Puerto Rico (PONS et al., 1961), Colombia (ALVAREZ et al., 1965), Wales (HYDE et al., 1949, 1956), and England (BARUAH, 1961; NOBLE and CLAYTON, 1963). VALLERY-RADOT et al., (1950) observed an increase in the number of spores during the winter months. NOBLE and CLAYTON (1963) isolated *A. fumigatus* and *A. niger* from the air in a London hospital and also demonstrated a hundred-fold increase of the number of spores during the autumn and winter months. The fungus was likewise shown to be present in the hospital blankets.

Occupational exposure has been stressed ever since DIEULAFOY et al. (1890) and RÉNON (1895) reported the disease in *pigeon-crammers and wig cleaners.* Fortunately, in this age of the "affluent society" these occupations and their inherent dangers have largely disappeared, although occasional cases are still reported (YESNER and HURWITZ, 1950). More danger seems to exist for farmers who very often come into contact with decaying vegetation or with the materials previously mentioned.

Industrial exposure may be significant in factories where molasses is fermented by *Aspergilli* for the production of citric or other acids. Such process is carried out in large open pans and, when finished, the layer of *Aspergillus* culture is removed by workers who at this moment are exposed to the dust containing great quantities of spores (HOREJSI et al., 1960).

Pathogenesis

In some cases the *Aspergillus* infection is primary but most often is secondary or opportunistic.[1]

Portals of Entry: The air-borne spores may gain entrance into the body in a variety of manners. The usual routes of infection are the ear canal, nose and sinuses, eye, skin and adnexa and respiratory tract, the latter being the most important. Open heart and major vascular surgery provide another portal of entry for a very ominous type of the disease (Porta, 1959; Newman et al., 1964; Darrell, 1967; Mahvi et al., 1968). Luke et al. (1963) have suggested the possibility of inoculation through exchange-transfusions and Mahvi et al. (1968) have indicated as an alternative the penetration of the fungus through a splinter wound. Other possible sites of entrance are a rectal fistula (Welsh and McClinton, 1954), the uterus after a septic abortion (Finegold et al., 1959), and traumatic injuries (Zimmerman, 1950).

The development of an infection depends on external as well as internal factors (Fig. 9). See Table 3.

External Factors: Among the external factors, the number of spores that enter the body, i.e. the/size of the inoculum, seems to be the most important (Austwick, 1965). This in turn is determined by the ability of the fungus to proliferate in the environment (Austwick, 1962a). Baruah (1961) calculated that the atmospheric concentration of Aspergillus-Penicillium spores in a cow-shed ranged from 1,300 to 12,390,000 spores/m³. If a constant concentration of 100,000 spores/m³ is assumed, a cow would inhale 600,000 spores/hour, or 14,400,000 in 24 hours. Under similar conditions a man would inhale 60,000 spores/hour, but under maximum concentration this inhalation would be in the order of 7,000,000 spores/hour.

Austwick and Appleby (1965) have estimated that at least 16,000,000 spores are needed to cause an infection in young chickens. Other observations (Sidransky and Friedman, 1959) suggest that extremely low concentrations of air-borne spores may be sufficient to induce pulmonary infections in cortisone-treated animals. The number of spores needed to produce an infection in man has not been precisely determined.

Internal Factors: The individual factors that may facilitate the onset of the fungal infection are:

1. Acute or chronic diseases that debilitate the individual's mechanisms of defense, such as leukemias, lymphomas, disseminated malignant tumors, leukopenic states and infectious diseases.

2. Therapeutic agents which may alter the patient's reactivity, including adrenal corticosteroids, cytotoxic drugs and radiation therapy, often given to treat the conditions listed above or as immunosuppressors.

3. Drugs that may produce changes in the individual's flora, i.e. wide-spectrum antibiotics.

4. Local disorders which facilitate the entry of the fungus, as tuberculosis, bronchiectasis, bronchial cysts, chronic bronchitis, asthma, silicosis and other pneumoconioses, histoplasmosis and bronchogenic carcinoma.

5. Traumatic injuries that facilitate the entry of the fungus, particularly in

---

[1] According to the Committee of the International Symposium on Opportunistic Fungus Infections, the term *opportunistic* should be used to denote fungi that invade the tissues of man or animals with predisposing conditions (Baker, 1962b).

cases of corneal infections and mycetoma pedis. In the following paragraphs some of the more important iatrogenic factors are discussed.

Antibiotics: These drugs may affect the host in a number of ways. There is some evidence that tetracyclines, dihydrostreptomycin and penicillin depress the synthesis of antibodies *in vivo* (STEVENS, 1953), and that chloramphenicol has a similar effect *in vitro* (AMBROSE and COONS, 1963). The possible effects of anti-biotics on phagocytosis are less clearly established, although some studies suggest that they may inhibit phagocytosis of bacteria by human leukocytes (MUNOZ and GEISTER, 1950).

Whether these factors, inhibition of antibody synthesis and inhibition of phagocytosis, are operative in human *Aspergillus* infections is not clear at the present time. In clinical practice the main effect of antibiotics is to alter the individual's microflora by allowing the proliferation of fungi in the absence of competing organisms. In addition many patients are already victims of bacterial infections that may also act as predisposing factors by producing local tissue damage.

Adrenal Corticosteroids: Increased levels of adrenal corticosteroids, whether spontaneously occurring (SAYLE et al., 1965) or therapeutically induced, favor the development of *Aspergillus* infections in humans. In the experimental field, SIDRANSKY and FRIEDMAN (1959) observed that cortisone rendered mice inhaling spores of *A. flavus* highly susceptible to fatal pulmonary aspergillosis. In the search for an explanation of this enhanced susceptibility, EPSTEIN et al. (1967) demonstrated, in a similar experiment, that there was a decreased peribronchial leukocytic infiltrate in the cortisone-treated mice as compared to control animals. FRENKEL (1962) has moreover demonstrated that cortisone inhibits inflammatory cellular responses, as well as proliferation of epithelioid and giant cells. At the ultrastructural level, it has been further observed that in cortisone treated animals the lysosomes of alveolar macrophages, unlike those of control animals, fail to attract and to fuse with the phagocytic vacuoles containing spores (MERKOW et al., 1968). This diminished lysosomal activity is considered to be an important factor in the increased susceptibility of cortisone treated animals.

Organ Transplantation and other Factors: The iatrogenic setting favoring mycotic infections reaches its ideal state (from the fungus' point of view) in patients undergoing immunosuppresive therapy for organ transplantation. Although the number of systematic studies is still small it is now clear that patients on such therapy are highly vulnerable to mycotic infections, just as they are to bacterial or viral diseases. Among RIFKIND et al's. 23 cases (1967) with systemic fungal infections complicating renal transplantation, 7 were found to have aspergillosis. The condition was associated in various cases with candidiasis, cytomegalic inclusion disease and *Pneumocystis* infection. In SAUNDERS and BIEBER's case (1968) of cardiac transplantation the lungs were the site of a diffuse *Aspergillus* infection that involved alveoli, bronchi, arteries and veins. The transplanted heart disclosed fungal invasion of the endocardium and a coronary artery branch, accompanied by focal myocardial necrosis. Fungus lesions were also present in the brain.

Neutropenia, spontaneously occurring or induced by cytotoxic drugs in the treatment of leukemias, lymphomas and other malignancies, has been shown to be frequently associated with fungal invasion (REED, 1935; BAKER, 1962a; FRANCOMBE et al., 1965).

Histopathogenesis: In humans, the incursion of spores, in the majority of cases, does not produce a pathologic process. If the person is debilitated or predisposed, the spores proliferate, and the mycelium invades the tissue to produce an acute necrotizing disease. In persons that repeatedly inhale spores hypersensitivity may result. In other instances, the fungus may find a pre-existing bronchopulmonary cavity, or perhaps create one, and proliferate to form a large mycelial mass constituting the condition known as aspergilloma.

The mechanisms by which the fungus produces tissue injury are less well known. Some strains of *A. fumigatus*, under suitable nutritional conditions, produce several substances known to be toxic to animals, namely fumigacin, fumigatin and gliotoxin (Forgacs and Carll, 1962). Whether these toxic meta-bolites are responsible for *in vivo* tissue injury is not clear. Microscopic study of newly developed pulmonary lesions reveals focal necrosis of individual alveolar septa. This *histolytic property* seems to be an important factor and certainly facilitates the invasion of the tissues. However, it seems somewhat incongruous that the most potent toxin-producing species is *A. flavus*, whereas the most commonly infecting one is *A. fumigatus*. It appears likely, therefore, that other factors must be operative.

Dissemination: *Aspergillus* disseminates along blood vessels and seems also to be able to spread along lymphatics, as well as intrabronchially. The fungus has a marked tendency to invade arteries and veins, producing a necrotizing angiitis, thus setting the stage for its hematogenous spread. The organs most frequently involved by metastatic propagation are the heart, brain, kidneys, gastrointestinal tract, liver, thyroid and spleen.

The involvement of lymph nodes is considered evidence for lymphatic spread.

Bronchogenic dissemination from a primary pulmonary focus does not seem to be rare, but little on this subject can be found in the literature. This mechanism seems to be operative in patients with active open lesions as recent abscesses. Gowing and Hamlin (1960) considered that the fungus can reach the alveoli by aspiration into the respiratory bronchioles with subsequent spread into the associated alveolar sacs.

General Morphology

The response of the human organism to the presence of *Aspergillus* varies from a very mild non-specific inflammatory reaction to a severe acute necrotizing lesion or to a granulomatous inflammation. Minimal responses usually occur when the fungus colonizes a cavity such as the external ear or a bronchus and are characterized by a mild polymorphonuclear or mononuclear leukocytic infiltration.

From the *histopathologic point of view*, the lesions observed in the tissues are of 3 types: 1. necrotizing; 2. suppurative; and 3. granulomatous. The *necrotizing lesions* exhibit a central zone of coagulative necrosis surrounded by a variable amount of polymorphonuclear leukocytes, often pyknotic (Fig. 11), and an outer zone of hemorrhage. The necrotic area often contains vessels displaying invasion by mycelial elements, necrosis of their walls and thrombosis. The suppurative lesions usually have the microscopic appearance of small abscesses with an exudate rich in neutrophils (Fig. 12).

Both necrotizing and *suppurative lesions* are seen most frequently in the lungs, but may be found in the brain, heart, liver, spleen, kidney and other organs. An absolute distinction between these two types of lesions is not always possible since some of them exhibit both necrotizing and suppurative components.

The *granulomatous lesions* are composed of epithelioid and giant cells accom-panied by polymorphonuclear and mononuclear leukocytic infiltration. This form

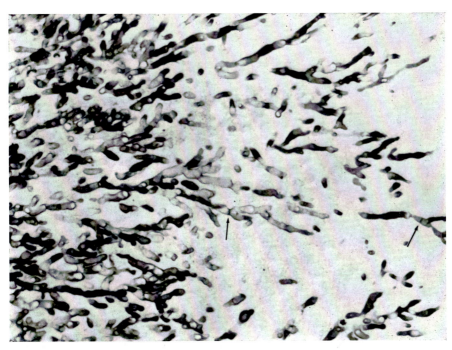

Fig. 4. Morphology of the fungus in tissues. The hyphae are septate (arrows) and exhibit dichotomous branching. Grocott-Gomori, × 450

of reaction is not necessarily chronic and has been observed in cases of acute
primary aspergillosis of the lungs (HERTZOG et al., 1949; STRELLING et al., 1966).
In other instances, the granulomatous lesions have a marked fibroblastic component. This type of inflammation occurs also in the paranasal sinuses, orbit and
cranial cavity.

AUSTWICK (1962b) described still another type of lesion, the *"asteroid"* body.
This formation, 50—80 μ in diameter, is composed of a central core of hyphae and
a peripheral rim of eosinophilic radiating club-like structures similar to those
observed in actinomycosis. The asteroids have been interpreted as the result of
the host's immunologic response to the fungus. They are frequently seen in the
lungs of cattle but apparently have not been observed in humans. SYMMERS (1962)
has observed eosinophilic amorphous deposits of fibrin which form club-like
expansions of the surface of human intracavitary aspergillomas. These structures
may, however, be of a different nature inasmuch as they are seen only in intraluminal masses.

Morphology of the Fungus in Tissues: The hyphae of the *Aspergilli* are usually
well stained with hematoxylin and eosin (H & E), but their morphology is better
appreciated with the use of special stains. The most frequently employed are the
periodic acid Schiff (PAS), the Gridley, and the Grocott-Gomori methenamine-
silver nitrate stains.

The hyphae are septate, have uniform caliber, measure about 7—10 μ in diameter, branch dichotomously at an angle of 45° and are basophilic with H & E
stains (Fig. 4). They often display a radial disposition, especially in intracavitary
lesions (Fig. 5). This type of hypha is sometimes referred to as "actinomycetoid". In

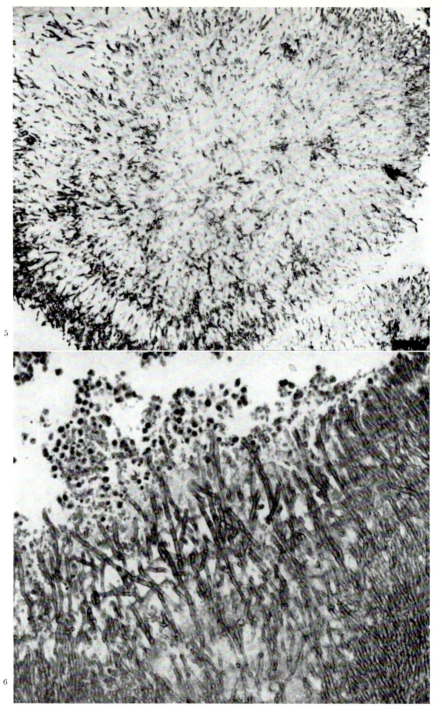

Fig. 5. Morphology of the fungus in tissues. Intrabronchial aspergillosis. The hyphae display a radiating arrangement. Grocott-Gomori. Approx. × 100

Fig. 6. Morphology of the fungus in tissues. Invasive hyphae exhibiting parallel growth. H & E, × 200

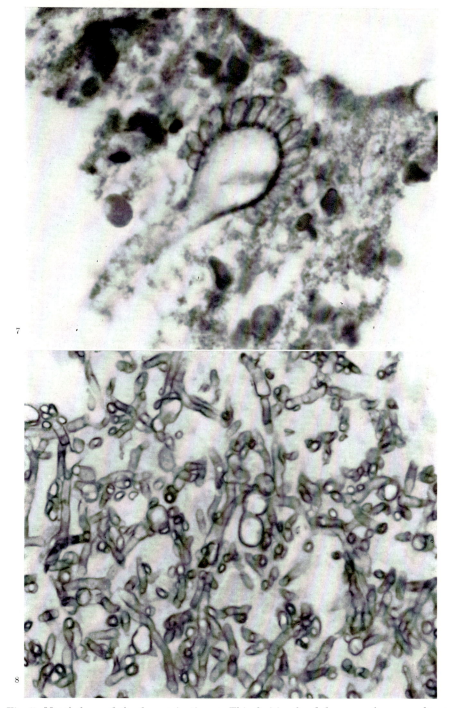

Fig. 7. Morphology of the fungus in tissues. This fruiting head from a pulmonary abscess displays a row of sterigmata. H & E, × 1000

Fig. 8. Morphology of the fungus in tissues. Some hyphae show degenerative changes consisting of irregularity and swelling. This appearance is reminiscent of that of a Phycomycete. Grocott-Gomori, × 450

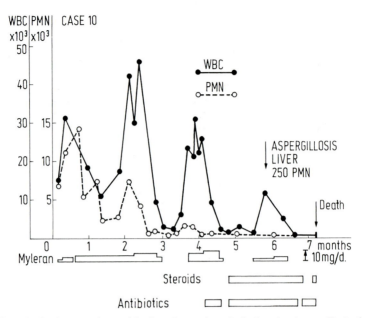

Fig. 9. Clinical plot in a patient with chronic myelocytic leukemia. Aspergillosis developed 6 weeks prior to death, at the time the patient had severe neutropenia. (Courtesy of Dr. R. D. Baker. Amer. J. clin. Path. **37**, 358 (1962), and The Williams & Wilkins Company)

other instances, especially in invasive lesions, the hyphae are straight, parallel and have very few branches (Fig. 6). Another type of hypha that may occasionally be encountered is an ovoid or somewhat irregular structure, 5—10 μ in diameter, which represents a germinating spore with its primary branch.

The *fruiting heads* of the *Aspergilli* are pathognomonic and, when observed, allow a definite histologic classification of the fungus (Fig. 7). In sections only the conidiophore, the vesicle and a row of sterigmata with variable degrees of brownish-yellow pigmentation can be seen. Spores are difficult to find. These fruiting heads are very rarely seen in tissues, but are often encountered in aerated cavities such as an aspergilloma or in the external ear canal.

The fungus may undergo degenerative changes. In some cases, the hyphae, although present in the tissues, are not stained with H & E. This is especially true in fibrosing granulomatous inflammation of the paranasal sinuses, orbit or cranial cavity. Stains for fungi usually reveal the presence of bizarre hyphal elements with irregular swellings and abortive branching.

In other instances, especially in the center of fungus balls hyphae are wider, somewhat irregular, less basophilic and lose their septa, resembling the hyphae of a *Phycomycete* (Fig. 8).

Differential Diagnosis. Aspergillus in tissues displays similarities with *Candida*, *Penicillium* and *Phycomycetes*.

The hyphae (pseudohyphae) of *Candida* are thinner than those of *Aspergillus* and exhibit septa at which level the hyphae are constricted. The presence of blastospores is also a distinguishing feature.

Penicillium organisms have uniformly cylindrical septate hyphae 2—5 μ in width that branch at an angle of 25°—45°. Characteristics helpful in distinguishing them from *Aspergilli* are the presence in their hyphae of clear vacuoles alternating with basophilic zones, and the occurence of chlamydospores. *Penicillium*, like *Aspergillus*, may have a radiating growth and invade blood vessels.

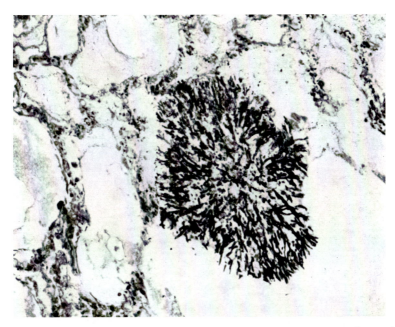

Fig. 10. Tissue changes. Adjacent to the fungus there is minimal necrosis and granulocytic infiltration of individual septa. The mycellium is in a respiratory bronchiole, probably as a result of intrabronchial spread from a pulmonary abscess

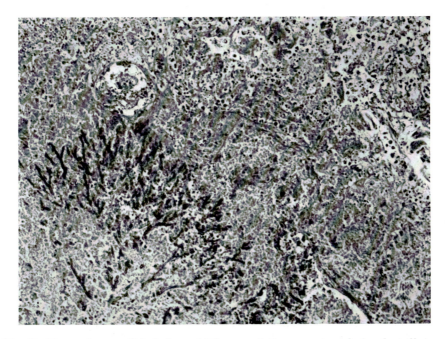

Fig. 11. Tissue changes. This lesion exhibits coagulative necrosis and abundant fibrinous exudate as well as numerous pyknotic neutrophils. H & E, × 100

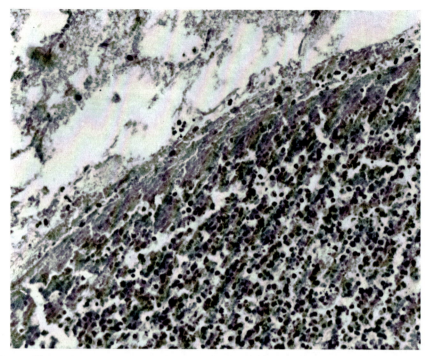

Fig. 12. Tissue changes. Purulent focus in the lung, displaying a sharp demarcation from the surrounding parenchyma. *Aspergillus* hyphae, not visible in the picture, were present in the center of the abscess

The *Phycomycetes* can be distinguished by their irregular wide hyphae that are usually non septate and branch at variable angles.

In spite of the characteristics mentioned the differential diagnosis of these fungi may be quite difficult or impossible unless the organism is identified by culture.

Biopsy. The diagnostic value of biopsies in aspergillosis (and other mycoses) has been discussed by CONANT et al. (1954) and by BAKER (1957). Most cases of aspergillosis in which a clinical diagnosis proves difficult are likely to be deeply seated in the thoracic, abdominal or cranial cavities and are difficult to reach. In infections localized in the nasal fossae, paranasal sinuses and orbit, the biopsy may be the single most important diagnostic procedure.

In these cases, the identification of a fibrosing granulomatous process, often with no visible hyphal elements in the routine stains, is a peremptory indication for the request of special stains. Other locations in which a biopsy may prove helpful are the ear, skin and bronchi. Cultures of the fungus must be done simultaneously. "How many regrets this procedure would save!" (BAKER, 1957).

Clinical Types and Morphologic Findings

Aspergillosis, usually a disease of the respiratory tract, may spread via the blood stream to the heart, central nervous system, liver, spleen and other organs. It may also be a localized infection of the nose and paranasal sinuses, eye, ear and skin.

This section will deal with aspergillosis of the different systems both from the clinical and from the morphologic points of view. Table 1 lists the main features and Table 2 the frequency of organ involvement in 81 cases of disseminated aspergillosis found in the literature.

General reviews on the subject include those of THOM and CHURCH (1926), CONANT et al. (1954), LANDAU et al. (1963), EMMONS et al. (1963), HILDICK-SMITH et al. (1964), BADER (1965), and AUSTWICK (1965).

Respiratory System

The lungs are the organs most frequently affected by the disease. Reviews have been published by WÄTJEN (1931), VADALA (1940), HINSON et al. (1952), FINEGOLD et al. (1959), NAJI (1959), GREER (1962), and WAHNER et al. (1963).

Pulmonary aspergillosis may be acute or chronic, primary or secondary, although this latter differentiation is not always possible (DES AUTELS et al., 1962).

In a number of instances reported the diagnosis has been made solely on the basis of the isolation of the fungus from the sputum and the data available are not sufficient to classify the case (MIERES, 1925; STEELE, 1926; SMITH, W.R., 1934; GARCIA-TRIVIÑO et al., 1935; NAVARRO-BLASCO, 1936; WAHL, 1936; TEIXEIRA, 1941; DONALDSON et al., 1941—1942), although sometimes the cases are claimed to be of primary nature (WAHL, 1928; SCHNEIDER, 1930; SÁNCHEZ-FREIJO, 1935; MOOLTEN, 1938—1939; STOLOW, 1939).

The predisposing disease may be systemic as with leukemias, or localized to the respiratory tract as in tuberculosis (KELMENSON, 1959; RODIN et al., 1963), bronchiectasis and primary or metastatic tumors (YOUNG, 1926; KAMPMEIER et al., 1934; UTZ et al., 1959). In some cases the fungal infection is superimposed on a terminal bacterial bronchopneumonia or on an organizing pneumonitis (FINE-GOLD et al., 1959). Other associated conditions reported are leukemic reticuloendotheliosis (VAITHIANATAN et al., 1962), amebic abscess of the liver (GONZÁLEZ-MENDOZA et al., 1962), coal workers pneumoconiosis (HEPPLESTON et al., 1949), kala-azar (MACKIE, 1922), a pneumonectomy space (SOCHOCKY, 1959) and dermatomyositis treated with steroids (STANLEY, 1965).

Clinical Manifestations: The symptomatology of pulmonary aspergillosis, especially the secondary form, is difficult to define. HEFFERNAN et al. (1966) and SIDRANSKY and PEARL (1961) have pointedly observed that no consistent set of symptoms or signs appear which may be helpful to the diagnosis. Most cases are secondary and the mycotic infection is usually overshadowed by the underlying disease.

Secondary Aspergillosis of the lungs is most often an acute process. The main symptoms are cough, purulent expectoration, fever, dyspnea, chest pain and blood-streaked sputum of recent onset, appearing in a patient with an underlying disease. Hemoptysis or blood-streaked sputum is an important symptom and has been related to fungal invasion of blood vessels (SEABURY and SAMUELS, 1963). Physical findings are variable and depend to a large extent on the characteristics of the mycosis as well as on the nature of the underlying local disease. They include wet rales, rhonchi and signs of consolidation which mimic a lobar pneumonia. Local tenderness of the thoracic wall can sometimes be elicited. Chest X-ray examination may reveal numerous foci of infiltration, usually bilateral and discrete, less frequently confluent and of lobar distribution. VAN ORDSTRAND (1940) observed a shadow radiating from the hilum which he compared with a "sun burst". Any or all of the above symptoms may be absent, and surprises in the autopsy room, or at the examination of surgical specimens are indeed common.

Table 1. *Disseminated. Aspergillosis Clinical and pathological findings of 81 cases gleaned from the literature*

Author and Year	Country	Author Case No.	Age Sex	Predisp. Factors	Organs Affected	Culture
LINCK (1939)	Germany	—	19, M	Not apparent	Lungs ? brain, leptomeninges	—
CAWLEY (1947)	U.S.	—	8, M	?	Lungs, brain, dura, mediastinum, heart, liver, spleen, ankle	A. fumigatus
GERSTL et al. (1948)	U.S.	2	62, M	Pneumonia, anemia, leukopenia	Lungs, skin	A. fumigatus
ZIMMERMAN (1950)	U.S.	2	25, M	Trauma with leg amputation	Heart, kidney	—
—	U.S.	3	32, F	Old rheumatic heart disease	Heart, adrenal	—
WELSH and McCLINTON (1954)	U.S.	—	64, M	Rectal fistula, necrosis of ischiorectal tissues, antibiotics	Lungs, duodenum	A. fumigatus
LEVY et al. (1955)	U.S.	—	24, F	Idiop. anemia, ACTH	Lungs, heart, brain	Asperg. sp.
ZIMMERMAN et al. (1955)	U.S.	1	Newborn M	Staph. sepsis, antibiotics, steroids	Lungs, brain, liver, pericardium	A. sydowi
WELSH et al. (1955)	U.S.	—	18, M	Idiop. neutropenia, S. cholera-esuis sepsis, ACTH, steroids, antibiotics	Lungs, heart	A. flavus, A. fumigatus, A. nidulans
KEYE et al. (1956)	U.S.	1	23, ?	Systemic lupus	Trachea, bronchi, lung, brain	A. fumigatus
—		3	4 mos., Sex ?	Neuroblastoma with metastasis	Lungs, meninges, brain	
SHERMAN and BOSHES (1956)	P. Rico	5	23, F	Atypical leukemia ? ACTH	Lungs, trachea, heart, brain, dura	Asperg. sp.
KIRSCHTEIN and SINDRANSKY (1956)	U.S.	—	50, M	Anemia, ACTH, antibiotics, leukopenia	Lungs, heart	A. flavus
AKKOYUNLU et al. (1957)	Turkey	—	20 days M	Not apparent	Lungs, bronchi, brain, leptomeninges	—
SATHMARY (1958)	U.S.	—	37, M	Ac. myeloid leukemia, B. subtilis pneumonia, antibiotics, steroids	Lungs, brain, heart, kidney, thyroid	A. fumigatus
GRCEVIC et al. (1959)	U.S.	1	36, M	Antibiotics, steroids	Lungs, bronchi, brain, heart	Asperg. sp.
—		2	13, M	Hepatitis, antibiotics, steroids	Lungs, brain, heart, kidneys, pancreas, thyroid, spleen, mediast. nodes	Asperg. sp.
FINEGOLD et al. (1959)	U.S.	3	22, M	Antibiotics, febrile disease	Lungs, heart, brain, thyroid, kidney	Asperg. sp.
PORTA (1959)	U.S.	9	33, F	Septic abortion, antibiotics	Lungs, heart, spleen, uterus, brain	A. fumigatus
—		—	14, M	Open-heart surgery (subaortic stenosis)	Heart (aortic valve), aorta, kidneys, periadrenal tissues, aortic embolus	
GOWING and HAMLIN (1960)	U.K.	2	44, M	Ac. myeloid leukemia, steroids, cytotoxics	Lungs, liver, spleen, kidneys, heart, thyroid	A. fumigatus
—		4	14, F	Ac. myeloid leukemia, steroids, cytotoxics	Lungs, brain, meninges	—

	Country	No.	Age, Sex	Underlying disease / therapy	Organs involved	Organism
Allan et al. (1960)	U.S.	—	18 days M	Not apparent	Lungs, liver, spleen, kidneys, heart, thyroid, jejunum, tongue, skin	A. fumigatus
Hadorn (1960)	Switzerland	—	25, M	Open-heart surgery (subvalvular aortic stenosis)	Suture line in aorta above valve, myocardium, embolus to femoral artery, brain	A. fumigatus
Marsalek et al. (1960)	CSSR	—	60, M	Tuberculosis, amyloidosis	Lungs, kidneys, heart, mediastinal lymph nodes, adrenals	A. restrictus
Utz et al. (1961)	U.S.	43	27, M	Not stated	Lungs, skin, prostate, probably kidneys	A. fumigatus
Baker (1962)	U.S.	9	70, M	Ac. myeloblastic leukemia, steroids, antibiotics	Brain	—
—		10	10, M	Chr. myeloid leukemia, neutropenia, cytotoxics, antibiotics	Lungs, liver	Asperg. sp.
Fraumeni and Fear (1962)	U.S.	—	41, M	Lymphoma and leukemia, steroids, antibiotics, X-ray, cytotoxics	Lungs, heart, spleen, kidney, stomach, psoas, thyroid, brain	A. fumigatus
Conen et al. (1962) (Hendrick et al., 1963)	Canada	—	7, F	?	Lungs, brain	A. fumigatus
Landau et al. (1963)	U.S.	2	3, M	Ac. lymphobl. leukemia, steroids, X-ray, cytotoxics, antibiotics	Lungs, brain, heart, pancreas, kidneys, thyroid	—
Paradis (1963)	U.S.	—	2 mos. F	Prematurity, cytomegalic incl. dis.	Lungs, brain, heart, eyes, mediast. nodes, small bowel, kidney	A. fumigatus
Gruhn (1963)	U.S.	20	68, F	Chr. granulocytic leukemia, neutropenia, steroids, cytotoxics, antibiotics	Lungs, intestine, heart, liver, kidney, brain	—
Luke et al. (1963)	U.S.	—	51, F	Exchange transfusion, antibiotics, steroids	Heart, kidney, thyroid, brain	A. fumigatus
Wahner et al. (1963)	U.S.	1	4, M	Staph. pneumonia, antibiotics	Lungs, heart, mediastinal nodes, kidney	A. fumigatus
Seabury and Samuels (1963)	U.S.	4	24, M	Sarcoidosis, anemia, steroids, antibiotics	Lungs, kidneys, liver, spleen	A. fumigatus
Carbone et al. (1964)	U.S.			7 cases of generalized aspergillosis are included. Underlying diseases were: ac. leukemia 4, lymphoma 2, myeloid metaplasia 1. Organs involved were: Lung 7, central nervous system 5, kidney 3, intestine 3, heart 2, liver 2, thyroid 2, spleen 1. Neutropenia, steroids, antibiotic and cytotoxic drug therapy were considered as possible pathogenic factors.		
Hutter et al. (1964)	U.S.	2	3, F	Ac. leukemia, steroids, ACTH, cytotoxics, antibiotics	Lungs, brain	—
—		6	8, M	Ac. leukemia, X-ray, cytotoxics, antibiotics	Lungs, spleen, kidneys, jejunum	—
—		7	10, M	Ac. leukemia, steroids, cytotoxics, antibiotics	Lungs, heart, kidney, thyroid	A. fumigatus

Table 1. Continuation

Author and Year	Country	Author Case No.	Age Sex	Predisp. Factors	Organs Affected	Culture
Hutter et al. (1964)	U.S.	8	10, M	Ac. myelog. leukemia, steroids, cytotoxics, antibiotics	Lungs, kidneys	—
—		10	12, M	Ac. lymph. leukemia, steroids, cytotoxics, antibiotics	Lungs, small bowel	—
—		16	43, M	Steroids, cytotoxics, antibiotics, X-ray, lymphosarcoma	Lungs, heart, kidneys, thyroid, muscle, brain	A. fumigatus
—		17	56, F	Ac. viral hepatitis, steroids, antibiotics	Lungs, heart	—
—		19	57, M	Ret.-cell sarcoma, steroids, antibiotics, X-ray, cytotoxics	Lungs, kidneys	—
—		28	68, M	Hypoplastic anemia, steroids, antibiotics	Lungs, stomach	—
—		30	69, M	Ac. myel. leukemia, steroids, antibiotics	Lungs, stomach	—
Soergel et al. (1964)	U.S.	—	55, M	Rheumatoid arthritis, steroids, antibiotics, neutropenia	Lungs, heart, kidney	—
Schumacher et al. (1964)	U.S.	24	4, M	Ac. lymphocytic leukemia, total body irradiation	Brain, oral cavity	—
—		27	26, M	Ac. monobl. leukemia, antibiotics, cytotoxics, total body irradiation	Lungs, liver	—
Louria et al. (1964)	U.S.	2	10, M	Ac. blastic leukemia, X-ray cytotoxics	Lungs, brain, heart, liver, kidney, thyroid	A. fumigatus
Sayle et al. (1965)	U.S.	1	62, F	Ca. of pancreas, Cushing's syndrome, antibiotics	Lungs, heart	—
Francombe et al. (1965)	Canada	—	80, M	Pancytopenia (idiopathic), steroids, antibiotics	Lungs, liver, spleen, kidney, bone	Asperg. sp.
Redmond et al. (1965)	U.K.	—	6, M	Not apparent	Lungs, ribs, vertebrae	A. nidulans
Buttrick et al. (1965)	U.S.	1	15 days F	Prematurity, cytomegalic incl. disease, antibiotics, steroids	Heart, brain, eyes, peritoneum, pleura, small bowel, lymph nodes, kidneys, thyroid	A. fumigatus
Heffernan (1966)	U.S.	7	60, F	Ac. myeloid leukemia	Lungs, pleura, mediast. nodes, stomach, liver, spleen, pancreas, kidney, heart, brain	—

Reference	Country	No.	Age, Sex	Predisposing condition	Organs involved	Species
—	—	11	78, M	Pernicious anemia, ac. myel. leukemia	Lungs, stomach (polyps)	—
—	—	19	17, F	Ac. lymph. leukemia	Lungs, esophagus	—
—	—	20	71, M	Ac. myel. leukemia	Lungs, myocardium	—
FISHER et al. (1966)	U.S.	—	54, M	T.B.C., pancytopenia, antibiotics, steroids	Lungs, coronary arteries, myocardium, liver, spleen, GI tract, peritoneum	A. fumigatus
HUGHES (1966)	U.S.	—	8, F	Staph. aureus and S. typhimurium sepsis	Lungs, brain	A. fumigatus
STRELLING et al. (1966)	U.K.	1	4, F	Not apparent	Lungs, mediastinal nodes, spleen, liver	A. fumigatus
—	—	2	1, F	Not apparent	Lungs, mediastinal nodes, spleen	A. fumigatus
KHOO (1966)	Singapore	—	2 mos. F	Not apparent	Lungs, brain, heart, kidney, pulmonary artery, small intest., diaphragm, thyroid	A. fumigatus
LEDERMAN et al. (1966)	U.S.	—	7, M	Recurrent pneumonitis	Lungs, brain, eye, heart, skin, vertebrae	A. fumigatus
DARRELL (1967)	U.S.	—	40, M	Prosthetic replacement mitral valve	Prosthetic mitral valve (thrombus), brain, eye	A. fumigatus
RIFKIND et al. (1967)	U.S.	7	25, M	Immunosuppresive therapy (renal transplantation)	Lung, kidney, brain, heart	—
		8	37, M	Immunosuppresive therapy (renal transplantation)	Lung, liver	—
		15	16, M	Immunosuppresive therapy (renal transplantation)	Lung, brain, heart	—
		19	28, M	Immunosuppresive therapy (renal transplantation)	Lung, kidney, brain, thyroid, heart	—
		21	17, M	Immunosuppresive therapy (renal transplantation)	Lung, brain, heart	—
		23	35, M	Immunosuppresive therapy (renal transplantation)	Lung, brain, heart	—
PEÑA et al. (1968)	Colombia	10	19, M	Intoxication by yellow P, antibiotics, steroids	Lungs, kidneys, eye, meninges	—
MAHVI et al. (1968)	U.S.	—	9, M	Open-heart surgery (congenital aortic stenosis), foot wound	Brain stem, aortic embolus	A. niger
SAUNDERS and BIEBER (1968)	U.S.	—	55, M	Immunosuppresive therapy (heart transplant)	Lungs, new heart, brain	Asperg. sp.

Table 2. *Frequency of Organ Involvement in 81 cases of Disseminated Aspergillosis*

Organ and Nos. of Cases		Organ and Nos. of Cases		Organ and Nos. of Cases	
Lungs	71	Stomach	5	Adrenal	1
Heart	46	Leptomeninges	5	Ankle	1
Brain	44	Dura	2	Chest Wall	1
Kidney	33	Eyes	4	Esophagus	1
Liver	16	Skin	4	Tongue	1
Thyroid	16	Bone	3	Uterus	1
Spleen	14	Skeletal Muscle	3	Oral Cavity	1
Intestine	12	Pancreas	3	Periadrenal Tissues	1
Mediastinal Nodes	8	Spinal Canal	2	Prostate	1

Table 3. *Pre-existing conditions in 81 cases of disseminated Aspergillosis*

Leukemia	25 cases
Lymphoma	5 cases
Immunosuppressive therapy	7 cases
Idiopathic anemia, neutropenia or pancytopenia	6 cases
Sepsis (*Staph.*, *choleraesuis*), pneumonitis	5 cases
Open heart surgery	4 cases
Viral hepatitis	2 cases
Malignant tumors	2 cases
Tuberculosis	2 cases
Prematurity with cytomegalic inclusion disease	2 cases
Systemic lupus erythematosus	1 case
Septic abortion	1 case
Sarcoidosis	1 case
Myeloid metaplasia	1 case
Rheumatoid arthritis	1 case
Yellow P intoxication	1 case
Traumatic amputation of leg	1 case
Rectal fistula	1 case
Exchange transfusion	1 case
Old rheumatic heart disease	1 case
Not apparent	11 cases
Total	*81 cases*

The isolation of *Aspergillus* sp. from the sputum is frequently reported (EDWARDS, 1935; FINEGOLD et al., 1959; FRAUMENI and FEAR, 1962; WAHNER et al., 1963) and, although not necessarily diagnostic, this finding is helpful. However, it must be kept in mind that *Aspergilli* in sputum may be non pathogenic saprophytes.

The infection may lead to death in a period of time ranging from 2 or 3 days to one or two months, or it may enter a chronic phase that exhibits a clinical picture similar to that of tuberculosis. The chronic form of the disease is characterized by a tendency to abscess formation (COOPER, 1946), fibrosis (SILVER et al., 1962), and pleural empyema (WAHNER et al., 1963). Under adequate treatment the patients may recover (CANNON, 1935; PEER, 1960; RUBINSTEIN, 1963).

Primary aspergillosis of the lungs evolves as an acute pneumonitis characterized by a sudden onset of chills, fever, cough, hemoptoic sputum, cyanosis and chest pain. Physical signs of consolidation my be present. The fungus may sometimes be identified in the sputum (DELIKAT and DYKE, 1945). Chest X-rays reveal a discrete or confluent nodular infiltrate of the lung fields. The condition may have a favorable outcome (DELIKAT and DYKE, 1945), may lead rapidly to a suppurative stage (TOIGO, 1960), or prove fatal (HERTZOG, 1949; TOIGO, 1960; STRELLING et al., 1966).

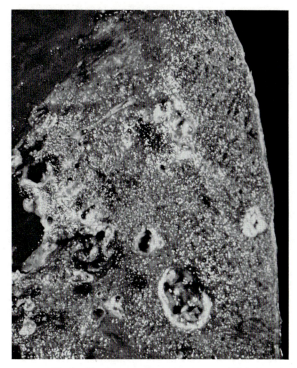

Fig. 13. Pulmonary aspergillosis. The lung parenchyma is consolidated and exhibits numerous well demarcated necrotic foci. (Presbyterian-University Hospital, Pittsburgh, Pa.)

Primary aspergillosis may also have a chronic evolution, with a clinical picture similar to tuberculosis (HETHERINGTON, 1943; HUNT et al., 1961). The main symptoms are cough, weakness, hemoptysis and weight loss. Abscess-like cavities (WILSON et al., 1967) or nodular infiltrations of the lungs are seen on X-rays and the fungus may be found in the sputum. Some patients are asymptomatic and X-ray alterations precede the symptoms by a number of years. In some instances there is a long term history of occupational exposure to grain or dust (COE, 1945).

Morphologic Findings: *Secondary aspergillosis* of the acute type most commonly presents as a necrotizing pneumonitis. The lungs are heavy, weighing 1200—1500 grams, and disclose multiple, poorly demarcated foci of consolidation that measure 2 or 3 cm in diameter. As a rule these foci do not have any specific distribution, and may be more abundant in any pulmonary lobe. On sectioning they typically have a bright white or yellow-colored necrotic center with a hemorrhagic halo (GOWING and HAMLIN, 1960; BAKER, 1962a). Sometimes the lesions have the gross appearance of pulmonary infarcts (CASTLEMAN et al., 1966). On occasion the process is more diffuse and the lungs exhibit consolidation of one or more lobes. There may also be numerous abscesses a few mililmeters in diameter. Large abscesses are not frequent, although they have been reported in a number of cases (ATKINSON et al., 1958; BECH, 1961; FRAUMENI and FEAR, 1962; REDMOND, 1965).

Microscopically the foci of consolidation show coagulative necrosis surrounded by an area of intra-alveolar fibrinous exudate and an outer zone of recent hem-

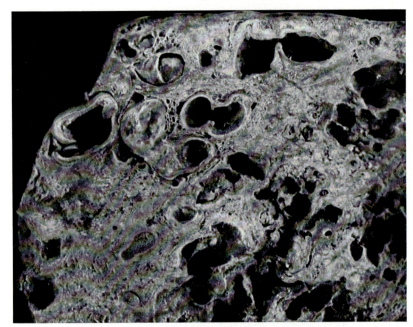

Fig. 14. Double pulmonary infection by *Aspergillus* and *Candida*. There are numerous ectatic bronchi, several intraparenchymatous abscesses and consolidation of the intervening parenchyma

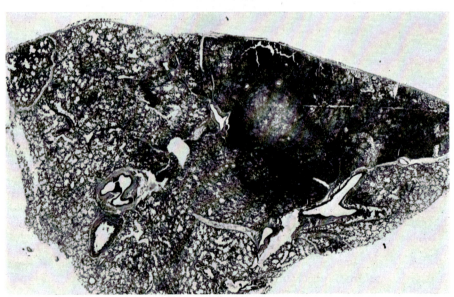

Fig. 15. Pulmonary aspergillosis. This focus reveals a necrotic center with remnants of alveolar septa surrounded by an area of recent hemorrhage. H & E, Approx. × 30

orrhage (Fig. 15, 16). Leukocytes, especially pyknotic neutrophils are found at the edge of the necrotic zone. Large areas of consolidation disclose only an intra-alveolar exudate composed mainly of neutrophils and macrophages.

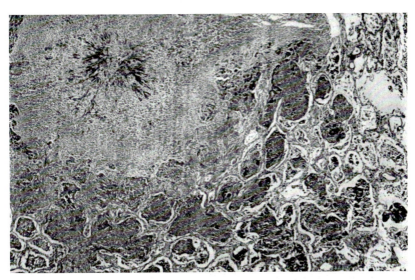

Fig. 16. Pulmonary aspergillosis. A sharply demarcated necrotic focus shows radiating hyphal elements. The non necrotic alveoli contain a proteinaceous material characteristic of pulmonary alveolar proteinosis. The patient also suffered from a chronic granulocytic leukemia. PAS. Approx. × 100. (Courtesy of Dr. R. Hellstrom, Pittsburgh, Pa.)

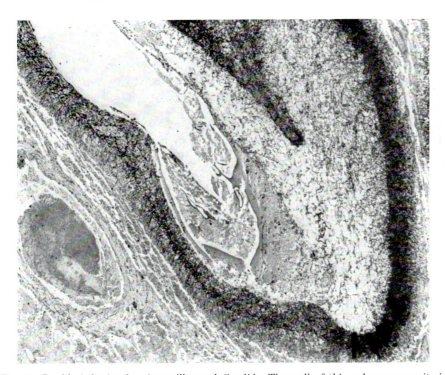

Fig. 17. Double infection by *Aspergillus* and *Candida*. The wall of this pulmonary cavity is lined by a massive fungal growth in which both *Aspergillus* and *Candida* hyphae may be identified at higher magnification. Typical fruiting heads were present in an area and *Candida* sp. was repeatedly isolated from the sputum. (Same case as Fig. 14)

Occasionally the inflammatory reaction is characterized by granulomas of giant and epithelioid cells (KIRSCHTEIN and SIDRANSKY, 1956; TORACK, 1957; REDMOND et al., 1965). Concurrent staphylococcal abscesses may be present (GOWING and HAMLIN, 1960). The inflammatory reaction may be modified by conditions that alter the reactivity of the host. In patients with leukemia and steroid therapy, the neutrophils around foci of coagulation necrosis may be absent, instead of which scattered mononuclear cells are found (GOWING and HAMLIN, 1960).

The chronic form of secondary aspergillosis has similar pathologic characteristics as the acute form, although a more marked tendency for fibrosis and abscess formation is manifest (Fig. 14, 17). In its terminal stages the lesion may be reduced to well demarcated isolated nodular residual lesions as observed by TAKANO et al. (1962).

Primary aspergillosis manifests itself as a granulomatous pneumonitis (HERTZOG, 1949; STRELLING et al., 1966). In these cases there is a diffuse consolidation of both lungs. On sectioning both discrete and confluent grayish-white nodules measuring from 0.1—3 cm in diameter are seen in all lobes. Microscopically they are composed of a center of neutrophils and a peripheral zone of epithelioid and giant cells. Numerous hyphae are present.

In cases having a chronic evolution there is a tendency to increased degrees of fibrosis around granulomas or abscesses (ROSS, 1951). Occasionally the lungs are studded with numerous ragged cavities (LIBRACH, 1957). The case reported by HUNT et al. (1961) was characterized by extensive fibrosis of the lungs that extended into the mediastinum and neck.

Pleura: The alterations of the pleura in all types of aspergillosis reflect the type of changes observed in the lung. In some instances there is a fibrinous pleuritis with variable degrees of organization which contains hyphae (KIRSCHTEIN and SIDRANSKY, 1956). Pleural empyema is occasionally encountered (WAHNER et al., 1963; SCHECHTER et al., 1960). In chronic cases fibrous adhesions may obliterate the pleural cavity to a variable degree. Occasionally, bronchopleural and pericardial fistulas are reported as a postoperative complication (WAHNER et al., 1963; HIDDLESTONE et al., 1954).

Larynx, Treachea, Bronchi: The fungus is sometimes found within normal or ectatic bronchi as 1—2 mm white or yellow granules. The mycelium may or may not invade the bronchial wall which may show little or no inflammatory reaction. In the latter instance it is assumed that the fungus is growing as a saprophyte. In invasive cases, *Aspergillus* often produces an acute necrotizing laryngo-tracheo-bronchitis with a marked mucosal inflammatory reaction and destruction of the cartilage plates. OKUDAIRA and SCHWARZ (1962) have described in detail a pseudomembranous tracheo-bronchitis previously mentioned in the literature only *en passant* (LARA, 1928). The pseudomembrane consisted of a compact mass of hyphae, mucus, nuclear debris, and white and red blood cells. The adjacent tissues were infiltrated by polymorphonuclear and mononuclear leukocytes. SMITH et al. (1965) described a case in which hemorrhagic ulcers were present in the larynx, trachea and bronchi.

Pulmonary Aspergilloma: *Aspergilloma* is the only form of aspergillosis that manifests itself as a well defined clinical syndrome. SCHWARZ et al. (1961), VILLAR et al. (1962), VILLAR (1963) and a Lancet Editorial (1968) have reviewed the subject. The discussion that follows is based upon the analysis of 126 cases gleaned from the literature.

This form of the disease has the highest incidence in the 4th, 5th and 6th decades with similar frequencies in each decade. The age limits reported are 10 (PIMENTEL, 1966) and 82 years (LEVIN, 1956). The condition is found more frequently in men than in women in the proportion of 2.8:1, although in a recent British Tuberculosis Association survey (B.T.A., 1968), females outnumbered males. Most cases of aspergilloma appear in patients suffering from an underlying disorder that has damaged the bronchopulmonary tree, especially by producing cavitation or necrosis of the parenchyma. The associated conditions are the following: proven tuberculosis (28 cases), bronchiectasis and bronchiectatic cysts (11), histoplasmosis (5), bacterial pneumonia (4), asthma (3), silicosis (2), pulmonary sarcoidosis (2), removed echinococcus cyst of lung (2), bronchiolar carcinoma (1), asbestosis (1), emphysematous bleb (1). Nineteen cases were claimed to be primary. In 47 cases the presence or absence of a previous disease could not be definitely established: in general terms, the authors tended to regard them as secondary, with tuberculosis suspected in a number of them. The predisposing causes may be multiple as in CORPE and COPE's case (1956) in which bronchogenic cystic disease was complicated by a *Salmonella choleraesuis* infection.

Table 4. *Species identified in 34 cases of disseminated Aspergillosis in which cultures were reported*

A. fumigatus	29 cases
A. flavus	2 cases
A. nidulans	2 cases
A. niger	1 case
A. sydowi	1 case
A. restrictus	1 case
Total	36 cases*

* The 2 extra cases are accounted for by a patient that disclosed a triple infection.

How often aspergillomas develop in pre-existing pulmonary cavities is not well known. In a prospective survey by the British Tuberculosis Assocation (B.T.A., 1968), positive precipitin serum reactions to *Aspergillus* antigens were obtained in 25% of patients with quiescent tuberculous cavities larger than 2.5 cm. The radiological appearance was compatible with aspergilloma in 44% of the positive reacting individuals (11% of the total).

Clinical Manifestations: The symptomatology is variable and the manifestations directly ascribable to aspergilloma are often difficult to separate from those of the underlying condition.

Hemoptysis, the most important symptom, and very often the presenting one, is encountered very frequently (76 cases, or 60%). It is generally recurrent and extends for periods of months or even years. Usually it is mild, but occasionally it may be severe (LEVIN, 1956; VANTRAPPEN et al., 1959) and even fatal (HUSEBYE, 1967). SALFELDER et al. (1961) have described the curious occurrence of postural hemoptysis in a young woman. Other common symptoms are, in order of frequency, cough, expectoration, fever, weakness and weight loss. Expectoration of small fragments of mycelium is infrequently observed (IKEMOTO, 1963—1964; WEENS and THOMPSON, 1950). Other symptoms encountered are chest pain (RUEDA et al., 1962), wheezing, night sweats and clubbing of the fingers. In many cases the general state of health is quite well preserved and the patient may even be asymptomatic when the aspergilloma is disclosed by a chest roentgenogram (VELLIOS et al., 1957). In those in which the general condition is poor this can usually be attributed to the underlying disease.

The physical examination is in most patients unrewarding. Signs can be elicited pointing to the presence of a pulmonary cavity or a focus of consolidation.

The prognosis is, in general terms, good, and only a relatively small number of deaths have occurred (17 cases, or 13%). The aspergilloma was the immediate cause of death in one patient (HUSEBYE 1967) and a contributor in 3 others through post-operative complications (DÉVÉ, 1938; FINEGOLD et al., 1959), and pneumonia (MONTES, 1963). In 6 cases the demise was related to the pre-existing diseases, which were cor pulmonale (MACARTNEY, 1964; FERNÁNDEZ-LUNA, 1958), acute respiratory infection (HINSON et al., 1952), cachexia (SCHWARZ et al., 1961), brain abscess (PIMENTEL, 1966), and generalized carcinomatosis (MAYS et al., 1967). In 2 other cases, death was unrelated to the underlying disease or to the fungal infection (PECORA et al., 1960; IKEMOTO, 1963—1964). In the remaining 5 cases the cause of death was not determined (PESLE et al., 1954; LEVIN, 1956; IKEMOTO, 1963—1964; AGUILAR-CELI, 1960).

It is quite difficult to assess the total *duration* of the process. Estimates vary from 3 months (ROBINSON, 1962) to 31 years (MONTES, 1963), but most fall between 1 and 3 years, although in BARIÉTY et al's. case (1957) the symptoms were present only 18 days. It is likely that, if left undisturbed, the process will remain stable for a long time.

The *clinical diagnosis* of pulmonary aspergilloma rests heavily upon the demonstration of the characteristic radiological picture. This is described as a round to oval thin walled cavity in an upper lobe containing a moderately dense mass. A thin air crescent separates the mass from the wall of the cavity. Usually the mass occupies about 80—90% of the cavity, but sometimes it fills only $1/3$ or $1/4$ of it. The intracavitary mass is typically movable and can be seen to change its position with the movements of the patient, an important diagnostic sign. ARGEN et al. (1962) observed mobility and plasticity of the ball in a case studied by cineradiography. In some cases the mass is not mobile (RILEY et al., 1962). The *X-ray picture*, although highly characteristic, is not absolutely pathognomonic of aspergilloma. Other conditions such as certain phases of a hydatid cyst, inspissated necrotic or purulent material in an abscess or bronchiectatic cavity, an intra-cavitary blood clot or a Rasmussen aneurysm can produce a similar appearance (WEENS and THOMPSON, 1950). In one case pulmonary angiography showed displacement of the segmental and lobar arteries near the lesion, reduction of their caliber, and retention of the contrast medium (SALFELDER, 1961). In rare occasions a fluid level may be observed (BRAATELIEN et al., 1961; FOUSHEE et al., 1958; GUILFOIL, 1964).

Most often the roentgenographic changes are evident on standard chest films although sometimes they are apparent (and certainly better seen) only on tomo-grams (COLLIE et al., 1965) (Figs. 18, 19). Occasionally there is calcification of the intracavitary mass, extensive enough to be seen in X-rays as focal nodules or as coral-like structures (PIMENTEL, 1966). Bronchography is not very helpful. In most cases the contrast medium does not enter the cavity (LEVIN, 1956). Occasion-ally it does, producing displacement of the intraluminal mass (VILLAR et al., 1962) or delineating the shape of a "glass of champagne" (GALUSSIO and MOSCA, 1963). SALFELDER et al. (1961) observed "amputation" of bronchi in one case. Associated bronchiectases can also be demonstrated by this technique (SCHWARZ et al., 1961; BARNOLA et al., 1961).

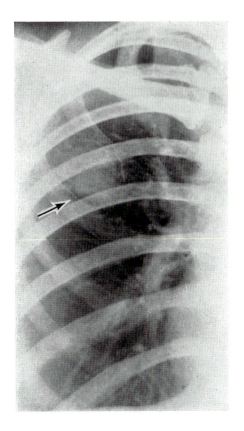

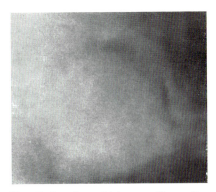

Fig. 19. Intrabronchial aspergilloma. Tomogram. The intracavitary mass, the air meniscus and the cavity wall are clearly visible. Same patient as Fig. 18. (Courtesy of Dr. M. Sánchez-Bertieri, Cali, Colombia). (Originally published in Mycopathologia 1968)

Fig. 18. Intrabronchial aspergilloma. Plain chest film. The upper right lung field displays a thin-walled cavity containing a dense mass, from which it is separated by an air meniscus (arrow). (Courtesy of Dr. M. Sánchez-Bertieri, Cali, Colombia). (Originally published in Mycopathologia 1968)

Bronchoscopy is most of the time non contributory (KESHISHIAN, 1961; ROBINSON et al., 1962; HAUSMANN, 1958). Minor degrees of non-specific inflammation may be observed in the lobar bronchus adjacent to the lesion (ROBINSON et al., 1962; HEMPHILL, 1946) or in the main bronchi (ROBINSON et al., 1962; WEENS and THOMPSON, 1950).

Laboratory Studies: Examination of the sputum directly or by culture, an important diagnostic step, is positive in most instances. Thus in 19 of the 23 cases studied by CAMPBELL and CLAYTON (1964), *A. fumigatus* was obtained.

Blood cell counts are usually not helpful. Among CAMPBELL and CLAYTON'S (1964) 23 cases of pulmonary aspergilloma, only one had more than 1000 eosinophils per cu. mm. This finding agrees with the generally held notion that eosinophilia is not a typical feature in patients with aspergilloma. In isolated cases there is moderate leukocytosis with neutrophilia (VILLAR et al., 1962).

Serum precipitins are an almost invariable finding in patients with aspergilloma (NICHOLSON, 1964; CAMPBELL and CLAYTON, 1964).

Etiologic Agent: *Aspergillus fumigatus* is the fungus most frequently found (34 cases), followed by *A. flavus* (2 cases, ARGEN et al., 1962; RAMIREZ, 1964), *A. niger* (3 cases, VILLAR et al., 1962; GALUSSIO et al., 1963; MONTES, 1963), *A. terreus* (2 cases, PLIHAL et al., 1964; WAHNER et al., 1963), and *A. versicolor* (1 case, CUEVA, 1965) (Table 5). Cultures can be made from the sputum, from bronchial secretions obtained at bronchoscopy, and from the surgical specimen. In many cases it is difficult to obtain any growth from the intraluminal mass after surgery, perhaps due to loss of viability of the fungus. With the possible exception of *Nocardia* (WILHITE, 1966) it is very doubtful that fungi other than *Aspergillus* are capable of producing the clinical-pathological picture of a "fungus ball", although in some early reports an *Actinomyces* (WEENS and THOMPSON, 1950) and a "*Monilia*-like" organism (GRAVES et al., 1951) were incriminated.

Table 5. *Species identified in 43 cases of Aspergilloma in which cultures were reported*

A. fumigatus	34 cases
A. niger	3 cases
A. flavus	2 cases
A. terreus	2 cases
A. versicolor	2 cases
Total	43 cases

Pathogenesis: The exact mechanism by which the fungus implants itself is not fully understood. It is supposed, however, that an airborne fragment of mycelium or spores can be brought into contact with the previously diseased tissue, whereupon it will proliferate and eventually acquire its full dimensions. Sequential chest X-rays have shown the appearance of mycelial masses in previously empty tuberculous cavities or abscesses (FINEGOLD et al., 1959; RILEY et al., 1962). In other cases a known aspergilloma has been observed to enlarge (LEVIN, 1956; RAMSAY, 1960; HUSEBYE, 1967). The lesion grows slowly as evidenced in one of Levin's cases in which the cavity enlarged from 2 to 3 cm and the mass from 1 to 2 cm in 3 years.

One of the conditions that seems necessary for the development and growth of aspergilloma is the presence of a free communication between the site of implantation of the fungus and the airway. The finding of bronchi communicating with the cavity in a great number of cases supports this view. The relationship of *aspergilloma and tuberculosis* is of particular interest. In some cases the fungus colonizes a pre-existing tuberculous cavern. However, this is not always the case, and perhaps because of the presence of bronchiectasis and poor drainage, the fungus may instead colonize an adjacent bronchus (VILLAR et al., 1962). The difficulties encountered in ascertaining this relationship is exemplified by a case that we had the opportunity to study (PEÑA et al., 1968). In this patient the existence of an aspergilloma and/or tuberculosis was suspected on the basis of the radiological picture. No other lesions were visible on chest X-rays. The finding of acid-fast bacilli in the sputum "confirmed" the existence of tuberculosis. Lobectomy showed, however, that the cavity wall was formed of bronchial elements (smooth muscle, respiratory epithelium and mucous glands) with only a moderate inflammatory infiltrate. No evidence of active or healed tuberculosis was present. The possibility was then entertained that atypical *Mycobacteria* could have been growing in an aspergilloma cavity, but definite cultural proof was unfortunately lacking. The case reported by GUILFOIL (1964), in which acid-fast bacilli were isolated twice, is remarkably similar.

MARTIN-LALANDE'S (1961) review of 20 cases of aspergillosis and tuberculosis culled from the literature suggests that *Aspergillus* and *Mycobacteria* are unable to grow simultaneously in the human lung. This investigator points out that when tuberculosis and aspergillosis appear in the same individual, active tuberculous lesions and *Aspergillus* lesions do not occur in the same area. Indeed, MARTIN-LALANDE'S (1961) experimental work indicates that the tubercle bacillus is initially destroyed *in vitro* by the *Aspergillus*. However, this is not an absolute rule, and SÉGRETAIN (1962) has illustrated the seemingly peaceful coexistence of *Mycobacterium* and *Aspergillus* in the same cavity.

Eighteen of the 126 cases reviewed were claimed to be of primary nature (DÉVÉ, 1938; MONOD et al., 1951; YESNER et al., 1950; ROBINSON et al., 1962; BRAATELIEN et al., 1961; ORIE et al., 1960; HOCHBERG et al., 1950; BARIÉTY et al., 1957; FOUSHEE et al., 1958; GALUSSIO et al., 1963; and MONTES, 1963). However, the possibility of occurrence of primary disease is still controversial and perhaps is more widely accepted in Europe than in the United States. MONOD et al. (1951), and PESLE and MONOD (1954) used the term *bronchiectasis — producing aspergilloma ("aspergillome bronchectasiant")* to denote a definite pathogenetic mechanism. A critical evaluation of some of the cases believed to be primary reveals that the evidence on which such an impression was built is often insufficient. However, several reports should be kept in mind. YESNER and HURWITZ's case (1950), a chicken farmer who had ample opportunity for contracting an infection by feeding his flock mouth to beak, did not exhibit evidence of any other disease, clinically or pathologically. BRAATELIEN et al's. 2 cases (1961) had a history of heavy exposure to grain dust; no other significant underlying condition could be detected either clinically or on examination of the resected pulmonary lobe, and the aspergilloma was considered to be primary. It seems, therefore, that aspergilloma occurs as a primary entity even though these cases are rare. It is thought that in the primary disease the repeated exposure to air-borne spores, perhaps of an occupational nature, is important. This would lead to the development of an intrabronchial mycelial mass that after attaining a certain size, would obstruct the airway and produce dilatation of the bronchus through a valve action mechanism.

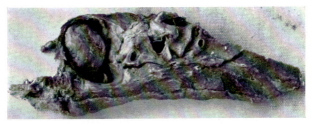

Fig. 20. Intrabronchiectatic aspergilloma. Resected right upper lobe from patient of Fig. 18. A smooth walled cavity contains an unattached ovoid mass. (Originally published in Myco-pathologia 1968)

Morphologic Findings: On gross inspection *the classical aspergilloma* appears as a medium sized, round or oval cavity measuring around 3 cm in diameter, located in the apical segment of the right or left upper lobes. Such a lesion has a very regular contour; its walls are white, firm, well defined and usually measure from 1—5 mm in thickness. The inner lining is usually smooth and grayish-white, The material found in the cavity is commonly a yellow-brown, friable, granular, ovoid mass that has a smooth or lobulated surface and does not adhere to the cavity wall (Fig. 20). In the majority of cases, one or several bronchi, measuring 2—3 mm in diameter open into the cavity. However, a great deal of variation exists. The lesion may affect the lower lobes. The size of the cavity varies from 1 (HINSON et al., 1952) to 19 cm (IKEMOTO, 1963—1964) in diameter. The inner surface is sometimes irregular, ragged and rugose and sometimes shaggy. Occasionally there is more than one cavity (SCHWARZ et al., 1961). The area most fre-

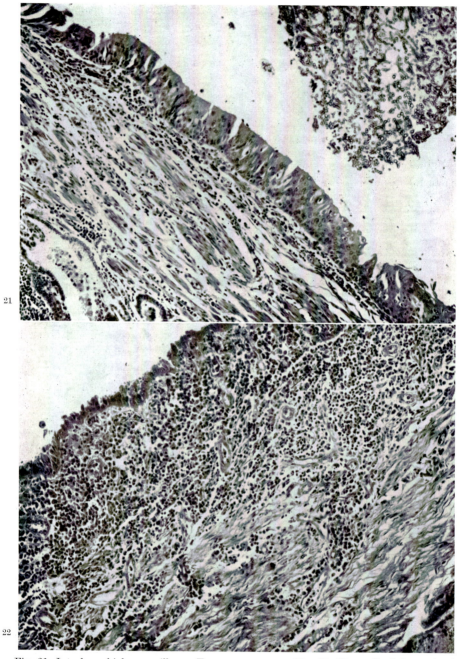

Fig. 21. Intrabronchial aspergilloma. From same case as Fig. 18. The wall of the cavity is composed of an epithelial lining, a smooth muscle layer and bronchial glands. In the right upper corner is a fragment of the mycelial mass. The inflammatory reaction is minimal. H & E, × 100

Fig. 22. Wall of pulmonary aspergilloma. In this case the cavity wall is composed of fibrous connective tissue with an abundant mononuclear leukocytic infiltration. This type of lesion probably develops from a healed tuberculous cavity. H & E, × 100

quently involved is the right upper lobe (52 cases), followed by the left upper lobe (40 cases). The condition may be bilateral, involving both upper lobes (6 patients). The lower lobes are less frequently involved (left, 5 cases; right, 4 cases). In 1 case it was located in an interlobar space. In the remaining 18 cases the exact location was not specified. Whether in the upper or in the lower lobes the lesion has a great predilection for an apical segment. The intracavitary contents may vary. There can be several masses of a dark-brown or grayish and pasty or crumbly material. Focal calcification is not unusual (GERSTL et al., 1948; PIMENTEL, 1966), but extensive calcification to the point of the mass becoming a cavernolith or a coral-like structure is rare (VILLAR et al., 1962). In some cases it is not possible to find a communication with a bronchus perhaps due to closure of the drainage by the inflammatory process. Communication of the aspergilloma cavity with the pleural space producing a hydro-pneumothorax has been reported (FERNÁNDEZ-LUNA, 1958).

Microscopically the wall of the cavity has a variable appearance according to its origin (Figs. 21—22). In some cases it exhibits bronchial elements as smooth muscle, cartilage plates and mucous glands. A respiratory epithelium with foci of squamous metaplasia forms the inner lining. This type of cavity certainly originates in saccular or cylindrical bronchiectases, or bronchial cysts. Another kind of cavity is that in which only a fibrotic wall can be identified, often lined by patches of respiratory epithelium. This kind originates probably from tuberculous caverns or other healed conditions. Both types of cavity may display a degree of inflammatory infiltrate varying from mild to marked, in which lymphocytes, plasma cells and monocytes are abundant. Sometimes eosinophils (HEMPHILL, 1946) and polymorphonuclear leukocytes are found. Infrequently, granulomas composed of giant and epithelioid cells are observed, which betray the origin of the cavity: tuberculosis (PECORA and TOLL, 1960; PIMENTEL, 1966), histoplasmosis (PROCKNOW et al., 1960), and sarcoidosis (ADELBERG et al., 1961). The intracavitary mass reveals upon microscopic examination an almost pure intertwining meshwork of hyphae with very little or no inflammatory exudate (Fig. 23). In many cases the hyphae have a radial disposition around several centers, as if growth was proceeding independently in separated colonies. The mycelium often exhibits broad concentric bands, each band having different staining characteristics. This disposition has been referred to as "zonal" growth and probably represents different periods of growth. In such cases the better preserved and more basophilic hyphae are usually located at the periphery, whereas the degenerating ones are located toward the center of the colony and tend to be eosinophilic. In some cases it is possible to identify the fruiting heads of the fungus. Only in rare instances are hyphae observed penetrating the cavity wall (PECORA and TOLL, 1960; ROBINSON et al., 1962; ENJALBERT et al., 1957; FOUSHEE et al., 1958; SNELLING et al., 1963). In 3 such cases (reported in the 3 last references) the presence of the hyphae was associated with a granulomatous reaction. In one case (MONTES, 1963), there was extensive invasion of the pulmonary parenchyma by numerous hyphae.

The lobe where the cavity lies is usually retracted, firm, covered by a thickened pleura, and may show some degree of peri-cavitary fibrosis and collapse. Other portions of the lobe, as well as the rest of the pulmonary parenchyma, may reflect the pre-existing condition, but very often are remarkably free of any pathological process.

Treatment: The treatment of choice for pulmonary aspergilloma seems to be a *lobectomy* (FRIEDMAN et al., 1956; VILLAR et al., 1962) or a segmental resection (KRASNITZ, 1957; LEVENE et al., 1965). IKEMOTO (1963—1964) and RAMIREZ (1964) have administered endobronchial instillations of amphotericin B and

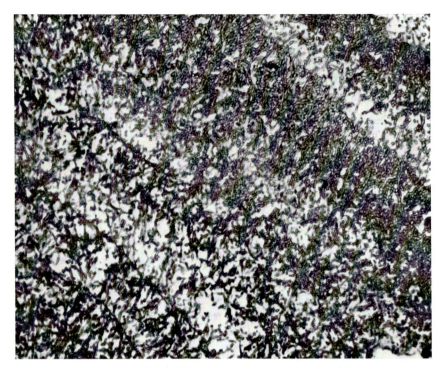

Fig. 23. Intracavitary aspergilloma. The intracavitary mass is composed of an almost pure growth of intertwining hyphae. Zonal growth of the mycelium, probably representing different periods of fungal growth is apparent. H & E, × 100

iodides with some success. More recently, HENDERSON and PEARSON (1968) have advocated local surgical evacuation of the cavity followed by irrigation with natamycin.

Allergic Bronchopulmonary Aspergillosis: *Aspergilli* posses complex antigenic factors, and repeated inhalation of its spores may lead to sensitization (BIGUET et al., 1962), usually manifested as bronchial asthma.

In 1930 BERNTON described the first case of an asthmatic syndrome associated with hypersensitivity to *A. fumigatus*.

Since then numerous reports have appeared illustrating various aspects of the condition (WEINER, 1960; ARGRABITE et al., 1963; ELLIS, 1965; SANERKIN et al., 1966; STARK, 1967; SPOTNITZ et al., 1967; AGBAYANI, 1967; PATTERSON, 1968). It is estimated that about 11% of patients with asthma have allergic pulmonary aspergillosis (HENDERSON et al., 1968). Studies of British workers, especially those of the Brompton group, have done a great deal to clarify the relationship between hyperreactive states, actual *Aspergillus* infection and the various types of antibody response encountered in affected individuals (PEPYS et al., 1964; LONGBOTTOM and PEPYS, 1964; CAMPBELL and CLAYTON, 1964). The subject has been reviewed by PEPYS (1966a, b, c), and by HENDERSON et al. (1968).

Clinical Manifestations: An asthmatic syndrome due to *Aspergillus* sensitization may be either simple or complicated by transient pulmonary infiltrations and blood eosinophilia, a syndrome that has been called "pulmonary eosinophilia".

Clinically, the former is similar to other types of asthma and manifests itself by paroxysms of dyspnea and wheezing followed by cough and expectoration of mucoid material. Symptoms of coryza may be present. The manifestations appear very often during the day, soon after the patient has come into contact with the material harboring the fungus (HINSON et al., 1952). The condition may be present for a long time before the patient seeks medical attention. Instances of occupational disease have been reported (WEINER, 1960).

PEPYS states that in Britain pulmonary eosinophilia associated with asthma is due, in the great majority of cases, to pulmonary aspergillosis (1966a). Clinically there are febrile episodes, wheezing, cyanosis, cough, and, not infrequently, hemoptysis. The sputum may contain characteristic plugs consisting of mucus, hyphae, eosinophils, CHARCOT-LEYDEN crystals and CURSCHMANN spirals (HINSON et al., 1952). Bronchoscopy reveals the presence of a thick mucous secretion blocking bronchi of various calibers. The resulting obstruction may lead to collapse of a pulmonary segment, a lobe, or the entire lung (ELLIS, 1965; SANERKIN, 1966). X-ray examination may disclose areas of collapse and/or consolidation, more frequently in the upper lobes (HENDERSON, 1968). The superimposed pneumonitis as well as the repeated exposure often lead to a chronic phase lasting for months or years, often accompanied by upper lobe contraction, as seen on X-rays (HENDERSON, 1968). A number of patients recover, although the disease is occasionally fatal, as in one of HINSON et al's. patients (1952) who died in status asthmaticus. The condition may be treated with apparent good results by desensitization with emulsified extracts of the fungus (ARGRABITE, 1963), by inhalations of fungistatics (STARK, 1967) or by the use of steroids (PATTERSON, 1968; HENDERSON, 1968).

Etiopathogenesis: Two types of antibodies seem to mediate these clinical manifestations:

1. a *reagin*, or *skin-sensitizing antibody* that is associated with an immediate hypersensitivity response. This antibody can be demonstrated by the production of immediate wheal reactions on skin testing and is responsible for the asthmatic symptoms (PEPYS, 1966a).

2. a *precipitin type* of antibody that can be demonstrated in the patient's serum with the appropriate test antigens.

In addition to the immediate skin hypersensitivity response there may exist a slower type of skin reaction that develops 3—4 hours after testing. This form of response is considered to be a precipitin-mediated reaction of the Arthus type. However, it probably also requires the presence of a reagin.

Although both types of antibodies may occur in simple asthma as well as in asthma with pulmonary eosinophilia, their incidence in the two syndromes is different. In non-selected, uncomplicated asthmatics the prick skin test (immediate) with *A. fumigatus* is positive in about 10% of cases, whereas in cases of asthma with pulmonary eosinophilia the frequency of positivity is about 90% (PEPYS, 1966a). Serum precipitins against *Aspergillus* antigens are present in about 9% of uncomplicated asthmatics (LONGBOTTOM and PEPYS, 1964; PEPYS, 1964), whereas in asthma with pulmonary eosinophilia they appear in 66% or more of the cases (PEPYS, 1966a). It seems that both reagins and precipitins are necessary for the appearance of pulmonary infiltrations (LONGBOTTOM and PEPYS, 1964). PATTERSON et al. (1968) have reported a very illustrative case in whom both reaginic and precipitating antibodies were present while the patient was harboring *A. fumigatus* in his respiratory tract. With treatment, the organism disappeared followed by the decrease of both types of antibodies.

Morphologic Findings: Grossly, the lungs are distended and show marked dilatation of the bronchi (HINSON et al., 1952). These are full of a tenacious mucus and have a thickened mucosa. Microscopically the material occluding the bronchi is composed of mucus, fibrin, Curschmann's spirals, Charcot-Leyden crystals, eosinophils or other inflammatory cells and hyphal elements. A striking change is the very abundant production of mucus by individual cells and by the bronchial glands. No alterations are described in the pulmonary parenchyma.

Farmer's Lung: According to DICKIE and RANKIN (1958) farmer's lung may be defined as an interstitial granulomatous pneumonitis occurring in agricultural workers. Although 25% of patients with this condition have serum precipitins against *A. fumigatus* (PEPYS et al., 1962) no definite relationship of this syndrome with *Aspergillus* has been conclusively demonstrated. On the other hand, it has been shown, on the basis of immunoelectrophoretic techniques, that the serum of approximately 90% of patients reacts with thermophylic *Actinomycetes (Thermopolyspora polyspora* and *Micromonospora vulgaris)* (PEPYS and JENKINS, 1965). This has led to the identification of these fungi as the most important cause of farmer's lung (PEPYS, 1966a, c).

Cardiovascular System

Heart: Involvement of the heart in aspergillosis may result from hematogenous spread, usually originating in the lungs, or from an initial endocardial colonization. The subject has been reviewed by MERCHANT et al. (1958), LANDAU et al. (1963), and NEWMAN et al. (1964). Among the 81 cases of generalized aspergillosis listed in Table 1, 46 had involvement of the heart. The symptomatology referable to the cardiovascular system varies according to the extent of the involvement of endocardium, myocardium and pericardium, and to whether the disease is metastatic or primary. Initial endocardial involvement is encountered in similar circumstances as those in which bacterial endocarditis occurs. They include old rheumatic endocarditis (ZIMMERMAN, 1950) and open-heart surgery either for rheumatic valvulitis with prosthetic replacement of the mitral valve (NEWMAN et al., 1964; DARRELL, 1967) or for congenital aortic or subaortic stenosis (PORTA, 1959; HADORN, 1960; MAHVI et al., 1968). Much more frequently the process is the result of a generalized hematogenous dissemination originating in the lungs. In some instances the portal of entry is a traumatic injury (ZIMMERMAN, 1950) and the infection involves a seemingly healthy endocardium. In rare cases the fungus may reach the pericardium through direct spread from an adjacent pulmonary abscess (FRAUMENI and FEAR, 1962).

Clinical Manifestations: *Endocarditis* tends to dominate the clinical picture in those cases in which the endocardium is initially involved. The clinical picture is similar to that observed in subacute bacterial endocarditis. The most important manifestations are embolization, fever, murmurs and heart failure. Less conspicuous are hematuria and splenomegaly. Embolisms involve quite often large arteries, which is perhaps related to the bulkiness of the mycotic vegetations. The most frequent sites are the aortic bifurcation (with production of a Lériche syndrome), the arteries of the lower extremities (femoral, popliteal), the kidneys, the spleen and the central nervous system (HADORN, 1960; NEWMAN et al., 1964; MAHVI, 1968; ZIMMERMAN, 1950). Embolism to the spleen produces flank pain and splenomegaly. Kidney involvement is manifested by hematuria. Embolism to the central nervous system is attended by the corresponding focal signs. Multiple petechiae of the skin, of the oral mucosa and of the conjunctiva are frequent, appear sometimes in crops, and may be extremely numerous. Osler's nodes of the toes and fingers may coexist. Ocular involvement with rapidly progressing amblyopia is not infrequent (PARADIS et al., 1963; LEDERMAN et al., 1966; DARRELL, 1967). Heart failure may be due to valvular or myocardial lesions and

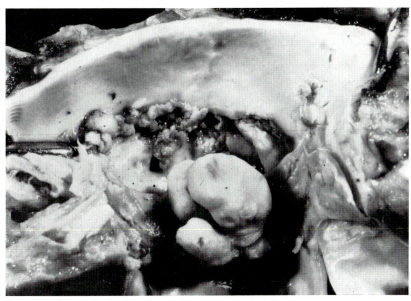

Fig. 24. *Aspergillus* endocarditis. This aortic valve homograft, apparently the primary site of infection, exhibits large polypoid vegetations. Premortem blood cultures were positive for *Aspergillus* sp. (Presbyterian-University Hospital, Pittsburgh, Pa.)

occasionally to pericardial involvement. The presence of murmurs is related to the valvular lesions produced by the *Aspergillus* infection or by the underlying disease. A loud diastolic murmur was present in NEWMAN et al's. case (1964) in which a tongue of thrombus protruded through the aortic valve making it insufficient. A widening of the pulse pressure reflects an aortic insufficiency. The disease is characterized by a rather fast evolution which can be estimated in weeks rather than in months. Terminal shock or sudden death are frequent.

Pericarditis is in some instances an important part of the clinical picture (FRAUMENI and FEAR, 1962), and is manifested by rapid enlargement of the cardiopericardial shadow, electrocardiographic changes, increased venous pressure and pulsus paradoxus.

Myocarditis is usually focal. On occasions it is manifested by heart failure.

With few exceptions (case observed at the Presbyterian-University Hospital of Pittsburgh, see Fig. 24), *Aspergillus* has not been cultured from the blood in life, although it has been recovered from heart blood after death (DARRELL, 1967; LEDERMAN et al., 1963).

Morphologic Findings: The disease affects myocardium and endocardium with approximately the same frequency. The pericardium is perhaps less frequently involved. *Myocardial* foci of necrosis measuring 1 or 2 mm are very frequently encountered. They are visible as white or yellow foci, often subendocardial or subepicardial, that involve the ventricles and sometimes the atria. Microscopically they display coagulative necrosis and variable numbers of hyphae (Fig. 26). Invasion of vessels, with subsequent thrombosis and myocardial necrosis is quite frequent.

Involvement of the *mural endocardium* is characterized by small abscesses and sometimes polypoid vegetations or thrombi in the atria or in the ventricles (LEVY et al., 1955; BUTTRICK et al., 1965; KHOO et al., 1966).

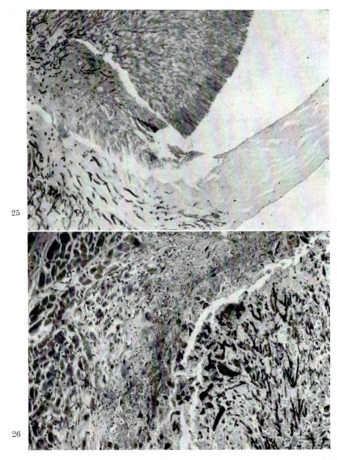

Fig. 25. Aortic valve. From same case as Fig. 24. The vegetation is composed of an almost pure growth of hyphae, some of which penetrate deeply into the valve tissue. Grocott-Gomori, × 100. (Presbyterian-University Hospital, Pittsburgh, Pa.)

Fig. 26. Myocardial aspergillosis. The mycelium is surrounded by necrotic myocardium containing pyknotic neutrophils. H & E, × 100

Valvular involvement is the most spectacular lesion of the disorder (Figs. 24, 25). Most frequently the aortic and the tricuspid valves are affected. The region of the mitral valve is less frequently affected, but cases have been reported following prosthetic replacement of the mitral valve (Newmann et al., 1964; Darrell, 1967) and disseminated pulmonary infection (Marsalek et al., 1960). Involvement of the pulmonary valve has apparently not been recorded. The process is characterized by bulky, friable or firm polypoid reddish-brown to gray vegetations which are much larger than those observed in bacterial endocarditis. Generally the vegetations measure 2 or 3 cm but sometimes they reach extremely large sizes (Kirchstein and Sidransky, 1956). There may also be destruction and perforation of the valves or of the interventricular septum (Zimmerman, 1950).

Microscopically the vegetations are composed of a massive mycelial growth (Zimmerman, 1950), sometimes mixed with large numbers of polymorphonuclear leukocytes (Luke et al., 1963), and covered by a fibrinous layer. The points of

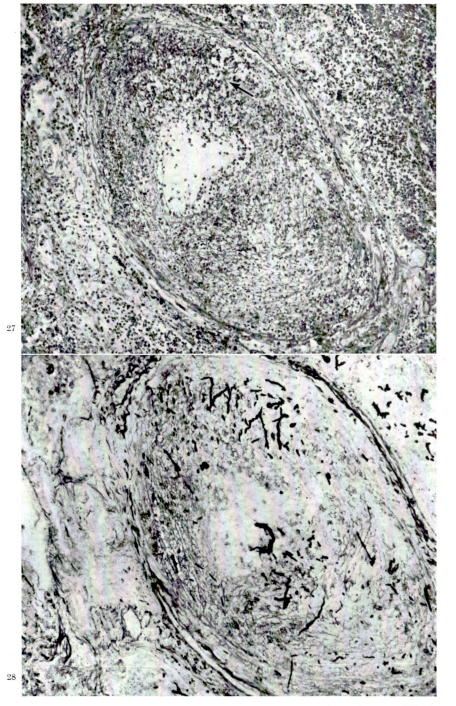

Fig. 27. Thrombosed necrotic vessel. Although hyphae are abundant, they are difficult to see (arrow). PAS, × 100

Fig. 28. Same vessel as in Fig. 27. The hyphae are clearly seen with the Grocott-Gomori stain. × 100

attachment of the vegetations to the valves exhibit necrosis of the collagen and granulocytic infiltration. The valves themselves are the site of edema, inflammatory infiltrate and sometimes show the stigmata of an old rheumatic process. In mural lesions the endocardium is covered by a fibrinous thrombus containing hyphae and neutrophils. The hyphae may extend into the underlying myocardium which shows inflammatory changes.

Pericarditis is frequently characterized by small abscesses that involve the epicardial surface. Occasionally there is purulent effusion and the pericardial membranes are covered by a shaggy fibrinous exudate (FRAUMENI and FEAR, 1962). Microscopically the epicardial abcesses or exudate contain variable numbers of hyphae surrounded by granulocytes and fibrin.

Vessels: As previously noted, one of the characteristics of *Aspergillus* is its tendency to invade small to medium sized arteries and veins, producing necrosis of their walls as well as thrombosis (Figs. 27, 28). This is a very frequent occurrence and GOWING and HAMLIN (1960) observed involvement of small vessels in all of their cases. The coagulative necrosis usually involves the entire circumference of the vessel, but sometimes is segmental. There is also reactive infiltration by polymorphonuclear leukocytes.

Subsequent *thrombosis* is an important factor in the character of the lesions and some of the more necrotizing ones are due to ischemia. In rare instances invasion and thrombosis of coronary branches leads to myocardial infarction (FISHER et al., 1966).

Involvement of large vessels such as the aorta is much more rare but has been reported following open-heart surgery for aortic stenosis (PORTA, 1959; MAHVI et al., 1968; HADORN, 1960). The lesion is characterized by thrombi or polypoid vegetations containing hyphae which adhere to the intima of the vessel and are located a few millimeters distal to the aortic valve.

Central Nervous System

Involvement of the central nervous system in aspergillosis is, in most instances, the result of generalized dissemination of the disease, with the lungs as the initial focus. Reviews on this subject have been published by SCHEIDEGGER (1958) and by FETTER et al. (1967). Among the 81 cases of generalized aspergillosis listed in Table 1, 44 (53%) have involvement of the central nervous system. In addition Table 6 lists 15 cases in which involvement of the central nervous system was apparently the result of direct extension from lesions in the orbit and paranasal sinuses, from self-administered narcotics, and from intrathecal penicillin therapy. In a small number of cases the original site of infection is unknown (DAVID et al., 1951). The routes of dissemination used by *Aspergillus* to reach the central nervous system from distant organs have not been conclusively demonstrated. However, there is little doubt that the blood stream is the pathway followed in cases of systemic spread originating in lung and heart, or in the cases attributed to self-administration of drugs (BURSTON et al., 1963), or to exchange transfusions (LUKE et al., 1963).

"Direct" extension from the orbit, nose or paranasal sinuses may be due to actual invasion and erosion of the bone plate of the cranial base, to extension through the anatomic orifices like the cribriform plate (SCHNYDER, 1948) and optic foramen, or to spread along anastomotic vessels that communicate between the cranial cavity and the orbit or sinuses via the ophthalmic vein. Definite proof of these various possibilities is lacking. However, in WÄTJEN's (1928) and in McKEE's cases (1950), the intracranial involvement was attributed to ethmoid

Table 6. *Aspergillosis of the central nervous system without systemic involvement**

Author and year	Age	Sex	Portal of Entry
OPPE (1897)	37	M	Sphenoid sinus
WATJEN (1928)	66	F	Ethmoid sinuses
MONIZ et al. (1931)	44	F	Eye
GUILLAIN et al. (1935) . . .	33	F	Orbit (?)
McKEE (1950)	60	M	Sphenoid sinus
DAVID et al. (1951)	42	F	Not apparent
WYBEL (1952)	40	F	Spinal canal (Intrathecal penicillin therapy)
IYER et al. (1952)	23	M	Unknown
IYER et al. (1952)	10 mos.	M	Unknown
JACKSON et al. (1955) . . .	36	M	Nasal sinuses or orbit
JACKSON et al. (1955) . . .	22	F	Orbit
ZISKIND et al. (1958) . . .	35	M	Malar region (?)
BURSTON et al. (1963) . . .	37	M	Self administration of drugs (?)
TVETEN et al. (1965) . . .	57	M	Orbit (?)
SCHNYDER (1948)	71	M	Nasal fossae

* Features of 15 cases culled from the literature.

and sphenoid sinusitis, and the bones of the base of the skull were involved by the mycotic process. Furthermore experimental evidence suggests that *Aspergillus* spores may spread from the nose into the cranial cavity and brain by way of emissary veins (EPSTEIN et al., 1968).

Clinical Manifestations: The clinical picture of aspergillosis of the central nervous system depends in great part on whether the disease is primary or meta-static, as well as on the location, extent and character of the lesions.

In some cases the clinical picture is that of a space-occupying lesion or of an abscess (SCHNYDER, 1948; IYER et al., 1952; JACKSON et al., 1955; BURSTON et al., 1963; TVETEN, 1965; SATHMARY, 1958; HENDRICK et al., 1963; DAVID et al., 1951).

The symptoms or signs more frequently encountered are headache, hemi-paresis and convulsions, but there is often fever, paralysis of cranial nerves, and abnormal plantar reflexes. Sometimes there is blurring of the optic discs, vomit-ing, coma and other signs of increased intracranial pressure. Occasionally loss of memory and personality changes (BOSHES et al., 1956) are present. In other instances the clinical picture is that of a meningitic process (LINCK, 1939; AKKO-YUNLU et al., 1957), manifested by fever, convulsions, nuchal rigidity, and in children, tense fontanelle. The neurologic signs are often non-specific (KHOO, 1966; McKEE, 1950).

In cases in which the disease is due to a direct extension from nose or eye lesions, the symptomatology related to these organs is prominent and precedes the intracranial involvement for months or even years (MONIZ et al., 1931; JACKSON et al., 1955; TVETEN, 1965).

In some instances *Aspergillus* infection of the central nervous system presents itself as rather bizarre syndromes, as a "neuroma" of the trigeminal nerve (ZIS-KIND et al., 1958), arteritis, thrombosis and rupture of the internal carotid artery with subarachnoid hamorrhage (McKEE, 1950), spinal block with quadriparesis (WYBEL, 1952), unilateral painless exophthalmos (JACKSON et al., 1955), and chronic encephalitis with progressive dementia and spastic paralysis (IYER et al., 1952).

Examination of the cerebrospinal fluid may show a moderate increase of protein (around 140—190 mg per 100 ml), and a moderate pleocytosis varying from a few cells to 600 or 700 per mm³, most of which are polymorphonuclear leukocytes. Rare cases (HUGHES, 1966) disclose counts over 1000 cells. In cases of spinal block the protein reaches high levels (WYBEL, 1952). The fungus has not been isolated from the cerebrospinal fluid during life, but post-mortem cultures of the cerebrospinal fluid are occasionally positive for *A. fumigatus* (LEDERMAN et al., 1966).

Carotid angiograms, ventriculograms and electro-encephalograms are useful adjuncts.

In the great majority of cases the prognosis is poor, although fluctuations and temporal improvement may appear for some time. Only two cases have been reported with apparent recovery following the removal of a cerebral *Aspergillus* abscess (DAVID et al., 1951; HENDRICK and CONEN, 1963, — same case reported by CONEN et al., 1962).

Morphologic Findings: The morphologic changes observed in aspergillosis of the central nervous system vary according to whether the infection is the result of hematogenous dissemination or of local spread. In the first instance, the lesions tend to be acute and necrotizing or purulent (Fig. 29). In the second case the process is usually chronic and has a tendency to fibrosis and granuloma formation.

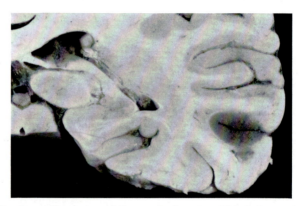

Fig. 29. Embolic *Aspergillus* lesion of the cerebral cortex. This lesion, quite similar to an infarct, is characterized by hemorrhage, necrosis and microscopically, by the presence of hyphae in and outside vessels. (Presbyterian-University Hospital, Pittsburgh, Pa.)

Hematogenous lesions most frequently take the form of multiple abscesses that measure between 0.1 and 2.5 cm (ZIMMERMAN, 1955; SATHMARY, 1958; FRAUMENI et al., 1962; LUKE et al., 1963; HUGHES, 1966), although sometimes they are quite large, measuring 4 or 5 cm (HENDRICK et al., 1963), and producing massive destruction of a hemisphere (LANDAU et al., 1963). The lesions may involve the cerebral cortex, white matter and basal ganglia, and do not have preference for any of the cerebral lobes. The cerebellar hemispheres are likewise frequently affected. A thick fibrous capsule is seen only in rare instances (HENDRICK et al., 1963). Microscopic examination discloses frank pus in the center of the lesion and abundant neutrophilic infiltration at the edges, sometimes accompanied by giant and epithelioid cell granulomas (Fig. 32). Lesions of necrotizing non suppurative type are also frequently seen. They are typically described as white or yellow multiple foci of necrosis with a hemorrhagic component, measuring from a few millimeters to several centimeters. They have a similar distribution to that observed in abscesses. Microscopically they consist of an area of coagulative necrosis with variable amounts of neutrophilic reaction and hemorrhage. Hyphae are commonly seen in the tissues. Vasculitis with thrombosis is quite common both in abscesses and in coagulative necrotic foci.

Brain lesions originating by *local spread* from the orbit, nose or sinuses are, in the majority of cases, of the fibrosing granulomatous type. The more typical examples have been described by IYER et al. (1952), JACKSON et al. (1955), and ZISKIND et al. (1958). These lesions are essentially masses of newly formed inflammatory tissue of rather large size that compress or infiltrate the brain parenchyma and often surround and compress groups of cranial nerves. On inspection they are somewhat irregular, lobulated, poorly demarcated, firm and are often mistaken for infiltrating neoplasms. They are found at the base of the brain, in the orbit, and in the right frontal lobe. On sectioning, these lesions reveal a yellow or gray-white to pink surface and are occasionally soft, cavitated or necrotic. Microscopic examination reveals the masses to be composed of more or less dense fibrous connective tissue infiltrated with collections of lymphocytes, mononuclear cells and eosinophils. The most important characteristic is the presence of foreign body giant cells and epithelioid cells, often arranged in well defined granulomas. Hyphal elements may not be easily found on routine stains. Sometimes the cytoplasm of giant cells contains ovoid or elongated spaces which upon staining with special techniques for fungi, will evidence fragments of hyphae (JACKSON et al., 1955).

The two types of inflammation discussed (purulent-necrotizing and granulomatous) are not unrelated, and may coexist. It seems, however, that the portal of entry of the infection is an important factor in determining the type of inflammatory reaction, which will, in turn, influence the clinical course of the disease.

Examination of the outer surface of the brain reflects the changes present in the cerebral tissues. In some instances there is swelling of the organ accompanied by the usual signs of increased intracranial pressure, as flattening of the convolutions, narrowing of the sulci, herniation of the cerebellar tonsils and uncal grooving. Hemorrhage of the pons and midbrain of the type associated with increased intracranial pressure is occasionally found (BURSTON et al., 1963).

The midbrain (BOSHES et al., 1956), the medulla (GRCEVIC et al., 1959; BUTTRICK et al., 1965) and the pons (IYER et al., 1952) as well as the cranial nerves are at times affected by direct invasion or by compression from an adjacent process.

The *leptomeninges* are frequently affected, although the extent and the importance of the process are quite variable (Fig. 30). In cases of metastatic cerebral infection the meningeal inflammation is often limited to those areas overlying parenchymatous foci. The meningeal inflammation tends to have the same histologic characteristics as the brain lesions. In some cases the meningitis is either generalized or mostly basilar and its symptoms become a prominent part of the clinical picture (LINCK, 1939). In such cases the leptomeninges are cloudy and contain gray or greenish exudate which upon microscopic examination is composed mostly of neutrophils (KHOO et al., 1966) or shows an admixture of inflammatory cells (AKKOYUNLU et al., 1957).

The *dura* may also be the site of focal inflammatory infiltrations in cases of generalized aspergillosis (CAWLEY, 1947; BOSHES et al., 1956). In instances of brain involvement by extension from a neighboring eye or sinus infection, the pachymeninges as well as the leptomeninges are, of necessity, at least focally involved.

The *ventricular system* is seldom the site of any changes. In rare cases, a necrotizing hemorrhagic lesion may rupture into the lateral ventricle (ZIMMERMAN, 1955).

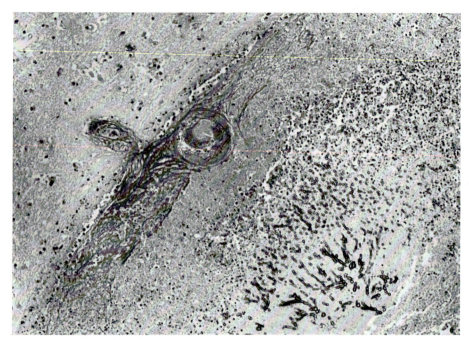

Fig. 30. *Aspergillus* meningitis. In the depth of a cerebral sulcus the leptomeninges are the site of necrosis, neutrophilic and fibrinous exudate and proliferation of the fungus. The molecular cell layer of the cerebral cortex also displays necrosis and leukocytic infiltrate. H & E, × 100 (Presbyterian-University Hospital, Pittsburgh, Pa.)

In cases of basal meningitis with obstruction there can be a moderate and uniform dilatation of the ventricles.

Involvement of the *spinal canal* is rare but has been occasionally reported (Wybel, 1952; Hughes, 1966; Redmond et al., 1965; Lederman et al., 1966) (Fig. 31). The blood-borne infection may affect the leptomeninges and form a well defined subdural mass. In other cases there is invasion of vertebrae, blockage of the spinal canal, and compression of the cord by an epidural mass.

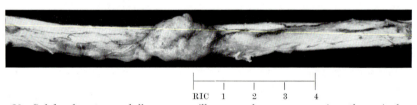

Fig. 31. Subdural extra-medullary aspergillar granuloma compressing the spinal cord. Microscopically the mass is composed mostly of a pure fungal growth and polymorphonuclear leukocytes. (Presbyterian-University Hospital, Pittsburgh, Pa.)

In cases in which the infection has followed intrathecal administration of penicillin there is marked thickening of the tissues around the cervical cord, attended by fibrosis and granulomatous inflammation (Wybel, 1952). In no instances, perhaps with the exception of Lederman et al's. patient on whom a precise description is not available, has actual mycotic involvement of the spinal cord been described.

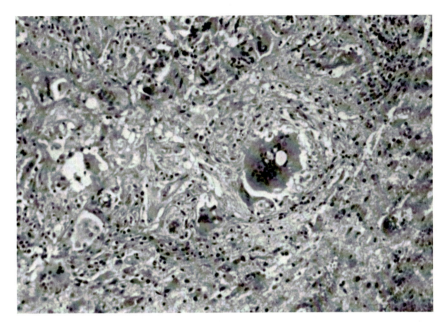

Fig. 32. Fibrogranulomatous reaction in the cerebrum. Foreign-body giant cells, histiocytes, lymphocytes and a moderate fibrous connective tissue proliferation are the main components. H & E, × 100

Involvement of small vessels in the central nervous system is as frequent as in other organs. Major cerebral vessels are rarely affected. In these cases there may be invasion, thrombosis and rupture of the internal carotid or middle cerebral arteries producing subarachnoid hemorrhage or brain infarction (McKEE, 1950; TVETEN, 1965). Another possibility of vascular injury to the brain is the compression of small or medium-sized arteries produced by tumor-like granulomas, leading to necrosis of the cerebral tissues (JACKSON et al., 1955).

Digestive System

Clinical Manifestations: Involvement of the liver (20% of the 81 cases of disseminated aspergillosis reviewed) is likely to produce few clinical manifestations and the majority of these lesions pass undetected. It may however, be manifested by local pain and moderate enlargement of the organ. In rare cases there is jaundice and a tender palpable liver mass due to a fungal abscess (BAKER, 1962a).

In a substantial number of cases the *intestine* (especially the *small bowel*), *stomach, esophagus* and *tongue,* in that order of frequency are affected. In most instances involvement of the gastrointestinal tract is not clinically apparent. However, the fungus may be present in ulcerations of the stomach (FRAUMENI and FEAR, 1962), or duodenum (WELSH and McCLINTON, 1954) and produce erosion of vessels followed by fatal hemorrhage. Rare cases of ulcerative *stomatitis,* with no apparent involvement of other organs, are reported (WHITAKER et al., 1933).

The *pancreas* is rarely involved.

Morphologic Findings: Infections of the *liver* and *pancreas* are likely to be of necrotizing or purulent character (Fig. 33). Grossly there are multiple white or yellow foci measuring from 0.1—2 or 3 cm sometimes accompanied by a zone of hemorrhage. Microscopically these foci show coagulative necrosis, a variable number of hyphae and polymorphonuclear leukocytic infiltration with abscess formation. Thrombotic vasculitis is common.

In the *stomach, duodenum, small bowel* and *esophagus* the lesions tend to be necrotizing, ulcerating and hemorrhagic. Microscopically, necrosis, neutrophilic infiltration, hemorrhage and infiltrating hyphae are the main features.

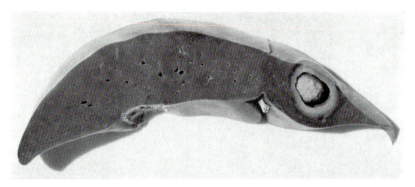

Fig. 33. *Aspergillus* abscess of the liver. The ball in the cavity consists of necrotic liver tissue covered with hyphae. The cavity wall is infiltrated with hyphae. From same patient as Fig. 9. (Courtesy of Dr. R. D. BAKER. Amer. J. clin. Path. **37**, 358 (1962), and The Williams & Wilkins Company)

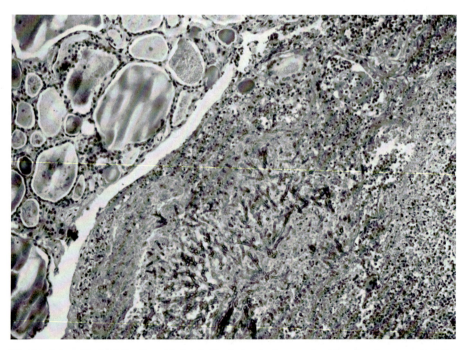

Fig. 34. Aspergillosis of the thyroid gland. The lesion is characterized by abundant neutrophilic infiltrate. H & E, × 100

Endocrine Glands

The *thyroid* is affected in a surprisingly large number of cases (16 out of 81 cases, or 20%), which is similar to that of the liver (Fig. 34). The *adrenal glands* are only rarely affected. No specific symptoms are described in these patients. From the histopathologic point of view the lesions are similar to those of other organs.

Genito-Urinary System

The kidney is frequently involved in generalized aspergillosis (33 out of 81 cases, or 40%). Symptoms are usually absent but there may be lumbar pain and hematuria.

Involvement of the *prostate* is manifested by enlargement and tenderness of the organ (UTZ et al., 1961).

Isolated intraluminal aspergillosis producing obstruction of the urinary tract occurs occasionally. The fungus may form a cast in the renal pelvis (COMMINGS et al., 1962) or lower ureter (FREIDELL et al., 1962). Growth of *Aspergillus* around a calculus of the urinary bladder has also been reported (BROUNST et al., 1963).

Aspergillus vaginitis is rarely observed. Clinically there is discharge and pruritus vulvae (GOLDSTINE, 1933). The vaginal wall exhibits gray-white nodules or a sooty-black pigmentation (WEINSTEIN et al., 1938—1939). Microscopic examination reveals hyphae and necrosis.

In rare instances a post-abortal *uterus* may be the portal of entry for a generalized aspergillosis (FINEGOLD et al., 1959).

Spleen and Lymph Nodes

Involvement of the *spleen* is relatively frequent (14 cases out of 81, or 17%) but does not as a rule produce significant clinical changes.

Involvement of *lymph nodes*, especially of the mediastinal groups is not rare (8 cases out of 81, or 10%) (GRCEVIC et al., 1959; MARSALEK et al., 1960; PARADIS, 1963; WAHNER et al., 1963; HEFFERNAN et al., 1966; STRELLING et al., 1966). No specific symptoms are described.

Grossly and microscopically the lesions are similar to those of other organs.

Musculo-Skeletal System

Clinical Manifestations: Bony structures are rarely affected in systemic aspergillosis. Bones that may be involved are vertebrae and ribs (REDMOND et al., 1965; HUGHES, 1966; SHAW et al., 1936; LEDERMAN et al., 1966), the maxilla (MEHROTRA, 1965), and the base of the skull (HUGHES, 1966).

The clinical manifestations of spinal involvement are kyphosis and destruction of vertebrae, as seen on X-rays. There is infraorbital swelling with invasion of the maxilla.

Skeletal muscles are rarely involved, although lesions of the psoas and diaphragm have been reported. Such processes are not easy to detect clinically and are usually autopsy findings.

Morphologic Findings: Bone lesions are of a destructive and purulent nature. Involved vertebrae frequently collapse. On microscopic examination there are abscesses containing hyphae, sometimes surrounded by groups of giant cells (REDMOND et al., 1965) and a variable degree of fibroblastic reaction. Necrosis is prominent in muscle lesions.

Treatment of Disseminated Aspergillosis: EVANS and BAKER (1959), UTZ et al. (1961), UTZ (1962, 1963a, b) and PROCKNOW (1962) have discussed the treatment of disseminated aspergillosis. It is the consensus that amphotericin B continues to be the drug of choice in cases of serious infection in spite of its toxic potential. Saramycetin (X-5079C) is also capable of significant anti-mycotic activity.

Eye, Adnexa and Orbit

Aspergillosis of the eye may be endogenous, usually the result of hematogenous spread from a distant organ, or exogenous, due to contamination following trauma or surgery.

Endogenous Intraocular Aspergillosis: This form of ocular aspergillosis occurs as a complication of a systemic infection. Well documented examples are rare. Cases based on autopsy studies have been observed by PARADIS et al. (1963), LEDERMAN et al. (1966), and DARRELL (1967). COGAN (1949) and HARLEY et al. (1959), have also reported 2 cases, based on clinical studies. The primary site of infection is usually the lung, but the heart has been implicated in instances following open-heart surgery (DARRELL, 1967).

Clinical Manifestations: Early symptoms include irritating sensation in the eye, tearing, pain, and partial loss of vision. Examination reveals injection of the conjunctiva, chemosis, normal or elevated intraocular tension, hypopion, and gray masses in the vitreous chamber. Usually the infection is unilateral or asymmetrical. Symptoms of involvement of other systems are often present, especially of the central nervous system. The condition has a rapid course and may lead to retinal detachment and extensive destruction of the uvea and retina with total loss of vision.

Morphologic Findings: Grossly there may be cloudiness of the anterior chamber, formation of synechiae and swelling, dislocation or destruction of the lens. The vitreous is frequently opaque and contains exudates. The retina is often detached. Microscopically almost every structure of the eye may be affected. The cornea is edematous or normal. The iris and ciliary body may show leukocytic infiltration. The lens is the site of variable degrees of destruction. Vitreo-retinal abscesses are an important finding (LEDERMAN et al., 1966; DARRELL, 1967). In addition to the necrosis and polymorphonuclear leukocytic infiltration characteristic of such lesion, an outstanding feature is the presence of numerous foreign-body giant cells around the purulent focus. Hyphae are often present in the abscess or in other locations as the anterior chamber or iris. They frequently display an atypical morphology. In some cases the abscesses are initially located between the sclera and the ciliary body, but subsequently extend into the retina and vitreous. The inflammatory process is sometimes diffuse and takes the form of multiple small necrotic foci that involve the iris, ciliary body, retina and vitreous.

Exogenous Aspergillosis: This form of the disease may be localized to the cornea or may be invasive, affecting intraocular structures. The latter usually follows penetrating trauma or intraocular surgery, but may also be due to extension of a corneal infection.

Keratitis: An extensive review of the literature dealing with *Aspergillus* keratitis was published by SCHOLER and SAUBERMAN (1959). The more general subject of mycotic keratitis has been surveyed by ZIMMERMAN (1962), and CHICK et al. (1962). The latter found that cases have been reported in substantial numbers in two periods: from 1879 to 1916 (42 cases), and from 1951 to the time of their writing (84 cases).

The cornea is the most frequent site of ocular aspergillosis, and *Aspergillus* is the most frequent cause of mycotic keratitis. In GINGRICH's compilation (1962) of 109 cases of keratomycosis studied by culture, *Aspergillus* sp. was the most common fungus (38 cases) followed by *Penicillium* (11 cases). *A. fumigatus* is the most frequent species, but *A. flavus, glaucus, niveus* and *versicolor* have also been found.

Aspergillosis of the cornea is almost always preceded by traumatic injury or corneal disease. The injury is usually minor, and often produced by fragments of vegetable matter that may themselves carry the contaminant fungus. The most frequent pre-existing ocular conditions are glaucoma with bullous keratitis, as well as various other ulcers (ZIMMERMAN, 1962). Occasionally, no trauma or predisposing factors are apparent (STERN and KULVIN, 1950). It is the consensus that the incidence of corneal aspergillosis has increased due to the topical use of steroids and perhaps also of antibiotics (MITSUI and HANABUSA, 1955; SCHOLER and SAUBERMAN, 1959; ZIMMERMAN, 1962; SUIE and HAVENER, 1963; FINE, 1965; ALLEN, 1966).

Clinical Manifestations: Corneal aspergillosis is characterized by the development of a corneal ulcer measuring 0.3—0.5 cm in diameter, accompanied by redness of the eye, pain and blurred vision. On examination, the ulcer has the appearance of a slightly raised ovoid, gray plaque with well-demarcated, slightly irregular, rolled or fragmented edges. Hypopion is frequently present. The fungus may be found by examination of smears from the ulcer edge and by culture. The latter method is positive more frequently.

Morphologic Findings: Histopathologic examination of an ulcer reveals necrosis and loss of substance of the cornea accompanied by polymorphonuclear leukocytic infiltration of the tissues. The hyphae may be present in the center of the defect, but are most often seen at the edges. They may penetrate deeply into the corneal stroma producing little or no necrosis. Descemet's membrane may for some time limit the fungal invasion, but is ultimately invaded. Rupture of the ulcer into the anterior chamber produces involvement of the iris and lens, although the inflammatory process occasionally penetrates more deeply.

Corneal ulcerative aspergillosis may be treated with nystatin, but the final result is all too often a corneal scar (MANGIARACINE and LIEBMAN, 1957; SAUBERMAN and SCHOLER, 1959) or sometimes a staphyloma (GINGRICH, 1962).

Exogenous Intraocular Aspergillosis: This form of the disease may be secondary to a mycotic keratitis (CASTROVIEJO and MUÑOZ-URRA, 1921) or to an intraocular surgical procedure. The latter type has become quite troublesome in recent years. Of particular interest is the infection following an intracapsular cataract extraction (FINE, 1962). Postsurgical intraocular fungal infections are an entity with distinctive clinical and histopathological features (FINE and ZIMMERMAN, 1959a, b). Clinically the condition is characterized by a long latent period of days, weeks or even months between operation and onset of symptoms. Pain, redness and blurred vision may appear suddenly. Examination reveals gray white masses in the anterior part of the vitreous, as well as good preservation of light perception. Histopathologic study discloses numerous well demarcated microabscesses located generally in the areas surgically manipulated, i.e. the anterior part of the vitreous and ciliary body. Branching hyphae can be demonstrated. DIAMOND and KIRK (1962) have reported a case following an intracapsular cataract extraction, characterized by massive granulomatous sclerochoroiditis.

Experimental intraocular *Aspergillus* infection has been treated by FINE and ZIMMERMAN (1960) by intraocular injections of nystatin, which they feel might occasionally be indicated in humans as a heroic procedure.

Orbit: The orbit may sometimes be involved by *Aspergillus* infections. Most of the cases are due to extension from processes involving the paranasal sinuses (ADAMS, 1933; WELLER et al., 1960; BAILEY and FULMER, 1961).

Clinical Manifestations: The lesions behave as intraorbital masses producing unilateral exophthalmos (JACKSON et al., 1955), diplopia and compression of the orbital structures. In some instances the process is extremely destructive (WRIGHT, 1927). Propagation into the cranial cavity is a dangerous possibility (BAILEY et al., 1961; JACKSON et al., 1955). The condition may last for years and is quite difficult to treat.

Morphologic Findings: On gross inspection the process is characterized by firm, poorly demarcated, inflammatory masses that compress the neighboring tissues and even produce erosion and destruction of the orbital floor or other bony structures. Microscopically there is a fibrosing granulomatous reaction with foreign body giant cells, neutrophils and mononuclear leukocytes and marked fibroblastic proliferation. The fungus may be difficult to demontrate and special stains should always be used in suspicious cases. *A. fumigatus* and *A. flavus* are cultured from such cases.

Eye Adnexa: Isolated granulomas presenting as an ulceration of the upper eyelid may be due to *A. fumigatus* (HARRELL et al., 1966). Microscopic examination reveals a granulomatous inflammatory reaction and hyphae. Cases of non-specific dacryocystitis, blepharitis, conjunctivitis (ROSENVOLD, 1942; MOSTAFA, 1966), chronic granulomatous blepharitis (BENNETT et al., 1962) and mycotic obstruction of the lacrimal canaliculi (DONAHUE, 1949), due to *A. niger* have also been recorded.

Nose and Paranasal Sinuses

Aspergillosis of the paranasal sinuses and nose is usually the result of an exogenous infection. The earliest reports are those of SCHUBERT (1885), MACKEN-ZIE (1893), HARMER (1913), and TILLEY (1914—1915).

The condition may affect the nose and the maxillary antrum as well as other paranasal sinuses. It usually begins in the maxillary antrum, from which it may extend into the ethmoid, sphenoid or frontal sinuses and into the orbit. Isolated involvement of the nose is apparently very rare.

Table 7 lists the areas involved, the responsible microorganisms and the type of histopathologic reaction observed in 23 cases of infection of the nose and paranasal sinuses found in a review of the literature.

Clinical Manifestations: For unknown reasons nasal and sinus aspergillosis affects women more frequently than men (5:1). It is most often unilateral and has a chronic course marked by periods of activity alternating with periods of quiescence. The usual symptoms are similar to those observed in other types of chronic sinusitis and include dull pain, sinus fulness, nasal obstruction, and nasal as well as postnasal secretion. Sometimes there is spontaneous discharge of tissue fragments that have a membranous appearance. If the frontal, sphenoid, or ethmoid sinuses are also involved, the sensations of fulness and pain are localized to the frontal or parietal areas.

Examination reveals tenderness on pressure over the maxillary antrum, enlargement of the inferior turbinate and opacity on transillumination of the antrum. On puncturing the maxillary sinus it may be difficult or impossible to syringe out its contents, although membranous fragments of tissue may be obtained. In the rare cases limited to the nose, a thick membrane may fill and occlude the nasal fossae (FELDERMAN, 1940). X-ray examination reveals increased density of the affected cavities.

Table 7. *Aspergillosis of nose and paranasal sinuses**

Author and Year	Age Sex	Etiol. Agent	Areas Involved	Histopath. Picture
SCHUBERT (1885) . . . — F		—	—	—
MACKENZIE (1893) . . — F		*Aspergillus sp.*	Rt. maxillary sinus	Chronic non-specific inflamm.
HARMER (1913) . . . — F		*A. fumigatus*	Rt. maxillary sinus	Not described
HARMER (1914—1915) — F		*Aspergillus*	Maxillary sinuses	Chronic non-specific inflamm.
HARMER (1914—1915) — F		*Aspergillus*	Maxillary sinuses	?
HARMER (1914—1915) — F		*Aspergillus*	Maxillary sinuses (bilaterally)	?
HARMER (1914—1915) — F		*Aspergillus*	Maxillary sinuses and ethmoid sinuses (bilaterally)	?
SKILLERN (1921) . . . 50 M		*Aspergillus*	Lt. maxillary sinus	Not described
ADAMS (1933) . . . . 32 F		*A. fumigatus*	Lt. frontal, ethmoid, sphenoid, maxillary sinuses and orbit. Rt. ethmoid and maxillary sinuses	Fibrosing granulomatous inflammation
KELLY (1934) . . . . 60 F		*Aspergillus sp.*	Rt. maxillary sinus	Not described
NASH (1938) . . . . 43 F		*Monilia or Aspergillus*	Lt. nose, ethmoid sinus, orbit.	Necrotizing inflammation
FELDERMAN (1940) . . 43 F		*Aspergillus sp.*	Nose (bilaterally)	Not described
BATT (1941) . . . . . 44 F		*Aspergillus sp.*	Lt. maxillary sinus	Not described
JACKSON et al. (1955) 22 F		*Aspergillus sp.*	Orbit, ethmoid, cranial cavity	Fibrosing granulomatous inflammation
MONTREUIL (1955) . . 34 F		*Aspergillus sp.*	Rt. maxillary sinus	Not described
ANDERSEN et al. (1956) 55 F		*A. fumigatus*	Lt. maxillary and ethmoid sinuses	Not described
ARNAUD et al. (1957) 29 F		*Aspergillus sp.*	Lt. maxillary and Rt. ethmoid sinuses	Not described
ARNAUD et al. (1957) 53 F		*Aspergillus sp.*	Maxillary and ethmoid sinuses (bilaterally), trachea	Not described
SAVETSKY et al. (1961) 53 F		*Aspergillus*	Lt. maxillary sinus	Chronic non-specific inflamm.
BAILEY et al. (1961) 65 M		*A. flavus*	Rt. maxillary sinus, orbit, base of brain	Granulomatous inflammation
WELLER et al. (1960) 31 M		*A. flavus*	Rt. maxillary and ethmoid sinuses, orbit, pterygo-maxillary fossa	Fibrosing granulomatous inflammation
HORA (1965) . . . . 39 M		*A. flavus*	Rt. maxillary and ethmoid sinuses	Chronic non-specific inflamm.
ARONS et al. (1966) . . 25 M		*Aspergillus sp.*	Soft tissue of Rt. pre-auricular and infra-orbital areas and Rt. maxillary sinus	Not described

* Features of 23 cases culled from the literature.

In some instances the condition spreads into the orbit and into the cranial cavity. Symptoms referable to these organs are then predominant. There may be exophthalmos, diplopia, paralysis of cranial nerves and signs of increased intracranial pressure (JACKSON et al., 1955; WELLER et al., 1960; BAILEY and FULMER, 1961). X-ray studies reveal destruction of the bony structures such as the floor of the orbit or the walls of the maxillary sinus.

Morphologic Findings: The maxillary sinuses, as they appear during surgery, have a thickened mucosa and sometimes thickened osseous walls. They contain a material variably described as fibrinopurulent (BAILEY and FULMER, 1961), whitish and solid and resembling a cholesteatoma (SAVETSKY and WALTNER, 1961), cheesy (SKILLERN, 1921), or flaky, friable and greenish (MONTREUIL, 1955). Many writers have been impressed by the presence of friable, grumous, gray membranous material, that has been described as "pseudodiphtheritic" (MACKENZIE, 1893).

Occasionally, the mucosal lining of the sinus has a polypoid appearance (BATT, 1941; ANDERSEN et al., 1956; ARNAUD et al., 1957).

Upon microscopic examination of cases of *Aspergillus* sinusitis, two main types of inflammatory response are found. The first is a chronic non-specific inflammation, characterized by a polymorphonuclear and mononuclear leukocytic infiltrate in the lamina propria of the mucosa. Sometimes the reaction is mostly purulent. The epithelium is often ulcerated or shows focal squamous metaplasia. Typical branching *Aspergillus* hyphae are often seen infiltrating the mucosa. Sometimes the pseudomembranous material obtained at curettage contains a layer of actively proliferating hyphae and fruiting heads. In rare instances the mass filling the antrum is a compact network of hyphae, reminiscent of that observed in intrabronchial aspergillomas (ARNAUD et al., 1957).

The second type of inflammatory response is a fibrosing granulomatous process. This was first observed by ADAMS in 1933 and is characterized by numerous multinucleated foreign body giant cells, occasionally arranged in groups. Accompanying them is a fibrosing process, usually quite marked, with mononuclear cells, fibroblasts and variable degrees of collagenization. The exact nature of the process may be difficult to recognize. In conventional stains, the cytoplasm of giant cells shows clear spaces that upon staining with the appropriate techniques reveals bizarre hyphal elements with abortive branching and bulbous dilatations (ADAMS, 1933; JACKSON et al., 1955).

The bony structures of the sinuses and orbit are usually well preserved or are moderately thickened. In invasive cases however, there may be actual destruction and necrosis of the osseous plates that separate the sinuses from the orbit or from the cranial cavity (WELLER et al., 1960; BAILEY and FULMER, 1961).

The prognosis varies according to the kind of inflammatory response. The chronic non-invasive, non-specific type has a good prognosis. It may be treated with gentian-violet or crystal-violet topically applied, and systemic or topical administration of fungistatics (mycostatin). Surgical procedures of the Caldwell — Luc or De Lima type are indicated. The results are good.

The fibrosing-granulomatous type may be treated with surgical procedures, topical application of mycostatin and systemic administration of amphotericin B or griseofulvin. The results are generally poor (WELLER et al., 1960; BAILEY and FULMER, 1961).

Ear

Aspergillosis of the external ear is one of the oldest known forms of the disease. The earliest works on the subject are those of WREDEN (1867), BURNETT (1874, 1879, 1889) and SIEBENMANN (1889).

The existence of aspergillosis of the ear as an entity is highly controversial. By denying its existence, in his article entitled "The Myth of Otomycosis", KINGERY (1965) creates some suspense about this subject. Perhaps not to be outdone in matters of suspense the Hitchcock Clinic group (McGONIGLE et al., 1967) refer to otomycosis as a "distinctive clinical entity" and proceed to report 5 cases. These widely divergent opinions illustrate the controversy that surrounds the role of *Aspergillus* and other fungi as primary agents of otitis externa.

In principle, two possibilities may be outlined concerning the role of *Aspergillus* in external ear infections. First, that the fungus is the primary etiologic agent of the disease. Second, that the fungus, acting as a saprophyte, invades ears already affected by other diseases as eczema or chronic otitis media. The problem is rendered somewhat more complex by the fact that a number of fungi, including *Aspergillus*, may be cultured from normal ears (LEA et al., 1958). The weight of the evidence indicates that *Aspergillus* may indeed produce primary inflammatory changes of the ear canal (McBURNEY et al., 1936; SIMMS, 1937; STUART and BLANK, 1955). However, the fungus sometimes acts as an opportunistic element and proliferates in pre-existing inflammatory processes as otitis media and eczema (STUART and BLANK, 1955). It must be stressed that only 15—20% of cases of otitis externa are due to fungi (CONANT et al., 1954). The most important bacterial agent is *Bacillus pyocyaneus* (LESHIN, 1953).

The fungi most frequently found in otomycosis are the *Aspergilli* although other fungi as *Candida, Penicillium, Mucor* and the dermatophytes may also be encountered (WOLF, 1947; GREGSON and LA TOUCHE, 1961). The most common species is *A. niger*. Thus in STUART and BLANK'S series (1955) of 29 cases of otomycosis, *A. niger* was found in 19 cases, *A. flavus* in 6, *A. fumigatus* in 2, *A. nidulans* in 1 and *A. flavipes* in 1. It is worth mentioning that in otitis externa the otherwise more prevalent *A. fumigatus* is not the most frequent species. To explain this phenomenon, SHARP and JOHN (1946) invoke the existence of a selective factor. GREGSON and LA TOUCHE (1961) believe that metabolic requirements are partially responsible for this selectivity.

Aspergillus thrives in cerumen and cellular debris that frequently accumulate in the aural canal. It is stated that otomycosis is more frequent in hot tropical climates (LESHIN, 1953) and some reports indicate a high prevalence in such regions (ISMAIL, 1962).

Clinical Manifestations: Aspergillosis of the ear attacks both sexes with the same frequency and is generally unilateral, although bilateral cases are not rare. A dermatitis of the lining membrane of the aural canal, sometimes with involvement of the pinna is the basic alteration. The disease may affect the ear drum, but rarely does it produce perforation of this membrane to involve the middle ear (WHALEN, 1938; REBOUÇAS, 1939). The clinical manifestations vary in intensity from asymptomatic eruptions of the canal to extensive, pruriginous and painful processes. The most important symptom is a dull, boring pain (PITTENGER, 1938). Other symptoms are itching, tinnitus and sensation of fulness. Wax, dried secretions and proliferating mycelium accumulate and sometimes block the ear canal with resulting impairment of hearing. Secondary bacterial infection may occur, which produces a more exudative, eczematoid and sometimes malodorous lesion. Treatment with topical applications of silver nitrate (IRIARTE, 1943), gentian violet (REBOUÇAS, 1939), Iodocloroquin (McGONIGLE et al., 1967), and nystatin (GREGSON and LA TOUCHE, 1961) has been used.

Mycotic infections of postoperative ear cavities following mastoidectomy or fenestration are a common problem. In POWELL et al's survey (1962), *A. terreus* was the fungus most commonly found (22 cases), whereas *A. niger* was rarely found (1 case). Although these data are difficult to evaluate (given the low frequency of *A. niger* infections) it is evident that fungi are usually associated with a significant quantity of debris in postoperative ear cavities, and that postoperative fungal infections of the mastoid are very common.

Morphologic Findings: On gross examination the aural canal is partially filled with a mass of wax, scales, dry secretions and a membranous substance that resembles pieces of sponge sometimes covered by tiny black dots, as if sprinkled with pepper (HOOVER, 1912; LANGERON, 1922; PITTENGER, 1938). If the material is removed, which is easily done, it leaves an inflamed congested surface. Characteristically, the material reaccumulates in 4 or 5 days (FELDERMAN, 1940). The membranous lining of the external ear may be superficially eroded, but is not deeply invaded. The pinna is oftentimes affected by a scaly dermatitis. Microscopic examination of the material obtained from the ear usually reveals cellular debris. The spongy masses are composed of an abundant mycelial growth in which fruiting heads are frequent.

Skin and Adnexa

Aspergillosis of the skin is not frequent. It may be endogenous, as a result of a blood-borne infection, or exogenous. Among the cases of generalized aspergillosis listed in Table 1, only 4 had involvement of the skin (LEDERMAN et al., 1966; ALLAN and ANDERSEN, 1960). Metastatic lesions may be suppurative encrusted papules that involve the scalp and extremities.

Exogenus aspergillosis of the skin is as a rule a chronic inflammatory process involving the dermis and subcutaneous tissues, sometimes accompanied by ulceration.

The species most frequently responsible for exogenous aspergillosis are *A. niger*, *A. fumigatus* and *A. terreus*. In contradistinction with the visceral forms of the disease *A. fumigatus* is not the most common species.

Most probably the fungus does not penetrate through an intact skin, but requires a previous break of the epidermis as exemplified by the cases of LYNCH (1923), FRANK et al. (1933), and CHEETHAM (1964). However, in some instances no history of a previous injury is apparent (LYNCH, 1925; MYERS et al., 1930; and BENNETT et al., 1962).

Clinical Manifestations: In *endogenous aspergillosis*, skin involvement is only a minor part of a generalized disease and its manifestations are superseded by the more important involvement of other organs.

Exogenous aspergillosis in the majority of cases involves only the skin and subcutaneous tissues and remains more or less localized near the portal of entry. However, in some instances, the disease spreads to more distant areas. Lesions encountered include subcutaneous abscesses (FRANK and ALTON, 1933; CHEETHAM, 1964) and raised ulcero-papular skin lesions (MYERS and DUNN, 1930; BALL, 1933; HARRELL et al., 1966). ROBINSON et al. (1935) observed a number of patients apparently with superficial infections of the skin, involving legs, hands, feet and anus, but the clinical picture was not clearly described. The case recorded by CAHILL et al. (1967) in an Egyptian farmer is unique. This patient exhibited a very large number of confluent skin nodules of the face, scalp, trunk and extremities, resembling lepromatous leprosy. However, biopsies and cultures demonstrated *A. niger*. Cases of *A. niger* infection of abdominal surgical incisions characterized by skin and suture-line abscesses are occasionally reported (FRANK and ALTON, 1933).

Morphologic Findings: In the skin as in other sites, *Aspergillus* evokes two basic types of inflammatory reaction, the purulent non-specific and the granulomatous forms. The role of *Aspergilli* as initial agents of purulent inflammation of the skin is controversial and some of these lesions may also yield pathogenic bacteria on culturing (MYERS and DUNN, 1930). However, it is the consensus that *Aspergilli* do indeed play a pathogenetic role. Grossly, the lesions are described as indurated ulcers with minute pustules along the edge (MYERS and DUNN, 1930), or as frank subcutaneous abscesses (CHEETHAM, 1964). Histopathologic findings include epithelial hyperplasia and intraepithelial or subcutaneous abscesses.

The granulomatous type of reaction may be observed in the eyelid, face, or throughout the entire skin surface. Grossly the lesions are described as an elevated skin ulcer, as large, irregular exophytic masses resembling a neoplasm or as nodular lesions. Microscopically they disclose giant cells either scattered or arranged in groups around necrotic foci, as well as an abundant leukocytic infiltration located in the dermis. Hyphae are often seen among the inflammatory infiltrate.

Nails

It is difficult to evaluate the etiologic role of *Aspergillus* in onychomycosis, although most writers believe that it can produce alterations of the nails (BERESTON et al., 1946; BERESTON, 1950; MOORE et al., 1948; MOORE, 1950). The earlier cases of *Aspergillus* onychomycosis were reported in France by EMILE-WEIL et al. (1918—1919), SARTORY (1920), and OTA (1923).

The species most frequently encountered, according to BERESTON et al. (1946) is *A.glaucus*. Other species found are *A.flavus*, *A.niger*, *A.nidulans*, *A.terreus*, *A.rubrum* and *A.onycophylus* (MOORE et al., 1948; BERESTON et al., 1941; BERESTON et al., 1945; GRECO et al., 1935; SMITH, L.M., 1934; PALDROCK et al., 1952).

The condition involves the nails of the fingers and toes approximately with the same frequency. It often starts at one of the margins. The nails are thickened, show pronounced vertical striations, crumble easily and show a greenish or whitish discoloration.

Direct examination and cultures of scrapings reveal the etiologic agent. The ultimate diagnosis rests upon the correlation of the clinical and mycological findings.

Mycetoma Pedis

Only in rare instances do *Aspergillus* infections produce mycetoma (PINOY, 1913; GAMMEL, 1927). Cases have been reported by NICOLLE and PINOY in Tunis (1906), Puestow in the United States (1929) (same case reported by FOERSTER and PUESTOW, 1927), FONSECA in Brazil (1930), and BOUFFARD (quoted by PINOY, 1913). The etiologic agents reported are *A.amstelodami* and *A.nidulans*. In general terms the clinical and anatomopathological features of this form of the disease do not differ from other types of mycetoma, although it may occasionally involve the face and upper extremities.

Aspergillosis in Children

In the young, the disease runs a faster course and disseminates more frequently. Most instances have been reported since 1947, although occasional cases had been previously recorded (PONCE, 1935). Reviews on this subject have been published by BERKEL et al. (1963), KHOO et al. (1966), STRELLING et al. (1966) and BLATTNER (1967).

As in the adult, the infection may be primary or secondary. The latter is more frequent and evolves as an acute disease. The pre-existing conditions as well as the morphologic findings are similar to those observed in adults.

Primary aspergillosis in children is rare, but a number of cases have been described (HERTZOG et al., 1949; AKKOYUNLU et al., 1957; ALLAN et al., 1960; DE LEON-ANTONI, 1962; STRELLING et al., 1966; KHOO, 1966). The disease takes the form of an acute bronchopneumonia, often causing death within a few days. Hertzog's 2 cases, a brother and a sister (one with no anatomopathologic study), and STRELLING et al's 2 cases, two sisters, are exceedingly interesting and do not leave any doubts as to the existence of an acute primary form. Each of these pairs of siblings came from farm families. In both reports, the infection of the second sibling developed shortly after that of the first and all died of an acute pneumonic process within 5—14 days after the onset of the disease. At autopsy, the lungs were very extensively infiltrated by a nodular granulomatous process, that yielded *A. fumigatus* on culture. Microscopically, the granulomas consisted of histiocytes and giant cells, many of which had a core of polymorphonuclear leukocytes.

Aspergillosis in Animals

Fungi of the genus *Aspergillus* may attack a wide variety of animals, including mammals, birds and insects. The subject has been reviewed by AINSWORTH and AUSTWICK (1959) and by AUSTWICK (1965). The three most important types of infection are: 1. mycotic abortion in cattle and mares; 2. pulmonary infection in mammals; and 3. respiratory tract infection in birds. In addition, *Aspergilli* may produce invasive disease of insects (MEDELIN, 1960) and infect incubating poultry eggs (LUCET, 1897; WRIGHT et al., 1961).

Mycotic Abortion

Mycotic abortion, a frequent disease in cows and mares, is due to inflammation and necrosis of the placenta (AINSWORTH and AUSTWICK, 1959; MAHAFFEY et al., 1964; HILLMAN, 1961). Among the various types of abortion in cattle, mycotic placentitis is found in 20% of the placentas examined histologically (HILLMAN, 1961). About 73% of these abortions are due to *Aspergillus* sp. (AUSTWICK and VENN, 1962). In cattle, most abortions occur around the 7th or 8th month of pregnancy, during the winter months. HILLMAN's experimental work (1961) in pregnant heifers suggests that the placental infection is blood-borne. In mares, the possibility of an initial endometrial infection as another portal of entry must be considered (MAHAFFEY et al., 1964).

Morphologic Findings: On gross examination the affected placentas reveal irregularly shaped areas of necrosis, sometimes with ulceration especially on the maternal surface. Microscopically there is chronic inflammation with presence of mononuclear cells, giant cells and neutrophils. Hyphae are seen among necrotic villi. Similar lesions may be present in the amnion.

Pulmonary Aspergillosis in Mammals

Pulmonary aspergillosis in mammals appears to be frequent and has been observed in horses (RANDALL, 1925), lambs (AUSTWICK et al., 1960), calves (EGGERT et al., 1960) and dairy cows (AUSTWICK, 1962b). It is probable that at least a number of infections in lambs and cows is subclinical. AUSTWICK's observations are of great importance, since they indicate that most dairy cows (66%) may harbor pulmonary *Aspergillus* infections.

Morphologic Findings: As described by AUSTWICK (1962b), the lungs of cows disclose subpleural or intraparenchymatous firm nodules measuring 0.1—2 mm and varying from very few to many hundreds. On microscopic examination, the nodules contain asteroid bodies measuring 50—80 μ, which are composed of refractile crystalline radiating structures. Hyphae are present in the majority of the asteroid bodies. Around most nodules there is a fibrous capsule and a moderate inflammatory reaction consisting of macrophages and polymorphonuclear leukocytes. Asteroids are not pathognomonic of aspergillosis and may be present in other conditions.

In lambs, pulmonary aspergillosis may be manifested by discrete purulent foci or by diffuse consolidation. Older lesions are composed of epithelioid cells and occasionally contain asteroid bodies similar to those observed in cows.

Avian Aspergillosis

Aspergillosis is encountered in chickens, ducks, turkeys, parrots (AINSWORTH and AUSTWICK, 1955), captive exotic birds (AINSWORTH and REWELL, 1949) and free living wild birds (McDIARMID, 1955). The fungus species most frequently responsible is *A.fumigatus*, but *A.flavus*, *A.niger*, and *A.nidulans* are also observed. The condition may acquire the form of an epizootic pneumonia especially in chickens, pigeons and turkeys, with a mortality rate as high as 90% (SAVAGE and ISA, 1933; TAYLOR, 1966; and WITTER et al., 1952). Under experimental conditions leukemic chickens exhibit an enhanced susceptibility to aspergillosis (CHICK, 1963).

Morphologic Findings: The organs most frequently involved are the air-sacs, followed by the lungs (AINSWORTH and REWELL, 1949). Other organs involved are the trachea, central nervous system and kidneys (AINSWORTH and AUSTWICK, 1955). Grossly the surfaces of the air-sacs are covered by raised white nodules which may coalesce to form a white or green lining of the entire sac. The fungus does not tend to penetrate tissues. Microscopically the inflammatory response is characterized by proliferation of granulation tissue, on the surface of which the fungus multiplies.

The lungs are the site of scattered, small nodules with a necrotic center that resemble those observed in tuberculosis. There may be consolidation of the parenchyma or formation of large abscesses. Microscopically there is a great variability in the inflammatory response, from focal bronchopneumonia, to a granulomatous nodular infiltration with epithelioid and giant cells.

Toxins

The importance of toxic metabolites produced by fungi of the genus *Aspergillus* in human pathology remains to be settled.

The earliest works on these toxic metabolites are those of CENI and BESTA (1902), BODIN and GAUTIER (1906), and HENRICI (1939). These investigators were able to isolate substances that exhibited neurotoxic properties for laboratory animals from *A.fumigatus*, *A.flavescens* and *A.niger*. These substances were not chemically identified.

More recently TILDEN et al. (1961) have obtained endotoxins from *A.fumigatus* and *A.flavus*, that possess nephrotoxic properties. The endotoxin from *A.fumigatus* has in addition dermonecrotic and hemolytic properties. It has been partially purified and found to be a protein (RAU et al., 1961).

FORGACS et al. (1954) have observed a toxigenic strain of *A.clavatus*. It is possible that toxic substances produced by this fungus and by *A.chevalieri* and *A.fumigatus* are responsible for some cases of bovine hyperkeratosis although this is still uncertain (FORGACS, 1962).

A. fumigatus strains, under certain conditions, produce antibacterial substances known to be toxic to animals. Among them are gliotoxin, fumigacin and fumigatin. Production of these substances under natural conditions deserves further study (Forgacs and Carll, 1962).

Wilson (1966) reviewed the toxic substances, other than aflatoxin, produced by *A. flavus*. These are more or less well defined from the chemical point of view, and include oxalic acid, kojic acid, aspergillic acid, beta-nitropropionic acid and a tremorgenic factor. Spontaneous occurrence of intoxication in man or animals due to exposure to *A. flavus* — produced toxins has not been conclusively demonstrated. Oxalic acid is a stomach irritant and kojic acid is a convulsant (Werch et al., 1957). Aspergillic acid and related compounds have antibiotic properties. Beta-nitropropionic acid shares with chloramphenicol a nitro compound in their structure and is a vasodilator. A tremorgenic factor of unknown chemical composition, recognized by Wilson and Wilson in 1964, produces tremors that last from 1—3 days when administered to mice in doses of 0.5 mg. A new metabolite, with toxic properties for chicken embryos, has been isolated by Rodricks et al. (1968), to which the name aspertoxin has been applied.

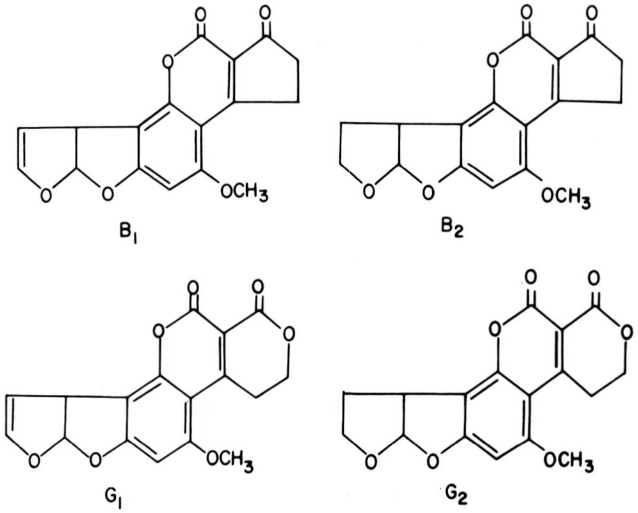

Fig. 35. Chemical structure of aflatoxins

Aflatoxins

The search for toxic metabolites produced by *Aspergilli* culminated recently with the discovery of aflatoxins (Fig. 35). Wogan (1966) and Phelps (1967) have published comprehensive reviews on the subject. In 1960 and 1961 a series of outbreaks of an unknown "X" disease, occurring in turkeys and other animals was observed in England. A Brazilian groundnut meal was incriminated (Blount, 1961) and a toxic factor was isolated from it (Allcroft et al., 1961). Siller and Ostler (1961) studied the histopathology of the disease in turkeys.

Sargeant et al. (1961) identified *A. flavus* as the toxin-producing agent. Smith and McKernan (1962) demonstrated that the chromatographically separated fractions of *A. flavus* extracts possessed hepatotoxic properties. Van der Zijden et al. (1962) isolated the toxin in crystalline form. By means of chromatographic analysis two components were obtained, one showing a blue fluorescence and the other a green fluorescence under ultra-violet light, which were called aflatoxins B and G (NESBITT et al., 1962). It was further demonstrated that there are two blue (B_1 and B_2) and two green (G_1 and G_2) components. Aflatoxin B_1 is the more abundant.

These compounds possess a furanocoumarin structure (ASAO et al., 1965). Aflatoxins B_2 and G_2 are the dihydroderivatives of B_1 (CHANG et al., 1963) and G_1, respectively.

Two main groups of tests, one biological, the other chemical, are available for the detection of aflatoxins (GOLDBLATT, 1967). The most commonly used biological test consists of the administration of extracts of the suspected substance to one-day-old ducklings for 7 days. The livers are then examined microscopically for characteristic lesions such as periportal necrosis and especially for bile duct hyperplasia. The chemical tests consist of extraction of the suspected substance with a solvent, followed by chromatographic analysis and ultraviolet light examination of the chromatograms. Using this method DE IONGH et al. (1965) were able to demonstrate aflatoxins in a sample of peanuts of the year 1922. C_{14} labelled aflatoxin has recently been produced (WOGAN, 1967) by culturing *A. flavus* in media enriched with C_{14} methionine.

Biological Effects

The biological effects of the aflatoxins depend on the amount of toxin administered, on the duration of the exposure, and on the species. Young animals are more sensitive than the mature. Turkeys and ducklings are very susceptible, while chickens are comparatively resistant. Pigs and calves are also quite susceptible. Sheep are remarkably resistant (ALLCROFT, 1965).

Acute Toxicity: The LD_{50} dose of aflatoxin B_1 varies between 0.36 mg/kg (per os), for day-old ducklings (CARNAGHAN et al., 1963), and 17.9 mg/kg (per os), for female rats (BUTLER, 1964a). The LD_{50} dose for male rats is 7.2 mg/kg (per os). Aflatoxin G_1 is somewhat less toxic and aflatoxins B_2 and G_2 are much less toxic.

Morphologic Changes: The acute changes produced by aflatoxin B_1 in ducklings and rats are found mainly in the liver (BUTLER, 1964a, 1964b). In 16—24 hours after administration of an LD_{50} dose to a rat there is loss of glycogen and of cytoplasmic basophilia in the periportal areas. In 48 hours there are well developed periportal areas of necrosis, which at 72 hours are being invaded by histiocytes; proliferation of biliary channels is manifest. At 7 days there is some increase in the amount of reticulin in the portal areas, which by 14 days is more marked and accompanied by an increasing biliary proliferation. By the end of the fourth week there is proliferation of fibrous connective tissue surrounding hyperplastic liver cell nodules, with resulting distortion of the parenchyma. The toxicity response of ducklings and rainbow trout is similar to that of rats. However, hemorrhage and necrosis appear to be somewhat more severe in trout (ASHLEY, 1967). Bile duct hyperplasia is more marked in ducklings and parallels closely the amount of aflatoxin B_1 administered (WOGAN and NEWBERNE, 1964). Other acute lesions in the rat include necrosis of the proximal convoluted tubules of the kidneys, hemorrhages of the corticomedullary junction of the adrenal glands, petechial hemorrhages of the lungs and focal necrosis of the myocardium. These lesions heal in a short period of time.

In cell cultures (LEGATOR, 1966) the earliest effect of a mixture of aflatoxins is the inhibition of DNA synthesis and suppresion of mitosis.

At the ultrastructural level (BUTLER, 1966), administration of aflatoxin B_1 to rats produces early dilatation of the rough endoplasmic reticulum cisternae,

dislocation of ribosomes and swelling of the mitochondria, especially in periportal liver cells. SHANK and WOGAN (1964) have observed that administration
of aflatoxin B_1 to ducklings and rats produces depletion of glycogen and increase
in total lipids of the liver. WOGAN and FRIEDMAN (1965) demonstrated that
aflatoxin B_1 in rats causes inhibition of trytophan pyrrolase induction, indicating
that the toxin alters the ability of the liver to respond to regulation of enzyme
production.

Chronic Toxicity — Carcinogenesis: Aflatoxin is one of the most potent *hepato-
carcinogenic substances* known (BUTLER and BARNES, 1963). BUTLER (1965) has
estimated that the daily dose for induction of liver tumors in rats is 10 μg per day,
whereas the dose of dimethylnitrosamine would be 750 μg/day and of butter
yellow 9000 μg/day. A total dose of 2—3 mg is capable of inducing liver tumors in
rats (NEWBERNE, 1967). Even before the toxic substance was identified LAN-
CASTER et al. (1961) demonstrated the marked carcinogenic properties of samples
of groundnuts in rats. These findings were confirmed by numerous other observations (LE BRETON et al., 1962; BUTLER and BARNES, 1963).

Aflatoxin is also a potent carcinogen for other species as the rainbow trout
(WOLF and JACKSON, 1963; ASHLEY et al., 1965; HALVER, 1965; FALK, 1967;
SINNHUBER, 1967). The incidence of carcinomas in animals seems to be directly
proportional to the amount of aflatoxin and to the lenght of exposure (NEWBERNE,
1965; SINNHUBER, 1967). Continuous administration is not necessary for the
induction of liver tumors (BARNES and BUTLER, 1964; WOGAN, 1966).

The cancerogenic properties of aflatoxins are not limited to the liver. DICKENS
and JONES (1963) have induced sarcomas by repeated subcutaneous injection of
aflatoxins in rats.

Morphologic Findings: The single non-cancerous aflatoxin induced lesion
common to all species studied, perhaps with the exception of the mouse, is a
proliferation of bile-duct cells in the portal spaces (NEWBERNE, 1967). A veno-
occlusive reaction of the liver seems on the contrary, to be specific for bovines.

The pathology of aflatoxin-induced hepatomas has been studied among others
by NEWBERNE (1965, 1967), ASHLEY (1967), WALES (1967), and SIMON et al.
(1967). The species more frequently investigated are rats, ducklings, mice and
trout. Although there are some individual differences, the basic changes are the
same in all species. The liver tumors are multicentric. On gross examination the
tumor nodules are soft, gray-yellow and hemorrhagic or necrotic. Sometimes
there are metastases to the lungs, or direct extension to the peritoneum. In
trout, occasional metastases may be found in the kidneys and gills (HALVER, 1967).

Microscopically, the earliest change observed is a bile-duct proliferation in the
portal areas that progresses to connect with other portal tracts. This lesion does
not seem to progress beyond the state of hyperplasia. Another early change is the appearance of large liver cells with large hyperchromatic nuclei and prominent nucleoli
(megalocytosis), mainly in the periportal areas. This is followed by a hyperplastic
stage, characterized by the appearance of liver-cell nodules (NEWBERNE, 1965).

In the fullblown state, a large portion of the liver parenchyma is replaced by
anaplastic hepatocytes that may be arranged in a trabecular pattern or in solid
sheets. Atypias and mitotic figures are frequent. In ducklings the induced tumors
appear benign and do not produce metastasis (NEWBERNE, 1965).

At the ultrastructural level the Golgi complex and the endoplasmic reticulum
of tumor cells are highly developed (SCARPELLI, 1967). The latter feature corre-
lates with marked cytoplasmic basophilia.

The importance of the aflatoxins in human pathology, and particularly their
carcinogenic potential, have not as yet been fully evaluated. The higher incidence

of hepatoma in the countries of Central and Southern Africa (Mozambique, Senegal, Congo Republic, Gambia, South Africa), particularly in the male negroid population, is well known but hard to explain. Aflatoxin has naturally been held suspect (LE BRETON et al., 1962). This hypothesis seems plausible but it has still to be shown that the incidence of liver carcinoma in a population rises parallel with its degree of exposure to aflatoxin (OETTLÉ, 1965).

References

ADAMS, N.F.: Infection involving the ethmoid, maxillary and sphenoid sinuses and the orbit due to *Aspergillus fumigatus*. Arch. Surg. **26**, 999 (1933). — ADELBERG, J.L., BERKOWITZ, G., SHIELDS, T.W.: Aspergillosis complicating sarcoidosis. Successful surgical resection. Quart. Bull Northw. Univ. med. Sch. **35**, 16 (1961). — AGBAYANI, B.F., NORMAN, P.S., WINKEN-WERDER, W.L.: The incidence of allergic aspergillosis in chronic asthma. J. Allergy **40**, 319 (1967). — AGUILAR-CELI, P.: Aspergillosis pulmonar. An. Fac. Med. (Lima) **43**, 544 (1960). — AINSWORTH, G.C., AUSTWICK, P.K.C.: A survey of animal mycoses in Britain: General aspects. Vet. Rec. **67**, 88 (1955). ~ Fungal diseases of animals (Commonwealth Bureau of Animal Health Review Series, No. 6), 148 pp. (England): Commonwealth Agricultural Bureaux, Farnham Royal 1959. — AINSWORTH, G.C., REWEL, R.E.: The incidence fo aspergillosis in captive wild birds. J. comp. Path. **59**, 213 (1949). — AKKOYUNLU, A., YUCEL, F.A.: Aspergillose broncho-pulmonaire et encéphaloméningée chez un nouveau-né de 20 jours. Arch. franç. Pédiat **14**, 615—622 (1957). — ALLAN, G.W., ANDERSEN, D.H.: Generalized aspergillosis in an infant 18 days of age. Pediatrics **26**, 432 (1960). — ALLCROFT, R.: Aspects of aflatoxicosis in farm animals. In: G.N. WOGAN (ed.), Mycotoxins in foodstuffs, p. 153. Cambidge, Mass.: M.I.T. Press 1965. — ALLCROFT, R., CARNAGHAN, R.B.A., SARGEANT, K., O'KELLY, J.: A toxic factor in Brazilian groundnut meal. Vet. Rec. **73**, 428 (1961). — ALLEN, J.C.: Drug usage and proper diagnosis in treatment of the red eye. Wis. med. J. **65**, 480 (1966). — ALVAREZ, R., REYES, M.A., MADRIÑÁN, C.D.: Encuesta sobre hongos ambientales en la ciudad de Cali. Antioquia méd. **15**, 497 (1965). — AMBROSE, C.T., COONS, A.H.: Studies on antibody production. J. exp. Med. **117**, 1075 (1963). — ANDERSEN, H.C., STENDERUP, A.: Aspergillosis of the maxillary sinus. Acta Oto-laryng. (Stockh.) **46**, 471 (1956). — ARGEN, R.J., LESLIE, E.V., LESLIE, M.B.: Intracavitary fungus ball — Pulmonary aspergillosis. Report of a case. J. Amer. med. Ass. **179**, 944 (1962). — ARGRABITE, J.W., MORROW, M.B., MEYER, G.H.: Allergic bronchial asthma and pulmonary infection due to *Aspergillus fumigatus* treated by infections of emulsified allergen. Ann. Allergy **21**, 583 (1963). — ARKLE, C.J., HINDS, F.: A case of pneumonomycosis. Trans. path. Soc. Lond. **47**, 8 (1895—1896). — ARNAUD, G., PESLE, G.D., DE ANGELIS: L'Aspergillose des sinus (A propos de 2 cas). Ann. d'Otol. **74**, 796 (1957). — ARONS, M.S., LYNCH, J.B., LEWIS, S.R., LARSON, D.L., BLOCKER, T.G.: Hemifacial resection for rare inflammatory diseases of the parotid gland: I. Aspergillosis. II. Pseudosarcomatous fasciitis. Amer. Surg. **32**, 496 (1966). — ASAO, T., BUCHI, G., ABDEL KADER, M.C., CHANG, S.B., WICK, E.L., WOGAN, G.N.: The structures of aflatoxin B_1 & G_1. In: G.N. WOGAN (ed.), Mycotoxins in foodstuffs, p. 265. Cambridge, Mass.: M.I.T. Press 1965. — ASHLEY, L.M.: Histopathology of rainbow trout aflatoxicosis. In: HALVER, J.E., MITCHELL, I.A. (ed.), Trout hepatoma research conference papers, p. 103. Research report 70. Washington, D.C.: U.S. Govermennt Printing Off. 1967. — ASHLEY, L.M., HALVER, J.E., GARDNER, W.K., WOGAN, G.N.: Crystalline aflatoxins cause trout hepatoma. Fed. Proc. **24**, 627 (1965). — ATKINSON, J.B., ATKINSON, G.R.: Lymphosarcoma with pulmonary aspergillosis. Penn. med. J. **61**, 1373 (1958). — AUSTWICK, P.K.C.: Ecology of *Aspergillus Fumigatus* and the pathogenic *Phycomycetes*. Recent Progr. Microbiol. **8**, 644 (1962a). ~ The presence of *Aspergillus fumigatus* in the lungs of dairy cows. Lab. Invest. **11**, 1065 (1962b). ~ Chapter on Pathogenicity. In: RAPER, K.B., FENNELL, D.I.: The Genus Aspergillus, p. 82. Baltimore: Williams & Wilkins Co. 1965. — AUSTWICK, P.K.C., APPLEBY, E.C.: Unpublished data. Quoted by AUSTWICK, P.K.C. (1965). — AUSTWICK, P.K.C., GITTER, M., WATKINS, C.V.: Pulmonary aspergillosis in lambs. Vet. Rec. **72**, 19 (1960). — AUSTWICK, P.K.C., VENN, J.A.J.: Mycotic abortion in England and Wales 1954—1960. Proc. 4th International Congress Animal Reproduct. **3**, 562 (1962). — BADER, G.: Die visceralen Mykosen. Pathologie, Klinik und Therapie, 423 pp. Jena: Gustav Fischer 1965. — BAILEY, J.C., FULMER, J.M.: Aspergillosis of orbit. Report of a case treated by the newer antifungal antibiotic agents. Amer. J. Ophthal. **51**, 670 (1961). — BAKER, R.D.: The diagnosis of fungus diseases by biopsy. J. chron. Dis. **5**, 552 (1957). ~ Leukopenia and therapy in leukemia as factors predisposing to fatal mycoses. Mucormycosis, aspergillosis, and cryptococcosis. Amer. J. clin. Path. **37**, 358 (1962a). ~ Foreword to the International Symposium on Opportunistic Fungus Infections. Lab. Invest. **11**, 1017 (1962b). — BALL, H.A.: Aspergillus dermatomycosis. Report of case. Calif. west. Med. **38**, 178 (1933). — BARIÉTY, M., POULET, J., MONOD,

O., DE BRUX, J.: Aspergillose aiguë, purement pulmonaire, à forme de cancer bronchique. Bull. Soc. méd. Hôp. Paris 73, 397 (1957). — BARNES, J.M., BUTLER, W.H.: Carcinogenic activity of aflatoxin to rats. Nature (Lond.) 202, 1016 (1964). — BARNOLA, J., ANGULO-ORTEGA, A.: Aspergilosis pulmonar. Mycopathologia (Den Haag) 15, 408 (1961). — BARUAH, H.K.: The air spora of a cowshed. J. gen. Microbiol. 25, 483 (1961). — BATT, F.: Aspergillosis and other mycoses in the sinuses of the nose. Acta otolaryng. (Stockh.) 29, 129 (1941). — BAUM, LITZMAN, EICHSTEDT: Quoted by VIRCHOW (1856). — BECH, A.O.: Diffuse broncho-pulmonary aspergillosis. Thorax 16, 144 (1961). — BENNETT, J.E., KIRBY, E.J., BLOCKER, T.G.: Unusual inflammatory lesions of the face. Plast. reconstr. Surg. 29, 684 (1962). — BENNETT, J.H.: On the parasitic vegetable structures found growing in living animals. Trans. roy. Soc. Edinb. 15, 277 (1844). — BERESTON, E.S.: Further studies on Aspergillus infections of the nails. Sth. med. J. (Bgham, Ala.) 43, 489 (1950). — BERESTON, E.S., KEIL, H.: Onychomycosis due to Aspergillus flavus. Arch. Derm. Syph. (Chic.) 44, 420 (1941). — BERESTON, E.S., WARING, W.S.: Onychomycosis and dermatomycosis caused by Trichophyton rubrum and Aspergillus nidulans. Arch. Derm. Syph. (Chic.) 52, 162 (1945). ~ Aspergillus infection of the nails. Arch. Derm. Syph. (Chic.) 54, 552 (1946). — BERKEL, I., SAY, B., TINAZTEPE, B.: Pulmonary aspergillosis in a child with leukemia. Report of a case and a brief review of the pediatric literature. New Engl. J. Med. 269, 893 (1963). — BERNTON, H.S.: Asthma due to mold-Aspergillus fumigatus. J. Amer. med. Ass. 95, 189 (1930). — BIGUET, J., TRAN VAN KY, P., CAPRON, A., FRUIT, J.: Annalyze immunochimique des fractions antigéniques solubles d' Aspergillus fumigatus. C. R. Acad. Sci. (Paris) 254, 3768 (1962). — BLATTNER, R.J.: Pulmonary aspergillosis in children. J. Pediat. 70, 139 (1967). — BLOUNT, W.P.: Turkey "X" disease. Turkeys 9, 52 (1961). — BODIN, E., GAUTIER, L.: Note sur toxine produite par l' Aspergillus fumigatus. Ann. Inst. Pasteur 20, 209 (1906). — BOSHES, L.D., SHERMAN, I.C., HESSER, C.J., MILZER, A., MacLEAN, H.: Fungus infections of the central nervous system. Experience in treatment of cryptococcosis with cycloheximide (actidione). Arch. Neurol. Psychiat. (Chic.) 75, 175 (1956). — BOUFFARD: Quoted by PINOY (1913). — BOYCE, R.: Remarks upon a case of aspergillar pneumomycosis. J. Path. Bact. 1, 163 (1893). — BRAATELIEN, N.T., PERLMUTTER, H.M.: Aspergillosis of the lung. Dis. Chest 39, 425 (1961). — British Tuberculosis Association: Aspergillus in persistent lung cavities after tuberculosis. Tubercle (Edinb.) 49, 1 (1968). — BROUNST, G., ALLAMÉ, F., BROUNST, S.: Un cas primaire d' aspergillome urinaire observé au Liban. Bull. Acad. nat. Méd. (Paris) 147, 50 (1963). — BRUNNER, A.: Das sogenannte Aspergillom. Schweiz. med. Wschr. 1958 499—563. — BRUSKIN, S.: A comprehensive survey of the incidence of fungus spores in the New Brunswick, New Jersey, area. Ann. Allergy 11, 15 (1953). — BURNETT, C.H.: A case of myringomycosis aspergillina. Arch. Ophthal. Otol. 4, 121 (1874). ~ Twenty cases of the growth of Aspergillus in the living human ear. Amer. J. Otol. 1, 10 and 93 (1879). ~ Aspergillus in the human ear. — With report of eleven cases. Med. Surg. Reporter 61, 539 (1889). — BURSTON, J., BLACKWOOD, W.: A case of Aspergillus infection of the brain. J. Path. Bact. 86, 225 (1963). — BUTLER, W.H.: Acute toxicity of aflatoxin B₁ in rats. Brit. J. Cancer 18, 756 (1964a). ~ Acute liver injury in ducklings as a result of aflatoxin poisoning. J. Path. Bact. 88, 189 (1964b). ~ Liver injury and aflatoxin. In: G.N. WOGAN (ed.), Mycotoxins in food-stuffs, p. 175. Cambridge, Mass.: M.I.T. Press 1965. ~ Early hepatic parenchymal changes induced in the rat by aflatoxin B₁. Amer. J. Path. 49, 113 (1966). — BUTLER, W.H., BARNES, J.M.: Toxic effects of groundnut meal containing aflatoxin to rats and guinea pigs. Brit. J. Cancer 17, 699 (1963). — BUTTRICK, D.D., ROBERTS, L.: Generalized cytomegalic inclusion disease. Report of two cases with associated fungal infection, one involving aspergillosis, the second with candidiasis. Amer. J. Dis. Child. 110, 319 (1965). — CAHILL, K.M., EL MOFTY, A.M., KAWAGUCHI, T.P.: Primary cutaneous Aspergillosis. Arch. Derm. 96, 545 (1967). — CAMPBELL, M.J., CLAYTON, Y.M.: Bronchopulmonary aspergillosis. A correlation of the clinical and laboratory findings in 272 patients investigated for bronchopulmonary aspergillosis. Amer. Rev. resp. Dis. 89, 186 (1964). — CANNON, G.D.: Secondary aspergillosis (Aspergillus Niger) superimposed upon bronchiectasis. Report of a case. J. thorac. Surg. 4, 533 (1935). — CARBONE, P.P., SABESIN, S.M., SIDRANSKY, H., FREI, E.: Secondary aspergillosis. Ann. intern. Med. 60, 556 (1964). — CARNAGHAN, R.B.A., HARTLEY, R.D., O'KELLY, J.: Toxicity and fluorescence properties of the aflatoxins. Nature (Lond.) 200, 1101 (1963). — CASTLEMAN, B., McNEELY, B.U. (editors): Case records of the Massachusetts General Hospital. New Engl. J. Med. 274, 1079 (1966). — CASTROVIEJO, R., MUÑOZ-URRA, F.: Aspergilosis ocular. Arch. Oftal. hisp.-amer. 21, 453 (1921). — CAWLEY, E.P.: Aspergillosis and the Aspergilli. Report of a unique case of the disease. Arch. intern. Med. 80, 423 (1947). — CENI, C., BESTA, C.: Über die Toxine von Aspergillus fumigatus und A. flavescens und deren Beziehungen zur Pellagra. Zbl. allg. Path. path. Anat. 13, 930 (1902). — CHANG, S.B., ABDEL KADER, M.M., WICK, E.L., WOGAN, G.N.: Aflatoxin B₂: Chemical identity and biological activity. Science 142, 1191 (1963). — CHARNEAU, A.: Contribution à l'étude de l'aspergillome bronchectasiant. Paris Diss. 1954, 60 S. — CHEETHAM, H.D.: Subcutaneous infection due to

References   823

Aspergillus terreus. J. clin. Path. **17**, 251 (1964). — CHICK, E.W.: Enhancement of asper-gillosis in leukemic chicken. Arch. Path. **75**, 81 (1963). — CHICK, E.W., CONANT, N.F.: Mycotic ulcerative keratitis: A review of 148 cases from the literature. Invest. Ophthal. **1**, 419 (1962). — COE, G.E.: Primary bronchopulmonary aspergillosis, an occupational disease. Ann. intern. Med. **23**, 423 (1945). — COGAN, D.G.: Endogenous intraocular fungous infection. Report of a case. Arch. Ophthal. **42**, 666 (1949). — COHNHEIM, J.: Zwei Fälle von Mykosis der Lungen. Virchows Arch. path. Anat. **33**, 157 (1865). — COLLIE, R.J., FIGIEL, L.S., FIGIEL, S.J., RUSH, D.K.: Pulmonary aspergilloma. Report of two cases. Dis. Chest **47**, 343 (1965). — COMINGS, D.E., TURBOW, B.A., CALLAHAN, D.H., WALDSTEIN, S.S.: Obstructive *Aspergillus* cast to the renal pelvis. Report of a case in a patient having diabetes mellitus and Addison's disease. Arch. intern. Med. **110**, 255 (1962). — CONANT, N.F., SMITH, D.T., BAKER, R.D., CALLAWAY, J.L., MARTIN, D.S.: Manual of Clinical Mycology. 2nd Edition, 456 pp. Philadelphia: W.B. Saunders Company 1954. — CONEN, P.E., WALKER, G.R., TURNER, J.A., FIELD, P.: Invasive primary aspergillosis of the lung with cerebral metastasis and complete recovery. Dis. Chest **42**, 88 (1962). — COOPER, N.S.: Acute bronchopneumonia due to *Aspergillus fumigatus* Fresenius. Report of a case, with a description of acute and granu-lomatous lesions produced by the fungus in rabbits. Arch. Path. **42**, 644 (1946). — CORNET, E., KERNEIS, J.P., MOIGNETEAU, C.R., DUPON, H., COIFFARD, P.: Un cas d'aspergillome bronchectasiant précocement infecté. Poumon **13**, 221—230 (1957). — CORPE, R.F., COPE, J.A.: Bronchogenic cystic disease complicated by unsuspected choleraesuis and *Aspergillus* infestation. Amer. Rev. Tuberc. **74**, 92 (1956). — CRAMER, C.: Über eine neue Fadenpilz-gattung: Sterigmatocystis Cramer. Vierteljahresschrift Naturforsch. Ges. Zürich. **4**, 325 (1859). — CUEVA, A.: Informe preliminar sobre micosis pulmonar. Rev. méd. hondur. **33**, 250 (1965).— DARRELL, R.W.: Endogenous *Aspergillus* uveitis following heart surgery. Arch. Ophthal. **78**, 354 (1967). — DAVID, M., CHARLIN, A., MORICE, J., NAUDASCHER, J.: Infiltration mycosique à *Aspergillus amstelodami* du lobe temporal simulant un abcès encapsulé. Ablation en masse. Guérison opératoire. Rev. Neurol. **85**, 121 (1951). — DE IONGH, H., VLES, R.O., DE VOGEL, P.: The occurrence and detection of aflatoxin in food. In: G.N. WOGAN (ed.), Mycotoxins in foodstuffs, p. 235. Cambridge, Mass.: M.I.T.Press 1965. — DE LEON-ANTONI, E., MARCIAL-ROJAS, R.A.: Pulmonary aspergillosis. Report of first case in Puerto Rico with necropsy findings. Bol. Asoc. méd. P. Rico **54**, 189 (1962). — DELIKAT, E., DYKE, S.C.: Acute pul-monary mycosis. Lancet **2**, 370 (1945). — DES AUTELS, E.J., HOFFMAN, O.R., MONTES, M.: Invasive pulmonary aspergillosis. Difficulties in establishing the diagnosis and distinguishing primary from secondary infection. Dis. Chest **42**, 208 (1962). — DESLONGCHAMP, E.: Note sur les moeurs du Canard Eider (Anas Mollissima Latham), et sur des moisissures developpées, pendant la vie, à la surface interne des poches aériennes d'un de ces animaux. Ann. Sci. nat. Zool. (Ser. 2) **15**, 371 (1841). — DÉVÉ, F.: Une nouvelle forme anatomo-radiologique de mycose pulmonaire primitive. Le Mégamycétome intrabronchectasique. Arch. méd.-chir. Appar. resp. **13**, 337 (1938). — DIAMOND, M.A., Kirk, H.Q.: Postoperative intraocular aspergillosis. Amer. J. Ophthal. **54**, 1124 (1962). — DICKENS, F., Jones, H.E.H.: The car-cinogenic action of aflatoxin after its subcutaneous injection in the rat. Brit. J. Cancer **17**, 691 (1963). — DICKIE, H.A., RANKIN, J.: Farmer's lung. An acute granulomatous inter-stitial pneumonitis occurring in agricultural workers. J. Amer. med. Ass. **167**, 1069 (1958). — DIEULAFOY, CHANTEMESSE, WIDAL: Une pseudo-tuberculose mycosique. Gaz. Hôp. (Paris) **63**, 821 (1890). — DONAHUE, H.C.: Unusual mycotic infection of the lacrimal canaliculi and conjunctiva. Amer. J. Ophthal. **32**, 207 (1949). — DONALDSON, J.M., KOERTH, C.J., Mc CLORKE, R.G.: Pulmonary aspergillosis. J. Lab. clin. Med. **27**, 740 (1942). — *Editorial:* Pulmonary Mycetoma. Lancet **2**, 439 (1968). — EDWARDS, J.C.: A baffling case of pulmonary carcinomatosis. New Engl. J. Med. **213**, 15 (1935). — EGER, W., KÜHRT, P.: Über akute Pilz-encephalitis (Aspergillose) beim Menschen und im Tierexperiment. Dtsch. Z. Nervenheilk. **171**, 370—387 (1954). — EGGERT, M.J., ROMBERG, P.F.: Pulmonary aspergillosis in a calf. J. Amer. vet. med. Ass. **137**, 595 (1960). — ELLIS. R.H.: Total collapse of the lung in asper-gillosis. Thorax **20**, 118 (1965). — EMILE-WELL, Y., GAUDIN, L.: Contribution a l'étude des onychomycoses. Onychomycoses à *Penicillium*, à *Scopulariopsis*, à *Sterigmatocystis*, à Spicaria. Arch. Méd. exp. Anat. Path. **28**, 452 (1918—1919). — EMMONS, C.W.: The Jekyll-Hydes of mycology. Mycologia **52**, 669 (1960). ~ Natural occurrence of opportunistic fungi. Lab. Invest. **11**, 1026 (1962). — EMMONS, C.W., BINFORD, C.H., UTZ, J.P.: Medical mycology, 380 pp. Philadelphia: Lea & Febiger, 1963. — ENJALBERT, L., SÉGRETAIN, G., ESCHAPASSE, H., MOREAU, G., BOURDIN, M.: Deux cas d'aspergillose pulmonaire. Etude anatomo-patholo-gique. Sem. Hôp. Paris **33**, 830—842 (1957). — EPSTEIN, S.M., MIALE, T.D., MOOSSY, J. SIDRANSKY, H.: Experimental intracranial aspergillosis. J. Neuropath. exp. Neurol. **27**, 473 (1968). — EPSTEIN, S.M., VERNEY, E., MIALE, T.D., SIDRANSKY, H.: Studies on the patho-genesis of experimental pulmonary aspergillosis. Amer. J. Path. **51**, 769 (1967). — EVANS, J.H., BAKER, R.D.: Treatment of experimental aspergillosis with amphotericin B. Antibiot. and Chemother. **9**, 209 (1959). — FALK, H.L.: Potential hepatocarcinogenesis for fish. In;

HALVER, J.E., MITCHELL, I.A. (ed.), Trout hepatoma research conference papers, pp. 175. Research report 70: Washington, D.C.: U.S. Government Printing Off. 1967. — FELDERMAN, L.: Infection with *Aspergillus niger*. Report of two cases. Arch. Otolaryng. **31**, 327 (1940). — FERNANDEZ-LUNA, D.: Aspergilosis pulmonar. Rev. bras. Tuberc. **26**, 431 (1958). — FETTER, B.F., KLINTWORTH, G.K., HENDRY, W.S.: Mycoses of the central nervous system, 214 pp. Baltimore: The Williams & Wilkins Co. 1967. — FINE, B.S.: Intraocular mycotic infections. Lab. Invest. **11**, 1161 (1962). ~ Mycotic keratitis. In the Cornea World Congress, p. 207. Washington: Butterworths 1965. — FINE, B.S., ZIMMERMAN, L.E.: Postoperative mycotic endophthalmitis diagnosed clinically and verified histopathologically. Brit. J. Ophthal. **43**, 753 (1959a). ~ Exogenous intraocular fungus infections with particular reference to complications of intraocular surgery. Amer. J. Ophthal. **48**, 151 (1959b). ~ Therapy of experimental intraocular *Aspergillus* infection. Arch. Ophthal. **64**, 849 (1960). — FINEGOLD, S.M., WILL, D., MURRAY, J.F.: Aspergillosis. A review and report of twelve cases. Amer. J. Med. **27**, 463 (1959). — FISHER, A.M., OSSMAN, A.G., SHAW WILGIS, E.F., KRAVITZ, S.C.: Generalized tuberculosis with pancytopenia. Report of a case with aspergillosis as a terminal event. Bull. Johns Hopk. Hosp. **119**, 355 (1966). — FOERSTER, O.H., PUESTOW, K.L.: Maduromycosis (due to *Aspergillus nidulans*). Arch. Derm. Syph. (Chic.) **16**, 91 (1927). — FONSECA, O.DA.: Mycetoma por "*Aspergillus amstelodami*". Rev. méd.-cirurg. Brasil **38**, 415 (1930). — FORGACS, J.: Mycotoxicoses in animal and human health. Proc. U.S. Livestock Sanitary Assoc., 66th Annual Meeting, p. 426, 1962. — FORGACS, J., CARLL, W.T.: Mycotoxicoses. Advanc. vet. Sci. **7**, 273 (1962). — FORGACS, J., CARLL, W.T., HERRING, A.S., MAHLANDT, B.G.: A toxic *Aspergillus clavatus* isolated from feed pellets. Amer. J. Hyg. **60**, 15 (1954). — FOUSHEE, J.H.S., NORRIS, F.G.: Pulmonary aspergillosis. A case report. J. thorac. Surg. **35**, 542 (1958). — FRANCOMBE, W.H., TOWNSEND, S.R.: Pancytopenia and disseminated aspergillosis. Canad. med. Ass. J. **92**, 81 (1965). — FRANK, L., ALTON, O.M.: Aspergillosis: A case of postoperative skin infection. J. Amer. med. Ass. **100**, 2007 (1933). — FRAUMENI, J.D., FEAR, R.E.: Purulent pericarditis in aspergillosis. Ann. intern. Med. **57**, 823 (1962). — FREIDELL, H.V., GERHART, W.F.: Rupture of abdominal aortic aneurysms complicated by acute renal failure and aspergillosis. Calif. Med. **97**, 80 (1962). — FRENKEL, J.K.: Role of corticosteroids as predisposing factors in fungal diseases. Lab. Invest. **11**, 1192 (1962). — FRESENIUS, G.: Beiträge zur Mykologie, 111 pp. Frankfurt: H.L. Bronner 1863. — FRIEDMAN, C., MISHKIN, S., LUBLINER, R.: Pulmonary resection for *Aspergillus* abscess of the lung. Dis. Chest **30**, 345 (1956). — FRIEDREICH, N.: Fall von Pneumomycosis aspergillina. Virchows Arch. path. Anat. **10**, 510 (1856). — FÜRBRINGER, P.: Beobachtungen über Lungenmycose beim Menschen. Virchows Arch. path. Anat. **66**, 330 (1876). — GALUSSIO, J.C., MOSCA, A.: Megamicetoma intracavitario (aspergiloma). A propósito de dos casos. Sem. méd. **123**, 570 (1963). — GAMMEL, J.A.: The etiology of maduromycosis. With a mycologic report on two new species observed in the U.S. Arch. Derm. Syph. (Chic.) **15**, 241 (1927). — GARCÍA-TRIVIÑO, CAMBRONERO, M., ESTEBAN, J.: Un caso interesante de aspergilosis pulmonar. Siglo méd. **95**, 30 (1935). — GAUCHER, E., SERGENT, E.: Un cas de pseudo-tuberculose aspergillaire simple chez un gaveur de pigeons. Bull. Mem. Soc. Med. Hôp. (Paris) Ser. III, **11**, 512 (1894). — GERSTL, B., WEIDMAN, W.H., NEWMANN, A.V.: Pulmonary aspergillosis: Report of two cases. Ann. intern. Med. **28**, 662 (1948). — GINGRICH, W.D.: Keratomycosis. J. Amer. med. Ass. **179**, 602 (1962). — GOLDBLATT, L.A.: Detection and elimination of aflatoxin. In: HALVER, J.E., MITCHELL, I.A. (ed.), Trout hepatoma research conference papers, p. 160. Research report 70. Washington, D.C.: U.S. Government Printing Off. 1967. — GOLDSTINE, M.T.: *Aspergillus fumigatus* vaginitis. Amer. J. Obstet. Gynec. **25**, 756 (1933). — GONZALEZ-MENDOZA, A., BRANDT, H., GONZALEZ-LICEA, A.: Coexistence of pulmonary mycosis and amebic abscess of the liver. Amer. J. trop. Med. **11**, 786 (1962). — GOWING, N.F.C., HAMLIN, I.M.E.: Tissue reactions to *Aspergillus* in cases of Hodgkin's disease and leukemia. J. clin. Path. **13**, 396 (1960). — GRAVES, C.L., MILLMAN, M.: Lobectomy for fungous abscess of the lung: effect of penicillin. J. thorac. Surg. **22**, 202 (1951). — GRAWITZ, P.: Über Schimmelvegetationen im thierischen Organismus. Experimentelle Untersuchung. Arch. Path. Anat. Physiol. Klin. Med. **81**, 355 (1880). — GRCEVIC, N., MATTHEWS, W.F.: Pathologic changes in acute disseminated aspergillosis. Amer. J. clin. Path. **32**, 536 (1959). — GRECO, N.V., BIGATTI, A.: Onicomicosis por *Aspergillus onycophylus*. Rev. Asoc. méd. argent. **49**, 509 (1935). — GREER, A.E.: Disseminating fungus diseases of the lung, 398 pp. Springfield Illinois: Charles C. Thomas 1962. — GREGORY, P.H., BUNCE, M.E.: Microfloral succession in hay. Rept. Rothamsted Exp. Sta. **1959**, 109 (1960). — GREGORY, P.H., LACEY, M.: Liberation of spores from mouldy hay. Trans. Brit. Mycol. Soc. **46**, 73 (1963). — GREGSON, A.E.W., LA TOUCHE, C.J.: Otomycosis: A neglected disease. J. Laryng. **75**, 45 (1961). — GREKIN, R.H., CAWLEY, E.P., ZHEUTLIN, B.: Generalized aspergillosis. Report of a case. Arch. Path. **49**, 387 (1950). (Case reported also by GRCEVIC and MATTHEWS, 1959). — GRUHN, J.G., SANSON, J.: Mycotic infections in leukemic patients at autopsy. Cancer **16**, 61 (1963). — GUILFOIL, P.H.: Pulmonary aspergillosis. A case report. Ohio St. med. J. **60**, 679 (1964). — GUILLAIN, G.,

BERTRAND, I., LEREBOULLET, J.: Etude anatomo-clinique sur un abscès mycosique du lobe frontal. Rev. Neurol. 64, 684 (1935). — GUISAN, M.: Sklerosierende posttraumatische Aspergillus-Meningitis. Schweiz. Arch. Neurol. Neurochir. Psychiat. 90, 235—254 (1962). — HADORN, W.: Aortenruptur durch *Aspergillus*infektion nach Operation einer Aortenstenose. Endaortitis polyposa mycotica. Schweiz. med. Wschr. 90, 929—934 (1960). — HALVER, J.E.: Aflatoxicosis and rainbow trout hepatoma. In: G.N. WOGAN (ed.), Mycotoxins in foodstuffs, p. 209. Cambridge, Mass.: M.I.T. Press, 1965. ~ Crystalline aflatoxin and other vectors for trout hepatoma. In: HALVER, J.E., MITCHELL, I.A. (ed.), Trout hepatoma research conference papers, p. 78. Research report 70. Washington, D.C.: U.S. Government Printing Off. 1967. — HARLEY, R.D., MISHLER, J.E.: Endogenous intraocular fungus infection. Trans. Amer. Acad. Ophthal. Otolaryng. 63, 264 (1959). — HARMER, D.: Suppuration of the antrum due to *Aspergillus fumigatus*. J. Laryng. Rhinol. Otol. 28, 494 (1913). — HARRELL, E.R., WOLTER, J.R., GUTOW, R.F.: Localized aspergilloma of the eyelid. Treatment with local amphotericin B. Arch. Ophthal. 76, 322 (1966). — HAUPTMANN, A., SANDER, C.: Ein hämatogen entstandenes solitäres Aspergillusgranulom bei einem Neunjährigen. Z. Kinderheilk. 90, 124—133 (1964). — HAUSMANN, P.F.: Pulmonary aspergilloma. J. thorac. Surg. 35, 538 (1958). — HEFFERNAN, A.G.A., ASPER, S.P.: Insidious fungal disease. A clinicopathological study of secondary aspergillosis. Bull. Johns Hopk. Hosp. 118, 10 (1966). — Hemphill, R.A.: Mycotic lung infection. Amer. J. Med. 1, 708 (1946). — HENDERSON, A.H.: Allergic aspergillosis: review of 32 cases. Thorax 23, 501 (1968). — HENDERSON, A.H., ENGLISH, M.P., VECHT, R.J.: Pulmonary aspergillosis. Thorax 23, 513 (1968). — HENDERSON, A.H., PEARSON, J.E.G.: Treatment of bronchopulmonary aspergillosis with observations on the use of natamycin. Thorax 2, 519 (1968). — HENDRICK, E.B., CONEN, P.E.: Recovery from a cerebral *Aspergillus* abscess metastatic from a pulmonary focus in the lung. Canad. J. Surg. 6, 352 (1963). (Case also reported by CONEN et al., 1962). — HENRICI, A.T.: An endotoxin from *Aspergillus fumigatus*. J. Immunol. 36, 319 (1939). — HEPPLESTON, A.G., GLOYNE, S.R.: Pulmonary aspergillosis in coal workers. Thorax 4, 168 (1949). — HERTZOG, A.J., SMITH, T.S., GIBLIN, M.: Acute pulmonary aspergillosis. Report of a case. Pediatrics 4, 331 (1949). — HETHERINGTON, L.H.: Primary aspergillosis of the lungs. Amer. Rev. Tuberc. 47, 107 (1943). — HIDDLESTONE, H.J.H., ROSSER, T.H.L., SEAL, R.M.E.: Pulmonary aspergillosis. Tubercle (Edinb.) 35, 15—18 (1954). — HILDICK-SMITH, G., BLANK, H., SARKANY, I.: Fungus diseases and their treatment. 494 pp. Boston: Little, Brown & Co., 1964. — HILLMAN, R.B.: A study of mycotic placentitis and abortion in cattle, 141 pp. Thesis: Ithaca, New York: Cornell University 1961. — HINSON, K.F.W, MOON, A.J., PLUMMER,. N.S.: Broncho-pulmonary aspergillosis. — A review and a report of eight new cases. Thorax 7, 317—333 (1952). — HOCHBERG, L.A., GRIFFIN, E.H., BICUNAS, A.D.: Segmental resection of the lung for aspergillosis. Amer. J. Surg. 80, 364 (1950). — HÖER, P.W., SCHWEISFURTH, R.: Chronische Lungenaspergillose mit metastatischen Aspergillusgranulomen in den parenchymatösen Organen und ihren Identifizierung im Tierversuch. Verh. dtsch. Ges. Path. 1960, 343, 346. ~ Chronische granulomatöse Form der generalisierten Aspergillose beim Menschen und ihre Identifizierung im Tierversuch. Frankfurt. Z. Path. 71, 56—81 (1961). — HOOVER, F.P.: Aspergillosis — Its diagnosis and treatment. Amer. Physician Med. Council (Phil.) 17, 106 (1912). — HORA, J.F.: Primary aspergillosis of the paranasal sinuses and associated areas. Laryngoscope (St. Louis) 75, 768 (1965). — HOREJSI, M., SACH, J., TOMSIKOVA, A., MECL, A.: A syndrome resembling farmer's lung in workers inhaling spores of *Aspergillus* and *Penicillia* moulds. Thorax 15, 212 (1960). — HUGHES, W.T.: Generalized aspergillosis. A case involving the central nervous system. Amer. Dis. Child. 112, 262 (1966). — HUNT, W., BRODERS, A.C., STINSON, J.C., CARABASI, R.J.: Primary pulmonary aspergillosis with invasion of the mediastinal contents and lymph nodes. Amer. Rev. resp. Dis. 83, 886 (1961). — HUSEBYE, K.O.: Serial studies in a case of pulmonary aspergillosis. Dis. Chest 51, 327 (1967).— HUTSON, L.R.: Bagasse litter as a contributory factor in avian aspergillosis. Canad. vet. J. 7, 117 (1966). — HUTTER, R.V.P., COLLINS, H.S.: The occurrence of opportunistic fungus infections in a cancer hospital. Lab. Invest. 11, 1035 (1962). — HUTTER, R.V.P., LIEBERMAN, P.H., COLLINS, H.S.: Aspergillosis in a cancer hospital. Cancer (Philad.) 17, 747 (1964). — HYDE, H.A., RICHARDS, M., WILLIAMS, D.A.: Allergy to mould spores in Britain. Brit. med. J. 1, 886 (1956). — HYDE, H.A., WILLIAMS, D.A.: A census of mould spores in the atmosphere. Nature (Lond.) 164, 668 (1949). — IKEMOTO, H.: Pulmonary aspergilloma or intracavitary fungus ball. Report of five cases. Sabouraudia 3, 167 (1963—1964). — IRIARTE, D.R.: Aspergilosis auricular por *Aspergillus fumigatus* (FRESENIUS, 1863). Arch. venez. Soc. Oto-rinolaring. 4, 33 (1943). — ISMAIL, H.K.: Otomycosis. J. Laryng. 76, 713 (1962). — IYER, S., DODGE, P.R., ADAMS, R.D.: Two cases of *Aspergillus* infection of the central nervous system. J. Neurol. Neurosurg. Psychiat. 15, 152 (1952). — JACKSON, I.J., EARLE, K., KURI, J.: Solitary *Aspergillus* granuloma of the brain. Report of two cases. J. Neurosurg. 12, 53 (1955).— JÄGER, G.F.: Über die Entstehung von Schimmel im Innern des thierischen Körpers. Dtsch. Arch. Anat. Physiol. (Meckel) 2, 354 (1816). — JANKE, D., THEUNE, J.: Zur Kenntnis der

Aspergillose mit besonderer Berücksichtigung ihrer granulomatösen Hautmanifestation. Hautarzt **13**, 145—152 u. 193—198 (1962). — KAMPMEIER, H., BLACK, H.A.: Pulmonary aspergillosis in association with bronchial carcinoma. Amer. Rev. Tuberc. **30**, 315 (1934). — KELLY, A.B.: Aspergillosis of the nose and maxillary antrum. J. Laryng. **49**, 821 (1934). — KELMENSON, V.A.: Treatment of pulmonary aspergillosis. Dis. Chest **36**, 442 (1959). — KESHISHIAN, J.M.: Solitary pulmonary aspergilloma. Amer. Surg. **27**, 729 (1961). — KEYE, J.D., MAGEE, W.E.: Fungal diseases in a general hospital. A study of 88 patients. Amer. J clin. Path. **26**, 1235 (1956). — KHOO, T.K., SUGAI, K., LEONG, T.K.: Disseminated aspergillosis. Case report and review of the world literature. Amer. J. clin. Path. **45**, 697 (1966). — KINGERY, F.A.: The myth of otomycosis. J. Amer. med. Ass. **191**, 129 (1965). — KIRSCHSTEIN, R.L., SIDRANSKY, H.: Mycotic endocarditis of the tricuspid valve due to *Aspergillus flavus*. Report of a case. Arch. Path. **62**, 103 (1956). — KRASNITZ, A.: Broncho-pulmonary aspergillosis. N.Y. St. J. med. **57**, 3852 (1957). — LAGÈZE, P., BÉRARD, M., GALY, P., TOURAINE, R.: Le mégamycétome pulmonaire ou aspergillome intra-cavitaire à propos de trois cas. J. franc. Méd. Chri. thor. **7**, 648—662 (1953). — LANCASTER, M.C., JENKINS, F.P., PHILP, J.M.: Toxicity associated with certain samples of groundnuts. Nature (Lond.) **192**, 1095 (1961). — LANDAU, J.W., NEWCOMER, V.D., SCHULTZ, J.: Aspergillosis; report of two instances in children associated with acute leukemia and review of the pertinent literature. Mycopathologia (Den Haag) **20**, 177 (1963). — LANGERON, M.: Sur un champignon d'une otomycose brésilienne: *Sterigmatocystis Hortai*. Bull. Soc. Path. exot. **15**, 383 (1922). — LARA, A.: Algunos casos de aspergilosis observados en la península de Yucatán. Rev. Med. Yucatán **15**, 41 (1928). — LEA, W.A., SCHUSTER, D.S., HARRELL, E.R.: Mycological flora of the healthy external auditory canal: A study of 120 human subjects. J. invest. Derm. **31**, 137 (1958). — LE BRETON, E., FRAYSSINET, C., BOY, J.: Sur l'apparition d'hépatomes "spontanés" chez le Rat Wistar. Role de la toxine de l'*Aspergillus flavus*. Intérêt en pathologie humaine et cancérologie experimentale. C. R. Acad. Sci. (Paris) **255**, 784 (1962). — LEDERMAN, I.R., MADGE, G.: Endogenous intraocular aspergillosis. Arch. Ophthal. **76**, 233 (1966). — LEGATOR, M.: Biological effects of aflatoxin in cell culture. Bact. Rev. **30**, 471 (1966). — LESHIN, N.: Correlation of clinical otitis externa with mycobacteriologic studies. Arch. Otolaryng. **58**, 716 (1953). — LEVENE, N., RIVAROLA, C., BLUE, M.E.: Surgical considerations in pulmonary tuberculosis complicated by bronchopulmonary aspergillosis. Amer. Rev. resp. Dis. **91**, 262 (1965). — LEVIN, E.J.: Pulmonary intracavitary fungus ball. Radiology **66**, 9 (1956). — LEVY, E.S., COHEN, O.B.: Systemic moniliasis and aspergillosis complicating corticotropin therapy. Arch. intern. Med. **95**, 118 (1955). — LIBRACH, I.M.: Primary pulmonary aspergillosis. Report of a fatal case. Antibiot. Med. Clin. Ther. **4**, 377 (1957). — LICHTHEIM, L.: Über pathogene Schimmelpilze. I. Die Aspergillusmykosen. Berl. Klin. Wschr. **19**, 129 und 147 (1882). — LINCK, K.: Tödliche Meningitis aspergillina beim Menschen. Virchows Arch. path. Anat. **304**, 408 (1939). — LINK, H.F.: Observations in ordines plantarum natureles. Ges. Naturf. Freunde Berlin Magazin **3**, 1 (1809). — LONGBOTTOM, J.L., PEPYS, J.: Pulmonary aspergillosis: diagnostic and immunological significance of antigens and C substance in *Aspergillus fumigatus*. J. Path. Bact. **88**, 141 (1964). — LOURIA, D.B., COLLINS, H.S.: Some aspects of pulmonary mycotic infections. Tuberculology **21**, 76 (1964). — LUCET, A.: De l'*Aspergillus fumigatus* chez animaux domestiques et dans les oeufs en incubation. Etude clinique et experimentale, 108 pp. Paris: Ch. Mendel 1897. — LUKE, J.L., BOLANDE, R.P., GROSS, S.: Generalized aspergillosis and *Aspergillus* endocarditis in infancy. Report of a case. Pediatrics **31**, 115 (1963). — LYNCH, K.M.: *Aspergillus* in scalp lesions following redbug (leptus) bites. Arch. Derm. Syph. (Chic.) **7**, 599 (1923). ~ Invasion of the hair of the scalp by *Aspergillus*. Sth. med. J. (Bgham, Ala.) **28**, 119 (1925). — McBURNEY, R., SEARCY, H.B.: Otomycosis: An investigation of effective fungicidal agents in treatment. Ann. Otol. (St. Louis) **45**, 988 (1936). — McDIARMID, A.: Aspergillosis in free-living wild birds. J. comp. Path. **65**, 246 (1955). — McGONIGLE, J.J., JILLSON, O.F.: Otomycosis: An entity. Arch. Derm. **95**, 45 (1967). — McKEE, E.E.: Mycotic infection of brain with arteritis and subarachnoid hemorrhage. Report of a case. Amer. J. clin. Path. **20**, 381 (1950). — MACARTNEY, J.N.: Pulmonary aspergillosis: A review and a description of three new cases. Thorax **19**, 287 (1964). — MACKENZIE, D.: Preliminary report on *Aspergillus* mycosis of the antrum maxillare. Bull. Johns Hopk. Hosp. **4**, 9 (1893). — MACKIE, F.P.: Visceral infections due to higher fungi. Indian J. med. Res. **9**, 781 (1922). — MEDELIN, M.F.: Internal fungal parasites of insects. Endeavour **19**, 181 (1960). — MAHAFFEY, L.W., ASAM, N.M.: Abortions associated with mycotic lesions of the placenta in mares. J. Amer. vet. med. Ass. **144**, 24 (1964). — MAHVI, T.A., WEBB, H.M., DIXON, C.D., BOONE, J.A.: Systemic aspergillosis caused by *Aspergillus niger* after open heart surgery. J. Amer. med. Ass. **203**, 520 (1968). — MANGIARACINE, A.B., LIEBMAN, S.D.: Fungus keratitis (*Aspergillus fumigatus*). Treatment with Nystatin (Mycostatin). Arch. Ophthal. **58**, 695 (1957). — MARSALEK, E., ZIZKA, Z., RIHA, V., DUSEK, J., DVORACEK, D.: Plicni aspergilloza s generalizaci vyvolana druhem *Aspergillus restrictus*. Čas. Lék. čes. **99**, 1285 (1960). — MARTIN-LALANDE, J.: Aspergillose et tuberculose pulmonaire associées. (Contribution à l'étude des modalités de coexistence). Rev. Tuberc. (Paris) **25**, 1235 (1961). — MAYER, A.C.: Verschimmelung (Mucedo) im lebenden Körper. Dtsch. Arch. Anat. Physiol. (Meckel) **1**, 310 (1815). — MAYS, E.E., HAWKINS, J.A.: Cavitary bronchiolar carcinoma with an intracavitary aspergilloma. Amer. Rev. resp. Dis. **95**, 1056 (1967). — MEHROTRA, M.C.: Aspergillosis of maxilla; an unusual case. Oral Surg. **20**, 33 (1965). — MERCHANT, R.K., LOURIA, D.B., GEISLER, P.H., EDGCOMB, J.H., UTZ, J.P.: Fungal endocarditis: Review of the literature and report of three cases. Ann. intern. Med. **48**, 242 (1958). — MERKOW, L., PARDO, M., EPSTEIN, S.M., VERNEY, E., SIDRANSKY, H.: Lysosomal stability during phagocytosis of *Aspergillus flavus* spores by alveolar macrophages of cortisone treated mice. Science **160**, 79 (1968). — MICHELI, P.H.: Nova plantarum genera juxta tournefortii methodum disposita. Florence, 1729, 234 pp. — MIERES, J.F.: Caso de seudotuberculosis causada por el *Aspergillus fumigatus*. Sem. méd. **1**, 370 (1925). — MITSUI, Y., HANABUSA, J.: Corneal infections after cortisone therapy. Brit. J. Ophthal. **39**, 244(1955).— MONIZ, E., LOFF, R.: Aspergillose cerebrale. Presse méd. **39**, 273 (1931). — MONOD, O., PESLE, G., SÉGRÉTAIN, G.: L'aspergillome bronchectasiant. Presse méd. **59**, 1557—1559 (1951). — MONOD, O., PESLE, G., MEYER, A.: L'aspergillome bronchectasiant. Sem. Hôp. (Paris) 3588—3602 (1957). — MONTES, M.: Pathologic study of a case of primary pulmonary aspergillosis. Amer. Rev. resp. Dis. **87**, 409 (1963). — MONTREUIL, F.: Fungus infection of the antrum. J. Laryng. **69**, 559 (1955). — MOOLTEN, S.E.: A case of primary broncho-pulmonary aspergillosis. J. Mt Sinai Hosp. **5**, 29 (1938—1939). — MOORE, M.: Discussion following paper presented by E.S. BERESTON. Sth. med. J. (Bgham, Ala.) **43**, 492 (1950). — MOORE, M., WEISS, R.S.: Onychomycosis caused by *Aspergillus terreus*. J. invest. Derm. **11**, 215 (1948). — MOSTAFA, M.S., EL-D.: *Aspergillus niger* infection of the eye. Amer. J. Ophthal. **62**, 1204 (1966). — MUNOZ, J., GEISTER, R.: Inhibition of phagocytosis by aureomycin. Proc. Soc. exp. Biol. (N.Y.) **75**, 367 (1950). — MYERS, J.T., DUNN, A.D.: *Aspergillus* infection of the hand. J. Amer. med. Ass. **95**, 794 (1930). — NAJI, A.F.: Bronchopulmonary aspergillosis. Report of two new cases, review of literature, and suggestion for classification. Arch. Path. **68**, 282 (1959). — NASH, C.S.: Fulminating infection of nose due to *Monilia* or *Aspergillus*. Report of a case. Arch. Otolaryng. **28**, 234 (1938). — NAVARRO-BLASCO, A.: Sobre aspergilosis pulmonar. Clin. Lab. **29**, 81 (1936). — NESBITT, B.F., O'KELLY, J., SARGEANT, K., SHERIDAN, A.: Toxic metabolites of *Aspergillus flavus*. Nature (Lond.) **195**, 1062 (1962). — NEWBERNE, P.M.: Carcinogenicity of aflatoxin-contaminated peanut meals. In: G.N. WOGAN (ed.), Mycotoxins in foodstuffs, p. 187. Cambridge, Mass.: M.I.T. Press, 1965. ~ Biological activity of the aflatoxins in domestic and laboratory animals. In: HALVER, J.E., MITCHELL, I.A., (ed.), Trout hepatoma research conference papers, p. 130. Research Report 70. Washington, D.C.: U.S. Government Printing Off. 1967. — NEWBERNE, P.M., CARLTON, W.W., WOGAN, G.N.: Hepatomas in rats and hepatorenal injury in ducklings fed peanut meal or aspergillus flavus extract. Path. vet. (Basel) **1**, 105—132 (1964). ~ Hepatomas in rats and hepatorenal injury in ducklings fed peanut meal or aspergillus flavus extract. (Leberzellcarcinome bei Ratten. Leber- und Nierenparenchymschäden bei Entenküken nach Fütterung mit Erdnußmehl oder Aspergillus flavus-Extrakten.) Path. vet. (Basel) **1**, 105—132 (1964). — NEWMAN, W.H., CORDELL, A.R.: *Aspergillus* endocarditis after open-heart surgery. Report of a case and review of literature. J. thorac. cardiovasc. Surg. **48**, 652 (1964). — NICHOLSON, H.: Infección aspergilar en tuberculosis pulmonar. Tórax **13**, 89 (1964). — NICOD, J.-L., SCHLEGEL, J.: Mycose pulmonaire double à Aspergillus fumigatus Fres. et à Mucor pusillus Lindt. Schweiz. Z. allg. Path. **15**, 307—321 (1952). — NICOLLE, C., PINOY: Sur un cas de mycetome d' origine aspergillaire, observé en Tunisie. Arch. de Parasitologie **10**, 437 (1906). — NOBLE, W.C., CLAYTON, Y.M.: Fungi in the air of hospital wards. J. gen. Microbiol. **32**, 397 (1963). — OEHLERT, W.: Autoradiographische Untersuchung bei der experimentellen Aspergillose der Ratte. (Größe des Eiweiß-Umsatzes verschiedener Zellen untersucht mit S_{35}-markierten Thioaminosäuren.) Acta histochem. (Jena) **6**, 315—332 (1959). — OEHLERT, W., DÜFFEL, F.: Experimentelle Untersuchungen über die Aspergillusinfektion mit Nachweis toxisch wirkender Stoffwechselprodukte des Aspergillus fumigatus. Zbl. allg. Path. path. Anat. **98**, 41—49 (1958). — OETTLÉ, A.G.: The aetiology of primary carcinoma of the liver in Africa. A critical appraisal of previous ideas with an outline of the mycotoxin hypothesis. S. Afr. med. J. **39**, 817 (1965). — OKUDAIRA, M.: Histopathological differentiation between Candida albicans and Aspergillus fumigatus in tissue sections. Acta path. jap. **5**, 117—124 (1955). — OKUDAIRA, M., Schwarz, J.: Tracheobronchopulmonary mycoses caused by opportunistic fungi, with particular reference to aspergillosis. Lab. Invest. **11**, 1053 (1962). — OLK, W.: Bronchogene generalisierte Aspergillose. Zbl. allg. Path. **97**, 361—371 (1958). — OPPE, W.: Zur Kenntniss der Schimmelmykosen beim Menschen. Zbl. allg. Path. **8**, 301 (1897). — ORIE, N.G.M., DE VRIES, G.A., KIKSTRA, A.: Growth of *Aspergillus* in the human lung: Aspergilloma and aspergillosis. Amer. Rev. resp. Dis. **82**, 649 (1960). — OSLER, W.: *Aspergillus* from the lung. Trans. path. Soc. Philad. **13**, 108 (1887). — OTA, M.: Sur une nouvelle espèce d'*Aspergillus* pathogène: *Aspergillus jeanselmei*. Ann. Parasit. hum. comp. **1**, 137 (1923). — PALDROK, H., HOLLSTROM,

E.: Onychomycosis due to *Aspergillus terreus* Thom. Acta Dermat. Venereol. **32**, 255 (1952). — Paradis, A.J., Roberts, L.: Endogenous ocular aspergillosis. Report of a case in an infant with cytomegalic inclusion disease. Arch. Ophthal. **69**, 765 (1963). — Patterson, R.: Hypersensitivity disease of the lung. Univ. Mich. med. Cent. J. **34**, 8 (1968). — Pecora, D.V., Toll, M.W.: Pulmonary resection for localized aspergillosis. New Engl. J. Med. **263**, 785 (1960). — Peer, E.T.: Case of aspergillosis treated with amphothericin "B". Dis. Chest **38**, 222 (1960). — Peet, M.M.: *Aspergillus fumigatus* infection of the cerebellum. Trans. Amer. neurol. Ass. **71**, 165 (1946). (Case also reported by Cawley, 1947). — Peña, C. E., Salazar, H.: Aspergilosis en Colombia. Estudio clinico-patológico de 15 casos. Mycopathologia (Den Haag) **34**, 65 (1968). — Pepys, J.: Possible role of precipitins against *Aspergillus fumigatus*. Amer. Rev. resp. Dis. **90**, 465 (1964). ∼ Pulmonary hypersensitivity disease due to inhaled organic antigens. Postgrad. med. J. **42**, 698 (1966a). ∼ Immunological aspects of respiratory disease. J. Laryng. **80**, 373 (1966b). ∼ Pulmonary hypersensitivity disease due to inhaled organic antigens. Ann. intern. Med. **64**, 943 (1966c). — Pepys, J., Jenkins, P.A.: Precipitin (F.L.H.) test in farmer's lung. Thorax **20**, 21 (1965). — Pepys, J., Longbottom, J.L., Jenkins, P.A.: Vegetable dust pneumoconioses. Immunologic responses to vegetable dusts and their flora. Amer. Rev. resp. Dis. **89**, 842 (1964). — Pepys, J., Ridell, R.W., Citron, K.M., Clayton, Y.M.: Precipitins against extracts of hay and moulds in the serum of patients with farmer's lung, aspergillosis, asthma, and sarcoidosis. Thorax **17**, 366 (1962). — Pesle, G.D., Monod, O.: Bronchiectasis due to aspergilloma. Dis. Chest **25**, 172 (1954). — Phelps, R.A.: Aflatoxins in feeds. A review. In: Halver, J.E., Mitchell, I.A. (ed.), Trout hepatoma research conference papers, p. 145. Research report 70. Washington, D.C.: U.S. Government Printing Off. 1967. — Pimentel, J.C.: Pulmonary calcification in the tumor-like form of pulmonary aspergillosis: pulmonary aspergilloma. Amer. Rev. resp. Dis. **94**, 208 (1966). — Pinoy, E.: Actynomycoses et mycetomes. Bull. Inst. Pasteur **11**, 929 and 977 (1913). — Pittenger, B.N.: Case reports of aspergillosis. Kentucky med. J. **36**, 161 (1938). — Plihal, V., Jedlickova, Z., Vickliky, J., Tomanek, A.: Multiple bilateral pulmonary aspergillomata. Thorax (Lond.) **19**, 104—111 (1964). — Ponce, G. de O.: Forma broncho-pneumonica da aspergillose pulmonar pura e primitiva? Rev. bras. Med. Pharm. **11**, 72 (1935). — Pons, E.R., Belaval, M.E.: A one-year aeroallergen survey of Puerto Rico. J. Allergy **32**, 195 (1961). — Porta, E.A.: Endocarditis micótica por *Aspergillus* en un caso de estenosis subaórtica. Rev. Hosp. Niños (B. Aires) **1**, 37 (1959). — Powell, D.E.B., English, M.D.: Clinical bacteriological and mycological findings in post-operative ear cavities. J. Laryng. **76**, 12 (1962). — Procknow, J.J.: Treatment of opportunistic fungus infections. Lab. Invest. **11**, 1217 (1962). — Procknow, J.J., Loewen, D.F.: Pulmonary aspergillosis with cavitation secondary to histoplasmosis. Amer. Rev. resp. Dis. **82**, 101 (1960). — Puestow, K.L.: A contribution to the study of maduromycosis, with report of a case of infection with *Aspergillus nidulans*. Arch. Derm. Syph. (Chic.) **20**, 642 (1929). — Ramirez, J.: Pulmonary aspergilloma. Endobronchial treatment. New Engl. J. Med. **271**, 1281 (1964). — Ramsey, B.H.: The upper lobe lesion — old or new, with reference to a case of aspergillosis (mycetoma). Dis. Chest **38**, 625 (1960). — Randall, R.: Aspergillosis. Vet. Bull. (Washington) **16**, 103 (1925). — Rankin, N.E.: Disseminated aspergillosis and moniliasis associated with agranulocytosis and antibiotic therapy. Brit. med. J. **4816**, 918—919 (1953). — Raper, K.B., Fennell, D.I.: The genus *Aspergillus*, 686 pp. Baltimore: Williams & Wilkins Co. 1965. — Rau, E.M., Tilden, E.B., Koenig, V.L.: Partial purification and characterization of the endotoxin from *Aspergillus fumigatus*. Mycopathologia (Den Haag) **14**, 346 (1961). — Rayer, Montagne: Mycose aspergillaire dans les poches aeriennes d'un bouvreuil. J. Inst. (Paris) In-4, 270 (1842). (Quoted by Robin, C., 1853). — Rebouças, J.: Aspergilose niger do conduto. Rev. bras. Oto-rino-laring. **7**, 169 (1939). — Redmond, A., Carre, I.J., Biggart, J.D., Mackenzie, D.W.R.: Aspergillosis (*Aspergillus nidulans*) involving bone. J. Path. Bact. **89**, 391 (1965). — Reed, J.A.: Aspergillosis and moniliosis. Sth. med. J. (Bgham., Ala.) **28**, 729 (1935). — Rénon, L.: Recherches cliniques et experimentales sur la pseudo-tuberculose aspergillaire. Thèse de Paris, 1893. ∼ Deux cas familiaux de tuberculose aspergillaire simple chez des peigneurs de cheveux. C. R. Soc. Biol. (Paris) **47**, 694 (1895). ∼ Etude sur l' Aspergillose chez les animaux et chez l' homme, 301 pp. Paris: Masson et Cie. 1897. — Rifkind, D., Marchioro, T.L., Schneck, S.A., Hill, R.B.: Systemic fungal infections complicating renal transplantation and immunosuppressive therapy. Clinical, microbiologic, neurologic and pathologic features. Amer. J. Med. **43**, 28 (1967). — Riley, E.A., Tennenbaum, J.: Pulmonary aspergilloma or intracavitary fungus ball. Report of five cases. Ann. intern. Med. **56**, 896 (1962). — Robin, C.: Histoire naturelle des vegetaux parasites qui croissent sur l'homme et sur les animaux vivants, 702 pp. Paris: Baillière 1853. — Robinson, C.L.N., McPherson, A.R.: Bronchopulmonary aspergilloma. Canad. J. Surg. **5**, 411 (1962). — Robinson, G.H., Grauer, R.C.: Use of autogenous fungus extracts in treatment of mycotic infections. Arch. Derm. Syph. (Chic.) **32**, 787 (1935). — Rodin, A.E., Hnatko, S.I.: Non-reactive tuberculosis. Canad. med. Ass. J. **89**, 817 (1963). — Rodricks, J.V., Henery-

LOGAN, K.R., CAMPBELL, A.D., STOLOFF, L., VERRETT, M.J.: Isolation of a new toxin from cultures of *Aspergillus flavus*. Nature (Lond.) **217**, 668 (1968). — RODRÍGUEZ-VILLEGAS, R., SCHENA, A.T.: Micosis pulmonar en una cavidad residual hidatídica. Sem. méd. **2**, 93 (1941). — ROMINGER, L., BÖHM, F.: Über einen Fall von generalisierender pyämischer Aspergillose. Beitr. Klin. Tuberk. **113**, 221—233 (1955). — ROSENVOLD, L.K.: Dacryocystitis and ble-pharitis due to infection by *Aspergillus niger:* report of cases. Amer. J. Ophthal. **25**, 588 (1942). — ROSS, C.F.: A case of pulmonary aspergillosis. J. Path. Bact. **63**, 409 (1951). — RUBINSTEIN, P.: Micosis broncopulmonares consecutivas al tratamiento antibiótico o corti-coide. Rev. Asoc. méd. argent. **77**, 53 (1963). — RUEDA, G., MEJÍA, A.: Micetoma pulmonar. (Revisión de literatura, presentación de un caso.) Trib. méd. (Bogotá) **1**, 1 (1962). — SALFELDER, K., CAPRETTI, C., HARTUNG, M., MONCADA-REYES, F.: Dos casos poco comunes de aspergilosis pulmonar y pleural. Mycopathologia (Den Haag) **14**, 78 (1961). — SANCHEZ-FREIJO, C.: La aspergilosis pulmonar primitiva (Un caso de forma aguda). Siglo méd. **95**, 222 (1935). — SANERKIN, N.G., SEAL, R.M.E., LEOPOLD, J.G.: Plastic bronchitis, mucoid impaction of the bronchi and allergic broncho-pulmonary aspergillosis, and their relationship to bronchial asthma. Ann. Allergy **24**, 586 (1966). — SARGEANT, K.A., SHERIDAN, A., O'KELLY, J., CARNAGHAN, R.B.A.: Toxicity associated with certain samples of groundnuts. Nature (Lond.) **192**, 1096 (1961). — SARTORY, A.: Sur un champignon nouveau du genre *Aspergillus* isolé dans un cas d'onychomycose. C. R. Acad. Sci. (Paris) **170**, 523 (1920). — SATHMARY, M.N.: *Bacillus subtilis* septicemia and generalized aspergillosis in a patient with acute myeloblastic leukemia. N.Y. St. J. Med. **58**, 1870 (1958). — SAUBERMANN, G., SCHOLER H.J.: Aspergillose der Hornhaut. I. Kasuistischer und experimenteller Beitrag zur Diagnose und Therapie, p. 1—22. Basel: S. KARGER 1959. — SAUNDERS, A.M., BIEBER, C.: Pathologic findings in a case of cardiac transplantation. J. Amer. med. Ass. **206**, 815 (1968). — SAVAGE, A., ISA, J.M.: A note on mycotic pneumonia in chickens. Sci. Agr. **13**, 341 (1933). — SAVETSKY, L., WALTNER, J.: Aspergillosis of the maxillary antrum. Report of a case and review of the available literature. Arch. Otolaryng. **74**, 695 (1961). — SAYLE, B.A., LANG, P.A., GREEN, W.O., BOSWORTH, W.C., GREGORY, R.: Cushing's syndrome due to islet cell carcinoma of the pancreas. Report of two cases: One with elevated 5-hydroxyindole acetic acid and complicated by aspergillosis. Ann. intern. Med. **63**, 58 (1965). — SCARPELLI, D.G.: Ultrastructural and biochemical observations on trout hepatoma. In: HALVER, J.E., MITCHELL, I.A. (ed.), Trout hepatoma research conference papers, p. 60. Research report 70. Washington, D.C.: U.S. Government Printing Off. 1967. — SCHECHTER, F.R., LEIVY, F.E., NIEDZWIEDZ, A.: Pulmonary aspergillosis complicating therapy for lymphoma with reversible uric acid uremia. J. Einstein Med. Cent. **8**, 153 (1960). — SCHEIDEGGER, S.: Pilzerkrankungen. In: HENKE, F., LUBARSCH, O. (ed.), Handbuch der speziellen pathologischen Anatomie und Histologie, Vol. 13, part 2, section A. Berlin-Göttingen-Heidelberg: Springer 1958. — SCHMIDT, E.L., BANKOLE, R.O.: Detection of *Aspergillus flavus* in soil by immuno-fluorescent staining. Science **136**, 776 (1962). — SCHNEIDER, L.V.: Primary aspergillosis of the lungs. Amer. Rev. Tuberc. **22**, 267 (1930). — SCHNYDER, H.K.: Aspergillose der Schädelbasis. Pract. oto-rhino-laryng. (Basel) **10**, 402—421 (1948). — SCHOLER, H.J., SAUBERMANN, G.: Aspergillose der Hornhaut. II. Diskussion von 90 Fällen der Literatur, p. 23—58. Basel: S. Karger 1959. — SCHUBERT, P.: Zur Casuistik der Aspergillusmykosen. Dtsch. Arch. Klin. Med. **36**, 162 (1885). — SCHU-MACHER, H.R., GINNS, D.A., WARREN, W.J.: Fungus infection complicating leukemia. Amer. J. med. Sci. **247**, 313 (1964). — SCHWARZ, J., BAUM, G.L., STRAUB, M.: Cavitary histoplasmosis complicated by fungus ball. Amer. J. Med. **31**, 692 (1961). — SEABURY, J.H., SAMUELS, M.: The pathogenic spectrum of aspergillosis. Amer. J. clin. Path. **40**, 21 (1963). — SÉGRETAIN, G.: Pulmonary aspergillosis. Lab. Invest. **11**, 1046 (1962). — SÉGRETAIN, G., VIEU, M.: Formes parasitarires des aspergillus dans l'aspergillome bronchique: Diagnostic biologique des aspergilloses broncho-pulmonaires. Sem. Hôp. Paris/Path. Biol./Arch. Biol. méd. **1957**, 421—429. — SHANK, R.C., WOGAN, G.N.: Effects of aflatoxin B$_1$ on some aspects of liver metabolism. Fed. Proc. **23**, 200 (1964). — SHARP, W.B., JOHN, M.B.: Pathogenicity of the *Aspergilli* of otomycosis. Tex. Rep. Biol. Med. **4**, 353 (1946). — SHAW, F.W., WARTHEN, H.J.: Aspergillosis of bone. Sth. med. J. (Bgham, Ala) **29**, 1070 (1936). — SHERMAN, I.C., BOSHES, L.D.: Some fungus infections of the central nervous system: experience with recent treatments. Bol. Asoc. méd. P. Rico **48**, 225 (1956). — SIDRANSKY, H., FRIEDMAN, L.: The effect of cortisone and antibiotic agents on experimental pulmonary aspergillosis. Amer. J. Path. **35**, 169 (1959). — SIDRANSKY, H., PEARL, M.A.: Pulmonary fungus infections associated with steroid and antibiotic therapy. Dis. Chest. **39**, 630 (1961). — SIEBENMANN, F.: Die Schimmelmykosen des menschlichen Ohres, 118 pp. Wiesbaden: J. F. Bergmann 1889. — SILLER, W.G., OSTLER, D.C.: The histopathology of an entero-hepatic syndrome of turkey poults. Vet. Rec. **73**, 134 (1961). — SILVER, M.D., MASON, W.E.H., ROBINSON, C.L.N., BLANK, F.: Pulmonary aspergillosis. Canad. med. Ass. J. **87**, 579 (1962). — SIMMS, R.F.: *Aspergillus* infection as the cause of external ear diseases. Sth. med. J. (Bgham, Ala.) **30**, 1224 (1937). — SIMON, R.C., DOLLAR, A.M., SMUCKLER, E.A.: Descriptive classification on normal and altered histology of trout livers. In: HALVER, J.E., MITCHELL, I.A. (ed.), Trout hepatoma research conference papers, p. 18. Research report 70. Washington, D.C.: U.S. Government Printing Off. 1967. — SINNHUBER, R.O.: Aflatoxin in cottonseed meal and liver cancer in rainbow trout. In: HALVER, J.E., MITCHELL, I.A. (ed.), Trout hepatoma research conference papers, p. 48. Research report 70. Washington, D.C.: U.S. Government Printing Off. 1967. — SKILLERN, R.H.: Aspergillos of the maxillary sinus. Laryngoscope (St. Louis) 31, 946 (1921). — SLUYTER, F.T.: De vegetabilibus organismi animalis parasitis, ac de novo epiphyto in pitryiasi versicolore obvio. Diss. Inaug. Berlin 1847. Quoted by VIRCHOW (1856). — SMITH, A.G., SCHULTZ, R.B.: Observeratsions in the disposition of Aspergillus fumigatus in the respiratory tract. Amer. J. clin. Path. 44, 271 (1965). — SMITH, L.M.: Aspergillus infection of the nails. Urol. cutan. Rev. 38, 783 (1934). — SMITH, R.H., McKERNAN, W.: Hepatotoxic action of chromatographically separated fractions of Aspergillus flavus extracts. Nature (Lond.) 195, 1301 (1962). — SMITH, W.R.: Aspergillosis. J. Tenn. med. Ass. 27, 407 (1934). — SNELLING, M.R.J., McGLADDERY, H.M., PONNAMPALAM, J.T.: Bronchopulmonary aspergillosis. Dis. Chest 44, 100 (1963). — SOCHOCKY, S.: Infection of pneumonectomy space with Aspergillus fumigatus treated by "nystatin". Dis. Chest 36, 554 (1959). — SOERGEL, K.H., COTE, R.A., TAUGHER, P.J.: Felty's syndrome and generalized aspergillosis. Marquette med. Rev. 30, 33 (1964). — SPOTNITZ, M., OVERHOLT, E.L.: Mucoid impaction of the bronchi associated with Aspergillus. Report of a case. Dis. Chest 52, 92 (1967). — STANLEY, P.: Pulmonary aspergillosis occurring in a patient receiving large doses of prednisolone. Tubercle (Edinb.) 46, 227 (1965). — STARK, J.E.: Allergic pulmonary aspergillosis successfully treated with inhalations. of nystatin. Report of a case. Dis. Chest 51, 96 (1967). — STEELE, A.E.: A case of infection with Aspergillus versicolor. Boston med. surg. J. 195, 536 (1926). — STEVENS, K.M.: The effect of antibiotics upon the immune response. J. Immunol. 71, 119 (1953). — STERN, S.G., KULVIN, M.M.: Aspergillosis of the cornea. Amer. J. Ophthal. 33, 111 (1950). — STOLOW, A.J.: Primary broncho-pulmonary aspergillosis. J. med. Soc. N. J. 36, 484 (1939). — STRELLING, M.K., RHANEY, K., SIMMONS, D.A.R., THOMSON, J.: Fatal acute pulmonary aspergillosis in two children of one family. Arch. Dis. Childh. 41, 34 (1966). — STUART, E.A., BLANK, F.: Aspergillosis of the ear. A report of twenty-nine cases. Canad. med. Ass. J. 72, 334 (1955). — SUIE, T., HAVENER, W.H.: Mycology of the eye: a review. Amer. J. Ophthal. 56, 63 (1963). — SWAEBLY, M.A., CHRISTENSEN, C.M.: Molds in house dust, furniture stuffing, and in the air within homes. J. Allergy 23, 370 (1952). — SYMMERS, W. St. C.: Histopathologic aspects of the pathogenesis of some opportunistic fungal infections, as exemplified in the pathology of aspergillosis and phycomycosis. Lab. Invest. 11, 1073 (1962). — TAKANO, J., CUELLO, C., HOFFMANN, E., CORREA, P.: Estudio de lesiones residuales pulmonares. Rev. lat.-amer. Anat. pat. 6, 63 (1962). — TAYLOR, P.A.: Mycotic pneumonia in pigeons. Canad. vet. J. 7, 262 (1966). — TEIXEIRA, L.: Um caso de aspergillose pulmonar. Rev. Flum. de Med. 6, 147 (1941). — THOM, C., CHURCH, M.B.: The Aspergilli, 272 pp. Baltimore: Williams & Wilkins Co. 1926. — THOM, C., RAPER, K.B.: A manual of the Aspergilli, 373 pp. Baltimore: Williams & Wilkins Co. 1945. — TILDEN, E.B., HATTON, E.H., FREEMAN, S., WILLIAMSON, W.M., KOENIG, V.L.: Preparation and properties of the endotoxins of Aspergillus fumigatus and Aspergillus flavus. Mycopathologia (Den Haag) 14, 325 (1961). — TILLEY, H.: Aspergillosis of the maxillary antrum. Proc. roy. Soc. Med. 8, (pt. 2), 14 (1914—1915). — TOBLER, W.W., MINDER, W.: Generalisierte chronische Aspergillose beim Kind und ihre Beziehung zur antibiotischen Therapie. Helv. paediatr. Acta, Ser. C., 9, 209—230 (1954). — TOIGO, A.: Pulmonary aspergillosis. Amer. Rev. resp. Dis. 81, 392 (1960). — TORACK, R.M.: Fungus infections associated with antibiotic and steroid therapy. Amer. J. Med. 22, 872 (1957). — TURHAN, B.: Aspergillosis der Lunge. Istanbul. Üniv. Tip. Fak. Meck. 15, 748—757 (mit engl. Zusammenfassung 1952) (Türkisch). — TVETEN, L.: Cerebral mycosis. A clinic-pathological report of four cases. Acta Neurol. Scand. 41, 19 (1965). — UTZ, J.P.: The spectrum of opportunistic fungus infections. Lab. Invest. 11, 1018 (1962). ∼ Chemotherapeutic agents for the systemic mycoses. New Engl. J. Med. 268, 938 (1963a). ∼ Systemic fungal infections amenable to chemotherapy. D.M. p. 1—52, September 1963b. — UTZ, J.P., ANDRIOLE, V.T., EMMONS, C.W.: Chemotherapeutic activity of X-5079 C in systemic mycoses of man. Amer. Rev. resp. Dis. 84, 514 (1961). — UTZ, J.P., GERMAN, J.L., LOURIA, D.B., EMMONS, C.W., BARTTER, F.C.: Pulmonary aspergillosis with cavitation — Iodide therapy associated with an unusual electrolyte disturbance. New Engl. J. Med. 260, 264 (1959). — VADALA, A.J.: Mycotic infection of the bronchopulmonary tract. Ann. Otol. (St. Louis) 49, 291 (1940). — VAITHIANATHAN, T., BOLONIK, S.J., GRUHN, J.G.: Leukemic reticuloendotheliosis. Amer. J. clin. Path. 38, 605 (1962). — VALLERY-RADOT, P., HALPERN, B.N., SÉGRETAIN, A., DOMART, A.: Etude de la nature et de la densité de la flore mycologique dans l'atmosphere de Paris durant l'année 1948. Acta allerg. (Kbh.) 3, 179 (1950). — VAN DER ZIJDEN, A.S.M., KOELENSMID, W.A.A.B., BOLDINGH, J., BARRETT, C.B., ORD, W.O., PHILIP, J.: Aspergillus flavus and turkey X disease. Nature (Lond.) 195, 1060 (1962). — VAN ORDSTRAND, H.S.: Pulmonary aspergillosis. Report of a case. Cleveland Clin. Quart. 7, 66 (1940). — VANTRAPPEN, G., SIMONS, C., VAN

DE WOESTIJNE, K.P., GYSELEN, A.: Intracavitary and intrabronchial fungus masses. Dis. Chest **35**, 528 (1959). — VEDDER, J.S., SCHORN, W.F.: Pulmonary aspergillosis with metastatic skin nodules. J. Amer. med. Ass. **209**, 1191 (1969). — VELLIOS, F., CRAWFORD, A.S., GATZIMOS, C.D., HAYNES, E.: Bronchial aspergillosis occurring as intracavitary "fungus ball". Amer. J. clin. Path. **27**, 68 (1957). — VILLAR, T.G.: The diagnosis of pulmonary aspergilloma. Geriatrics **18**, 883 (1963). — VILLAR, T.G., CORTEZ-PIMENTEL, J., COSTA, M.F.E.: The tumour-like forms of aspergillosis of the lung (pulmonary aspergilloma). A report of 5 new cases and a review of the Portuguese literature. Thorax **17**, 22 (1962). — VIRCHOW, R.: Beiträge zur Lehre von den beim Menschen Vorkommenden pflanzlichen Parasiten. Virchows Arch. path. Anat. **9**, 557 (1856), — WAHL, E.F.: Pneumomycosis. Trans. Amer. ther. Soc. **35**, 36 (1936). — WAHL, E.F., ERICKSON, M.J.: Primary pulmonary aspergillosis. J.M.A. Georgia **17**, 341 (1928). — WAHNER, H.W., HEPPER, N.G.G., ANDERSEN, H.A., WEED, L.A.: Pulmonary aspergillosis. Ann. intern. Med. **58**, 472 (1963). — WALES, J.H.: Degeneration and regeneration of liver parenchyma accompanying hepatomagenesis. In: HALVER, J.E., MITCHELL, I.A. (ed.), Trout hepatoma research conference papers, p. 56. Research report 70. Washington, D.C.: U.S. Government Printing Off. 1967. — WÄTJEN, J.: Zur Kenntnis der Gewebsreaktionen bei Schimmelmykosen. Virchows Arch. path. Anat. **268**, 665 (1928). (with complete reference of the older European Lit.). ~ Durch Schimmel- und Sproßpilze bedingte Erkrankungen der Lungen. In: HENKE, F., LUBARSCH, O. (ed.), Handbuch der speziellen pathologischen Anatomie und Histologie, vol. 3, part 3. Berlin: Springer 1931. — WEENS, H.S., THOMPSON, E.A.: The pulmonary air meniscus. Radiology **54**, 700 (1950). — WEINER, A.: Occupational bronchial asthma in a baker due to *Aspergillus*. A case report. Ann. Allergy **18**, 1004 (1960). — WEINSTEIN, L., LEWIS, R.M.: A case of fungus infection of the vagina. Yale J. Biol. Med. **11**, 85 (1938—1939). — WELLER, W.A., JOSEPH, D.J., HORA, J.F.: Deep mycotic involvement of the right maxillary and ethmoid sinuses, the orbit and adjacent structures. Laryngoscope (St. Louis) **70**, 999 (1960). — WELSH, R.A., BUCHNESS, J.M.: *Aspergillus* endocarditis, myocarditis and lung abscesses. Report of a case. Amer. J. clin. Path. **25**, 782 (1955). — WELSH, R.A., McCLINTON, L.T.: Aspergillosis of lungs and duodenum with fatal intestinal hemorrhage. Arch. Path. **57**, 379 (1954). — WERCH, S.C., OESTER, Y.T., FRIEDEMANN, T.E.: Kojic acid — a convulsant. Science **126**, 450 (1957). — WHALEN, E.J.: Fungous infections of the external ear. J. Amer. med. Ass. **111**, 502 (1938). — WHEATON, S.W.: Case primarily of tubercle, in which a fungus (*Aspergillus*) grew in the bronchi and lung, simulating actinomycosis. Trans. path. Soc. Lond. **41**, 34 (1890). — WHITAKER, L.W., JACKSON, B.F.: Buccal infection with *Aspergillus niger*. Med. Bull. Veterans' Adm. (Wash.) **10**, 162 (1933). — WILHITE, J.L., COLE, F.H.: Invasion of pulmonary cavities by *Nocardia asteroides*. Amer. Surg. **32**, 107 (1966). — WILSON, B.J.: Toxins other than aflatoxins produced by *Aspergillus flavus*. Bact. Rev. **30**, 478 (1966). — WILSON, B.J., WILSON, C.H.: Toxin from *Aspergillus flavus*: Production on food materials of a substance causing tremors in mice. Science **144**, 177 (1964). — WILSON, J.A.S., MUNRO, D.D.: Surgical treatment of mycotic infections of the lung. Canad. med. Ass. J. **97**, 166 (1967). — WITTER, J.F., CHUTE, H.L.: Aspergillosis in turkeys. J. Amer. vet. med. Ass. **121**, 387 (1952). — WOGAN, G.N.: Chemical nature and biological effects of the aflatoxins. Bact. Rev. **30**, 460 (1966). ~ Isolation, identification, and some biological effects of aflatoxins. In: HALVER, J.E., MITCHELL, I.A. (ed.), Trout hepatoma research conference papers, P. 121. Research report 70. Washington, D.C.: U.S. Government Printing Off. 1967. — WOGAN, G.N., FRIEDMAN, M.A.: Effects of aflatoxin B_1 on tryptophan pyrrolase induction in rat liver. Fed. Proc. **24**, 627 (1965). — WOGAN, G.N., NEWBERNE. P.M.: Characteristics of the bile duct hyperplastic response to aflatoxin in ducklings. Fed. Proc. **23**, 200 (1964). — WOLF, F.T.: Relation of various fungi to otomycosis. Arch. Otolaryng. **46**, 361 (1947). — WOLF, H., JACKSON, E.W.: Hepatomas in rainbow trout: Descriptive and experimental epidemiology. Science **142**, 676 (1963). — WREDEN, R.: Recherches sur deux nouvelles especes de vegetaux parasites (*Aspergillus flavescens* et *Aspergillus nigricans*) de l'home. C. R. Acad. Sci. (Paris) **65**, 368 (1867). — WRIGHT, M.L., ANDERSON, G.W., McCONACHIE, J.D.: Transmission of aspergillosis during incubation. Poultry Sci. **40**, 727 (1961). — WRIGHT, R.E.: Two cases of granuloma invading the orbit due to an *Aspergillus*. Brit. J. Ophthal. **11**, 545 (1927). — WYBEL, E.R.: Mycosis of cervical spinal cord following intrathecal penicillin therapy. Report of a case simulating cord tumor. Arch. Path. **53**, 167 (1952). — YESNER, R., HURWITZ, A.: A report of a case of localized broncho-pulmonary aspergillosis successfully treated by surgery. J. thorac. Surg. **20**, 310 (1950). — YOUNG, F.H.: Two cases of neoplasms of the mediastinum with unusual complications. Lancet **210**, 1196 (1926). — ZIMMERMAN, L. E.: *Candida* and *Aspergillus* endocarditis. With comments on the role of antibiotics in dissemination of fungus disease. Arch. Path. **50**, 591 (1950). ~ Fatal fungus infections complicating other diseases. Amer. J. clin. Path. **25**, 46 (1955). ~ Mycotic keratitis. Lab. Invest. **11**, 1151 (1962). — ZISKIND, J., PIZZOLATO, P., BUFF, E.E.: Aspergillosis of the brain: Report of a case. Amer. J. clin. Path. **29**, 554 (1958).

Mucormycosis

(Opportunistic Phycomycosis)

Roger D. Baker, New Brunswick/New Jersey, USA

With 43 Figures

Definition

Mucormycosis is an acute, frequently fatal, fungus disease characterized by the occurrence of broad, non-septate (coenocytic) hyphae in tissues which tend to grow into arteries and produce thrombosis and infarction. The infection nearly always develops in a person whose resistance is lowered by a metabolic disorder, a blood dyscrasia, corticosteroid therapy, or malnutrition. Mucormycosis complicates diabetic acidosis and leukemia.

Mucormycosis assumes cranial, pulmonary, gastrointestinal, disseminated, cutaneous and focal forms.

In the *cranial form* the fungus enters the nose and spreads rapidly, producing vascular thrombosis and infarcts of the nasal mucous membrane, the hard palate, the orbit, the tissues of the face, and the brain and meninges. In the *pulmonary form* the fungus proliferates in the main bronchi and then enters the hilar tissues and pulmonary arteries to produce infarcts of the lung. In *gastrointestinal mucormycosis* the fungus enters from the lumen and causes gangrene (infarction) of portions of the digestive tract. In *disseminated mucormycosis* the infection spreads from the lungs or head and causes lesions in many organs. Usually in *primary cutaneous mucormycosis* an ulcer develops on the leg of a diabetic patient. In *focal mucormycosis*, a single lesion occurs, as, for example, mucormycosis of the kidney.

The organism most frequently causing mucormycosis is a species of the genus *Rhizopus* (Fig. 1). This organism is ubiquitous in nature and a saprophyte, growing on bread and fruit and causing spoilage (Fig. 2). As it grows in nature or on culture it produces stolons (runners), rhizoids (stick-tights), sporangiaphores (bearers of sporangia), and sporangia (sacs full of red-blood-cell-sized spores). Species of the genera *Mucor* and *Absidia* have also been reported as causal agents of mucormycosis. *Rhizopus, Mucor* and *Absidia*, belonging to the family Mucoraceae of the order Mucorales, cause mucormycosis. Because of the component Mucor- in these designations of family and order, the term mucormycosis is appropriate, and should be retained. However, the order Mucorales belongs to the class Phycomycetes characterized by non-septate hyphae, and mucormycosis might be termed opportunistic phycomycosis to indicate that it is a phycomycosis usually found in a person of lowered bodily resistance. The unmodified name phycomycosis includes not only mucormycosis but also two other phycomycosis, subcutaneous phycomycosis and rhinoentomophthoromycosis which are found in persons without predisposing diseases, in Indonesia, Africa and Latin-America (see Chapter by Clark and Edington 15).

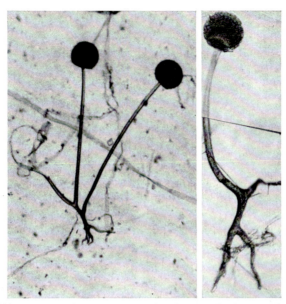

Fig. 1. To left, *Rhizopus oryzae* in a wet preparation, unstained, photographed at 200×. Note the stolon and rhizoids below, the sporangiophores and the sporangia. To right, at 300×, the columella is clearly visible and the spores can just be seen. The rhizoids show clearly. (From BAKER, 1957a)

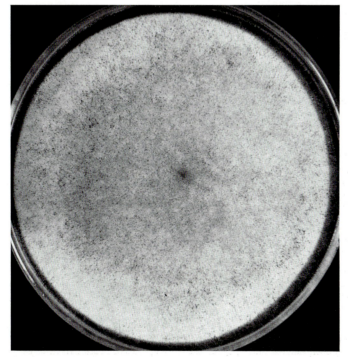

Fig. 2. Culture of *Rhizopus oryzae* two days after inoculation of Sabouraud's glucose agar. The white cottony growth is developing a brownish tinge due to the pigment in the sporangia and endospores

The History of Mucormycosis

Barthelat published an account of the pathogenic *Mucors* and the mucormycoses of animals and man in 1903, and reviewed the literature and the published cases up to that time. He illustrated his account with line-drawings of the filamentous mycelium without cross-septa in the hyphae and the spores in sporangia or sacs on the ends of stalks or sporangiophores. He pictured the rhizoids of *Rhizopus*.

These organisms did not frequently infect animal or man, Barthelat wrote. Sluyter may have described a *Mucor* in a pulmonary cavity in 1847. In 1855 Küchenmeister described a *Mucor* in a cancer of the lung. His figure shows a sporangium with a non-septate mycelium. There is no indication that the fungus was more than a contaminant. Many of the cases of "mucormycosis" reported before 1900 are dubious because of failure to demonstrate the fungus in tissue sections. The Mucoraceae are ubiquitous saprophytes and frequently contaminate pathologic lesions. Two cases of Cohnheim had been mentioned by some as mucormycosis, but the organisms are more like those of *Aspergillus*, according to Barthelat.

In 1876, Fürbringer published 2 new cases of mucormycosis. In the first the patient died of disseminated cancer and the right lung showed a hemorrhagic infarct with fungus hyphae and a few sporangia.

In the second case there was pulmonary emphysema and chronic gastro-enteritis. At the apex of each lung there was an infarct the size of a nut. Behind the infarct situated in the left apex there was a similar nodule surrounded by an infiltrated and indurated zone which contained mycelium.

In the two cases, the fungus showed the same features, except that in the second the sporangia seemed to be less mature. Fürbringer considered the two fungi as being *Mucor mucedo*, but he added that they looked also like *M. circinelloides*. Lindt thought it was M. *corymbifer*.

I am willing to accept Fürbringer's cases as the earliest reported examples of pulmonary mucormycosis (See Table 3).

In 1885, Paltauf published the case of a 52-year-old man who died after having presented the symptoms of an infectious disease. Histologically Paltauf found fungus filaments in the pus of an abscess of the pharynx and larynx, and in lesions of the brain, lung and intestine. There was no culture but Paltauf thought the fungus was *Mucor corymbifer*.

In 1886 Bostroem demonstrated 2 preparations from the tuberculous lungs of a 30-year-old subject with the simultaneous presence of *Aspergillus* and a *Mucor*. These were probably contaminants.

Obraszow and Petrov, in 1890, reported the case of a girl who died with lesions of actinomycosis. In her right lung there were foci with fungus filaments with the appearance of *Mucor* or *Penicillium*. No cultures of the parasite were made.

Herla in 1895 observed a *Mucor* in a pulmonary cavity in a woman who died with a cancer of the liver.

In 1899 Podack published a treatise on mucormycosis. He reported a case of endothelioma of the right pleural cavity, associated with which there were numerous fungus filaments, sporangia, and sporangiophores in the subpleural pulmonary tissue. These filaments were seen not only in the alveoli but also in the interstitial tissue and in the walls of veins. There were lesions rich in mycelium on the surface of the pleura. Podack called the fungus *Mucor corymbifer*. I have accepted Podack's case as the third example of pulmonary mucormycosis (See table of pulmonary mucormycosis).

In 1901, Lucet and Constantin reported a case observed by Lambry which came from a woman with a pulmonary affliction. In the sputum of the patient these authors found mycelial filaments which were cultured and characterized as a new *Mucor* to which they gave the name *Rhizomucor parasiticus*. Subjected to treatment with arsenic and potassium iodide, as recommended for aspergillosis, the patient improved and, 2 months later, her condition was considered satisfactory. I have not included this case in the table of pulmonary mucormycosis because there were no tissue studies.

In summary, according to Barthelat, if one viewed all the publications relative to mucormycosis in animals and man before 1903, they could be arranged in 4 groups: (1) Those in which a fungus was mentioned and named arbitrarily. The majority were insufficiently described and without scientific value. (2) Those publications concerning tumors from which a fungus had been isolated and considered to be a species of *Mucor*. In these cases the parasite had not been proved to be the cause of the neoplasm. (3) Those reporting mucormycoses of the respiratory tract. The fungus grew on a pre-existing lesion. Nearly all were in autopsies and it was impossible to determine whether the fungus was a saprophyte or a parasite. (4)

The fourth group of publications concerned the cases of primary mycoses (FÜRBRINGER, PALTAUF, LUCET and CONSTANTIN, and PODACK). These cases demonstrated that *Mucors* could play an active infectious role like other living agents of disease.

In his review, BARTHELAT devoted much attention to otomycosis and nasopharyngeal lesions "caused" by *Mucors*. He cited 53 cases of otomycosis of which 2 were attributed to *Mucors*. My own review of these cases suggests that the fungus was growing as a saprophyte in the ear wax and was not causing a lesion.

EMMONS (1964) believes that PALTAUF's (1885) case of generalized mucormycosis should be accepted as the first genuine example of the disease. He refers to earlier cases, but believes that the diagnosis of these was based upon the growth of an organism in culture rather than the demonstration of a fungus in the tissues. *Mucor, Absidia* and *Rhizopus* are common saprophytes which grow rapidly and their spores may contaminate ulcers, collected sputum, exudates and cultures made from clinical specimens.

If Fürbringer's cases of pulmonary mucormycosis (1876) were the first, then in 1969 the disease would be 93 years old. Throughout this time mucormycosis has been recognized as a very rare disease of sporadic occurrence. Though still rare, it is appearing more frequently since 1943.

My attention was first drawn to the disease by an account of 3 fatal cases in diabetic patients, reported in the Johns Hopkins Hospital Bulletin by GREGORY et al., in 1943. It was an amazing story for a fungus disease. The course of the disease was rapid, only two to five days to death, and the lesions of the head and brain were infarcts caused by the growth of the broad, coenocytic (non-septate), hyphae into arteries where they formed thrombi.

The first case of pulmonary mucormycosis in the United States was reported in 1948 by BAKER and SEVERANCE. This was in a white female child, 3 years old, with diabetes, who at postmortem had hemorrhagic lesions in the lungs and infarcts in the spleen and brain, all due to vascular thromboses caused by broad coenocytic hyphae. It appeared that the pulmonary lesions were secondary to a primary cranial mucormycosis.

ZIMMERMAN in 1955 called attention to the manner in which mucormycosis complicates other diseases. MOORE et al. in 1949 published the first well-documented case of mucormycosis of the digestive tract. In 1959 HUTTER published a comprehensive review of mucormycosis and emphasized this mycosis as a complication of the therapy of leukemia.

Mycology

Among the 255 reported cases of mucormycosis the results of cultures were positive in 43 cases (Table 1). *Rhizopus* was reported as having been cultured in 32 instances, *Mucor* in 10, *Absidia* in 2, and a fungus of the Mucorales order in 1. *Rhizopus* predominated in the cranial and gastrointestinal cases, and *Mucor* in the pulmonary cases.

The genera *Rhizopus, Mucor* and *Absidia* belong to the family Mucoraceae, the order Mucorales, the class Phycomycetes (non-septate hyphae), the superclass Eumycetes (true fungi), the subphylum Fungi (absence of chlorophyll) and the phylum Thallophyta (comparatively simple plants) (PROCKOP and SILVA-HUTNER).

The class Phycomycetes contains the orders Mucorales and Entomophthorales. This chapter on mucormycosis deals with infection by the family Mucoraceae of the order Mucorales. The chapter on subcutaneous phycomycosis and rhino-entomophthoromycosis deals with infections of the family Entomophthoraceae of the order Entomophthorales.

The class Phycomycetes is characterized by coenocytic (non-septate) hyphae, and by zygospores.

The genus *Rhizopus* is characterized by sporangiophores which arise singly or in clusters opposite rhizoids and bear spherical sporangia with amber spores between sporangial wall and columella (Fig. 1).

The small size and shape of the rhizoids, sporangia (30 μ—70 μ), sporangiophores (300 μ—600 μ long by 5 μ—12 μ wide), and the small columellae (10 μ—25 μ) and spores (4 μ—8 μ × 3 μ—7 μ), and their ridged markings, identified the species of the fungus derived from the case of cephalic mucormycosis of PROCKOP and SILVA-HUTNER as *Rhizopus arrhizus*. This was confirmed by Dr. H. HESSEL-

Table 1. *Fungi cultured from 43 cases of mucormycosis diagnosed on the basis of characteristic non-septate hyphae in tissues. From 1 gastrointestinal case 3 cultures were obtained*

	Total	Cranial	Pulmonary	G. I.	Disseminated	Cutaneous	Focal
Rhizopus cultures (32)							
Rhizopus oryzae	9	8	1	—	—	—	—
Rhizopus arrhizus	5	4	—	—	1	—	—
Rhizopus nigricans	5	2	—	3	—	—	—
Rhizopus rhizopodiformis . .	1	—	—	—	—	1	—
Rhizopus microsporus . . .	4	—	—	4	—	—	—
Rhizopus	8	8	—	—	—	—	—
Mucor cultures (10)							
Mucor corymbifer(a)	2	—	2	—	—	—	—
Mucor hiemalis	1	—	—	1	—	—	—
Mucor ramosissimus . . .	1	—	—	—	—	1	—
Mucor	6	2	3	—	1	—	—
Absidia cultures (2)							
Absidia lichtheimi	1	1	—	—	—	—	—
Absidia ramosa	1	—	—	—	—	—	1
Non-specified cultures (1)							
Fungus of Mucorales order .	1	1	—	—	—	—	—
Total	45	26	6	8	2	2	1

TINE of the Northern Regional Research Laboratories, Peoria, Illinois, where the culture was entered as No. A-11, 715 in his collection.

Rhizopus grows rapidly and fills the petri dish in 5 days with a dense, cottony aerial mycelium which is at first white, then dark gray (Figs. 2 and 3). *Rhizopus arrhizus* was cultured from the case of HARRIS which is presented in detail later in this chapter. In case 2 of BAUER et al. *Rhizopus oryzae* was cultured and identified as such by Dr. HESSELTINE.

In the case of BAKER et al. (1962) *Rhizopus rhizopodiformis* was the species identification given by Dr. HESSELTINE. In his thesis, Hesseltine cites two instances in which this species was recovered from a mycosis in animals, in one case from a dog and in another from a horse. *R. rhizopodiformis* has very close affinities with the genus *Mucor* and is distinguished from other species of *Rhizopus* chiefly by the branched sporangiophores, the presence of occasional pyriform columellae, and the lack of striations in the walls of the sporangiospores.

It is apparent that the species identification of *Rhizopus* is beyond the scope of the usual hospital or even medical school microbiologist or mycologist.

The species terminology of *Rhizopus* apparently varies according to the expert who makes the identification, for none of the species mentioned above are included in the list of species recovered by NEAME and RAYNER from cases of mucormycosis involving the digestive system. The Commonwealth Mycological Institute of England reported *Rhizopus microsporus* van Tiegh from 3 of their cases. *Rhizopus stolonifer* (Syn. *R. nigricans*) from 2 cases, and *Rhizopus stolonifer*, *Rhizopus microsporus* van Tiegh, and *Mucor hiemalis* Wehm from 1 case.

The genus *Mucor* is also a rapidly growing fungus which fills the petri dish in days with an abundant growth of floccose aerial mycelium which is at first white, then dark gray (CONANT et al., 1954). The non-septate vegetative mycelium of *Mucor* gives rise to numerous unequalled length sporangiophores which branch irregularly and bear terminal globose, spore-filled sporangia. The wall of the

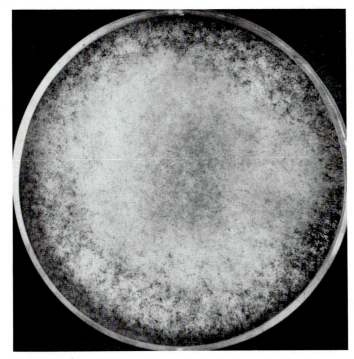

Fig. 3. Culture of *Rhizopus oryzae* 4 days after inoculation of Sabouraud's glucose agar. The aerial mycelium has become browner. *Rhizopus* will grow on to the cover of the Petridish attaching itself by the rhizoids

sporangium is easily broken, scattering the elliptical spores, leaving a fragment of the sporangial wall (collarette) at the base of the spherical columella. This structure is the swollen end of the sporangiophore which extends into the sporangium and is seen only when the sporangial wall ruptures and the mass of spores are dispersed.

The genus *Absidia* has rhizoids which resemble those of *Rhizopus*, but come from the stolons between the sporangiophores, rather than opposite them as is characteristic of *Rhizopus*.

EMMONS et al. give no description of *Mucor* but include a description of *Absidia corymbifera* (Cohn) SACCARDO and TROTTER (1912), and give as the synonymy: *Mucor corymbifer* 1884; *Lichtheimia corymbifera* VUILLEMIN (1903). *A. corymbifer* grows rapidly, they write, covering a Petri dish in a few days. The colony is a coarse, gray, wooly, coenocytic mycelium with numerous upright branched sporangiophores. Sporangia are pearshaped and are borne on aerial hyphae *between* systems of branching root-like hyphae which are called rhizoids. With a lens the rhizoids can be seen attached to the inner wall of a culture tube. The origins of the sporangiophores *between* these rhizoids are more difficult to find.

I wonder, as I record the diagnosis of *Rhizopus*, *Mucor*, and *Absidia* in Tables 2—7, whether the distinctions between the three genera have always been clear to the person who diagnosed the fungus. Certainly it would be easy to diagnose as *Rhizopus* a fungus with rhizoids, without regard to whether these "rootlets" came from an origin opposite the sporangiophores or between them.

In the subsequent reporting of new cases of mucormycosis, I hope that cultures may be obtained more frequently, that the fungus will be fully described in the

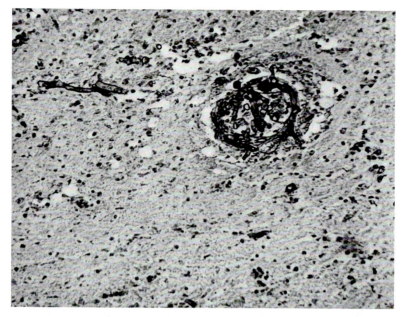

Fig. 4. The coenocytic (non-septate) hyphae of mucormycosis in the brain of one of the cases of GREGORY et al. (1943). Note the growth in the vessel wall and lumen, the right-angle branching and the devitalized (infarcted) cerebral tissue. The hyphae can be confused with capillaries (H & E, × 200)

case report, and that the identification of the fungus will be corroborated by an expert in the field of the Phycomycetes.

EMMONS mentions another problem in connection with the identification of Phycomycetes and in relating them to disease in man and animals. The order Mucorales contains not only the family Mucoraceae (which includes *Rhizopus*, *Mucor* and *Absidia*), but also the families Cunninghamellaceae and Mortierellaceae; and phycomycete diseases in addition to mucormycosis, subcutaneous phycomycosis and rhinoentomophthoromycosis have been described in animals. For man, Emmons mentions that one case of lymphosarcoma reported by HUTTER (1959) had disseminated mycosis and *Cunninghamella elegans* was cultured. *Mortierella* has also been isolated from cutaneous ulcers, according to EMMONS.

Appearance of Mucoraceae in Tissues

The members of the family Mucoraceae are seen in paraffin sections stained with hematoxylin and eosin as broad (6—50 μ) coenocytic (non-septate) hyphae which branch at right angles or nearly at right angles (Fig. 4). *Aspergillus* is easily confused with the Mucoraceae but the hyphae have cross septa, are narrower, and branch at an acute angle. It may grow in colonies in the tissues. *Candida* may be confused with the Mucoraceae, but the filaments are much narrower, are often composed of pseudohyphae, and frequently accompanied by small oval spores.

The Mucoraceae can be distinguished from the Entomophthoraceae (*Basidiobolus meristosporus* and *Entomophthora coronata*) because the latter have eosin-staining hyaline material around the hyphae in tissue.

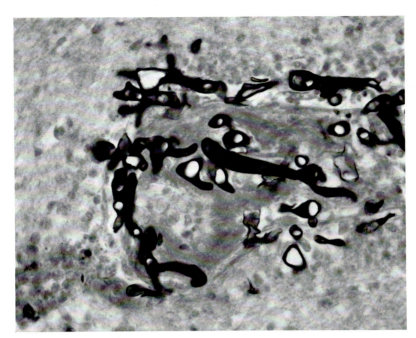

Fig. 5. Hyphae of mucormycosis in and about a thrombosed cerebral blood vessel. Grocott-Gomori methenamine silver stain (G.M.S.), × 500. (From BAKER, 1957a, Fig. 5)

The circumstances of the case also assist in the differential diagnosis. The Mucoraceae are usually found in vessel walls or infarcts within the tissues of a person suffering from a debilitating disease such as diabetes or leukemia. They are found in the internal organs, and cause fatalities. The Entomophthoraceae may be found in an otherwise healthy individual who has a localized subcutaneous lesion or one which involves the air sinuses or bony structure of the face. These infections are usually non-fatal. Infections with the Entomophthoraceae have been observed only in Indonesia, Africa and Latin America, with a few exceptions, whereas the infections with the Mucoraceae have been observed in all parts of the world and where predisposing diseases and conditions exist favoring the invasion of a usually non-pathogenic or opportunistic fungus.

The organisms of mucormycosis are fairly well demonstrated in tissue with hematoxylin and eosin. The Gomori methenamine silver method is much better (BAKER, 1957b). If study with hematoxylin and eosin suggests an organism of mucormycosis, the Gomori methenamine silver stain with a green or blue counterstain should be obtained (Fig. 5). The indigo-carmine-picric acid stain (BAKER, 1956) stains the hyphae of mucormycosis in tissues, but is less valuable than the G. M. S. stain. The periodic acid Schiff and hematoxylin stain (P. A. S. H.) does not color the organisms of mucormycosis well, nor does the Gram stain.

The hyphae of mucormycosis often present an internal structure which is separated slightly from the delicate wall. Rarely the hyphae present swellings or enlargements. The hyphae when cut crosswise may suggest spores to the inexperienced observer.

Usually only hyphae are seen in tissues, but sporangia have been reported in several cases. BAUER et al. found sporangia in an air sinus at postmortem and LA TOUCHE et al. demonstrated sporangia in the mucosa of the left middle tur-

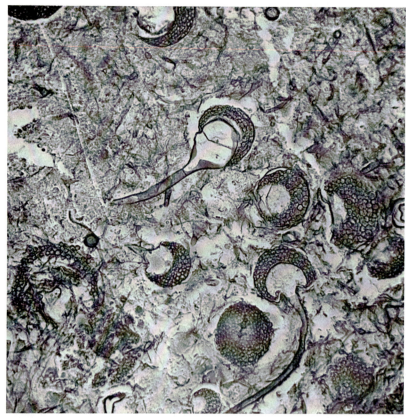

Fig. 6. Phycomycete organism causing mucormycosis in the left middle turbinate of the case of La Touche et al. (1963) (Fig. 2). Note the sporangia, the contained spores, the columellae and the sporangiophores (H & E, × 400)

binate (Fig. 6). Possibly the formation of sporangia is dependent on proximity to a cavity containing air.

The tables show that the disease is world-wide, with a preponderance of cases reported from the United States. Whether the *Rhizopus* organism is more prevalent in the United States or not, I cannot say, for the greater frequency in the United States may be due to better diagnosis, to more reports in medical journals, to more diabetic and treated leukemic patients.

Epidemiology

Mucormycosis is clearly not transmissible from person to person. The organisms live on the ground, in houses, and are abundant on old bread and spoiling fruit. The organisms are saprophytes which must be inspired frequently by normal persons. In the person with a predisposing condition, such as diabetic acidosis or leukemia, the fungus proliferates in the mucosa of the nose, air sinuses or bronchi and spreads locally. *In vitro* studies indicate that the serum from a normal person inhibits the growth of *Rhizopus* (Gale and Welch). In the several cases of secondary infection of cutaneous burns, the burn, for an unknown reason, acted like the abnormally receptive mucosa of the nose or bronchus.

Predisposing Diseases and Conditions

Mucormycosis is usually a secondary or opportunistic mycosis. The normal human organism resists infection with the ubiquitous *Rhizopus, Mucor* and *Absidia*. How the normal body effects this, and what the essence of the change is which permits the fungus to enter, is not understood.

Diabetes is the most frequent antecedent disease in cranial and focal mucormycosis, leukemia in the pulmonary and disseminated forms, and malnutrition in the gastrointestinal form. Diabetes may also predispose to the pulmonary, gastrointestinal and disseminated forms of the disease. Diabetes and blood diseases are the antecedent conditions in most of the reported cases of human mucormycosis. Why was mucormycosis not reported more frequently before 1943, the date of publication of the paper by GREGORY et al. concerning diabetic patients ? Why was the pulmonary and disseminated form not reported more frequently before the papers of BAKER, in 1957, and of HUTTER in 1959, which emphasized diseases of the hematopoetic system, especially leukemia, as antecedent conditions ?

Apparently mucormycosis was not a frequent disease before the publication dates just cited. The organisms in the tissues are readily seen in hematoxylin and eosin sections of postmortem or surgically removed tissues, and competent histopathologists have been active since 1885.

At Johns Hopkins Hospital the autopsy reports of 1902 are on file with protocols by OPIE, WHIPPLE and MCCALLUM. At Duke Hospital the files of autopsy protocols date from 1930 and there was minute review of each case by FORBUS, SPRUNT and BAKER. In Boston, Chicago, Philadelphia, and in medical centers of Europe, particularly in Germany, mucormycosis could not have gone unrecognized at postmortem examination as a complication of diabetes or leukemia.

In the three cases of cranial mucormycosis reported by GREGORY et al. an individual with diabetes mellitus developed diabetic acidosis, then mucormycosis of the face and head, and died with cerebral mucormycosis within two to five days.

In my tabulation of 255 reported cases of mucormycosis I have listed diabetes 46 times and diabetic acidosis 46 times. Therefore diabetes was present in 36% of the cases of mucormycosis. Certainly the well-regulated diabetic is less likely to develop this severe mycosis than the poorly-regulated one. Probably the acidotic complication of diabetes was necessary to permit the infection but had not been recognized in the patients. HUTTER (1959) speaks of steroid diabetes in connection with patients dead of pulmonary mucormycosis who had received corticosteroids in the therapy of leukemia.

It is a curious observation that *blood diseases* are complicated by the pulmonary and disseminated forms of mucormycosis while diabetes mellitus plays a minor role in these forms of the fungus infection. The blood dyscrasias predisposing to mucormycosis were as follows: leukemia, 39; neutropenia, 8; aplastic anemia, 3; lymphosarcoma and Hodgkin's disease, 4; myeloma, 2. The leukemias were acute or chronic, myelogenous or lymphogenous. Corticosteroids were listed as predisposing factors in 30 of these disorders of the hematopoetic system.

In my study of fatal mycoses complicating leukemia (BAKER, 1962), I concluded that neutropenia, drug therapy, hypogammaglobulinemia and splenectomy were probably factors accessory to the leukemia in permitting the development of the mycosis. In leukemia a neutropenia may develop as a phase in the course of the disease or as a result of anti-leukemic drugs, and the mycosis becomes established after the neutropenia has been severe and prolonged (Fig. 7). *Corticosteroid therapy*, as I have demonstrated in normal monkeys, has a powerful spreading factor for *Rhizopus*, and it is probable that leukemia, neutropenia and

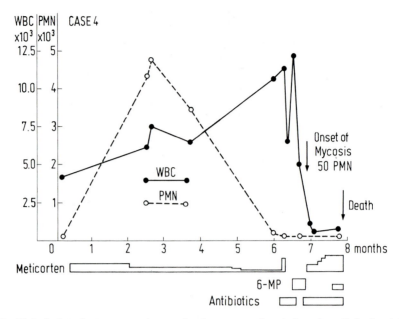

Fig. 7. Clinical plot of mucormycosis complicating a case of acute lymphocytic leukemia. The onset of the mycosis occurred when there was severe neutropenia and after corticosteroids had been administered for a long time

corticosteroid therapy provide an ideal triad of circumstances for the development of complicating mucormycosis (Baker, 1964).

Renal disease or renal insufficiency were mentioned as possible predisposing conditions in 16 cases: glomerulonephritis 3 times, acute renal failure and renal insufficiency 5 times, hydronephrosis with uremia twice; renal cortical necrosis once, the nephrotic syndrome once and uremia alone in 4 cases. Uremia also complicated some of the cases with renal diseases. Renal disease appears to lower resistance by a metabolic change induced by uremia.

Malnutrition in the form of kwarshiorkor was given as a predisposing factor in the development of the gastro-intestinal form of mucormycosis in many of the cases reported from South Africa by Neame and Raynor.

Diarrhea, or diarrhea and vomiting, with acidosis, was thought to have been the forerunner of some of the cranial and gastrointestinal cases of mucormycosis.

Extensive *body burns* preceded the development of disseminated mucormycosis in 4 cases (Baker, 1956; Rabin et al.; Straatsma et al.) and focal mucormycosis, of the hand only, in 1 case (Foley and Shuck). In the cases of Rabin et al. the bones of the face became necrotic where the fungus had proliferated.

Of the miscellaneous preceding or associated conditions mention was made of carcinomas, postoperative status, congenital heart disease, amebiasis, cirrhosis, prematurity, hepatic failure, infectious hepatitis, pancreatitis, septic abortion, and fracture.

In all of the anatomical forms of mucormycosis there were between 5 and 50% of the cases in which no predisposing condition or associated disease appeared to be present. Apparently *Rhizopus* and possibly *Mucor* and *Absidia* can sometimes act as primary pathogens rather than secondary invaders or opportunists.

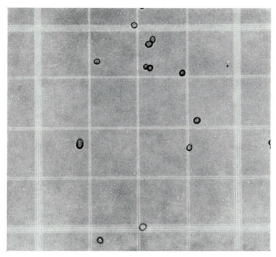

Fig. 8. Endospores of *Rhizopus oryzae* from a ruptured sporangium, in a blood-counting chamber, being enumerated for intravenous animal inoculation. They resemble erythrocytes in size and shape

Experimental Mucormycosis

A large number of reports on experimental mucormycosis have appeared since 1955 (Fig. 8). These have been directed toward the hypothesis that the predisposition to mucormycosis is a metabolic disturbance (BAUER et al., 1956).

Acute alloxan diabetes permitted a fulminating mucormycosis to develop in rabbits (BAUER et al., 1955a, b; ELDER and BAKER, 1956; BAKER et al., 1956). However, chronic alloxan diabetes, like human non-acidotic diabetes, failed to modify host resistance (SCHOFIELD and BAKER, 1956). In acute alloxan diabetes the inflammatory response is by no means paralyzed (SCHAUBLE and BAKER, 1957) though phagocytosis may be diminished (WERTMAN and HENNEY, 1962). The induction of acute alloxan diabetes activated quiescent mucormycotic granulomata in rabbits (SHELDON and BAUER, 1958).

The role of predisposing factors in experimental fungus infections is reviewed by SHELDON and BAUER (1962). Other papers on the subject are by BAUER et al. (1956) and BAUER and SHELDON (1957), BAUER et al. (1957), OSSWALD and SEELIGER (1958), SHELDON and BAUER (1959), and PAPLANUS and SHELDON (1965). But experimental mucormycosis can be produced in the healthy rat (JOSEFIAK and FOUSHEE, 1958).

The most spectacular indication of the spread of *Rhizopus* in the monkey pretreated with the corticosteroid prednisolone was displayed in the form of kidneys swollen by infection and gastric ulcers due to vascular thromboses. This contrasted with the absence of these findings in the monkeys injected with *Rhizopus* intravenously but not pretreated with prednisolone (BAKER et al., unpublished).

To round out the subject of experimental mucormycosis, mention is made here of the preventive and curative effect of Amphotericin B in experimental *Rhizopus oryzae* infection (CHICK et al., 1958a, b).

Cranial Mucormycosis

Cranial mucormycosis begins in the nasal mucosa and extends to the palate, the paranasal sinuses, the orbit, the face and the brain (Table 2). The manifestations of this progression of the disease have been termed the classical central nervous system syndrome of mucormycosis. This was a uniformly fatal condition prior to 1955, as observed in the 3 cases of GREGORY et al., LE COMPTE and MEISSNER, BAKER and SEVERANCE, WOLF and COWEN, STRATEMEIER, KURREIN, MARTIN et al., the 2 cases of BAUER et al., and the case of GUNSON and BOWDEN, 13 cases reported from 1943 to 1955.

Table 2. *Cranial Mucormycosis (107 cases)*

Authors and Case Number	Location of Case Age, Sex, Race	Predisposing Factors	Anatomic Involvement	Cultures	Duration	Treatment	Status of Patient
OPPE (1897)	Dresden/Germany 37, M, W	None	Base of brain	No	?	None	Dead (nodule found at autopsy)
HAFSTROM et al. (1941)	Stockholm/Sweden 69, M, W	None	Brain, left central	No	10 years	Surgical removal	Survived
GREGORY et al. (1943) Case 1	Baltimore/USA 43, F, N	Diabetic coma	Orbit, face, brain, carotid artery, cavernous sinus	No	4 days	For shock and acidosis	Dead, mucormycosis
— Case 2	Baltimore/USA 52, F, N	Diabetic coma. Chronic sinusitis	Nose, ethmoid sinus, eye, brain	No	5 days	For diabetic coma. Enucleation of eye	Dead, mucormycosis
— Case 3	Baltimore/USA 75, M, W	Diabetes	Eye, brain, cervical cord	No	2 days		Dead, mucormycosis
LeCOMPTE and MEISSNER (1947)	Boston/USA 57, M, W	Diabetes Hemochromatosis	Orbit, brain	No	2 days	Insulin	Dead, mucormycosis
BAKER, SEVERANCE (1948) BAKER (1956), Case 4 BAKER (1957), Case 2	San Antonio/USA 3, F, W	Diabetic coma	Left orbit, brain, left internal carotid artery, lung	No	10 days	Insulin	Dead, mucormycosis
WOLF, COWEN (1949) BURNS (1959), Case 1	New York/USA 42, M, N	Diabetes	Left ethmoid, orbit, eye, brain, cavernous sinus	No	10 days	Antibiotics, anticoagulants	Dead, mucormycosis
STRATEMEIER (1950)	Philadelphia/USA 32, F, N	Diabetic coma	Nose, left turbinate, orbit, brain	No	2 days		Dead, mucormycosis
WADSWORTH (1951)	New York/USA 10, M	None	Right bulbus oculi	No	4 years and 8 m.	Enucleation	Well
KURRELN (1954)	Worcester/Engl. 5, M	Glomerulonephritis, pneumonia, diarrhea	Left frontal lobe of brain, meninges	No	14 days	Penicillin	Dead, mucormycosis
MARTIN et al. (1954)	Texas/USA 2.5 mos., M, W	Diarrhea, acidosis	Left orbit, face, brain, internal carotid artery, esophagus, lungs, pancreas, marrow	No	8 days	Antibiotics	Dead, mucormycosis

Reference	Location, age, sex	Underlying disease	Site	Organism	Duration	Treatment	Outcome
Bauer et al. (1955) Case 1	Atlanta/USA 25, F, W	Diabetes	Left orbit, brain	No	5 days	Intravenous fluids, insulin	Dead, mucormycosis
— Case 2	Atlanta/USA 40, M, N	Diabetes	Ethmoid, right orbit, brain, pituitary, carotid artery	*Rhizopus oryzae*	2 days	Insulin, antibiotics	Dead, mucormycosis
Gunson and Bowden (1955)	Toronto, Canada 8, F, W	Chronic glomerulonephr., uremia	Brain, left internal carotid artery, left middle cerebral artery	No	10 days	Not stated	Dead, mucormycosis
Harris (1955) Georgiade et al. (1956), Case 1 Baker (1957), Case 2 Dillon and Sealy (1962), Case 3	Durham/USA 14, F, N	Diabetes	Palate, left paranasal sinuses, left orbit	*Rhizopus arrhizus* 2 mos.		Insulin, iodides, desensitization	Well in 1968
Foushee and Beck (1956)	Winston-S./USA 65, F, W	Cholecystect. Carc. of kidney	Right cheek, brain, meninges	No	4 days	Aureomycin	Dead, mucormycosis
Georgiade et al. (1956), Case 2	Durham/USA 16 mos., M, W	Diabetes	Left side of palate	No	6 mos.	Plastic repair	Living
Keye and Magee (1956), Case 1	St. Louis, Mo./USA Infant	—	Brain, duodenum	—	—	—	Dead, mucormycosis
— Case 2	St. Louis, Mo./USA Infant	—	Brain	—	—	—	Dead, mucormycosis
— Case 3	St. Louis, Mo./USA Adult	—	Brain	—	—	—	Dead, mucormycosis
Clinicopathologic conference (1956)	Sydney/Australia 53, F	Diabetic acidosis	Right eye, brain, lung	No	10 days	Insulin, penicillin, fluids	Dead, mucormycosis
Baker (1957) Case 1	Durham/USA 62, M, W	Cirrhosis	Sphenoid and ethmoid sinuses, left eye, brain, internal carotid artery	No	14 days	Penicillin	Dead, mucormycosis
— Case 3	Durham/USA Adult, M, W	Diabetic acidosis	Left ethmoid, orbit	*Rhizopus*	—	Insulin	Cured
Jackson and Karnauchow (1957)	Ottawa/Canada 20 days, F	Congenital heart disease	Brain, meninges, ileum	No	13 days	Descrysticin, chloramphenicol	Dead, mucormycosis

Table 2. Continuation

Authors and Case Number	Location of Case Age, Sex, Race	Predisposing Factors	Anatomic Involvement	Cultures	Duration	Treatment	Status of Patient
McCall and Strobos (1957)	Winston-S./USA 18, F, W	Diabetes	Left eye, face	*Rhizopus oryzae*	—	Enucleation of left eye	Living, with hemiparesis and aphasia caused by mucormycosis
Merriam and Tedeschi (1957)	Boston/USA 57, M, W	Diabetic acidosis	Orbit, left eye, cavernous sinus	*Rhizopus oryzae*	14 weeks	Insulin, enucleation, antibiotics	Cured
Bryan et al. (1958)	Iowa City/USA 34 months, F	Diabetic acidosis	Right orbit, palate, face, ear, internal carotid artery, brain, intestines, lungs, aorta	No	6 days	Insulin, hydrocortisone	Dead, mucormycosis
Dwyer and Changus (1958)	Norwalk/USA 46, F, W	Diabetic acidosis	Left facial gangrene, nose, palate, sinuses, orbit, brain, cavernous sin.	No	9 days	Insulin, antibiotics	Dead, mucormycosis
Smith et al. (1958)	San Francisco/USA 38, M, W	Diabetes	Right orbit, both internal carotid arteries, cavernous sinuses, sphenoid sinus	No	9 days	Antibiotics	Dead, mucormycosis
Smith and Kirchner (1958) Gabriele (1960), Case 1 Case 2	New Haven/USA 72, M, W	Diabetes	Right facial gangrene, turbinates, sinuses, orbit, internal carotid, brain	No	20 days	Antibiotics	Dead, mucormycosis
Smith and Kirchner (1958) Gabriele (1960), Case 2 Case 2	New Haven/USA 6.5 years	Diabetes	Turbinates, sinuses, left orbit, internal carotid artery, brain, pituitary	No	4 days	Antibiotics	Dead, mucormycosis
Smith and Kirchner (1958) Gabriele (1960), Case 3 Case 3	New Haven/USA 50, F, W	Diabetes	Turbinates, oral cavity, maxillary sinus and bone, right orbit	No	44 days	Antibiotics, mycostatin, Amphotericin B	Dead, mucormycosis
Borland (1959)	Kansas City/USA 7 mos., M, N	Diarrhea, acidosis	Face, ethmoid, right orbit, brain	No	7 days	Hydration	Dead, mucormycosis

Burns (1959) Case 2	New York/USA 60, M, N	Diabetic acidosis	Ethmoid, left orbit, brain	Rhizopus	13 days	Intravenous Amphotericin B	Dead, mucormycosis
Dolman and Herd (1959)	Vancouver/Canada 15, F	Acute pancreatitis, renal cortical necrosis, diabetes	Left face, orbit, cavernous sinus, internal carotid artery, brain, pituitary	No	10 days	Insulin, Levophed, hydrocortisone, antibiotics	Dead, mucormycosis
Faillo et al. (1959)	Fort Benning/USA 50, M, W	Diabetes	Left face, maxillary sinus, orbit	No	2 mos.	Operative	Living
Lie-Kian-Joe et al. (1959)	Indonesia 15, F	Diabetes	Orbit, left nostril, turbinate, brain	No	16 days	—	Dead, mucormycosis
Smith and Yanagasawa (1959) Gabriele (1960), Case 4	New Haven/USA 39, M, N	Diabetes	Right eye and sinus, turbinate, carotid artery, brain	Rhizopus	6 days	Opening of air sinuses	Dead, mucormycosis
Long and Weiss (1959)	Washington/USA 24, F	Diabetes	Left orbit, brain, pituitary, vessels of lung	No	5 days	Insulin, intravenous fluids, Levarterenol	Dead, mucormycosis
Muresan (1960)	Bucharest/R. 18, M	None	"Tumor" of left parietal lobe of brain	No	Many weeks	Surgical removal	Well 2.5 years postoperative
Neame (1960), Case 7	Durban/S. Africa 3 weeks, M	Gastroenteritis	Inferior surface, frontal lobe, brain	No	7 days	—	Dead, mucormycosis
— Case 11	Durban/S. Africa 27, M	Uremia, chron. glomerulonephritis	Inferior surface, frontal lobe, brain	No	2 days	—	Dead, mucormycosis
Banker (1961), Case 2	Boston/USA 3.5 years, M	Nephrotic syndrome	Orbit, sinuses, internal carotid artery, brain	Mucor	1 month	Not stated	Dead, mucormycosis
Berk et al. (1961)	Oakland/USA 49, M	Chronic pancreatitis with diabetes	Left nasal cavity, orbit, sinuses, internal carotid artery, cavernous sinus	Rhizopus	16 days	U-0178	Dead, mucormycosis
Gass (1961) Case 1	Baltimore/USA 44, M	Diabetic acidosis	Nose, sinus, left orbit	No	2 months	Amphotericin B, exenteration of left eye and sinuses	Well
— Case 2	Baltimore/USA 13, M, N	Diabetic acidosis	Nasal tissues, frontal sinuses, orbit, brain	No	—	—	Dead, mucormycosis

Table 2. Continuation

Authors and Case Number	Location of Case Age, Sex, Race	Predisposing Factors	Anatomic Involvement	Cultures	Duration	Treatment	Status of Patient
HOAGLAND et al. (1961), Case 1	Fort Benning/USA 50, M	Diabetes, pancreatitis	Palate, right orbit, antrum, sphenoid	No	1 month	Extirpation of right face	Well
— Case 2	Fort Benning/USA 33, M Amer. Indian	Diabetic acidosis	Left palate, maxillary and ethmoid sinuses	*Rhizopus nigricans*	18 days	Extirpation of left face; Amphotericin B	Well
TURPIN et al. (1961)	Paris/France 13, M	Acute leukemia	Brain	No	10 days	Transfusions	Dead, mucormycosis
WASSERMAN et al. (1961), Case 1	Richmond/USA 59, M, N	Diabetic acidosis	Palate, sinuses, orbits, internal carotid artery, brain (no autopsy)	*Rhizopus*	7 days	Insulin, Amphotericin B	Dead, mucormycosis
— Case 2	Richmond/USA 45, M, N	Diabetic acidosis	Palate, sinuses, left orbit, internal carotid artery, brain	No	4 days	Insulin, fluids, Amphotericin B	Dead, mucormycosis
— Case 3	Richmond/USA 65, F, N	Diabetic acidosis	Nose, palate, sinuses, right orbit	No	42 days	Fluids, insulin, iodides	Living, with defect
BANK et al. (1962)	Israel 60, M	Diabetic acidosis	Right orbit	*Rhizopus arrhizus*	—	Insulin, antibiotics	Survived
EGGENSCHWILER (1962)	Basel/Switzerland 48, M	None	Right antrum with bony involvement, ethmoids	*Absidia lichtheimi*	Chronic	Operation: Caldwell-Luc	Well
LANDAU and NEWCOMER (1962)	Los Angeles/USA 15, F, W	Diabetic acidosis	Palate, left paranasal sinuses, orbit	*Rhizopus arrhizus*	44 days	Amphotericin B	Cured
RINALDI and ASHBY (1962)	Newport News/USA 53, M, N	Diabetes	Face, right orbit, palate (no autopsy)	No	12 days	Insulin	Dead, mucormycosis
STRAATSMA et al. (1962), Case 1	AFIP Accession No. 575574; F	Diabetic acidosis	Classic C.N.S. syndrome	—	—	—	
— Case 2	AFIP Accession No. 580752 21, F, N	Hodgkin's disease	Classic C.N.S. syndrome	—	—	—	

— Case 3 Reeves et al. (1965)	AFIP Accession No. 694863 St. Barbara/USA 30, F, N	Diabetic acidosis, renal insufficiency	Left orbit, face, ethmoids, internal carotid artery, meninges	No	6 days	Antibiotics	Dead, mucormycosis
Straatsma et al. (1962), Case 4	AFIP Accession No. 864638 26, F, N	Diabetic acidosis, renal insufficiency	Classic C.N.S. syndrome	—	—	—	
— Case 5	AFIP Accession No. 989662 39, M, N	Diabetic acidosis, renal insufficiency	Classic C.N.S. syndrome	—	—	—	
— Case 25	AFIP Accession No. 216244 30, M, N	Brain tumor and crainiotomy	Brain	—	—	—	
— Case 26	AFIP Accession No. 532008 25, M, N	None	Nasal cavity	—	—	—	
— Case 27	AFIP Accession No. 542127 47, F, N	Hypertension	Brain	—	—	—	
— Case 28	AFIP Accession No. 682762 55, M, N	Renal insufficiency	Antrum, face	—	—	—	
— Case 30	AFIP Accession No. 734644 38, F, N	Diabetic acidosis	Antrum, orbit	—	—	—	
— Case 32	AFIP Accession No. 909312 65, F, Race ?	Renal insufficiency, disseminated cryptococcosis	Brain	—	—	—	
— Case 33	AFIP Accession No. 982789; 32, M (Amer. Ind.)	Diabetic acidosis	Nose, ethmoid, antrum, orbit	—	—	—	
Suprun (1962)	Tel Aviv/Israel 46, F	Diabetic acidosis	Left orbit, skin of nose, brain	No	2 days	—	Dead, mucormycosis

Table 2. Continuation

Authors and Case Number	Location of Case Age, Sex, Race	Predisposing Factors	Anatomic Involvement	Cultures	Duration	Treatment	Status of Patient
Agrest et al. (1963) Case 1	B. Aires/Argentina 19, F	Abortion, acute renal failure, hyperglycemia	Right orbit, cerebral arteries, brain	No	7 days	Insulin, Levaphed	Dead, mucormycosis
— Case 2	B. Aires/Argentina 59, F	Diabetic acidosis	Brain, middle and anterior cerebral arteries	Rhizopus	5 days	Insulin, dialysis	Dead, mucormycosis
Burrow et al. (1963)	New Haven/USA 47, M	Diabetic acidosis	Turbinate, right face, orbit	Rhizopus nigric.	60 days	Amphotericin B	Cured
Fuentes (1963), Case 1	Mexico City/Mex. 9, M	Diabetic acidosis	Left naris, orbit, brain, lung	No	9 days	Corticoids and antibiotics	Dead, mucormycosis
— Case 2	Mexico City/Mex. 10, M	Diabetes	Right orbit, palate, brain	No	4 days	Insulin, para-metasona	Dead, mucormycosis and candidosis
— Case 3	Mexico City/Mex. 22 months, F	Amebiasis	Left orbit, brain	No	3 days	Antibiotics	Dead, mucormycosis and amebiasis
— Case 4	Mexico City/Mex. 11, F	Infectious diarrhea	Brain and meninges	No	—	Antibiotics	Dead, mucormycosis, and Klebsiella septicemia
La Touche et al. (1963, 1964)	Leeds/England 58, F	Diabetic acidosis	Orbit, palate, left antrum, pons	Rhizopus oryzae	54 days	Amphotericin B	Cured
Suga (1963)	Keio/Japan 38, F	Agranulocytosis	Paranasal sinuses, orbit, bulbus oculi, brain, lungs, endocardium, colon	No	78 days	—	Dead, mucormycosis
Frágner and Rokas (1964)	Czechoslovakia 55, M	Hyperglycemia, pulmonary tuberculosis	Ethmoids, internal carotid artery, pituitary	Rhizopus oryzae	—	—	Dead, mucormycosis

				Mucor			
Lubbe and Pennington (1964)	Melbourne/Austr. 41, F	Renal failure	Nasal cavity, palate, right face, orbit, brain	*Mucor*	11 days	Antibiotics	Dead, mucormycosis
Rowe and Payne (1964)	Sydney/Austr. 48, F	Diabetic acidosis	Right face, palate, ethmoids, orbit	No	7 days	Insulin, antibiotics	Dead, mucormycosis
Taylor et al. (1964)	USA 40, F	Diabetes	Left palate, left maxillary sinus	*Rhizopus*	—	Amphotericin B, regulation of diab.	Well
Weisskopf (1964) Case 1	San Francisco/USA 68, F	Diabetes	Left nostril, turbinates, orbit, face, internal carotid artery	No	14 days	Antibiotics, Amphotericin B	Dead, mucormycosis
— Case 2	San Francisco/USA 45, M	Diabetes	Face, arteries	No	Not stated	Antibiotics, cortisone	Dead, mucormycosis
— Case 3	San Francisco/USA 23, F	Diabetes	Palate, sinuses, left orbit, internal carotid artery, cavernous sinus	No	25 days	Antibiotics, ACTH	Dead, mucormycosis
De Weese et al. (1965), Case 1	Portland/USA 1.5, M	Acidosis from diarrhea	Nares, right orbit, ethmoids	No	3 days	Amphotericin B	Well
— Case 2	Portland/USA 25, F	Diabetes	Nose, right eye, palate	No	3 mos.	Amphotericin B	Well
Gordon and Little (1965), Case 1	Albany/USA 40, M, N	Diabetic acidosis	Nose, left orbit, sinuses, brain (no autopsy)	No	4 mos.	Amphotericin B Surgical explorat.	Dead, mucormycosis
— Case 2	Rochester/USA 44, M, W	Diabetes	Sinus, right orbit, brain, cavernous sinus	*Rhizopus oryzae*	5 days	—	Dead, mucormycosis
Hurtado et al. (1965)	Santiago/Chile 58, F	Diabetic acidosis	Right orbit, face, palate, ethmoids, brain	Fungus of *Mucorales* order	8 days	Insulin, antibiotics	Dead, mucormycosis
Parmentier et al. (1965)	Brussels/Belgium 75, F	Diabetes	Right orbit, ethmoids	No	3.5 weeks	Insulin	Dead, mucormycosis
Peña and Dorado (1965), Case 2	Palmira/Colombia 5 months, M	Diarrhea, acidosis	Orbit, meninges, brain	No	—	Amphotericin B	Dead, mucormycosis
Stehbens (1965) Case 2	Sydney/Australia 35, F	Acute leukemia, cortis.	Branch of right internal carotid artery	No	—	Antibiotics, purinethol	Dead, subarachnoid hemorrhage

54*

Table 2. Continuation

Authors and Case Number	Location of Case Age, Sex, Race	Predisposing Factors	Anatomic Involvement	Cultures	Duration	Treatment	Status of Patient
Sun et al. (1965) Case 11	Peking/China 11, M	Uremia, glo-merulonephr.	Cerebellum	No	—	Antibiotics	Dead, uremia
Tomiyasu and Baker (1965)	Los Angeles/USA 65, M, W	Diabetic acidosis	Right orbit, arteries, brain	No	—	Amphotericin B	Dead, mucormycosis
Ginsberg et al. (1966)	Cincinnati/USA 76, M, W	Diabetic acidosis	Nose, sinuses, orbit, palate, brain	*Rhizopus oryzae*	14 days	Antibiotics	Dead, mucormycosis
Grover et al. (1966)	Nagpur/India 16, M, Hindu	Diabetic acidosis	Nasal mucosa, ethmoids, orbit, internal carotid artery, brain	*Rhizopus oryzae*	18 days	Insulin, penicillin	Dead, mucormycosis
Perez et al. (1966)	Ponce/P. Rico 43, F, W	Diabetes	Orbit, brain	*Rhizopus*	5 days	Amphotericin B	Dead, mucormycosis
Tinaztepe and Tinaztepe (1966)	Ankara/Turkey 4.5, M	Hydro-nephrosis, ure-mia, acidosis	Orbit, brain	No	23 days	Gantrisin	Dead, mucormycosis
Abramson et al. (1967), Case 1	Boston/USA 38, M, N	Diabetes	Right orbit, sphenoid	No	60 days	Amphotericin B	Dead, rup-tured internal carotid artery
— Case 2	Boston/USA 40, F, N	Diabetic acidosis	Palate, right orbit	No	55 days	Amphotericin B	Living
Baum (1967)	New York/USA 53, M, W	Diabetes	Left turbinate, left orbit	—	7 weeks	Amphotericin B	Living
Green et al. (1967)	Philadelphia/USA 45, M, N	Diabetic acidosis	Turbinates, palate, ethmoids, right orbit, brain	No	18 days	Control of diabetes	Dead, mucormycosis
Miyake and Okudaira (1967), Japan; Claim 3 cases							
Pastore (1967)	Richmond/USA 59, M, W	Diabetes	Left maxillary sinus	No	27 days	Surgical removal of mucous membrane	Survived
Prokop and Silva-Hutner (1967)	New York/USA 46, F	Diabetic acidosis	Right antrum, orbit, right carotid, cranial nerves	*Rhizopus arrhizus*	2 mos.	Insulin, anti-biotics, nystatin, Amphotericin B	Survived

The case of HARRIS was the first survival of a patient with all of the features of the classical central nervous system syndrome of mucormycosis, except for a pronounced involvement of the central nervous system itself. That is, there was involvement of the palate, the paranasal sinuses, the orbit and several of the cranial nerves, but the advance of the fungus ceased before it reached the brain and meninges and the patient survived. There were two other cases of survival of patients with cranial mucormycosis before the report of HARRIS (Table 2), but they did not show the syndrome of classical central nervous system mucormycosis. In one, the case of HAFSTROM et al., there was an inactive nodule in the brain of 10 years duration removed surgically and in the other, the case of WADSWORTH, there was an inactive mucormycosis in an enucleated eye.

As the case of HARRIS was the first survival in the classic central nervous system syndrome of mucormycosis, as the patient was thoroughly studied clinically and followed after the cure, and as the case demonstrated the lesions of mucormycosis so well, I am recording the clinical story here, in full detail.

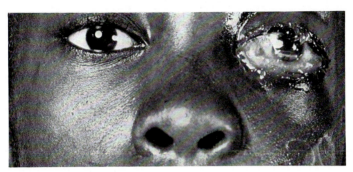

Fig. 9. Cranial mucormycosis. Note the proptosis of the left eye 1 week after admission to hospital of this 14-year-old diabetic patient of HARRIS (1955) (Fig. 1)

Case Report (HARRIS). History: Constance M., a 14-year-old colored girl, was admitted to Duke Hospital, Durham, N.C./USA, January 29, 1954 (Fig. 9). For a month she had noted polyuria, polydypsia, weakness and weight loss. For a week she had had nasopharyngitis, soreness of the roof of her mouth and pain in the left side of her head. She entered another hospital 6 days previously in impending diabetic coma. The blood sugar concentration was 500 mg/100 ml, and the carbon dioxide combining power 24 volumes per cent. Treatment of diabetic acidosis and diabetes was begun. The next day the left eye become injected, proptosed and fixed. Her temperature rose to 103° F and her leukocyte count to 18,000. Penicillin and dihydrostreptomycin were prescribed. She developed paralysis of the left side of the face, weakness of the left side of the soft palate, weakness on swallowing and drooling from the left side of her mouth.

Physical Findings: There was fever (39.2° C). The left side of the face was swollen. The left eye was proptosed and there was a complete internal and external ophthalmoplegia on that side. The conjunctivae on the left were edematous and injected. Corneal clouding and ulceration were present and there was some greenish-yellow purulent exudate. The left fundus showed severe venous congestion. The left ear canal was macerated and contained white cheesy-looking material. The left ear drum was white and thickened, and the landmarks were obscured. The nasal turbinates on the left were swollen. The breath was foul.

At the junction of the soft and hard palate on the left side, there was an ulceration 3 by 3 cm which was partly covered by a brownish-yellow cheesy material (Fig. 10). In the center of the ulcer there was a perforation (1 by 1 cm) of the palate which revealed the nasal cavity. The bare pterygoid plate on the lateral side of the nasal cavity could be seen through the perforation. The entire area was covered with a whitish cheesy necrotic material and a serosanguinous exudate oozed from the perforation. On the left lateral aspect of the tongue there was a firm, white mass (0.5 by 0.5 cm). The neck resisted passive movement and was painful, particularly on flexion.

There was almost complete blindness on the left. The left third, fourth and sixth nerves were completely paralyzed, the left pupil was moderately dilated and fixed. There was complete anesthesia of the maxillary division of the left fifth nerve and partial anesthesia of its orbital division with absent corneal sensation. There was weakness of the left side of the face but this might have been more apparent than real because of the swelling. The left side of the tongue showed diffuse atrophy. The tongue deviated to the left on protrusion and the palate deviated to the right on gagging. The lower jaw deviated to the left on opening the mouth and there was weakness of the muscles of mastication on the left, and of the left sternocleidomastoid and trapezoid muscles.

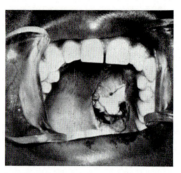

Fig. 10. Cranial mucormycosis. Note the large perforation of the left side of the palate. Patient of Harris (1955) (Fig. 1)

Laboratory Findings: The hemoglobin was 12 g. The total white count and the proportion of neutrophils were increased during the first 4 days. On admission the urine showed ketone bodies, a trace of protein, 3 plus sugar, 12—15 leucocytes, and rare erythrocytes. The fasting blood sugar was 225 mg/100 ml; the carbon dioxide combining power, 66 vol.-%; the serum chloride, 95 m Eq./l; serum sodium, 143 m Eq./l; and serum potassium, 4.4 m Eq./l. The total protein was 7.4 g/100 ml with A/G ratio of 1.0. Intradermal tuberculin skin test was negative in 1:1000 dilution. The histoplasmin, Frei and coccidioidin skin tests were negative but that for blastomycosis showed a slight transient erythema. There was a mildly positive reaction to intradermal Rhizopus vaccine in 1:1000 dilution and a very intense, 3 plus, indurated reaction to the 1:100 dilution.

A biopsy from the ulcer of the palate on February third showed necrotic fatty areolar tissue without nuclear staining but with maintenance of tissue structure.

Broad, branching, non-septate hyphae, 4—14 μ in thickness and up to 180 μ in length, occurred in the walls and lumina of blood vessels and lymphatics, and in nerves and other tissues. The hyphae were those of the coenocytic phycomycetes. No bacteria were stainable deep in the tissue though gram-positive cocci, gram-positive and gram-negative bacilli and a yeast suggestive of *Candida* were adherent to the surface. A biopsy on February eighth showed healthy granulation tissue free of organisms, but with broad branching hyphae in the pus on the surface.

Cultures of these biopsied lesions showed *Rhizopus arrhizus*. Cultures for acid-fast organisms were negative. On March 11, the nasal mucosa was biopsied. One fragment showed lymphoid tissue covered on all sides by stratified squamous epithelium. The other was a fragment of skeletal muscle heavily infiltrated by acute inflammatory cells but without fungi. On March 18, *Rhizopus arrhizus* was again cultured from the palatal lesion.

Electroencephalographic findings were interpreted as suggestive of a fronto-temporal dysfunction.

Roentgenograms of the chest on January 29 showed an area of increased density in the left lower lung field associated with shift of the heart to the left and elevation of the left diaphragm, indicating atelectasis of segments of the left lower lobe.

Roentgenograms of the skull, sinuses and orbits showed cloudiness of all sinuses on the left side but no evidence of bone destruction (Fig. 11). On February 6 the lungs were normal. On February 20 the sinuses on the left side still appeared clouded without bone destruction. On March 25 the left antrum, ethmoid and frontal sinuses were still markedly clouded. Similar dense clouding of the left sinuses and thickening of the membrane on the left side of the sphenoidal sinus were noted on April 14. On April 22 haziness but no definite bone destruction was found in the left mastoid cells.

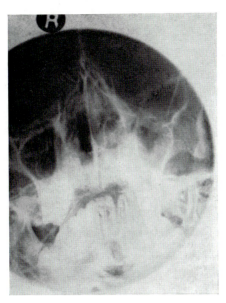

Fig. 11. Cranial mucormycosis. Note the cloudiness of the sinuses on the left. Patient of HARRIS (1955), shown in Figs. 9 and 10. Photograph of X-ray from BAKER (1957a)

Course: The admission diagnosis was diabetes complicated by either tumor or infection causing bronchopneumonia and extensive involvement of the left side of the head and face. The child was thought to have left pansinusitis, cavernous and left lateral sinus thrombosis with extension to the jugular vein and inflammation around the hypoglossal foramen. The diagnosis of mucormycosis was suggested shortly after admission and was verified by biopsy and culture.

Therapy was directed toward rigid control of the diabetes, elimination of secondary bacterial contamination, symptomatic relief and the possibility of specific action against the invading fungus.

The diabetes was controlled with diet and insulin. Therapy against the fungus consisted of iodides and desensitization. After March 16, the patient was afebrile save for 2 spikes to 39°C on March 28 and April 4. A very marked improvement in general condition occurred during the first week probably due to the control of the diabetes and bacterial infection. She was ambulatory after 10 days and showed slow, steady improvement during the remainder of her hospital stay. There were occasional and fairly severe headaches referred to the left ear with lancinating pains deep in the left ear.

Shortly after admission, loss of vision in the left eye progressed to complete blindness. The conjunctivitis and corneal ulceration responded rapidly to hot saline compresses and medication with chlortetracycline eye drops and ointment. A left tarsorrhaphy was done on February 13 because of the child's proptosis, corneal anesthesia and inability to close the eye. The proptosis slowly receded. Towards the end of the hospital stay, slight movement of the eyeball on attempted lateral gaze could be detected. There was no light perception through the closed lids.

A left myringotomy was done on February 9 and a small amount of purulent material obtained. No organisms were seen and cultures did not show growth of fungi or bacteria. Another culture for fungi on April 3 was negative. The otitis externa slowly subsided and the canal was clear by April 16. At that time the left drum appeared thick, edematous and white, particularly in the inferior portions, an appearance ascribed to chronic otitis media possibly of fungal origin.

Under local therapy the white cheesy necrotic material disappeared in 3 weeks, leaving a healthy edge to the palatal perforation. The ulceration filled in from the periphery and by the end of hospitalization was only one-half the size on admission. The perforation into the left nasopharynx remained unchanged. The medial pterygoid plate was exposed and the structures distorted.

On admission there was swelling of the left orbit, left cheek and area in front of the left ear. The left anterolateral aspect of the neck was also swollen with moderate tenderness along the course of the left internal jugular vein. The latter was firm and cordlike to palpation. As the left-sided facial swelling slowly subsided, two small, firm, non-tender subcutaneous nodules (2 by 3 cm and 1 by 1 cm in size) could be felt beneath the left eye. These nodules slowly diminished in size and had disappeared by the time of discharge. The swelling around the left ear and in the neck likewise disappeared, but the left internal jugular vein remained thickened to palpation.

Dysarthria, dysphagia and difficulty in chewing diminished. The left facial paresis improved. Weakness and atrophy of the left tongue, palate and masseters remained unchanged. However, there was a return of sensation to portions of the left side of the face. The complete anesthesia which originally extended from forehead to jaw gradually receded so that, by discharge, the area extended from the lower forehead to the upper lip and from the front of the ear to the lateral side of the nose.

At the time of discharge, June 2, 1954, the child felt well. The perforation remained unchanged. Many neurological abnormalities persisted: blindness of the left eye, left ophthalmoplegia, deafness on left, left facial weakness, left palatal weakness, atrophy and paresis of the left side of the tongue, weakness of the left mastication muscles, diminished to absent sensation of the left side of the face and weakness of the left trapezius. Roentgenograms showed clouding of the sinuses on the left.

The child was seen on November 19, 1954, at which time she was feeling well and going to school. The urine had been consistently free from sugar on the same dose of insulin. The exophthalmos of the left eye had completely receded. External ophthalmoplegia was still present. The area of anesthesia was somewhat smaller but extended from the lips to the forehead on the left face. The perforation of the palate was clean and less than one-half of its original size. The patient was re-examined on January 26, 1955, one year after admission. She has continued to do well.

Discussion of Case of Dr. HARRIS: The case demonstrated an extensive invasion of *R. arrhizus* in an individual predisposed to infection by uncontrolled diabetes mellitus. The portal of entry of the fungus was apparently the nasal cavity or the accesory nasal sinuses on the left. The fungus then invaded the palate where a perforation developed. Invasion of blood vessels, lymphatics and nerves together with necrosis and inflammation were demonstrated in biopsies. The necrosis was probably in part infarction, as thrombosis was undoubtedly present. The dense clouding of all the nasal sinuses on the left side was probably due to mucosal invasion by hyphae as has been seen in other cases. The fungus organisms extended from the palate and sinuses directly through the tissues and along the vessels and nerves. The proptosis and ophthalmoplegia were due to retro-orbital inflammation and the involvement of vessels and nerves entering and leaving the orbit. The involvement of the fifth, seventh, ninth, eleventh and twelfth nerves suggested an extensive invasion along the left side of the base of the skull through blood vessels so that the left posterior jugular outflow was involved. The cord-like thickening of the left internal jugular vein indicated invasion and thrombosis of that vein. The nodules in the cheek demonstrated local invasion with abscess or with infarcted foci.

In the light of the frequency of fatal cerebral involvement in the literature it was amazing that the child recovered from the acute phase of her disease and a year later seemed to be well except for the neurological residue and a relatively clean palatal perforation. The vascular thrombi organized and recanalized, the organisms died and necrotic tissue became fibrotic.

This case of HARRIS cannot be tabulated exactly as one of classical central nervous system mucormycosis, for the brain was largely spared. The facial features place it within the cranial category and it may be termed rhinoorbital mucormycosis.

Nasal Mucormycosis

In cranial mucormycosis there is usually a lesion of the nasal cavity on physical examination or at postmortem or a history of bloody discharge from the nose. The involvement is most frequently unilateral, though it may be bilateral, and palatal, sinus, orbital or facial involvement tend to be on the same side as the unilateral nasal involvement.

Examination of the interior of the nostril may reveal a bloody discharge and a black, dry-looking infarcted region. The turbinates may be black and gangrenous, due to vascular obstruction. In most case reports it has apparently been taken for granted that the fungus entered via the nose and the nasal mucous membranes, but the appearances suggest that it could be those of infarction secondary to vascular obstruction. Presumably the fungus could enter a paranasal sinus or the conjunctival sac of the eye and produce the nasal lesions.

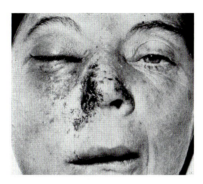

Fig. 12. Mucormycosis of the face. Note the proptosis of the right eye, the infarction of the nose and the effect of nerve paralyses on the eyelids and mouth. There was infarction of the right side of the palate and necrotizing ethmoiditis due to the fungus. From LUBBE and PENNINGTON (Fig. 1). Courtesy of authors and the Medical Journal of Australia

SMITH and YANAGISAWA say that the most important physical sign of rhinomucormycosis is the gray-black appearance of the nasal mucosa, which resembles dried clotted blood; and that the gray-black discoloration of the nasal mucosa is unlike that seen in any other nasal disease.

Two of the cases of GREGORY et al. showed nasal lesions. In one patient there was a dark, discolored mucosa and necrosis of the nasal septum.

BAUM described a swollen middle turbinate with overlying easily bleeding friable tissue. A biopsy of the turbinate revealed the hyphae of mucormycosis in areas of necrosis with scant neutrophils. The hyphae were invading blood vessels.

In GASS' patient there had been epistaxis from the left nares two days before admission. Dried blood was present in the left nares when the patient was brought to the hospital. On the third hospital day an otolaryngological consultant described peculiar, almost black mucous membrane in the left nares. The nasal septum was ulcerated and perforated.

In the case of DWYER and CHANGUS the left nostril contained hemorrhagic exudate, and the left side of the nose was gangrenous.

BERK et al. found a black and soft nasal septum at autopsy and microscopically there were hyphae in the nasal septum. In Case 1 of FUENTES there was, at autopsy, a congested and hemorrhagic inflammatory area with a gangrenous aspect, in the left nostril. WEISSKOPF mentions a crust in the left nostril and red, dry and atrophic turbinates.

DE WEESE and ROBINSON report 2 cases of mucormycosis of the nose and sinuses with recovery following treatment. In the first case nosebleed was the first event and a perforation of the septum was discovered. Biopsies of the nasal lesions showed hyphae. In their second case there was a depression of the cartilaginous part of the nasal septum, a foul nasal discharge, necrotic dehiscence of the right lateral wall of the nose and posterior nasal septum.

SMITH and KIRCHNER illustrate the autopsy specimen of black thrombosed turbinate from their Case 2 (Fig. 15).

Review of these case reports impresses one with the gangrenous nature of the nasal lesions, based on ischemia. Bone and cartilage share in the process and become soft, and the nasal septum may be perforated.

Palatal Mucormycosis

Harris, as already mentioned, reported a case of mucormycosis with a palatal perforation on the left at the junction of the hard and soft palate. The perforation, 1×1 cm, was in the center of an ulcer 3×3 cm in diameter, partially covered by a brownish-yellow, cheesy material. The bare pterygoid plate of the lateral side of the nasal cavity could be seen through the perforation. With healing the ulcer filled in from the periphery, but the perforation into the nasopharynx remained unchanged.

Georgiade et al. described and illustrated the palatal slough in the case of Harris and reported an infant case of palatal slough which they thought might have been mucormycotic in origin.

Dwyer and Changus described the left side of the palate of their case as escharotic. Hoagland et al. described as gray the right half of the palate in a non-fatal case. In their second case, also non-fatal, they mention an abnormality of the palate on the left. In case 1 of Wasserman et al. there was a black eschar in the midline of the palate. Rinaldi and Ashby mention a lesion of the hard palate in their case. Lubbe and Pennington have an illustration of a large, right-sided lesion of the palate. This was probably gangrenous, as there was gangrene of the face in this case. Taylor et al. report the case of a 40-year-old diabetic woman with necrosis of the palatal bone proved to be mucormycotic in cultures and tissue sections. Successful treatment consisted of the use of Amphotericin B and regulation of the diabetes. Weisskopf describes ulceration of the palate in his case 3. De Weese et al. describe ulceration of the roof of the mouth in their second case. It was located posteriorly and to the right. In the autopsy report of their case, Hurtado et al. observed incipient gangrene of the palatal arch on the right. In the nonfatal case of Abramson et al., the necrotic palatal bone was removed and later a prosthesis was adapted to the defect.

In Case 3 of Smith and Kirchner there was a sinus tract from the hard palate and alveolus of the maxilla leading to the maxillary sinus.

In summary, the palatal lesions of cranial mucormycosis tend to be unilateral in location and ischemic in nature, that is, they are regions of gangrene due to infarction. Hyphae were demonstrated in the tissues and blood vessels of the palate. The affected palate bone became necrotic and softened and in a few cases perforations developed with the formation of a permanent communication between the oral and nasal cavity.

Paranasal Mucormycosis

The case reports of cranial mucormycosis indicate that the maxillary, ethmoid, and occasionally sphenoidal and frontal sinuses are involved and act as way-stations on the route of the fungus to the orbital cavity and the brain.

The sinusitis is usually unilateral and on the side on which the nose, palate and eye are affected. The left side is said to be affected more frequently than the right.

In one of the cases of Gregory et al. there was purulent ethmoiditis with necrosis of bone, and perforation into the orbit and beneath the dura, and into the nose. Stratemeier's case had chronic empyema of the anterior ethmoids. Bauer et al. found the mucosa of the ethmoids and frontal sinuses red and necrotic. There was necrosis of bone, and the fungus was demonstrated in it. Merriam et al. describe dark brown contents of the sphenoid and ethmoid sinuses with demonstrable fungi in the contents. In Harris' case the antrum had a thickened mucous membrane, as seen in X-ray, and there was no bony involvement.

In most cases the sinuses do not contain fluid and the majority of X-ray studies fail to show a fluid level.

In one of Gass' cases, however, there was clouding of the left ethmoidal sinuses and a questionable fluid level in the left antrum was found on X-ray examination. On the fifth hospital day the ethmoidal bone biopsy was reported as showing mucormycosis. On the 33rd hospital day a rhinotomy, debridement of the left nasal cavity, exenteration of the left sinus complex, and left eye enucleation were done. At operation much of the frontal process of the maxillary bone, the entire left ethmoidal labyrinth, nasal septum, the turbinates, the anterior wall of the sphenoid sinus, the bone comprising the optic foramen, and the floor and medial wall of the orbit were necrotic. The necrosis extended to the cribriform plate and was thought to extend through the plate into the anterior cranial fossa. The patient was discharged from the hospital 27 days following his admission, and 3 months after the onset of his disease the activity of the fungus had ceased and the patient appeared to be "well."

In Case 1 of BURNS the sinuses on the affected side were cloudy in X-ray. In his Case 2 there were mycelia in tissue from the ethmoid sinus at operation and *Rhizopus sp.* was cultured from the contents. In Fig. 1 of ROWE and PAYNE hyphae are pictured in the necrotic wall of an ethmoid sinus. REEVES et al., in an autopsy report, describe ethmoiditis and sphenoiditis.

SMITH and YANAGISAWA described and illustrated a fluffy growth of white fungus on the skin of the face at the operative site following an external operation on a mucormycotic sinusitis. The fungus was growing at the inner angle of the eye close to the nose and resembled an early culture of *Rhizopus*. Apparently the organism had extended from the sinus and had spread to the skin surface adjacent to the incision.

In the case of SMITH and KIRCHNER there was a peculiar perforation extending from the right maxillary alveolar ridge and hard palate to the maxillary sinus.

In Case 2 of BAUER et al. (1955a) the postmortem examination revealed, in addition to hyphae in the tissues of the mucosa of the right ethmoid sinus, sporangia attached to their sporangiophores and containing spores. Scattered spores were present in the tissues.

Mucormycotic Otitis Media

HARRIS described otitis media during the course of the mucormycosis of his patient, but the fungus could not be cultured from pus from the middle ear or from the contents of the external ear canal. Later, the left ear drum appeared thick as though from chronic otitis media, possibly of fungal origin.

REEVES et al. reported a suppurative left otitis media observed at autopsy in a case of mucormycosis of the central nervous system. There was also ethmoiditis and sphenoiditis.

In the case of BRYAN et al., that of a 34-month-old infant, a moderate inflammation of the right tympanic membrane was seen clinically. At autopsy the right middle ear contained red-brown fluid. Microscopically, hyphae of mucormycosis were observed in the Haversian system and intertrabecular spaces of the bone around the right middle ear.

Orbital Mucormycosis

Orbital or rhinoorbital mucormycosis consists of unilateral orbital cellulitis with proptosis, ptosis, internal and external ophthalmoplegia, optic neuritis, posterior uveitis and obstruction of the central retinal artery (GINSBERG et al.). Marked visual impairment is usual and the ocular signs tend to be permanent.

This dramatic disease usually presents as a well-defined clinical syndrome (BAUM). The typical story is that of an adult with uncontrolled diabetes, usually in acidosis, who suddenly develops facial pain and headache, rhinitis with epistaxis, lid edema, and the other features mentioned above (Fig. 12). The patient lapses into coma, and death commonly ensues within two weeks. To date, almost all cases of orbital mucormycosis have occurred in patients with some type of debilitating disease, usually diabetic acidosis.

GASS and FERRY, and STRAATSMA et al. have written excellent reviews of rhinoorbital mucormycosis.

There are 77 cases (68%) of orbital and ocular mucormycosis among the 107 cases of cranial mucormycosis listed in Table 2. (The 4 cases listed as classic CNS mucormycosis are presumed to have had orbital disease and are included in the figure of 77.)

The predisposing disease in 68 (88%) of the 77 cases of orbital mucormycosis was diabetes, almost always in an acidotic state. The other predisposing conditions were hydronephrosis, uremia, and acidosis; diarrhea and acidosis (2 cases); the nephrotic syndrome; renal failure; cirrhosis; Hodgkin's disease; agranulocytosis; and amebiasis. Orbital mucormycosis, therefore, can be considered an important and frequently lethal complication of diabetes mellitus. The importance of keeping the diabetic patient from becoming acidotic cannot be overemphasized. Particularly, the diabetic patient should avoid extended overindulgence in alcohol, as this has led to acidosis and mucormycosis in several of the reported cases.

The causative fungus, usually a *Rhizopus* species, probably reaches the tissues of the orbital cavity from the nasal cavity or the paranasal sinuses, especially the

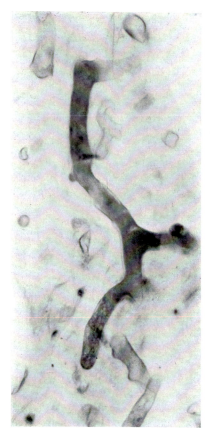

Fig. 13. Hypha of mucormycosis from the orbital fatty tissue. Note the broad non-septate hyphae with right-angle branching. From case of BAKER and SEVERANCE (1948). H & E, × 350. Photograph from BAKER (1966)

ethmoid air cells or the maxillary sinus. A direct infection of the conjunctival sac or cornea cannot be excluded. Infection of the soft tissues of the orbital cavity may be complicated by infection of the bulbus oculi, the bony orbit and the tissues of the face and nose. The infection may extend through the roof of the orbit to the anterior fossa of the cranial cavity and to the meninges and parenchyma of a frontal lobe of the brain producing mucormycotic meningitis and mucormycosis of the brain.

The infection of the orbit may involve the ophthalmic artery causing it to become thrombosed. The mucormycotic thromboarteritis may extend to the artery of origin, the internal carotid artery and to the circle of Willis and its branches.

Of the 77 cases of orbital mucormycosis death has ensued in the majority (77%). The 18 which are listed as survivals (23%) together with the factor apparently responsible for survival are listed as follows:

WADSWORTH, self-limited; HARRIS, insulin; BAKER (1957), insulin; McCALL and STROBOS, enucleation of eye; MERRIAM and TEDESCHI, insulin, enucleation; FAILLO et al., operation; GASS (case 1), Amphotericin B and exenteration of eye and sinuses; HOAGLAND et al. (case 1), extirpation of right face; WASSERMAN et al. (case 3), insulin and iodides; BANK et al., insulin; LANDAU and NEWCOMER, Amphotericin B; BURROW et al., Amphotericin B; LA TOUCHE et al., Amphotericin B; DE WEESE et al. (case 1), Amphotericin B; DE WEESE et al. (case 2), Amphotericin B; ABRAMSON et al. (case 2), Amphotericin B; BAUM, Amphotericin B; PROKOP and SILVA-HUTNER, insulin and Amphotericin B.

All of the factors of survival are not included in the above listing. Some listed as having Amphotericin B had insulin and other therapeutic agents. A factor of considerable importance in survival may be the shorter period of diabetic acidosis occasioned by prompt diagnosis and therapy of the uncontrolled diabetes. The spread of the infection to the brain is halted.

Apparently Amphotericin B has been a factor in improving the prognosis of orbital mucormycosis.

Pathologic Findings. Examination of the orbital contents at postmortem from within the cranial cavity discloses hemorrhagic, grayish, infarcted tissues. Numerous hyphae are free in the tissues and within arteries and nerves.

Ocular Mucormycosis

GINSBERG et al. in 1966 described the eyes removed at autopsy from a fatal case of cerebral mucormycosis, making clear why there is blindness and ophthalmoplegia in these cases.

The partially collapsed left globe, the mucormycotic one, had numerous fragments of adherent muscle and fatty tissue. A horizontal section revealed the vitreous to be diffusely

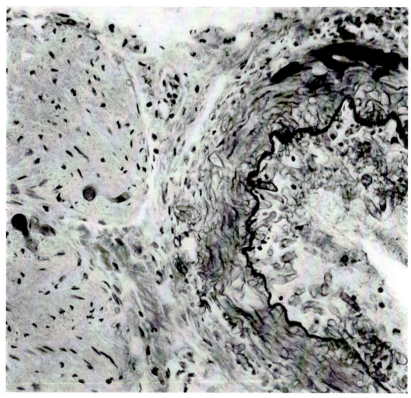

Fig. 14. Mucormycosis, with hyphae in a nerve (left) and in the wall and lumen of an artery (right) (H & E, × 145). Hyphae also may travel along lymphatic vessels. Photograph from BAKER (1966)

cloudy. Microscopically a disseminated cellular infiltrate, predominantly neutrophilic, was present in the posterior choroid, sclera, episclera, extraocular muscles and orbital tissues. Anteriorly, the inflammation extended to the edge of the choroid, the tendons of the horizontal rectus muscles, the limbal episclera and the bulbar conjunctiva. The amount of cellular exudation varied considerably, being moderate within the eye and quite severe in the orbit where there was considerable necrosis with moderate edema.

Leukocytic infiltration was mainly perivascular but also surrounded foci of extravascular hyphae in necrotic tissue. Although some areas of suppuration appeared to reflect the direct effect of the fungus, most of the necrosis was attributable to infarction. The inflammatory reaction appeared most intense in relation to small or medium-sized arteries, especially the choroidal, short and long ciliary vessels and those of the extraocular vessels. The infiltrate in extensively necrotic extraocular muscle with intense reaction around a thrombosed vessel is sufficient to explain the ophthalmoplegia.

As for the loss of vision, although the optic nerve was unaffected, there was vascular invasion, chiefly arterial, with and without thrombosis, and hyphae were identified in blood vessels of the uveal tract, optic meninges, conjunctiva and orbit.

STRAATSMA et al. give particular attention to ocular disorders in 5 cases with the classic central nervous system syndrome of mucormycosis. Three patients had proptosis, with edema and limitation of mobility indicative of orbital cellulitis. Three patients demonstrated extraocular muscle paralysis, and one showed retinal hemorrhages. Three developed unilateral or bilateral occlusion of the central retinal artery as shown by pallor of the fundus, a cherry-red spot in the macula, and a fixed, dilated pupil.

Histologically, the hyphae were present throughout the soft tissues of the orbit and showed a predilection for invasion of the major vessels with resultant thrombosis and infarction (Fig. 14). Involvement of the optic and ciliary nerves was frequent, and in a few cases panophthalmitis was observed.

In Wadsworth's case of ocular mucormycosis (1951) the eye was removed surgically. There was massive fibrosis of the retina in the posterior portion of the globe and the retina was completely detached. Under high magnification one could see bone formation in the region of fibrosis, and old hemorrhage with cholesterol crystals. Incorporated in scar near the optic nerve were branching, non-septate, phycomycete hyphae. There was none of the surrounding eosin-staining material characteristic of infection by Entomophthora and infiltrations of eosinophils were not present. The walls of the hyphae are so sharp, and in places so thickened, in Fig. 3 of Wadsworth's article, that one wonders whether calcification has not occurred.

The active infection must have occurred months or years before the enucleation of the eye, because the fungi were embedded in scar tissue. The clinical story indicates increase in size of the lesion by ophthalmologic examination and the development of acute secondary glaucoma about 4 months before enucleation. Probably there was a subclinical orbital and ocular infection from the nose at a former time or, less likely, a blood-born deposit in the eye from pulmonary mucormycosis. There was no associated diabetes or other predisposing condition.

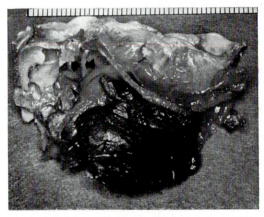

Fig. 15. Autopsy specimen of black thrombosed turbinate from case 2 of Smith and Kirchner (1958) (Fig. 4)

Facial Mucormycosis: The first case of facial mucormycosis was reported by Gregory et al. in 1943.

It was that of a diabetic patient with acidosis who died of cerebral mucormycosis. Two days before death the face became edematous, especially about the eyes, and then dark blue over the bridge of the nose. There were no microscopic sections of the affected skin, but undoubtedly fungi would have been found in the subcutaneous or cutaneous tissues and blood vessels.

The second case, of Martin et al., was one in which sections were obtained (Fig. 16). This was the case of a $2^{1}/_{2}$ month old diabetic infant who died of cerebral mucormycosis with thrombosis of the carotid artery. Four days before death, gangrene of the left side of the face developed and hyphae were observed in tissue sections of the left side of the face and its underlying tissues.

McCall and Strobos, Dwyer and Changus, Faillo et al. and Borland report similar cases. Of the 6 patients just mentioned, 4 died and 2 recovered.

The location of the facial lesion varied from case to case. For example, in the case of Smith and Kirchner (Fig. 17), the gangrene was a round region, about 6 cm in diameter, just

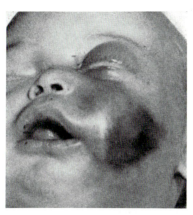

Fig. 16. Cranial mucormycosis. Infarction (gangrene) of left orbit and cheek. Case of MARTIN et al. (1954). Photograph by courtesy of Dr. J.M. LUKEMAN

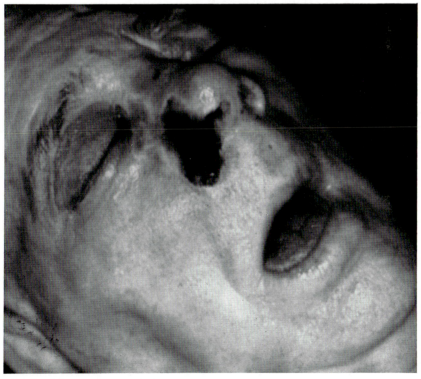

Fig. 17. Cranial mucormycosis. Note the black necrotic region of infarction of the cheek and nose adjacent to the right nostril, and also the periorbital swelling with discoloration. Case 1 of SMITH and KIRCHNER (1958) (Fig. 1)

to the right of the right nostril. In the case of LUBBE and PENNINGTON (Fig. 12), it was a little larger and elongated, running parallel to, and just to the right of the nose. In the case of HURTADO et al., the area of reddish induration extended from the nose well out on the right cheek.

Other cases are described by Rinaldi and Ashby, Foushee and Beck, Hoagland et al., Weisskopf, and De Weese and Robinson.

In summary, mucormycosis of the face, of a gangrenous, infarcted nature, occurs in about a fourth of the cases of cranial mucormycosis. It is not as common as orbital edema and proptosis, but occurs on the same side and is usually unilateral, though in a few cases it has spread across the upper part of the nose to involve both sides of the nose and adjacent cheeks. A whole cheek may be red, indurated and swollen, or livid regions may occur next to a nostril or between the eye and the nose, fanning out onto the cheek. The majority of the lesions are not ulcerated. One lesion was reported as an abscess of the right naso-labial fold (Gabriele). The coldness of the infarcted area of the cheek during the life of the patient was mentioned by one observer.

Mucormycosis of the Brain: The tables include 64 cases of mucormycosis of the central nervous system, 1 of which had spinal cord as well as cerebral lesions and 2 of which had mucormycosis of the spinal cord without involvement of the brain.

My Table 2 of cranial mucormycosis includes all cases of mucormycosis with lesions in the head or face, except 5 cases listed as disseminated. In the 5 tables of mucormycosis cases there is no duplication of listing.

If the classic central nervous system syndrome is defined as combined orbital and cerebral involvement, the following cases qualify for this designation:

Cases 1, 2 and 3 of Gregory et al., Lecompte and Meissner, Baker and Severance, Wolf and Cowan, Stratemeier, Martin et al. (Fig. 16); cases 1 and 2 of Bauer et al., Sydney Hospital (1956a, b), Bryan et al., Dwyer and Changus; cases 1 and 2 of Smith and Kirchner (Figs. 15, 17), Borland, Dolman and Heard, Lie Kian-Joe et al., Smith and Yanagasawa, Long and Weiss, Banker; case 2 of Gass; cases 1 and 2 of Wasserman et al.; cases 1, 2 and 3 of Straatsma et al., Suprun, Agrest et al.; cases 1 and 2 of Fuentes, Suga, La Touche et al., Lubbe and Pennington (Figs. 12, 27); case 1 of Gordon and Little, Hurtado et al.; case 2 of Peña and Dorado, Tomiyasu and Baker, Ginsberg et al., Grover et al., Pérez et al., and Tinaztepe and Tinaztepe (Figs. 22—26).

In a small number of cases, the orbit was not affected, but there were *lesions* of the *nose, paranasal sinuses* or other portions of the face which suggested that the infection of the brain had come from the region of the face.

In the remaining group of cases of cranial mucormycosis, with lesions of the brain or meninges and sometimes of the internal carotid artery, it is not clear how the cerebral lesion developed, whether from the face region or through the blood stream, or from the lungs or elsewhere. Some of these cases have a single, solitary tumor-like mass in the brain.

This group comprises the cases of Oppe, Hafstrom et al., Kurrein, Gunson and Bowden, Foushee and Beck, Keye and Magee (3 cases), Jackson and Karnauchow, Muresan, Turpin et al., Straatsma et al. (cases 5, 27 and 32), Agrest et al., and Fuentes (cases 3 and 4).

Allied to this last group, but with a high probability that the brain lesion has developed as part of a disseminated mucormycosis with the primary lesion in the lung or elsewhere, are the brain lesions listed in Table 5 of disseminated mucormycosis.

These are the cases of Paltauf, Torack (case 7), Hutter (case 4), Rabin et al. (cases 1 and 2) and Baker (1962) (case 11).

In 32 cases of the classical central nervous system syndrome of mucormycosis the prosector examined the brain in detail and his observations have found their way into print and into published illustrations.

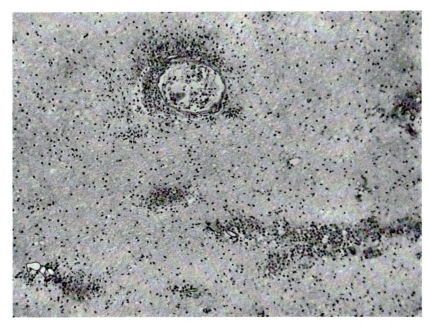

Fig. 18. Cerebral mucormycosis, to show cellular infiltrate, mostly neutrophilic, about blood vessels. Hyphae are just visible in the wall of the largest vessel. Swollen hyphae are seen elsewhere (H & E, × 100)

The classical central nervous system lesions of mucormycosis were described by GREGORY et al. in 1943 (Figs. 4, 18). A patient in diabetic acidosis developed nasal, paranasal, or orbital mucormycosis and the infection spread to infect the brain.

In 29 of the 32 cases the *Rhizopus* hyphae appeared to enter the brain directly from the nasopharynx, paranasal sinuses or orbit by invading the bone of the floor of the anterior fossa of the skull, the dura, the leptomeninges, and finally the cortex and white matter of a frontal lobe of the brain. During the advance the fungus invaded vessels and caused thrombosis and infarction. Bone and brain were softened. Microscopically, hyphae, thrombosis, necrosis, and cells of acute inflammation were described.

I will review the findings in the first case of GREGORY et al., and then those of the subsequent cases:

This historic case of medical mycology was that of a 43-year-old colored woman who developed diabetic acidosis and then pain and loss of vision in the left eye. She soon showed gangrene of the left orbit and of the bridge of the nose, and died only 4 days after the onset of this peculiar infection. There was infarction (gangrene) of the left side of the nasal septum and the turbinates, mycosis of the eyeball, thrombosis of the left cavernous sinus, the left internal carotid artery, the anterior cerebral artery, the middle cerebral, the posterior cerebral and the inferior cerebellar. There was meningovascular mucormycosis of the base of the brain as shown by dull, opaque and blood-stained leptomeninges. This appearance extended over the tips of the frontal lobes.

There was infarction of the inferior portions of the frontal lobes, with minimal inflammatory reaction, and infarction, early, of the left cerebral hemisphere. Coronal sections of the frontal lobes showed softening of the orbital surfaces to a depth of 2—3 cm. There was mucormycosis of the pituitary gland.

The authors suggested that the infection started in the nose and extended through the angular vein and its branches which reach the orbit and empty into the cavernous sinus by way of the ophthalmic vein.

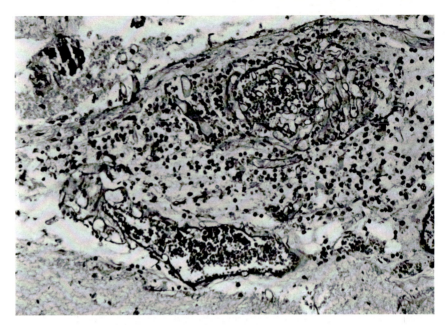

Fig. 19. Mucormycotic meningitis. Note the polymorphonuclear inflammatory edudate in the edematous leptomeninges and the hyphae both free and within vessels (H & E, × 130)

This is a possibility, and there has been cavernous sinus thrombosis in at least six of the 32 reported cases.

In the second case of GREGORY et al. there was no thrombus in any dural sinus. The patient, a diabetic who had been on an alcoholic bout for several weeks, was brought to the hospital with a proptosis, i.e. forward projection, of the right eye. Apparently the disease began with mucormycotic ethmoiditis and there was direct extension to the right orbit and to the floor of the anterior cranial fossa to form an abscess beneath the dura and to involve the frontal lobes of the brain. The protocol states that after the brain was removed, purulent material was seen beneath the dura on both sides of the crista galli. On the inferior surfaces of the frontal lobes of the brain the tissue was destroyed and ragged. On coronal sectioning the necrosis was found to extend 4 cm inward from the orbital surfaces and posteriorly to the corpus callosum. There was osteomyelitis of the bony plates forming the medial border of the right orbital cavity.

In the third case of GREGORY et al. the right orbit and the pons of the brain showed severe mucormycosis at autopsy. Could the process have begun in the right conjunctival sac? It is not clear that the nose and paranasal sinuses were examined at autopsy. Here was a case apparently without inferior frontal lobe necrosis.

There are only two other cases in which the evidence for a direct spread from below to the frontal lobes is not adequate. I will give the findings in these two cases, LE COMPTE and MEISSNER, and STRAATSMA et al., Case 3, and then the findings in the remainder of the cases, in which the evidence for direct spread was good.

In the case of LE COMPTE and MEISSNER the right eye was swollen and inflamed and the pupil was larger than on the left. There was no movement in the left arm or leg. At autopsy, note was made of the great tendency of the fungus to grow in vessels. The brain showed petechial hemorrhages of the cerebellum, pons and medulla. There was acute mucormycotic meningoencephalitis with an intense polymorphonuclear reaction in many places. The orbital surfaces of the frontal lobes seemed to be no more involved than any other portion of the brain. My comment was that the disease appeared to begin in the conjunctival sac of the right orbit, but that the left hemiplegia indicated that the fungus was already in the right motor tracts of the brain affecting the left motor tracts of the cord and that both the eye and central nervous system involvement might have developed from an undiscovered focus, as from the ethmoid air cells.

In the third case of STRAATSMA et al., which is the case later reported in more detail by REEVES et al., there was, in a diabetic woman of 30, gangrene of the eyelids and left side of the bridge of the nose. Suppurative ethmoiditis and sphenoiditis developed. There was bilateral cavernous sinus thrombosis, and thrombosis of the left anterior and middle cerebral arteries, the intracranial portion of the left internal carotid artery, and both ophthalmic arteries. There was basilar fibrinopurulent meningitis. An interesting finding was an acute suppurative left otitis media.

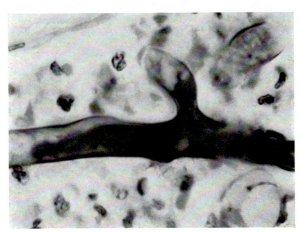

Fig. 20. Hypha in meningeal mucormycosis. Note the right-angle branching and the neutrophils and red cells in the leptomeninges (H & E, × 800)

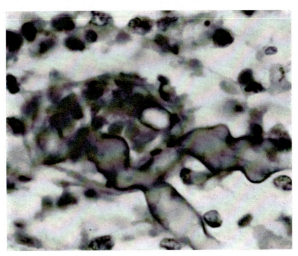

Fig. 21. Meningeal mucormycosis. Note the hyphae penetrating a minute vessel and stimulating the conglomeration of platelets and the agglutination of blood cells as the process of thrombosis is initiated (H & E, × 1000)

As nothing was said about the orbital surface of the left frontal lobe of the brain, I conclude that a venous spread was possible as was described in the first case of GREGORY et al.

The abstracts of the cases in which there is evidence for a direct spread of infection from the nose, paranasal sinuses or orbit to the brain, through bone and

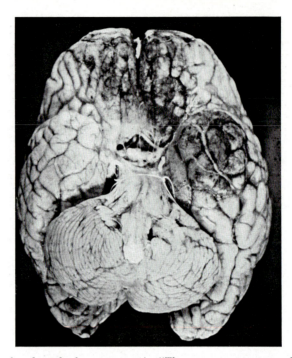

Fig. 22. Meningeal and cerebral mucormycosis. "There was an opaque, red-grey thickening of the meninges of the inferior surface of the frontal and temporal lobes," wrote the Doctors TINAZTEPE, and they continued: "The lepto-meninges over the cerebral convexities appeared thin and transparent except in the depth of the cerebral sulci where they had a slight gray-white appearance, suggesting exudate, around the blood vessels. Basilar and anterior cerebral arteries showed thrombosis." Previously unpublished photograph. Courtesy of Drs. TINAZTEPE and TINAZTEPE

dura will now follow. The neuropathologic findings are included in these abstracts, and the cases are arranged chronologically.

Case of BAKER and SEVERANCE (1948). A 3-year-old girl with diabetes had hemorrhage in the left eye, and the left pupil was larger than the right. At postmortem examination the fat of the left orbit was congested and red. Microscopically there were hyphae in the fat, arteries, veins, perineurial lymphatics, edematous muscle and bone. The thrombus in the left internal carotid artery showed numerous hyphae. On the orbital surfaces of the frontal lobes of the brain, more pronounced on the left, were regions of injection and softening. Frontal sections through these areas showed necrosis of brain extending through the gray matter and into the white matter. Microscopically there was minimal acute inflammation. The bony wall of the orbit and the capsule of the pituitary contained hyphae.

My comment on this case was that the mycosis first appeared in the orbit and conjunctiva, that the under surface of the brain was infected, probably by the fungus coming up from the orbits or paranasal sinuses below and that the fungus disseminated from the cranium to the lung.

Case of WOLF and COWEN (1949). A 42-year-old colored male diabetic developed left proptosis with redness and swelling of the lids. The left pupil was larger than the right. The left nasal cavity was edematous and full of discharge. An external right ethmoidectomy showed hyphae. There were hyphae in the eyeball. There was left cavernous sinus thrombosis, lepto-meningitis over the orbital surfaces of the frontal lobes, more on the left, and necrosis of the frontal lobes far into the white matter.

In this case the infection could have entered the cranial cavity via veins to the cavernous sinus or it could have penetrated upward through the orbital roofs to the frontal lobes of the brain.

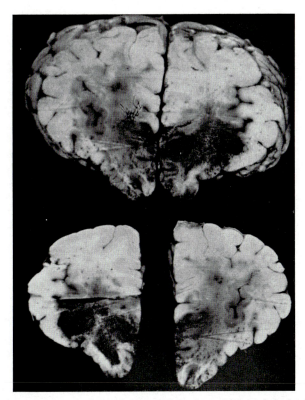

Fig. 23. Cerebral mucormycosis. Coronal section of the frontal lobes of the brain shown in the previous figure. There is bilateral hemorrhagic necrosis and infarction. The fungus has come up through the floor of the anterior fossa of the skull from the orbits and paranasal sinuses invading the meninges and brain, and causing thromboses of arteries. Case of TINAZTEPE and TINAZTEPE (1966) (Fig. 2)

Case of STRATEMEIER (1950). A 33-year-old colored woman developed diabetic coma after a heavy alcoholic bout. The left eyelid was swollen and ptosed.

At postmortem examination there was chronic empyema of the anterior ethmoid cells. The left posterior nares showed a thickened, necrotic and hemorrhagic membrane. The left turbinate bone and the nasal septum were necrotic. Microscopically the mucosa of the middle turbinate on the left side was deeply infiltrated with lymphocytes and occasional fungi and spores.

There were thrombosed vessels on the orbital surfaces of the frontal lobes and microscopically these vessels were blocked by masses of leucocytes, fibrin and hyphae. There was infarction of the orbital surface of the frontal lobes. Coronal cuts showed this infarction to extend into the frontal lobes a short distance.

The author's interpretation was that the fungus had spread from the nares to the brain.

Case of MARTIN et al. (1954). An infant of two and one half months with diarrhoea and acidosis developed necrosis of the left orbit including the globe, and gangrene of the left cheek. At autopsy there was thrombosis of the left ophthalmic and left internal carotid arteries. There was meningovascular mucormycosis. The orbital surface of the left frontal lobe was necrotic. The fungus disseminated to the lungs, pancreas and bone marrow.

Case 1 of BAUER et al. (1955). A 25-year-old white woman developed diabetic acidosis and left periorbital edema with a fixed pupil, larger than that on the right. At autopsy the under surfaces of the frontal lobes of the brain were adherent to the dura and the leptomeninges here and at the base of the brain were more opaque than normal. The inferior portions of both frontal lobes and the tips of both temporal lobes were softer than normal. A coronal section through the anterior half of the brain showed an infarct of the superior and lateral portion of the left cerebral hemisphere extending to include the basal ganglia on the left, Microscopically sections

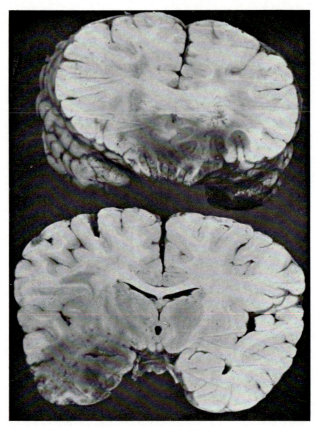

Fig. 24. Cerebral mucormycosis. Coronal section of the brain showing extension of the hemorrhagic necrosis. Case of Tinaztepe and Tinaztepe (Fig. 3)

from the infarct showed hyphae, necrosis, polymorphonuclear neutrophils and gitter cells.
There were a few hyphae in the pons. There were hyphae in the dura about the pituitary gland
but the dura itself was free.

Interpretation: The infection spread from the orbits through the orbital roofs to the dura
of the anterior cranial fossa and into the leptomeninges. The infarct suggests a thrombosis of
the middle cerebral artery, and the arteries and veins of the brain and meninges were involved.

Case 2 of Bauer et al. A 40-year-old colored person with diabetic acidosis had mucormycosis of the paranasal sinuses and orbit on the right. The dura overlying the roof of the right
orbit was roughened and adherent to the leptomeninges of the right frontal lobe. There was
necrotic bone in the walls of the ethmoid air cells and the right frontal sinus. The diaphragma
sellae and the coverings of the pituitary stalk contained hyphae.

The area of necrosis at the base of the right frontal lobe extended into the adjoining white
matter. There were numerous minute mucormycotic infarcts throughout the cortex and particularly in the floor of sulci. This showed grossly as areas of discoloration 0.5—1.2 cm in diameter. They had a red pinpoint center surrounded by a ring of gray tissue with a pink halo.
The right internal carotid artery was thrombosed.

In this case mucormycosis developed in the right nostril and paranasal sinuses and orbit
and passed upward to involve the dura and right frontal lobe of the brain. The leptomeningitis
and vasculitis became general over the brain and caused minute infarcts.

The thrombosis of the internal carotid artery can be explained on the basis of a probable
thrombosis of the ophthalmic artery, via such tributaries as the anterior and posterior ethmoidal arteries and frontal arteries. Also it is well to realize that thrombosis of the inferior orbital
branch of the anterior cerebral could produce infarction of the inferior portion of the frontal
lobe, perhaps similar to what is observed in these cases of mucormycosis.

Case at Clinical Pathological Conference of the Sydney Hospital, Australia, 1956. This was a case of orbito-cerebral mucormycosis with frontal lobe involvement and metastatic lesions in the lungs. On the medial surface of the anterior pole of each frontal lobe there was an area of congestion with underlying petechial hemorrhages and softening. Conspicuous petechial hemorrhages were present throughout both cerebral hemispheres and in the brain stem and pons. Microscopically in the frontal lobe there was acute hemorrhagic meningoencephalitis, with hyphae in blood vessels and gray and white matter. Many were surrounded with well-preserved polymorphonuclear neutrophils indicating that the infection occurred during life and was of short duration. In other parts of the brain there were petechial hemorrhages but no mycelium.

In the middle and lower lobes of the right lung and in the left lung were round, pale brown regions 1—3 cm in diameter. Near one lesion a firm thrombus was found in a vessel.

Case of BRYAN et al. (1958). This 3-year-old girl had orbito-cerebral mucormycosis. Clinically there was muscular weakness of the left side of the body.

The infection appeared to begin in the nose and involve the right-sided structures of the face, the palate, the ear and then the frontal and temporal lobes of the brain. The fungus spread to the lungs and intestines. The author called the case disseminated. It is a cranial case with dissemination.

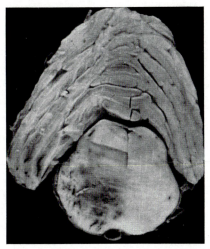

Fig. 25. Mucormycosis of the brain. Section of the pons showing thrombosis of the basilar artery with hemorrhagic necrosis (infarction) of the left side. Case of TINAZTEPE and TINAZTEPE (Fig. 4)

The meningeal vessels were congested. The inferior portions of both frontal lobes and of the tip of the right temporal lobe were red and soft. These changes were more extensive in the right frontal lobe than in the left. The opposing surfaces of the dura mater were soft and red.

The pituitary gland was red and soft. The right middle ear contained red brown fluid. Fungi were found in the Haversian system and intertrabecular spaces of the bone around the right middle ear, in the pituitary gland and in the lungs. There was patchy infarction of the small intestine.

The right internal carotid artery was occluded by thrombus. There was recent thrombotic occlusion of the aorta below the origin of the inferior mesenteric artery and into the common iliac artery.

Case of DWYER and CHANGUS (1958). The authors write: "The route of spread was demonstrated from the maxillary sinus into adjacent bone, along vessels, especially through the perineural vessels of the branches of the maxillary nerve, into the sphenopalatal ganglion involving the periorbital tissues, both cavernous sinuses, meninges, brain."

The frontal lobes were not involved but the left temporal lobe was.

The above should be a sufficient number of case reports to indicate the usual route of access of the fungus to the brain and the types of cerebral pathology produced.

There appeared to be evidence for the direct spread of the fungus from the paranasal sinuses and orbit, through the softened bone of the floor of the anterior fossa of the brain and

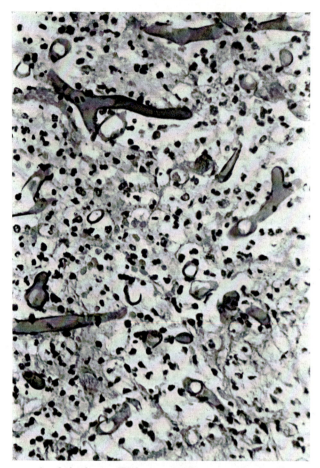

Fig. 26. Mucormycosis of the brain. High power microscopy showing hemotoxophilic, large nonseptate fungi (Fig. 7). Case of Tinaztepe and Tinaztepe, a $4^1/_2$-year-old boy with uremia and acidosis complicating bilateral hydronephrosis

through dura to the orbital surfaces of the frontal lobe or lobes of the brain in the case of Kurrein (1954), the cases 1 and 2 of Smith and Kirchner (1958), Borland (1959), case 2 of Burns (1959), Dolman and Herd (1959), Lie-Kian-Joe (1959), Long and Weiss (1959), Gass' case 2 (1961), case 1 of Wasserman (1961), Suprun (1962), Agrest (1963), case 2 of Fuentes (1963), La Touche et al. (1963), case 1 and 2 of Gordon (1965), Hurtado et al. (1965), Perez et al. (1966) and Tinaztepe and Tinaztepe (1966) (Figs. 22—26).

In summary, the changes in the brain frequently encountered at autopsy in cases of the classical central nervous system syndrome of mucormycosis may be:

1. Softening of the orbital surface of one of the frontal lobes corresponding to a region of localized pachymeningitis and necrosis of bone above a paranasal sinus or the orbit (Figs. 22, 23). At times the process is bilateral.

2. A diffuse acute meningovascular mucormycosis (Figs. 19, 20, 21).

3. Multiple minute infarcts throughout the brain.

4. Infarcts of the pons, the temporal lobes or even an entire hemisphere (Figs. 24, 25, 26, 27).

The general change is an acute meningo-encephalitis with infarcts of various sizes secondary to mucormycotic arteritis and thrombosis. Abscesses scarcely

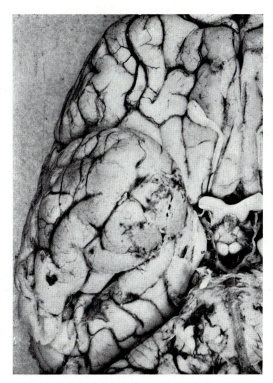

Fig. 27. Mucormycosis of the base of the right temporal lobe. The lesion corresponded to a region of thickened dura in the right middle fossa. This plaque of thick dura was firm, adherent to the meninges and brain, 3 cm in diameter, 3 mm in height and sharply outlined. Hyphae were demonstrated in the temporal lobe lesion Fig. 3 of LUBBE and PENNINGTON, courtesy of authors and Medical Journal of Australia

occur. Areas of encephalomalacia may simulate abscesses. The inflammatory response to the presence of the hyphae of *Rhizopus* is at times nil or minimal. The hyphae may stimulate microabscess formation very rarely. Much of the inflammatory reaction in the brain is secondary to the necrotic cerebral tissue caused by ischemia. Accompanying bacterial infecton is reported, but rarely.

Cerebral Lesions from the Systemic Blood Stream

Not all mucormycosis of the brain originates in the nose, paranasal sinuses or the orbit. In some cases the infection begins in the lung and there is secondary hematogenous dissemination to the brain. Two cases illustrate this occurrence.

Case 11 of BAKER (1962), was one of acute lymphoblastic leukemia with pulmonary mucormycosis. The brain contained a swollen red region, 3 cm in diameter, which was softer than normal, and which occupied the internal capsule, the caudate and lentiform nuclei, and the thalamus (Fig. 28). This region broke away easily from the surrounding cerebral tissue.

Case 23 of GRUHN and SANSON is remarkably similar to BAKER's case. They picture a coronal brain slice with a rounded lesion in the corpus striatum and basal ganglia.

Mucormycotic lesions of the brain which are secondary to primary pulmonary infection are rounded and deep in the brain, contrasting with mucormycotic lesions which have developed on the inferior aspect of the frontal lobe as a result of extension of the infection upward.

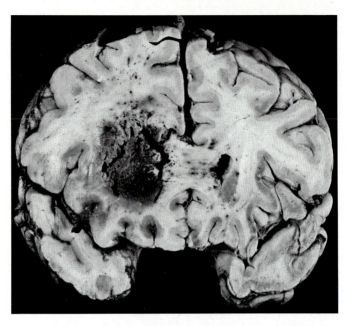

Fig. 28. Mucormycotic infarct in acute lymphoblastic leukemia. The primary lesion in this case 11 of Baker (1962) was in the lower lobe of the right lung; and the cerebral lesion is metastatic from the lung

Mucormycotic Mycotic Aneurysms

In 3 cases of cranial mucormycosis in the literature mucormycotic aneurysms have developed. As with other infectious agents such as the tubercle bacillus or *Streptococcus viridans*, the organism grows into the wall of an artery and weakens it. An aneurysm or swelling may develop, and may rupture, causing hemorrhage. This is a mycotic aneurysm no matter what the living agent causing the disease may be. Here the term mycotic does not refer to a fungus infection but to any living agent. Three illustrative cases are pertinent.

A white male of 62 years, a non-diabetic, had had a portacaval shunt operation performed 2 years antemortem (Table 2, Baker, 1957a, case 1). Three days before death he became comatose and spinal tap revealed xanthochromic, bloody spinal fluid. The carotid angiograms showed obstruction of the left internal carotid artery, and there was an aneurysmal dilatation of this artery just proximal to the origin of the left anterior cerebral artery, and the aneurysm filled from the right. At autopsy, a massive subarachnoid hematoma was found in the left middle fossa, extending through the comminuted tissue of the left temporal lobe into the lateral ventricle. Embedded in the hematoma was the left internal carotid artery, the free basal end of which was expanded into a ragged, saccular dilatation 1 cm in diameter, suggesting the distal half of an aneurysm. Obstruction of the remaining extracranial portion of the artery in the neck was demonstrated by the injection of water into the aortic end of the common carotid and by noting that water did not escape from the internal carotid artery inside the skull.

Microscopically, fungus invasion of cerebral arteries was strikingly evident in sections of the left internal carotid, both middle cerebrals, both posterior communicating arteries, and the basilar artery. The fungus extended along small blood vessels and nerves into the left orbit where it was limited to those trunks, not being found free in the areolar tissue. The mycelium was most abundant in the lumina and subendothelial tissues of arteries, frequently obstructing them with a tangle of filaments rich in neutrophils and embedded in fibrin. Occlusion of the left internal carotid artery was due to such a mass. A satisfactory section of the aneurysm was not obtained, but sections of this segment of the internal carotid artery showed ulcerations of the artery wall extending from the luminal surface through to the adventitia.

The wall of the left cavernous sinus was invaded by fungus, as was the pituitary capsule in its entirety, with some extension of the mycelium into the posterior lobe of the gland. The remaining dural sinuses were uninvolved. Intra-arterial extension of the fungus into the brain was evident, with involvement of small areas of the left frontal cortex, left insular cortex and left caudate nucleus. Hyphae penetrated freely into the brain substance and evoked very little inflammatory response. Pial vessels overlying the left temporal lobe, cerebellum, and pyramids also bore their load of fungus and had excited remarkably little meningeal reaction.

The immediate cause of death was considered to be massive intracranial hemorrhage due to rupture of an aneurysm of the left internal carotid artery, the origin of which is still not clear. From its location, it may well have been congenital rather than mycotic. Rupture may have been precipitated by invasion of the wall of the aneurysm by the fungus.

In brief, there was an aneurysm, which may have been a congenital aneurysm to begin with and then became a mycotic aneurysm and ruptured. Or, possibly the aneurysm was entirely fungal in origin. In any event, the case illustrates the affinity the fungus has for arteries and its ability to ulcerate the inner surfaces and to penetrate and weaken the walls of the artery.

In an article entitled "atypical cerebral aneurysms", STEHBENS (1965) of Australia reported the case of a woman of 35 years who had developed acute lymphoblastic leukemia and had received cortisone, antibiotics, purinethol and multiple transfusions. The cortisone therapy favored the entrance and spread of the fungus. Autopsy confirmed the diagnosis of acute leukemia with widespread hemorrhages. A large subdural hematoma was found over the anterior half of the left cerebral hemisphere, with an extensive subarachnoid hemorrhage at the base of the brain. Blood clot was firmly adherent to the right internal carotid artery at the origin of the posterior communicating artery. An aneurysmal sac was not seen, but was believed to be embedded in blood clot and fibrin. Another small artery embedded in clot nearby had a fusiform dilatation over a length of 4 mm. The second, third, fourth, and fifth cranial nerves on the right side were incorporated in the organizing blood clot.

Serial paraffin sections were cut of the fusiform aneurysm and of the right internal carotid artery. On microscopic examination, the architecture of their walls was grossly disturbed by arteritis with extensive infiltration of polymorphonuclear leucocytes, many of which were necrotic. Some loose fibroblastic reaction had occurred, and giant cells were present. Numerous broad branching hyphae, mostly non-septate, had infiltrated the arterial wall and were present in thrombus and inflammatory exudate in the lumen. No sporangia were seen. The diagnosis was made on histological grounds, and meningeal involvement was also found.

In this case there was a fusiform unruptured mucormycotic mycotic aneurysm, and possibly another one which had ruptured.

ABRAMSON et al. (1967), reported from Boston, Massachusetts, a terminal hemorrhage arising from a ruptured mycotic aneurysm of the internal carotid artery, in the carotid canal of the petrous portion of the temporal bone. There were hemorrhagic infarctions in the right parietal and occipital areas. Extensive granulation tissue was present around the cranial nerves at the apex of the right orbit, but no fungi were present in that region. In this case at autopsy there was also necrosis involving the sphenoid bone and adjacent temporal, occipital and frontal bones and superior nasopharynx. Typical large, rarely septate hyphae were present in the necrotic material. The patient was a 38-year-old Negro man with diabetes for many years who developed acidosis and orbital mucormycosis and a mucormycotic mass in the nasopharynx.

Further information than that given in the published report is obtained through the courtesy of Dr. RONALD A. ARKY and Dr. KAROLY BOLOGH of Boston (ABRAMSON et al.). Dr. V. SANGALANG diagnosed thrombosis with aneurysmal rupture of the petrous portion of the right internal carotid artery, secondary to direct extension from mucormycotic infection of the nasopharynx. Longitudinal sections of the thrombosed petrous segment of the right internal carotid artery showed an abrupt transition from the intact to the degenerated segment, especially well demonstrated by elastic tissue stains. The wall was totally replaced by necrotic inflammatory debris with mural thrombosis. Micro-organisms were not seen.

The failure to find hyphae in the wall of the vessel suggested that the necrosis was of ischemic origin due to obstruction of vessels by the mucormycotic process elsewhere.

The above three cases indicate that infiltration and weakening of the walls of arteries by hyphae of mucormycosis may produce aneurysms and rupture of arteries.

Table 3. *Pulmonary Mucormycosis (46 cases)*

Authors and Case Number	Location of Case Age, Sex, Race	Predisposing Factors	Anatomic Involvement	Cultures	Duration	Treatment	Status of Patient
Fürbringer (1876) Case 1	Europe 66, M	Metastatic carcinoma	2 walnut-sized foci, right upper lobe	No	—	—	Dead, mycosis incidental
— Case 2	Europe 31, M	Gastrointestinal catarrh	3 apical walnut-sized nodules	No	—	—	Dead, mycosis incidental
Podack (1899)	Europe 39, M	Carcinoma of pleura	Subpleural nodules	No	—	—	Dead, mycosis incidental
Lang and Grubauer (1923)	Europe 56, F	Tuberculous pulmonary cavity	Wall of pulmonary cavity	Mucor corymbifer	—	—	Dead, mucormycotic and coccal pneum.
Wätgen (1929)	Graz/Austria 34, F	Sarcoma	Hemorrhagic infarcts of lung	No	Not stated	Not stated	Dead, mycosis incidental
Gukelberger (1938)	Bern/Switzerland 46, M	Pneumonia, mild diabetes	Lung	No	2 mos.	Iodides	Living
Lloyd et al. (1949)	Boston/USA 26, F, N	Pregnancy, macerated fetus, dehydration	Lung: infarct of right upper lobe	No	13 days	For dehydration	Dead, mucormycosis
Baker (1956), Case 1 Baker (1962), Case 2	Durham, N.C./USA 47, M, W	Leukemia, cortisone, ACTH	Right lung	No	30 days	Antibiotics	Dead, mucormycosis
— Case 2	Chapel Hill/USA 23, M, W	Leukemia, cortisone	Right lung, right pleura, spleen	No	19 days	6-MP-antibiotics, cortis.	Dead, mucormycosis
— Case 3	Greenwood/USA 51, M, W	Diabetes	Hilus and base of left lung	No	13 days	Antibiotics, insulin	Dead, mucormycosis
— Case 5	Durham/USA 50, M, N	Diabetic acidosis, syphilis	Upper lobes of both lungs	No	8 days	—	Dead, mucormycosis
Keye and McGee (1956), Case 1	St. Louis/USA 38	Hodgkin's disease	Lungs	—	—	—	Dead, mucormycosis

Reference / Case	Location / Age, Sex, Race	Predisposing condition	Organs involved		Duration	Treatment	Outcome
— Case 2	St. Louis/USA 23	Leukemia	Lung	—	—	—	Dead, mucormycosis
— Case 3	St. Louis/USA 1.5	Leukemia	Lung	—	—	—	Dead, mucormycosis
— Case 4	St. Louis/USA 38	Hodgkin's disease	Lung and esophagus	—	—	—	Dead, mucormycosis
— Case 6	St. Louis/USA Age unknown ?	Leukemia	Lungs	—	—	—	Dead, mucormycosis
MAYFIELD and CONDIE (1957)	Seattle/USA 24, M, W	Leukemia, cortisone	Left lung, pulmonary artery	No	23 days	6MP, amethopterin, cortisone	Dead, mucormycosis
STEFANINI (1957)	Boston, USA 35, M	Leukemia, ACTH, steroids	Lungs, pulmonary arteries	No	2 weeks	ACTH, corticosteroids, penicillin	Dead, mucormycosis
TORACK (1957) Case 11	New York/USA 50, F	Leukemia, meticorten	Lung	No	18 days	Urethane, meticorten	Dead, mucormycosis
DILLON et al. (1958) DILLON and SEALY (1962), Case 1	Durham/USA 20, F, N	Diabetic acidosis	Right bronchus intermedius	No	30 days	Resection of right, middle and lower lobes	Cured
BLANKENBERG and VERHOEFF (1959)	Huntersville/USA 23, F, N	None (Diabetes appeared 1 year after operation)	Right, middle, and lower lobes	No	3 mos.	Operative removal	Living
BURNS (1959) Case 3	New York/USA 36, M, N	Diabetic acidosis, prednisone, splenectomy	Right lung, pulmonary arteries, meninges	No	3 days	Prednisone	Dead, mucormycosis
HUTTER (1959) Case 1	New York/USA 13, M, W	Leukemia, Meticorten	Left lower lobe of lungs, heart	No	23 days	6-MP, antibiotics	Dead, mucormycosis
— Case 2	New York/USA 62, M, W	Leukemia, Meticorten	Right upper and lower, and left lower lobes, spleen	No	10 days	6-Chloropurine, antibiotics	Dead, mucormycosis

Table 3. Continuation

Authors and Case Number	Location of Case Age, Sex, Race	Predisposing Factors	Anatomic Involvement	Cultures	Duration	Treatment	Status of Patient
— Case 3	New York/USA 8, M	Lymphosarcoma, Meticorten	Lungs, larynx, heart, esophagus, stomach, ileum	*Mucor*	21 days	Antibiotics, mycostatin	Dead, mucormycosis
SHANKLIN (1959)	Syracuse, USA 54, M, W	Cushing's syndrome	Left upper and lower, and right upper lobes of lungs, thyroid	No	34 days	Antibiotics	Dead, mucormycosis
CUADRADO et al. (1961), Case 2	Dallas/USA 65, F, W	Leukemia	Upper lobes of lungs, main pulmonary artery	No	10 days	6-MP, cortico-tropin, antibiotics	Dead, mucormycosis and leukemia
GLOOR et al. (1961) Case 1	Basel/Switzerland 63, M	Leukopenia, corticosteroids	Right upper lobe, entire left lung	*Rhizopus oryzae*	17 days	Antibiotics, corticosteroids	Dead, mucormycosis
BAKER (1962) Case 4	Durham/USA 20, M, W	Leukemia, neutropenia, Meticorten	Lung, liver	No	4 weeks	Meticorten	Dead, mucormycosis
— Case 9	Durham/USA 70, M, W	Leukemia, neutropenia, prednisone	Right middle lobe of lungs	*Mucor*	6 weeks	Antileukemics, prednisone, antibiotics	Dead, mucormycosis and aspergill.
DILLON and SEALY (1962), Case 2	Durham/USA 15, F	Diabetic acidosis	Right middle lobe	*Mucor*	3 mos.	Lobectomy	Cured
STRAATSMA et al. (1962), Case 15	AFIP Accession No. 545672 55, M, W	Carcinoma and renal insufficiency	Pulmonary	—	—	—	
— Case 16	AFIP Acc. No. 561012; 67, M, W	Leukopenia	Pulmonary	—	—	—	
— Case 17	AFIP Acc. No. 732623; 25, M, W	Leukemia	Pulmonary	—	—	—	
— Case 18	AFIP Accession No. 755869 69, M, W	Carcinoma, diabetes, renal insufficiency	Pulmonary	—	—	—	

			Site	Disseminated	Duration	Treatment	Outcome
— Case 19	AFIP Acc. No. 758019; 67, M, N	Carcinoma	Pulmonary	—	—	—	Dead, mucormycosis
— Case 20	AFIP Acc. No. 846871; 32, M, W	Leukemia	Pulmonary	—	—	—	Dead, mucormycosis
— Case 21	AFIP Acc. No. 915355; 45, M, W	Leukemia	Pulmonary	—	—	—	Dead, mucormycosis
BALASUBRAHMANYAN, CHAUDHURI (1963)	Pondicherry/India 5, M	Uremia of hydro-nephrosis	Both lungs	No	7 days	Antibiotics	Dead, mucormycosis
DARJA and DAVY (1963)	Saskatoon/Canada 72, M, W	Leukemia, steroids	Upper left lobe, right upper and middle lobes of lungs	*Mucor corymbifera*	21 days	Antibiotics, total body irradiation	Dead, mucormycosis
DOUROV and DUSTIN (1964)	Belgium 65, F	Leukemia	Vessels of lungs	No	Not stated	Not stated	Dead, mucormycosis
HUTTER et al. (1964) Case 22	New York/USA 62, M, W	Leukemia, hypogammaglobulinemia, steroid-induced diabetes	Right middle lobe of lungs	No	9 days	Transfusions, X-ray to spleen and prednisone	Dead, aspergillosis and mucormycosis
SUN et al. (1965) Case 8	Peking/China 42, F	Uremia, hydrocortisone	Right upper lobe of lungs, bronchi and vessels	No	Not stated	Antibiotics, hydrocortisone	Dead, uremia, mucormycosis
WALL and MADISON (1965)	Winston-Salem/USA; 36, M, W	Leukemia, prednisone	Right lung and right pulmonary artery	No	3 weeks	Hydroxy urea, prednisone	Dead, mucormycosis, hemoptysis
WINSTON (1965)	England 29, M	Diabetes	Left main bronchus, pulmonary artery	No	35 days	—	Dead, mucormycosis, hemorrhage
ELLIS (1966)	London/England 55, M	Diabetes	Right upper lobe of lungs	No	3 days	Insulin, intravenous fluids, aramine	Dead, mucormycosis

Mucormycosis of the Spinal Cord

There are 3 cases in which spinal cord lesions are mentioned.

In case 3 of Gregory et al. the mucormycosis affected the cervical cord.

In the postmortem examination of case 3 of Banker the hyphae of mucormycosis were identified in the walls and lumens of thrombosed arteries and veins surrounding the thoracic, lumbar and sacral segments of the spinal cord and in the subarachnoid space. The spinal cord was infarcted and had probably been so for 5 days. There was no inflammation or glial reaction. This case was that of a 12-year-old boy with erythroleukemia of a year's duration treated with steroids for 6 months. One month before death he developed spastic paraplegia and a sensory level at the mid-thoracic region. Hyphae were identified in the lungs and kidneys at autopsy as well as in the spinal canal. The infection originated in the lung, and the spinal cord involvement is the result of dissemination of the organisms. The case is listed in Table 6 of disseminated mucormycosis (Banker, 1961).

In case 5 of Parkhurst and Vlahides the spinal cord from T-1 to T-4 was infarcted, with thrombi and hyphae present in adjacent vessels. The autopsy also presented a large hemorrhagic infarct of the left lung with infarction of the pulmonary arteries supplying the infarct. Moreover, in the heart there was an infarct in the right anterior ventricular wall with an adherent mural thrombus. The thrombus and many vessels contained numerous nonseptate hyphae (see Table 6, Parkhurst and Vlahides, 1967). The patient had leukemia and had been treated with steroids and cytotoxic drugs.

Thus, mucormycosis does invade the spinal cord. In one instance it was an extension of the process from the brain in a cranial case, and in two instances a metastatic lesion from pulmonary mucormycosis.

Primary Pulmonary Mucormycosis

Table 3 lists 49 reported cases of pulmonary mucormycosis, but does not indicate 29 cases of disseminated mucormycosis which originated in the lung and displayed primary pulmonary mucormycosis (Table 5). In Table 4 of gastrointestinal mucormycosis there are two cases with pulmonary lesions, but it appears more probable that the infection passed from the digestive tract to the lung, rather than vice versa. Thus there are 78 cases of primary pulmonary mucormycosis in the world literature. This compares with 107 cases of cranial mucormycosis or about 70% as many.

In slightly less than half of the cases of primary pulmonary mucormycosis there was antecedent leukemia and many of the leukemic patients had received corticosteroids. About 10% of the cases developed in diabetic patients and 4% in patients with Hodgkin's disease. There was a variety of other predisposing conditions, and in a few cases, specifically in those of the early German literature, no predisposing condition was cited.

Cultures in the pulmonary cases were reported by Lang and Grubauer (1923) as *Mucor corymbifer*, by Hutter, case 3 (1962) as *Mucor*, by Gloor et al. (1961) as *Rhizopus oryzae*, by Baker (1962) as *Mucor*, by Dillon and Sealy (1962) as *Mucor*, and by Darja and Davy (1963) as *Mucor corymbifera*.

Among the disseminated cases which may have begun in the lungs, cultures were reported by McBride et al. (1960) as *Rhizopus arrhizus*, and by Baker (1962) as *Mucor*.

In summary, *Mucor* was reported 5 times, *Rhizopus* twice, and *Absidia* once. This is in contrast to cranial mucormycosis, in which the reports of cultures listed *Rhizopus* as first and *Mucor* and *Absidia* less frequently. It appears that *Mucor* is the predominant organism in pulmonary cases and *Rhizopus* in cranial cases. However, it would be interesting to analyze the evidence for the diagnosis of *Mucor* and *Absidia* in all of these cases. In many reports there is simply the statement that such and such an organism was cultured and there is no description, illustration, or indication that the organism was submitted to a mycologist with a special interest in the Mucoraceae.

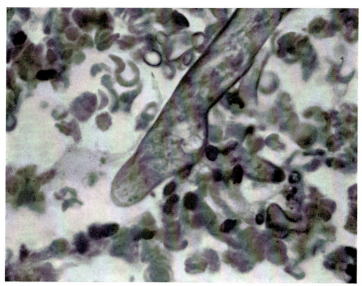

Fig. 29. Pulmonary mucormycosis. Growing tip of nonseptate hypha entering an alveolus (H & E, × 1,000)

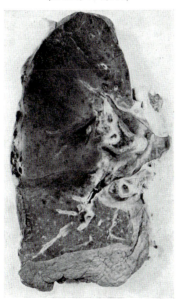

Fig. 30. Pulmonary mucormycosis. Massive mucormycotic infarct of the upper lobe and the upper portion of the lower lobe of the right lung. Note the enormous mucormycotic thrombus of the pulmonary artery and its main branches, and the pleurisy on the lateral aspect of the upper lobe. Duke Hospital autopsy No. 8775

Fürbringer (2 cases) (1876), and Podack (1899) described walnut-sized pulmonary foci and subpleural nodules as instances of mucormycosis of the lung. Lang and Grubauer (1923) found the fungus in the wall of a tuberculous cavity and cultured *Mucor corymbifer*.

Wätjen (1929) described infarcts of the lung.

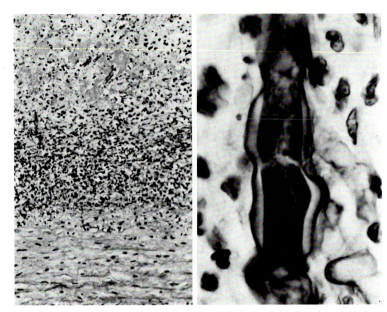

Fig. 31 (left). Mucormycotic thrombosis of an artery of the lung. Media of artery below, neutrophilic infiltrate at periphery of thrombus, and hyaline thrombus with fungus hyphae, at the top. H & E, × 200. Figure 3 of Case 1 of Baker (1956)
(Right). Segment of hypha in the wall of a pulmonary blood vessel. Iron hematoxylin. H & E, × 1487. Figure 4 of Case 1 of Baker (1956)

In the case of pulmonary mucormycosis described by Lloyd et al. (1949), the pleural surfaces of the right lung were pinkish red to purple, with fibrin on the upper lobe, especially posteriorly. This upper lobe was rubbery in consistency. On the pleural surface there were scattered, fine cystic blebs measuring 0.1 cm in diameter, none of which was ruptured. The cut surface of the right upper lobe showed a red, homogeneous, wet surface which oozed large amounts of fluid on pressure. The medial aspect of the right upper lobe just above the interlobar fissue revealed a black, homogeneous-looking area of softening occupying about one third of the lobe, which was in contrast to the firm surrounding red area. The right lower and middle lobes were of a dark red color and had a wet red surface which oozed large amounts of fluid on pressure. The whole lung was subcrepitant to firm in consistency, the upper lobe giving an impression of early consolidation, the middle and lower lobes giving an impression more consistent with atelectasis, congestion, and edema. The pulmonary vessels were dissected to their third and fourth branches. A questionable firm reddish-yellow thrombus was noted at the second bifurcation of the right lower lobe vessel. After fixation, a moderate sized, gray, friable, adherent thrombus was found in the artery leading to the softened area in the right upper lobe.

The left lung was congested.

The bronchial mucosa was a deep reddish pink and edematous. The lumen contained tenacious, reddish gray, mucopurulent material. The hilar nodes showed moderate anthracosis.

Microscopically, Lloyd et al. examined 18 sections of lung. Sections from the soft, black, homogeneous area of the right upper lobe showed broad fungal hyphae devoid of cross septa. In the lung tissue where the mycelia were numerous there was preservation of the alveolar pattern but the cellular detail was blurred. There was abundance of cellular debris and edema fluid in the alveolar spaces. The pleura was markedly thickened and edematous. There was a fibrinopurulent exudate on the surface containing many polymorphonuclear neutrophils. One section showed a definite, recent, pulmonary infarct with the characteristic microscopic findings. Section of the pulmonary artery supplying the area of the infarct showed a large, antemortem thrombus with massive invasion of the thrombus and of the vessel walls by mycelial hyphae.

This careful examination and description of Lloyd et al. indicates clearly that the lesion of the right upper lobe was an antemortem infarct dependent upon vascular thrombosis stimulated by the intraluminal growth of the fungus. This pulmonary picture is presented in the majority of the cases subsequently reported.

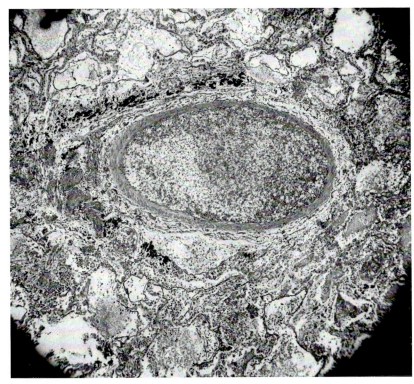

Fig. 32. Mucormycotic thrombus of an artery in the mucormycotic infarct of the lower lobe of the right lung in case 11 of BAKER (1962). The pulmonary infection gave rise to the metastatic infarct of the brain illustrated previously. H & E, × 60. Hyphae are hardly visible in the thrombus. In G.M.S. stain they would be easily visible. Figure 14, case 11 of BAKER (1962)

MURPHY and BORNSTEIN (1950) obtained a calcified nodule of the lung at operation and reported it as an example of mucormycosis. The cross section of the excised specimen shows concentric rings and there is a thin peripheral capsule. The appearance suggests histoplasmosis. The photomicrographs are not sharp, and the appearances of the organisms of mucormycosis are not clearly shown. A *Mucor* was grown from the calcified material and injected into a rabbit. The photomicrograph of the section of kidney from the rabbit shows non-septate hyphae like those of mucormycosis. The cultured fungus was identified as *Absidia italiana* (COST and PERIN) Dodge. The case must be listed as doubtful because of the uncharacteristic appearance of the fungus in the human tissue preparations.

The case of NICOD et al. (1952), reported as a double pulmonary infection with *Aspergillus fumigatus* and *Mucor pusillus*, also lacks documentation with respect to histopathology.

BAKER (1956) reported four cases of primary pulmonary mucormycosis, two in patients with leukemia and two in patients with diabetes (Figs. 30—36). The pulmonary lesions were as follows:

Case 1: Thrombosis, massive infarct, pneumonia, pleurisy, right lung; mycotic bronchitis.

Case 2: Thrombosis, infarct, right lower lobe; mycotic bronchitis.

Case 3: Thrombo-arteritis, thrombo-phlebitis, mycotic pneumonia, left lung; mycotic bronchitis.

Case 4: Thrombo-arteritis, mycotic pneumonia, right upper lobe.

MAYFIELD and CONDIE (1957) reported mucormycotic thrombosis of intrapulmonic arteries with pulmonary infarcts. An interesting feature of their case was the presence of a mucormycotic mural thrombus of the main pulmonary artery close to the pulmonary valve.

DILLON et al. (1958) reported a case, in a diabetic patient, of mucormycosis of the bronchus successfully treated by lobectomy. Biopsies of the distal portion of the right bronchus intermedius had shown the broad nonseptate hyphae in the necrotic wall of the bronchus. There

56*

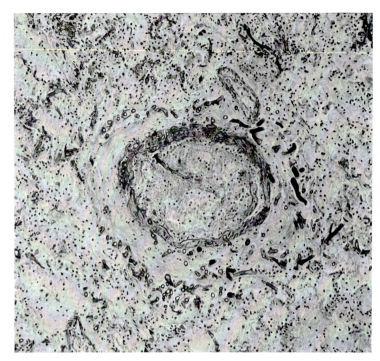

Fig. 33. Pulmonary mucormycosis. Hyphae in and about a thrombosed blood vessel within a pulmonary infarct. H & E, × 150. From CONANT et al. (1954) (Fig. 105)

was an abscess in the removed right lower lobe, but without fungus organisms. The mucormycosis of the bronchus apparently had led to the development of the pulmonary abscess of other cause. Or, the abscess could have been a softened infarct.

In the case of BLANKENBERG and VERHOEFF (1959) there was a cavity measuring 6 by 5 by 4 cm in the resected right lower lobe and another cavity measuring 4 by 4 by 4 cm in the resected right middle lobe. The cavities were surrounded by thick layers of grayish-brown fibrinous hemorrhagic material and thick layers of indurated whitish-gray necrotic tissue. Many branches of the medium-sized bronchi were completely obliterated and filled with necrotic whitish-brown firm material. Cross sections of the lung showed many foci of yellowish-gray, firm, and soft friable areas near the large cavity. Microscopically there were areas of liquifaction necrosis surrounded by thick layers of eosinophilic, amorphous, or granular material with mild infiltration of neutrophils, lymphocytes and plasma cells. Many multinucleated foreign body giant cells were seen. In the necrotic area numerous basophilic, irregularly shaped structures were observed. Around the necrotic spaces many large blood vessels and bronchi showed almost complete necrosis of the wall. Other blood vessels showed hyalinization of the wall or recent thrombus of the lumen, characterized by obliteration with spindle shaped cells with hyperchromatic large nuclei. Occasionally even small bronchi contained much foreign material. The foreign material was characterized by broad branching coenocytic hyphae of varying thickness. When the fungus appeared to be growing luxuriantly, it was thick; in regions in which infarction had occurred or the tissues were necrotic, hyphae were shrunken and irregular. A marked tendency to invade vessels was noted.

It is my opinion that the cavities represented liquifaction of infarcts. The clinical history suggested that the process in the lungs might have begun more than three months prior to lobectomy when a non-productive cough began. Nearly six weeks before lobectomy she developed what she described as a chest cold. Nineteen days before lobectomy she began to produce about one ounce of blood-streaked sputum daily and developed a fever. There was some evidence at this time that there was an associated bacterial infection, and there was x-ray evidence of some form of pneumonia in the left lung. However, I would think it likely that the cavities in this case, and in the case reported by DILLON et al., represented liquifaction necrosis of *pulmonary infarcts* caused by mucormycosis. These would represent late stages of pulmonary infarcts.

In Case 3 of BURNS (1959) there was *thrombosis of the pulmonary artery* branches to the left upper and lower lobes with pulmonary infarction. The thrombosis was due to invasion of the pulmonary artery by mycelia of mucormycosis. In addition, mycelia were in the pulmonary alveoli. In this case there was a history of slight left ptosis, and it may be that the case is primarily of cranial type. I have, however, classified it as primarily pulmonary because the pulmonary findings were so striking, but may be in error in so doing.

Case 1 of HUTTER (1959) was that of a boy with acute leukemia. In each upper lobe of the lungs there were yellowish-gray bulging zones, 1 cm in diameter, surrounded by congestion. The artery to the posterior basal segment of the left lower lobe was thrombosed and was surrounded by congestion. Microscopically this vessel contained a fungus with large, coenocytic (nonseptate) hyphae with branching at obtuse angles. These hyphae were present in other smaller vessels and extended through their walls and into the parenchyma, where there was infarction. Alveoli contained hyaline membranes, and smaller vessels had pale hyaline material appearing like loose white thrombi. Aspiration pneumonitis, clumps of bacteria, and leukemic infiltrate were also noted in the lungs. Dr. HUTTER's comment was: "This child had pulmonary mucormycosis with mycotic embolization to the myocardium. There was also histological evidence of bacterial infection in the lungs. Although the infecting fungi may have been airborne, the possibility of infection from draining maxillary sinuses exists. Possible predisposing factors were leukemia, chemotherapy (steroids and antibiotics) and metabolic alterations (steroid-induced diabetes).

In HUTTER's case 2, at autopsy, the infarct in the right upper lobe measured 5 by 5 by 3 cm, the one in the right lower lobe, 3 cm in diameter. An infarct in the left lower lobe was small and was not measured. The vessels adjacent to the hemorrhagic areas contained antemortem clots. Microscopically there were branching, nonseptate hyphae in these clots as well as in smaller arteries and venules. The fungi extended through vessel walls and were plentiful in the alveoli as well as in the bronchioles. Pulmonary mucormycosis with mycotic embolization to the spleen were the essential features of this case.

In Case 3 of HUTTER the lungs (the right 600, and the left 300 g in weight) had numerous nodular hemorrhagic infarcts that on section showed central yellow pinhead-sized foci. There were also ulcerations of the major branches of the right main stem bronchus and granular reddish tan exudate on the vocal cords. Microscopically, there was marked bronchial and bronchiolar infestation with the organisms of mucormycosis. Two observations were of note: (1) the hyphae appeared to penetrate intact mucosal epithelium in places; and (2) sporangia were noted in the lumina of the bronchi. There were mucormycotic thrombi of large and small arteries and veins; red and white cells, and fibrin and platelets were present. The fungi penetrated the walls of bronchi and vessels and were present in alveoli in the surrounding zone of hemorrhagic infarction. Alveoli at the periphery of the infarct contained fibrin deposits. The vocal cords were ulcerated, and numerous hyphae of mucormycosis were penetrating into the tissue. In the aerated lumen sporangia were forming. In addition, there were numerous blastospores and pseudomycelia, characteristic of *Candida*, present on the surface of the vocal cords.

In the case of pulmonary *mucormycosis* complicating *Cushing's syndrome* reported by SHANKLIN, his Fig. 1 shows the posterior halves of the lungs with a cavity 5—7 cm in diameter in the left lower lobe, containing soft, friable, caseous material. In other parts of the left lower lobe there were several smaller cavities, 1—2 cm in diameter of a similar type. Other similar areas were found in the left upper lobe. In the apex of the right upper lobe there was a similar area, sharply demarcated by scar tissue. Microscopically, he describes foci of infarction, abscesses with hyphae and thrombosed vessels. Grossly, the lesions in the lungs are not wedge-shaped and do not extend to the pleura at the level of section, but are rounded and look like abscesses. The microscopic description suggests that they are truly infarcts with disintegration of the infarcted tissue, simulating abscesses.

In case 2 of CUADRADO et al. (1961) there were numerous wedge-shaped, dark red infarcts in the upper lobes of the lungs. The main pulmonary artery contained a premortem thrombus that occluded the main branch to the right upper lobe. Microscopically, organisms of mucormycosis were numerous in thrombi and infarcts.

In case 1 of GLOOR et al. (1961) there were, in both lungs, numerous large and small arteries occluded with fresh thrombi. In both upper lobes and in the left lower lobe there were larger hemorrhagic infarcts. In addition, there were foci of terminal bronchopneumonia in the lower lobes.

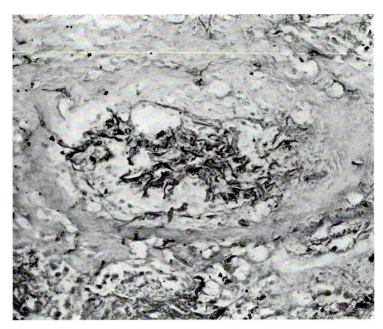

Fig. 34. Shrunken hyphae in the thrombosed lumen of a pulmonary vessel in an infarct of long duration. H & E, × 100

In illustration of his case 4, BAKER (1962) pictures a gray, firm, infarct of the right middle lobe, of 4 weeks' duration. There was a brown, thick exudate in the right pleural cavity, and fibrous adhesions overlay the right pleural cavity. Microscopically, the vessels and pulmonary parenchyma of the infarct contained thrombi and nonseptate hyphae. In the peripheral region there was granulation tissue and fibrosis.

At the postmortem examination of case 9 of BAKER there was hemorrhagic consolidation of the upper portion of the right lower lobe and the lower portion of the left lower lobe. In these consolidated areas there were yellow nodules, measuring from 0.5—1.5 cm in diameter. Microscopically, thrombi with non-septate hyphae were observed in the lesions of the lung.

In DILLON and SEALY's case 2 a right middle lobe was removed surgically. Mucormycotic organisms were found in sections of the wall of an abscess in this middle lobe. One wonders if this abscess represented disintegration of an infarct.

In the case of BALASUBRAHMANYAN and CHAUDHURI (1963) there were small, firm areas scattered throughout the middle and upper lobes of the right lung and both lobes of the left lung.

On section, these were firm and congested and looked like small areas of necrosis. Microscopically, these nodules showed edema of the alveoli with small areas of necrosis around which dense collections of inflammatory cells were visible. The lesions were close to blood vessels which showed invasion of their walls and lumina by non-segmented mycelia.

These foci apparently represented scattered nodules of infarction dependent upon thrombosis.

In DARJA and DAVY's case there was a raised, purple area 7 cm in diameter in the base of the upper lobe of the left lung, and another such area 11 cm in diameter in the base of the right middle lobe. The pulmonary artery divisions leading to the upper lobe of each lung and to the right middle lobe were occluded by thrombi. On section, the indurated areas were well-circum-

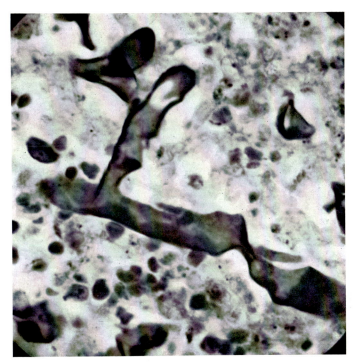

Fig. 35. Thrombus of a pulmonary blood vessel containing hyphae of mucormycosis. From a case of leukemia complicated by the cenocytic fungus infection. G.M.S., × 800

scribed, purplish-red and centrally necrotic. Multiple blood vessels within these hemorrhagic areas were thrombosed. Small amounts of mucus were present in the bronchi. Microscopically tangles of broad non-septate hyphae occupied many air-spaces and infiltrated the alveolar septa. Penetration of hyphae into the walls of arteries with thrombosis and infarction was conspicuous. Hyphae were incorporated in the thrombi. Tissue necrosis was extensive.

In case 8 of SUN et al. (1965) the lesion was in the right upper lobe. Hyphae of mucormycosis were seen in bronchial lumina and blood vessels of this region. There was acute suppurative inflammation and the formation of small abscesses in the surrounding pulmonary tissue.

This description is different in two respects from that in the previous cases. Infarction is not mentioned and abscess formation is a prominent feature. However, there were hyphae in bronchi and in blood vessels. If there were hyphae in blood vessels, there were certainly thrombi and probably infarcts. The author does not illustrate the appearances. Infarction may be attended with pronounced neutrophilic infiltrates.

In the case of WALL and MADISON (1965), fatal pulmonary phycomycosis complicating leukemia, there was adherent, occlusive, dark red thrombotic material 3 cm proximal to the hilar bifurcation of the right pulmonary artery. Distally, the lung was mottled dark red. Microscopically, hematoxylinophilic coenocytic hyphae permeated and apparently colonized the thrombotic material and were scattered through the disrupted internal elastic membrane of the artery. In addition, there was associated arteritis and early organization of the thrombus. Focal ischemic necrosis was present in the upper and lower right lung lobes; in viable tissue there was pulmonary edema.

WINSTON (1965) reported a case of mucormycosis in a 29-year-old diabetic man in whom death was due to hemorrhage from a lesion of the right main bronchus and adjacent pulmonary artery. The right main brochus was almost completely blocked by a soft grayish-purple mass. On section a spherical mass $1^{1}/_{2}$ cm in diameter infiltrated the bronchus and the pulmonary artery. The lesion was an ischemic infarct of the bronchus and pulmonary artery surrounded by polymorphonuclear neutrophils. Rupture had occurred at the edge of the infarct and here there was fibrosis. Hyphae were plentiful in the infarct.

This rupture of an artery of the lung, with hemorrhage, is reminiscent of the similar process in the cranial cavity when the internal carotid becomes weakened by the mycotic arteritis and forms an aneurysm and ruptures.

Summary of Primary Pulmonary Mucormycosis

From this review of the findings in the lungs in reported cases of pulmonary mucormycosis there emerges a picture of the pathology of this condition.

It becomes clear that the usual initial process is the proliferation of the fungus in the bronchi at the hilus of the lung. These *penetrate* into the hilar structures but especially into the *arteries*. It is not clear why the fungus prefers arteries to veins, but it is clear that arteritis is much more frequent than phlebitis. The fungus, once within the artery, produces thrombosis. There may be huge thrombi in the main pulmonary artery to a lung, or in the smaller branches to capillary size. An infarct develops, possibly because of concomitant involvement of veins and lymphatics. This thought is interjected because, in general, infarcts of the lung do not develop except in the presence of chronic passive congestion due to congestive failure.

The infarcts may be massive, involving two or more lobes or they may be small and multiple, only a centimeter or so in diameter. They are not always wedge-shaped.

The early infarcts are hemorrhagic and they may remain this type for, certainly, a week or so. At a later stage they are gray and homogeneous, and often there is scar tissue about them and thickening of the pleura.

A later stage is softening of the infarct to form a cavity often erroneously interpreted as an abscess cavity. Possibly some of these cavities are abscess cavities due to secondary bacterial infection.

The lesions of the lung almost always have the vascular obstructive features mentioned. There is certainly an element of acute edematous and fibrinous bronchopneumonia, accompanying or complicating the infarction.

The only other form of primary involvement is ulceration of a main bronchus by the fungus. There is usually also involvement of the larger arteries. The last case cited was of this type, and fatal hemorrhage ensued.

Hematogenous Pulmonary Mucormycosis

We have seen, in our consideration of cranial mucormycosis, that the fungus can gain a foothold in the orbit or paranasal sinuses and disseminate through the systemic circulation to the lungs. The case of BAKER and SEVERANCE, reported in more detail in BAKER (1956) is pertinent:

On the day before the death of this child of 3 years, the left pupil was much larger than the right pupil, and there was hemorrhage in the left eye. At autopsy the left orbital fat was congested and red in contrast to the ordinary yellow fat of the right orbit. On the inferior surface of the left frontal lobe of the brain there was an area of injection and softening which measured 4 by 2.5 cm. The left internal carotid artery presented a thrombus at the level where it was severed in removing the brain and there were thrombi in vessels of the left middle fossa.

These findings indicate that the infection began in the cranial region of this diabetic child. At the *postmortem examination* the lower lobe of the left lung was congested and edematous on cut section, and there was a dark purple area, 4 cm in diameter, in the middle of the lobe with thrombi in branches of the pulmonary artery. The bronchi contained thick, brown, mucoid material. The upper lobe on the left was pink and air-containing. The upper right lobe was congested and edematous on cut section, with a severely congested area 2 cm in diameter. There was a thrombosed vein leading from this lobe. The middle lobe was dark purple, but air-containing. The lower lobe was pink, edematous, and rubbery. The bronchi on the right contained more of the thick, brown, mucinoid material noted on the left.

The *microscopic findings* supported the gross observations and clinical story indicating that the case was primarily cranial. Branching hyphae were numerous in the orbital tissues.

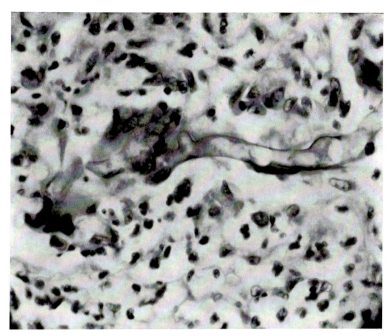

Fig. 36. Giant cell response to a hypha in case 7 of BAKER (1956), a disseminated case of 3 to 4 months duration. Giant cell response is very uncommon (H & E, × 700)

Microscopically, sections of bronchi of all sizes contained branching hyphae, 4—18 μ thick and up to 100 μ long, with occasional neutrophils and red cells. The wall of the largest bronchus was necrotic. The pulmonary parenchyma was not necrotic and contained numerous hyphae like those in the bronchi. Alveolar exudate consisted of edema fluid, hemorrhage, fibrin, and small numbers of neutrophils. The larger hilar blood vessels presented hyphae everywhere, including, especially, permeation of walls. Thrombi estimated to be of several day's duration, also showed hyphae. They occluded all but an axial pathway for fluid blood. Organization of thrombi was not observed. Many of the smaller vessels contained fluid blood. Lymph vessels in edematous pulmonary fibrous septa contained hyphae and neutrophils. Since all of the numerous sections of lung showed hyphae, it was presumed that the infection involved all lobes of both lungs (Fig. 29). There were fungi in hilar lymph nodes, fat, connective tissue, perineurial lymphatics, nerve trunks and pleura.

Thus we see how completely the metastatic fungus permeated the tissues of the lungs, including the bronchi and pleura. The pulmonary lesions were early infarcts and edematous pneumonia.

Similar cases of pulmonary lesions resulting from hematogenous dissemination from primarily cranial mucormycosis are reported by MARTIN et al., BRYAN et al., LONG and WEISS, FUENTES (case 1), and SUGA. The ages of their patients were 2½ months, 34 months, 24 years, 9 years, and 38 years. Including the case of BAKER and SEVERANCE, 4 of the cases were in the pediatric age group and 2 in the adult group. This suggests that hematogenous, systemic, dissemination from cranial mucormycosis may be more frequent in children and infants than in adults.

In the 34-month-old diabetic girl reported by BRYAN et al. (1958) the metastatic lesions of the lung were described as follows: The upper and lower lobes of the right lung and the lower lobe of the left lung were bluish, firm and non-aerated; the remaining lobes were congested. Histologically, fibrin thrombi occluded the vessels of the lungs and these thrombi showed fungi. There was an associated fibrinous, hemorrhagic, fluid exudate in the air spaces. This was thought to be more an effect of infarction than of the direct toxic effect of the fungi.

Table 4. *Esophageal and Gastrointestinal Mucormycosis*

Authors and Case Number	Location of Case Age, Sex, Race	Predisposing Factors	Anatomic Involvement	Cultures	Duration	Treatment	Status of Patient
Marchand (1910)	Leipzig, Germany 18, F, W	Mushroom poisoning	Stomach, ulcer	No	15 days	Not stated	Dead
Beneke (1911)	Marburg/Germ. 33, M, W	None	Stomach, ulcer	No	Few days	Not stated	Dead, pneumonia
Ljubimowa (1913)	St. Petersburg/Russia; 46, F, W	None	Stomach	No	1 day	Exploratory operation	Dead, peritonitis
Teutschländer (1917)	Heidelberg/Germ. 64, M, W	None	Stomach	No	7 days	Gastroenter-ostomy	Dead, pneumonia
Löhlein (1920) Case 2	Germany Male	War prisoner. Malnutrition?	Stomach	No	—	—	Dead
Moore et al. (1949)	Milwaukee/USA 37, F, W	None	Large intestine with perforation of cecum	No	15 days	Sulfonamide	Dead, generalized peritonitis
Lie Kian Joe and N. Eng (1956)	Java 48, F, Chinese	None	Stomach; ulcer of lesser curvature	No	6 months	Resection	Well
Baker et al. (1957) Case 1	Durham/USA 43, M, W	Cortisone, Toxic hepatitis	Small and large intestines, stomach and liver	No	3 days	Cortisone, tetracycline	Dead, gangrene of intestine and intestinal hemorrhage
— Case 2	Jackson/USA 75, M, W	None	Cecum and ascending colon	No	12 days	Intravenous fluids	Dead, mucormycosis and bronchopneum.
Clark (1957)	Cleveland/USA 59, M, W	Diabetes, leukemia (?)	Duodenum with extension to left lobe of liver and cecum	No	5 weeks	Antibiotics	Dead, mucormycosis; terminal pneumonia
Torack (1957) Case 10	New York/USA 65, M, W	Aplastic anemia	Stomach	No	4 days	Corticosteroids, antibiot.	Dead, mucormycosis
Watson (1957)	Natal/Afr. 26 mos., M, N	Kwashiorkor	Anterior stomach wall, perforation	No	4 weeks	High-protein diet	Dead, mucormycosis

GATLING (1959)	Roanoke/USA 16 days, F, W	Otitis media	Entire stomach wall, extension to adjacent organs	No	11 days	Antibiotics, nystatin	Dead, mucormycosis
MONTENEGRO et al. (1959) Case 1	São Paulo/Brazil 10 months, F	Malnutrition	Small intestine	—	3 days	Nystatin	Dead, bronchopneumonia
— Case 2	São Paulo/Brazil 1 F	Malnutrition	Colon	—	30 days	—	Dead, intestinal hemorrhage
LEVIN and ISAACSON (1960)	Johannesburg/Afr. Premature, N	Prematurity	Descending colon with perforation	No	5 days	Antibiotics	Dead, meconium peritonitis
NEAME, RAYNER (1960), Case 1	Durban/S. Afr. 20, M	Amebic colitis, hepatitis	Stomach	—	—	—	—
— Case 2	Durban/S. Afr. 52, M	Pellagra	Esophagus, colon	—	—	—	—
— Case 3	Durban/S. Afr. 47, M	Uremia	Stomach	—	11 days	—	—
— Case 4	Durban/S. Afr. 23, F	Uremia, peritonitis	Stomach, colon, liver	—	13 days	—	—
— Case 5	Durban/S. Afr. 36, F	Uremia	Stomach	—	27 days	—	—
— Case 6	Durban/S. Afr. 2, F	Amebic colitis and liver abscess	Colon	—	28 days	—	—
— Case 8	Durban/S. Afr. 30, M	Amebic colitis, renal tuberculosis	Colon	—	14 days	—	—
— Case 9	Durban/S. Afr. 3, F	Kwashiorkor, pulm. tuberculosis	Stomach	—	15 days	—	—
— Case 10	Durban/S. Afr. 1, F	Kwashiorkor	Colon, stomach, liver, gall bladder	—	70 days	—	—
— Case 12	Durban/S. Afr. 2, M	Kwashiorkor, empyema	Stomach, colon	—	9 days	—	—
— Case 13	Durban/S. Afr. 11 months, F	Kwashiorkor	Stomach	Rhizopus microsporus van Tiegh	15 days	—	—

Table 4. Continuation

Authors and Case Number	Location of Case Age, Sex, Race	Predisposing Factors	Anatomic Involvement	Cultures	Duration	Treatment	Status of Patient
— Case 14	Durban/S. Afr. 6 days, M	Prematurity	Stomach, colon. liver	—	3 days	—	—
— Case 15	Durban/S. Afr. 2, M	Kwashiorkor	Esophagus, rectum	*Rhizopus stolonifer* (Syn. *R. nigricans*)	14 days	—	—
— Case 16	Durban/S. Afr. 27, F	Typhoid, peritonitis	Colon	*Rhizopus microsporus* van Tiegh	8 days	—	—
— Case 17	Durban/S. Afr. 11 months, M	Kwashiorkor	Colon	*Rhizopus stolonifer* (Syn. *R. nigricans*)	35 days	—	—
— Case 18	Durban/S. Afr. 26, M	Amebic dysentery with peritonitis	Colon	—	12 days	—	—
— Case 19	Durban/S. Afr. 50, F	Amebic dysentery with peritonitis	Stomach	*Rhizopus stolonifer, Rhiz. micro- sporus, Mucor hiemalis*	4 days	—	—
— Case 20	Durban/S. Afr. 2, F	Kwashiorkor	Stomach	*Rhizopus microsporus*	56 days	—	—
— Case 21	Durban/S. Afr. 35, M	Typhoid	Ileum	—	12 days	—	—
— Case 22	Durban/S. Afr. 37, F	Hepatic failure	Stomach	—	—	—	—
Sutherland and Jones (1960)	Acornhoek/Transv. 50, M, N	None	Greater curvature of stomach near cardia, 5 × 8 cm. "tumor"	No	1 month	Penicillin	Dead, terminal pneumonia

Cuadrado et al. (1961), Case 3	Dallas/USA 8, M, W	Leukemia, steroids	Right colon and lung	No	Not stated	6-MP, aminopterin, steroids	Dead, mucormycosis
De Feo (1961)	Schenectady/USA 51, M	Leukemia, hydrocortisone	Descending colon, branch of pulmonary artery	No	3 weeks	Antibiotics, hydrocortisone	Dead, peritonitis, mucormycotic perforation
Trujillo (1961)	Medellin/Colombia 7 months, M, W	Enteritis, dehydration	Stomach and duodenum	No	—	Operative exploration	—
Straatsma et al. (1962), Case 22	AFIP Accession No. 571372 36, M, Mongolian	Gastroenteritis	Gastrointestinal mucormycosis	—	—	—	—
— Case 23	AFIP Acc. No. 955878; 37, M, N	Diabetic acidosis and renal failure	Gastrointestinal mucormycosis	—	—	—	—
— Case 24	AFIP Acc. No. 996826; 70, M, N	Renal insufficiency	Gastrointestinal mucormycosis	—	—	—	—
Kahn (1963)	South Africa 17, F, N	Diabetes, puerperium	Stomach and esophagus	No	—	—	Dead
Abramowitz (1964)	South Africa 35, M, N	None	Stomach and colon	No	13 days	Hydrocortis., antibiotics	Dead, peritonitis
Kubo (1965)	Japan	—	Stomach and duodenum	—	—	—	—
Stein and Schmaman (1965), Case 1	Johannesburg/SA 35, M, N	Malnutrition	Stomach and duodenum	No	9 days	Antibiotics, operation	Dead, peritonitis
— Case 2	Johannesburg/SA 35, M, N	—	Stomach with pyloric ulcer, 3 cm diameter	No	4 days	Surgical	Dead, peritonitis
Sun et al. (1965) Case 6	Peking/China 23 days, M, Chin.	Prematurity, Hydrocortisone	Pyloric antrum of stomach	No	24 days	Surgical	Dead, post-operative
Calle and Klatsky (1966)	Baltimore/USA 23, F, N	None	Infarcts, ulcers, terminal ileum and cecum	No	28 days	Antibiotics	Dead, generalized peritonitis
Peña (1967)	Colombia Newborn	Prematurity	Small intestine	No	15 days	—	Dead, mucormycosis

In the 24-year-old pregnant diabetic patient of Long and Weiss (1959) the metastatic pulmonary lesions were in the posterosuperior portion of the lower right lobe where there was a poorly demarcated pyramidal acrepetant lesion. There was a thrombus in an artery leading to this infarct. Microscopically there were phycomycetes in vessels of the lung and in the pulmonary tissue. Their Fig. 1 shows the fungus in the pulmonary vessel with destruction of the vessel wall and thrombosis.

In the 9-year-old diabetic boy reported by Fuentes the thoracic cavities showed no macroscopic alterations of importance except for severe congestion of organs. Microscopically colonies of fungi were observed with the production of focal chronic inflammation. This disposition of organisms and this type of inflammation is extraordinary and peculiar in a case with a short clinical course.

These are sufficient examples to indicate that the metastatic pulmonary lesions from cranial mucormycosis are less striking and well-defined than in primary pulmonary mucormycosis, probably because they develop late in the course of the infection.

In summary, pulmonary lesions of mucormycosis may be encountered in postmortem examination of cases dying of primary cranial infection. Such dissemination appears to be more frequent in infancy and childhood than in adult life. The fungus comes to lie in the vascular bed of the lungs. It produces thromboses of vessels, and swarms into the pulmonary parenchyma and hilar structures including the main bronchi. Infarction develops and there is an edematous pneumonia as well. The lesions are like those of primary pulmonary mucormycosis, but less advanced.

In some of the cases of gastrointestinal mucormycosis (Table 4), there were also lesions in the lung, and the question is whether the fungus infected the digestive tract first and spread to the lung, or vice versa. In some of the cases of disseminated mucormycosis (Table 5). the infection may have begun in the gastrointestinal tract and spread to the lung.

Esophageal Mucormycosis

Esophageal mucormycosis is much less common than esophageal candidosis (Table 4). The instances of mucormycosis of the esophagus mentioned in the literature follow:

In Case 3 of Hutter (1959) the lower end of the esophagus was eroded, and hemorrhage extended throughout all layers. Histologically there were numerous hyphae and sporangia of "*Mucor*" in the lumen. Hyphae extended interstitially through all walls and penetrated vessels. Blastospores and pseudomycelia of *Candida* were present superficially without deep penetration. This then, was a double mycotic infection of the esophagus.

In case 4 of Hutter there were gross ulcers of the esophagus. On microscopic examination, the esophageal ulcers contained submucosal "*Mucor*" thrombi with infarction of the overlying mucosa. There were fibrin clots and hemorrhagic dissection through the muscle wall, with intramural *Mucor* thrombi in small vessels. Hyphae were also present interstitially. On the surface of the mucosa there were large clusters of blastospores of *Candida* (no pseudohyphae) and colonies of bacteria.

In both of Hutter's cases the esophageal mucormycosis was probably blood-borne because the lesions were deep in the wall of the esophagus and because the lesions in the body were disseminated, indicating mycemia. However, in the first case, with hyphae of "*Mucor*" in the esophageal lumen, the fungus may have spread directly into the wall.

In case 1 of McBride et al. the distal third of the esophagus was black and ulcerated. The necrotic membranous inflammation of the distal esophagus was sharply separated from the uninvolved esophagus above and the stomach below, as shown in Fig. 2 of the article. Microscopically in the wall of the distal segment of the esophagus there were many hyphae and extensive areas of necrosis, hemorrhage, neutrophilic infiltration and vascular thrombosis.

Two of the cases of Neame and Rayner (1960) had esophageal lesions. One case had multiple small ulcers and the other large ulcers.

Kahn (1963) reported an esophageal and gastric mucormycosis.

Miyake and Okudaira (1967) tabulate mucormycosis of the esophagus in one or two cases in which the infection was in multiple organs.

Mucormycosis of the Stomach

For cases in which the mucormycosis of the stomach is the only mucormycotic lesion in the body, or when it is clearly the primary lesion, the descriptions of the gross and microscopic features follow in chronologic sequence (See Table 4).

BENEKE (1911) described a small, elongated, gray-white ulcer close to the pylorus of the stomach. Microscopically, thick, largely non-septate hyphae were growing into blood vessels and there was thrombosis. Bacilli were present. Death in this case was not due to mucormycosis but to a terminal pneumonia and the lesion of the stomach was an incidental finding. It was not unlike a chronic peptic ulcer.

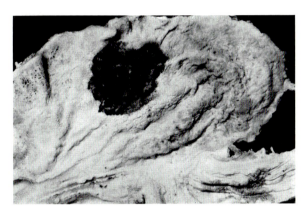

Fig. 37. Mucormycosis of stomach in chronic lymphocytic leukemia. The black slough is an infarct caused by fungal thrombosis. From case 5 of BAKER (1962), which also had lesions in the lung, liver, and kidney. The gastric lesion is secondary

LIE KIAN JOE and NJO-INJO TJOIE ENG (1956) described a surgical specimen of gastric mucormycosis. Roentgenograms of the stomach had showed a large defect filled with barium on the lesser curvature. It was noted during the operation that the stomach was thickened along the lesser curvature. Partial gastrectomy was performed. The removed tissue showed an ulcer. Eighty sections were cut of a block from the stomach wall. The slides showed an ulcer with overhanging edges. The ulcer extended to the muscular layer. The base of the ulcer consisted of three zones, a thin one of necrotic tissue, a zone of granulation tissue with many dilated blood capillaries and a broad zone of fibrous or scar tissue which contained blood vessels with thick walls. This scar tissue reached to the peritoneum. It had almost entirely destroyed the muscular coat under the ulcer. Small pieces of muscular tissue, remnants of the muscular coat, were seen in the scar tissue. Numerous neutrophils were present in the zone of granulation tissue. The inflammatory reaction in the scar tissue was chronic. A feature was the presence of many eosinophils diffusely scattered throughout the granulation tissue, giving it a reddish appearance. In the scar tissue the eosinophils were around blood vessels with plasma cells and round cells. The submucosa at the margin of the ulcer was thickened by the same fibrous tissue as that found at the base of the ulcer. Cross and longitudinal sections of large hyphae were found in the necrotic zone and in the zone of granulation tissue at the base of the ulcer, not in the scar tissue. The hyphae had a thin wall and were blue-violet in the H and E slides. They contained a granular mass, reddish brown in color. No septate divisions were seen. Their diameter varied from 3.5—34 μ and they were present in the necrotic zone singly or in small groups. From here they grew into the zone of living granulation tissue where they were often found in small abscesses. One doubtful giant cell was found in one of the slides. The hyphae showed no tendency to grow into the blood vessels. Groups of bacteria were seen in the necrotic zone. No culture could be made.

In discussion of their case, LIE KIAN JOE and NJO-INJO TJOEI ENG refer to the presence of many eosinophils and say that as far as they know there is only one fungus among the Phycomycetes which provokes a prominent tissue eosinophilia in man, i. e. *Basidiobolus ranarum*, a saprophytic fungus found in the digestive tract of frogs and lizards and in beetles which feed upon the excrement of these animals and are in turn eaten by them. This fungus was found to cause induration and swelling of the subcutaneous tissue in Indonesian boys. Marked tissue eosinophilia was also found in pigs which were infected with *Absidia racemosa* or *Rhizopus equinus*, both members of the family Mucoraceae (CHRISTIANSEN, 1929). However, it seemed unlikely to the authors that the fungus in their case was identical with one of these, or with *Basidiobolus ranarum*, because of a marked difference in diameter of the hyphae.

In addition to this reason against the fungus being *Basidiobolus ranarum* is the fact that there is no hyaline substance adjacent to the fungus, as is so characteristic of cases of subcutaneous phycomycosis caused by *Basidiobolus ranarum*. The tissue response is rather like that of a case of mucormycosis of the arm reported by BAKER et al. (1962), from which *Rhizopus rhizopodiformis* was grown, in that in both cases the fungus lies within microabscesses. However, the failure of the fungus to invade blood vessels is peculiar for a Mucoraceae. From all the evidence, I am willing to accept this case as one of mucormycosis.

WATSON (1957) described a mucormycotic gastric perforation in a child with kwashiorkor. When the abdomen was opened at postmortem there was found to be a black, necrotic-looking piece of omentum adherent to the anterior aspect of the stomach. There was no general peritonitis. On the omentum being removed from the stomach a large perforation of the anterior wall of the viscus was found. This consisted of a complete sloughing of an area about 5 cm in diameter. The lower edge of the perforation extended as far as the greater curvature and the upper edge was about 1 cm from the lesser curvature. The margins of the perforation consisted of black, ragged, necrotic tissue, surrounding which was a zone of reaction with small hemorrhagic spots. The stomach wall was edematous and exhibited a red flare about 1 cm in width. Microscopic sections through the stomach wall showed a wide-spread inflammatory exudate with numerous polymorphonuclear and round cells. There was destruction of the mucosa in the necrotic edge of the perforated area, and the adjacent mucosa was edematous. Numerous fungal hyphae were present in the stomach wall. These were particularly noticeable in the walls of the blood vessels in the submucosa, and in places the hyphae were found encroaching on the lumen of the vessels. The hyphae were non-septate and showed considerable variation in size. The average diameter was 10 μ but some were as large as 20 μ. Many of the blood vessels appeared to be thrombosed and this probably accounted for the extensive necrosis. The appearances were typical of those described in mucormycotic infections. No cultures were made before the viscus was fixed with formalin. Since no lesions were found in the body anywhere other than in the stomach, it is reasonable to assume that the fungus entered the stomach wall from the lumen of this viscus because the tissues were devitalized by malnutrition. The location of the lesion was not at all that of a chronic peptic ulcer.

GATLING (1959) reported a case of gastric mucormycosis occurring in an otherwise apparently healthy newborn infant who died of the infection on the 16th day. At autopsy, the wall of the stomach, from the cardia to within 0.5 cm proximal to the pylorus, was greatly thickened and indurated. The mucosa of the stomach was ragged and tan-brown and opaque. The serosal surface was covered with fibrin. Microscopically large numbers of nonseptate hyphae were present within the mucosa of the stomach and extended through the entire stomach wall. There was extensive vascular invasion. The infection had extended within the wall beneath the intact mucosa at the pyloric end. Many gram-negative bacilli and occasional gram-positive cocci were demonstrated in the superficial portion of the necrotic mucosa. Cultures of the gastric contents and a subdiaphragmatic abscess were overgrown by Friedländer's bacillus. The anatomical diagnosis was acute necrotizing phlegmonous, mucormycotic gastritis, with extension to the liver, spleen, pancreas, colon, diaphragm and left lung.

The report of NEAME (1960), concerning gastric mucormycosis is the most comprehensive of the entire literature. He reports 11 cases from Durban, South Africa, eight of which are limited to the stomach. He gives a description of the histopathology which applies to any part of the digestive tract, as follows:

Under low magnification, the most striking feature was necrosis and hemorrhage. In less advanced lesions, only the mucosa and part of the submucosa were affected, while, in more advanced cases, the remainder of the submucosa, the muscle layer, and even the serosa, were involved. There was perforation in 5 cases. In most cases, thrombosis was apparent in submucosal and serosal vessels. Under higher magnification, numerous pleomorphic hyphae could be seen in the necrotic tissue, invading the lumina and vessel walls, where thrombi were often present. The hyphae were nonseptate, averaged 15—20 μ in width, and had a well-defined edge and a cytoplasm showing areas of lighter, vacuolated and darker, granular staining, which could, on occasion, give the impression that the hyphae were septate. They showed numerous lateral branches, while sporangia were seen in a number of sections. In his case 9 what was presumed to be a columella of *Rhizopus* was found. Neutrophils were numerous in most sections, many around vessels and in hemorrhagic and necrotic areas.

NEAME described the morbid anatomy applicable to the entire digestive system as follows: The disease presented in three ways: (1) as small ulcers approximately 1 cm in diameter; (2) as larger ulcers with well-circumscribed borders; and (3) as more diffuse and often perforated necrotic lesions. Each is a further stage in the progression of the disease.

1. The small ulcers were superficial and consisted of a central portion of yellow slough, surrounded by a zone of erythema. A greenish-black discoloration was noted on the undersurface of the serosa. The lesions could easily be mistaken for amebic ulceration. Ulcers of this type were found in the descending or sigmoid colon of three cases and the ileum of one case, while multiple ulcers were found in the colon and esophagus of another.

2. Larger ulcers averaged 3—4 cm in diameter, the central 1.5 cm being black and necrotic. The peripheral 1 cm was raised, edematous, and gray in color. Surrounding this was a zone of intense erythema. On the serosal surface, blackish discoloration could be seen, deep to the peritoneum. This type of lesion was found most frequently at the pyloric antrum, as in 6 of the gastric cases, but occurred in the colon of 3 cases and the rectum and esophagus of 1 case.

3. A typical example of the more diffuse lesion occurred in a 6-day-old child who had necrosis of the whole thickness of the stomach, with sloughing and perforation, and the peripheral part of the lesion showed a zone of erythema. Another case showed a diffuse hemorrhagic necrotic lesion involving 8 cm of the transverse colon. On the mucosal surface, there were multiple areas of ulceration, one of which had perforated. On one occasion ulceration was diffuse but superficial with a velvety surface. Diffuse lesions of the stomach were present in four cases and of the colon in two.

The lesions of the digestive tract, excluding the small-ulcer type, were easily discernible, and of the last 15 cases, 12 were recognized at autopsy.

Because NEAME was remarkably successful in demonstrating the causative organism in his cases, data concerning the mycology and his methods of taking materials are included here.

Mycology: Swabs were taken from all lesions where fungal invasion was suspected and were submitted to the Bacteriology Department for direct examination and culture. 1. Direct Examination: A wet preparation was made in 20% KOH solution, allowed to stand overnight, and examined the next day. By this method, nonseptate hyphae of the family Mucoraceae were found in nine cases. 2. Culture: No positive swab cultures occurred until a medium in a Petri dish was used, consisting of Sabouraud's glucose agar on which white bread, which had been sterilized by autoclaving at 15 lb. for 15 min, and by dry heat in a hot air oven at 160 C. was placed. In eight cases there was a profuse growth of *Rhizopus*, while two cases were overgrown with various molds. It is of interest that all the cases of mucormycosis from which culture was obtained were of *Rhizopus* species.

Pathogenesis: Following ingestion and given the right environment, the fungus invaded the alimentary wall, causing local infarction and subsequent ulceration. Contiguous spread from stomach to liver and transverse colon was noted. "Kissing ulcers" on opposing walls of the stomach developed in two cases. In one case spread via the portal vein to the liver occurred, judging from the appearance at autopsy and on microscopic sectioning.

Site: An outstanding feature of Neame's series was the predominance of mucormycosis of the digestive tract. Two of his cases involved the central nervous system and the remainder the digestive system.

Associated Disease: Among the associated diseases of the 12 cases of Neame involving the stomach there were the following: Kwashiorkor in 6 cases, amebiasis in 2, hepatic disease in 2, uremia in 3.

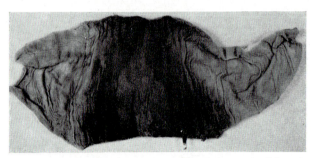

Fig. 38. Intestinal mucormycosis. Hemorrhagic necrosis (infarction) of ileum with central area of ulceration of necrotic mucosa. Case 1 of Baker et al. (1957)

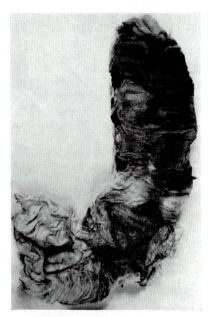

Fig. 39. Intestinal mucormycosis. Terminal ileum (above), ileocecal valve, and proximal cecum (lower left), showing areas of hemorrhagic necrosis. Case 1 of Baker et al. (1957)

It is interesting that there was so much digestive tract mucormycosis in South Africa and one wonders if *Rhizopus* is particularly prevalent there, possibly growing on ingested food. There are other areas of the globe where malnutrition is prevalent, as in Latin America and India, but no such incidence of mucormycosis of the digestive tract.

Neame noted that *cortisone* has been mentioned in the literature as a predisposing factor, and stated that no cortisone had been used prior to the development of the infection in the patients of his series. On the other hand, antibiotics had been given to all.

The author noted, further, the difficulty of diagnosis in digestive tract mucormycosis. None of his cases was diagnosed clinically. However, diagnosis could be made on the basis of knowledge of the predisposing factors and pathogenesis, sensitivity tests and biopsy, and the finding of numerous non-septate hyphae in the gastric aspirate or stool, -though the last could be merely saprophytic.

SUTHERLAND and JONES (1960), of Eastern Transvaal, Africa, reported a case of gastric mucormycosis in a Swazi of about 50 years. At postmortem examination there was a grayish white mass 8 by 5 cm along the greater curvature near the cardia. The surface of the mass was elevated one centimeter above the surrounding mucosa and was covered with a gelatinous exudate. Microscopically the mass was composed of necrotic and hemorrhagic material which was diffusely infiltrated with numerous non-septate hyphae of mucormycosis. Vascular invasion was prominent. The presence of a tumor-like mass in gastro-intestinal mucormycosis may signify an infection of longer duration than usually occurs. The authors suggested that the fermented foods and beer of the Bantu may possibly be factors in gastro-intestinal fungus infections by the introduction of excessive numbers of spores.

TRUJILLO's (1961) case was in an infant of 7 months. At operation the pyloric portion of the stomach was enlarged and palpable. A biopsy included the pylorus and a part of the duodenum. Microscopically there was ulceration of the mucosa of the pylorus, and the entire gastric and duodenal wall was invaded by thick, non-septate hyphae.

KAHN (1963) reported a case in South Africa involving the stomach and esophagus, found at the postmortem examination of a 17-year-old, puerperal, diabetic Negro girl.

ABRAMOWITZ (1964) reported fatal mucormycotic perforations of the stomach in a 35-year-old Bantu. There was peritonitis at postmortem examination. Two ulcers of the stomach had perforated, one into the greater sac through the anterior stomach wall, the other into the gall-bladder. There were areas of superficial ulceration throughout the colon. Histological sections of the stomach at the sites of the perforations and of the bowel at the areas of colonic ulceration showed a marked hemorrhagic and inflammatory reaction, with large branching non-septate fungal hyphae.

In case 1 of STEIN and SCHMAMAN there was, at surgical exploration, a rent along the lesser curvature of the stomach extending from the cardia to the pyloric sphincter. The posterior wall was adherent to the pancreas and completely covered by an exudate. The duodenum was edematous and had a perforation 0.7 cm in diameter in the anterior wall. The posterior wall of the stomach was freed, and found to have some very hard areas in it. A biopsy was taken. The rest of the mucosa appeared normal. The stomach was repaired. The duodenum was extremely friable and could not be sutured. The patient died and there was no postmortem examination. The biopsies taken from the stomach and duodenum, however, showed the characteristic features of mucormycosis. There were varying degrees of necrosis with only slight infiltration with neutrophils. Numerous broad, non-septate, branching, fungal hyphae were present. Several blood vessels in the sections showed penetration of their walls by these hyphae, which were also present in the lumen accompanied by thrombosis. A remarkable feature was the virtual absence of inflammatory reaction in the walls of the vessels where they were infiltrated by the fungal hyphae. As mucormycosis was not suspected during the surgical procedure, specimens were not taken for culture.

In case 2 of STEIN and SCHMAMAN (1965) there was a perforated ulcer about 1 cm in diameter on the lesser curvature of the stomach. A biopsy was taken and the perforation sutured. Microscopic examination of the gastric biopsy showed acutely inflamed granulation tissue in which there were numerous broad, non-septate, branching hyphae. At autopsy on the sixth postoperative day there was generalized peritonitis. The stomach was distended and contained altered blood. At the pyloric end of the lesser curvature there was an ulcer measuring 3 cm in diameter, to which omentum had been sutured. Numerous fungal hyphae were present even on the peritoneal surface.

BAKER (1962) has an excellent photograph of mucormycosis of the stomach in chronic lymphocytic leukemia (Fig. 37). Figure 3 of that article shows the black slough, the size of a silver dollar towards the greater curvature and about half way between the cardia and pylorus. It was an infarct caused by fungus thrombosis. This case 5 of this article had mucormycotic lesions also in the lung, liver, and kidney, and represented a disseminated mucormycosis. The infarct of the stomach was a hematogenous lesion, the primary lesion being in the right lung.

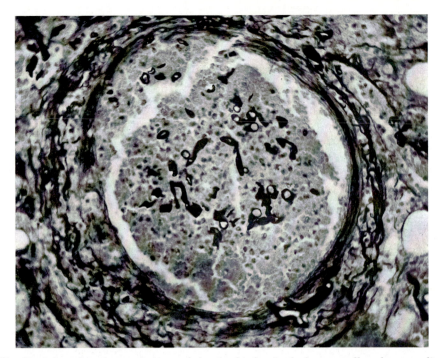

Fig. 40. A thrombosed mesenteric vessel showing hyphae in the lumen, wall, and surrounding tissue. Methenamine silver nitrate stain, × 160. Case 1 of Baker et al. (1957)

In case 7 of this same article a similar, but less conspicuous gastric mucormycosis, is described. There was a hemorrhagic indurated region, 2.5 by 2 cm in the fundus of the stomach involving the mucosa and extending to the serosa. Hyphae hematogenously borne from the primary pulmonary lesion had stimulated the formation of thrombi in vessels of the stomach, producing the hemorrhagic infarct.

From the foregoing extensive descriptive anatomic pathology, one obtains a concept of the characteristic changes in gastric mucormycosis.

Most of the reported cases have been primary infections of the stomach and most have been reported from South Africa and in subjects with kwarshiorkor. This may devitalize the gastric mucosa and permit the fungus to enter. Possibly the gastric mucosa exhibits nutritional edema and develops fissures permitting access of the fungus. Possibly the food eaten by these subjects is overgrown with *Rhizopus*. Neame showed that *Rhizopus* is the Mucoraceae usually involved in gastric mucormycosis.

Rhizopus is especially important as a cause of spoilage of fruits and stored potatoes, especially sweet potatoes (Skinner et al., 1947). The small fruits, especially strawberries, are particularly susceptible. The disease in strawberries is known as leak, because of the softening and dripping of the fruit. It is a source of considerable loss in shipment and is prevented by refrigeration. In sweet potatoes, a characteristic soft rot is produced.

The fungus entering the mucosa of the stomach penetrates the blood vessels and stimulates thrombosis and consequent infarction (gangrene). With the necrosis of the mucosa an ulcer is produced. Later there may be gangrene of the wall and a perforation.

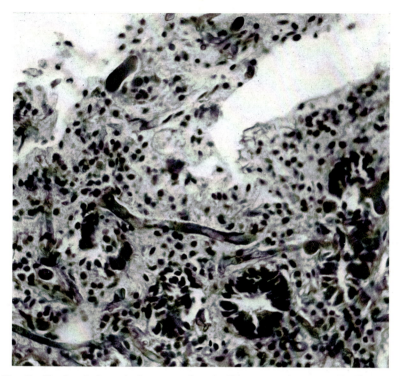

Fig. 41. Hyphae in intestinal mucosa. Case 2 of Baker et al. (1957). H & E, × 160

The lesions occur in various parts of the stomach. The entire stomach wall may be thickened and necrotic. Ulcers may develop along the lesser curvature of the stomach in the prepyloric region, suggesting chronic peptic ulcers, but it is not clear that any mucormycotic lesions in this region begin as chronic peptic ulcers.

Finally, attention is called to the possibility of regions of gastric infarction or gangrene developing from organisms reaching the stomach in the blood stream. The lesions would not be ulcerated at first, but would soon become so.

Intestinal Mucormycosis

Baker et al. (1957) reported two cases of intestinal mucormycosis (Figs. 38, 39, 40, 41) and tabulated two previously reported cases as follows: (1) Paltauf (1885): A 52-year-old white male in Austria had the mycosis for 17 days, died with mycotic septicemia and showed lesions in the terminal ileum; Moore et al. (1949): A 37-year-old white woman in Wisconsin, U.S.A., had mucormycosis for 15 days, dying of peritonitis, and showed lesions in the large bowel (See Table 4).

Case 1 of Baker et al. (1957) was that of a 43-year-old white man who developed hepatitis and jaundice while under therapy for cavitary tuberculosis of the right lung. At postmortem examination there was extensive mucormycosis of the gastrointestinal tract, minimal mucormycosis of the liver, and none elsewhere in the body.

Apparently the fungus invaded the intestinal wall from the lumen and produced thrombosis of small mesenteric vessels of the serosa. The fungus reached the liver by the portal blood stream and produced a small focus of infection there. The absence of fungus infection in other parts of the body indicated that the fungus was not disseminated to the gastrointestinal tract via the mesenteric arteries. Intramural hemorrhage of the intestine due to hepatic insufficiency

Table 5. *Disseminated Mucormycosis (37 cases)*

Authors and Case Number	Location of Case Age, Sex, Race	Predisposing Factors	Anatomic Involvement	Cultures	Duration	Treatment	Status of Patient
PALTAUF (1885)	Graz/Austria 52, M	None stated	Brain, lungs, pharynx, ileum	No	8 days	None stated	Dead, mucormycosis
CRAIG and FARBER (1953)	Boston/USA	Leukemia	Disseminated visceral	—	—	—	Dead, mucormycosis
ZIMMERMAN (1955) Case 6	Washington/USA 53, N	Myeloma, hemosiderosis, hepatoma	Lung, heart, kidney	No	—	Urethane, cortisone, X-ray	Dead, mucormycosis
BAKER (1956) Case 6	Durham/USA 3, F, N	75% of body burned	Lung, spleen, liver	No	3 days	Penicillin	Dead, mucormycosis
— Case 7	Phoenix/USA 4, M, W	—	Lung, liver, kidney	No	30 days	—	Dead, mucormycosis
TORACK (1957) Case 7	New York/USA 64, M, W	Myeloma, anemia, corticosteroids	Lungs, brain, stomach, spleen, heart	No	20 days	Corticosteroids, antibiotics	Dead, mucormycosis
HUTTER (1959) Case 4	New York/USA 8, M, W	Leukemia, steroid diabetes	Brain, lungs, spleen, digestive tract, thyroid, diaphragm	No	21 days	Antileukemics, antibiotics, steroids	Dead, mucormycosis
McBRIDE et al. (1960) Case 1	Nova Scotia/Canada 32, F, W	Septic abortion, renal cort. necrosis, anuria and uremia	Intestines, lungs, liver, kidneys, spleen, larynx	No	7 days	Antibiotics	Dead, mucormycosis
— Case 2	Boston/USA 26, M, W	Hepatitis, uremia	Lungs, esophagus, stomach, ileum, colon	*Rhizopus arrhizus*	10 days	Antibiotics	Dead, mucormycosis
BANKER (1961) Case 3	Boston/USA 12, M	Erythroleukemia, steroids	Lung, kidney, spinal cord	No	1 month	Steroids	Dead, mucormycosis
CUADRADO et al. (1961), Case 1	Dallas/USA 31, M, W	Diabetic acidosis, uremia	Lung, liver, spleen, pleura	No	30 days	Heparin, femoral vein ligation	Dead, mucormycosis
GLOOR et al. (1961), Case 2	Basel/Switzerland 69, M	Myeloblastic leukemia, corticosteroids	Aortic valve, myocardium, lung, kidney, spleen	No	21 days	Ilotycin, corticosteroids	Dead, mucormycosis
BAKER (1962) Case 5	Durham/USA 49, M, N	Chron. lymphocytic leukemia, neutrop., steroids	Right lung, stomach, kidney, liver	*Mucor*	4 weeks	Antileukemics, steroids, antibiotics	Dead, mucormycosis, aspergillosis

— Case 7	Durham/USA 45, M, W	Acute myeloblastic leukemia, neutrop.	Both lungs, stomach, right kidney	No	1 week	Antileukemics, antibiotics	Dead, mucormycosis
— Case 11	Durham/USA 58, M, W	Acute lymphoblastic leukemia, neutrop., steroids	Lungs, brain, thyroid	No	1 week	BW 57-323, steroids	Dead, mucormycosis
STRAATSMA et al. (1962), Case 6	AFIP Acc. No. 336851; 55, M, W	Aleukemic leukem., renal insufficiency	Disseminated mucormycosis	—	—	—	—
— Case 7	AFIP Acc. No. 486865; 66, M, W	Subleukemic myelogen. leukemia	Disseminated mucormycosis	—	—	—	—
— Case 8	AFIP Acc. No. 557484; 68, M, W	Chronic myelogenous leukemia	Disseminated mucormycosis	—	—	—	—
— Case 9	AFIP Acc. No. 565089; 28, M, N	Cutaneous burns	Disseminated mucormycosis	—	—	—	—
— Case 10	AFIP Acc. No. 729137; 62, M, W	Renal insufficiency	Disseminated mucormycosis	—	—	—	—
— Case 11	AFIP Acc. No. 801945; 62, M, W	Diabetes, agranulocytosis	Disseminated mucormycosis	—	—	—	—
— Case 12	AFIP Acc. No. 840049; 64, M, N	Postoperative status	Disseminated mucormycosis	—	—	—	—
— Case 13	AFIP Acc. No. 847623; 28, M, W	Chronic pulmonary disease	Disseminated mucormycosis	—	—	—	—
— Case 14	AFIP Acc. No. 856793; 43, M, W	Chronic myeloid leukemia	Disseminated mucormycosis	—	—	—	—
ERIKSEN (1963)	Copenhagen/Denmark; 23, M	Lymphogranulomatosis	Lungs, cerebrum, kidneys, myocardium	No	†	Antitumor drugs, prednisone, antibiotics	Dead, mucormycosis
GRUHN and SANSON (1963), Case 23	Chicago/USA 50, F	Chronic lymphocytic leukemia	Lung and brain	No	—	Steroids, antibiotics	Dead, mucormycosis
BRUNSON (1964)	Jackson/USA 63, M, N	Leucopenia and neutropenia	Lungs, liver, stomach, kidney, brain	No	—	Antibiotics	Dead, mucormycosis

Table 5. Continuation

Authors and Case Number	Location of Case Age, Sex. Race	Predisposing Factors	Anatomic Involvement	Cultures	Duration	Treatment	Status of Patient
SIMON et al. (1964)	Evanston/USA 76, M	Splenectomy, steroids, anemia	Lungs, liver, kidneys, duodenum, brain	No	4 days	Stilbestrol, steroids	Dead, mucormycosis
CUSSEN (1965)	Melbourne/Aust. 13, F, W	Hypopituitary dwarfism, Fanconi's syndrome, renal hypertension, prednisolone	Brain, thyroid, lungs	No	1 week	Prednisolone, antibiotics	Dead, mucormycosis
SUN et al. (1965) Case 6	Peking/China 23 days, M	Hydrocortisone	Pylorus, jejunum, liver, gall bladder, pancreas, lungs	No	21 days	Antibiotics, hydrocortisone	Dead, mucormycosis
— Case 7	Peking/China 56, M	Infectious hepatitis	Heart, kidney, lungs	No	—	Antibiotics, steroids	Dead, mucormycosis and bacterial infection
McMILLAN (1967) CPC Ohio	Columbus/USA 49, M, W	Acute leukemia, prednisone	Pulmonary vessels, appendix, kidneys	No	—	Transfusions, cytoxine, prednisone	Dead, mucormycosis
PARKHURST and VLAHIDES (1967), Case 1	Schenectady/USA 62, F	Aplastic anemia, steroids	Disseminated mucormycosis	—	—	Antibiotics, steroids	Dead, mucormycosis
— Case 2	Schenectady/USA 51, M	Lymphoblastic leukemia, steroids	Disseminated mucormycosis	—	—	Antibiotics, steroids	Dead, mucormycosis
— Case 3	Schenectady/USA 84, F	Acute stem cell leukemia, steroids	Disseminated mucormycosis	—	—	Antibiotics, steroids, cytotoxics	Dead, mucormycosis
— Case 4	Schenectady/USA 28, F	Acute myeloblastic leukemia, steroids	Disseminated mucormycosis	—	—	Antibiotics, steroids, cytotoxics	Dead, mucormycosis
— Case 5	Schenectady/USA 67, F	Chronic myelocytic leukemia, steroids	Lung, heart, spinal cord	No	1 week	Antibiotics, steroids, cytotoxics	Dead, mucormycosis

may have been the first event, followed by secondary infection of devitalized tissues. The extension of the infection to small mesenteric vessels then led to intestinal infarction. Death was due to massive intraluminal hemorrhage. Figure 1 of the paper of BAKER et al. (1957) is that of a segment of ileum showing a focal area of hemorrhagic necrosis with a central area of ulceration of the necrotic mucosa. Figure 2 shows the intestinal mucormycosis just above and below the ileocecal valve, with areas of hemorrhagic necrosis.

CALLE and KLATSKY (1966), report another case of mucormycosis of the terminal ileum and cecum with death due to generalized peritonitis. An interesting feature was the presence, at the margin of a lesion, of giant cells containing the non-septate hyphae of mucormycosis, presumably *Rhizopus*. This is probably to be correlated with the relatively long duration of the mycosis, estimated at 28 days.

CALLE and KLATSKY also present an excellent tabulation of the 14 cases of intestinal mucormycosis in the literature, including their own case. Not included in their table are cases in which involvement of the intestine was only part of a disseminated mucormycosis. The table includes the case of MOORE et al., the two cases of BAKER et al. (1957), the case of CLARK, the two cases of MONTENEGRO, five cases of NEAME and RAYNER, a case of LEVIN and ISAACSON and finally the case of CALLE and KLATSKY. Half of these 14 cases were from South Africa, 2 from Brazil and 5 from the United States of America. This paper also contains a valuable table showing the subdivisions of the Phycomycetes and indicating the *Rhizopus* and *Absidia* species isolated from cases of human phycomycosis and the species of *Rhizopus* and *Absidia* used to produce experimental phycomycosis in animals. This data refers to mucormycosis in general, and is not restricted to intestinal mucormycosis. It is interesting that no *Mucors* are listed.

The case of intestinal mucormycosis by CLARK, listed in the table of CALLE and KLATSKY, deserves special mention, because of the manner in which the fungus extended from the duodenum into the liver forming a tumor-like mass in the liver. There was also a mucormycotic carcinoma-like mass in the cecum. The case illustrates that occasionally mucormycosis of the gastrointestinal tract may take the form of tumor-like masses, in addition to infarction and ulceration.

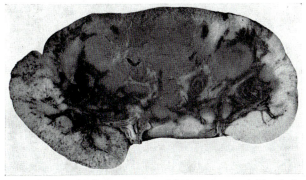

Fig. 42. Hematogenous mucormycotic infarct of kidney in myeloblastic leukemia. Mucormycosis also in lung (the primary site) and stomach. Case 7 of BAKER (1962)

Disseminated Mucormycosis

Table 5 includes 40 cases of disseminated mucormycosis which complicated leukemia, myeloma, septic abortion, body burns, diabetic acidosis, cortisone therapy, and renal insufficiency (Fig. 42). Leukemia, treated with modern drugs, is the most frequent antecedent of disseminated mucormycosis.

Each case of mucormycosis reported in this chapter is entered in only one of the five tables. In several of the cases of cranial mucormycosis there was dissemination to the lungs and elsewhere. Moreover, some of the cases listed as gastrointestinal and esophageal disseminated or were part of a dissemination from the cranial region or lung. In gastrointestinal mucormycosis the infection may spread centrifugally to the diaphragm, liver and omentum without regard to anatomic boundaries. A similar spreading, not along vascular channels but directly through the tissues, occurs in cranial mucormycosis and at the hilus of the lung in pulmonary mucormycosis. However, the fungus has such an attraction to blood vessels that these are invariably involved in the instances of direct spread of *Rhizopus*.

Pulmonary mucormycosis and mucormycosis of body burns constitute important primary sites for disseminated mucormycosis.

Cutaneous and Subcutaneous Mucormycosis

Secondary cutaneous and subcutaneous mucormycosis has already been discussed in the section on the cranial form of the disease. The infarct or gangrene of the skin of the face or nose is secondary to vascular obstruction by thrombi of arteries, veins and lymphatics caused by hyphae growing in the lumina of these vessels.

Cases of this type were reported by BRYAN et al., SMITH and KIRCHNER, DOLMAN and HERD, RINALDI and ASHBY, SUPRUN, BURROW et al., REEVES et al., STRAATSMA et al. (case 28), LUBBE and PENNINGTON, WEISSKOPF (case 1 and 2), and HURTADO et al.

The eight cases of primary cutaneous and subcutaneous mucormycosis are listed in Table 6. The predisposing factors were diabetes in 3 cases, cutaneous burns in 3, and there was no predisposing factor in two. The infection was on the leg in 3 cases, on an upper extremity in two, and on the face in 3. Abstracts of the eight cases follow.

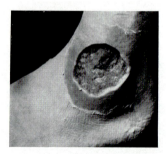

Fig. 43. Cutaneous mucormycosis. An ulcer which developed spontaneously in a diabetic patient. The ulcer healed in $4^1/_2$ months. (From JOSEFIAK et al.)

The lesion of the case of JOSEFIAK et al. developed *de novo* in a diabetic of 26 years (Fig. 43). A region of black gangrene appeared above the malleolus of the leg. The necrotic tissues sloughed out leaving a deep ulcer. Biopsies showed the characteristic broad hyphae in abscesses and in the walls of vessels. With the control of the diabetes, and the administration of potassium iodide, the ulcer healed in $4^1/_2$ months. It was not clear whether the fungus was implanted locally or reached the leg *via* the blood stream.

The case of KNOTH-BORN involved both legs of a 50-year-old farm woman. The illustrations in the report show organisms which are coenocytic and compatible with those of mucormycosis.

In the two cases reported by RABIN et al. the patients had sustained extensive thermal cutaneous burns involving the face, and the facial tissues became infected with an organism of mucormycosis. This led to gangrenous necrosis of the central and midportion of the face and to systemic mucormycosis. The fungus caused softening of the nasal cartilages and bones and

Table 6. *Primary cutaneous and subcutaneous Mucormycosis (8 cases)*

Authors and Case Number	Location of Case Age, Sex, Race	Predisposing Factors	Anatomic Involvement	Culture	Duration	Treatment	Status of Patient
JOSEFIAK et al. (1958)	Winst.-Salem/USA; 26, M	Diabetes	Lower left leg	No	4½ mos.	Diabetic control	Well
KNOTH-BORN (1959)	Gießen/Germany 50, F, W	—	Skin of legs	No	—	—	—
RABIN et al. (1961) Case 1	Ft. Sam Houston/USA; 22, M	Body burns, 64%	Face, nasal cavity, brain, lungs, kidney, spleen, heart	No	12 days	Antibiotics	Dead, mucormycosis
RABIN et al. (1962) Case 2	Ft. Sam Houston/USA; 20, M, N	Body burns, 45%	Face, nasal cavity, left orbit, meninges, heart, kidneys	No	8 days	Antibiotics	Dead, mucormycosis
BAKER et al. (1962)	New Orleans/USA 79, F, W	Diabetes	Right arm	*Rhizopus rizopodiformis*	8 days	Antibiotics	Dead, mucormycosis
ROBERTS (1962)	West Palm Beach/USA; 24, M, N	Diabetic acidosis	Right leg	No	17 days	Control of diabetes	Recovery
VIGNALE and MACKINNON (1964)	Bagé/Brazil 39, F	None	Face, neck, nasal septum	*Mucor ramosissimus*	24 days	Amphotericin B	Cured
FOLEY and SHUCK (1968)	Ft. Sam Houston/USA; 20, M, N	Burn	Hand	No	7 days	Amputation	Cured

these structures were removed by debridement. In these two cases the burn represented the predisposing factor and there was no diabetes.

The case of Baker et al. (1962) was that of a 79-year-old white woman admitted to the Louisiana State University Medical Service of Charity Hospital on September 22, 1961, because of fever and stupor. A diabetic for many years, she had been hospitalized at Charity Hospital for 2 weeks for the same complaints 1 month previously.

During the first admission she was treated with penicillin, chloramphenicol, diet and insulin. She was discharged on an 1800-calorie diabetic diet and 1 tablet of chlorpropamide daily.

The patient's course at home was satisfactory for 1 week only. She then developed temporary loss of motor power and sensation in the left leg. She became lethargic, unstable in her movements, and intermittently refused food and fluids. A carbuncle appeared over the right scapula on September 15, and was incised and drained the next day. Intramuscular penicillin was administered for several days.

From September 17 until the day of admission she refused her chlorpropamide, food, and most fluids. She complained of pain, stiffness of the neck, and headache, and became unresponsive on September 21.

Significant findings at admission on September 22 were: brachial blood pressure, 190 mm of mercury, systolic, and 80, diastolic; dehydration; bilateral cataracts; stiff neck which appeared painful on attempted movement; draining carbuncle over the right scapula; absence of abnormal reflexes; and fever of 102° F. Acetone was absent from the urine and serum, and only 1 plus glycosuria was present. The hematocrit was 44.5%, and the white blood cell count and differential were normal. Examination of the cerebrospinal fluid was normal chemically and cytologically.

Although the patient was intermittently responsive, treatment did not alter her fever or progressive deterioration. It was necessary to cannulate several veins in order to administer intravenous fluids and antibiotics. Transfusions with whole blood, regulation of electrolytes, digitalization, and insulin did not improve her status.

She was treated as if she had staphylococcal and gram-negative rod septicemia, because these organisms were grown from the carbuncle. The absence of positive blood cultures may have been due to antibiotic treatment which was instituted on the night of admission.

Multiple decubiti developed. On October 3 the right forearm above the venous cannula was swollen, purplish, and firmly nodular. The arm became progressively more dusky and edematous. On October 5 the epidermis became elevated by a large vesicle which contained serosanguineous fluid. The material from the unbroken vesicle revealed *Rhizopus rhizopodiformis* and *Aerobacter aerogenes*. Melena was observed on the same day and was intermittently present thereafter.

The right arm was incised and packed on October 8, and material from the subcutaneous tissues was obtained for laboratory study. The tissue contained hyphae which were recognized as belonging to the phycomycetes. Cultures of the tissue and of deep exudate the following day grew *A. aerogenes* and *Rhizopus rhizopodiformis*.

At postmortem examination the remnants of the carbuncle were represented by an ulcer of the back, 4 by 4 cm in diameter, with healthy-looking granulation tissue in its base.

On the dorsum of the right arm there were incisions over an area 9 by 3.5 cm. There were foci of yellow and white opacity in the subcutaneous tissue which represented fat necrosis and minute abscesses. There was no enlargement of lymph nodes at the elbow or axilla.

In the right globus pallidus of the brain there were minute foci of old encephalomalacia, each 3—4 mm across. The heart (340 g) had no infarct or severe coronary arteriosclerosis. The aorta was rigid and calcified in its terminal third. The left pleural cavity contained 600 cc of clear yellow fluid, and the right, 400 cc. There was atelectasis of the lower lobe of each lung. The liver weighed 1980 g and the spleen 220 g.

There was an ulcer, 2 by 1 cm in diameter and 1.5 cm deep, in the first portion of the duodenum, with hemorrhagic foci in the base. The terminal ileum contained small amounts of tarry blood, and there were brown feces in the colon. Five pedunculated polypi were found along the large bowel. The right kidney weighed 110 g and the left, 120 g. The trigone of the bladder was red and swollen. The pancreas was of normal size. The thyroid was atrophic (7 g) and contained colloid nodules. The right adrenal weighed 10 g, the left 11 g.

Microscopically, there were broad (8—15 μ), branching, coenocytic hyphae in the skin and underlying tissues of the right forearm. They were in abscesses and necrotic fat, bordered in some instances by giant cells, and in the walls of blood vessels. Bacilli were found in the incised necrotic fat close to the hyphae but not in the abscesses or giant cells. There was mild fibroblastic response near the muscle. Fungi were not found in other tissues of the body.

Microbiologically, an antemortem culture from the arm grew rapidly at room temperature as a fluffy growth, at first white and later dark brown or black. Dr. C. W. Hesseltine of Peoria, Illinois, identified it as *Rhizopus rhizopodiformis*. The following description appears in Hesseltine's thesis, 1950:

"Colonies at first white, then black-plumbeus, nearly as black in reverse, little or no sterile mycelium, less than 3 mm in height; odor sometimes strong; stolons hyaline; rhizoids poorly developed, hyaline or brown-colored; sporangiophores branched, especially near the surface of the medium, from stolens, or from swellings of the hyphae or opposite the rhizoids; septations only above a branch, up to 800 μ in height (mostly less than 500 μ), up to 15 μ in width; sporangia spherical, white, then a glistening black, finally a gray-black, averaging 90—120 μ, exceptionally to 140 μ, columellae hyaline or colored, variable in shape from pyriform or oblong to globose, reaching 72 μ in diameter. Sporangiospores non-striate, smooth, heavy-walled, spherical, nearly hyaline singly but black in mass, averaging 4—5 μ; chlamydospores cylindrical or spherical or oval, up to 25 μ in diameter; zygospores unknown."

R. rhizopodiformis is rarely encountered as a saprophytic contaminant and only a few isolates have been described in the literature. In his thesis Hesseltine cites two instances in which the species was recovered from a mycosis in animals, in one case from a dog and in another from a horse. The organism has very close affinities with the genus *Mucor* and is distinguished from other species of *Rhizopus* chiefly by the branched sporangiophores, the presence of occasional pyriform columellae, and the lack of striations in the walls of the sporangiospores.

Undoubtedly *diabetes* predisposed to the subcutaneous infection of the arm by *R. rhizopodiformis*. Also, it is reasonably certain that the fungus entered the tissues around the cannula used in intravenous therapy. The fungus must have been present in the arm for at least a week, as there was giant cell and localized abscess production in response to its presence. The *Rhizopus* penetrated vessel walls, as in cerebral and pulmonary mucormycosis. The presence of microabscesses, however, indicated that the organism exerted its effect as a direct inflammatory agent as well as by vessel invasion, thrombosis, and ischemia. The necrosis of fat may have been due to ischemia or to the presence of bacteria.

In the local tissue reaction in the arm, *A. aerogenes* appeared to play a minor role, as no bacteria could be found in the abscesses or giant cells. However, a bacillus was visible in necrotic fat in the neighborhood of hyphae, and this may have represented a *Proteus* organism.

The fungus infection of the arm, possibly reinforced by a bacillary infection, may have been responsible for the fever which the patient had during her hospital stay. No other satisfactory cause of fever was demonstrated at postmortem and, while Gram-negative rod septicemia was postulated, it was never proved by blood culture. There was evidence of mild gastrointestinal bleeding at autopsy, not sufficient to be the main cause of death. It is reasonable to conclude, therefore, that the fungus infection of the arm was a major contributing factor in the causation of the death of this patient.

The case of ROBERTS was similar to that of JOSEFIAK et al. An ulcer developed in the right lower leg of a 24-year-old Negro diabetic. He survived following excision of the ulcer, rigid diabetic management, and supportive nutritional measures.

The case of VIGNALE et al. is unique in the annals of mucormycosis. The case differs from classical cranial, pulmonary, digestive tract and disseminated mucormycosis with respect to the type of lesion, the length of the course of the disease, and the absence of diabetes or other predisposing factor. The case resembles somewhat the African cases of entomophthoromycosis. If it were not that the fungus agent was a *Mucor*, I would have been inclined to regard the case as one of entomophthoromycosis or subcutaneous phycomycosis. VIGNALE et al. note that subcutaneous phycomycosis described in horses by BRIDGES and EMMONS (1961) and BRIDGES, ROMAINE and EMMONS (1962) offers a number of features common to those described in this case: extreme chronicity, extensive destruction and failure to cure spontaneously.

At the age of 15 years the girl from South Brazil noticed a flat, faintly erythematous lesion on the left cheek; it measured 1 cm in diameter and had undefined boundaries and a soft consistence. There was no history of trauma or local infection. After a few months the lesion became slightly raised and remained stationary for about 5 years. By the end of 10 years, the lesions had spread centrifugally forming a papulose, congestive, infiltrated plaque.

When the patient was 39 the process had extended to involve the cartilage and bone of the nose and face. The nasal bridge was absent, the nasal orifices appearing at the same level as the remaining surrounding skin. At the level of the hard and soft palates there was a 15 by 20 mm perforation, slightly towards the left. The uvula had disappeared. In the neck, as on some portions of the face there were papules from 2—4 mm in diameter.

Numerous biopsies showed a fibrosing and granulomatous inflammatory process made up of histiocytes, lymphocytes and a few giant cells and irregularly distributed mycelial filaments.

Cultures of biopsy material were made on Sabouraud glucose agar. In every case, within a few days, yellowish white mycelium developed forming little raised colonies. The microscopic features were characteristic of a phycomycete and sporangia indicative of the genera *Mortierella* or *Mucor* were present. Repeated isolation of the same species as well as morphological similarities in tissues and in cultures were indications of its pathogenicity. On four occasions cultures of biopsy samples yielded the same fungus which Hesseltine and Ellis (1964) regard as *Mucor ramosissimus* Samutsevitsch. Treatment with amphotericin B was apparently successful.

Foley and Shuck (1968) report the case of a 20-year-old Negro man whose right hand, together with 65% of his body surface, was burned after a mine explosion in Vietnam. On the eleventh post burn day his right hand became swollen and tender over the thenar area. Topical chemotherapy had been used, and in some way this may have contributed to the infection. At exploratory operation the hand appeared to be gangrenous and was disarticulated. Histopathologic examination revealed ischemic necrosis of the subcutaneous, muscle and connective tissue at all levels sampled. There was invasion through unhealed burn by broad, non-septate, irregularly branching hyphae characteristic of Phycomycetes. The hyphae infiltrated the wall and lumen of small vessels that were infected and thrombosed. There was a cellulitis and abscess of the thenar area with necrosis, and hyphae invading blood vessels.

Focal Mucormycosis

This table of 6 cases is a miscellany of isolated lesions of mucormycosis. There is one lesion of the tibia, one of a fracture site, one of the larynx, two of the kidney, and one of the aorta (See Table 7).

The lesions of the larynx and of the fracture site in the leg were reported in tabular form by Straatsma et al., and no detailed data are available. Eriksen et al. (1962) reported mucormycosis of a fracture of a tibia and the recovery of *Absidia ramosa* from the lesion.

Diriart et al. (1963) reported renal mucormycosis. There are no illustrations.

Prout and Goddard (1960) reported a case of renal mucormycosis in a surgically removed kidney. There were non-septate hyphae and thrombosed arteries. Giant cells formed part of the cellular response. Amphotericin B was used in treatment and the patient lived.

Fienberg and Risley (1959) reported the first case of mucormycosis limited to the aorta. The fungus infection occurred in a 45-year-old woman with controlled diabetes. The source of the infection on the basis of autopsy data was considered to be a ruptured appendix with extruded fecal material. Complete occlusion of the lumen of the abdominal aorta was the result of the fungal infection.

Spontaneous Mucormycosis in Animals

Gisler and Pitcock described 2 cases of intestinal mucormycosis in monkeys (*Macaca mulatta*). In the first case there were ulcers of the cecum and ascending colon. Hyphae were demonstrated in them and in a focus in the liver. These were thrombosed vessels. The case resembles those of intestinal mucormycosis in man. In the second case there was neutropenia of 1,330 cells per cubic millimeter. There was ulcerative colitis of the ascending and transverse portions of the large intestine. There were hyphae of mucormycosis and also *Endameba histolytica* in the lesions. The mucormycosis seemed to be incidental.

Lucke and Linton reported the case of an 11-year-old mandrill which had been in the Bristol Zoological Gardens for 4 years. It died after 3 days of illness. At autopsy ulcerative lesions were found in the stomach and intestines and granulomatous lesions were found involving the lungs, heart, kidneys, liver, spleen and

Table 7. *Focal Mucormycosis (6 cases)*

Authors and Case Number	Location of Case Age, Sex, Race	Predisposing Factors	Anatomic Involvement	Cultures	Duration	Treatment	Status of Patient
FTENBERG and RISLEY (1959)	Beverly/USA 45, F	Diabetes, abscess of appendix	Abdominal aorta	No	5 days	Penicillin, cortisone	Dead, mucormycosis
PROUT and GODDARD (1960)	Miami/USA 51, M	Alcoholism, pulmonary tuberculosis	Kidney	No	—	Nephrectomy, Amphotericin B	Survived
ERIKSEN et al. (1962)	Copenhagen/Denmark	Fracture	Tibia	*Absidia ramosa*	—	—	Well, fungus disappeared
STRAATSMA et al. (1962) Case 29	AFIP Acc. No. 705571 40, F, N		Larynx	—	—	—	—
STRAATSMA et al. (1962) Case 31	AFIP Acc. No. 787760 45, F, N		Fracture site, leg	—	—	—	—
DIRIART et al. (1963)	Paris/France 8 months	Mucoviscidosis, azotemia	Kidney	No	5 weeks	Antibiotics	Dead

occasional lymph nodes, and there was a discharging ulcer in the skin of the right shoulder. Large non-septate hyphae were seen in all the lesions but the fungus was not isolated.

Hessler et al. described mucormycosis in a rhesus monkey.

Thus the occurrence of intestinal lesions in primates is as in man. The disseminated granulomatous lesions of Lucke and Linten are of a different nature than the disseminated lesions of man except that one of Baker's (1956) cases had giant cell response to the fungus.

Ainsworth and Austwick published a book entitled *Fungal Diseases of Animals* (1959). They discuss mucormycosis occurring in pigs, cattle, horses, dogs, mink, guinea pigs, fowls, and mice, and state that the lesions may be ulcerative and confined to the gastric and intestinal mucosa. A granulomatous form involves lymph nodes and is thus unlike mucormycosis in man. Occasionally the granulomatous lesions become generalized. In their section on bovine mycotic abortion they mention many cases of infection of the placenta with fungi of the *Mucoraceae*.

Austwick and Venn (1957, 1961) found 12.3% of 638 cases of mycotic abortion associated with mucoraceous fungi, and 64% with *Aspergillus*.

Nicolet et al., reporting on bovine abortion, found 14 cases of mucormycosis and 19 of aspergillosis. *Absidia corymbifera* was the most prevalent species.

Mahaffey and Adams reported phycomycetous mycotic lesions of the placenta in mares.

Ainsworth and Austwick, Gitter and Austwick, and Shirly report abomasal ulcers containing phycomycete hyphae.

Christiansen (1929) described chronic granulomatous lesions in cattle. Momberg-Jorgensen described subcutaneous lesions in the mink. Gleiser reported a renal lesion in a dog, a stomach lesion in another dog, and lymph node lesions in a heifer.

Davis et al. described pulmonary and lymph-nodal lesions in cattle and pigs. Gitter and Austwick (1959) described mucormycosis in a litter of sucking pigs. Kaplan et al. described mucormycosis in a harp seal, Marcato and Dimon in a gazelle, Morquer et al. in cattle and swine, Turner in bovine foetuses, Mehnert in young pigs, Mostafa et al. in goats, Tewari in buffaloes, Hewer in an okapi, Sauer in a squirrel.

A case of mucormycosis in the uterus and rumen of a cow was considered in a clinicopathologic conference at the New York State Veterinary College.

Diagnosis: The clinical and postmortem diagnosis of the cranial form of mucormycosis should offer no difficulty to the physician or pathologist who knows that unilateral proptosis, gangrene of the face, black mucosa of the nose, and gangrene of the palate proclaim mucormycosis. The diagnosis of the other forms of the disease are, in contrast, exceedingly difficult, as a mucormycotic infarct of the lung might pass for pneumonia in X-ray and gangrene of the bowel for mesenteric thrombosis.

Mucormycosis should be kept in mind as a possible complicating infection in diabetic and leukemic patients.

Biopsy has proved to be the most effectice means of making a diagnosis in the reported cases of mucormycosis. Smears are of less value than wet preparations, i. e., placing material in a drop of normal saline and placing a cover-slip on the fluid, and examining in the microscope with the light cut down. The hematoxylin and eosin stain of the biopsy is usually sufficient for a diagnosis.

To grow the fungus in *culture* is difficult, and many reports indicate failure even though the samples of material seemed ample. The method of Neame should be tried. He simply took material on a swab and inoculated it into Sabouraud glucose agar to which had been added autoclaved and heat-dried white bread. By this method he grew *Rhizopus* from several gastro-intestinal lesions. If pathologists are to obtain cultures of the Mucoraceae at postmortem, they must resist the all-too-frequent practise of fixing tissues in formalin without saving material for culture. A mucormycotic infarct of the lung or bowel may resemble infarcts due to thrombosis or embolism of other nature.

There is usually little difficulty in differential histologic diagnosis. *Aspergillus*, however, may be confused with *Rhizopus*.

Prevention: Mucormycosis might be prevented by keeping diabetics in optimal regulation, by avoiding the use of corticosteroids in leukemic patients, and by avoiding the use of antileukemic drugs which induce neutropenia. There is probably no means of keeping the infecting fungus from the patient, but studies along these lines are indicated.

Treatment: Regulation of the acidotic diabetic patient, the use of Amphotericin B and the surgical resection of gangrenous tissue appear to have been curative measures in surviving patients (PROCKNOW, UTZ).

References

ABRAMOWITZ, M. B.: Fatal perforations of the stomach due to mucormycosis of the gastrointestinal tract. S. Afr. med. J. **38**, 93 (1964). — ABRAMSON, E., WILSON, D., ARKY, R. A.: Rhinocerebral phycomycosis in association with diabetic ketoacidosis. Ann. intern. Med. **66**, 735 (1967). — AGREST, A., MANUEL, A., BARCAT, J. A., EJDEN, J.: Cerebral mucormycosis. Medicina (B. Aires) **23**, 102 (1963). — AINSWORTH, G. C., AUSTWICK, P. K. C.: Fungal diseases of animals. Commonwealth Agricultural Bureaux (Farnham Royal, Bucks, 1959). — AUSTWICK, P. K. C., VENN, J. A. J.: Mycotic abortion in England and Wales 1954—1960. Proceedings of the IV International Congress on Animal Reproduction, p. 562. The Hague 1961. ∼ Routine investigation into mycotic abortion. Vet. Rec. **69**, 488 (1957). — BADER, G.: Die visceralen Mykosen (Pathologie, Klinik und Therapie), 423 pp. Jena: Gustav Fischer 1965. ∼ BADER, G., STILLER, D., RUFFERT, K.: Fluorochrome stains for histological diagnosis of visceral mycoses. Nature (Lond.) **208**, 796 (1965). — BAKER, R. D.: Pulmonary mucormycosis. Amer. J. Path. **32**, 287 (1956). ∼ Mucormycosis, a new disease? J. Amer. med. Ass. **163**, 805 (1957a). ∼ The diagnosis of fungus diseases by biopsy. J. chron. Dis. **5**, 552 (1957b). ∼ Diabetes and mucormycosis. Diabetes **9**, 143 (1960). ∼ Essential pathology. Baltimore: Williams & Wilkins Co. 1961. ∼ Leukopenia and therapy in leukemia as factors predisposing to fatal mycoses. Mucormycosis, aspergillosis, and cryptococcosis. Amer. J. clin. Path. **37**, 358 (1962). ∼ Drug-induced mycoses. In: Proceedings of the Second Symposium on Drug-Induced Diseases, State University of Leyden, October 1964, pp. 50—60. Excerpta Medica International Congress Series No. 85. ∼ Fungus infections. Chapter in Pathology. Ed. by W.A.D. ANDERSON. St. Louis: C.V. Mosby Co. 1966. — BAKER, R. D., BASSERT, D. E., FERRINGTON, E.: Mucormycosis of the digestive tract. Arch. Path. **63**, 176 (1957). — BAKER, R. D., SCHOFIELD, R. A., ELDER, T. D., SPOTO, A. P.: Alloxan diabetes and cortisone as modifying factors in experimental mucormycosis (Rhizopus infection). Fed. Proc. **15**, 506 (1956). — BAKER, R. D., SEABURY, J. H., SCHNEIDAU, J. D.: Subcutaneous and cutaneous phycomycosis. Lab. Invest. **11**, 1091 (1962). — BAKER, R. D., SEVERANCE, A. O.: Mucormycosis with report of acute mycotic pneumonia. Amer. J. Path. **24**, 716 (1948). — BALASUBRAHMANYAN, M., CHAUDHURI, S.: A case of pulmonary mucormycosis. Indian J. Path. Bact. **6**, 60 (1963). — BANK, H., SHIBOLET, S., GILAT, T., ALTMANN, G., HELLER, H.: Mucormycosis of head and neck structures. A case with survival. Brit. med. J. **1**, 766 (1962). — BANKER, B. Q.: Cerebral vascular disease in infancy and childhood. I. Occlusive vascular diseases. J. Neuropath. exp. Neurol. **20**, 127 (1961). — BARTHELAT, G.-J.: Les mucorinées pathogénes et les mucormycoses chez les animaux et chez l'homme. Arch. parasitol. **7**, 1 (1903). — BAUER, H., AJELLO, L., ADAMS, E., HERNANDEZ, D.: Cerebral mucormycosis. Pathogenesis of the disease. Amer. J. Med. **18**, 822 (1955a). — BAUER, H., FLANAGAN, J. F., SHELDON, W. H.: Experimental cerebral mucormycosis in rabbits with alloxan diabetes. Yale J. Biol. Med. **28**, 29 (1955a). ∼ Experimental cerebral mucormycosis in diabetic rabbits. Amer. J. Path. **31**, 600 (1955). ∼ The effects of metabolic alterations on experimental Rhizopus oryzae (mucormycosis) infection. Yale J. Biol. Med. **29**, 23 (1956). — BAUER, H., SHELDON, W. H.: Leukopenia with granulocytopenia in experimental mucormycosis (Rhizopus oryzae infection). J. exp. Med. **106**, 501 (1957). — BAUER, H., WALLACE, G. L., SHELDON, W. H.: The effects of cortisone and chemical inflammation on experimental mucormycosis (Rhizopus oryzae infection). Yale J. Biol. Med. **29**, 389 (1957). — Baum, J. L.: Rhino-orbital mucormycosis occurring in an otherwise apparently healthy individual. Amer. J. Ophthal. **63**, 335 (1967). — Beneke, R.: Ein Fall von Schimmelpilzgeschwür in der Magen- schleimhaut. Frankfurt. Z. Path. **7**, 1 (1911). — Berk, M., Fink, C. I., Uyeda, C. T.: Rhino- mucormycosis. J. Amer. med. Ass. **177**, 511 (1961). — Bernard, P. N.: Sur un Rhizopus pathogene de l'homme: Rhizopus equinus (1) Lucet et Constantin 1903, variété annamensis (2) Noel Bernard 1914. Bull. Soc. Path. exot. **7**, 430 (1914). — Bianchi, L., Della Torre, B.: A fatal case of phycomycosis. Mycopathologia (Den Haag) **19**, 145 (1963). ~ Rara forma di ficomicosi umana a decorso piemico. Minn. Med. **53**, 2462 (1962). — Bianchi, L., Della Torre, B., Martinazzi, M.: Fatal pancreatic necrosis in human phycomycosis. Path. et Microbiol. (Basel) **30**, 15 (1967). — Bianchi, L., Magrassi, B.: Osserrazioni su una rara forma di ficomicosi piemica con localizzazioni scheletriche multiple. Chir. Organi Mov. **53**, 160 (1964). — Blankenberg, H. W., Verhoeff, D.: Mucormycosis of the lung. Amer. Rev. Tuberc. **70**, 357 (1959). — Borland, D. S.: Mucormycosis of the central nervous system. Amer. J. Dis. Child. **97**, 852 (1959). — Bostroem: Demonstration mikroskopischer Präparate von Schimmel- pilzen. Berl. klin. Wschr. **23**, 232 (1886). — Boyd, W.: A textbook of pathology. Structure and function in diseases. Seventh edition, 1378 pp. Philadelphia: Lea and Febiger 1961. — Brunson, J. G.: Clinicopathologic conference conducted by the Department of Pathology, University of Mississippi School of Medicine, Jackson, Mississippi. J. Miss. med. Ass. **5**, 95 (1964). — Brown-Thomsen, J.: Phycomycosis vulneris. Ugeskr. Laeg. **128**, 17 (1966). — Bryan, G. T., Read, C. H., Zimmermann, G. R.: Disseminated mucormycosis in a child with diabetes mellitus. A case report. J. Iowa St. med. Soc. **48**, 193 (1958). — Burns, R. P.: Mucor- mycosis of the sinuses, orbit and central nervous system. Trans. Pacif. Cst otoophthal. Soc. **40**, 83 (1959). — Burrow, G. N., Salmon, R. B., Nolan, J. P.: Successful treatment of cerebral mucormycosis with Amphotericin B. J. Amer. med. Ass. **183**, 370 (1963). — Calle, S., Klatsky, S.: Intestinal phycomycosis (mucormycosis). Amer. J. clin. Path. **45**, 264 (1966). — Chick, E. W., Evans, J., Baker, R. D.: Treatment of experimental mucormycosis (Rhizopus oryzae infection) in rabbits with Amphotericin B. Antibiot. et Chemother. (Basel) **8**, 394 (1958). ~ The inhibitory effect of amphotericin B on localized Rhizopus oryzae infection (mucormycosis) utilizing the pneumoderma pouch of the rat. Antibiot. et Chemother. (Basel) **8**, 506 (1958). — Christiansen, M.: Chronic lesions in cattle-granulomatous. Virchows Arch. path. Anat. **273**, 879 (1929). — Clark, R. M.: A case of mucormycosis of the duodenum, liver, and cecum. Gastroenterology **33**, 985 (1957). — *Clinical Pathological Conference. New York State Veterinary College*, Cornell vet. **57**, 308 (1967). — *Clinicopathological Conference* from the Ohio State Univ. Hosp., Columbus/Ohio. Ohio St. med. J. **63**, 494 (1967). — Cohnheim: Zwei Fälle von Mykosis der Lungen. Virchows Arch. path. Anat. **33**, 157 (1865). — Conant, N. F., Smith, D. T., Martin, D. S., Calloway, J. L., Baker, R. D.: Manual of clinical mycology. Philadelphia and London: W. B. Saunders Co. 1954. — Craig, J. M., Farber, S.: Development of disseminated visceral mucormycosis during therapy for acute leukemia. Amer. J. Path. **29**, 601 (1953). — Cuadrado, S. P., Haberman, S., Race, G. J.: Visceral mucormycosis (phycomycosis). Tex. St. J. Med. **57**, 712 (1961). — Cussen, I. J.: Primary hypopituitary dwarfism with Franconi's hypoplastic anemia syndrome, renal hypertension and phyco- mycosis. Report of a case. Med. J. Aust. **2**, 367 (1965). — Darja, M., Davy, M. I.: Pulmonary mucormycosis with cultural identification. Canad. med. Ass. J. **89**, 1235 (1963). — Davis, C. L., Anderson, W. A., McCrory, B. R.: Mucormycosis in food-producing animals. J. Amer. vet. med. Ass. **126**, 261 (1955). — Defeo, E.: Mucormycosis of the colon. Amer. J. Roentgenol. **86**, 86 (1961). — Deweese, D. D., Robinson, L. B.: Mucormycosis of the nose and paranasal sinuses. Trans. Amer. laryng. rhin. otol. Soc., p. 452 (1965). — Deweese, D. D., Scheuning, A. J., Robinson, L. B.: Mucormycosis of the nose and paranasal sinuses. Laryngoscope (St Louis) **75**, 1398 (1965). — Dillon, M. L., Sealy, W. C.: Surgical aspects of opportunistic fungus infections. Lab. Invest. **11**, 1231 (1962). — Dillon, M. L., Sealy, W. C., Fetter, B. F.: Mucormycosis of the bronchus successfully treated by lobectomy. J. thorac. Surg. **35**, 464 (1958). — Diriart, H., Poujol, J., Schneider, J., Isidor, P.: Mucoviscidose à localisation rénale dominante parasitée par une mucoracée. Arch. franç. Pédiat. **20**, 220 (1963). — Dolman, C. L. A., Herd, J. A.: Acute pancreatitis in pregnancy complicated by renal cortical necrosis and cerebral mucormycosis. Canad. med. Ass. J. **81**, 562 (1959). — Dourov, N., Dustin, P.: Fréquence des mycoses dans les hemopathies malignes traitées. Intl. Colloquium on Medical Mycology. Ann. Soc. belge Méd. trop. **44**, 909 (1964). — Dwyer, G. K., Changus, G. W.: Rhinomucormycosis resulting in fatal cerebral mucormycosis. Arch. Otolaryng. **67**, 619 (1958). — Eggenschwiler, E.: Die Mucormykose der Nasennebenhöhlen und ihre Komplikationen (sog. craniale Form der Mucormykose). Pract. oto-rhino-laryng. (Basel) **24**, 166 (1962). — Elder, T. D., Baker, R. D.: Pulmonary mucormycosis in rabbits with alloxan diabetes. Arch. Path. **61**, 159 (1956). — Ellis, P. A.: Mucormycosis. A cause of abscess of the hilum of the lung. Brit. J. Dis. Chest **60**, 203 (1966). — Emmons, C. W., Binford, C. H., Utz, J. P.: Medical mycology, 380 pp. Philadelphia: Lea & Febiger 1963. — Emmons, C. W.: Phycomycosis in man and animals. Riv. Pat. Veg. (Pavia) **4**, 329 (1964). — ERIKSEN, K.R.: Dissemineret mucormykose. Ugeskr. Laeg. **125**, 1849 (1963). — ERIKSEN, K.R., CHRISTENSEN, A.M., HORNBAK, H.: Localized mucormycosis. Ugeskr. Laeg. **124**, 1700 (1962). — ERNST, H.C.: Case of mucor infection. J. med. Res. **39**, 143 (1918, 1919). — FAILLO, P.S., SUBE, H.P., ANDERSON, N.H.: Mucormycosis of the paranasal sinuses and the maxilla. Oral Surg. **12**, 304 (1959). — FANKHAUSER, R., KELLER, H., LANZ, E.: Granulomatose Entzündung von Zwischen-wirbelscheiben beim Rind. Morphologische Mucormykose. Schweiz. Arch. Tierheilk. **108**, 699 (1966). — FEGELER, F.: Medizinische Mykologie in Praxis und Klinik, 125 pp. Berlin-Heidel-berg-New York: Springer 1967. — FEJER, E.: Medizinische Mykologie und Pilzkrankheiten, 987 pp. Budapest: Akadémai Kiadó 1966. — FERRY, A.P.: Cerebral mucormycosis (phyco-mycosis). Surv. Ophthal. **6**, 1 (1961). — FETTER, B.F., KLINTWORTH, G.K., HENDRY, W.S.: Mycoses of the central nervous system, 214 pp. Baltimore: Williams and Wilkins 1967. — FIENBERG, R., RISLEY, T.S.: Mucormycotic infection of arteriosclerotic thrombus of the ab-dominal aorta. New Engl. J. Med. **260**, 626 (1959). — FOLEY, F.D., SHUCK, J.M.: Burn-wound infection with Phycomycetes requiring amputation of hand. J. Amer. med. Ass. **203**, 596 (1968). — FOUSHEE, S., BECK, W.C.: Mucormycosis of central nervous system. N.C. med. J. **17**, 26 (1956). — FRÁGNER. P., ROKOS, J.: Prípad mukormykózy (*Rhizopus oryzae*). Čas. Lék. čes. **103**. 1084 (1964). — FRANKS, A.G., GUIDUCCI, A.: Mucormycosis. In: Medical mycology, ed. by R.D.G. PH. SIMONS, chapter 36. Amsterdam: Elsevier Publ. Co. 1954. — FRENKEL, J.K.: Role of corticosteroids as predisposing factors in fungal diseases. Lab. Invest. **11**, 1192 (1962). — FREYCON, M.T.: La mucormycose ou phycomycose. Pédiatrie **18**, 109 (1963). — FUENTES OLANO, C.: Cuatro casos de mucormicosis cerebral. Bol. méd. Hosp. infant. (Méx.) **20**, 571 (1963). — FÜRBRINGER, P.: Beobachtungen über Lungenmycose beim Menschen. Virchows Arch. path. Anat. **66**, 330 (1876). — GABRIELE, O.F.: Mucormycosis. Amer. J. Roentgenol. **83**, 227 (1960). — GALE, G.R., WELCH, A.M.: Studies of opportunistic fungi. I, Inhibition of Rhizopus oryzae by human serum. Amer. J. med. Sci. **241**, 604 (1961). — GASS. J.D.M.: Ocular manifestations of acute mucormycosis. Arch. Ophthal. **64**, 226 (1961). ~ Acute orbital mucormycosis. Report of 2 cases. Arch. Ophthal. **65**, 214 (1961). — GATLING, R.R.: Gastric mucormycosis in a newborn infant. Arch. Path. **67**, 249 (1959). — GEORGIADE, M., MAGUIRE, C., CRAWFORD, H., PICKRELL, K.: Mucormycosis and palatal sloughs in diabetics. Plast. reconstr. Surg. **17**, 473 (1956). — GINSBERG, J., SPAULDING, A.G., LAING, V.O.: Cerebral phycomycosis (mucormycosis) with ocular involvement. Amer. J. Ophthal. **62**, 900 (1966). — GISLER, D.B., PITCOCK, J.A.: Intestinal mucormycosis in the monkey (*Macaca mulatta*). Amer. J. vet. Res. **23**, 365 (1962). — GITTER, M., AUSTWICK, P.K.C.: Mucormycosis and Moni-liasis in a litter of sucking pigs. Vet. Rec. **71**, 6 (1959). ~ The presence of fungi in abomasal ulcers of young calves. A report of 7 cases. Vet. Rec. **69**, 924 (1957). — GLEISER, C.A.: Mucor-mycosis in animals. A report of three cases. J. Amer. vet. med. Ass. **123**, 441 (1953). — GLOOR, F., LÖFFLER, A., SCHOLER, H.J.: Mucormykosen. Path. et Microbiol. (Basel) **24**, 1043 (1961). — GORDON, M.A., LITTLE, G.N.: Annual report of the division of laboratories and research for 1964. Albany, New York State Dep. of Health, p. 98 (1965). — GREEN, W.H., GOLDBERG, H.I., WOHL, G.T.: Mucormycosis infection of the craniofacial structures. Amer. J. Roentgenol. **101**, 802 (1967). — GREER, A.E.: Disseminated Fungus diseases of the Lung. Springfield/Ill.: Charles C. Thomas 1962. — GREGORY, J.E., GOLDEN, A., HAYMAKER, W.: Mucormycosis of the central nervous system. A report of three cases. Bull. Johns Hopk. Hosp. **73**, 405 (1943). — GROCOTT, R.G.: A stain for fungi in tissue sections and smears using Gomori's methenamine-silver nitrate technic. Amer. J. clin. Path. **25**, 975 (1955). — GROVER, S., NAIDU, A., JUNNAR-KAR, R.V.: Rhinocerebral phycomycosis. A case report. Indian J. Path. Bact. **9**, 264 (1966). — GRUHN, J.G., SANSON, J.: Mycotic infections in leukemic patients at autopsy. Cancer (Philad.) **16**, 61 (1963). — GUENIOT, M.: La mucormycose chez les diabetiques. Sem. Hôp. Path. Biol. (Paris) **7**, 1077 (1959). — GUKELBERGER, M.: Pneumomykosis Mucarina als Sekundärinfektion einer Bronchopneumonie. Dtsch. Arch. klin. Med. **182**, 28 (1938). — GUNSON, H.H., BOWDEN, B.H.: Cerebral mucormycosis. Report of a case. Arch. Path. **60**, 440 (1955). — HAFSTROM, T., SJÖQUIST, O., HENSCHEN, F.: Zur Kenntnis der mykotischen Veränderungen des Gehirns. Acta chir. scand. **85**, 115 (1941). — HARRIS, J.S.: Mucormycosis. Report of a case. J. Pediat. **16**, 857 (1955). — HAWKER, L.E., ABBOTT, P.M.: Fine structure of vegetative hyphae of Rhizopus. J. gen. Microbiol. **30**, 401 (1963). — HERLA, V.: Note sur un cas de pneumomycose chez l'homme. Bull. Acad. roy. Med. Belg. **9**, 1021 (1895). — HESSELTINE, C.W.: Revision of the Mucorales based especially upon a study of the representatives of this order in Wisconsin. Thesis. University of Wisconsin, Madison, Wisconsin, 1950. ~ Survey of the mucorales. Trans. Acad. Sci. **14**, 210 (1952). — HESSLER, J.R.: Mucormycosis in a Rhesus monkey. J. Amer. vet. med. Ass. **151**, 909 (1967). — HEWER, T.F.: Aspergillosis and Mucormycosis in an okapi. A clinical-pathological conference. Bristol med.-chir. J. **79**, 121 (1964). — HILDICK-SMITH, G., BLANK, H., SARKANY, I.: Fungus diseases and their treatment. Boston: Little, Brown & Co. 1964. — HOAGLAND, R.J., SUBE, J., BISHOP, R.H., jr., HOLDING, B.F., jr.: Mucormycosis. Amer. J. med. Sci. **242**, 415 (1961). — HÖER, P.W., BLÄTTNER, G.: Pulmonale Mucormykose

(Phycomykose) beim Neugeborenen. Frankfurt. Z. Path. **74**, 13 (1964). — HÜCKEL, A.: Zur Kenntnis der Biologie des Mucor corymbifer. Beitr. path. Anat. **1**, 115 (1886). — HURTADO, R., INNER, R. S., POZO, S., VEIT, Y. O.: Mucormycosis cerebral. Rev. méd. Chile **93**, 179 (1965). — HUTTER, R. V. P.: Phycomycetous infection (mucormycosis) in cancer patients. A complication of therapy. Cancer (Philad.) **12**, 330 (1959). — HUTTER, R. V. P., COLLINS, H. S.: The occurrence of opportunistic fungus infections in a cancer hospital. Lab. Invest. **11**, 1035 (1962). — HUTTER, R. V. P., LIEBERMAN, P. H., COLLINS, H. S.: Aspergillus in a cancer hospital. Cancer(Philad.) **17**, 747 (1964). — JACKSON, J. R., KARNAUCHOW, P. N.: Mucormycosis of central nervous system. Canad. med. Ass. J. **76**, 130 (1957). — JOSEFIAK, E. J., FOUSHEE, J. H. S.: Experimental mucormycosis in the healthy rat. Science **127**, 1442 (1958). — JOSEFIAK, E. J., FOUSHEE, J. H. S., SMITH, L. C.: Cutaneous mucormycosis. Amer. J. clin. Path. **30**, 547 (1958). — KAHN, L. B.: Gastric mucormycosis. Report of a case with a review of the literature. S. Afr. med. J. **37**, 1265 (1963). — KAPLAN, W., GOSS, L. J., AJELLO, L., IVANS, S.: Pulmonary mucormycosis in a harp seal caused by mucor pusillus. Mycopathologia (Den Haag) **12**, 101 (1959, 1960). — KEENEY, E. L.: Practical medical mycology. Springfield/Ill.: Charles C. Thomas 1955. — KEYE, J. D., MAGEE, W. E.: Fungal diseases in general hospital. A study of 88 patients. Amer. J. clin. Path. **26**, 1235 (1956). — KNOTH-BORN, R. C.: Cutane Mucorinfektion bei einer 50-jährigen Bäuerin. Z. Haut- u. Geschl.-Kr. **26**, 348 (1959). — KUBO, T.: Tumor of small intestine (mucormycosis). Jap. J. clin. Path. **13**, 710 (1965). — KÜCHENMEISTER, G. F. H.: Die in und an dem Körper des lebenden Menschen vorkommenden Parasiten. Ein Lehr- und Handbuch der Diagnose und Behandlung der tierischen und pflanzlichen Parasiten des Menschen. Leipzig (Germany): B. G. Teubner 1855. — KURREIN, F.: Cerebral mucormycosis. J. clin. Path. **7**, 141 (1954). — LANDAU, J. W., NEWCOMER, V. D.: Acute cerebral phycomycosis (mucormycosis). A report of a pediatric patient successfully treated with amphotericin B and cycloheximide and review of the pertinent literature. J. Pediat. **61**, 363 (1963). — LANG, F. J., GRUBAUER, F.: Über Mucor- und Aspergillusmykose der Lunge. Virchows Arch. path. Anat. **245**, 480 (1923). — LATOUCHE, C. J., SUTHERLAND, T. W., TELLING, M.: Histopathological and mycological features of a case of rhinocerebral mucormycosis (phycomycosis) in Britain. Sabouraudia **3** (pt. 2), 148 (1964). ∼ Rhinocerebral mucormycosis. Lancet **1963 II**, 811. — LECOMPTE, P. M., MEISSNER, W. A.: Mucormycosis of the central nervous system associated with hemochromatosis. Amer. J. Path. **23**, 673 (1947). — LEVIN, S. E., ISAACSON, C.: Spontaneous perforation of the colon in the newborn infant. Arch. Dis. Childh. **35**, 378 (1960). — LICHTHEIM, L.: Über pathogene Mucorineen und die durch sie erzeugten Mykosen des Kaninchens. Z. klin. Med. **7**, 140 (1884). — LIE-KIAN-JOE, ENG, N. T., TJOKRONEGORO, S., SCHAAFMA, S., EMMONS, C. W.: Phycomycosis of the central nervous system, associated with diabetes mellitus in Indonesia. Amer. J. clin. Path. **32**, 62 (1959). — LJUBIMOWA, W. J.: Ein Fall von Ulcus ventriculi verursacht durch Schimmelpilze. Virchows Arch. path. Anat. **214**, 432 (1913). — LLOYD, J. B., SEXTON, L. I., HERTIG, A. T.: Pulmonary mucormycosis complicating pregnancy. Amer. J. Obstet. Gynec. **58**, 548 (1949). — LÖHLEIN, M.: Über Schimmelmykosen des Magens. Virchows Arch. path. Anat. **227**, 86 (1920). — LONG, E. L., WEISS, D. L.: Cerebral mucormycosis. Amer. J. Med. **26**, 625 (1959). — LOPEZ, H., HURTADO, H., CORREA, E.: Las micosis profundas en el Hospital de San Juan de Dios (Anos 1959—1962). Cali, Colombia: Publ. Hosp. S. Juan de Dios **16**, 1 (1964). — LUBBE, T. R., PENNINGTON, Orbital mucormicosis. Med. J. Aust. **1**, 681 (1964). — LUCET, A., CONSTANTIN, J.: Contributiona à l'étude des mucorinées pathogénes. Arch. parasit. **4**, 362 (1901). — LUCKE, M., LINTON, A. H.: Phycomycosis in a Mandrill (*Mandrillus sphinx*). Vet. Rec. **77**, 1306 (1965). — MAHAFFEY, L. W., ADAM, N. M.: Abortions associated with mycotic lesions of the placenta in mares. J. Amer. vet. med. Ass. **144**, 24 (1964). — MARCATO, P. S., DIMOU, D.: Su un caso di mucormycosi del rumine in una gazzella. Nuova Vet. **38**, 279 (1962). — MARCHAND, F.: Ein eigentümlicher Magenbefund (Ulcus gangraenosum durch Fadenpilzwucherung) nach Vergiftung durch verdorbene Steinpilze. Verh. dtsch. Ges. Path. **14**, 183 (1910). — MARTIN, F. P., LUKEMAN, J. M., RANSON, R. F., GEPPERT, L. J.: Mucormycosis of the central nervous system associated with thrombosis of the internal carotid artery. J. Pediat. **44**, 437 (1954). — MAYFIELD, G. R., CONDIE, F.: Paradoxical mucorthrombosis in thrombocytopenic purpura. Arch. Path. **63**, 260 (1957). — McBRIDE, R. A., CORSON, J. M., DAMMIN, J. J.: Mucormycosis. Two cases of disseminated disease with cultural identification. Review of literature. Amer. J. Med. **28**, 832 (1960). — McCALL, W., STROBOS, R. R. J.: Survival of a patient with central nervous system mucormycosis. Neurology (Minneap.) **7**, 290 (1957). — MEHNERT, B.: The role of fungi in diseases of young pigs. Zbl. Vet.-Med. (B) **13**, 201 (1966). — MERRIAM, J. C., jr., TEDESCHI, C. G.: Cerebral mucormycosis, a fatal fungus infection complicating other diseases. Neurology (Minneap.) **7**, 510 (1957). — MIYAKE, M., OKUDAIRA, M.: A statistical survey of deep fungus infection in Japan. Acta path. jap. **17**, 401 (1967). — MOMBERG-JORGENSEN, A. C.: Enzoötic mycosis in mink. Amer. J. vet. Res. **11**, 334 (1950). — MONTENEGRO, M. R., DEBRITO, T., LOMBARDI, J., LACAZ, C. S.: Mucormicose intestinal; Registro de dois casos. Rev. Hosp. Clin. Fac. Med. S. Paulo **14**, 59 (1959). — MOORE, M., ANDERSON, W. A. D., EVERETT, H. H.: Mucormycosis of large bowel. Amer. J. Path. **25**, 559 (1949). — MORQUER, R., LOMBARD, C., BERTHELON, M., LACOSTE, L.: Pathogénie de quelques Mucorales pour les animaux. Une nouvelle mucormycose chez les Bovidés. Bull. trim. Soc. mycol. Fr. **81**, 421 (1965). — MOSS, E.S., McQUOWN, A.L.: Atlas of medical mycology, 335 pp. Baltimore: Williams & Wilkins Co. 1960. — MOSTAFA, I.E., CERNA, J., CERNY, L.: Mucormycosis in goats. Report of two cases. Ceylon vet. J. **14**, 79 (1966). — MURESAN, A.: A case of cerebral mucormycosis diagnosed in life, with eventual recovery. J. clin. Path. **13**, 34 (1960). — MURPHY, J.D., BORNSTEIN, S.: Mucormycosis of the lung. Ann. intern. Med. **33**, 44 (1959). — NARASIMHAN, M.J., GANLA, V.G., DEODHAR NAR N.S.: Epidemic polyuria in man caused by a phycomycetous fungus (the Sassoon hospital syndrome). Lancet 1967 I, 760. — NEAME, P., RAYNER, D.: Mucormycosis. Report on 22 cases. Arch. Path. **70**, 261 (1960). — NICOD, J.L., FLEURY, C., SCHLEGEL, J.: Mycose pulmonaire double à Aspergillus fumigatus Fres. et à mucor pusillus. Lindt .Schweiz. Z. allg. Path. **15**, 307 (1952). — NICOLET, J., LINDT, S., SCHOLER, H.J.: L'avotemente mycosique de la vache. Considérations sur le diagnostic de routine. Path. et Microbiol. (Basel) **29**, 644 (1966). — OBRASZOW, E.S., PETROV, N.V.: Fall gleichzeitiger Aktinomykose und Schimmelmykose. Russ. Med. **7**, 457 (1889). — OPPE: Zur Kenntnis der Schimmelmykosen beim Menschen. Zbl. allg. Path. path. Anat. **8**, 301 (1897). — OSSWALD, H., SEELIGER, H.: Tierexperimentelle Untersuchungen mit antimycotischen Mitteln. Arzneimittel-Forsch. **8**, 370 (1958). — PALTAUF, A.: Mycosis mucorina. Virchows Arch. path. Anat. **102**, 543 (1885). — PAPLANUS, S.H., SHELDON, W.H.: The inflammatory response of hypothyroid rats to subcutaneous *Rhizopus oryzae* infection. Bull. Johns Hopk. Hosp. **117**, 140 (1965). — PARKHURST, G.F., VLAHIDES, G.D.: Fatal opportunistic fungus diseases. J. Amer. med. Ass. **202**, 279 (1967). — PARMENTIER, N., BALASSE, E., MEUR, G., PIRART, J., VANDERHAEGEN, J.J.: Etude anatomo-clinique d'un cas de phycomycose de l'étage craniofacial. Bull. Soc. belge Ophthal. **139**, 304 (1965). — PASTORE, P.N.: Mucormycosis of the maxillary sinus and diabetes mellitus. Report of a case with recovery. Sth. med. J. (Bgham, Ala.) **60**, 1164 (1967). — PEÑA, C.E.: Deep mycotic infections in Colombia. A clinicopathologic study of 162 cases. Amer. J. clin. Path. **47**, 505 (1967). — PEÑA, C.E., DORADO, J.A.: Mucormycosis (ficomicosis) en Colombia. Presentación de dos casos. Rev. Fac. Med. (Bogotá) **33**, 2 (1965). — PEREZ ARZOLA, M., GARCÍA SORIA, M., RIVIERA, E.: Cerebral mucormycosis. Bol. Asoc. méd. P. Rico **58**, 374 (1966). — *Phycomycosis* (Editorial): Actualid. pediát. **24**, 501 (1963). — PIRILA, P.: Eine Mucormykose der äußeren Genitalien. Acta derm.-venereol. (Stockh.) **22**, 377 (1941). — PLAUT, H.C., GRÜTZ, O.: Mucoraceen, pp. 159—163, and Die Schimmelpilze, pp. 156. In: W. KOLLE and A.V. WASSERMANN **5**, 1 (1928). — PODACK, M.: Zur Kenntnis des sog. Endothelkrebses der Pleura und die Mucormycosen im menschlichen Respirationsapparat. Dtsch. Arch. klin. Med. **63**, 1 (1899). — POLEMANN, G.: Klinik und Therapie der Pilzkrankheiten, 396 pp. Stuttgart: Georg Thieme 1961. — PROCKNOW, J.J.: Treatment of opportunistic fungus infections. Lab. Invest. **11**, 1217 (1962). — PROCKOP, L.D., SILVA-HUTNER, M.: Cephalic mucormycosis (phycomycosis). A case with survival. Arch. Neurol. (Chic.) **17**, 379 (1967). — PROUT, G.R., jr., GODDARD, R.: Renal mucormycosis. New Engl. J. Med. **263**, 1246 (1960). — RABIN, E.R., LUNDBERG, G.D., MITCHELL, E.T.: Mucormycosis in severely burned patients. Report of 2 cases with extensive destruction of face and nasal cavity. New Engl. J. Med. **264**, 1286 (1961). — REEVES, D.L., DICKSON, D.A., BENJAMIN, E.L.: Phycomycosis (mucormycosis) of the central nervous system. Report of a case. J. Neurosurg. **23**, 82 (1965). — RINALDI, I., ASHBY, S.F.: Facio-cranial mucormycosis. Report of a case. Virginia med. Mth. **89**, 595 (1962). — ROBERTS, H.J.: Cutaneous mucormycosis. Report of a case, with survival. Arch. intern. Med. **110**, 108 (1962). — ROWE, P.B., PAYNE, W.H.: Rhino-cerebral mucormycosis. Med. J. Aust. **2**, 960 (1964). — SAUER, R.M.: Cutaneous mucormycosis (phycomycosis) in a squirrel (*Sciureus carolinensis*). Amer. J. vet. Res. **27**, 380 (1966). — SCHAUBLE, M.K., BAKER, R.D.: The inflammatory response in acute alloxan diabetes. Arch. Path. **64**, 563 (1957). — SCHOFIELD, R.A., BAKER, R.D.: Experimental mucormycosis (Rhizopus infections) in mice. Arch. Path. **61**, 407 (1956). — SHANKLIN, D.R.: Pulmonary mucormycosis complicating Cushing's syndrome. Arch. Path. **68**, 262 (1959). — SHELDON, W.H., BAUER, H.: Activation of quiescent mucormycotic granulomata in rabbits by induction of acute alloxan diabetes. J. exp. Med. **108**, 171 (1958). ～ The development of the acute inflammatory response to experimental cutaneous mucormycosis in normal and diabetic rabbits. J. exp. Med. **110**, 845 (1959). ～ The role of predisposing factors in experimental fungus infections. Lab. Invest. **11**, 1184 (1962). — SHIRLEY, A.G.H.: Two cases of phycomycotic ulceration in sheep. Vet. Rec. **77**, 675 (1965). — SIMON, R., HOFFMAN, G.G., HARDING, H.B.: Phycomycosis. Aerospace Med. **35**, 668 (1964). — SLUYTER: De vegetabilibus organismi animalis parasitis ac de novo epiphyto in pityriasi versicolore obvio. Inaug. Diss. Berlin (Germany) 1847. — SMITH, D.T.: Miscellaneous fungus diseases. J. chron. Dis. **5**, 528 (1957). — STEVENSON, H.N.: Mucormycosis of maxillary sinus. Arch. Otolaryng. **18**, 775 (1933). — SMITH, H.W., KIRCHNER, J.A.: Cerebral mucormycosis. Report of 3 cases. Arch. Otolaryng. **68**, 715 (1958). — SMITH, H.W., YANAGISAWA, E.: Rhinomucormycosis. Report of a fatal case. New Engl. J. Med. **260**, 1007 (1959). — SMITH, M.E., BURNHAM, DEW.K., BLACK,

M.B.: Cerebral mucormycosis. Arch. Path. 66, 468 (1958). — STEHBENS, W.E.: Atypical cerebral aneurysms. Med. J. Aust. 1, 765 (1965). — STEFANINI, M., ALLEGRA, S.: Pulmonary mucormycosis in acute histocytic leukemia. New Engl. J. Med. 256, 1026 (1957). — STEIN, A., SCHMAMAN, A.: Rupture of the stomach due to mucormycosis. S. Afr. J. Surg. 3, 123 (1965). — STRAATSMA, B.R., ZIMMERMANN, L.E., GASS, J.D.: Phycomycosis. A clinicopathologic study of 51 cases. Lab. Invest. 11, 963 (1962). — STRATEMEIER, W.P.: Mucormycosis of central nervous system. Report of a case. Arch. Neurol. Psychiat. (Chic.) 63, 179 (1950). — SUGA, J., HAGAL, A., KASHIMA, H.: Autopsy case of disseminated mucormycosis with ocular involvement. J. clin. Ophthal. (Tokyo) 17, 365 (1963). — SUIE, T., HAVENER, W.H.: Mycology of the eye. A review. Amer. J. Ophthal. 56, 63 (1963). — SUN, H.L., WANG, T., MA, W., KAO, H.: A study of the pathology and morphology of deep mycosis. China med. J. 84, 125 (1965). — SUPRUN, H.: Mucormycosis infection. A post-mortem case report with a summarized survey of the literature. Israel med. J. 21, 40 (1962). — SUTHERLAND, J.C., JONES, T.H.: Gastric mucormycosis. Report of a case in a Swazi. S. Afr. med. J. 34, 161 (1960). — SUTHERLAND-CAMPBELL, H., PLUNKETT, O.A.: Mucor paronychia. Syph. 30, 651 (1934). — Sydney Hospital: Clinicopathological conference. Med. J. Aust. 2, 98 (1956a). ~ Clinicopathological conference. Med. J. Aust. 11, 30 (1956b). — SYMMERS, W. ST.C.: Histopathologic aspects of the pathogenesis of some opportunistic fungal infections, as exemplified in the pathology of aspergillosis and phycomycetoses. Lab. Invest. 11, 1073 (1962). ~ The tissue reactions in deep-seated fungal infections. The role of histological examination in mycological diagnosis. Ann. Soc. belge Méd. trop. 44, 869 (1964). ~ The occurrence of deep-seated fungal infections in general hospital practice in Britain today. Proc. roy. Soc. Med. 57, 405 (1964). — TAKAHASHI, Y.: A critical survey of medical mycology for the years 1946—1956 in Japan. Mycopathologia (Den Haag) 19, 105 (1963). — TAYLOR, R., SHKLAR, G., BUDSON, R., HACKETT, R.: Mucormycosis of the oral mucosa. Arch. Derm. 89, 419 (1964). — TEUTSCHLAENDER, O.: Mucormykose des Magens. Mitt. Grenzgeb. Med. Chir. 29, 127 (1916, 1917). — TEWARI, R.P.: Studies on some mycotic infections of domestic animals and poultry. Agra Univ. J. Res. 12, 163 (1963). — TINAZTEPE, B., TINAZTEPE, K.: Cerebral mucormycosis in a child. Turk. J. Pediat. 8, 207 (1966). — TOMIK, F.: Histologische und histochemische Diagnose der Systemmykosen. Zbl. allg. Path. path. Anat. 104, 189 (1963). — TOMIYASU, U., BAKER, R.N.: Phycomycosis (mucormycosis) of the orbital apex and cavernous sinus. Bull. Los Angeles neurol. Soc. 31, 177 (1966). — TORACK, R.M.: Fungus infections associated with antibiotic and steroid therapy. Amer. J. Med. 22, 872 (1957). — TRUJILLO, S.H.: Monografia sobre la mucormicosis en pediatrica. Anot. pediát. 4, 296 (1961). — TURNER, P.D.: Simultaneous infection of a bovine foetus by 2 fungi. Nature (Lond.) 205, 300 (1965). — TURPIN, R., BOCQUET, L., CAILLE, B., DEFRANOUX, A.: Mucormycose cérébral. Épisode terminale d'une leucose aiguë. Sem. Hôp. Ann. Péd. (Paris) 37, 2134 (1961). — UTZ, J.P.: The spectrum of opportunistic fungus infections. Lab. Invest. 11, 1018 (1962). ~ Systemic fungal infections amenable to chemotherapy. DM (Chic.) 1, 1963. — VIGNALE, R., MACKINNON, J.E., CASELLA DE VILA BOA, E., BURGOA, F.: Chronic destructive, mucocutaneous phycomycosis in man. Sabouraudia 3, 143 (1964). — WADE, J.L., MATTHEWS, A.R.K.: Cutaneous mucor infection of face. J. Amer. med. Ass. 114, 410 (1940). — WADSWORTH, J.A.C.: Ocular mucormycosis. Report of a case. Amer. J. Ophthal. 34, 405 (1951). — WALL, G.H., MADISON, W.N., jr.: Fatal pulmonary phycomycosis complicating leukemia. A case report. N. C. med. J. 26, 66 (1965). — WASSERMAN, A.J., SNIELS, W.S., SPORN, I.N.: Cerebral mucormycosis. Sth. med. J. (Bgham, Ala.) 54, 403 (1961). — WÄTJEN, J.: Pathologisch-anatomische Demonstrationen. Klin. Wschr. 8, 280 (1929). ~ Durch Schimmel und Sproßpilze bedingte Erkrankungen der Lungen. In: Handbuch der speziellen pathologischen Anatomie und Histologie Hrsg. von HENKE-LUBARSCH. Vol. 3, part 3, p. 397. Berlin: Springer 1931. — WATSON, K.C.: Gastric perforation due to fungus Mucor in a child with kwashiorkor. S. Afr. med. J. 31, 99 (1957). — WATSON, K.C., NEAME. P.B.: In vitro activity of Amphotericin B on strains of Mucoraceae pathogenic to man. J. Lab. clin. Med. 56, 251 (1960). — WEISSKOPF, A.: Mucormycosis, a rhinologic disease. Ann. Otol. (St. Louis) 73, 16 (1964). — WELLER, W.A., JOSEPH, D.J., HORA, J.F.: Deep mycotic involvement of the right maxillary and ethmoid sinuses. Laryngoscope (St. Louis) 70, (2), 999 (1960), — WERNER, H.J., WRIGHT, P., BAKER, R.D.: Electron microscope observations of Rhizopus rhizopodiformis. J. gen. Microbiol. 37, 205 (1964). — WERTMAN, K.F., HENNEY, M.R.: The effects of alloxan diabetes on phagocytosis and suceptibility to infection. J. Immunol. 89, 314 (1962). — WILSON, J.W., PLUNKETT, O.A.: The fungus diseases in man. Berkeley and Los Angeles: University of California Press 1965. — WINSTON, R.M.: Phycomycosis of the bronchus. J. clin. Path. 18, 729 (1965). — WOLF, A., COWEN, D.: Mucormycosis of central nervous system (abstr.). J. Neuropath. exp. Neurol. 8, 107 (1949). — WRIGHT, P., SYMMERS, W. ST. C.: Systemic pathology. New York: Elsevier Press 1967. — ZIMMERMAN, L.E.: Fatal fungus infections complicating other diseases. Amer. J. clin. Path. 25, 46 (1955).

Geotrichosis

J. **MORENZ**, Magdeburg, Germany (DDR)

With 12 Figures

A. Definition

Geotrichosis is a world-wide mycosis caused by *Geotrichum candidum*. The oral, bronchial and bronchopulmonary geotrichoses are endogenous in origin and have little tendency to hematogenous dissemination. The cutaneous geotrichoses are mostly exogenous in origin, limited to the skin, chronic, occur in superficial and deep forms, and sometimes are accompanied by allergic skin reactions in the form of geotrichids. Mycetemia without lesions in the organs, ulcerative keratitides, and a mycetoma have been observed.

B. Geographical Extent and Epidemiology

Geotrichum candidum is world-wide and ubiquitous. It is in soil and sewage, on damaged or dying plants and almost always present in sour milk and sour milk products. It grows especially well in sour vegetable liquid, moist food for farm animals, mash, spoiled wine, manure, and other animal excreta.

Although geotrichosis is of world-wide occurrence most of the cases have been observed in Europe and North America, probably because of the better diagnostic possibilities in these regions. SMITH (1949) gave data on the frequency of geotrichosis in the United States. He reported that among 250,000 admissions to Duke Hospital (Durham, North Carolina, USA) there were 207 patients with systemic mycoses and among them 4 with geotrichosis.

With regard to the age incidence of the cases of geotrichosis, there appears to be no predilection of the disease as a whole, or of the various forms, for any particular age period. The extremes of occurrence are in a 2-month-old infant and an 80-year-old man. The ratio of men to women is about 2:1. This difference may be fortuitous because of the small number of cases. Occupational predispositions are not evident.

As *G. candidum* can be isolated from the sputum and stool of healthy persons, that is, it is normally already present on the mucous membranes of the respiratory and digestive tract, therefore bronchopulmonary, bronchial and oral geotrichoses are endogenous infections. There are also exogenous infections. These are illustrated by the two corneal infections described by PERZ (1964) after mud, evidently containing *G. candidum* splashed into the eye, and injured the cornea. The mycetoma of the foot described by NICOLAU et al. (1957) apparently developed after a wound from a nail in the sole of a shoe. In cutaneous geotrichosis the manner of infection is, to some extent, still unclear. In the superficial forms, and in the deep forms which begin with an epidermal lesion, the concept of an exogenous infection (an injury mycosis) can be accepted. In contrast to this, in the patient of THIERS et al. (1953) the infection began with subcutaneous nodules, and the epidermis was implicated later.

C. Geotrichum Candidum - Occurrence in Humans

1. Intestinal Tract

G. candidum can be demonstrated most frequently in the stool, in 25—30% of persons without intestinal disorders, and in 50—60% of patients with intestinal disorders, especially in the region of the colon. In the latter group the quantity of excreted fungus is significantly greater.

Schnoor (1939) isolated *G. candidum (G. sp.)* from 29% of 314 normal stools. Swartz and Jankelson (1941) found *G. candidum (G. versiforme)* in 67% of 24 cases of nonspecific ulcerative colitis and in only 21% of the control group of 24 cases of healthy persons and patients with diarrhea due to other causes. Quantitatively, almost pure cultures were obtained from the colitis group, while in the control group there were generally only a few colonies. Golay and Wyss-Chodat (1942) isolated *G. candidum (G. sp.)* in only 3% of 102 stools of healthy persons and of patients with various skin lesions, but they obtained 54% positive stools in 28 patients with psoriasis. As there were 83% positives in the more severe psoriasis cases, the authors thought there might be a relationship between psoriasis and the presence of *G. candidum* in the stool. This observation was corroborated by Ettig (1965) who was able to demonstrate *G. candidum* in 98% of 125 psoriasis patients and in only 41% of 138 healthy persons and persons with other skin diseases. *G. candidum* grew luxuriantly in 22% of the stool cultures of the psoriasis patients in contrast to 4% of the control group. Ettig related the increased occurrence of the fungus in psoriasis to a dysfunction of the intestinal mucous membrane. The psoriasis was not influenced in 5 patients treated for 3 weeks with nystatin. The stools were fungus free in 5 days. Also, the geotrichin test was negative in the psoriasis patients. A larger research series comes from Felsenfeld (1944). He isolated *G. candidum (G. sp.)* in 27% of 900 cases without intestinal disturbances and in 26% of 100 carriers of typhoid bacteria. However, he isolated the fungus in 56% of 103 cases with diarrhea of recent onset. A study of 47 untreated bacterial diarrheas yielded 53% with *G. candidum* while in 51 cases treated with sulfathiazole only 6% were positive for *G. candidum*. Marselou and Paschali-Pavlatou (1956) demonstrated *G. candidum (G. sp.)* in 6% of rectal smears from 105 women. Saëz (1957) found *G. candidum* in 30% of 62 persons (both ill and healthy), Kärcher (1953) in 15% of 124 patients with various illnesses and Galinovic-Weisglass (1959) in 56% of 100 patients with various intestinal disorders and in 33% of 100 healthy subjects. In the patients the fungus was present in larger quantities than in the healthy subjects. Péter and Horváth (1959) established an increasing case frequency with age. In 119 children under a year of age, *G. candidum (G. sp.)* could be isolated in only 5% and these were bottle-fed infants. In the age period of 1—3 years 15% of 168 infants and children had isolates of *G. candidum* from their stools; in the age period of 6—12 years 37% of 184, and in the age period above 20 years 53% of 176 were positive. The average frequency of demonstration was 22% in 342 healthy subjects in contrast to 39% in 305 patients treated with antibiotics. Caretta (1961) isolated *G. candidum* from the stools in 10% of 135 patients more than 15 years old, Tzamouranis and Crimbithis (1962) in 13% of 155 patients, Heidenbluth (1963) in 40% of 50 subjects without skin diseases, Ott (1963) in 31% of 300 patients with various skin diseases, Ariyevich et al. (1963) in 28% of 107 patients suspected of having candidosis, and Morenz (1963) in 38% of 577 stools submitted for the investigation of pathogenic intestinal bacteria. Péter et al. (1967) could demonstrate *G. candidum* in 30% of 674 stool specimens from healthy persons and in 52% of 802 stools from patients with various diseases, such as epidemic hepatitis, etc.

Because of the frequent occurrence of *Geotrichum candidum* in the stool and its increased elimination in many intestinal disturbances, the relationship of this fungus to afflictions of the digestive tract, especially to diarrheal disorders, is discussed.

G. candidum was isolated by Castellani (1914; *Monilia asteroides*) in enteritis and sprue, by Mattlet (1926; *Mycoderma issavi, M. muyaga* and *M. kieta*) in enteritis and dysentery, and viewed as a possible etiological agent. Jannin (1913) found *G. candidum* twice in hyperacidic gastric juice in gastric dilatation. Although he did not accept the idea of an invasion of the mucosa, he considered the fungi to foster chronic bacterial processes. Ciferri et al. (1938) considered a *G. candidum* strain (*G. matalense*) isolated from an enterocolitis of 3 years duration to be not the cause but to play a secondary role. According to Swartz and Jankelson (1941), in spite of the frequent and abundant occurrence of *G. candidum* in the stool in colitis cases, there is no reason to consider it causal. Colonnello (1944) rejects an etiologic role for *G. candidum* in intestinal diseases. He found no difference between 30 healthy persons and 30 patients with various intestinal disorders with respect to the occurrence of *G. candidum*. *G. candidum* was isolated from rectal ulcerations by ALMEIDA and LACAZ (1940) and COLONNELLO (1944). Two patients of COUDERT et al. (1958) developed a feeling of abdominal fullness and anal itching in the course of tetracycline therapy, and also there were large numbers of the fungus in smears of the stool. As there was a diminution of the number of fungi with the disappearance of symptoms, the authors ascribed a causal relation to the fungus. In the 2 enterocolitis cases of KÄRCHER (1963) that had been treated with aureomycin, *G. candidum* was present in the stool in large quantity. After oral therapy with gentian violet there was a rapid improvement and a decrease in the numbers of *G. candidum* in the stool.

ARIYEVICH et al. (1963) reported 14 patients with various underlying lesions (5 cases of dysentery, 5 of chronic colitis, 2 of ulcerative colitis, one of pleuropneumonia and one of virus-grippe) who had been treated unsuccessfully with antibiotics concurrently or successively. Microscopically and culturally abundant *G. candidum (G.sp.)* was demonstrated as the only fungus or in combination with *Candida*. Therapy with *Candida*-vaccine and an acid-milk-bacteria preparation and later with nystatin was relatively successful. An intestinal geotrichosis or an infection with a combination of *Geotrichum* and *Candida* was postulated. The fungus infections were regarded as super-infections of a condition of disturbed bacterial flora due to antibiotics. The intestinal symptoms corresponded in general to the symptoms of the underlying disease. In some patients there were inconstant bowel movements, in others a chronic obstipation with moderate periodic abdominal pain. In all patients, after high dosages of antibiotics there was a worsened condition, especially with meteorism, severe girdle pains, increased bowel movements and occasionally with subfebrile temperatures and pruritus ani. In these cases the pathogenetic significance of *G. candidum* is difficult to appraise and can not be considered as completely certain. ABRAMOVA et al. (1964) described very completely a case regarded as intestinal geotrichosis (in relation to antibiotic therapy), in a 3 months old, male infant. The child was treated, shortly after birth, with various antibiotics for pneumonia, otitis and gastroenteritis. There was subnormal temperature; the infant was restless and the stools (4 to 17 a day) were pasty and mucoid. Pathogenic intestinal bacteria could not be demonstrated, but there was abundant *G. candidum (G.sp.)* microscopically and culturally. After the giving of colistin the condition was worse, whereas two courses of nystatin over 3 week periods and an intensive treatment with blood transfusions lead to healing and the elimination of the fungus. Also in this case the original significance of the *G. candidum* is not clear as the related general treatment could have accounted for the improvement.

G. and M. NEAGOE (1967) reported the cases of two 22—23-year-old patients, who, in the course of glutamic acid treatment of asthenia, developed a chronic diarrhea with weight loss of 8—10 kg and a large content of *G. candidum* in their stools. After discontinuing the glutamic acid therapy and after the giving of iodine, gentian violet or methylene blue, the intestinal symptoms improved and the content of *G. candidum* in the stools decreased. A renewal of the glutamic acid therapy lead to relapses. The authors believe that the increased growth of fungus caused by glutamic acid may lead to enterocolitis.

From a study of these cases, a conclusive judgment concerning the occurrence of intestinal geotrichosis is still not possible. Apparently there are geotrichoses of the mucous membranes of the respiratory and upper digestive tracts. These develop when the fungus proliferates in an altered terrain, and infection ensues. As the increase in the amount of *G. candidum* in the stool might be only an indication of an altered condition in the intestine, the success of therapy with fungistatic agents comes to have great diagnostic significance. However, one must bear in mind the possibility of an underlying disease or predisposing condition.

2. Respiratory Tract

Geotrichum candidum can be isolated from the sputum of from 1—6% of the population and of 25% of patients with pulmonary tuberculosis.

ALMEIDA and LACAZ (1940) isolated 4 strains of *G. candidum (G.sp.)* from 422 sputa. Among 124 sputum examinations KÄRCHER (1953) found *G. candidum (G.sp.)* once. COUDERT et al. (1957) was able to demonstrate *G. candidum* in 25% of 151 cases of pulmonary tuberculosis in a sanatorium. The presence of the fungus could not be correlated with the therapy of the tuberculosis or with the presence of the tubercle bacillus in the sputum. CARETTA (1961) found *G. candidum* in the sputum of 2 of 135 patients. VÖRÖS-FELKAI and NOVÁK (1961) demonstrated *G.candidum (G.sp.)* 17 times in the pharyngeal, laryngeal, and bronchial secretions and gastric juice of 1200 patients suspected of having mycoses. Among 143 isolates of fungi from the sputum and oral cavity MONTEMAYOR and GAMERO (1961) found *G.candidum (G.sp.)* 10 times. MORENZ (1963) isolated *G.candidum* in 14% of 262 sputa submitted for a search for the tubercle bacillus, and in only 6% of 326 other sputa. ARIYEVICH et al. demonstrated *G.candidum (G.sp.)* three times in 105 sputa and twice in 100 tongue smears of patients suspected of having candidosis. PÉTER et al. (1967) were able to culture *G.candidum* 6 times in 120 sputa and 3 times in 279 throat swabs from healthy persons, and 34 times in 279 sputa, 6 times in 121 throat swabs and once in 33 bronchial washings from patients, mainly patients with tuberculosis. REIERSÖL (1953) found *G.candidum (G.sp.)* twice in 250 laryngeal smears, TZAMOURANIS and CRIMBITHIS (1962) once in 155 pharyngeal smears, and OTT (1963) once in tongue smears from 300 dermatologic patients, while KOURKOUMELI-KONTOMICHALOU et al. (1961) were able to demonstrate *G.candidum* in 6% of the pharyngeal specimens from 240 healthy persons (hospital personnel). Among 6 fungi isolated from bronchial washings by MONTEMAYOR and GAMERO (1961) *G.candidum (G.sp.)* was isolated once. Among 580 bronchoscopic specimens GERNEZ-RIEUX (1960) found *G.candidum (G.sp.)* 5 times, twice in patients with pulmonary tuberculosis, twice in patients with tumors, and once in a patient with mega-esophagus. In 4 of these cases *G.candidum* was visible in direct preparations. From the lungs of 71 autopsies HALEY and McCABE isolated *G.candidum* once.

3. Skin

Geotrichum candidum occurs on the skin only accidentally. However, GUÉGUEN (1913) mentioned the more frequent occurrence of *G.candidum (Oidium lactis)* on the skin of persons working in milk plants.

CIFERRI and REDAELLI (1935) describe a strain of *G.candidum* isolated from eczema. REDAELLI and CIFERRI (1943) cite two additional strains, one from normal skin and one, with another fungus, from a lesion of the foot. FRÁGNER and SVATEK (1956) found *G.candidum* twice among 170 fungi isolated from the interdigital spaces of miners. PINKERTON et al. (1957) were able to demonstrate *G.candidum (G.sp.)* more often with *Trichophyton mentagrophytes* or *T.rubrum* in tinea pedis and tinea cruris. COUDERT et al. (1958) isolated *G.candidum* five times from scrapings and nail clipping among 128 specimens, but only from moist skin areas. MONTEMAYOR and GAMERO (1961) among 12 fungi isolated from intertrigo and 10 from onychomycosis found in each group a single strain of *G.candidum (G.sp.)*. DVOŘÁK and OTČENÁŠEK (1966) were able to demonstrate *G.candidum* 8 times culturally (4 times together with *Candida albicans*) and 3 times by direct microscopic observation among 2500 lesions of skin and nails. The material came from nails four times, four times from skin scrapings from between the toes, and from between the fingers and from the back of the hand. As *G.candidum* was demonstrated microscopically and in heavy growth of pure culture in a finger nail and in an interdigital lesion in these two cases, a *G.candidum* infection of a previously pathologically altered area was conjectured. The clinical picture and the course of the condition are unknown.

4. Urogenital Tract

G.candidum is only occasionally present in the urogenital tract and may be considered a nonsignificant contaminant.

FRÁGNER et al. (1955) isolated *G.candidum* from the vaginal secretions of 2 patients without giving the finding a clinical meaning. SAËZ (1957) was unable to isolate *G.candidum* in 64 samples from the vagina. PÉTER et al. (1967) isolated the fungus from 2 of 19 vaginal smears from patients with various disorders, but none from 50 smears from healthy subjects.

In urine *G.candidum* was present with bacteria once in the experience of DUNCAN et al. (1951) and COUDERT et al. (1958), but SAËZ (1957) could not demonstrate *G.candidum* in urines obtained aseptically. PÉTER et al. (1967) found *G.candidum* once in 43 urines and MORENZ (1963) twice in 877 urines. Both urines were, however, not taken aseptically nor were the majority of investigated specimens. ARIYEVICH et al. (1963) isolated *G.candidum (G.sp.)* four times from 168 urines from patients suspected of having candidosis but without disease of the urinary tract. On the other hand, *G.candidum (G.sp.)* in great quantity was demonstrated microscopically and culturally in the urine of a 32-year-old patient (from Moscow) with agranulocytosis and symptoms of cystitis who had been treated with penicillin, streptomycin, and other antibiotics. Cystoscopically a white coating was seen on the mucosa of the bladder. Also there were similar plaques on the oral mucosa, but they consisted of *Candida* elements.

D. Mycology

The mycologic diagnosis is relatively simple, as *G.candidum* is the only *Geotrichum* which occurs in man, apart from some insignificant exceptions (MORENZ, 1963—1964). There may be confusion with *Trichosporon* BEHREND (Synonyms: *Geotrichoides*, *Neogeotrichum*) which is mentioned because even in recent times mycoses caused by *Trichosporon* have been called geotrichoses.

The causal agents of the mycoses described by VRIJMAN (1933), CASTELLANI (1942), VOLK and CAÑAS (1942), PÉTOURAUD and COUDERT (1953), GAUVREAU and GRANDBOIS (1954), LOFGREN (1955) and BREDNOW (1958, Case O. BU.) do not belong to the genus *Geotrichum*.

Geotrichum candidum Link is known by about 100 synonyms (CARMICHAEL, 1957; MORENZ, 1963). Most often this fungus is listed among the genera *Oidium*, *Oospora*, and *Mycoderma*. The synonyms of the strains found in cases are given in Tables 1—5. The synonyms used in the text are placed in parentheses.

1. Micromorphology

Geotrichum candidum is a filamentous fungus with a hyaline, ramifying mycelium which breaks up into arthrospores (Fig. 1). They are 1.5 to 11×2 to 40 μ in size, and of a rectangular shape. From the arthrospores originate germ tubes, which grow out to form mycelium. In contrast to the *Trichosporon*, reproduction takes place by fission only. *Geotrichum candidum* belongs to the fungi imperfecti, as a sexual development is not known. The micromorphology can be observed best in slide cultures. The medium is poured on to a slide and the fungus is inoculated in streaks. Then a coverglass is put on and the preparation is incubated in a moist chamber for 3 days at room temperature. *Trichosporon* and *Coccidioides* may be mistaken for *Geotrichum*. However, *Trichosporon* propagates by forming arthrospores and blastospores that can be clearly demonstrated by slide culture and in fluid media. The mycelium formed by *Coccidioides immitis* fragments differently from that of *Geotrichum candidum*, not into arthrospores but into thick-walled chlamydospores, which are separated from one another in a characteristic way by empty hyphae. *C.immitis*, moreover, grows as a mold.

2. Direct Preparations

Sputum, bronchus aspirate, pus, ulcer scrapings or material from mucus membranes or from biopsies is placed directly on a glass slide. When there is much cellular material, a drop of physiological NaCl solution or of 20% sodium hydroxide solution is added and a coverglass is applied. The preparation can be seen by reduced illumination, unstained, for the mycelium of the fungus is relatively strongly light refracting. *Geotrichum candidum* stains very well with methylene blue, fuchsin, gentian violet, or PAS. Young mycelium is Gram positive, older mycelium is partly Gram negative. In sputum, feces and mucus there are rectangular arthrospores and mycelial fragments (Fig. 2) while in pus and tissue sections the fungus elements are frequently rounded off (4—12 μ in diameter) and are found in small numbers only. Round forms are not to be mistaken for yeast or *Blastomyces dermatitidis*, in which, in contrast to *Geotrichum candidum*, budding can always be demonstrated. Moreover, in *B.dermatitidis* there are never arthrospore-like structures in the tissue. However, with *Geotrichum candidum* peculiar shaped formations may occur, which look like budding cells. Cases in doubt can be easily clarified by culture. The strongly rounded or irregular forms, as well as

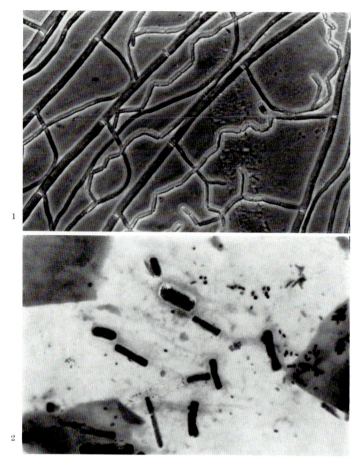

Fig. 1. *Geotrichum candidum*. Branching and septate mycelium with hyphae breaking up into arthrospores. Slide culture. Phase contrast, × 200

Fig. 2. Smear of sputum. *Geotrichum candidum* arthrospores, bacteria and epithelial cells. Gram stain, × 1000

the structures hard to stain, are involution changes in the fungus, determined by an inadequate environment in the interior of the tissue and by unfavorable cultural conditions.

3. Culture

The unpretentious fungus grows on all the usual media at room temperature, and not as well at 37°C (Fig. 3). Old specimens at times do not grow at 37°C, but can be adapted again to this temperature. The growth is strongly promoted by 2% glucose. Vitamins have no influence. The most commonly used medium is Sabouraud's glucose agar. Antibiotics are recommended to suppress bacterial growth. A mold fungus inhibitor for this relatively fast growing fungus is not necessary. In 2—4 days, at the latest, relatively large, shallow, yeast-like, greyish-white to cream colored colonies form with a predominantly flour-like, irregular surface. On liquid media *Geotrichum candidum* produces thick pellicles. Under the microscope one sees typical arthrospores and non-fragmented hyphae (Fig. 4).

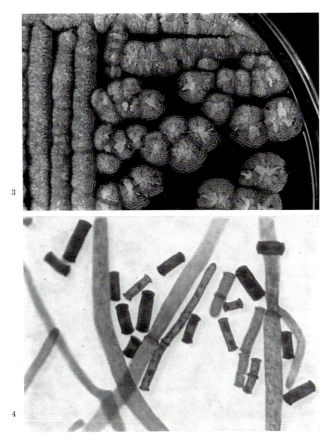

Fig. 3. *Geotrichum candidum.* Colonies on Sabouraud-glucose agar after 3 days at room temperature

Fig. 4. *Geotrichum candidum.* Septate hyphae and arthrospores. Smear of culture. PAS stain, × 1000

4. Physiology

Fermentation and assimilation are tested with the media commonly used in yeast diagnosis (LODDER and KREGER-VAN RIJ, 1952). The assimilation test can always be read clearly, when the strain is inoculated on to the surface of the test agar. The reading is done after 5—10 days of incubation at room temperature. Testing methods which prove the carbohydrate splitting by formation of acids are not appropriate, since the acids are only intermediate products.

Geotrichum candidum assimilates (without gas formation) glucose and galactose. However, erythritol, xylose, maltose, cellobiose, lactose, melibiose and saccharose are not assimilated. Sometimes strains are found which possess a low proportion of population, which can utilize sugars listed above as not assimilated. The biochemical behavior is an important feature for the differentiation of the *Geotrichum* species. Here they are serving only for the confirmation of the *Geotrichum candidum* diagnosis, which is determined, for all practical purposes, for isolates from human beings by means of micromorphology.

E. Pathogenesis and Immunology

1. Pathogenesis

As in other endogenous infections, factors which reduce resistance can initiate infection with *Geotrichum*. Bronchopulmonary geotrichosis has appeared with tuberculosis of the lungs, with typhoid fever, with bronchiectasis, and after acute febrile infections of the upper respiratory tract. Mycetemia has also been observed with miliary tuberculosis and diabetes. A membrane of *G. candidum* has appeared in the mouth cavity with pertussis, with gastroenteritis and with tonsillitis. Cases of geotrichosis have also been described without any predisposing disease. Disturbance of the intestinal flora caused by antibiotic treatment does not seem to play a role in the pathogenesis of geotrichosis. Only the cases reported by Wegmann (1954) and Grimmer (1954) can be explained in this way. Apart from tubercle bacilli, only one genuine mixed infection (with *Klebsiella*) was reported by Webster in 1959 and only one probable infection (with *Proteus* and *Coli*) were described by Nagy et al. (1958). The prognosis is variable with individual manifestations. An oral geotrichosis is a harmless secondary infection. The mucous membranes may not even show inflammation. Bronchopulmonary geotrichosis can, in spite of extensive infection of the lungs, be present without affecting the general condition. Other cases have been fatal, the patients having died of respiratory or circulatory failure. In addition to the functional disturbances of the lungs and heart, due directly or indirectly to injury to the lungs, animal experimentation suggests an additional pathogenic factor, a chronic intoxication by fungal degradation products, the intoxication being recognized by cachexia. Histologically parenchymal degenerations may occur in the liver and in the kidneys. Nothing is known about spontaneous cure in cases of bronchopulmonary and bronchial geotrichosis for all patients have either been treated with iodine or the further progress of the disease has not been stated. Of the cases of cutaneous geotrichosis, there are no resistance-reducing factors reported, though doubtless there are unknown predisposing factors. Attempts to infect human beings have been futile. In 1901, Ricketts scarified the skin and rubbed in *G. candidum (Oidium aceticum)*. However, the skin healed promptly. In 1884, Hueppe was unsuccessful when he inoculated *G. candidum (Oidium lactis)* repeatedly into his own skin. Tzamouranis, in 1962, reported that the infant he was observing, three months prior to the development of geotrichosis, was suffering from intertrigo due to *Candida*. In 1964, Perz (Case 2) reported that in the course of geotrichosis of the cornea, on the face, and on the hands and feet, there were desquamate skin changes with rhagades, from which *Candida albicans* could be isolated. In 1952, Bendove and Ashe reported that in a geotrichosis case *C. albicans* was found in the urine. These findings point to the presence of resistance-reducing factors which are of importance for the genesis of geotrichosis as well as candidosis. Favorable external factors were assumed for the patient of Balzer et al. (1912), as the localization of the skin lesions partly corresponded to the pressure spots on the patient's body from carrying a basket. Although spontaneous healing has not been observed, the prognosis of cutaneous geotrichosis is good, as the internal organs are not affected.

2. Immunology

a) **Agglutination and Complement Fixation Reaction:** In 1912, Balzer et al. determined an agglutination titer of 1:100 in their patient with cutaneous geotrichosis. In 1958, Seeliger found among 47 healthy persons: a titer of 1:40 or less 36 times, a titer of 1:80 4 times, and a titer of 1:160 7 times. Out of 200 sera examined by SCHABINSKI in 1960, 0.5% had an agglutinin titer of 1:100. MORENZ, in 1963, in an examination of 2, 284 sera, which were sent for the diagnosis of lues, found a normal distribution of the agglutinin titer. In a serum dilution of 1:85, 1%, and in a serum dilution of 1:120, 0.5% were positive. In 1935, MARTIN examined 3 blastomycosis patients with respect to the complement fixation reaction, using *Geotrichum* antigen (fungus suspension). The result was negative. The complement fixation test was positive with culture autolysate antigen, in the case of CHIALE (1937), a patient with geotrichids, but negative in the case of WEGMANN (1954). THJÖTTA and URDAL (1949) found the complement fixation test positive in a dilution of 1:60 in one of their cases and negative in another. Of ten patients, thought by ARIYEVICH et al. (1963) to have intestinal geotrichosis, 5 showed complement fixation.

SEELIGER (1958) studied 52 normal persons, in whom only 4 showed complement fixation in a serum dilution of 1:2 and only one in a serum dilution of 1:4. In more recent research SEELIGER (1962) tested 1, 334 sera, finding 16 positive in a dilution of 1:2 to 1:10 and 2 positive in greater dilutions. These 18 persons showed no clinical indication of geotrichosis, nor could *G.candidum* be demonstrated in the feces among 14 of them. MORENZ (1963) had negative tests on 565 sera at a dilution of 1:5.

In summary, from the foregoing results, positive agglutination tests in titers of 1:100 to 1:200, and positive complement-fixation tests in titers of 1:5 or higher point to geotrichosis in the presence of clinical symptoms, although a negative reaction in these dilutions does not rule out geotrichosis.

b) The Geotrichin Test: CHIALE (1937) was the first to have succesfully applied the intracutaneous injection of a culture autolysate of *G.candidum* in a case of geotrichosis of the skin. KUNSTADTER et al. (1950—1951) found the geotrichin test strongly positive in two patients with *Geotrichum* pneumonia, using bouillon culture filtrates of 1:10 and 1:100 dilutions, but also in 3 other members of the family who were not ill. Furthermore, two of 63 children with pneumonia gave a positive geotrichin skin test. The bronchopulmonary and bronchial cases of geotrichosis of WEGMANN (1954) and WEBSTER (1957/1959) were geotrichin-positive. However the two patients of SUNDGAARD et al. (1950) reacted negatively. SKOBEL et al. (1956) found the geotrichin test positive in 2% of adults. Their antigen consisted of an autoclaved suspension in physiological salt solution of 100,000 fungus cells per milliliter. A positive reaction was an erythema of at least 5 mm diameter of the tuberculin type. CANITROT-ARAUJO (1957) found a similar percentage of positives (2.8%) in more than 100 children tested with a culture filtrate of *G. candidum (G. pulmoneum)*.

From these scanty observations it appears that only about 2—3% of healthy persons or persons with unrelated diseases have a positive geotrichin test. If, on the other hand, the test should prove positive in every case of all or some disease types of geotrichosis, it will have value in differential diagnosis.

F. Symptomatology, Diagnosis, and Therapy

Because of the small number of described cases of geotrichosis, generalizations are possible only to a limited extent. As there are only sketchy pathologic-anatomic and histologic studies of geotrichosis, a consideration directed chiefly toward the morphological aspects of the disease is not possible. Complete studies by biopsy and autopsy are necessary in future cases. However, the casuistic representation of the various forms of geotrichosis and the symptomatology and diagnostic features will be given. Here let it be stated that, especially with bronchopulmonary and bronchial geotrichosis, a sure diagnosis requires more than the demonstration of the fungus. Moreover, not in every case cited in this chapter have all of the criteria for the diagnosis of geotrichosis been fulfilled yet considering all the evidence geotrichosis appears to be the appropriate diagnosis.

1. Bronchopulmonary Geotrichosis

The x-ray usually shows widespread, disseminated, partly confluent, irregularly delimited, soft, small spotty infiltrates in all or in some lung fields, without especial preference for particular segments. Less commonly there are large circumscribed tumor-like, non-homogeneous shadows in a lung field. In a quarter of the cases there are one or several thin-walled cavities. In children there may also be an enlargement of the hilar lymph nodes. There is slight, or no, tendency to fibrosis. Calcification is not observed.

The physical findings may not be prominent even with considerable x-ray changes. The percussion note is, at the most, slightly dulled, and the vocal fremitus is infrequently increased. Usually bronchial sounds are to be heard, and increased vesicular breathing, with dry rales, and also moist, rattling rales. Less frequently musical rales and pronounced bronchial breathing are indicative of pulmonary infiltrates. Especially annoying to the patients is a regularly present, often severe cough, even tormenting, and productive. The sputum, which may amount to 80 ml daily, is white to gray, thick and mucoid, and in some cases purulent. In a third of the cases it is tinged with blood. Occasionally there are hemoptyses. The temperature may be normal, subfebrile, or febrile (38—39°C, seldom higher). The sedimentation-rate is normal or slightly elevated (25—45 mm in an hour), seldom greatly increased (over 100 mm). The leucocyte count is normal or moderately elevated (up to 15,000 white cells per cubic mm, rarely higher). The red blood cell count and the hemoglobin are normal; at times there is a mild anemia.

The disease continues chronic or subacute for months, even for years, occasionally with acute phases, which possibly are caused by bacterial superinfection. With an acute onset the geotrichosis may be related to another acute infection, especially of the upper respiratory tract. The patients often complain of weakness, shortness of breath on exertion, loss of appetite and loss of weight. The prognosis can be characterized as good, especially when there is treatment with iodides. In spite of occasional mycetemias, lesions in other organs are seldom observed. However, there are 4 cases (not treated with iodides), with a fatal outcome. Postmortem examinations were performed on the cases of Şerban and Taşcă (1962) and Peninou-Castaing et al. (1964).

Bronchopulmonary geotrichosis, like the other forms of geotrichosis, has no typical clinical symptoms. In differential diagnosis pulmonary tuberculosis must be excluded and the pulmonary mycoses, especially candidosis, coccidiodomycosis, histoplasmosis, cryptococcosis and North American blastomycosis. Moreover, pulmonary neoplasms may be suspected, although in geotrichosis the infiltrate is usually non-homogeneous and irregularly demarcated.

A consideration of the following points of view permits a secure diagnosis.

1. *G. candidum* is demonstrable constantly and in large quantity in fresh sputum from a patient not being treated with iodine or nystatin. In healthy persons *G. candidum* is often present in the sputum, but microscopically it is present only in an isolated fashion and only a few colonies grow. Also in other pulmonary mycoses, in contrast to pulmonary tuberculosis, an increase in the

Table 1. *Bronchopulmonary Geotrichosis*

Author	Age and Sex	Occupation	Location	Organism
1. Bennett (1842)	M		Great Britain	Cryptogamic plant
2. Linossier (1916)	26 M	Soldier	France	*Oidium lactis A*
3. Martins (1928)	13 M		Portugal	*Zymonema pulmonalis membranogenes*
4. Smith (1934)	25 M	Student	Puerto Rico and North Carolina, USA	*Geotrichum* species
5. Smith (1934)	18 F		South Carolina, USA	*Geotrichum* species
6. Moore (1934)	22 M	Chemist	Missouri, USA	*Geotrichum* species
7. Smith (1945, Fig. 10)				*Geotrichum* species
8. Kunstadter et al. (1946)	22 M	Soldier	Texas, USA and North Africa	*Geotrichum* species
9. Thjötta and Urdal (1949)	37 F	Farm house-wife	Norway	*Geotrichum* species
10. Thjötta and Urdal (1949)	31 F	Farm house-wife	Norway	*Geotrichum* species
11. Kunstadter et al. (1950, Case 1)	6 M		Illinois, USA	
12. Kunstadter et al. (1950, Case 2)	4 F		Illinois, USA	
13. Good (1951, Fig. 4c)			Minnesota, USA	
14. Dávalos and Arcos (1954)	47 M	Civil official	Ecuador	*Geotrichum candidum*
15. Hauser (1954)	67 M	Farmer	Germany	*Geotrichum candidum*
16. Wegmann (1954)	55 F		Switzerland	*Geotrichum* species
17. Mahoudeau et al. (1955)	47 M		France	*Geotrichum candidum*
18. Webster (1957)	46 M	Truck driver	Tennessee, USA	*Geotrichum candidum*
19. Webster (1959, Case 2)	64 M	Locomotive engineer in retirement	Tennessee, USA	*Geotrichum candidum*
20. Webster (1959, Case 3)	66 M	Merchant in retirement	Tennessee, USA	*Geotrichum candidum*
21. Webster (1959, Case 4)	52 M	Farmer	Tennessee, USA	*Geotrichum candidum*
22. Bell et al. (1962)	57 M	Laborer	Great Britain	*Geotrichum* species
23. Nicolescu (1962)	23		Rumania	*Geotrichum* species
24. Peninou-Castaing et al. (1964)	54 M	Mason	France	*Geotrichum candidum*

occurrence of *G.candidum* is unknown. In association with *G.candidum* other fungi may occasionally be present, but only in small numbers. The sputum should be examined shortly after it is expectorated, as *G.candidum* can greatly increase in sputum preserved for a long time.

2. The geotrichin test is presumably positive in all pulmonary geotrichoses. As only 2—3% of healthy persons react positively, the negative geotrichin test permits the exclusion of geotrichosis.

3. A successful therapy with iodides or nystatin permits a non-mycotic pulmonary condition to be excluded.

4. Evidence against the diagnosis of tuberculosis is based on the failure to demonstrate tubercle bacilli, a negative tuberculin test and lack of improvement following treatment with anti-tuberculosis drugs. However, there are descriptions of cases of pulmonary geotrichosis combined with pulmonary tuberculosis.

5. Evidence against other pulmonary mycoses consist of negative results with skin tests, for example the coccidiodin and histoplasmin tests.

A plentiful growth of *G.candidum* from the sputum, a positive geotrichin test and successful iodide therapy are diagnostic of bronchopulmonary geotrichosis.

The first time *G.candidum* was demonstrated in a patient was in 1842 by Bennett. The patient suffered from phthisis with pneumothorax. The fungus was so plentiful in the thick, purulent sputum that it was macroscopically visible on the sides of the sputum container. At postmortem examination the left lung contained numerous cavities of various sizes. Some were filled with a soft tuberculous material in which the fungus was present as abundantly as in the sputum. Apparently there was secondary infection of cavitary pulmonary tuberculosis.

Linossier (1916) described a case thought to be tuberculous. However, tubercle bacilli could not be demonstrated in the sputum. Instead, *G.candidum* was present in large amounts, along with staphylococci and pneumococci. The patient died after the rapid development of cavities. There was no autopsy.

Martins (1928) found *G.candidum* microscopically and culturally in every examination of sputum from a 13-year-old youth who had suffered from a pneumonic condition and had frequent and severe hemoptyses. His general condition was poor and his temperature varied between 37 and 39 degrees centigrade. There was no support for the diagnosis of tuberculosis.

Smith (1934, 1947; see also Conant et al., 1954, Fig. 97) reported two cases of pulmonary geotrichosis. The first was that of a 25-year-old student who had two small cavities in the upper portion of the right lung and a large one in the left upper lung field (Fig. 5). The sputum was mucopurulent, frequently blood-tinged and without fetid odor, and totalled 15—30 ml per day. Tubercle bacilli could not be demonstrated, but present microscopically and culturally were numerous *G.candidum* and some Friedländer bacilli. Two weeks after the beginning of iodine therapy the cavities became smaller and one disappeared. After 7 months only residual fibrosis was visible in x-ray. The other case was that of an 18-year-old girl with small infiltrates in the lower two-thirds of both lungs. *G.candidum* was demonstrated in the sputum. After a year of iodine therapy the condition was not completely cured. The x-ray picture of another case (Smith, 1945, Fig. 10) showed numerous small thinwalled cavities in the lower halves of both lungs. No further details were given.

Moore (1934) reported the case of a man of 22 years who had had chronic pulmonary disease in the form of bronchiectasis for 7 years. He developed fever and increased expectoration and infiltrates in the left lung. *G.candidum* was demonstrated in relatively large amounts in the sputum. With three months of iodine therapy there was much improvement in the condition of the patient and it was thought there had been a bronchopulmonary geotrichosis complicating the bronchiectasis.

Kunstadter et al. (1946) reported the case of a 22-year-old solider who developed left-sided pleurisy and then bilateral spotty infiltrates (Fig. 6). On three consecutive occasions *G.candidum* was demonstrated in the sputum and gastric juice. With iodine therapy for three months the pulmonary infiltrates disappeared. The *G.candidum* disappeared from the sputum after the first week of iodine therapy.

Sundgaard et al. (1950; see also Thjötta and Urdal, 1949) isolated *G.candidum* from the sputum of 8 of 11 members of a farm family. Three sisters of this family gave evidence of pulmonary disease. A 37-year-old sister had apparently suffered from tuberculosis of the hip from age 14 to 26, although tubercle bacilli had not been found in discharge from the fistulae of the hip and the tuberculin reaction was negative. There were delicate, small, spotty, partly

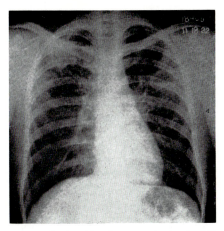

Fig. 5. Bronchopulmonary geotrichosis with a large cavity in the left upper lung field and two smaller cavities in the right upper lung field. (From SMITH, 1934)

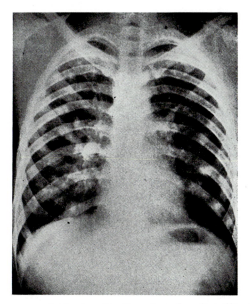

Fig. 6. Bronchopulmonary geotrichosis with disseminated, soft, infiltrates in all lung fields. (From KUNSTADTER et al., 1946)

confluent infiltrates in both lungs, particularly in the middle and subclavicular regions. The serum of this patient gave a positive complement-fixation reaction in a dilution of 1:60 with a suspension of a *G.candidum* from the patient, and also with the *G.candidum* of Case 2, although the scrum of Case 2 reacted negatively with both strains. As the geotrichin test in the two patients was negative, in contrast to all other tested cases of bronchopulmonary geotrichosis, and as no iodine treatment was carried out, the diagnosis rests only on the demonstration of *Geotrichum candidum* in the sputum. One can not be sure of the diagnosis of geotrichosis in these two cases, particularly in Case 2 which had a negative complement fixation reaction. The 31-year-old sister (Case 2) had a similar pulmonary picture with soft, indistinct, partly confluent, infiltrations in both lungs from the apices to the bases, especially in the central fields. The hilar lymphnodes were not enlarged, the tuberculin test was negative and tubercle bacilli were not demonstrable. The blood picture was normal, the sedimentation-rate

59*

24 mm. Both sisters were in good general condition and had no fever. For silicosis and carcinomatosis there was no support. The clinical symptoms, which were rather mild, consisted of moderate cough with a rather watery expectoration in which white firm flecks were present. Moreover, *G.candidum* was found in large quantities microscopically. The findings in the third sister were not characteristic of geotrichosis.

The author described 3 further cases (Cases 4, 5, and 6) in which the patients were found to have *G.candidum* in the sputum. In Case 4 there was pulmonary tuberculosis. For a pathognomonic meaning of the moderate quantity of fungus in the sputum, even as a secondary infection, there was little diagnostic proof except the positive geotrichin test. Nor is the evidence sufficient in the two cases with negative geotrichin tests to accept them as instances of geotrichosis.

Kunstadter et al. (1950; see also Whitcomb et al., 1949) describe 2 cases in whom the demonstration of *G.candidum* was not successful, apparently because of the early giving of iodine therapy. The geotrichin test was positive, although the test with histoplasmin, blastomycin, coccidiodin, torulin, and tuberculin were negative. In favor of geotrichosis was the success of iodine therapy. A 6-year-old boy became acutely ill with sore throat, rhinitis and fever. Except for low fever, all symptoms improved in a few days. Three weeks later the x-ray showed spotty infiltrates in both lungs and a pronounced hilar adenopathy. In spite of streptomycin treatment the fever persisted and in three months a severely productive cough had developed. The sputum was whitish, mucoid and often flaky though not bloody. The patient lost considerable weight and tired easily. Leucocytes 9,900, sedimentation-rate 32 mm, temperature 37.1°C. Tubercle bacilli and other pathogenic bacteria could not be demonstrated. The x-ray after six months still showed extensive, soft irregularly spotty infiltrates. With iodine therapy the cough disappeared in a few weeks. The x-ray showed a distinct clearing of the infiltrate with regression of the hilar lymphadenopathy. The patient felt well and put on weight. After a year, in spite of subjective freedom from complaints, the x-ray abnormalities had not completely faded out. However the iodine therapy was discontinued.

The 4-year-old sister of the above patient became ill shortly after her brother did, and had a mild acute upper respiratory infection, which lasted only 2 or 3 days. The x-ray, except for a mild enlargement of the hilar lymph nodes, was not remarkable. Although she had normal laboratory findings and only a mild cough, she showed after 6 months, as did her brother, a definite hilar adenopathy and a diffuse, spotty infiltrate, which affected the hilar regions and extended into the lower lobes. After 6 months of iodine therapy the lung fields were again clear and the enlargement of the hilar lymph nodes had subsided. In the other 3 members of this family, in whom the geotrichin reaction was likewise positive, no abnormal changes were noted in x-rays.

Good (1951) cited a case of geotrichosis which was limited to the right pulmonary apex when first studied. The continuing investigation showed a disseminated infiltrate of the left lower lobe field, and a hilar lymphadenopathy. After 2 months of iodides and antibiotics the x-ray changes and the clinical findings had disappeared.

Dávalos and Arcos (1954) reported the case of a 47-year-old man who complained of weakness and weight loss of 4 months duration, and of cough and whitish expectoration of 2 months duration. Roentgenologically there were infiltrates of both lung bases suggestive of tuberculosis. Tubercle bacilli and tumor cells could not be demonstrated. The general condition of the patient was good, leukocytes 12,000. The sputum cultures yielded *Penicillium*, *Aspergillus*, *Geotrichum* and *Acladium* at first, later only *G.candidum*. Although the iodine treatment was continued for only 3 weeks because the patient developed an intolerance for the drug, within a week the cough and expectoration had improved, and the laboratory findings became normal. A year later the x-rays showed only areas of fibrosis in the lower lung fields.

Hauser (1954) reported the case of a 67-year-old farmer who had suffered from a dermatitis herpetiformis Duhring for 4 years. In addition, he had cough and white, mucoid expectoration for years. His temperature was occasionally subfebrile. Leucocytes were 11,000 and sedimentation-rate 110 mm. In x-ray there was the picture of a "bilateral productive, cirrhotic, pulmonary tuberculosis" in the apical and subapical regions. In both middle lung fields there were small, punctate, infiltrates, and in the lower lung fields moderately dense shadows with clearing toward the periphery. In the tomogram a cavity was identified in the right upper lung field. In sputum, *G.candidum* could be demonstrated microscopically and culturally in large quantities and tubercle bacilli could not be found. Therapy with INH and streptomycin was unsuccessful.

Wegmann (1954/1957; see also Rossier, 1952) described a fatal geotrichosis of both lungs. The 55-year-old female patient had chronic cough with episodes of choking, and gelatinous expectoration for two years. Because of the suspicion of bronchiectasis she was treated continuously with penicillin and aureomycin. Moist musical and non-musical rales were

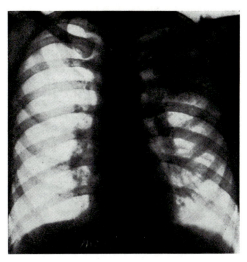

Fig. 7. Bronchopulmonary geotrichosis with a large round shadow in the left upper lung field. (From MAHOUDEAU et al., 1955)

audible in both lung bases. In x-ray there were pinhead-sized, thickly beset, rather sharply demarcated foci, increasing in number in the inferior portions of the lungs. Leukocytes 4,900; tuberculin and blastomycin tests negative; tubercle bacilli not demonstrable; oidiomycin and geotrichin test positive; *Geotrichum* complement fixation and precipitin test negative. In the sputum *G. candidum* was demonstrable in large quantities microscopically and culturally. Later, a spontaneous pneumothorax formed on the right, and this was treated with suction. Death from increasing circulatory insufficiency. No postmortem examination.

WEGMANN (1961; Fig. 103) shows, without further explanation, the x-ray of another case with pneumoperitoneum and a large thin-walled cavity.

MAHOUDEAU et al. (1955) described a tumor-like geotrichosis of the lung. The 47-year-old patient became ill with pain on the left side of the chest, cough, and bloody sputum. He lost weight and then had low grade fever. In x-ray there was a large, non-homogenous shadow in the upper left lung field (Fig. 7). Tubercle bacilli and tumor cells were not demonstrable. However, material obtained by bronchoscopy grew out *G. candidum* in pure culture. Iodine therapy produced rapid improvement. The x-ray changes disappeared completely and the patient was discharged cured.

WEBSTER (1957) described a pulmonary geotrichosis with cavity formation and mycetemia in a 46-year-old truck driver. The patient became ill three weeks previously with a shaking chill and high fever. Twenty-four hours before admission he had a relapse with persisting cough and thick, mucoid, rusty, earthy-smelling sputum. Shortly thereafter he coughed up bright red blood. The patient was acutely ill and very dyspneic. Temperature: 40.8°C. Leukocytes 24,600. X-ray showed a thin walled cavity and infiltrates in the upper portion of the left lower lobe. *G. candidum* was demonstrated in the sputum, gastric contents, stool, bronchial aspirate, and twice in the blood. The geotrichin reaction was strongly positive. Tubercle bacilli and other pathogenic bacteria were not demonstrable. Skin tests with tuberculin, coccidioidin, and histoplasmin were negative. He was first treated with tetracycline, and after clarification of the diagnosis, with iodine. Thereupon there was an involution of the infiltrates and a stepwise closing of the cavity. After six months only some peribronchial infiltrates could be seen.

WEBSTER (1959) described three brochopulmonary cases in addition to one bronchial geotrichosis. A 64-year-old locomotive engineer, who had suffered from Parkinsonism for five years, complained of cough with gray mucoid expectoration, shortness of breath and fever of three weeks duration. Temperature 38.8°C. Leukocytes 13,400. The x-ray showed a lobar pneumonia of the right upper lobe. In the sputum there were Friedländer bacilli, and *G. candidum*. There were no tubercle bacilli demonstrable. The tuberculin, histoplasmin, and coccidioidin tests were negative. Bronchoscopically there was no support for the diagnosis of neoplasm. In the exudate from the right upper lobe there were large quantities of the fungus and *Klebsiella*. After 9 months of treatment with streptomycin, aureomycin, sulphadiazine, and iodine, the pulmonary changes disappeared, and no bacteria or fungi were demonstrable. According to Webster, it was a double infection, with both organisms playing an important role.

A 66-year-old merchant in retirement suffered with a chronic cough, with gray gelatinous sputum, and dyspnea. Temperature 36.9°C, and leukocytes 6,050. In x-ray there was emphysema, and infiltrates in both lungs. In the sputum there were *G.candidum* and no tubercle bacilli. The geotrichin test was strongly positive, the tuberculin and histoplasmin tests were negative. Treatment with iodine improved the condition. An x-ray after 6 months showed less infiltrate, although *G.candidum* could still be cultured.

A 52-year-old farmer complained of increasing cough of two months duration, with thick gray gelatinous sputum, evening fever, night sweats, weakness and weight loss. For two weeks he had vomited blood. Temperature 38°C and leukocytes 12,000. In x-ray, the left upper lobe of the lungs showed a spotty infiltrate and cavity formation. Tubercle bacilli could not be demonstrated. The tuberculin, histoplasmin, and coccidioidin tests were negative, but the geotrichin test was positive. *G.candidum* was demonstrable in all cultures of sputum, in bronchial aspirates, and once in the blood. After oral iodine and intravenous gentian violet treatment the symptoms disappeared. In a later x-ray, no changes were recognizable. However *G.candidum* could still be demonstrated in the sputum.

Bell et al. (1962) reported the case of a 57-year-old laborer who, for four months, had complained of shortness of breath, weight loss, and a productive cough with 50—80 ml daily of a purulent sputum. Temperature normal, leukocytes 12,500. In the sputum *G.candidum* was constantly present in large quantities. *B.coli* and staphylococci were present in some examinations. Tubercle bacilli were never found. With nystatin and iodine the condition improved considerably and the fungus disappeared from the sputum.

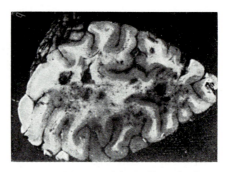

Fig. 8. Bronchopulmonary, metastasizing geotrichosis. Foci of softening containing *Geotrichum*, in the white substance of the brain. (From Şerban and Taşcă, 1962)

Nicolescu (1962) reported the case of a patient with chronic hepatitis who, in the course of cortisone treatment, developed fever, dyspnea and cough. The x-ray showed irregular and nodular foci in both lungs. The patient died in 6 days of a generalized infection. The pathologic-anatomical findings were described by Şerban and Taşcă (1962). The grayish-white broncho-pneumonic foci were rounded and sharply defined. The centers of these nodules were purulent or granulomatous with giant cells which sometimes contained fungi. At the periphery of the necrotic zones, there were clusters of the fungus. The thickness of hyphae was 6—12 μ and the diameter of the free-lying arthrospores, 12—15 μ. *G.candidum* was cultured. The white substance of the brain contained softenings with a diameter up to one cm (Fig. 8). Necrotic infarcted nodules were found in the kidneys and spleen. In the myocardium of the heart there were microinfarcts of 2—3 mm diameter. Microscopically the microabscesses of the myocardium showed the fungus (Fig. 9).

Peninou-Castaing et al. (1964) described a fatal cavitary pulmonary geotrichosis, which at first was associated with pulmonary tuberculosis. The 54-year-old brick layer became ill 18 months before his death, lost weight and developed a cough with mucoid and purulent sputum, in which tubercle bacilli and much *G. candidum* were demonstrated. The x-ray showed bilateral infiltrates with a large thick walled cavity at the right apex and another cavity in the left subapical region. There was a shadow on the right next to the pericardium. In the aspirate from the bronchus there were tubercle bacilli and numerous *G. candidum*. With antituberculous treatment with drugs for six months the tubercle bacilli disappeared from the sputum. The cavity at the right apex closed and the general condition improved. However, in spite of an extensive treatment with nystatin, there was a relapse with more cavities. The patient became cachectic and died. At autopsy, the right upper lobe was scarred, without a cavity. The cavities in the lower lobes had no granulation tissue wall. There was only fibrin containing fungus and a mucoid fluid with arthrospores in necrotic collections of neutrophils (Fig. 10). The tuberculosis was histologically cured. However *G.candidum* was isolated in culture in large quantities. The shadow next to the pericardium turned out to be large cysts of the emphysematous lung containing pus in which the fungus was also visible.

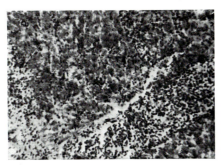

Fig. 9. Bronchopulmonary, metastasizing geotrichosis. Interstitial myocarditis with fungus containing microabscesses. H & E, × 56. (From ŞERBAN and TAŞCĂ, 1962)

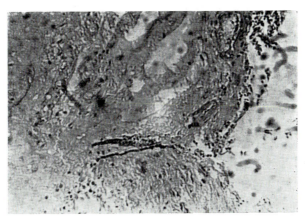

Fig. 10. Bronchopulmonary geotrichosis. Bizarre forms of arthrospores in necrotic masses of fibrin and polymorphonuclear cells at the edge of a pulmonary cavity. (From PENINOU-CASTAING et al., 1964)

2. Bronchial Geotrichosis

Bronchial geotrichosis has essentially no involvement of the lung itself, and is chronic or subacute. Persistent cough is a prominant feature. The diagnosis is made as in bronchopulmonary geotrichosis by demonstrating the fungus in the sputum. Especially convincing is the demonstration of *G.candidum* in material obtained by bronchoscopy, and improvement with iodine therapy. Concerning the geotrichin test in bronchial geotrichosis nothing is known.

The first report of the presence of *G. candidum* (*Monilia asteroides, Oidium matalense*) in bronchitis came from CASTELLANI and CHALMERS (1919). The next mention was that of MATTLET in 1926. In his case *G.candidum* was isolated repeatedly. SMITH (1934) reported two cases in which *G.candidum* could be demonstrated in the sputum. One case was that of a

Table 2. *Bronchial Geotrichosis*

Author	Age and Sex	Occupation	Location	Organism
1. Mattlet (1926)	F		Urundi, Africa	*Mycoderma nyabisi*
2. Smith (1934)	35 F		New York, USA	*Geotrichum* species
3. Smith (1934)	30 M		New York, USA	*Geotrichum* species
4. Reeves (1941)	25 F		North Carolina, USA	
5. Reeves (1941)	25 M		North Carolina, USA	
6. Minton et al. (1954, Case 1)	53 M	Painter	Panama	*Geotrichum* species
7. Minton et al. (1954, Case 2)	54 M		Panama	*Geotrichum* species
8. Mándi and Berencsi (1954, Case 1)	39 M		Hungary	*Geotrichum* species
9. Webster (1959, Case 1)	22 F	Housewife	Tennessee, USA	*Geotrichum candidum*

35-year-old woman without changes in the pulmonary parenchyma. After iodine therapy there was rapid cure. The other case was similar, with improvement of the condition in a man of 30 with the use of iodine. Reeves (1941) found two cases of geotrichosis amoung 79 bronchomycoses. There were symptoms of bronchitis for two to three years in both patients.

Minton et al. (1954) described two cases of endobronchial geotrichosis. A 53-year-old painter had had, for 4 years, several spontaneously self-limited episodes of coughing with bright red sputum. During a relapse there was coughing and hemoptyses. The daily amount of the dark or light red sputum was 60—120 ml. In bronchoscopic examination white exudative easily bleeding foci were observed in both main bronchi. Material from this region revealed *G.candidum*, microscopically and culturally. With iodine for two weeks, the blood disappeared from the sputum and the fungus was no longer present in the material from bronchoscopy. The second case was that of a 54-year-old man who had countless arthrospores in his sputum with positive *G.candidum* cultures. With iodine therapy the fungus disappeared from the sputum. The patient died of a heart attack. At autopsy the lungs and bronchi appeared normal. Mándi and Berencsi (1954) described an endobronchial geotrichosis in a 39-year-old man who had cavernous pulmonary tuberculosis of three years duration and a tuberculous pleurisy of one year. A pneumothorax was performed and INH and PAS were given. The mucosa of the trachea and the main bronchi showed numerous yellowish white foci relatively well attached which culturally gave *G.candidum*. With the thought that *G.candidum* was related to *Candida albicans*, the patient was treated for two months with a vaccine of *C.albicans*, with which the skin test was positive. During this period the coughing stopped. Bronchoscopically only a few gray white fungus foci were seen in the right bronchi. The tuberculosis had greatly improved during this time.

Webster in 1959 reported the case of a 22-year-old housewife who complained of weakness and cough of 4 months duration, and a yellow mucoid sputum with small gray flecks. There was no hemoptysis. In the mouth and throat, there was a white exudate suggestive of thrush. The x-ray of the lung showed increase in the peribronchial markings. From the exudate of the mouth, and from the sputum and stool, *G.candidum* was repeatedly cultured. The blood culture was negative. Tubercle bacilli were not demonstrable. Tuberculin, histoplasmin and coccidioidin tests were negative. With iodine therapy the symptoms improved. Two years later there was exacerbation of the bronchitis. Bronchoscopically, an exudate was seen bilaterally from which *G.candidum* was grown, but no tubercle bacilli. A year later the patient developed a pulmonary tuberculous cavity. Both tubercle bacilli and *G.candidum* were isolated from the sputum. As this fungus also occurs in the sputum of healthy people, the relationship between the two infections was not clear.

3. Oral Geotrichosis

In oral geotrichosis a membrane occurs on the mucosa of the oral cavity or pharynx, and is composed of arthrospores and fungus mycelium. A definite differention from the membranes of other causes (for example, those due to

Table 3. *Oral Geotrichosis**

Author	Age and Sex	Location	Organism
a) Thrush			
1. CASTELLANI and CHALMERS (1919)		Tropics	*Monilia asteroides*, *Oidium matalense*
2. BACHMANN (1921)	1	Germany	*Oospora* species
3. CASTELLANI (1928)	25 M	Ceylon	*Oidium matalense*
4. COLONNELLO (1944)	4	Italy	*Geotrichum candidum*
b) Tonsillar mycosis			
1. CASTELLANI (1928)			*Oidium matalense*, *Oidium asteroides*
2. MOTTA (1931)	F	Italy	*Oospora lactis*
3. CORTESE (1933)	37 F	Italy	*Geotrichum candidum*
c) Black Hairy Tongue			
1. SCHAEDE (1934)	21 M	Germany	*Oospora catenata*, *Oospora fragilis*
2. GRIMMER (1954)		Germany	*Endomyces lactis*
3. CARTEAUD and DROUHET (1955, Case 2)	79 M	France	*Geotrichum* species
4. CARTEAUD et al. (1957)		France	*Geotrichum* species
5. ARRIGHI and DROUHET (1957)	80 M	France	*Geotrichum* species

* The occupations of the patients were not known.

Candida albicans) is possible only microscopically or culturally. In thrush caused by *G.candidum*, grayish yellow, mostly loosly adherent patches develop on the reddened mucous membrane of the mouth, throat and esophagus. Tonsillar mycosis (in the narrower sense) is characterized by small gray-white or brown fungal foci on the tonsils without there being an inflammatory reaction. In black hairy tongue there is an easily removed, dark brown or blackish coating on the back of the tongue. This coating consists of a thick layer of arthrospores and mycelium. Except for a hypertrophy of the papillae of the tongue there are no signs of inflammation. Black hairy tongue is caused more frequently by bacteria or other fungi than by *G.candidum*. All types of coatings with *G.candidum* appear to develop on the basis of some unrelated previous pathologic change in the mucosa. The diagnosis is made by microscopic and cultural investigation of the membrane. Concerning the geotrichin test in oral geotrichosis nothing is known.

Thrush: The first indication that oral thrush could be caused by *G.candidum* came from CASTELLANI and CHALMERS (1919), who had observed it in the tropics. BACHMANN (1921) found at the autopsy of a year-old child with whooping cough pneumonia a gray white or gray yellow coating on the tip of the tongue, on the entire pharynx, throughout the esophagus and in the stomach, which histologically and culturally consisted of *G.candidum*. Under the coating, which was in part firmly and in part loosly attached, was a grayish-white, granularity on a reddish base. The tongue and pharynx were also reddened.

CASTELLANI (1928) mentioned a 25-year-old man with acute tonsillitis, severe sore throat, difficulty in swallowing and temperature up to 40°C. After 12 hours both tonsils were covered with a white exudate from which *G.candidum* and not diphtheria bacilli were isolated. COLONNELLO (1944) mentioned the appearance of thrush membranes on the tonsils and the mucous membranes of the cheeks as a complication of an acute gastroenteritis in a 4-year-old child. This coating consisted of *G.candidum*. The fungus was also in the stool in large quantities as long as the membranes persisted.

Ariyevich et al. (1963) reported the appearance of membranes on the tongue and in the pharynx of a 23-year-old female patient who had been treated with penicillin and ACTH for lupus erythematosus disseminatus. As both *G.candidum (G.sp.)* and *Candida* were isolated from the membranes, and the numbers of organisms were not stated, it is not clear whether the condition was oral geotrichosis or candidosis. Genuine mixed infections of *G.candidum* and other fungi are not known.

Tonsillar Geotrichosis: Castellani (1928) cited *G.candidum* as the cause of a lesion which he termed spinous tonsillar mycosis. On the tonsils there were numerous white, gray or brown, erect spicules generally originating in the crypts. These spicules consisted of fungal mycelia. Cortese (1933) described a similar case in a 37-year-old woman who complained of slight pain on swallowing. On the mucous membranes of the enlarged tonsils were several dozen grayish-white flecks firmly attached to the tonsils, and these consisted of *G.candidum*. Histologic examination showed fungal filaments among epithelial cells extending to the lymph follicles, but without appreciable inflammation. Also, in the case described by Motta (1931), there were similar, white, nodules on the gums and lingual tonsils. The histologic picture was like that described by Cortese.

Black Hairy Tongue: Schaede (1934) published a case in the lingual membrane of which two strains of *G.candidum* were isolated. In a healthy 21-year-old man there developed a black color of the tongue. A year later almost the entire tongue was covered with a 3 mm thick, dark brown coating. The superficial part of this covering could be easily removed. The edges of the tongue were red and moist. There was fetid odor. Microscopically the papillae of the tongue were covered with arthrospores. Also, a mycelium could be recognized, and this clung to the papillae and extended downward or upward from the surface. There were, also, numerous bacteria and occasional *Penicillium* mycelium. The prescribed iodine therapy was not regularly followed by the patient. A half year later the coating suddenly disappeared. The region of the former coating could be recognized by a slight elevation and a velvety pale white character of the mucous membrane.

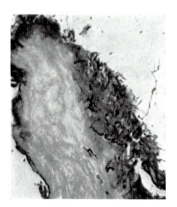

Fig. 11. Black hairy tongue. Coating of arthrospores and mycelium on a papilla of the tongue. PAS stain, × 350. (From Carteaud et al., 1957)

Grimmer (1954) reported the case of a black hairy tongue which developed after prolonged penicillin treatment of a secondarily infected tinea barbae profunda. *G.candidum* was microscopically and culturally demonstrable in great quantity. Carteaud et al. (1955/1957) in 15 cases of black hairy tongue were able to isolate *Candida* 7 times, *Geotrichum* 3 times, and both fungi together 5 times. *G.candidum* without *Candida* was demonstrated in a 79-year-old man with symptoms of two months duration. In the other cases no clinical data were given.

A histological preparation showed a coating of hyphae and arthrospores on a hypertrophied papilla (Fig. 11). In another histologic preparation the surface of the papilla bears a mixture of bacteria, *Candida* and *Geotrichum*. The papillae were not edematous or infiltrated with cells.

ARRIGHI and DROUHET (1957) reported the case of an 80-year-old man in whom a black hairy-tongue had appeared two weeks before without obvious cause. It consisted of a considerable papillary hypertrophy with a shaggy coating which could be easily scraped off. *G.candidum* was demonstrated culturally.

4. Cutaneous Geotrichosis

Cutaneous geotrichosis is a chronic fungus infection of the skin which untreated may last for many years. The skin lesions appear gradually, and may be disseminated, and may be accompanied by geotrichids. Areas of predilection are not recognized. The single or confluent lesions consist either of superficial erythematous, pustular, and squamous eruptions or as deeper infiltrates, mostly with miliary abscesses or small nodules. In some patients the infiltrated regions ulcerate superficially and later form scars. In others, extensive lesions occur, with central scarring, but with ulcerative, verrucous vegetations at the periphery. Geotrichids are polymorphous, erythematous-squamous, or eczematoid lesions. The infection is confined to the skin. The internal organs, draining lymph vessels and the lymph nodes are not affected. There are no large subcutaneous abscesses. The general condition is not affected. The skin lesions are indolent or slightly painful on pressure.

In the deeper forms, one or another of the following reactions may be observed. 1. A proliferation of the connective tissue tending toward fibrosis; 2. Diffuse, histiocytic and lymphocytic infiltrates; 3. Microabscesses with polymorphonuclear neutrophiles; 4. Granulomas with central necrosis surrounded by giant cells and histiocytes.

The epidermis tends to be hyperplastic. Fungus elements are found, in pus microscopically even if in small numbers. In tissue sections the fungi are hard to find, but special staining has been little used. Usually *G.candidum* is markedly rounded in tissue, and differentiation from yeast-like fungi may be difficult. Yet the regularly positive culture leaves no doubt as to the etiology of the skin lesions. The demonstration of the causative agent, preferably together with a biopsy, also permits a differential diagnosis, especially in ruling out verrucous skin tuberculosis, nodular and ulcerative syphilids, fungating epitheliomas, epidermal sporotrichosis, cutaneous North American blastomycosis and primary cutaneous coccidioidomycosis. In the superficial forms, *G.candidum* can be culturally demonstrated in the pus of the pustules and probably also microscopically in tissue sections. As *G.candidum* occasionally occurs on the normal skin, it is important to demonstrate it repeatedly and to rule out other causal agents, especially dermatophytes, yeasts, and staphylococci. The geotrichin test was positive in the one case of geotrichosis of the skin in which it was applied.

Deep Forms: RICKETTS (1901, Case 3; see also HYDE and RICKETTS, 1901, Case 12) described the case of a 33-year-old farmer with a skin lesion of the left lower eyelid and the adjacent portions of the cheek and temple. The condition had begun 2 years earlier as a "carbuncle". After it was opened, it failed to heal. The process became larger and twice it was scraped but without success. The clearly defined, reddish-brown, painless lesion consistend of irregular, raised, in part excoriated nodules with minor areas between, of non-involved skin. Histologic examination showed a pronounced epithelial hyperplasia and distinct, interepithelial and subcutaneous microabscesses with polymorphonuclear neutrophils and occasional giant and plasma cells.

Table 4. *Cutaneous Geotrichosis*

Author	Age and Sex	Occupation	Location	Organism
a) Deep Forms				
1. Ricketts (1901, Case 3)	33 M	Farmer	Illinois, USA	*Oidium aceticum*
2. Balzer et al. (1912)	37 M	Vegetable carrier	France	*Mycoderma pulmoneum*
3. Gougerot (1920)	24 M		France	*Mycoderma pulmoneum*
4. Gougerot (1936)			France	*Mycoderma pulmoneum*
5. Gougerot (1936)			France	*Mycoderma pulmoneum*
6. Thiers et al. (1953)	63 F	Teacher in retirement	France	*Geotrichum candidum*
7. Rousset et al. (1957)	54 M	Colonial official	France	*Geotrichum candidum*
8. Tzamouranis (1962)	4/12 F		Greece	*Geotrichum candidum*
b) Superficial Forms				
1. Chiale (1937, Case 3)	54 F		Italy	*Geotrichum candidum*
2. Canellis (1959)	50 M		Greece	*Geotrichum candidum*
3. Heidenbluth (1963)			Germany	*Geotrichum candidum*

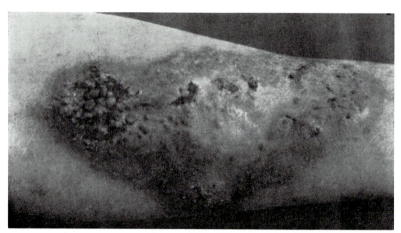

Fig. 12. Cutaneous geotrichosis. Ulcerous-verrucous, proliferating and centrally irregular, scarred lesions on the right lower arm. (From Balzer et al., 1912)

The surrounding tissue was diffusely infiltrated with the same cells. The sparse fungal elements in and about the abscesses were mostly round (12 μ in diameter), at times elongated, and with a double-contoured wall. They were stainable with methylene blue, carbol toluidin blue and acid orcein, except for old cells without recognizable protoplasm. From pus and from tissue scrapings *G.candidum* could be cultured, and in pus it could also be demonstrated microscopically. Tubercle bacilli were not demonstrable. Iodine treatment brought prompt improvement. The process was not completely healed at the time of the report.

Balzer et al. (1910/1912) described as "dermatomycose végétante disséminée" a geotrichosis of the skin in a 37-year-old male patient (Fig. 12).

The first ulcerations, which after treatment with calomel powder for 1—2 months became scarred, appeared 7 and 4 years before on the right lower arm and right lower leg. A year previously there was recurrence in the form of a disseminated ulcerative-vegetative process. Ulcers now appeared on the back, in the lumbar region and on the right shoulder. With a one month treatment with potassium iodide and arsenic, the patient was almost completely cured. After 9 months the lesions were again active and now also affected the left foot and the right temple. The general condition of the patient was always good. The internal organs were not affected, and there was no support for the diagnosis of lues or tuberculosis. The affected skin regions consisted of isolated lesions, "1 to 5 franc piece sized" and of confluent ulcers which in part formed long bands.

The lesions began as pustules which spread, ulcerated and became crusted. They finally developed into plaques. In the center of the plaque there was smooth, firm, irregular scarring. At the borders there were red-violet, firm infiltrates, which gave rise to drops of pus when pressed upon. With renewed iodine and arsenic medication the ulcers were largely healed in two months, but a month later they were again partly ulcerated. The complete scarring lasted more than three months. The further course is unknown. Histological examination gave a mixture of the following reaction types with all intermediate steps. There was, in one type, an inflammation of the connective tissue, with macrophages, plasma cells and lymphocytes which tended toward fibrosis. In another type there were tubercle-like structures and giant cells. In still another type there were micro-abscesses with neutrophils, macrophages and some eosinophils. The fungus was seen with difficulty and in small numbers in sections and smears. The fungus cells were round, oval or pear-shaped ($5 \times 7\ \mu$) or longer filaments (2—3 by 9—$17\ \mu$). G. candidum could be regularly isolated, often in pure culture, but at other times associated with bacteria.

GOUGEROT (1920) reported a second case of dermatomycosis vegetans with verrucous-ulcerative and gummous lesions, in which G. candidum was demonstrated microscopically and culturally. The disease began during the first year of life of the 24-year-old male patient. As the lesions were not influenced by iodine, they were excised and cauterized. In spite of almost complete healing, recurrences occurred. The right foot had two ulcerosquamous lesions, and the popliteal space had verrucous lesions. On the hands were scars which appeared to arise from abscesses. GOUGEROT (1936) reported two additional cases with numerous disseminated foci on all four extremities.

THIERS et al. (1953) wrote concerning disseminated, nodular lesions of geotrichosis with geotrichids in a 63-year-old woman teacher. The cutaneous changes developed gradually for a year, first on the face, then on the extremities and trunk. The firm, indolent, non-itching, pea-sized nodules arose subcutaneously and later affected the dermis which was slightly reddened. Over the nodules there formed small, dry, yellowish crusts which came off spontaneously, leaving a sunken, white scar. Between these nodules and scars there were poly-morphous, erythematous and squamous changes with slight subcutaneous edema which in places resembled a moist eczema. These lesions, from which the fungus could not be cultured, were regarded as geotrichids, and the nodules in which G. candidum was demonstrated micro-scopically and culturally were regarded as the related foci of infection. In biopsy, the nodules consisted of granulation tissue, one zone with prominent histiocytes and giant cells and a central, necrotic focus with polymorphonuclear leukocytes. The giant cells contained rounded, yeast-like, elements 4—$8\ \mu$ in size which could be stained with toluidin blue and erythrosin. The patient was treated with INH for 45 days with good results, although the fungus was resistant to INH in vitro. No new nodules appeared. The geotrichids healed. Later the patient was completely cured. Preceding therapy with penicillin, streptomycin, tetracycline, chloram-phenicol and fongeryl were ineffective.

ROUSSET et al. (1957) reported the case of a 54-year-old colonial official, in whom the disease began with a conjunctivitis (reddened eye, lacrimation), and a small, white, epithelioma-like induration on the mucous membrane of the lower lid, which later ulcerated superficially. After a month there appeared on the mucous membrane of the lower lip (later on the upper lip), a vesicle, which was accompanied by a progressing leukoplakia-like infiltrate, with central superficial ulceration. Except for the sensation of foreign body, the patient was free of pain. The biopsy showed a granuloma with foreign-body giant cells and yeast-like elements, which were embedded in thick histiocytic-plasma cell infiltrates and less frequently (together with filamentous elements) in the interstitial tissues. G. candidum could be cultured from the lesions in pure form. Although a 15-day treatment with intramuscular lipiodol brought only slight improvement, there developed, after a 10-day oral nystatin therapy, considerable improvement, but with scarring. Local treatment with argyrol, methylene blue and aureomy-cin was unsuccessful.

Tzamouranis (1962) described a cutaneous geotrichosis in a 4-month-old infant. On the right cheek was a small reddening and infiltrate, which spread in a few days to nearly the entire cheek. At the periphery there appeared new isolated papules which soon became confluent. Small lesions appeared on the forehead, the neck and the left cheek. Little scaling and itching occurred. In direct preparations, on two occasions, there were single, round to oval, double-contoured, non-budding elements and culturally numerous *G.candidum* colonies and some streptococcal and aerobic spore forms. After treatment with nystatin ointment, the lesions healed rapidly, as did a recurrence which appeared a month later. The first attempted treatment with chloramphenicol and penicillin was unsuccessful.

Superficial Forms: Chiale (1937) viewed the foot lesions of the following case as foci from which the hypersensitivity of the organism developed and led to a geotrichid. In a 54-year-old woman, who suffered from an erythematous, vesicular and squamous exzematoid lesion of the foot for 10 years, there suddenly developed on both legs and on the lower arms, small, diffusely scattered, spotty, slightly scaling, herpetic, somewhat itchy lesions. From the old foci on the foot and, rarely, from the new cutaneous lesions, *G.candidum* could be isolated, but not from the blood. The geotrichin test and the *Geotrichum* complement fixation reaction were positive.

Canellis (1959) described a folliculitis decalvans of the scalp due to *G.candidum*. In a 50-year-old man there developed, over the course of 5 years, several disseminated, pin-head sized, follicular pustules and crusts, and small, erythematous and squamous foci in the region of the temples, and in the region of the hair-part, several sharply circumscribed, bald places with smooth, whitish or erythematous surfaces and atrophy of the skin. At the edge of the bald areas and in the hairy scalp there were also numerous pustules related to the follicles. In the pus *G.candidum* was demonstrated microscopically and culturally. The serologic test for syphilis and the blood sugar test were negative. After 25 days of local and oral nystatin treatment the skin lesions were cured. Nine months later the patient was free of lesions.

Heidenbluth (1963) was able to demonstrate *G.candidum* microscopically and culturally in a series of patients who suffered from persistent anal eczema. The fungus was recovered from the stool and from scrapings from the perianal region. The cutaneous appearances and the subjective symptoms of the patients disappeared rapidly under nystatin therapy.

5. Other Geotrichoses

In this section cases of geotrichosis will be described which do not fit into the categories of bronchopulmonary, bronchial, oral, or cutaneous geotrichosis.

Mycetemia due to Geotrichum: In the two cases to be described there was a mycetemia due to *G.candidum* without a demonstrable geotrichosis of other organs. The portal of entry of the fungus was not ascertainable. Apparently the invasion, without appreciable local proliferation of the fungus, was via the digestive or upper respiratory tracts.

Bendove and Ashe (1952) reported on a 79-year-old man with diabetes who, because of dietary negligence, developed hyperglycemia and glycosuria and a greatly reduced general condition. Furthermore he acquired pharyngitis. With the use of penicillin, chloramphenicol and aureomycin he became free of fever. Later, fever of 37.8—39.2°C. appeared which could not be influenced. The blood sugar reached 380 mg%, the glycosuria 70 grams per day. Red blood cells were 3.4 millions, leukocytes 12,150, sedimentation-rate 90 mm. By X-ray the lungs showed no lesions. Although the glycosuria was controlled, the patient lost weight and appeared cachectic. In the blood *G.candidum* was demonstrated four times culturally, and also in the sputum. Thereupon the patient was treated with neomycin, which, however, had to be abandoned after 12 days, as difficulty in hearing developed which, moreover, was enduring. Although the *in vitro* effect of neomycin on the strain isolated was slight, the temperature slowly returned to normal. *G.candidum* could no longer be demonstrated in the blood or the sputum, and the patient soon recovered.

Kaliski et al. (1952) reported the case of a 2-month-old infant with miliary tuberculosis, in whom shortly before death abundant *G.candidum* could be cultured from blood samples. Even in smears of the blood, typical rectangular arthrospores were visible. The portal of entry could not be determined. Also, in sections of the lung no fungi were found.

Table 5. *Other Geotrichoses*

Author	Age and Sex	Occupation	Location	Organism
a) *Geotrichum* mycetemia				
1. BENDOVE and ASHE (1952)	79 M		New York, USA	*Geotrichum* species
2. KALISKI et al. (1952)	2/12 M		Texas, USA	*Geotrichum* species
b) *Geotrichum* mycetoma				
1. NICOLAU et al. (1957)	37 F	Farmwife	Rumania	*Geotrichum candidum*
c) *Geotrichum* wound infection				
1. NAGY et al. (1958)	64 M		Hungary	*Geotrichum* species
d) Geotrichosis of the cornea				
1. PERZ (1964, Case 1)	53 M	Mechanic	Poland	*Geotrichum candidum*
2. PERZ (1964, Case 2)	60 M	Farmer	Poland	*Geotrichum candidum*

Geotrichum Mycetoma: NICOLAU et al. (1957, 1958, 1959, 1964) described a mycetoma of the foot with bony changes caused by *G. candidum*. The lesion was cured with INH.

A 37-year-old farm woman developed a firm, plum-sized swelling on the sole of the left foot which was operatively removed, as was a recurrence which developed two years later. After a year there was again a recurrence, which, in the course of another year, led to the development of a painful, unwieldy swelling of the foot. The reddish-brown, dry skin, without ulcers or fistulae, showed numerous reddish nodules of millet-seed size, partly confluent. Nodules which were opened mechanically were found to consist of an oily mass with numerous white pinhead sized granules in which *G. candidum* was demonstrated microscopically and culturally. Roentgenologically the posterior half of the 5th metatarsal bone and the posterior end of the 4th metatarsal were thickened, the bony structure deformed and the cortex dentated. The general condition of the patient was good. Erythrocytes were 3,600,000, leukocytes 4,600, sedimentation-rate 60 mm. The biopsy showed a nodular infiltrate in the corium and partly also in the upper layers of the subcutaneous tissue, which were separated from one another by young connective tissue. The infiltrate in the edematous connective tissue consisted largely of plasma cells. Between them, isolated or in clusters, there were polymorphonuclear neutrophils, lymphocytes, histiocytes and individual giant cells. Furthermore, there were some interstitial, hemorrhagic foci. Capillaries were rich in the granulation tissue. In the infiltrate there were numerous round or oval fungus granules composed of an amorphous or slightly granulated mass without clubshaped projections. In the granule, by Gram stain, one could see relatively thin fungal hyphae (1 μ in diameter), but not in the PAS stain, because the matrix of the granule was PAS positive. In the infiltrate and especially in the neighborhood of the granules there were numerous cells with PAS-positive Russell bodies. With oral and local treatment with INH there was healing in four months and this was complete at the end of a year. Two months after the beginning of therapy no granules could be demonstrated. The bony lesions showed no change at four months but after a year they had healed, with calcification. In the following six years there was no recurrence.

Geotrichum Wound Infection. NAGY et al. (1958) described a suppurative and metastasizing wound infection in a 64-year-old man who, because of left-sided renal tuberculosis, had a nephrectomy. Three weeks later a thrombophlebitis appeared in both legs. From the region of the operation thick yellow pus escaped and *Proteus* and colon bacilli were cultured from it. There was no fever, but the white cells numbered 17,400 and the sedimentation-rate 102 mm in one hour. On the extremities appeared bean-sized abscesses which contained hemorrhagic pus in some instances. A week later the patient died. He had received streptomycin, INH, penicillin and aureomycin. At the postmortem examination, numerous microabscesses were found, in the corium, lungs, pancreas and retroperitoneal tissues. *G. candidum* could be demonstrated culturally in pus from the pustules of the skin and from the retroperitoneal abscesses. Microscopically there were Gram-positive, round or oval elements, single or in groups, in the region of the micro abscesses, in the lymphocytic infiltrate of the mucosa of the air passages, in the wall of the abscess cavity, and in the liver. The abscess wall was infiltrated with lymphocytes, leukocytes and giant cells in many places, but the picture was not that of tuberculous granulation tissue. Nor were tubercle bacilli demonstrable.

Apparently in this case there was a secondary infection of a bacterial process in the form of disseminated geotrichosis.

Geotrichosis of the Cornea. Perz (1964) described two local infections of the cornea. A 53-year-old locksmith received a squirt of mud in his right eye. In spite of thorough washing, pain and lacrimation developed the following day. A chronic, ulcerative keratitis ensued. The edges of the grayish yellow ulcers were undermined and the neighboring cornea was slightly dull. The conjunctiva was more or less injected, the iris severely injected, the corneal reflex diminished and precipitates were visible on Descemets membrane. Temporarily there was a hypopyon. Local treatment with antibiotics, iodine and Nipagin were unsuccessful. A smear of the ulcer showed *G.candidum* in pure culture. In the eye itself there spread a network of fungus mycelia from the ulcer into the neighboring corneal tissues. After three months vascularization began. Further ulceration had occurred. In six months there was healing with corneal scars. The patient could appreciate only strong light through this eye.

In the second case, a 60-year-old farmer got hay dust into his eyes. The next day an acute inflammation of the left eye developed, with severe pain and lacrimation. At first, serpigenous corneal ulcer with hypopyon was diagnosed. The conjunctiva was injected, and the lower half of the cornea presented grayish-yellow ulcers with undermined edges. The iris had a washed-out appearance and showed posterior synechiae. Local treatment was with atropine, sulfathiazole and silver nitrate. After a month the edge of the ulceration began to vascularize. After three months the whole process healed. The light sensitivity of the eye was maintained. From two excisional biopsies of the infiltrated cornea *G.candidum* could be grown in pure culture.

6. Specific Therapy

In the treatment of bronchopulmonary geotrichosis iodine is still the drug of choice. After several weeks of iodine therapy there is a lessening of the amount of sputum, a stopping of the troublesome cough and subjective feeling of well-being with increase in weight. Also dense pulmonary shadows clear in a few months and hilar lymph nodes become smaller. Even cavities disappear but some residual fibrosis remains. The fungus is no longer demonstrable in stool or sputum, or it occurs in smaller quantity. As a rule, oral potassium iodide is effective (Conant et al., 1954, page 71). Additionally or by itself sodium iodide can be given intravenously. Also ethyl-iodide inhalations are possible (Swartz and Jankelson, 1941). Acute reactions or disseminations which occasionally can develop as an expression of strong hypersensitivity to the iodine therapy in North American blastomycosis are not seen in the iodine therapy of geotrichosis. For complete cure, iodine therapy may be continued some months, or a year or longer. In bronchial geotrichosis one can count on cure or much improvement after several weeks of iodine therapy.

Nystatin was used in two cases of pulmonary geotrichosis (3—4 months by mouth, daily 3—9 mill. units and as an aerosol) by Bell et al. (1962) with success, and by Peninou-Castaing et al. (1954) without success. With cutaneous geotrichosis treated with nystatin in ointment and/or by mouth (2—5 mill. units daily) for 10—25 days, the lesions healed with scar formation. With cutaneous geotrichosis treated with iodine, recurrences appeared in the case of Balzer et al. (1912), in spite of extensive healing, and in the case of Rousset et al. (1957) there was, only with the following nystatin treatment, a significant improvement. The fungistatic dose of nystatin according to Drouhet (1955) and Dobins and Hazen (1961) is 6—16 units/ml. Also with nystatin, after a few days, there is a cessation or considerable diminution in the excretion of the fungus. As Duncan et al. (1951) found *G.candidum* moderately sensitive to neomycin, Bendove and Ashe (1952) treated their patient intramuscularly for three days with daily doses of 1000 units per kg and 10 days more with half doses. The infection could be dominated with that. There was, however, a persisting deafness. NICOLAU et al. (1958) were able to cure completely a mycetoma of the foot with bony change by the use of INH. By mouth daily 500—600 mg (altogether 35 grams) of INH were given and in addition 33 local injections of 5—10 ml of a 2% INH solution. The fungistatic INH dose for *G.candidum* is 50—100 μg/ml. Also in the patient of THIERS et al. (1953) there was improvement, with 250 mg of INH daily for 45 days, of the cutaneous lesions and they later healed completely, although the *G.candidum* strain isolated was, *in vitro*, resistant to INH. The pulmonary geotrichosis of HAUSER (1954) and PENINOU-CASTAING et al. (1964) was not influenced by INH. Concerning the therapy of oral geotrichosis there is only one example, that of CARTEAUD and DROUHET (1955), who saw the coating of a black hairy tongue disappear after the use of sodium bicarbonate mouth washings. If a therapy is necessary, oral geotrichosis can be treated with gentian violet etc. as is oral candidosis. The customary antibiotics, like penicillin, streptomycin, chloramphenicol and tetracycline, are ineffective against *G.candidum*. According to HEIDENBLUTH (1963) *G.candidum* is resistent to griseofulvin. Treatment with Amphotericin B was recommended by PROCKNOW and LOOSLI (1958) and WEGMANN (1961). The therapeutic use of *G.candidum* vaccine has not been studied.

G. Geotrichum Candidum Infections in Animals

Natural Infections: In spontaneously dying white mice which during life displayed weakness of the extremities, ACOSTINI (1932) found the lungs beset with small white pustules. In the lung and liver there were microscopically fungus filaments and culturally a bacteria-free pure culture of *G.candidum*. To test the pathogenicity of the isolated strain, healthy mice were injected intravenously, and they died in 3—4 months. *G.candidum* was demonstrable in their lungs and liver. Then a second passage was carried out, and the animals died after 1—2 months and finally, with the third passage, after 1—3 days. The last mice also showed changes in the intestines. TORRES et al. (1942) reported a gastritis in normally nourished white mice. The histologic investigation of 19 animals showed a thin coating on the stomach mucous membrane, which in seven mice extended into the crypts and gland lumina. From the membrane *G.candidum (G.sp.)* could be isolated. The mucosa itself showed a mild acute catarrhal inflammation.

MORQUER et al. (1955) described a caseous adenitis in pigs, which for ten years was repeatedly observed in the slaughter house of Oran. From the caseous, but not calcified, pinhead-sized to pea-sized lesions of lymph nodes *G.candidum* could be isolated. The spleen showed no changes and there was no lymphangitis. With the isolated strain, guinea pigs, white mice and piglets were experimentally inoculated. An acute, non-caseous adenitis was produced by subcutaneous injection and inoculation of the inguinal lymph nodes. Oral infections were not obtained in the pigs, nor were infections obtained from intratracheal and nasal instillations with another strain (*G.versiforme*).

AINSWORTH and AUSTWICK (1955) mentioned three mastitis cases in cows, in whom *G.candidum* was the only agent isolated, and two abortions, in which as a cause a *G.candidum* infection was considered possible. *G.candidum* could be found in abnormally large quantity in the feces of a pig and of a dog, both of whom had severe diarrhea. HEYN (1958) described in a 6-month aborted fetus of a cow a purulent and necrotizing dermatitis with pronounced parakeratosis. The skin changes consisted of foci the size of 5-Mark pieces, extending 1 cm above the surface of the skin, the slimy coating of which could be easily removed. A collection of lymphocytes with occasional leukocytes and histiocytes extended to the subcutaneous tissues. Especially intense were the infiltrates in and about the hair follicles. Within the hair follicles were isolated, segmented and branching hyphae stained by the method of Giemsa. On the basis of the histologic picture an infection with *G.candidum (Oospora lactis)* was predicated. A cultural investigation was not possible.

Experimental Infections: Hueppe (1884) reported that in cats, rabbits, rats, and mice, after giving them *G.candidum* (Oidium lactis) by mouth, or intracutaneously, subcutaneously or intravenously, no disease process appeared. Lang and Freudenreich (1893) and Linossier (1916) got the same results with the intravenous infection of rabbits. Also, Thjötta and Urdal (1949) could see no pathological change after intravenous, intraperitoneal and intramuscular injections in rabbits and guinea pigs. The *G. candidum* strain isolated by Nicolau et al. (1957) from a mycetoma was not pathogenic for mice, guinea pigs and rats. Also the extensive research of Coudert et al. (1958) with different strains of *G.candidum* in rats, guinea pigs and mice was negative. They infected the animals intraperitoneally and by mouth. The lowering of the resistence by antibiotics, cortisone and streptokinase did not lead to infection. No changes were seen in animals, macroscopically or microscopically, in the period between three weeks and two months after the injections. Nor could the organism be cultured from the internal organs. Vieu and Segretain (1959) injected mice intraperitoneally with various strains of *G.candidum (G.candidum, G.versiforme* and *G.asteroides)*. The infections did not cause the death of the animals, nor were there changes in the organs at autopsy 45 days after injection. Caretta and Martinazzi (1960) injected 2, 10, and 20 mill. *G.candidum* arthrospores in rabbits without there being demonstrable clinical or histological changes after 30 days. Only in one further animal, which had received a considerably higher dose could there be found in the lung a diffuse, interstitial, microinfiltrate of polymorphonuclear neutrophils, eosinophils, lymphocytes and epithelioid cells. There were scattered foreign-body giant cells and foci of remnants of mycelium, bordered by connective tissue, to be seen. The fungus could, however, not be isolated. Brain, heart, liver, spleen, kidneys and adrenals were histologically unchanged. Caretta (1960) obtained the same result with a broader series of experiments. He injected eight strains of *G.candidum* in three different doses intravenously into 24 rabbits. According to Bader (1965) whose experimental infections likewise were unsuccessful, the fungus cells were taken up by macrophages and rendered harmless, after intravenous injections. In the liver, spleen, bone marrow and lymph nodes there appeared numerous cells whose cytoplasm contained large PAS-positive inclusions consisting of fungus break-down products.

Cao (1900) injected *G. candidum (Oidium lactis)* intravenously. A pregnant animal passed a dead fetus ten days later, and from its kidneys *G.candidum* in large quantity could be cultured, although visible pathologic changes were not present. The mother rabbit died after 25 days having been in very poor condition. There were no macroscopic lesions to be seen. However, the fungus could be demonstrated microscopically in the kidneys and culturally from the brain and kidneys. Another animal died, cachectic, after 42 days. Except for atrophy of the renal cortex there was macroscopically no finding of lesions. The cultural evidence was successful only from the brain. A third animal, which was injected with the strain isolated from the first animal died, somewhat emaciated, after 14 days. The left kidney showed a white cortical infarct, the right one 5 white nodules with purulent contents. The culture from kidney and brain was positive. Martins (1928) injected his strain *(Zymonema pulmonalis membranogenes)* into rabbits, dogs and guinea pigs. The intravenously injected rabbit and the intraperitoneally injected guinea pig showed no changes. An intravenously inoculated dog lost weight and a subcutaneously inoculated guinea pig developed a knotty infiltrate at the site of injection. CIFERRI and REDAELLI (1935) found a mild, generalized, miliary infection with prominent renal changes, after they injected a strain of *G.candidum* (Colombo Pasini Nr. 4) in a rabbit. CIFERRI et al. (1938), in four rabbits, injected a thick suspension of *G.candidum* (*G.matalense*) intravenously. Only the animal injected with 10 ml of suspension died after 23 days. The other animals survived and those receiving 3 and 5 ml showed no changes while those receiving 8 ml were emaciated. The dead, severely emaciated animal showed somewhat hyperemic lungs, a slightly enlarged liver and spleen of decreased consistency, numerous enlarged abdominal lymph nodes and distinctly enlarged kidneys. The microscopic renal finding was that of well-maintained glomeruli. The capsular spaces were, in some cases, filled with coagulated protein. The vessels of medium caliber contained numerous fungus elements, mostly in the form of foci of various size. Fungal foci were also found in the renal parenchyma. The tissue surrounding the fungal elements was partially necrotic. In part there was a slight, nodular, non-proliferating inflammation present (slight exudate with few cells). The tubular epithelium showed a diffuse albuminoid degeneration. Fungus elements could be found only in the kidneys. The other organs were normal or showed signs of a slight inflammation with parenchymatous degeneration. The rabbit injected with 8 ml and sacrificed two months later, also showed the same changes, even if in lesser degree. Here, also, the changes in the kidneys were prominent. But not every strain of *Geotrichum* produced lesions, as two other rabbits, injected with other *G.candidum* strains (*Pseudomycoderma matalense* and *Oidium* sp. CHAPMAN) in the same quantities as above did not become ill. These strains were old ones, from the culture collection, while the successfully injected strain had been freshly isolated from the stool of a patient ill with enteritis.

VÖRÖS-FELKAI and NOVÁK (1961) reported, without details, fatal intraperitoneal infections (within 7—10 days) in mice injected with 17 strains of *G.candidum* (*G.sp.*) isolated from humans. ARIYEVICH et al. (1963) injected rats. With the intravenous injection of 75 mill. arthrospores the animals, sacrificed after three days, showed grayish white nodules on the surface of the kidneys and histologically numerous renal abscesses with fungus elements. Also in the lungs there were small nodules with central, fungus-containing giant cells which were surrounded with lymphocytes and leukocytes. Also in the brain fungus elements and mild infiltrates near vessels could be demonstrated. With the subcutaneous injection of 50 million arthrospores abscesses formed after one or two days and these contained numerous hyphae. Intranasally injected fungus cells, 50 million of them, under light ether anesthesia, led, after one or two days, to exudative, leukocyte-rich foci in the lungs having fungus elements with right angled and rounded corners. In 3-day-old rats a part of the tongue surface was chemically traumatized and then brushed with a suspension of arthrospores. After one or two days one could see, histologically, numerous microabscesses with fungus filaments. The process later involved the non-traumatized portion of the tongue and also the esophagus. PERZ (1964) injected intraperitoneally two guinea pigs with 1 ml each and two mice with 0.5 ml each, using a strain of *G.candidum* isolated from a corneal ulceration in a suspension of 1 million arthrospores per ml. In the guinea pigs infection was unsuccessful. The mice died after 9 days, after they had been apathetic and without appetite for a day. At autopsy only a hyperemia of the liver and dilatation of the small intestine could be seen grossly but microscopically there were small thrombi and arthrospores in the coronary vessels. The fungus could not be cultured. SCHIEFER (1967) described, in mice, arthrospore-containing abscesses and epithelioid cell granulomas with a tendency toward caseation, and there were collections of foam cells with arthrospores.

In the following investigations of Ricketts, Balzer et al., and Nagy et al., a bacterial contamination of the *G.candidum* strain, sometimes difficult to recognize, cannot be definitely ruled out. Ricketts (1901) injected several animals with his strain (*Oidium aceticum*) isolated from cutaneous abscesses. In guinea pigs the intraperitoneal infection was negative. After subcutaneous injection into the skin of the belly there developed, after 5 days, abscesses with spontaneous rupture (Staphylococcal?). With injection into the back there was elevation of temperature, but no abscess formation. Subcutaneous injection in mice and intraperitoneal and subcutaneous injection in white rats had negative results. Also there were no effects following the subcutaneous injection of a dog. Another dog injected intravenously and sacrificed after a month showed only miliary, subcapsular, renal nodules consisting of young connective tissue and plasma cells. The causal agent was not demonstrable. An intravenously injected rabbit died, after 5 min, of a pulmonary embolus. Another died after two days without the fungus being demonstrated culturally. The kidneys were enlarged and pale with the features of fatty degeneration, as was also the liver. In the lungs there were small foci with epithelioid cell, lymphocytic and leukocytic infiltrates. The other organs were normal.

Balzer et al. (1912) carried out investigations with a strain isolated from a skin lesion (*Mycoderma pulmoneum*). The intraperitoneally and subcutaneously injected guinea pigs died of septicemia after 2 days. An intravenously injected rabbit died of septicemia after 8 days, having suffered rapid emaciation. Two subcutaneously injected rats died in very poor condition after 3 months, one with a large ulcer of the anus.

Nagy et al. (1958) injected two mice intraperitoneally with the *G.candidum* (*G.* sp.) isolated from their patient. Both animals succumbed to purulent peritonitis at 6—7 weeks. In smears of the peritoneal exudate there were numerous arthrospores with rounded ends and short hyphae. The internal organs also contained fungi.

The investigations described were carried out with living cultures. But also from intravenous injection of dead suspensions, for example in the immunizing of rabbits, fatal cases have been observed. This occurs not only after *G.candidum* inoculations, but often when large quantities of relatively bulky fungus material is injected intravenously (Thjötta et al., 1951; Seeliger, 1958; Torheim, 1963; Morenz, 1963). The long thick hyphae can block small vessels and induce microinfarcts.

There appears to be a special concentration of the fungus elements in the kidney, perhaps related to the excretion function of the kidneys. If the pulmonary capillaries are rapidly blocked, there can be the so-called rapid death situation with the picture of a pulmonary embolism. The organ changes are not dependent on the particulate nature of the fungus alone, but also on the toxic effect of the fungus. With homogenized *G.candidum* material immunized animals after several injections may become emaciated and finally succumb. In this way the degradation products of the fungus may lead to parenchymal degenerations, especially in the kidneys and the liver.

In summary, it is possible to say that under certain unknown circumstances *G.candidum* may also be pathogenic for animals, as the already described natural infections show. Moreover, an increase in virulence with animal passage may occur. Experimental infections were possible, as a rule, only with very large doses of infectious material. As the same symptoms also appeared with the killed fungus, the reactions are related to the large size of mycelial fragments (emboli, micro-infarcts) and to the toxic fungal degradation products (microinfiltrates, foreign body granulomas, parenchymal degenerations) without an increase in the number of fungi being necessary. For saprophytic and pathogenic types within the *Geotrichum candidum* species there is no support. The "pathogenic differences" in experimental infections with different strains can be explained by differences in fragmentation of the mycelium, as immunization with completely arthrospore-containing cultures or mechanically fragmentated hyphae is better tolerated by the animals.

References

ABRAMOVA, E. V., KRYLOV, L. M., SOKOLOVA, T. S.: Intestinal geotrichosis in a three-month-old child. (Russian). Vopr. Ochr. Mat. (Moskva) 9/2, 87 (1964). — ACOSTINI, A.: *Geotrichum candidum* Link, patogeno del mus. Boll. Soc. ital. Biol. sper. 7, 727 (1932). — AINSWORTH, G.C., AUSTWICK, P.K.C.: A survey of animal mycosis in Britain: general aspects. Vet. Rec. 67, 88 (1955). ~ A survey of animal mycosis in Britain: mycological aspects. Trans. Brit. Mycol. Soc. 38, 369 (1955). — ALMEIDA, F. de, LACAZ, C.S.: Considerações micólogicas sobre 4 amostras de *Geotrichum* isoladas do escarro. Folia clín. biol. (S. Paulo) 12, 41 (1940). ~ Cogumelo do genero *Geotrichum* isolado de lesoes ulcerativas do reto. Folia clín. biol. (S. Paulo) 12, 57 (1940). — ARIEVICH, A. M., KRYLOV, L. M., STEPANISHCHEVA, Z.G.: Geotrichosis of mucous membranes and internal organs (clinical and experimental investigation). (Russian). Klin. Med. (Moskva) 41, 14 (1963). — ARRIGHI, F., DROUHET, E.: Langue noire villeuse à *Geotrichum*. Bull. Soc. franç. Derm. Syph. 64, 753 (1957). — BACHMANN, W.: Ein Fall von Soorvarietät. Zbl. Bakt., I. Abt. Orig. 86, 129 (1921). — BADER, G.: Die viszeralen Mycosen (Pathologie, Klinik und Therapie). Jena: Gustav Fischer 1965. — BALZER, F., BURNIER, R., GOUGEROT, H.: Dermatite végétante et ulcéreuse due un champignon filamenteux constaté dans le pus, isolé par la culture et encore indéterminé. Bull. Soc. franç. Derm. Syph. 21, 342 (1910). — BALZER, F., GOUGEROT, H., BURNIER, R.: Dermatomycose végétante disséminée due au *Mycoderma pulmoneum*. Ann. Derm. Syph. (Paris), Sér. V, 3, 461 (1912). — BELL, D., BRODIE, J., HENDERSON, A.: A case of pulmonary geotrichosis. Brit. J. Dis. Chest 56, 26 (1962). — BENDOVE, R.A., ASHE, B.I.: *Geotrichum* septicemia. Arch. intern. Med. 89, 107 (1952). — BENNETT, J.H.: On the parasitic fungi found growing on the bodies of living animals. Proc. roy. Soc. Edinb. 1, 356 (1832—1844). ~ On the parasitic vegetable structures found growing in living animals. Trans. roy. Soc. Edinb. 15/II, 277 (1842). — BREDNOW, W.: Zur Klinik der Lungenmykosen. Med. Klin. 53, 622 (1958). — CANELLIS, P.: Geotrichosis der Kopfhaut unter dem Bilde einer Folliculitis decalvans. Hautarzt 10, 43 (1959). — CANITROT-ARAUJO, M.: Aportación al estudio de la alergia cutánea a diversos hongos patógenos. An. Fac. Med. Santiago de Compostela 1, 453 (1957). (Quoted from Rev. Med. vet. Myc. [Kew] III/1958). — CAO, G.: Oiden und Oidiomykose. Z. Hyg. 34, 282 (1900). — CARETTA, G.: Isolamento comparativo da escreti umani del *Geotrichum candidum* e saggi di patogenicità. Atti Ist. Bot. Lab. Critt. Pavia, Ser, V, 17, 293 (1960). ~ Reperti simultanei di *Candide e Geotrichi* in sputi e in feci umane. Nuovi Ann. Ig. 12, 309 (1961). — CARETTA, G., MARTINAZZI, M.: Aspetti morfologici delle candidosi, aspergillosi e geotricosi sperimentali. Pathologica 52, 245 (1960). — CARMICHAEL, J.W.: *Geotrichum candidum.* Mycologia 49, 820 (1957). — CARTEAUD, A.J.-P., DROUHET, E.: Étude mycologique à propos de six observations typiques de langue noire. Bull. Soc. franç. Derm. Syph. 62, 162 (1955). — CARTEAUD, A.J.-P., DROUHET, E., VIEU, M.: Les langues noires villeuses. Presse méd. 65, 966 (1957). — CASTELLANI, A.: Notes on the hyphomycetes found in sprue: with remarks on the classification of fungi of the genus "*Monilia Gmelin* 1791". J. trop. Med. Hyg. 17, 305 (1914). ~ Fungi and fungous diseases. Lecture II. Arch. Derm. Syph. (Chic.) 17, 61 (1928). ~ Dermatite eczematose micotica delle dita dei piedi dovuta probabilmente al *Geotrichum rotundatum* CASTELLANI 1911 ed al *Geotrichum rotundatum var. gallicum* n. v. Arch. ital. Sci. med. colon. 23, 1 (1942). — CASTELLANI, A., CHALMERS, A.J.: Manual of Tropical Medicine. London: Baillière, Tindall & Cox 1919. — CHIALE, G.F.: In tema di "foci" cutanei micotici. G. ital. Derm. Sif. 78, 771 (1937). — CIFERRI, R., REDAELLI, P.: Contribuzioni alla sistematica delle Torulopsidaceae. XV—XXXIII. Arch. Mikrobiol. 6, 9 (1935). — CIFERRI, R., VERONA, O., SAGGESE, V.: Reisolamento della *Pseudomycoderma matalense* e revisione del gruppo. Mycopathologia (Den Haag) 1, 212 (1938). — COLONNELLO, F.: Il *Geotrichum candidum* quale ospite dell' organismo umano. Atti Ist. Bot. Lab. Critt. Pavia, Ser. V, 3, 197 (1944). — CONANT, N.F., SMITH, D.T., BAKER, R.D., CALLAWAY, J.L., MARTIN, D.S.: Manual of Clinical Mycology. Philadelphia-London: W. B. Saunders Comp. 1954. — CORTESE, F.: Tonsillomicosi da "*Geotrichum candidum*." Valsalva 9, 149 (1933). (Quoted from COLONNELLO, 1944.) — COU-

Dert, J., Despierres, G., Saëz, H., Hollard, J.: Recherches sur la flore levuriforme bronchique en milieu sanatorial. Sem. Hôp. Paris **33**, 2978 (1957). — Coudert, J., Garin, J.-P., Saëz, H.: Quelques aspects de la géotrichose humaine. J. méd. Lyon **38**, 189 (1958). — Dávalos, R., Arcos, L.: Geotricosis pulmonar. Gac. méd. (Guayaquil) **9**, 155 (1954). — Dobias, B., Hazen, E.L.: Nystatin. Chemotherapia **3**, 108 (1961). — Drouhet, E.: Action de la nystatine (fungicidine) in vitro et in vivo sur *Candida albicans* et autres champignons levuriformes. Ann. Inst. Pasteur (Paris) **88**, 298 (1955). — Duncan, G.G., Clancy, C.F., Wolgamot, J.R., Beidleman, B.: Neomycin: results of clinical use in ten cases. J. Amer. med. Ass. **145**, 75 (1951). — Dvořák, J., Otčenášek, M.: *Geotrichum candidum* Link 1809 in einer Haut- und Nagelläsion. Derm. Wschr. **152**, 1183 (1966). — Ettig, B.: Das Vorkommen von *Geotrichum candidum* Link im Stuhl Psoriasiskranker. Hautarzt **16**, 491 (1965). — Felsenfeld, O.: Yeast-like fungi in the intestinal tract of chronically institutionalized patients. Amer. J. med. Sci. **207**, 60 (1944). — Frágner, P., Petrů, M., Vojtěchovská, M.: *Geotrichum candidum* při vaginálním fluoru. Čsl. Hyg. Epid. Mikrobiol. **4**, 434 (1955). — Frágner, P., Svatek, Z.: Mykosy kladenských havířů. Čsl. Hyg. Epid. Mikrobiol. **5**, 75 (1956). — Galinovic-Weisglass, M.: *Geotrichum* u intestinalnom traktu čovjeka. Higijena (Beograd) **11**, 316 (1959). — Gauvreau, L., Grandbois, J.: Un cas de mycose cutanée causée par un champignon de l'ordre des arthrospores. Laval méd. **19**, 59 (1954). — Gernez-Rieux, C.: Les pneumopathies fongiques. Rev. Tuberc. (Paris) **24**, 1088 (1960). — Golay, J., Wyss-Chodat, F.: De la présence fréquente d'un champignon du genre *géotrichum* (Link) dans l'intestin des psoriasiques. Rev. méd. Suisse rom. **62**, 961 (1942). — Good, C.A.: Fungus diseases of the lungs. Review of roentgenologic manifestations. Tex. St. J. Med. **47**, 817 (1951). — Gougerot, H.: Mycodermose cutanée due au "*Mycoderma pulmoneum*." Bull. Soc. franç. Derm. Syph. **27**, 185 (1920). ~ Mycodermoses (ou géotrichoses). In: Darier, J. et al.: Nouvelle Pratique Dermatologique, T. II. p. 569—579. Paris: Masson 1936. — Grimmer, H.: Antibiotika und Pilzerkrankungen der Haut und Schleimhaut. Antibiot. et Chemother. (Basel) **1**, 180 (1954). — Guéguen, F.: Méconnaissance fréquente de *l'Oidium lactis* Fresenius, saprophyte facilement identifiable de l'homme et des animaux. C. R. Soc. Biol. (Paris) **74**, 943 (1913). — Haley, L.D., McCabe, A.: A mycologic study of seventy-one autopsies. Amer. J. clin. Path. **20**, 35 (1950). — Hauser, W.: Geotrichose der Lunge. Ärztl. Wschr. **9**, 244 (1954). — Heidenbluth, J.: Über *Geotrichum candidum* und *Oospora lactis* und ihr Vorkommen beim Analekzem. Z. Haut- u. Geschl.-Kr. **34**, 222 (1963). — Heyn, W.: Hautmykose bei einem Rinderfetus. Dtsch. tierärztl. Wschr. **65**, 561 (1958). — Hueppe, F.: Untersuchungen über die Zersetzung der Milch durch Mikroorganismen. Mitt. kaiserl. Gesundheitsamt **2**, 309 (1884). — Hyde, J.N., Ricketts, H.T.: A report of two cases of blastomycosis of the skin in man, with a survey of the literature of human blastomycosis. J. cutan. Dis. **19**, 44 (1901). — Jannin, L.: Les "Mycoderma". Leur rôle en pathologie. Thése Fac. Méd. No. 1001, Nancy, 1913. — Kaliski, S.R., Beene, L.M., Mattman, L.: *Geotrichum* in blood stream of an infant. J. Amer. med. Ass. **148**, 1207 (1952). — Kärcher, K.H.: Neue Gesichtspunkte zur Klinik und Pathogenese der Hefeerkrankungen. Arch. Derm. Syph. (Berl.) **197**, 51 (1953). ~ Die Geotrichose. In: Jadassohn, J.: Handbuch der Haut- und Geschlechtskrankheiten, Ergänzungswerk Bd. IV/4, p. 197—203. Berlin-Göttingen-Heidelberg: Springer 1963. — Kourkoumeli-Kontomichalou, P., Papadakis, E., Daikos, G.: Nasopharyngeal flora of personnel of "Alexandra" hospital. (Greek). Acta microbiol. Hellen. **6**, 150 (1961). — Kunstadter, R.H., Milzer, A.: Incidence of mycotic infections in children with acute respiratory tract disease. Amer. J. Dis. Child. **81**, 306 (1951). — Kunstadter, R.H., Milzer, A., Whitcomb, A.: Bronchopulmonary geotrichosis in children. Amer. J. Dis. Child. **79**, 82 (1950). — Kunstadter, R.H., Pendergrass, R.C., Schubert, J.H.: Bronchopulmonary geotrichosis. Amer. J. med. Sci. **211**, 583 (1946). — Lang, M., Freudenreich, E. v.: Über *Oidium lactis*. Landwirtsch. Jahrb. Schweiz **7**, 229 (1893). — Linossier, G.: Contribution à l'étude des mycoses bronchopulmonaires. Étude biologique d'un "*Oidium lactis*" parasite de l'homme. Bull. Soc. méd. Hôp. Paris, Sér. III, **40**, 575 (1916). — Lodder, J., Kreger-Van Rij, N.J.W.: The Yeasts: A Taxonomic Study. North-Holland, Amsterdam, 1952. — Lofgren, R.C.: Oospora-like fungus found pathogenic to man. Arch. Derm. Syph. (Chic.) **71**, 56 (1955). — Mahoudeau, D., Lemoine, J.M., Poulet, J., Dubrisay, J.: Mycoses respiratoires pseudo-tumorales. (Aspergillose et géotrichose). J. franç. Méd. Chir. thor. **9**, 53 (1955). — Mándi, L., Berencsi, G.: Adatok a tüdömykozis kérdéséhez két eset kapcsán. Orv. Hetil. **27**, 742 (1954). — Marselou, U., Paschali-Pavlatou, M.: Fréquence des levures du genre *Candida* dans le vagin, le rectum et le pharynx. (Greek). Acta microbiol. Hellen. **1**, 239 (1956). — Martin, D.S.: Complement-fixation in blastomycosis. J. infect. Dis. **57**, 291 (1935). — Martins, C.: *Zymonema pulmonalis membranogenes* isolé d'un crachat de pneumopathie grave et mortelle. C. R. Soc. Biol. (Paris) **98**, 1162 (1928). — Mattlet, G.: Mycoses dans l'Urundi. Ann. Soc. belge Méd. trop. **6**, 1 (1926). — Minton, R., Young, R.V., Shanbrom, E.: Endobronchial geotrichosis. Ann. intern. Med. **40**, 340 (1954). — Montemayor, L. de, Gamero, B.H. de: Aislamiento y determinacion de 300 cepas del genero *Candida*.

Mycopathologia (Den Haag) **15**, 343 (1961). — MOORE, M.: A new *Geotrichum* from a bronchial and pulmonary infection, *Geotrichum versiforme* MOORE, *n. sp.* Ann. Missouri Botan. Garden **21**, 349 (1934). — MORENZ, J.: *Geotrichum candidum* Link. Taxonomie, Diagnose und medizinische Bedeutung. Mykol. Schriftenreihe (Leipzig) **1**, 1 (1963). ∼ Taxonomische Untersuchungen zur Gattung *Geotrichum* Link. Mykol. Schriftenreihe (Leipzig) **2**, 33 (1964). — MORQUER, R., LOMBARD, C., BERTHELON, M.: Pouvoir pathogène de quelques espèces de *Geotrichum.* C. R. Acad. Sci. (Paris) **240**, 378 (1955). — MOTTA, R.: Micosi benigna della tonsilla linguale da *Oospora lactis.* Valsalva **7**, 599 (1931). (Quoted from COLONNELLO, 1944). — NAGY, L., MOLNÁR, L., FLÓRIÁN, E.: Geotrichosis. Zbl. allg. Path. **98**, 374 (1958). — NEAGOE, G., NEAGOE, M.: Enterokolitis durch *Geotrichum candidum* nach Therapie mit Glutaminsäure. Dtsch. Z. Verdau.- u. Stoffwechselkr. **27**, 205 (1967). — NICOLAU, S.G., AVRAM, A.: Der gegenwärtige Stand der Behandlung des Myzetoms im Lichte eigener Erfahrung. Derm. Wschr. **140**, 792 (1959). ∼ Cas de mycétomes observés en Roumanie. Arch. Union Méd. Balkan. (Bucureşti) **2**, 597 (1964). — NICOLAU, S.G., AVRAM, A., COLINTINEANU, L., BĂLUŞ, L., STOIAN, M.: Efect favorabil al hidrazidei acidului izonicotinic asupra leziunilor osoasc dintr-un caz de micetom al piciorului cu grăunţi albi, provocat de *Geotrichum candidum.* Derm.-Vener. (Buc.) **3**, 263 (1958). — NICOLAU, S.G., HULEA, A., AVRAM, A., COLINTINEANU, L., BĂLUŞ, L.: Studiu clinic şi micologic asupra unei forme tuberoase de micetom cu grăunţi albi al piciorului produs de *Geotrichum candidum.* Derm.-Vener. (Buc.) **2**, 217 (1957). — NICOLESCU, N.: Aspecte radiologice în micozele pulmonare. Viaţa med. **9**, 707 (1962). — OTT, E.: Über das Vorkommen von Hefen im Magen-Darm-Trakt unter besonderer Berücksichtigung quantitativer Unterschiede. Mykosen **6**, 7 (1963). — PENINOU-CASTAING, J., COLLAS, R., BATTESTI, M.R.: Géotrichose pulmonaire d'évolution fatale associée a une tuberculose pulmonaire. Poumon **20**, 287 (1964). — PERZ, M.: Drożdżyca ragówki spowodowana przez *Geotrichum candidum.* Klin. oczna **34**, 273 (1964). — PÉTER, M., HORVÁTH, G.: Cercetări clinico-micologice privind frecvenţa genului *Geotrichum.* Rev. Medicală **5**, 430 (1959). — PÉTER, M., HORVÁTH, G., DOMOKOS, L.: Date referitoare la frecvenţa genului *Geotrichum* în diferite produse biologice umane. Med. Internă **19**, 875 (1967). — PÉTOURAUD, C., COUDERT, J.: Blastomycose cutanée à "*Geotrichum cutaneum*" de Beurmann et Gougerot (1909) localisée, chez un employé dans une fromagerie. Bull. Soc. franç. Derm. Syph. **60**, 299 (1953). — PINKERTON, M.E., MULLINS, J.F., SHAPIRO, E.M.: The ecology of superficial fungus infections in Galveston, Texas. A five year survey. Tex. Rep. Biol. Med. **15**, 26 (1957). — PROCKNOW, J.J., LOOSLI, C.G.: Treatment of the deep mycoses. Arch. intern. Med. **101**, 765 (1958). — REDAELLI, P., CIFERRI, R.: Relazione sul primo quinquennio (1938—1943) di attività del Centro Micologia Umana e Comparata della R. Università di Pavia. Atti Ist. Bot. Lab. Critt. Pavia, Ser. V, **3**, 1 (1943). — REEVES, R.J.: The incidence of bronchomycosis in the South. Amer. J. Roentgenol. **45**, 513 (1941). — REIERSÖL, S.: An investigation of the occurrence of fungi in 250 laryngeal swabs from tuberculous patients. Acta path. microbiol. scand. **32**, 500 (1953). — RICKETTS, H.T.: Oidiomycosis (blastomycosis) of the skin and its fungi. J. med. Res. **6**, 373 (1901). — ROSSIER, P.H.: Antibiotica und Mykosen. Helv. med. Acta **19**, 261 (1952). — ROUSSET, J., COUDERT, J., GARIN, J.P.: Blastomycose superficielle des muqueuses à foyers multiples. Bull. Soc. franç. Derm. Syph. **64**, 316 (1957). — SAËZ, H.E.: Le *Geotrichum candidum* Link. Caractéristiques morpho-biologiques; fréquence chez l'homme. Bull. Soc. Myc. Fr. **73**, 343 (1957). — SCHABINSKI, G.: Grundriß der medizinischen Mykologie. Jena: Gustav Fischer 1960. — SCHAEDE, R.: Über zwei neue Oosporaarten bei „schwarzer Haarzunge". Derm. Wschr. **98**, 521 (1934). — SCHIEFER, B.: Pathomorphologie der Systemmykosen des Tieres. Jena: Gustav Fischer 1967. — SCHNOOR, T.G.: The occurrence of *Monilia* in normal stools. Amer. J. trop. Med. **19**, 163 (1939). — SEELIGER, H.P.R.: Mykologische Serodiagnostik. Leipzig: J.A. Barth 1958. ∼ Serodiagnostik der Pilze und mykotischen Infektionen. Zbl. Bakt., I. Abt. Orig. **184**, 203 (1962). — ŞERBAN, P., TAŞCĂ, C.: Aspecte privind diagnosticul morfologic al unor micoze generalizate, în practica prosecturală. Morfol. norm. si pat. (Buc.) **7**, 257 (1962). — SKOBEL, P., SCHABINSKI, G., ESSIGKE, G.: Untersuchungen über die Immunitätslage und den Wert der Serodiagnostik bei *Candida*-Mykosen. Ärztl. Wschr. **11**, 317 (1956). — SMITH, D.T.: Oidiomycosis of the lungs. Report of a case due to a species of *Geotrichum.* J. thorac. Surg. **3**, 241 (1934). ∼ Pulmonary mycoses. Clinics **4**, 994 (1945). ∼ Fungus diseases of the lungs. Springfield: Thomas 1947. ∼ Fungous infections in the United States. J. Amer. med. Ass. **141**, 1223 (1949). — SUNDGAARD, G., THJÖTTA, T., URDAL, K.: Familiaer opptreden av geotrichosis pulmonum. Nord. Med. **43**, 434 (1950). — SWARTZ, J.H., JANKELSON, I.R.: Incidence of fungi in the stools of non-specific ulcerative colitis. Amer. J. dig. Dis. **8**, 211 (1941). — THIERS, H., GOUDERT, J., COLOMB, D.: Lésions nodulaires disséminées (*geothricum candidum*) avec allergides. Efficacité remarquable de l'Isoniazide. Bull. Soc. franç. Derm. Syph. **60**, 165 (1953). — THJÖTTA, T., RASCH, S., URDAL, K.: Preparation of fungous antigens for immunization and for serological reactions. Acta path. microbiol. scand. **28**, 132 (1951). — THJÖTTA, T., URDAL, K.: A family endemic of geotrichosis pulmonum. Acta path. microbiol. scand. **26**, 673 (1949).

— Torheim, B.J.: Immunochemical investigations in *Geotrichum* and certain related fungi. III. Gel-precipitation studies of reactions between rabbit immune sera and polysaccharides extracted from fungi. Sabouraudia **2**, 292 (1963). — Torres, C.M., Leão, A.E.A., Salles, J.F.: Gastrite espontânea do camondongo e cogumelos do gênero *Geotrichum* Link. Mem. Inst. Osw. Cruz **39**, 97 (1942). — Tzamouranis, N.: Sur un cas de géotrichose cutanée. Arch. Inst. Pasteur hellén. **8**, 49 (1962). — Tzamouranis, N., Crimbithis, E.: La fréquence de *Geotrichum* et des levures dans les selles et la cavité buccopharyngée de l'homme en Grèce. Arch. Inst. Pasteur hellén. **8**, 119 (1962). — Vieu, M., Segretain, G.: Contribution à l'étude de *Geotrichum* et *Trichosporum* d'orgine humaine. Ann. Inst. Pasteur (Paris) **96**, 421 (1959). — Volk, R., Cañas, E.: Un caso de blastomicosis. Medicina (Méx.) **22**, 615 (1942). — Vörös-Felkai, G., Novák, E.K.: Incidence of yeasts in human material. Acta microbiol. Acad. Sci. hung. **8**, 89 (1961). — Vrijman, L.H.: *Geotrichum*-infectie. Ned. T. Geneesk. **77**/II, 2129 (1933). — Webster, B.H.: Pulmonary geotrichosis. Amer. Rev. Tuberc. **76**, 286 (1957). ∼ Bronchopulmonary geotrichosis: A review with report of four cases. Dis. Chest **35**, 273 (1959). — Wegmann, T.: Pilzerkrankungen der inneren Organe als Folge von Behandlung mit Antibiotica, unter besonderer Berücksichtigung des Respirationstraktes. Antibiot. et Chemother. (Basel) **1**, 235 (1954). ∼ Mykosen der inneren Organe. Ergebn. inn. Med. **8**, 457 (1957). ∼ Pilzkrankheiten der inneren Organe. In: Polemann, G.: Klinik und Therapie der Pilzkrankheiten. Stuttgart: Georg Thieme 1961. — Whitcomb, F.C., Milzer, A., Kunstadter, R.H.: Incidence of mycotic infections in children with acute respiratory disease. J. Pediat. **35**, 715 (1949).

Miscellaneous Uncommon Diseases Attributed to Fungi and Actinomycetes

JOSEPH C. PARKER JR., Boston/Mass., USA and GORDON K. KLINTWORTH, Durham/N. C., USA

With 60 Figures

Adiaspiromycosis
(Haplomycosis)

In 1942, a thick-walled, spherical fungus was discovered in the lungs of wild rodents in Arizona, USA, and designated *Haplosporangium parvum* (EMMONS, 1942; EMMONS and ASHBURN, 1942). The genus *Emmonsia* was proposed for this organism by CIFERRI and MONTEMARTINI (1959), but CARMICHAEL (1951, 1962) considers that the fungus should be included in the genus *Chrysosporium* Corda. Four species have been described (Table 1).

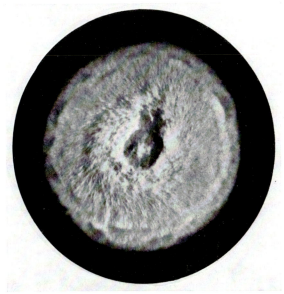

Fig. 1. Colony of *Emmonsia parva* on modified Sabouraud's glucose agar after two weeks at 30°C. (After EMMONS, C.W., and JELLISON, W.L.: Ann. N.Y. Acad. Sci. 89, 91—101, 1960)

The fungus grows slowly on Sabouraud's agar at room temperature producing a white colony, whose appearance varies with the species and strain (Fig. 1). Conidia (aleurospores) that are almost spherical (2—14 μ in diameter) are borne on simple or compound conidiophores, which arise at right angles from delicate branching septate hyphae (0.5—2 μ in diameter). The spores are borne singly or rarely in chains of two. When the fungus is incubated at 37°C, the conidia and

Table 1. Comparison between different species of *Emmonsia* (Modified from Thirumalachar et al., 1965)

	E. brasiliensis *	E. ciferrina *	E. crescens	E. parva
Conidia	(1) 7—10 × 5—7 μ (2) Hyaline smooth	(1) 7—14 × 4.8 μ (2) Hyaline smooth	(1) 2—4 × 2.5—4.5 μ (2) Hyaline smooth	(1) 2.4 × 2.5—4.5 μ (2) Hyaline smooth
Adiaspores in culture	(1) Produced at 37°C (2) 20—25 μ in diameter (3) Wall 1.5—2.7 μ thick (4) Multinucleate	(1) Produced on blood agar and several other media at 28 to 37°C (2) 20—45 μ in diameter (3) Wall 1.5—2 μ thick (4) Multinucleate	(1) Produced at 37°C on blood agar (2) 250—480 μ in diameter (3) Wall up to 70 μ in thickness (4) Multinucleate	(1) Produced at 40°C on blood agar (2) 15—25 μ in diameter (3) Wall 2 μ thick (4) Uninucleate
Adiaspores in lung tissue	20—25 μ in diameter	(1) 15—25 μ in diameter (2) Wall thickness 1.5—2 μ	250—480 μ in diameter	15—40 μ in diameter
Mycelium		Septate and branching, in later stages forming arthrospores in alternate cells as in *Coccidioides immitis*	Septate and branching	Septate and branching

* Padhye and Carmichael (1962) have drawn attention to the fact that *E. brasiliensis* and *E. ciferrina* are almost identical in colonial and microscopic morphology to *Chrysosporium pruinosum*.

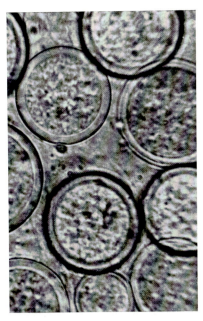

Fig. 2. Adiaspores of *Emmonsia ciferrina* on oatmeal tomato paste agar. × 1000. (After THIRUMALACHAR, M.J., PADHYE, A.A., and SRINIVASAN, M.C.: Mycopathologia (Den Haag) 26, 323—332, 1965)

some of the hyphal cells enlarge and form large spherules (adiaspores) comparable to those that develop in the host (Fig. 2). These adiaspores like other fungal spores do not reproduce by budding or endosporulation. In some species such as *E. crescens* they are multinucleated, while in others, such as *E. parva*, they possess a single nucleus. Following isolation of the fungus from the host at room temperature, or after the removal of colonies from 37° C to room temperature, hyphae develop from the adiaspores. The number of emerging hyphae is directly proportional to the number of nuclei in the adiaspores. For example, a single germ tube arises with *E. parva*, while there are multiple germ tubes with *E. crescens* (Fig. 3). Arthrospores develop in the mycelium of at least some species, including *E. ciferrina* (THIRUMALACHAR et al., 1965). At culture the fungus resembles *Histoplasma capsulatum* but differs in not producing macroconidia. In tissue *Emmonsia* is not only larger than *Histoplasma*, but does not reproduce by budding. Though the fungus was originally discovered while investigating the natural history, host range, and ecology of *Coccidioides immitis*, and was often associated with coccidioidomycosis, the fungus differs in morphology and colonial characteristics from *C. immitis*.

EMMONS and JELLISON (1960) designated the large spherules in the lungs as "adiaspores" and proposed the term "adiaspiromycosis" for the resultant pulmonary disease.

Since the condition first became recognized, it has been detected in numerous small mammals throughout the world (BAKERSPIGEL, 1956, 1957, 1965; DOWDING, 1947a, b; DVŎRAK et al., 1965, 1967; ERICKSON, 1949; JELLISON, 1947, 1950, 1954, 1956, 1958; JELLISON and LORD, 1964; JELLISON and PETERSON, 1964; McDIARMID and AUSTWICK, 1954; PROKOPIČ et al., 1965; SMITH and LANCASTER, 1965; TAYLOR et al., 1967; TEVIS, 1956). The fungus has been isolated not only from animals, but also from soil and air (BATISTA and SHOME, 1963; MENGES and HABERMANN, 1954; THIRUMALACHAR et al., 1965).

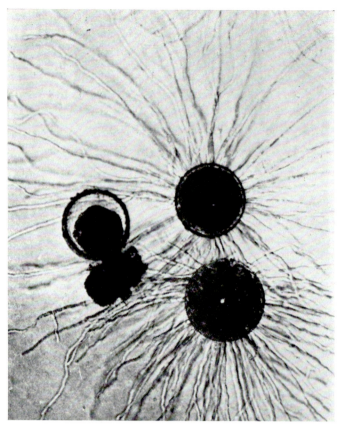

Fig. 3. Multiple germ tubes have arisen from adiaspores of *Emmonsia crescens* that were incubated for three weeks at 37°C on blood agar and then removed to room temperature. × 337. (After Emmons, C. W., and Jellison, W. L.: Ann. N. Y. Acad. Sci. 89, 91—101, 1960)

Reports of the organism in man have appeared in Brazil, France, and India (Batista et al., 1963a, b; Chevrel et al., 1964; Doby-Dubois et al., 1964; Misra et al., 1966). Though the fungus has been associated with pulmonary disease in man, further documentation is necessary in order to evaluate its role in the genesis of the lesions.

Following inhalation, the individual fungal spores increase in size from the original diameter of 2—4.5 μ to enormous thick-walled cells (the adiaspores) that are many times their initial dimensions. These may become 500 μ in diameter, with cell walls reaching a thickness of 70 μ in *E. crescens*. The walls stain well with the periodic acid Schiff technique. The organism appears to be incapable of reproduction in the host and apparently dies without budding or undergoing endosporulation. The giant fungal spores are surrounded by a minimal, but definite, cellular reaction (Fig. 4).

Allescheriosis

(Monosporiosis)

The fungus *Allescheria boydii* belongs to the class Ascomycetes. In the perfect or ascocarpic stage the organism forms brown, thin-walled, spherical bodies (cleistothecia) which contain transparent, ovoid asci with eight yellow-brown

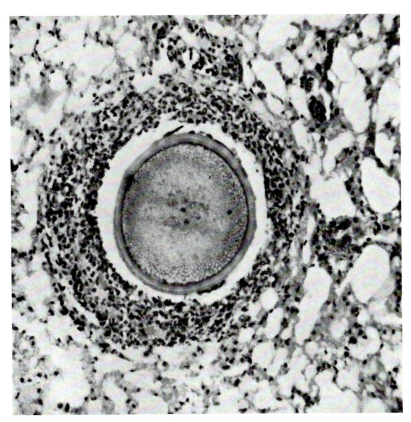

Fig. 4. Adiaspore of *Emmonsia parva* in the lung of a wild rodent (*Sorex cinereus*) × 300. (After BAKERSPIGEL, A.: Canad. J. Microbiol. 7, 676, 1961)

ascospores (Fig. 5). The binomium *Monosporium apiospermum* refers to the conidial or imperfect form of the fungus. This form possesses conidiophores with single, terminal conidia (Fig. 6), and lacks cleistothecia, characterizing the sexual stage. The fungus has a worldwide distribution, and is a common soil saprophyte (AJELLO, 1952). It grows rapidly on artificial media at both room temperature and 37° C and forms a white cottony colony which later turns dark smoky gray (Fig. 7). The reverse side of the colony is usually black. The majority of isolates do not produce ascocarps in culture but form the imperfect stage (EMMONS, 1944).

Allescheria boydii was first isolated in 1921 by BOYD and CRUTCHFIELD from a mycetoma in man. Since that time, the organism has been cultured from similar lesions on numerous occasions. In most instances the imperfect form of the same fungus has been described, perhaps because most isolates do not produce the perfect stage in culture. Most cases of mycetoma due to *A. boydii* have been reported from the United States, though the organism has been isolated from such lesions in many parts of the world. The fungus is the commonest isolate from mycetoma in the *United States* and continental *Europe:*

(ARVEIRA-NEVES, 1942; AVRAM, 1967; AVRAM et al., 1968; BATTISTINI et al., 1958; BOL'SHAKOVA et al., 1960; BORELLI, 1957; BOYD and CRUTCHFIELD, 1921; BRICENOMAAZ, 1967; CAMAIN et al., 1957; CARRION and KNOTT, 1944; CIFERRI and REDAELLI, 1950; COCKSHOTT, 1957; CONVIT et al., 1961; COURTOIS et al., 1954; DE ALMEIDA and SIMOES BARBOSA,

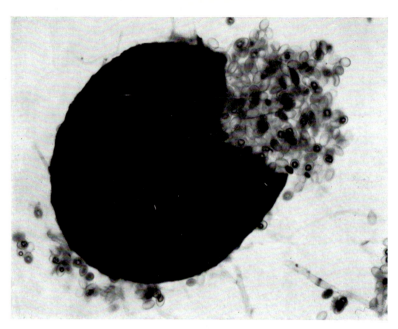

Fig. 5. A ruptured cleistothecium with ascospores (perfect stage of *Allescheria boydii*). Lacto-phenol cotton blue preparation. × 475

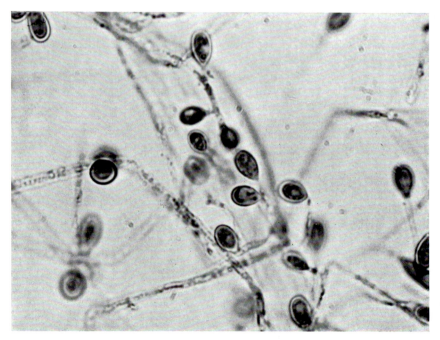

Fig. 6. Imperfect form of *Allescheria boydii* showing single, terminal conidia. Lacto-phenol cotton blue preparation. × 1000

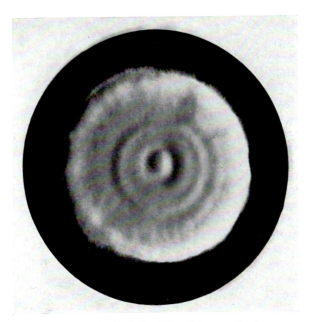

Fig. 7. Colony of *Allescheria boydii* on Sabouraud's glucose agar

1940; DESTOMBES et al., 1966; DOWDING, 1935; DROUHET, 1955; EL-MOFTY et al., 1965; EMMONS and GREENHALL, 1962; FIENBERG, 1944; GAY and BIGELOW, 1930; GELLMAN and GAMMEL, 1933; GREEN and ADAMS, 1964; HANLON et al., 1955; HAUKOHL and SADOFF, 1954; HERRERO et al., 1955; JONES and ALDEN, 1931; JORGE et al., 1941; JOSEFIAK and KOKITO, 1959; KATSNEL'SON et al., 1962; LATAPÍ, 1963; LAPATÍ and ORTIZ, 1963; MACKINNON, 1963; MAHGOUB, 1964; MARIAT, 1963; MEYERDING and EVERT, 1947; MOHR and MUCHMORE, 1958; MONTPELLIER and GUILLON, 1921; NIÑO, 1941, 1949, 1953; NIÑO et al., 1962; NIÑO and FREIRE, 1966; REES, 1962; SEABURY et al., 1959; SHAW and MACGREGOR, 1935; TAYLOR et al., 1964; THEODORESCU et al., 1959; TWINING et al., 1946; VANBREUSEGHEM, 1967; VERGHESE and KLOKKE, 1966).

As with mycetoma produced by other fungi (see Chapter 12, Mycetoma), granules consisting of matted mycotic elements are common in both the lesions and the purulent discharge. The granules are up to 1 cm in diameter and possess a white to yellow color. In tissue sections they are eosinophilic and readily demonstrated with Grocott's methenamine silver and the periodic acid Schiff stains. The granules are composed of a central mass of septate hyphae (4—5 μ) and chlamydospores (Figs. 8, 9). The cellular infiltrate consists predominantly of polymorphonuclear leukocytes, lymphocytes, and plasma cells. Granulomas and multinucleated giant cells are rarely observed. Mycetomata with granules have been produced in guinea pigs, hamsters, and mice following inoculation with *Allescheria boydii* (AVRAM, 1967; SCHMITT et al., 1963).

Several examples of pulmonary infection with *Allescheria* have been described (CREITZ and HARRIS, 1955; DROUHET, 1955; LOURIA et al., 1966; MISRA et al., 1966; SCHARYJ et al., 1960; STOECKEL et al., 1960; TRAVIS et al., 1961). The organism has not only been isolated from sputa and pulmonary lesions, but also has been identified in tissue from the lung (CREITZ and HARRIS, 1955; TRAVIS et al., 1961). In most instances there has been an associated disease in the respiratory system. The latter has included sarcoidosis, chronic bronchitis, emphysema, and a benign bronchogenic cyst. The pulmonary lesions resemble those of myce-

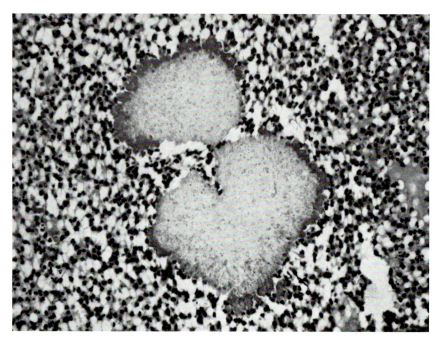

Fig. 8. Granule in subcutaneous tissue from a mycetoma due to *Allescheria boydii*. Hematoxylin and eosin stain. × 240

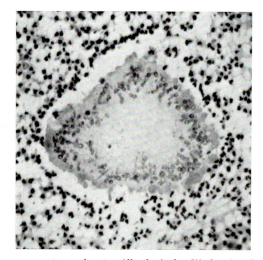

Fig. 9. Granule from a mycetoma due to *Allescheria boydii* showing fungal elements in its periphery. Modified periodic acid Schiff stain. × 240

toma in the extremities and are characterized by a purulent exudate and yellow to white granules.

Allescheria boydii has been isolated from corneal ulcers (ERNEST and RIPPON, 1966; GORDON et al., 1959; LEY, 1956; NAUMANN et al., 1967; PAULTER et al., 1955). In some such instances fungal elements have also been identified in corneal

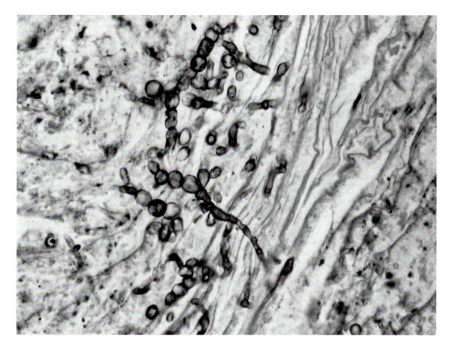

Fig. 10. Hyphal elements and chlamydospores of *Allescheria boydii* in tissue from the eye.
Grocott's methenamine silver stain. × 550

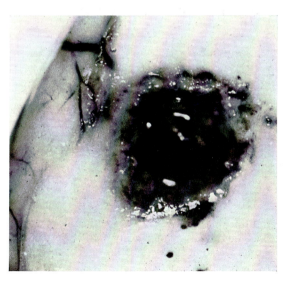

Fig. 11. A cerebral abscess due to *Allescheria boydii*. (After ROSEN, F., DECK, J.H.N., and
REWCASTLE, N.B.: Canad. med. Ass. J. 93, 1125—1127, 1965)

scrapings or histologic sections (ERNEST and RIPPON, 1966) (Fig. 10). In most
cases there has been a past history of corneal injury and antecedent therapy with
steroids and/or antibiotics.

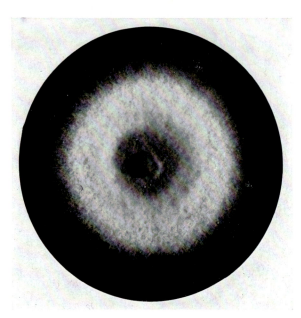

Fig. 12. Colony of *Alternaria sp.* on Sabouraud's glucose agar

Other sites have rarely been infected by *Allescheria boydii*. The organism accompanied a chronic meningitis in a middle-aged woman from Trinidad (ARONSON et al., 1953; BENHAM and GEORG, 1948; WOLF et al., 1947). The patient developed signs of meningitis after a previous spinal anesthetic. Cultures of the cerebrospinal fluid yielded *A. boydii* on multiple occasions. After a course of eight months the patient died. At post-mortem examination a granulomatous meningitis was found over the spinal cord and around the brainstem and cerebellum.

The fungus has rarely produced disseminated lesions in man. ROSEN et al. (1955) documented abscesses in the brain and thyroid due to *A. boydii* in a patient who had been treated with both steroids and immunosuppressive agents for subacute glomerulonephritis (Fig. 11).

Allescheria has occasionally been cultured from urine and prostatic secretions (MEYER and HERROLD, 1961), a crust in the external auditory canal (BELDING and UMANZIO, 1935), and blood (ZAFFIRO, 1938).

Alternariosis

One of the ubiquitous plant pathogens which has been associated with human disease is *Alternaria*. The fungus grows readily on a variety of media which it may contaminate. The round colonies may be white early in their growth, but later become dark olive-green or brown to gray-black. With age they are covered by a loose, light colored, aerial mycelium (Fig. 12). The dark hyphae are septate and the conidiophores contain simple or branched chains of inverted, clavate, olivaceous to brown macroconidia with an elongated, lighter tip and with longitudinal and/or transverse septa. These muriform conidia possess apices that are often attenuated in long simple chains (Fig. 13).

As early as 1930, HENRICI suggested that *Alternaria* may cause suppurative lesions, but the evidence was inconclusive. Since then, the fungus has been isolated

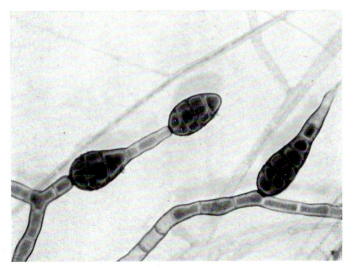

Fig. 13. *Alternaria tenuis* with attenuated macroconidia. Lacto-phenol cotton blue preparation.
× 1000

from many different sources in man, including the bile, cerebrospinal fluid, conjunctival sac, and skin (AINSLEY and SMITH, 1965; BORSOOK, 1933; BOTTICHER, 1966; OHASHI, 1960). As *Alternaria* is a common contaminant of laboratory media, it has generally been discarded as insignificant when cultured from clinical material. However, it is questionable whether the organism is always non-pathogenic to man. For example, *A.tenuis* has been repeatedly cultured from a lesion in the hand produced by a splinter (BORSOOK, 1933). BOTTICHER (1966) also raised doubt about the non-pathogenic nature of *Alternaria* when she isolated *Alternaria sp.* on 121 occasions from 2,381 specimens of suspected superficial mycoses of the skin, hair, and nails. Broad pigmented septate hyphae and/or muriform spores resembling those of *Alternaria* were identified in most potassium hydroxide preparations from the lesions. In six skin scrapings of typical mycotic lesions, *Alternaria* was the only fungus isolated and identified in the tissue. At the Duke University Medical Center *Alternaria sp.* was cultured on four separate occasions from an ovoid 8.5 cm × 5 cm, denuded, cutaneous lesion on the lower calf of a woman with discoid lupus erythematosus and leukopenia (MILLER and TINDALL, 1967). This lesion, which was studded with black granules, followed a scratch with a tree limb. Rare fungal elements characterized by hyphal structures and oval bodies unlike those usually seen were identified in the patient's tissue. They were associated with an inflammatory reaction that was composed of both abscesses and discrete granulomas (Figs. 14, 15).

Besides invading tissue, *Alternaria* has been implicated as an allergen in some individuals (BOTTICHER, 1966; HARRIS, 1941; HOPKINS et al., 1930; HYDE and WILLIAMS, 1949; PRATT et al., 1954; PRINCE et al., 1949, 1961; WALTON, 1949).

Arthrodermosis

Several investigators have described a cutaneous disease due to *Arthroderma simii (Epidermophyte simii, Trichophyton simii)* in dogs, monkeys, poultry, and even man, who may become infected through contact with diseased animals

61*

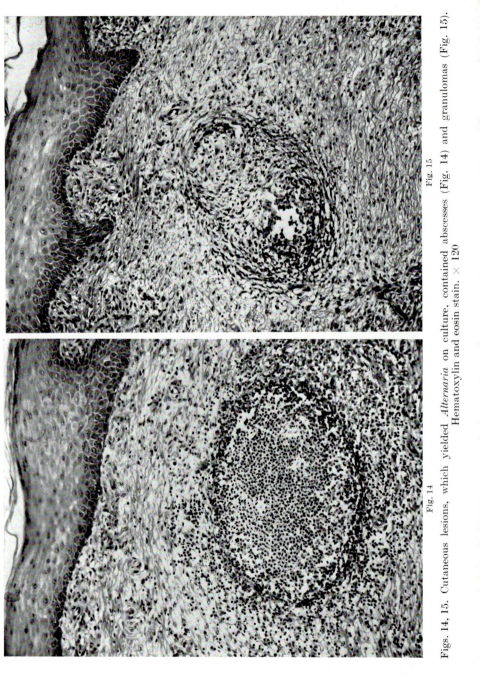

Figs. 14, 15. Cutaneous lesions, which yielded *Alternaria* on culture, contained abscesses (Fig. 14) and granulomas (Fig. 15). Hematoxylin and eosin stain. × 120

Fig. 15

Fig. 14

(EMMONS, 1940; GUGNANI et al., 1967a; KLOKKE and DURAIRAJ, 1967; PINOY, 1912a, b; RIPPON et al., 1968; SINGH, 1963; STOCKDALE et al., 1965). This heterothallic fungus, called *Trichophyton simii* in its imperfect stage and *Arthroderma simii* in its perfect stage, appears to have a restricted geographic distribution. All infections, for which a locality is known, have originated from India, where the

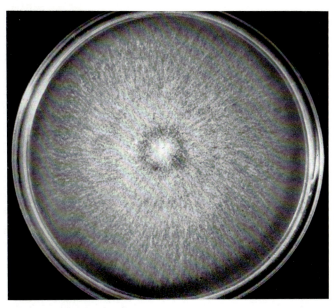

Fig. 16. *Arthroderma simii* on malt agar extract. (After STOCKDALE, P.M., MacKENZIE, D.W.R., and AUSTWICK, P.K.C.: Sabouraudia 4, 112—123, 1965)

fungus has been isolated from the soil and hair of several, healthy small mammals (GUGNANI et al., 1967b; RIPPON et al., 1968; STOCKDALE et al., 1965).

The morphology of the fungus and its colonial characteristics have been thoroughly described by STOCKDALE et al. (1965). The organism grows rapidly on numerous media and produces colonies that are white to very pale buff or rose-buff in color. They are uniformly and finely granular and possess a diffuse margin and central, white, conical, velvety umbo. The reverse side of the colony is non-pigmented at first, but later has a red-yellow discoloration (Fig. 16). Numerous

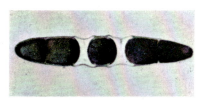

Fig. 17. Chlamydospores of *Arthroderma simii*. × 960. (After STOCKDALE, P.M., MacKENZIE, D.W.R., and AUSTWICK, P.K.C.: Sabouraudia 4, 112—123, 1965)

macroconidia, borne terminally on complexly branched hyphae, are hyaline and cylindrical to fusiform. They measure 6—11 μ × 35—85 μ with up to 10 septa. Thick-walled spores formed by one or more of the cells may be contained by empty intercalary cells (Fig. 17). Clavate to pyriform (1.5—3 μ × 2—6.5 μ) microconidia are rare in young cultures, but more abundant in old ones. They are borne along the sides of simple hyphae. Cleistothecia (closed sporebearing structures) characteristic of the genus *Arthroderma* have been produced on soil and other media (STOCKDALE et al., 1965).

In the monkey the lesions consist of small, superficial, silvery desquamating scales with some inflammation of the underlying dermis (EMMONS, 1940; STOCK-DALE et al., 1965) (Fig. 18). Hair loss is not a feature in the monkey, and though some hair follicles may be invaded, the hair shaft is not penetrated (EMMONS, 1940; PINOY, 1912a, b). Alopecia does, however, occur in the guinea pig and mouse in whom the disease can readily be produced experimentally. Infection can also be transmitted to chickens, monkeys, and rabbits, and the resulting lesions are indistinguishable from those occurring naturally (EMMONS, 1940; GUGNANI et al., 1967b; STOCKDALE et al., 1965).

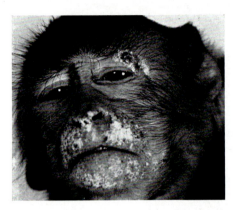

Fig. 18. Rhesus monkey with desquamating lesions on the face due to *Arthroderma simii* (After STOCKDALE, P.M., MacKENZIE, D.W.R., and AUSTWICK, P.K.C.: Sabouraudia 4, 112—123, 1965)

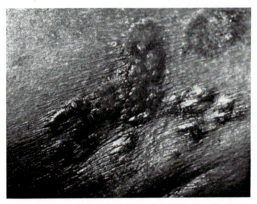

Fig. 19. Human skin lesions due to *Arthroderma simii*. (After KLOKKE, A.H., and DURAIRAJ, P.: Sabouraudia 5, 153—158, 1967)

The pathogenicity of the fungus for man was demonstrated experimentally by EMMONS in 1940. Later, the organism was isolated from cutaneous lesions in a laboratory technician, who handled infected guinea pigs, and in a poultry attendant (STOCKDALE et al., 1965). Since then, the fungus has also been isolated from numerous superficial cutaneous lesions in individuals from India (GUGNANI et al., 1967a; KLOKKE and DURAIRAJ, 1967; RIPPON et al., 1968) (Fig. 19).

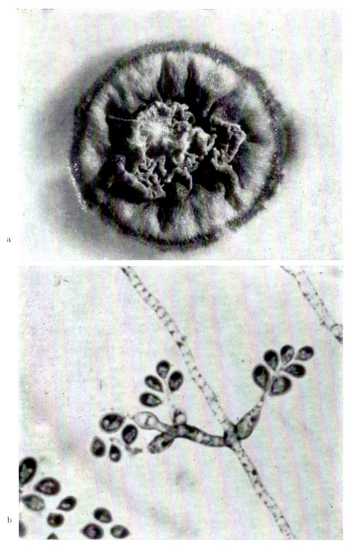

Fig. 20. a) Colony of *Beauveria tayeaui* on Sabouraud's agar (Courtesy of Dr. M. LAHOURCADE). b) and c) Filaments and spores of *Beauveria tayeaui*. (After FRÉOUR, P., LAHOURCADE, M., and CHOMY, P.: Presse med. 74, 2317—2320, 1966)

Beauveriosis

In 1835 a micro-organism first became recognized as a cause of disease. This occurred when the fungus *Beauveria bassiana* (formerly termed *Botrytis bassiana*) was found to produce muscardine, a contagious disease of silkworms (BASSI, 1835). Subsequently, this fungus was found to be widespread in nature and pathogenic to many insects (ELLINGBOE et al., 1957; MADELIN, 1963).

For more than a century *Beauveria sp.* was generally regarded as non-pathogenic for man and other vertebrates. However, pulmonary infection by *B. bassiana* has been documented in giant tortoises that were kept in captivity (GEORG et al.,

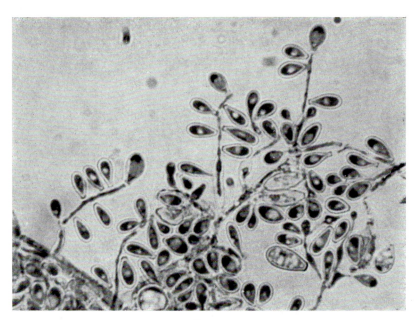

Fig. 20c

1962). Though Langeron (1934) repeatedly isolated *Beauveria brumpti* from an infected human eye, fungal elements were not demonstrated in the affected tissues. Recently Fréour et al. (1966a, b, c) incriminated the entomogenous fungus *Beauveria tayeaui* (originally described as *Beauveria bassiana*) in a pulmonary infection in man (Lahourcade, 1966). They reported a 22-year-old woman who developed a dry, persistent cough associated with debility, anorexia, loss of weight, and a mild pyrexia. Prior to the onset of the disease, the patient had always lived in North Africa and at the age of 11 she manifested ulcerative cervical lymphadenopathy thought to be tuberculosis. Subsequent radiological examination demonstrated a thick-walled pulmonary cavity and discrete disseminated lesions in the lungs of variable size. *Beauveria bassiana* was isolated from her bronchial aspirations. She was later treated with amphotericin B followed by pneumonectomy. Fungal elements were seen in the pulmonary tissue, and *B. bassiana* was the only organism cultured from the surgically excised specimen (Fig. 20). Following surgery, the patient's health was stable.

Cephalosporiosis

The cephalosporia are widely dispersed throughout the world, and have been isolated from soil, air, and sewage. Some species have been associated with disease in insects and a variety of plants, including trees, wheat, corn, and sugar cane (Pisano, 1963). In addition *Cephalosporium spp.* are also important to man, as a source of antibiotics.

Most species of *Cephalosporium* are readily grown on many artificial media, including Sabouraud's dextrose agar (Fig. 21). At the tips of slender or swollen conidiophores, the fungus produces conidia that are usually hyaline and nonseptate. The spores vary in size with the species and usually measure up to 8 μ wide and 15 μ long (Fig. 22).

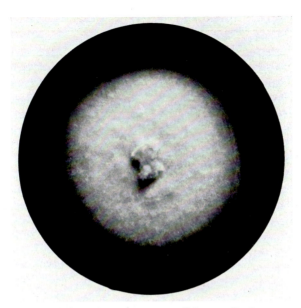

Fig. 21. *Cephalosporium sp.* grown on Sabouraud's glucose agar

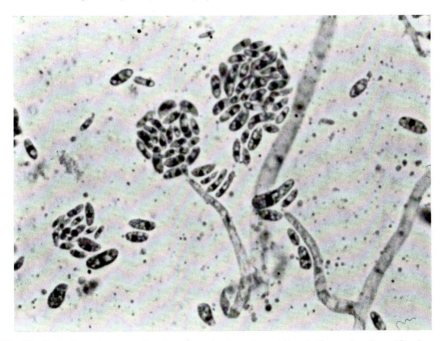

Fig. 22. *Cephalosporium sp.* showing masses of oval conidia at the ends of conidiophores. Lacto-phenol cotton blue preparation. × 1000

A wide variety of species have been implicated in human disease.

These include *C. acremonium* (ARIEVITCH et al., 1966; BATISTA et al., 1960; BOMMER et al., 1961; CABRINI and REDAELLI, 1929; CATANEI, 1944; COUTELEN and COCHET, 1945; COUTELEN et al., 1948; DEBUSMANN, 1939; GRÜTZ, 1925; MURRAY and HOLT, 1964; PITOTTI, 1932),

Table 2. *Mycetoma Produced by Cephalosporium sp.*

Species	Color of granules	Country	References
I. *Cephalosporium acremonium*	Colorless	West India	MURRAY and HOLT (1964)
II. *Cephalosporium falciforme*	White	Brazil Malaya Puerto-Rico Roumania Senegal	ALMEIDA et al. (1948) PONNAMPALAM (1964) CARRIÓN (1939, 1951) AVRAM (1964a, 1966) AVRAM et al. (1968) BAYLET et al. (1961)
III. *Cephalosporium*[1] *granulomatis*	Not mentioned	USA	WEIDMAN and KLIGMAN (1945)
IV. *Cephalosporium infestans*	Black	India	GAIND et al. (1962) PADHYE et al. (1963)
V. *Cephalosporium madurae*[2]	Black	India	PADHYE et al. (1962, 1963)
VI. *Cephalosporium recifei*	White	Brazil Senegal Venezuela	ARÊA-LEÃO and LÔBO (1934a, b) LÔBO (1943, 1963) ALMEIDA and SIMÔES-BARBOSA (1940b) BAYLET et al. (1961) BASTARDO (1963/1964)
VII. *Cephalosporium* sp.		Cameroon Chad Mexico Venezuela	GAMET et al. (1964) MARIAT (1963) LATAPÍ and ORTIZ (1963) GONZALEZ-OCHOA and RUITOBA (1944) BORELLI (1962)

1 This species was studied by MACKINNON (1951, 1954) who considered it to be a contaminant and synonymous with *Cephalosporium acremonium*.

2 MURRAY and HOLT (1964) pointed out that the description of the species *C. madurae* is not precise enough to be substantiated.

C. ballagii (BALLAGI, 1932), *C. cinnabarinum* (ARIEVITCH et al., 1966; KUKOLEVA and MALKUHA 1967), *C. cordoniformis* (SIMÔES-BARBOSA, 1941), *C. doukourei* (BOUCHER, 1918), *C. falciforme* (ALMEIDA et al., 1948; AVRAM 1964, 1966a, 1967; AVRAM et al., 1968; BAYLET et al., 1961; BORELLI, 1962; CARRION, 1939; DESTOMBES and SEGRETAIN, 1962; MACKINNON, 1963; PANNAMPALAM, 1964), *C. granulomatosis* (WEIDMAN and KLIGMAN, 1945), *C. griseum* (GOUGEROT et al., 1933), *C. infestans* (GAIND et al., 1962; PADHYE et al., 1963), *C. keratoplasticum* (BATISTA et al., 1960; HARADA and USUI, 1960), *C. madurae* (PADHYE et al., 1962), *C. nigrum* (KAMBAYASHI, 1937), *C. niveolanosum* (BENEDEK, 1927b), *C. onychophilum* (BATISTA et al., 1960), *C. pseudofermentum* (CIFERRI, 1932), *C. recifei* (ALMEIDA and SIMÔES-BARBOSA, 1940a; ARÊA-LEÃO and LÔBO, 1934a, b; BASTARDO DE ALBORNOZ, 1963/1964; BAYLET et al., 1961; LÔBO, 1943, 1963), *C. roseo-griseum* (WARD et al., 1961; ZAIAS, 1966), *C. rubrobrunneum* (HARTMANN, 1926), *C. serrae* (BATISTA et al., 1960; GINGRICH, 1962; FOCOSI, 1932a, b; MAFFEI, 1929), *C. spinosus* (NEGRONI, 1933a, b), *C. stühmeri* (SCHMIDT and VAN BEYMA, 1933), *C. tomskianum* (MATRUCHOT, 1948). In most instances where *Cephalosporium* has been cultured from lesions in man, the fungus has not been identified within lesions, so the significance of the isolates is equivocal.

The association of *Cephalosporium* with mycetoma has been reported by numerous investigators including:

ALMEIDA and SIMÔES-BARBOSA (1940a, b), ALMEIDA et al., (1948) ARÊA-LEÃO and LÔBO (1934a, b), AVRAM (1966a), BASTARDO DE ALBORNOZ (1963/1964), BAYLET et al. (1961), BORELLI (1962), CARRIÓN (1939, 1951), COUTELEN et al. (1948), DESTOMBES and SEGRETAIN (1962), GAIND et al. (1962), GAMET et al. (1964), GONZALEZ-OCHOA and RUILOBA (1944), LACAZ and FAVA NETTO (1954), LATAPÍ and ORTIZ (1963), LÔBO (1943, 1963), MACKINNON (1951, 1954, 1963), MARIAT (1963), MURRAY and HOLT (1964), NAKAMURA (1933), PONNAMPALAM (1964), SEGRETAIN (1962), VERGHESE and KLOKKE (1966), and WEIDMAN and KLIGMAN (1945).

Six species have been isolated from mycetomas (*C. acremonium* CORDA, *C. falciforme* CARRIÓN, *C. granulomatis* WEIDMAN and KLIGMAN, *C. infestans* GAIND and THIRUM, *C. madurae* PADHYE, SUKA, and THIRUM, and *C. recifei* LEÃO and LÔBO)[1]. The color of the granules in the draining sinuses have varied with the isolated species (Table 2) (Fig. 23). AVRAM (1966b, 1967) has produced comparable granules in mice, hamsters, and guinea pigs following inoculation with *Cephalosporium falciforme*.

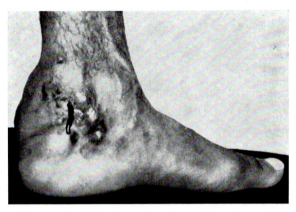

Fig. 23. Multiple draining sinuses due to *Cephalosporium madurae* in an ankle. (After PADHYE, A.A., and THIRUMALACHAR, M.J.: Sabouraudia 1, 230—233, 1961/1962)

In addition to mycetomas, species of *Cephalosporium* have been implicated as etiologic agents of gummato-ulcerative and superficial cutaneous lesions and onychomycosis.

(ASCHIERI, 1932; ARIEVITCH et al., 1964, 1966; BALLAGI, 1932; BENEDEK, 1927a, b; BOMMER et al., 1961; BOUCHER, 1918; CATANEI, 1944; COUTELEN and COCHET, 1945; COUTELEN et al., 1948; DuBOIS, 1942; GOUGEROT et al., 1933; GRÜTZ, 1925; HAENSCHE, 1957; HARADA and USUI, 1960; HARTMANN, 1926; JANKE, 1949; KAMBAYASHI, 1937; KESTEVEN, 1939; LEHNER, 1932; MALE and TAPPEINER, 1965; MILLER and MORROW, 1932; MOORE, 1955; NEGRONI, 1933a, b; PITOTTI, 1932; SCHMIDT and VAN BEYMA, 1933; SIMÔES-BARBOSA, 1941; WALSHE and ENGLISH, 1966; ZAIAS, 1966).

Occasionally, cases of cutaneous cephalosporiosis may spread to the regional lymphatics and produce a lymphangitis reminiscent of sporotrichosis (BALLAGI, 1932). In some cases, it has been suggested that the organism may become disseminated by auto-inoculation to other parts of the body. This may have occurred in a patient with cephalosporiosis at the knee in whom the infection spread to other parts of the skin (JANKE and ROHRSCHNEIDER, 1951). It has been suggested that *Cepahalosporium* may occasionally spread to other parts of the body by the blood stream. Although this is rare, systemic cephalosporiosis has been reported (BOMMER et al., 1961; HAENSCH, 1957).

Besides cutaneous disease, *Cephalosporium* has been implicated as a pathogen of the mouth, tonsils, and pharynx (CABRINI and REDAELLI, 1929; CIFERRI, 1932; COUTELEN et al., 1948; COWEN, 1965; COWEN and DINES, 1964; COWEN et al., 1965; DEBUSMANN, 1939). A midline granuloma eroding the hard palate, and resulting in destruction of the maxilla and mandible was described by COWEN and

---

1 The isolate designated *C.granulomatosis* by WEIDMAN and KLIGMAN (1945) was studied by MACKINNON (1951, 1954) who regarded it as *C.acremonium*. MURRAY and HOLT (1964) have pointed out that the description of *C.madurae* is not precise enough to be substantiated.

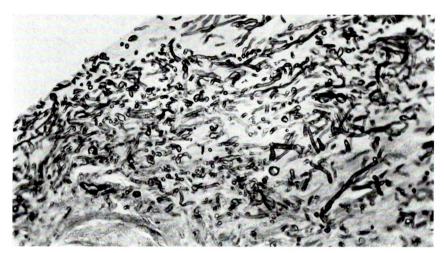

Fig. 24. *Cephalosporium sp.* in the corneal tissue. Periodic acid Schiff stain. × 305. (After ZIMMERMAN, L. E.: Survey Ophthal. 8, 1—25, 1963)

his colleagues (COWEN, 1965; COWEN and DINES, 1964; COWEN et al., 1965). Fungal hyphae and spores were identified in the latter lesion and *Cephalosporium* was cultured from it. *Cephalosporium* has also been associated with cystitis (MÜHLENS, 1938).

Ocular infection with *Cephalosporium* has been reported by several investigators. In most instances, the fungus was cultured from corneal ulcers (BEDELL, 1946, 1947; BYERS et al., 1960; FOCOSI, 1932b; GINGRICH, 1962; HOFFMANN and NAUMANN, 1963; KÜPER, 1962; MAFFEI, 1928; NAUMANN et al., 1967; ZIMMERMAN, 1962, 1963). In some of these cases, the organism was not only isolated from the corneal lesion, but demonstrated within tissue removed at keratoplasty (ZIMMERMAN, 1962) (Fig. 24). *Cephalosporium serrae* has most often been implicated in corneal lesions (GINGRICH, 1962; FOCOSI, 1932b; MAFFEI, 1928). The fungus is reported to have a potent proteolytic enzyme, which produces corneal ulceration and opacification in rabbits in 2—4 h (BURDA and FISHER, 1960). In addition to the keratitis, endophthalmitis following cataract extractions and other ocular surgery has been attributed to *Cephalosporium* (FINE, 1962; FINE and ZIMMERMAN, 1959; GREEN et al., 1965; KÜPER, 1962; THEODORE et al., 1961). The fungus has also been implicated in chronic dacryocystitis (FOCOSI, 1932a) and dacryocanaliculitis (JANKE and ROHRSCHNEIDER, 1951).

A chronic meningitis due to a *Cephalosporium* was reported by DROUCHET et al. (1965). While living in central Africa, a 33-year-old woman underwent a caesarean section under a spinal anesthetic. A left sciatica subsequently ensued and was treated with corticosteroids. A second pregnancy followed soon thereafter, during and after which the patient developed neurologic and psychiatric disturbances. At a surgical exploration a granulomatous meningitis was found, and hyphae were identified in the surgically excised meninges. *Cephalosporium sp.* was cultured from the ventricular and spinal fluids. The patient, who failed to respond to therapy (including actidione and amphotericin B), died approximately 15 months after the onset of neurological symptoms and about 4 months after surgical intervention. At autopsy examination hyphae were visualized in the meninges, but not in other parts of the body. *Cephalosporium sp.* was isolated from the brain and antibodies to the organism were detected in the blood after death.

Arthritis involving a major joint has been attributed to *Cephalosporium roseo-griseum* Saksena. WARD et al. (1961) isolated this species from the synovium and fluid from an arthritic knee following two traumatic injuries and treatment with corticosteroids.

Cephalosporium has been cultured from the bile, blood, gastric juice, pleural fluid, and sputum of human patients in the absence of tissue diagnoses (BATISTA et al., 1960; DEBUSMANN, 1939; DOUGLASS and SIMPSON, 1943; MATRUCHOT, 1948; MÜHLENS, 1938; VERKHOLOMOV, 1961).

In most instances of cephalosporiosis the organism appears to have been inoculated into the tissues. This has been described, for example, following an injury with palm leaves (WARD et al., 1961), a cow's tail (BEDELL, 1946, 1947), and a cotton stalk (ZIMMERMAN, 1963). Infection has also followed ocular surgery (FINE, 1962; FINE and ZIMMERMAN, 1959; GREEN et al., 1965; THEODORE et al., 1961), a tooth extraction (GRÜTZ, 1925), a compound fracture contaminated with soil (ARIEVITCH et al., 1966), an incised wound (GAIND et al., 1962), and a spinal anesthetic (DROUCHET et al., 1965).

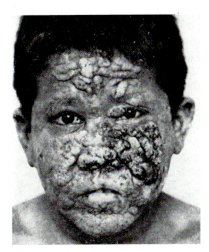

Fig. 25. Facial lesion which contained an unusual dematiaceous fungus. (After EMMONS, C. W., LIE-KIAN-JOE, NJO-INJO TJOEI ENG, POHAN, A., KERTOPATI, S., and VAN DER MEULEN, A.: Mycologia 49, 1—10, 1957)

Cercosporamycosis

The possibility that human disease may result from a fungus which causes leaf spots on plants was raised following the investigation of a patient in Indonesia (EMMONS et al., 1957, 1963; LIE-KIAN-JOE et al., 1957). The patient, a 12-year-old boy, suffered from extensive, indurated, verrucous and ulcerated, cutaneous and subcutaneous lesions of the face (Fig. 25). The lesions began many years before as a small nodule on the cheek, that could not be related to injury by thorns or insect bites. The nasal mucosa was also infected, and the nasal septum was perforated with a resultant saddle nose. The condition was not associated with any fever or regional lymphadenopathy. The ulcerated areas became crusted and the lesions subsequently extended to other areas, such as the thorax and thigh. Affected regions increased in extent and severity until the patient died, possibly from the mycosis. Unfortunately, an autopsy was not performed.

During life multiple biopsies of the lesions revealed hyperkeratosis, epithelial hyperplasia, keratin pearl formation and intraepithelial abscesses. Subcutaneous granulomas extended beyond the ulcerated regions. Brown septate hyphae (4—8 μ in diameter) were observed in unstained sections of all surgically excised lesions and were present throughout the skin and within subcutaneous granulomas. A fungus which did not resemble any known human pathogen was recovered repeatedly from multiple biopsy specimens, nasal secretions, and crusts from nasal mucosal ulcers. The cultured organism grew slowly at room temperature and at 30°C. An olive-gray colony (15 mm in diameter) possessed a luxuriant growth, dome-shaped tuft, and very short aerial hyphae after only 10-days growth on corn meal agar. On Sabouraud's medium the dark colony had a higher central dome. The fungus did not grow at 37°C. Sporulation occurred on corn meal agar and Sabouraud's agar. The conidiophores and conidia were brown and varied markedly in size and shape. Many conidiophores, most of which had poorly-differentiated hyphal elements, had barely discernible lateral and terminal scars from which conidia were readily detached. The conidia were clavate or acicular and possessed a truncated (usually convex) base and a rounded or greatly enlarged whip-like tip. Some immature conidia were unicellular, whereas the mature conidia (4—6 μ by 26—120 μ) had three to several septa. No muriform spores occurred. The fungus was identified as *Cercospora apii* Fresenius, a phytopathogen found throughout the world where celery is grown (LIE-KIAN-JOE et al., 1957; EMMONS et al., 1957, 1963). The isolate produced leaf spots on lettuce, tomatoes, and potatoes following its inoculation onto these plants.

The experimental production of lesions in animals using spore suspensions of this fungus was attempted, but without success. However, the fungus could be recovered in culture from the peritoneum of mice inoculated some weeks previously. Several attempts at self-inoculation by intradermal injection of conidia were made by some investigators (LIE-KIAN-JOE et al., 1957). Most of the intradermal injections produced a small nodule which resolved within a few days. One injection (using the inoculum from which leaf spots were produced in lettuce) was followed by the appearance of a slightly raised, brown papule (1.5 mm in diameter) which persisted for about 4 months. Mild pressure and friction produced an area of edema extending about 2 mm beyond the papule. The lesion slowly regressed and disappeared without any sequelae.

CHUPP (1957), who has extensive experience with the genus *Cercospora*, studied the isolate. Although Chupp could not specifically identify the fungus, he disagreed with the identification of the causal agent as *Cercospora apii* for the following reasons: (1) the colonies and the shape of the conidia did not resemble any of the species of *Cercospora* which he had seen; (2) the conidia of the fungus were pale brown whereas *Cercospora apii* has colorless conidia; (3) the bases of the conidia described by EMMONS et al. (1957) were convex whereas in *C. apii* they are clearly truncate; (4) EMMONS et al. (1957) did not report the inoculation of celery, which is maintained to be the only plant infected by *C. apii*; and (5) *C. apii* is worldwide in distribution and yet its pathogenicity for man has never been incriminated before.

Cryptostromosis
(Coniosporiosis or Maple-Bark Disease)

In 1932 TOWEY et al. described an acute respiratory disease in 35 bark peelers in Northern Michigan, USA. The condition was characterized by cough, dyspnea, fever, night sweats, and substernal pain. The disease was considered to result from the inhalation of spores of the fungus *Coniosporium corticale* (currently termed *Cryptostroma corticale*), which could be identified in the dust on maple logs from which the bark was peeled. Affected individuals had positive skin tests to extracts of the spore, whereas unaffected individuals gave negative results. They recovered following their removal from the contaminated environment.

The fungus, *Cryptostroma corticale (Coniosporium corticale)*, which may be pathogenic to trees (GREGORY and WALLER, 1951), grows on logs, especially hard

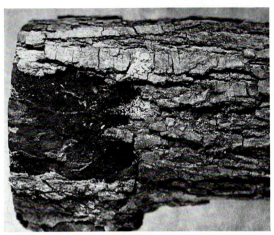

Fig. 26. Log from a maple tree with a pigmented area containing numerous spores of *Cryptostroma corticale*. (After WENZEL, F. J., and EMANUEL, D.A.: Arch. environm. Hlth 14, 385—389, 1967)

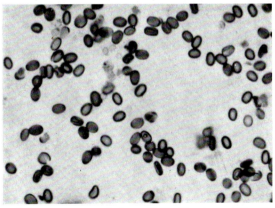

Fig. 27. Spores of *Cryptostroma corticale*. × 1225. (Courtesy of DR. D.A. EMANUEL)

wood such as maple, elm, ash, oak, and hickory. Maple logs appear to be more frequently involved than the other wood (Fig. 26). Although the wood and bark of infected trees appears healthy, a fine black dust is evident after the outer bark is removed.

Cryptostroma corticale grows on Sabouraud's medium at room temperature, but not at 37°C. Within three days, a white pleomorphic mycelium which is hyaline, septate, and profusely branched develops. The spores are ovoid and measure 4—5 μ in their greatest diameter (Fig. 27). In large masses, these spores

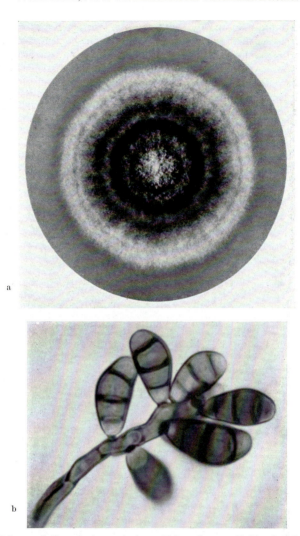

Fig. 28. (a) Colony of *Curvularia geniculata*. (After Georg, L.K.: J. Med. Ass. Ala. 33, 234—236, 1964). (b) Conidiophore with conidia of *Curvularia geniculata*. (After Nityananda, K., Sivasubramaniam, P., and Ajello, L.: Arch. Ophthal. 71, 456—458, 1964)

are black, although each individual one appears red-brown (Emanuel et al., 1962, 1966; Wenzel and Emanuel, 1967).

Thirty years after the fungus was first incriminated in human disease, other cases were recognized in a paper mill in Wisconsin, USA (Emanuel et al., 1962, 1966). Surgically excised lung tissue in these cases, which contained small oval bodies, revealed prominent pulmonary changes with interstitial fibrosis, inflammatory exudates, and occasional granulomas with multinucleated giant cells. *C.corticale* was isolated from this tissue. Those patients with overt respiratory disease had positive skin reactions and circulating antibodies to an extract from the spores of *C.corticale*. In addition, some of the other workers in the same paper mill manifested radiological alterations, positive serological tests or positive skin tests (Wenzel and Emanuel, 1967).

In unstained tissue sections the ovoid, thick-walled spores (3—5 μ in diameter) appear red-brown and are neither associated with hyphal elements nor evidence of replication (EMANUEL et al., 1966). The organism resembles *Histoplasma capsulatum* not only in its size and shape but also in the host's reaction to the fungus (EMANUEL et al., 1966).

It has been suggested that this disease is a hypersensitivity reaction to the inhaled spores of *Cryptostroma corticale* (EMANUEL et al., 1962, 1966; TOWEY et al., 1932).

Curvulariosis

Curvularia is a common fungal saprophyte of soil, and some species are phytopathogens of grasses (SPRAGUE, 1950). Two species have been implicated in human disease, namely *C.geniculata* and *C.lunata*.

The colony of *Curvularia* is dark brown to black and has a fluffy surface with many aerial hyphae and a reverse black pigmentation (Fig. 28a). The hyphae, conidiophores, and conidia have a natural light brown discoloration. *Curvularia* closely resembles *Helminthosporium*, but differs in possessing curved conidia with a prominent distal medial cell. In *C. geniculata* the conidiophore contains several cells with a diameter of 4—5 μ (Fig. 28b). The flat scars, which mark the sites of attachment of the spores to the conidiophore, project from the latter

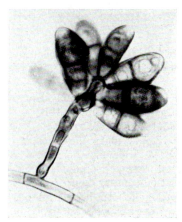
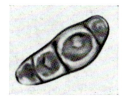

Fig. 29   Fig. 30

Fig. 29. Conidiophore with conida of *Curvularia lunata*. × 600. (After NITYANANDA, K.,
    SIVASUBRAMANIAM, P., and AJELLO, L.: Sabouraudia 2, 35—39, 1962)

Fig. 30. Curved septate conidium of *Curvularia lunata*. × 1150. (After NITYANANDA, K.,
    SIVASUBRAMANIAM, P., and AJELLO, L.: Sabouraudia 2, 35—39, 1962)

structure and give it the appearance of a knobby stick. The septate conidia vary in shape and size (21—50 μ × 10—15 μ in diameter), possess thick walls, and usually consist of 3—5 cells of which the distal medial cell is enlarged. The conidial attachment protrudes from the basal cell when the spore is released from the conidiophore (GEORG, 1964). *C.lunata* is microscopically similar to *C.geniculata*, except the point of conidial attachment is inserted into the conidiophore and does not protrude from it. Its conidia measure 19—25 μ by 8—14 μ (NITYANANDA et al., 1962; PARMELEE, 1956) (Figs. 29, 30).

Curvularia has been isolated from mycetomas of man and other animals. BAYLET et al. (1959) described a Senegalese patient with a mycetoma that dischar-

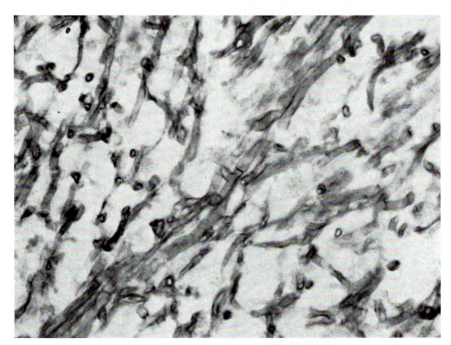

Fig. 31. *Curvularia geniculata* in corneal scrapings. Gridley stain. × 400. (After Nityananda,
K., Sivasubramaniam, P., and Ajello, L.: Arch. Ophthal. 71, 456—458, 1964)

ged black grains in the purulent exudates from its draining sinuses. The grains
contained pigmented hyphae and chlamydospores and cultures of them yielded
pure colonies of *C.lunata*. Bridges (1957) isolated *C.geniculata* from mycetomas
of a dog's feet that contained brown hyphae and chlamydospores in granules
within the tissue. Dematiaceous hyphae and chlamydospores, which may have
been *Curvularia*, have also been observed in nasal granulomata and mycetoma in
cattle, but were not culturally identified (Bridges, 1960; Roberts et al., 1963).

Curvularia geniculata and *C.lunata* have both been isolated from corneal
ulcers that contained brown, branched, septate hyphae (3—5 μ in diameter) in
scrapings and smears (Nityananda et al., 1962, 1964; Warren, 1964) (Fig. 31).
C.lunata was also repeatedly isolated, but not identified in scrapings, from another
patient with a corneal ulcer (Anderson et al., 1959).

Dermatophilosis
(Cutaneous Streptothricosis)

In 1915 Van Saceghem described a disease in cattle in the Republic of the
Congo (formerly known as the Belgium Congo) due to an organism that he designated *Dermatophilus congolensis*. Since then, it has become apparent that the
pathogen has a world-wide distribution, (Dean et al., 1961; Kaplan, 1966;
Smith et al., 1967; Vandermaele, 1961), and the resulting disease (dermatophilosis or cutaneous streptothricosis), is of considerable economic importance
in countries where livestock raising is an important industry.

The organism, a facultative anaerobe, is an actinomycete and requires a
medium which is rich in nutrients, such as brain-heart infusion agar or blood agar

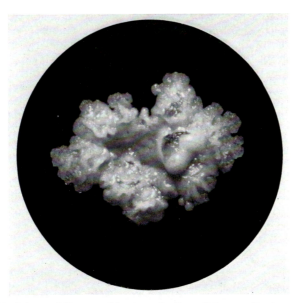

Fig. 32. Colony of *Dermatophilus congolensis* on Sabouraud's glucose agar

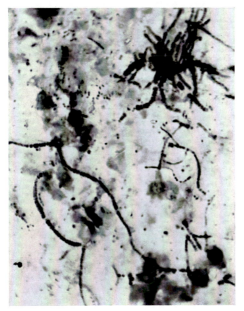

Fig. 33. Beaded filaments of *Dermatophilus congolensis*. Giemsa stain. × 1250. (After KAPLAN, W.: Southwest. Vet. 20, 14—19, 1966)

for growth. *D.congolensis* does not grow on common mycological media, such as Sabouraud's dextrose agar, and numerous antibiotics inhibit its growth (KAPLAN, 1966). On solid media, growth is apparent within 24—48 h, depending upon the temperature of incubation. The organism grows more rapidly at 37°C than at room temperature. Colonies vary in appearance depending upon numerous environmental factors. They may possess rough or smooth, shiny or dull surfaces, and are initially grey-white, later becoming yellow-orange (Fig. 32). In liquid media, growth is rapid at 37°C and small, fuzzy, round colonies are evident within the depths of the medium. Cultures that are less than 2 days old possess branched, septate hyphae which measure 0.5—1.5 μ in diameter, and later increase to 3—5 μ in width. These filaments divide transversely into narrow segments which form clusters of coccoid spores up to eight cells in width (Figs. 33, 34). Mature hyphae break up and release flagellated, mobile, coccoid zoospores (Gordon and Edwards, 1963; Gordon, 1964; Kaplan, 1966) (Fig. 35). These zoospores do not replicate, but germinate to form mycelium that later produces more zoospores. Formerly, Austwick (1958) suggested that three distinct species of Dermatophilus existed (D.congolensis, D.dermatonomus, and D.pedis), but after a morphological and biochemical investigation Gordon (1964) concluded that there was only one species, namely D.congolensis. Roberts (1965c) later confirmed this on serological evidence. Synonyms for Dermatophilus congolensis include: Actinomyces dermatonomus, Dermatophilus dermatonomus, Dermatophilus pedis, and Nocardia dermatonomus (Hart, 1967).

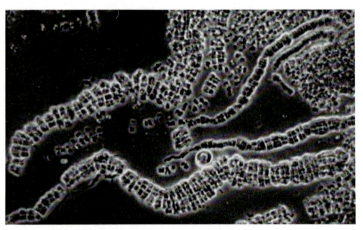

Fig. 34. Wet mount and dark phase contrast of Dermatophilus congolensis showing broad, beaded hyphae. × 500. (After Gordon, M.A.: J. Bact. 88, 509—522, 1964)

The cutaneous disease caused by D.congolensis has been reported in several animals, including cattle, deer, horses, goats (Hudson, 1937; Kaplan, 1966; Kaplan and Johnston, 1966; Le Riche, 1968; Pier et al., 1963; Searcy and Hulland, 1968a, b; Vandemaele, 1961; Van Saceghem, 1915). This actinomycete causes superficial cutaneous lesions with cellular infiltration and serous exudate after invasion of the epidermis (Dean et al., 1961, Roberts, 1965a—c; Roberts, 1967). The organism readily infects hair follicles, but does not invade hair or wool.

A number of possible modes of transmission of dermatophilosis have been suspected. Trauma and ticks have been implicated in the spread of this disease in livestock (Le Riche, 1968; Macadam, 1964). In sheep, the transmission of the actinomycete occurs especially by contact between wet animals (Le Riche, 1968; Roberts, 1963; Zlotnik, 1955). Dermatophilus congolensis has been transmitted from infected to normal rabbits by both stable flies (Stomoxys calcitrans) and by house flies (Musca domestica). No disruption of the skin was necessary to infect

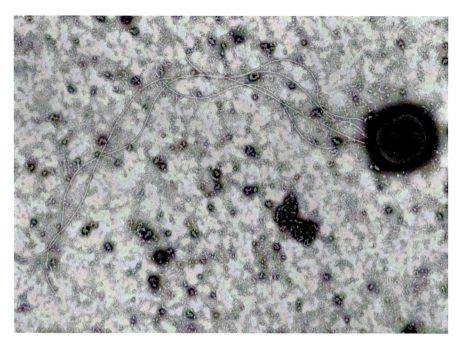

Fig. 35. Electron micrograph of an encapsulated, flagellated zoospore of *Dermatophilus congolensis*. × 30,000. (After GORDON, M.A.: J. Bact. 88, 509—522, 1964)

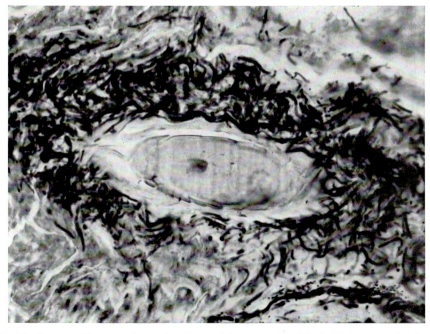

Fig. 36. *Dermatophilus congolensis* in skin showing numerous black filamentous organisms around the hair (center) but not involving it. Grocott's methenamine silver stain. × 220

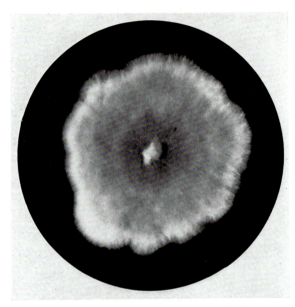

Fig. 37. Colony of *Fusarium sp.* on Sabouraud's glucose agar

them, but moistening of the animal's skin enhanced the transmission (Richard and Pier, 1966).

Dermatophilosis has been reported in four humans who handled an infected deer (Dean et al., 1961). Two to seven days after exposure to the organism, multiple, non-painful vesicles developed on their hands. The lesions were 2—5 mm in diameter, contained a serous or purulent exudate, and those which remained active for less than two weeks, healed spontaneously with brown scabs and later red-purple scars. The patients had no systemic effects from the infection. No human to human transmission was evident.

Dermatophilosis can be readily diagnosed in the host by microscopic examination of stained smears of exudates, scabs, or crusts. In tissue *D. congolensis* has a similar morphology to the cultured organism and appears as branching thin filaments. The organism is Gram-positive, not acid fast, and stains well with the Giemsa and Grocott's methenamine silver stains (Figs. 33, 36). In specimens from acute lesions, elements of *D. congolensis* are abundant and can be readily noticed (Kaplan, 1966). In material from healing lesions, the actinomycete may be sparse and careful search may be necessary to detect them. The fluorescent antibody technique may be of value in observing the organism in clinical material (Pier et al., 1964). The use of rabbits for recovery of *D. congolensis* has also been recommended (Kaplan, 1966).

Fusariosis

The ubiquitous *Fusarium* which has antibiotic properties (Arnstein et al., 1946; Boissevain, 1946; Cajori et al., 1954; Cook et al., 1947; Lacey, 1950) contains numerous species that are phytopathogens (Wollenweber et al., 1925; Wollenweber and Reinking, 1935). The organism grows rapidly on Sabouraud's dextrose agar at room temperature, but only slowly at 37°C. The colony, which appears fuzzy and diffuse, is initially white and later becomes gray or brightly colored. It may be slightly granular and elevated. The reverse side may have an orange-yellow to brown-gray pigment (Fig. 37). Several species of *Fusarium* produce pigment, and these particularly resemble *Trichophyton rosaceum* (EMMONS, 1944). On blood agar the colonies manifest a clear zone of hemolysis around each colony (beta hemolysis). Spider-like flocculi appear in broth. The colorless, multiseptate macroconidia, which may occur in clusters, are 30—70 μ by 4—10 μ and sickle-shaped (Fig. 38). Smaller fusiform microconidia (6—9 μ by 3—5 μ) are occasionally present, too. In young cultures the conidiophores are not branched, but in older ones they are. Many smooth or tuberculate layers of spores are produ-

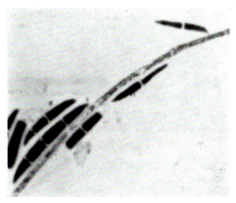

Fig. 38. *Fusarium sp.* with its elongated conidia. Lacto-phenol cotton blue preparation. $\times$ 1000

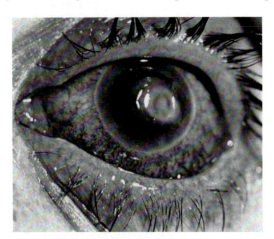

Fig. 39. Corneal ulcer due to *Fusarium sp.* (After ZIMMERMAN, L. E.: Surv. Ophthal. 8, 1—25, 1963)

ced (pionnotes). The widest septate hyaline hyphae (2—6 μ in width) are found in the older cultures. They are branched and contain intercalary chlamydospores.

The relatively few isolates of *Fusarium* in human disease usually have been identified as *Fusarium oxysporum*. The fungus has been associated with cutaneous, corneal, and urinary tract infections. Occasionally, the organism has been cultured from corneal ulcers, within which nonpigmented septate hyphae have sometimes been identified (ANDERSON and CHICK, 1963; ANDERSON et al., 1959; CHICK and CONANT, 1962; GILLESPIE, 1963; GINGRICH, 1962; LYNN, 1964;

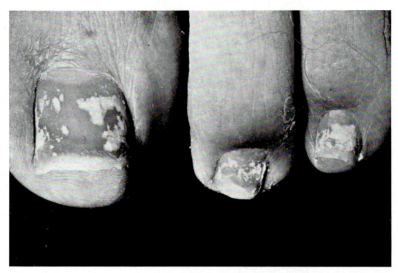

Fig. 40. Extensive involvement of the nail by *Fusarium oxysporum*. (Courtesy of Dr. N. ZAIAS)

MIKAMI and STEMMERMANN, 1958; PERZ, 1966; SIGTENHORST and GINGRICH, 1957; STOKES, 1959; ZIMMERMAN, 1963) (Fig. 39).

Fusarium has been cultured from cutaneous lesions in man (BOTTICHER, 1966; GAMET et al., 1964; HOLZEGEL, 1964; MIKAMI and STEMMERMANN, 1958; MING and YU, 1964; PETERSON and BAKER, 1959). The fungus has also been isolated from and observed in diseased nails (ZAIAS, 1966) (Figs. 40, 41).

On several occasions the fungus has been cultured from the urine of different patients. In some instances banana-shaped cells were observed in urine that

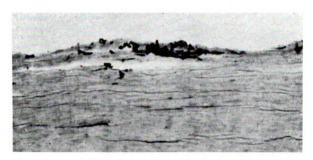

Fig. 41. Cross-section of a toe nail showing superficial fungal elements of *Fusarium oxysporum*. Periodic acid Schiff stain. × 120.(After ZAIAS, N.: Sabouraudia 5, 99—103, 1966)

yielded *Fusarium* on culture (FREI, 1925; LAZARUS and SWARTZ, 1948). The presence of *Fusarium* in the urine has usually been accompanied by leukocytes and often bacteria. FREI (1925) described a patient with small, white, star-shaped lesions in the posterior urethra from which *Fusarium sp.* was isolated.

Besides the above, toxins of *Fusarium* have been implicated in human disease. Outbreaks of a condition have been described in man and domesticated animals in rural populations of the U.S.S.R,. The disease, which has been referred to as alimentary toxic aleukia, has been attributed to a mycotoxin produced by *Fusarium sporotrichoides*. This species was identified in overwintered grain which affected individuals had ingested (JOFFE, 1960, 1962, 1963; SARKISOV and KVASH-NINA, 1948). The clinical course was characterized by three distinct phases (FORGACS, 1962a, b; MAYER, 1953a). Initially, there was an acute onset of diarrhea, vomiting, and an epigastric burning sensation. In several days, even if the subject continued to ingest the contaminated grain the initial symptoms subsided. Subsequently, the peripheral blood demonstrated a pancytopenia yet the patient felt well. About 2—8 weeks later, bone marrow aplasia was evident and necrotic skin lesions appeared (FORGACS and CARLL, 1962). Large populations died from secondary infections or hemorrhages due to this disease. Disease has been reproduced experimentally with this fungus in cats, domestic swine, and other animals (JOFFE, 1963, 1965; MAYER, 1953b). *Fusarium sporotrichoides* is capable of both proliferating and forming toxin at 0—10 °C (MAYER, 1953b). A toxin, *sporofusariogenin*, with a steroid configuration has been isolated from the fungus and found to cause the condition (JOFFE, 1965). This toxin withstands, like many other mycotoxins, storage for a prolonged period (2—6 years), acid and alkaline denaturation, and autoclaving at 125 °C for 30 min or 110 °C for 18 h (MAYER, 1953b). An additional species of *Fusarium* has also been implicated in food poisoning in the U.S.S.R.. Food prepared from grains that are contaminated with *Fusarium graminearium* produces abdominal pain, nausea, diarrhea, and ataxia. The disease is commonly called "Drunken Bread". Once ingestion of the toxin is discontinued, the symptoms subside (FORGACS, 1962a, b).

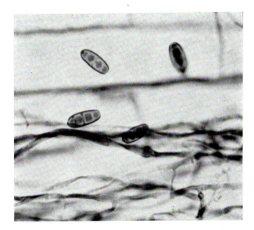

Fig. 42. *Helminthosporium sp.* with straight conidia. Polyvinyl alcohol cotton blue stain. × 320. (Courtesy of DR. C.T. DOLAN)

Helminthosporiosis

The ubiquitous species of *Helminthosporium* grow readily on standard mycological media, including Sabouraud's. The colonies become brown-gray and filamentous and then gray-brown to black with a velvety surface. The reverse side of the colony is brown-black. The occasionally racquet-shaped, septate hyphae (2.5—5.5 μ in width) possess branched conidiophores with terminal or laterally arranged black-brown, smooth-walled, cylindrical conidia (10 μ by 30 μ). Three or four septa are evident on these conidia which are straight (Fig. 42) and, therefore, readily distinguished from the curved conidia of *Curvularia* with their prominent distal medial cell.

Helminthosporium, a well known phytopathogen, has rarely been identified in mammalian tissue. The organism has been observed in and isolated from lesions in bovine nasal mucosa (ROBERTS et al., 1963). It has also been cultured from a mycetoma on a dog's foot, that contained numerous black granules of brown hyphae and chlamydospores (GEORG, 1964).

In man the fungus is frequently isolated from the sputum and skin, and may produce hypersensitivity reactions (WALTON, 1949). DOLAN et al. (1968, 1970) have evidence of *Helminthosporium* in human pulmonary tissue. They cultured *Helminthosporium sp.* from the lungs of two patients with chronic respiratory disease manifested by purulent sputum, hemoptysis, and fever. Multiple abscesses in pulmonary tissue were surrounded by lymphocytes, histiocytes, plasma cells, granulocytes, and fibrosis. Septate branching hyphae were observed in the lesions as well as the bronchi, bronchioles, and alveoli. The fungal elements appeared light brown in unstained sections and were readily demonstrated after silver impregnation (Fig. 43).

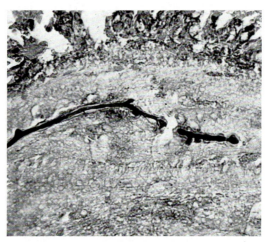

Fig. 43. *Helminthosporium sp.* in a pulmonary lesion. Silver chromate stain. × 350. (Courtesy of DR. C.T. DOLAN)

Keratomycosis

The first known case of mycotic keratitis is that of LEBER (1879). Since this report numerous fungi, as well as the actinomycetes, *Actinomyces bovis*, *Nocardia asteroides*, and *Streptomyces sp.*, have been cultured in many parts of the world from patients with keratitis. The fungal isolates have included *Acremonium sp.*, *Acrostalagmus cinnabarensis*, *Alliescheria boydii*, *Alternaria sp.*, *Aspergillus spp.*, *Blastomyces dermatitidis*, *Botrytis sp.*, *Candida spp.*, *Cephalosporium spp.*, *Cryptococcus neoformans*, *Curvularia spp.*, *Fusarium spp.*, *Fusidium spp.*, *Gibberella fujikurae*, *Glenosporium spp.*, *Hormodendrum sp.*, *Mucor sp.*, *Penicillium spp.*, *Periconia keratitidis*, *Rhizopus sp.*, *Scopulariopsis spp.*, *Sporotrichum schenckii*, *Sterygmatocystis nigra*, *Trichosporon sp.*, *Verticillium spp.* (AINLEY and SMITH, 1965; ANDERSON and CHICK, 1963; ANDERSON et al., 1959; BEDELL, 1946, 1947; BYERS, et al., 1960; CHICK and CONANT, 1962; ERNEST and RIPPON, 1966; FAZAKAS, 1959; FOCOSI, 1932; GEORG, 1964; GILLESPIE, 1963; GINGRICH, 1962;

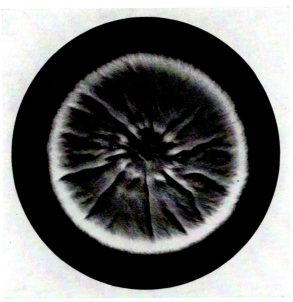

Fig. 44. Colony of *Paecilomyces* on Sabouraud's glucose agar

GORDON et al., 1959; HAGGERTY and ZIMMERMAN, 1958; HILDICK-SMITH et al., 1964; HOFFMAN and NAUMANN, 1963; KINNAS, 1965; LEY and SAUNDERS, 1956; LYNN, 1964; MAFFEI, 1928; MANCHESTER and GEORG, 1959; MANGIARACINE and LIEBMAN, 1957; MENEDELBLATT, 1953; MIKAMI and STEMMERMANN, 1958; MINODA, 1957; MITSUI and HANABRUSA, 1955; NAUMANN et al., 1967; NITYANANDA et al., 1962; PAUTLER et al., 1955; PERZ, 1966; ZIMMERMAN, 1962, 1963). Most isolates have not been accompanied by the identification of fungal elements within the excised tissue, and as many of these fungi are ubiquitous, their role in the genesis of the corneal lesions is often open to question. However, in many instances fungi such as *Allescheria boydii*, *Aspergillus spp.*, *Candida spp.*, *Cephalosporium sp.*, and *Curvularia spp.*, have been cultured from the involved tissue, which contained fungal elements.

Previous corneal trauma and the topical application of broad spectrum antibiotics and/or corticosteroids have been significantly associated with mycotic keratitis in man. Experimental evidence supports the clinical impression that corticosteroids and broad-spectrum antibiotics not only alter the normal flora of the eye, but also enhance fungal infection of the cornea (AGARWAL et al., 1963; SELIGMANN, 1952, 1953). Corticosteriods by altering the host's inflammatory response not only increase the relative virulence of recognized pathogens, but may allow other species that are general commensals to become pathogenic (AGARWAL et al., 1963; SUIE and HAVENER, 1963). Some fungi may cause corneal lesions in the absence of predisposing factors, for example *Cephalosporium sp.* has been reported to produce corneal ulceration and opacification in rabbits within 2—4 h (BURDA and FISHER, 1960).

Otomycosis

A wide variety of fungi have been cultured from the external ear of man in most parts of the world, but especially in the tropics (BRICEÑO-MAAZ and BRICEÑO-MAAZ, 1964; LAKSHMIPATHI and MURTI, 1960; SHARP et al., 1946). Some cases

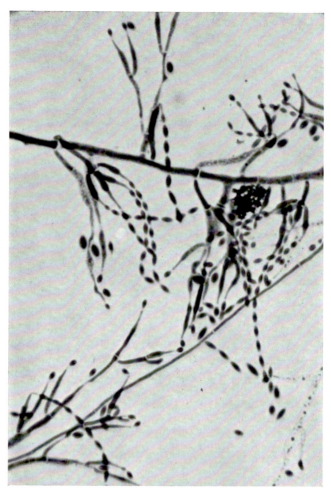

Fig. 45. *Paecilomyces sp.* showing chains of elliptical conidia arising from the tip of flask-shaped phialides. Lacto-phenol cotton blue preparation. × 1000. (After FETTER, B.F., KLINTWORTH, G.K., and HENDRY, W.S.: *Mycoses of the Central Nervous System.* Baltimore: Williams and Wilkins 1967)

have been associated with itching, pain, redness, scaling, and discharges of the external auricle, meatus, and auditory canal, but other isolates have been from seemingly normal external ears (HALEY, 1950; LEA et al., 1958; SOOD et al., 1967). The fungi that have been cultured have included numerous dermatophytes.

(ENGLISH, 1957; STUART and BLANK, 1955), as well as *Allescheria boydii* (BELDING and UMANZIO, 1935; BLANK and STUART, 1955), *Aspergillus spp.* (ANANTHANARAYAN, 1951; BEANEY and BROUGHTON, 1967; DURCAN et al., 1968; SOOD et al., 1967), *Candida albicans* (TOMIC-KAROVIC and POPADIC, 1953), *Cryptococcus neoformans* (GILL, 1947; WOLF, 1947), *Mucor spp.* (McBURNEY and GULLEDGE, 1955; SOOD et al., 1967), *Penicillium spp.* (ARIEVITCH and STEPANISCHEVA, 1964; KIRK, 1959; KUNEL'SKAIA, 1964; KUNEL'SKAIA and STEPANI-SCHEVA, 1964; McBURNEY and GULLEDGE, 1955; MOHAPATRA, 1961; SMYTH, 1961; SOOD et al., 1967), *Scopulariopsis spp.* (SMYTH, 1961), and *Waldemaria pernambucensis* (BATISTA et al., 1960; SMYTH, 1961).

As most of these fungi have only been cultured from the external ear and not identified in lesions, they simply may be saprophytes. However, fungi have

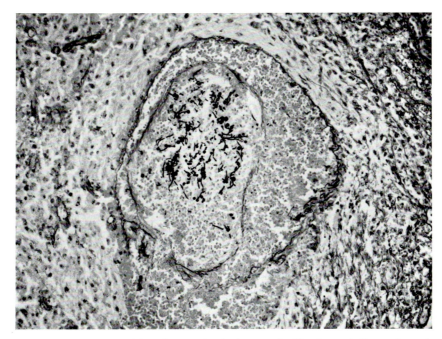

Fig. 46. Fungal elements of *Paecilomyces* in the lumen of a blood vessel. Grocott's methenamine silver stain. × 110

sometimes been observed in tissue scrapings and discharges and may be important in the genesis of the aural lesion. Moreover, lesions have been produced in the ear canals of man with fungi isolated from patients with otomycosis (Soop et al., 1967).

Paecilomycosis

Paecilomyces has a worldwide distribution and is a common saprophyte of fruits and vegetables. The fungus, which consists of several species, grows readily on numerous culture media including Sabouraud's medium. It produces a thin colony which becomes yellow-brown and powdery following the production of conidia (Fig. 44). The mycelium has broad, branching septate hyphae. Chains of ovoid spores (2—4 μ by 6—8 μ) arise from flask-shaped phialides that have long tapering necks at an angle to the main axis of the sterigmata (Fig. 45).

The fungus has rarely caused human disease. Uys et al. (1963) described a patient who died a year after the surgical correction of an incompetent mitral valve. The terminal clinical manifestations included emaciation, pyrexia without leucocytosis, and signs of cardiac failure and embolization. *Paecilomyces varioti*, which was isolated from several blood cultures three weeks before death, was also cultured from a thrombus overlying the mitral valve and from an embolus in an iliac artery after death. On post-mortem examination the fungus was demonstrated microscopically within thrombi in the region of the mitral valve and emboli in the iliac and cerebral arteries. An area similar to a tuberculoma with caseous necrosis, epithelioid cells, and multinucleated giant cells was present in the vessel wall overlying a thrombus in the iliac artery. This lesion as well as others contained hyphae (1.5—2 μ in diameter) with and without rounded bodies

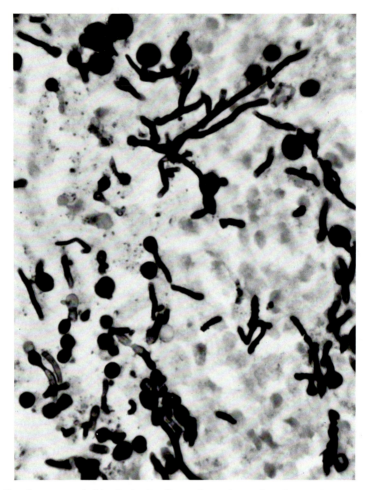

Fig. 47. *Paecilomyces varioti* in the brain. Grocott's methenamine silver stain. $\times$ 1000. (After FETTER, B.F., KLINTWORTH, G.K., and HENDRY, W.S.: *Mycoses of the Central Nervous System*. Baltimore: Williams and Wilkins 1967)

connected to them. The fungus was readily demonstrated with Grocott's methenamine silver technique (Figs. 46, 47).

Species of *Paecilomyces* have been cultured from a postoperative scleral lesion (PODEDWORNY and SUIE, 1964) and infected nails (ŠAULOV, 1965). The fungus was not identified in the tissue in these cases, and therefore they remain equivocal examples of paecilomycosis.

Penicilliosis

The genus *Penicillium*, commonly known as the blue or green mold, contains more than 200 different species that are widespread in nature. The fungus is often observed on decaying organic matter, and frequently contaminates laboratory media. Numerous species of *Penicillium* produce the antibiotic penicillin.

All species of *Penicillium* grow rapidly at room temperature on Sabouraud's glucose agar, producing a variety of pigmented colonies (Fig. 48). The aerial

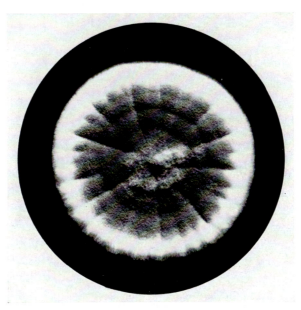

Fig. 48. *Penicillium sp.* on Sabouraud's glucose agar

mycelium forms a complex system of branches (metulae), from which the flask-shaped phialides radiate, like the bristles of a brush (*penicillus*). The conidia occur in unbranched chains from the tips of the latter structures (Fig. 49). The various species differ in the size, texture, and color of the colonies.

Penicillium has rarely been found to be pathogenic to plants or animals. It is commonly cultured from man in the abscene of disease. Several species have been implicated in disease, including *P. bertai, P. bicolor, P. citrinum, P. commune, P. crustaceum, P. glaucom, P. marneffei, P. mycetogenum,* and *P. spinulosum.* Most of the isolates are, however, of uncertain significance, as the fungus has usually not been observed in tissue from which it was cultured. Indeed, *Penicillium* is a frequent constituent of the conjunctival flora of healthy individuals (AINLEY and SMITH, 1965), and a common isolate of bronchial secretions (GERNEZ-RIEUX, 1964). Moreover, as the fungus is so widely dispersed in nature, even the repeated isolation of the *Penicillium* is of equivocal status.

Penicillium spp. have been isolated from patients with broncho-pulmonary disease.

(AIME et al., 1933; BUGYI, 1958; CASTELLANI, 1920; DaSILVA LACAZ, 1937; DeLORE et al., 1955; GARRETÓN, 1945; GIORDANO, 1918; HǒREJŠÍ et al., 1960; HUANG and HARRIS, 1963; JACKSON and YOW, 1961; NIÑO, 1932; NUSSBAUM and BENEDEK, 1927; PEZZALI, 1921; SOUCHERAY, 1954; TALICE and MacKINNON, 1929), keratitis (AINLEY and SMITH, 1965; ANDERSON et al., 1959; CHICK and CONANT, 1962; FAZAKAS, 1959; GINGRICH, 1962; MINODA, 1957; MITSUI and HANABUSA, 1955), chronic ear infections (ARIEVITCH and STEPANISCHEVA, 1964; KIRK, 1959; KUNEL'SKAIA, 1964; KUNEL'SKAIA and STEPANISCHEVA, 1964; McBURNEY and GULLEDGE, 1955; MOHAPATRA, 1961; SMYTH, 1961; SOOD et al., 1967), urinary tract infection (CHUTE, 1911; GILLIAM and VEST, 1951; SALISBURY, 1868), vaginitis and vulvo-vaginitis (CASTELLANI, 1920), lesions of nails and skin (ANDREEV, 1964; KESTEN et al., 1932; ŠAULOV, 1965), a post-operative mastoid cavity (SMYTH, 1962), black hairy tongue (LINEBACK, 1959), and a temporal lobe abscess (POLYANSKIY, 1938).

When *Penicillium* has been isolated from patients with respiratory disease there has usually been an underlying pulmonary disorder such as bronchiectasis,

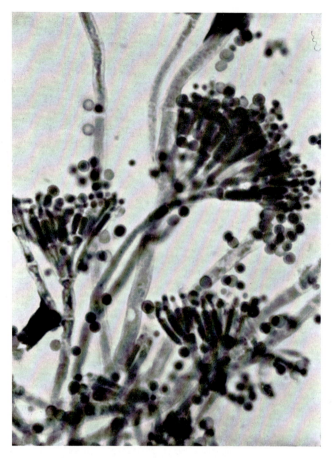

Fig. 49. *Penicillium sp.* showing typical brush-like conidia. Lacto-phenol cotton blue preparation. × 1000

tuberculosis, and lung abscesses. In most of these cases adequate proof of disease being caused by *Penicillium* is lacking. Sometimes a large mass of matted mycelia accumulates in a pulmonary cyst or cavity caused by an associated disease. Such lesions are occasionally characterized roentgenographically by a narrow zone of radiolucency between radio-opaque zones. Histologically, there is generally little or no reaction to the fungus and the organisms seem to be saprophytes. Occasionally, when the isolates have been associated with non-specific manifestations such as cough, hemoptysis, weight loss, and pyrexia, the etiology of the respiratory disease has not been clear.

P.mycetogenum has been isolated from a mycetoma that contained black granules. This species was found to be pathogenic to the pigeon, but not to the guinea pig (Mantelli and Negri, 1915).

Huang and Harris (1963) described a rare example of disseminated penicilliosis. The patient had acute leukemia complicated by pulmonary and cerebral penicilliosis and gastrointestinal candidosis. Antibiotics and steroid therapy anteceded the onset of the mycotic infection. *P.commune* was cultured from the pulmonary lesions at autopsy and observed within and around blood vessels. The

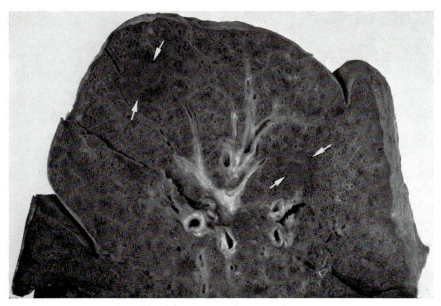

Fig. 50. Lung with hemorrhagic nodular lesions containing *Penicillium commune* (arrows) and secondary to a *Penicillium* thromboangiitis. (After HUANG, S.N., and HARRIS, L.S.: Amer. J. clin. Path. 39, 167—174, 1963)

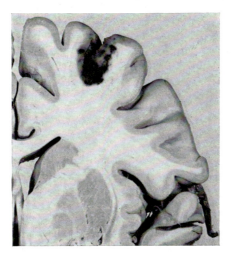

Fig. 51. Infarct in the brain caused by *Penicillium commune*. (After HUANG, S.N., and HARRIS, L.S.: Amer. J. clin. Path. 39, 167—174, 1963)

fungus had also invaded the adjacent tissue around infarcts in the lungs and brain (Figs. 50—52).

It has been suggested that sensitization to *Penicillium* may cause asthma and allergic rhinitis (DE MONTEMAYOR et al., 1965; SHELLEY, 1964; WALTON, 1949).

One species of *Penicillium* (*P.marneffei*) is known to cause spontaneous disease in the Bamboo rat (*Rhizomys sinensis*) that lives in the high plateaus of Vietnam. In this rodent the fungus produces a systemic infection manifested by

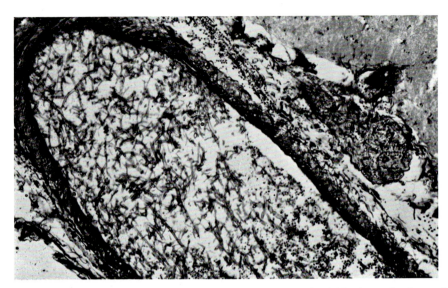

Fig. 52. Numerous hyphae of *Penicillium commune* within cerebral blood vessels. Grocott's methenamine silver stain. × 120

ascites, splenomegaly, hepatomegaly, lymphadenopathy, and intestinal lesions involving the Peyer's patches. The fungus is evident within macrophages and to a lesser extent in polymorphonuclear leukocytes, particularly in the liver, spleen, and lymph nodes. Though a clear case of infection with *P.marneffei* has not yet been documented in man, an investigator is reported to have developed a nodule in a finger 10 days after its accidental inoculation. The lesion was followed by palpably enlarged regional lymph nodes. All symptoms disappeared after treatment with Nystatin (CAPPONI et al., 1956; SEGRETAIN, 1959, 1962).

In tissue sections most species of *Penicillium* appear as branching septate hyphae. Though they can be seen in hematoxylin and eosin preparations, the hyphae are more readily demonstrated with special stains, such as Grocott's methenamine silver and the modified periodic acid Schiff stains (Figs. 53, 54). Histologically, *Penicillium* closely resembles *Aspergillus* and these two genera usually cannot be differentiated with certainty in the absence of culture. The flask-shaped phialides may aid in distinguishing between *Aspergillus* and *Penicillium*, but these are rarely observed in tissue. Unlike other species of *Penicillium*, *P.marneffei* does not produce prominent hyphae in lesions, but intracytoplasmic rounded bodies which superficially resemble *Histoplasma capsulatum* and *Leishmania donovanii*. However, with *P.marneffei* elongated fungal elements (20 μ), often with septate hyphae are sometimes evident.

Different toxins produced by *Penicillium spp.* cause disease in cattle, rodents, and other animals (KOBAYASHI et al., 1958, 1959 a, b; MIYAKE et al., 1955, 1959, 1960; OHMORI et al., 1954; SAKAI, 1955; SAKAI and URAGUCHI, 1955; SAKAKI, 1891; TSUNODA, 1953, 1963; URAGUCHI et al., 1961 a—c).

There has been evidence to suggest that toxins for *Penicillium* sp. produce gastrointestinal distubances in man. Lesions have not been adequately documented in humans, but the toxins produced by *Penicillium spp.* (Table 3) have been associated in rodents with such variable features as cirrhosis, hepatomas, nephrosis, and respiratory paralysis (ENOMOTO, 1959; ISHIKO, 1957; KOBAYASHI et al., 1958,

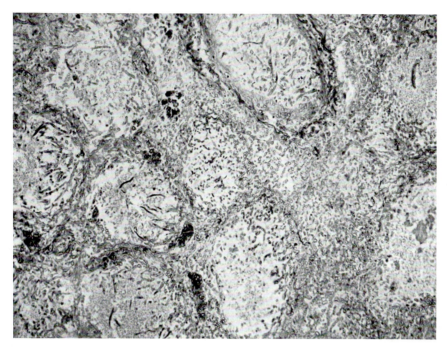

Fig. 53. Numerous hyphae of *Penicillium commune* in the lung. Grocott's methenamine silver stain. × 120

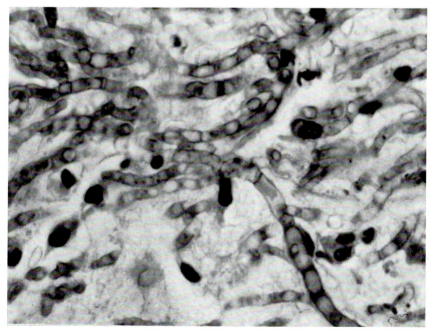

Fig. 54. Hyphae of *Penicillium commune*. Modified periodic acid Schiff stain × 1000

Table 3. Toxins of *Penicillium*

Species	Toxins
Penicillium brunneum	rugulosin, emodin, and skyrin
P.citreo-viride	citreoviridin
P.citrinum	citrinin
P.frequentans	frequentic acid
P.islandicum	islanditoxin
	luteoskyrin
P.notatum	notatin
P.ochrosalmoneum	citreoviridin
P.rugulosum	rugulosin
P.tardum	rugulosin
P.urticae	patulin
P.viridicatum	viridiatin

1959a, b; MIYAKE et al., 1955, 1959, 1960; OHMORI et al., 1954; SAITO, 1959; SAKAKI and URAGUCHI, 1955; TSUNODA, 1953, 1963; URAGUCHI et al., 1961a—c). Death of cattle has also been attributed to the toxins, patulin and viridiatin.

Rhodotorulosis

Rhodotorula, a red yeast-like organism, grows readily on Sabouraud's glucose agar and other common microbiological media at both room temperature and 37°C (Fig. 55). The colony possesses a prominent orange-red color and a dull, smooth surface. Though the fungus contains a red carotenoid pigment, the individual organisms generally appear colorless. The yeast-like cells are ovoid in shape, possess thin capsules, and replicate by budding. Pseudohyphae are produced in some instances. Like *Cryptococcus*, the organism hydrolyzes urea. Several species of *Rhodotorula* have been described, and include: *R.flava, R. glutinis, R.mucilaginosa*, and *R.saccharomyces*.

The organism has generally been regarded as nonpathogenic, but has been cultured from numerous sources in human patients including skin and nails, bronchial secretions, urine, blood, aortic valve, ascitic fluid, vulvovaginal area, cerebrospinal fluid, pharynx, and feces (AHEARN et al., 1966; BERGMANN and LIPSKY, 1964; CARETTA, 1961; CHAKRAVARTY, 1966; GERNEZ-RIEUX et al., 1964; LEEBER and SCHER, 1969; LINEBACK, 1959; LOURIA et al., 1960, 1967; MIGUENS, 1960; MÜLLER et al., 1967; SHELBOURNE and CAREY, 1962; SILVEIRA, 1959; VIEIRA and BATISTA, 1962; WILSON, 1965). Though the pathogenicity of *Rhodotorula* for man and other animals has yet to be established, several investigators have suggested that the organism may have adverse effects in man. They have drawn attention to the importance of not discarding isolates of this fungus as contaminants of culture media. The organism has not only been repeatedly isolated from multiple sources, including the cerebrospinal fluid, pharynx, feces, urine, and skin in the same patient (RIOPEDRE et al., 1960), but has also been cultured on several separate occasions from the blood and/or the urine in other patients (LEEBER and SCHER, 1969; LOURIA et al., 1967; SHELBOURNE and CAREY, 1962). Whether the fungus lives in man as a saprophyte or parasite remains to be established. It has usually been isolated in patients with some serious disease and has not been associated with any specific clinical features. Intravenous therapy appears to have been an important predisposing factor in the development of fungemia due to *Rhodotorula* (LEEBER and SCHER, 1969; LOURIA et al., 1967).

The organism has not been adequately demonstrated in tissue sections. Relatively few post-mortem examinations have been performed on patients from

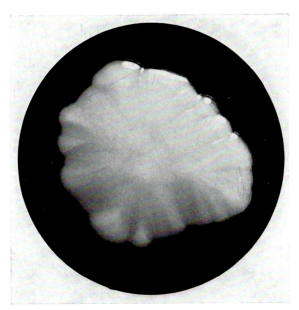

Fig. 55. Colony of *Rhodotorula sp.* on Sabouraud's glucose agar

whom *Rhodotorula* was cultured during life. In these cases the fungus could not be identified in the tissues (LOURIA et al., 1960, 1967). However, the patients had been treated with amphotericin B, and this may have accounted for the lack of histologic confirmation (LOURIA et al., 1960, 1967). Attempts to produce disease in laboratory animals with *Rhodotorula* have been inconclusive (LOURIA et al., 1960, 1967; RIOPEDRE et al., 1960).

Streptomycosis

Of all the genera of the Actinomycetes, *Streptomyces* is represented in nature by the largest number of species and varieties. Many of these play an extremely important role in medicine, not because of their pathogenicity, but on account of their importance in chemotherapy. Thus far, more than 350 species of *Streptomyces* produce numerous antibiotics, that are used in the treatment of infectious diseases, in the prevention of plant diseases, in the preservation of food, and for the promotion of animal growth (UMEZAWA et al., 1967).

Streptomyces spp. are aerobic, and grow readily at room temperature in ordinary media and at the ordinary atmosphere. The colonies of most *Streptomyces* on artificial media are smooth or lichenoid, hard and tensely textured, raised and adherent to the medium. They are usually covered completely or partially (in the form of spots or concentric rings) by an aerial mycelium, which may be pigmented (Fig. 56). The nature and intensity of the pigment depend on the species and on the composition of the media. The hyphae vary greatly in length; some are long with limited branching, others are short and profusely branched. They usually have a diameter of 0.7—0.8 μ (Fig. 57). The mycelium does not segment into bacillary and coccoid forms. Reproduction occurs by the formation of chains of spores (conidia) in spore-bearing hyphae (sporophores) that arise from the aerial mycelium either monopodially or in the form of small clusters of whorls. The sporophores may be straight or curved with curvatures ranging from waves to

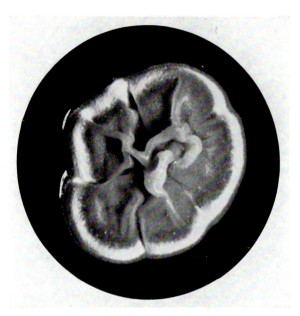

Fig. 56. Colony of *Streptomyces sp.* on Sabouraud's glucose agar

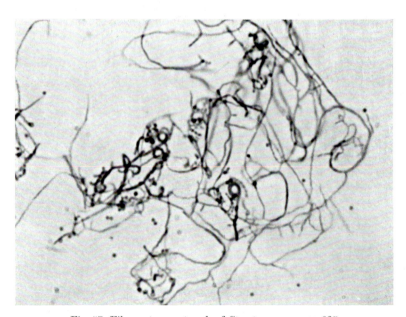

Fig. 57. Filamentous network of *Streptomyces sp.* × 625

spirals (Fig. 58). The marked variation in spore size and shape is of limited usefulness in taxonomical differentiation.

The *Streptomyces spp.* grow in soil or upon organic residues and often contaminate culture media. They are sometimes present on the skin, or in feces, saliva or sputum. Very few are pathogenic to either animals or plants. Some

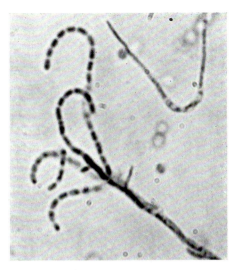

Fig. 58. *Streptomyces sp.* showing chains of conidia arising from a terminal sporophore. Lacto-phenol cotton blue preparation. × 2500

species of *Streptomyces*, including *S.scabies*, produce the common potato scab, the most important plant disease caused by the actinomycetes (WAKSMAN, 1967).

Three species of *Streptomyces* (*S.madurae* Vincent, *S.pelletieri* Laveran, and *S.somaliensis* Brumpt) cause mycetomas (see Chapter 12, Mycetoma). In some parts of the world the resulting disease is endemic with the pathogenic species differing in the various countries.

(ABBOTT, 1956; ADAMI and KIRKPATRICK, 1895; ANDRÉ, 1958; BLANC and BRUN, 1919; BRAULT, 1906; BRUMPT, 1960; CARTER, 1860, 1861; CATANEI, 1934, 1942, 1943; CATANEI and GOINARD, 1934; CATANEI et al., 1927; CATANEI and LEGROUX, 1931; CHADLI et al., 1963; CONVIT et al., 1961; CORNWALL and LA FRENAIS, 1922; DESTOMBES and ANDRÉ, 1958; DESTOMBES et al., 1965, 1966; DEY, 1962; DIOUF et al., 1965; GAMET et al., 1964; GUICHARD and JAUSION, 1923; GEMY and VINCENT, 1892, 1896; GONZALEZ-OCHOA and AHUMADA PIDALLA, 1958; HALDE and RINGROSE, 1958; HOMEZ, 1963; HYDE, 1896; LATAPÍ, 1959; LATAPÍ et al., 1961; LATAPÍ and ORTIZ, 1963; LE DANTEC, 1894; LEGRAIN, 1898; LINCOLN et al., 1965; LOBO, 1963; LYNCH, 1964; LYNCH and MOGHRABY, 1961; MACKINNON, 1954; MACKINNON and ARTAGAVEYTIA-ALLENDE, 1956; MAEGRAITH, 1963; MARIAT, 1963; MONT-PELLIER and LACROIX, 1921; NICOLAU and AVRAM, 1959; ORIO et al., 1963; PORRITT, 1962; PROCTOR, 1966; RAYNAUD et al., 1922; REMLINGER, 1912, 1913; REY, 1961; SAUL, 1961; SEGRETAIN and DESTOMBES, 1963; SEGRETAIN and MARIAT, 1958; SYMMERS and SPORER, 1944; VANBREUSEGHEM, 1958; VERGHESE and KLOKKE, 1966; VICTORIA et al., 1967; VINCENT, 1894) (Table 4). In countries where *S.madurae*, *S.pelletieri*, and *S.somaliensis* have all been isolated, the incidence of disease produced by each of the species is not the same. For example, *Streptomyces somaliensis* is the commonest species of the actinomycetes that has been cultured from mycetoma in the Sudan, being more than ten times as common as *S.madurae* and *S.pel-letieri* (LYNCH, 1964).

The mycetomata produced by *Streptomyces*, like those due to other organisms, are characterized by sinus formation, a granulomatous reaction, and grains. The granules, whose color varies with the species (Table 4), are dispersed throughout the diffuse and ill-defined lesions. *S.pelletieri* has the greatest polymorphonuclear leukocytic response. Multinucleated giant cells are generally evident in older lesions due to *S.somaliensis*, but rarely with infections by *S.madurae* and *S.pelle-tieri* (CAMAIN et al., 1957; LYNCH, 1964). After several years regional lymph node involvement may accompany the streptomycotic mycetoma (LYNCH, 1964). The rate of progression of mycetoma due to *Streptomyces* is stated to be more rapid

Table 4. *Geographic Distribution of Mycetomas due to S. madurae, S. pelletieri, and S. somaliensis and the Characteristics of their Granules*

Geographic Distribution	S. madurae	S. pelletieri	S. somaliensis
Algeria	+	—	—
Arabia	—	—	+
Brazil	+	+	—
Cameroon	—	+	—
Chad	+	+	+
Democratic Republic of the Congo	+	—	—
India	+	+	—
Israel	+	—	+
Mauritania	+	+	+
Morocco	+	—	—
Mexico	+	+	+
Nigeria	+	+	+
Roumania	+	—	—
Senegal	+	+	+
Somaliland	+	+	+
Sudan	+	+	+
Tanzania	—	+	+
Tunisia	+	—	—
United States of America	+	+	+
Upper Volta	+	+	—
Venezuela	+	+	+
Vietnam	+	—	—
Yemen	—	—	+

+ = organism identified
— = organism not identified

Characteristics of Granules:

Color:	Usually white or yellowish, occasionally reddish	Red	White or yellowish
Size:	1—5 mm	0.1—0.5 mm	0.5—2 mm
Staining:	Margins stain deeply with hematoxylin	Stains deeply and uniformly with hematoxylin	Eosinophilic

than those due to *Madurella*, and infections caused by *S. pelletieri* seem to be the most virulent of the actinomycetes (Lynch, 1964).

Extra-pedal sites may be involved with any of the *Streptomyces* that cause mycetoma. Even the testis may be affected (Clarke, 1953). In an extensive investigation of mycetoma, Rey (1961) found that *S. pelletieri* affected sites other than the feet more frequently than other organisms.

There is some evidence to suggest that different species of *Streptomyces* vary in their affinity for bone. It is generally agreed that osseous lesions are common, with infection by *S. pelletieri* (Delahaye et al., 1962; Klüken et al., 1964; Lynch, 1964; Rey, 1961). Lesions of the bone commonly accompany mycetomas that have been present for more than one year. The time that elapses between infection and the production of bone lesions depends, aside from the species, on the distance of the lesion from the bone (Klüken et al., 1965). The bone undergoes osteolysis and develops a reticulated appearance. Sometimes the periosteum is primarily involved. Under such circumstances there may be swelling without sinus formation, and the disease may simulate an osteogenic sarcoma, both clinically and radiologically.

The roentgenographic "sun ray" appearance that commonly occurs with osteogenic sarcomas may be present. Even a "sabre" tibia may be produced (LYNCH, 1964).

LYNCH (1964) inoculated *Streptomyces somaliensis* subcutaneously into guinea pigs, rabbits, rats, and monkeys, with or without acacia thorns and Freund's adjuvant, but was unable to produce lesions comparable to those in man. Collagenase activity has been demonstrated with *S.madurae* and the enzyme has been implicated in the pathogenicity of the species (RIPPON and LORINCZ, 1964; RIPPON and PECK, 1967).

Besides mycetoma, species of *Streptomyces* have rarely been incriminated in other human lesions. KOHN et al. (1951) described a patient with a pulmonary infection from whose blood *Streptomyces sp.* was cultured three times. Species of *Streptomyces* have been cultured from ulcerative keratitis (CHICK and CONANT, 1962). CLARK et al. (1964) isolated *Streptomyces griseus* from a cerebellar abscess of a patient who had a past history of frontal sinusitis, but no other associated disease. A pre-operative lumbar cerebrospinal fluid analysis revealed 2,240 neutrophils per cu-mm, 43 mg sugar per 100 ml and 195 mg protein per 100 ml with an increased globulin level. Culture of the fluid revealed no organisms. The ventricular fluid contained 650 erythrocytes per cu-mm, 4 lymphocytes per cu-mm, 80 mg protein per 100 ml, 70 mg sugar per 100 ml and 203 mEq/L chloride. An apparent cure followed treatment with antibiotics and aspiration of the abscess.

Streptomyces is readily demonstrated in tissue sections with bacterial stains, such as the Brown and Brenn or MacCallum-Goodpasture, and Grocott's methenamine silver stain, but are poorly visualized in hematoxylin and eosin stained preparations. The fungus forms a delicate Gram-positive mycelium which is morphologically indistinguishable from *Actinomyces* and *Nocardia*. Granules are generally present in tissue with infection by *S.madurae*, *S.pelletieri*, and *S.somaliensis*. Fibrin may resemble *Streptomyces* in tissue sections, but it can be readily differentiated from the actinomycete with suitable stains. For example, fibrin is Gram-negative, but *Streptomyces* is Gram-positive with the Brown and Brenn bacterial stain. Fibrin and *Streptomyces* are both Gram-positive with the McCallum-Goodpasture bacterial stain. *Streptomyces* is not acid-fast and does not tend to break up into rod-shaped and coccus-like bodies as species of *Actinomyces* and *Nocardia* sometimes do.

Torulopsiosis

Torulopsis, a genus belonging to the Cryptococcaceae, is closely related to *Cryptococcus* and *Candida* and reproduces by budding, but does not form pseudohyphae (SILVA-HUFNER, 1970; WICKERHAM, 1957). The fungus which is widely distributed in nature has been cultured from the sputum, stools and urine of apparently healthy humans, but the only species of this generally saprophytic genus that has been incriminated consistently in human disease is *T.glabrata*. Its nonhemolytic colonies, which are pasty and colorless or white to cream colored, become gray-brown with age. The organism is very sensitive to elevated pH and grows only in an acid medium (pH < 6.5) (EDEBO and SPETZ, 1965).

Torulopsis has been recovered from the bile, blood bone marrow, peritoneal fluid and pleural fluid as well as wound exudates and lesions of the oral cavity, fallopian tubes, vagina, nails, skin and subcutaneous tissue.

(AHEARN et al., 1966; ARTAGAVEYTIA-ALLENDE et al., 1961; BATISTA and PEREIRA, 1960; BATISTA et al., 1958, 1961; BERGMAN and LIPSKY, 1964; BERNHARDT, 1960; BLACK and FISHER, 1937; BRUNNER, 1964; CARETTA, 1961; CERNIK and DOANHOAG-HOA, 1963; COHEN et al., 1963; DAGLIO and MARTINEZ-MONTES, 1957; EDEBO et al., 1966; EDEBO and SPETZ, 1965; FÖLDVARI and FLORIAN, 1965; GUZE and HALEY, 1958; HALEY, 1961; HERMANEK, 1964; HURLEY and MORRIS, 1964; HOLMSTRÖM et al., 1959; KATZ and PICKARD, 1967; KEARNS

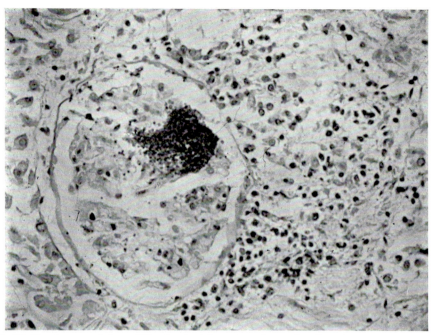

Fig. 59. Focal accumulation of *Torulopsis glabrata* in a glomerulus. Periodic acid Schiff stain. × 82. (After Edebo, L., Jönsson, L. E., Hallén, A., and Linbom, G.: Acta chir. scand. 131, 473—480, 1966)

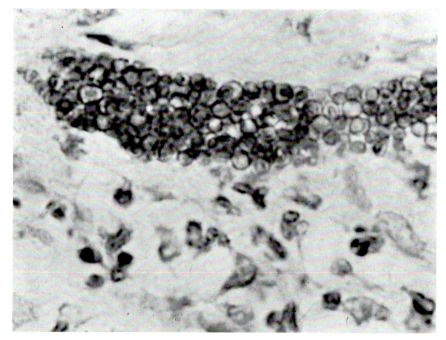

Fig. 60. Rounded yeast organisms of *Torulopsis glabrata* in the kidney. Periodic acid Schiff stain. × 400. (Courtesy of Dr. L. Edebo)

and GRAY, 1963; LOURIA, 1960; LOURIA et al., 1960, 1967; MALICKE, 1964; MARKS et al., 1970; MIQUENS, 1960; MINKOWITZ et al., 1963; MÜLLER et al., 1967; NEGRONI et al., 1966; OLDFIELD et al., 1968; PASSOS, 1961; PEREZ and GIL, 1960; PERRY, 1964; PLAUT, 1950; REIERSÖL, 1958; RIDDELL and CLAYTON, 1958; ŠAULOV, 1965; SILVEIRA, 1959; SMITH et al., 1963; VIEIRA and BATISTA, 1962). In some instances palely eosinophilic, 2—3 μ by 1—2 μ, yeast-like cells with thin refractile capsules were also evident in tissue sections (Figs. 59, 60) (EDEBO et al., 1966) and were associated with variable inflammatory patterns, most commonly mononuclear (MARKS et al., 1970).

Underlying debilitating diseases and chemotherapeutic agents like antibiotics, immunosuppressive drugs, and steroids appear to predispose to infections with this fungus (GRIMLEY et al., 1965; LOURIA et al., 1967; MARKS et al., 1970; MINKOWITZ et al., 1963; OLDFIELD et al., 1968). The possibility of contaminated intravenous catheters contributing to the entry of *T. glabrata* has been raised by LOURIA et al. (1960) and ROSE and HECKMAN (1970).

The pathogenicity of the organism has been investigated in guinea pigs, mice, rabbits, and rats (HASENCLEVER and MITCHELL, 1962; LÓPEZ-FERDINÁNDEZ, 1952). Following intravenous or intraperitoneal injections of *T. glabrata*, abscesses and lesions consisting predominantly of yeast-like cells in macrophages occurred in these animals.

Ustilagosis
(Ustilagomycosis)

An important phytopathogen affecting the corn industry is the smut fungus (*Ustilago zeae*), which parasitizes corn and closely related teosinte. The fungus affects the various parts of corn plants that are above the ground and characteristically causes excrescences and black smutty leaves on the host. The excrescences contain black chlamydospores and may attain a diameter of several inches. The fungus only causes local infection and does not pervade the entire plant. It is not seedborne and does not infect the germinating seedlings. Eventually, the black lesions release myriads of dark spores, which remain viable for some time in the soil. With favorable conditions the chlamydospores germinate and produce sporidia, which multiply by budding. The wind and other agents spread the spores to young, susceptible corn plants.

For some time *Ustilago* has been of interest to investigators of human disease, because it occasionally contaminates culture media. Though the pathogenicity of the fungus for man has yet to be established, it has been associated with human disease on rare occasions. For example, PREININGER (1937) described a 31-year-old farmer who developed cutaneous lesions at sites of contact with wet clothing after spending the night in a cornfield in a drizzling rain. Spores of *Ustilago* were identified in scrapings from the cutaneous lesions on the patient. Moreover, *Ustilago* has been cultured from the cornea of a patient with keratitis (ANDERSON et al., 1959). In neither of these instances was the fungus identified in the tissue, and its role in the genesis of the lesions is questionable. MOORE et al. (1946) believed that *U. zeae (U. maydis)* was the etiologic agent of a chonic granulomatous meningitis and ependymitis. Lesions with multinucleated giant cells and macrophages contained and surrounded many peculiar structures that resembled the sprout mycelium and spiny or echinulate spores of *U. zeae*. However, the fungus was not cultured and the identity of the pathogen remains speculative. In sensitized individuals spores of *Ustilago* may cause allergic reactions such as asthma (LE COULANT and LOPES, 1957).

Acknowledgements: This chapter could not have been completed without the assistance of numerous individuals, and especially DRS. L. AJELLO, P. K. C. AUSTWICK, A. BAKERSPIGEL, E. H. BOSSEN, N. F. CONANT, C. T. DOLAN, L. EDEBO, D. A. EMANUEL, C. W. EMMONS, B. F. FETTER, L. K. GEORG, M. A. GORDON, W. L. JELLISON, W. KAPLAN, A. H. KLOKKE, M. LAHOURCADE, H. S.

Neilsen, Jr., N.B. Rewcastle, P.M. Stockdale, J.E. Tindall, C.J. Uys, N. Zais, and L.E. Zimmerman, who supplied us with information, tissue sections, cultures, and illustrative material; Mr. Carl Bishop for photography; Miss Margaret F. Jones and the Duke Medical Center Library for reference service; the Williams and Wilkins publishing company; and the editors of the *American Journal of Clinical Pathology, Annals of the New York Academy of Science, Archives of Environmental Health, Archives of Ophthalmology, Canadian Journal of Microbiology, Journal of Bacteriology, Journal of the Medical Association of Alabama, Mycologia, Mycopathologia et Mycologia Applicata, La Presse Medicale, Sabouraudia, Southwestern Veterinarian*, and the *Survey of Ophthalmology* for permission to reproduce previously published illustrations.

References
Adiaspiromycosis

Bakerspigel, A.: *Haplosporangium* in Saskatchewan rodents. Mycologia 48, 568 (1956). ~ *Haplosporangium* in an additional rodent host *Microtus pennsylvanicus* Drumondi. Nature (Lond.) 179, 875 (1957). ~ Additional cases of adiaspiromycosis in Canadian rodents. Sabouraudia 4, 176 (1965). — Batista, A.C., De Lima, J.A., Pessoa, F.P., Shome, S.K.: Adiaspiromycose humana doença pulmonar causada por *Emmonsia brasiliensis* n. sp. Rev. Fac. Med. Univ. Ceara 3, 24 (1963a). ~ *Emmonsia brasiliensis* n. sp. um Hifomiceto de interesse para a mycopatologia humana. Rev. Fac. Med. Univ. Ceara 3, 45 (1963b). — Batista, A.C., Shome, S.K.: Isolation of *Emmonsia brasiliensis* from soil. Rev. Fac. Med. Univ. Ceara 3, 42 (1963). — Carmichael, J.W.: The pulmonary fungus *Haplosporangium parvum*. II. Strain and generic relationships. Mycologia 43, 604 (1951). ~ *Chrysosporium* and some other aleuriosporic Hyphomycetes. Canad. J. Botany 40, 1137 (1962). — Chevrel, M.L., Souquet, R., Ferrand, B., Richier, J.L., Doby, J.M., Doby-DuBois, M., Louvet, L.: Polyparasitisme pulmonaire mycosique: premier cas humain d'adiaspiromycose associée à une aspergillose. Ann. Anat. path. 9, 463 (1964). — Ciferri, R., Montemartini, A.: Taxonomy of *Haplosporangium parvum*. Mycopathologia (Den Haag) 10, 303 (1959). — Doby-Dubois, M., Chevrel, M.L., Doby, J.M., Louvet, M.: Premier cas humain d'adiaspiromycose, par *Emmonsia crescens* Emmons et Jellison 1960. Bull. Soc. Path. exot. 57, 240 (1964). — Dowding, E.S.: *Haplosporangium* in Canadian rodents. Mycologia 39, 372 (1947). ~ The pulmonary fungus *Haplosporangium parvum*, and its relationship with some human pathogens. Canad. J. Res., Sect. E 25, 195 (1947b). — Dvořák, J., Otčenášek, M., Prokopič, J.: The distribution of adiaspiromycosis. J. Hyg. Epidem. (Praha) 9, 510 (1965). ~ Seasonal incidence of adiaspores of *Emmonsia crescens* Emmons and Jellison 1960 in wildly living animals. Mycopathologia (Den Haag) 31, 71 (1967). — Emmons, C.W.: Coccidioidomycosis. Mycologia 34, 452 (1942). — Emmons, C.W., Ashburn, L.L.: The isolation of *Haplosporangium parvum* n. sp. and *Coccidioides immitis* from wild rodents: their relationship with coccidioidomycosis. Publ. Hlth. Rep. (Wash.) 57, 1715 (1942). — Emmons, C.W., Jellison, W.L.: *Emmonsia crescens* n. sp. and adiaspiromycosis (haplomycosis) in mammals. Ann. N.Y. Acad. Sci. 89, 91 (1960). — Erickson, A.B.: The fungus (*Haplosporangium parvum*) in the lungs of the beaver (*Castor canadensis*). J. Wildlife Management 13, 419 (1949). — Jellison, W.L.: An undetermined parasite in the lungs of a rock rabbit, *Ochotona princeps* Richardson (Lagomorpha: Ochotonidae). Proc. helminth. Soc. Wash. 14, 75 (1947). ~ Haplomycosis in Montana rabbits, rodents and carnivores. Publ. Hlth. Rep. (Wash.) 65, 1057 (1950). ~ The presence of pulmonary fungus in Korean rodents. Publ. Hlth. Rep. (Wash.) 69, 996 (1954). ~ Haplomycosis in Sweden. Nord. Vet.-Med. 8, 504 (1956). ~ Haplomycosis in Japan and Africa. Mycologia 50, 580 (1958). — Jellison, W.L., Lord, R.D.: *Adiaspiromycosis* in Argentine mammals. Mycologia 56, 374 (1964). — Jellison, W.L., Peterson, R.S.: *Emmonsia* a fungus, and *Besnoitia* a protozoan, reported from S. America. Bot. Chileno-Parasitol. 15, 46 (1964). — McDiarmid, A., Austwick, P.K.C.: Occurrence of *Haplosporangium parvum* in the lungs of the mole (*Talpa eutopaea*). Nature (Lond.) 174, 843 (1954). — Menges, R.W., Habermann, R.T.: Isolation of *Haplosporangium parvum* from soil and results of experimental inoculations. Amer. J. Hyg. 60, 106 (1954). — Misra, S.P., Shende, G.Y., Yerawadekar, S.N., Padhye, A.A., Thirumalachar, M.J.: *Allescheria boydii* and *Emmonsia ciferrina* isolated from patients with chronic pulmonary infections. Hindustan Antibiot. Bull. 9, 99 (1966). — Padhye, A.A., Carmichael, J.W.: *Emmonsia brasiliensis* and *Emmonsia ciferrina* are *Chrysosporium pruinosum*. Mycologia 60, 445 (1968). — Prokopič, J., Dvořák, J., Otčenášek, M.: Adiaspiromycosis (haplomycosis) in Czechoslovakia: preliminary report. Sabouraudia 4, 35 (1965). — Smith, J.M.B., Lancaster, M.C.: Adiaspiromycosis in the brush opossum, *Trichosurus vulpecula*, in New Zealand, Sabouraudia 4, 146 (1965). — Taylor, R.L., Miller, B.E., Rust, J.H., Jr.: Adiaspiromycosis in small mammals of New Mexico. Mycologia 59, 513 (1967). — Tevis, L.: Additional records of *Haplosporangium parvum* in mammals in Britain. Nature (Lond.) 177, 437 (1956). — Thirumalachar, M.J., Padhye, A.A., Srinivasan, M.C.: *Emmonsia ciferrina*, a new species from India. Mycopathologia (Den Haag) 26, 323 (1965).

Allescheriosis

AJELLO, L.: The isolation of *Allescheria boydii* Shear: an etiologic agent of mycetomas from soil. Amer. J. trop. Med. **1**, 227 (1952). — AROEINA-NEVES, J.: Contribucae ao estudo dos micetomas em Minas Georis, Brasil, *Monosporium apiospermum* Saccardo, 1911. Rev· bras. Biol. **2**, 305 (1942). — ARONSON, S.M., BENHAM, R., WOLF, A.: Maduromycosis of the central nervous system. J. Neuropath. exp. Neurol. **12**, 158 (1953). — AVRAM, A.: Grains expérimentaux maduromycosiques et actinomycosiques à *Cephalosporium falciforme, Monosporium apiospermum, Madurella mycetomi et Nocardia asteroides*. Mycopathologia (Den Haag) **32**, 319 (1967). — AVRAM, A., COJOCARU, I., DULĂMIȚĂ, L.: Le pied de madura à *Monosporium apiospermum*. A propos de 3 cas roumains. Dermatologica (Basel) **136**, 176 (1968). — BATTISTINI, F., BRICEÑO-MAAZ, T., DEBRICEÑO-MAAZ, C.: Caso de pie de madura producido por el *Monosporium apiospermum*. Gac. méd. Caracas **67**, 181 (1958). — BAXTER, M., MURRAY, I.G., TAYLOR, J.J.: A case of mycetoma with serological diagnosis of *Allescheria boydii*. Sabouraudia **5**, 138 (1966). — BELDING, D.L., UMANZIO, C.B.: A new species of the genus *Monosporium* associated with chronic otomycosis. Amer. J. Path. **11**, 856 (1935). — BENHAM, R.W., GEORG, L.K.: *Allescheria boydii*, causative agent in a case of meningitis. J. invest. Derm. **10**, 99 (1948). — BLANK, F., STUART, E.A.: *Monosporium apiospermum* Sacc., 1911, associated with otomycosis. Canad. med. Ass. J. **72**, 601 (1955). — BOL'SHAKOVA, G.M., STEPANISHCHEVA, Z.G.: [On Madura foot]. Vestn. Derm. Vener. **34**, 40 (1960) (Russian). — BORELLI, D.: Madurella mycetomi: fialides, fialosporos, inoculacion al raton. Bol. Venez. de Lab. Clin. **2**, 1 (1957). — BOYD, M.F., CRUTCHFIELD, E.D.: A contribution to the study o mycetoma in North America. Amer. J. trop. Med. **1**, 215 (1921). — BRICENOMAAZ, T.: [Mycetoma caused by *Monosporium apiospermum*.]. Derm. Venez. **6**, 155 (1967). — Camain, R., SEGRETAIN, G., NAZIMOFF, O.: Les mycétomes du Sénégal et de la Mauritanie: apercu épidémiologique et étude histopathologique. Sem. Hôp. Paris **33**, 771 (1957). — CARRION, A.L., KNOTT, J.: Mycetoma by *Monosporium apiospermum* in St. Croix, Virgin Islands. Puerto Rico J. publ. Hlth. **20**, 84 (1944). — CIFERRI, R., REDAELLI, P.: Probabilo sinonimi di *Allescheria boydii (Monosporium apiospermum)*. Mycopathologia (Den Haag) **5**, 120 (1950). — COCKSHOTT, W.P.: The therapy of mycetoma. W. Afr. med. J. **6**, 101 (1957). — CONANT, N.F., SMITH, D.T., BAKER, R.D., CALLAWAY, J.L., MARTIN, D.S.: *Manual of Clinical Mycology*, Ed. 2, pp. 240—252. Philadelphia: W.B. Saunders Company 1962. — CONVIT, J. BORELLI, D., ALBORNOZ, R., RODRÍQUEZ, G., HÓMEZ, J.: Micetomas, Cromomicosis, esporotricosis y enfermedad de Jorge Lobo. Mycopathologia (Den Haag) **15**, 394 (1961). — COURTOIS· G., DELOOF, C., THYS, A., VANBREUSEGHEM, R., BURNETTE, A.: Neuf cas de pied de Madura congoleus par *Allescheria boydii, Monosporium apiospermum et Nocardia madurae*. Ann. Soc. belge Méd. trop. **34**, 371 (1954). — CREITZ, J., HARRIS, H.W.: Isolation of *Allescheria boydii* from sputum. Amer. Rev. Tuberc. **71**, 126 (1955). — DE ALMEIDA, F., SIMOES BARBOSA, F.A.: Mycetomas brasileiros. An. Fac. Med. S. Paulo **235** (1940). — DESTOMBES, P., MARIAT, F., ROSATI, L., SEGRETAIN, G.: *Mycetomata in the Republic of Somaliland*. C. R. Acad. Sci. (Paris) Ser. D. **263**, 2062 (1966). — DOWDING, E.S.: *Monosporium apiospermum*, a fungus causing madura foot in Canada. Canad. med. Ass. J. **33**, 23 (1935). — DROUHET, M.: The status of fungus diseases in France. In: *Therapy of Fungus Diseases: An International Symposium*, p. 43. Boston: Little, Brown, and Company 1955. — EL-MOFTY, A.M., ISKANDER, I.D., NADA, M., ZAKI, S.M.: "Madura foot" in Egypt. Brit. J. Derm. **77**, 365 (1965). — EMMONS, C.W.: *Allescheria boydii* and *Monosporium apiospermum*. Mycologia, **36**, 188 (1944). — EMMONS, C.W., GREENHALL, A.M.: *Histoplasma capsulatum* and house bats in Trinidad. Sabouraudia **2**, 18 (1962). — ERNEST, J.T., RIPPON, J.W.: Keratitis due to *Allescheria boydii (Monosporium apiospermum)*. Amer. J. Ophthal. **62**, 1202 (1966). — FIENBERG, R.: Madura foot in a native American. Amer. J. clin. Path. **14**, 239 (1944). — GAY, D.M., BIGELOW, J.B.: Madura foot due to *Monosporium apiospermum* in a native American. Amer. J. Path. **6**, 325 (1930). — GELLMAN, M., GAMMEL, J.A.: Madura foot: a third case of monosporiosis in a native American. Arch. Surg. **26**, 295 (1933). — GORDON, M.A., VALLOTTON, W.W., CROFFEAD, G.S.: Corneal allescheriosis: a case of keratomycosis treated successfully with nystatin and amphotericin B. Arch. Ophthal. **62**, 758 (1959). — GREEN, W.O., ADAMS, T.E.: Mycetoma in the United States: a review and report of seven additional cases. Amer. J. clin. Path. **42**, 75 (1964). — HANLON, T.J., GEPHARDT, M.C., HOPPS, H.C.: Mycetoma in the U.S.: review with report of a case from new area. J. Okla. med. Ass. **48**, 299 (1955). — HAUKOHL, R.S., SADOFF, H.B.: Mycetoma: report of case due to *Monosporium apiospermum* in a native of Minnesota. Wis. med. J. **53**, 477 (1954). — HERRERO, F.J., USABEL, E.J., SIRENA, A.: Primer case en Tucumán (Argentina) de micetoma podal por *Monosporium apiospermum*. Pren. méd. argent. **42**, 3652 (1955). — JONES, J.W., ALDEN, H.S.: Maduromycotic mycetoma (Madura foot): report of case occurring in American Negro. J. Amer. med. Ass. **96**, 256 (1931). — JORGE, J.M., INTROZZI, A.S., NIÑO, F.L.: Micetoma podal maduromicósico con granos blancos por *Monosporium apiospermum*. Bol. Trab. Acad. Argent. Cir. **25**, 508 (1941). — JOSEFIAK, E.J., KOKIKO, G.V.: Mycetoma of the hand: report of a case. Arch. Path. **67**, 55 (1959). — KATSNEL'

SON, I.I., LEVKOV, A.A.: [A deep mycosis with mycetoma type skin damage]. Vestn. Derm. Vener. **36**, 78 (1962). (Russian). — LAPATÍ, F.: Das Mycetom. In: *Die Pilzkrankheiten der Haut durch Hefen. Schimmel, Aktinomyceten und verwandte Erreger*, p. 479. MARCHIONNI, A., and GÖTZ, H. (Eds.). Berlin-Göttingen-Heidelberg: Springer 1963. — LAPATÍ, F., ORTIZ, Y.: Los micetomas en Mexico. Memorias del primer congreso de dermatologia. 126 (1963). — LEY, A.P.: Experimental fungus infections of the cornea: Preliminary report. Amer. J. Ophthal. **42**, 59 (1956). — LOURIA, D.B., LIEBERMAN, P.H., COLLINS, H.S., BLEVINS, A.: Pulmonary mycetoma due to *Allescheria boydii*. Arch. intern. Med. **117**, 748 (1966). — PILLAY, V.K.G., WILSON, D.M., ING, T.S., KARK, R.M.: Fungus infection in steroid treated systemic lupus erythematosus. J. Amer. med. Ass. **205**, 261 (1968). — MACKINNON, J.E.: Causal agents of maduromycosis in the neotropical region. An. Fac. Med. Montevideo **48**, 453 (1963). — MAHGOUB, E.S.: The value of gel diffusion in the diagnosis of mycetoma. Trans. roy. Soc. trop. Med. Hyg. **38**, 560 (1964). — MARIAT, F.: On the geographic distribution and spread of the agents of mycetomas. Bull. Soc. Path. exot. **56**, 35 (1963). — MEYER, E., HERROLD, R.D.: *Allescheria boydii* isolated from a patient with chronic prostatitis. Amer. J. clin. Path. **35**, 155 (1961). — MEYERDING, H.W., EVERT, J.A.: Mycetoma or Madura foot: report of cases including one case of maduromycosis of the hand. Minn. Med. **30**, 407 (1947). — MISRA, S.P., SHENDE, G.Y., YERNADEKAR, S.N., PADHYE, A.A., THIRUMALACHAR, M.J.: *Allescheria boydii* and *Emmonsia ciferrina* isolated from patients with chronic pulmonary infections. Hindustan Antibiot. Bull. **9**, 99 (1966). — MOHR, J.A., MUCHMORE, H.G.: Maduromycosis due to *Allescheria boydii*. J. Amer. med. Ass. **204**, 335 (1968). — MONTPELLIER, J., GUILLON, P.: Mycétome du pied (type pied de Madura) du à *l'Aleuvisma apiospermum*. Bull. Soc. Path. exot. **14**, 285 (1921). — NAUMANN, G., GREEN, W.R., ZIMMERMAN, L.E.: Mycotic keratitis. Amer. J. Ophthal. **64**, 668 (1967). — NIÑO, F.L.: Micetoma podal maduromicósico con granos blancos por *Monosporium apiospermum* en la Republica Argentina. Bol. Inst. Clín. quir. (B. Aires) **17**, 483 (1941). ~ *Allescheria boydii* Shear, 1921, agents etiológicos del micetoma maduromicósico a granos blancos en la Argentina. Pren. méd. argent. **36**, 314 (1949). ~ Estudio micologico de la segunda observación argentina de micetoma podal por, *Monosporium apiospermum*. Pren. méd. argent. **40**, 764 (1953). — NIÑO, F.L., FREIRE, R.S.: Maduromycotic mycetoma in Chaco province. Mycopathologia (Den Haag) **28**, 95 (1966). — NIÑO, F.L., FREIRE, R.S., SALICA, P.: El mícetoma maduromicosico en la provincia del Chaco. Rev. Asoc. méd. argent. **76**, 359 (1962). — PAUTLER, E.E., ROBERTS, R.W., BEAMER, P.R.: Mycotic infection of the eye: *Monosporium apiospermum* associated with corneal ulcer. Arch. Ophthal. **53**, 385 (1955). — REES. W.H.: A case of mycetoma in the New Hebrides., Trans. roy. Soc. trop. Med. Hyg. **56**, 538 (1962). — ROSEN, F., DECK, J.H.N., REWCASTLE, N.B.: *Allescheria boydii*: unique systemic dissemination to thyroid and brain. Canad. med. Ass. J. **93**, 1125 (1965). — SCHARYJ, M., LEVINE, N., GORDON, H.: Primary pulmonary infection with *Monosporium apiospermum*. J. infect. Dis. **106**, 141 (1960). — SCHMITT, J.A., ZABRANSKY, R.J., JANIDLO, A.S., PEARSONS, J.E.: Experimental maduromycosis in the laboratory mouse. Mycopathologia (Den Haag) **18**, 164 (1963). — SEABURY, J.H., KROLL, V.R., LANDRENEAU, R.: A conservative method of treatment for maduromycosis. South med. J. (Birmingham, Ala.) **52**, 1176 (1959). — SHAW, R.M., MacGREGOR, J.W.: Maduromycosis: with the report of a case due to *Monosporium apiospermum*. Canad. med. Ass. J. **33**, 23 (1935). — STOECKEL, H., ERMER, C.: Ein Fall von *Monosporium*-mycetom der Lunge. Beitr. Klin. Tuberk. **122**, 130 (1960). — TAYLOR, W.W., RADCLIFFE, F., VAN PEENEN, P.F.D.: The isolation of pathogenic fungi from the soils of Egypt, the Sudan, and Ethiopia. Sabouraudia **3**, 235 (1964). — THEODORESCU, ST., VULCAN, P., AVRAM, A., STOICA, I.: Micetom cugraunti albi al piciorului determinat *Monosporium apiospermum*. Derm. Vener. (Buc.) **1**, 114 (1956). — TONG, J.L., VALENTINE, E.H., DURRANCE, J.R., WILSON, G.M., FISHER, D.A.: Pulmonary infection with *Allescheria boydii:* report of a fatal case. Amer. Rev. Tuberc. **78**, 604 (1958). — TRAVIS, R.E., ULRICH, E.W., PHILLIPS, S.: Pulmonary allescheriasis. Ann. intern. Med. **54**, 141 (1961). — TWINING, H.E., DIXON, H.M., WEIDMAN, F.D.: Penicillin in the treatment of Madura foot: report of 2 cases. U.S. nav. med. Bull. **46**, 417 (1946). — VANBREUSEGHEM, R.: Early diagnosis, treatment, and epidemiology of mycetoma. Rev. Med. Vet. Mycol. **6**, 49 (1967). — VERGHESE, A., KLOKKE, A.H.: Histologic diagnosis of species of fungus causing mycetoma. Indian J. med. Res. **54**, 524 (1966). — WOLF, A., BENHAM, R., MOUNT, L.: Maduromycotic meningitis. J. Neuropath. exp. Neurol. **7**, 112 (1947). — ZAFFIRO, A.: Forma singolare di mycosi cutanea da *Monosporium apiospermum* a sviluppo clinicamete setticemo: Considerazioni diagnostiche deduzioni mediocolegali. Giorn. ital. Med. Milit. **86**, 636 (1938).

Alternariosis

AINSLEY, R., SMITH, B.: Fungal flora of the conjunctival sac in healthy and diseased eyes. Brit. J. Ophthal. **49**, 505 (1965). — BORSOOK, M.E.: Skin infection due to *Alternaria tenuis* with the report of a case. Canad. med. Ass. J. **29**, 479 (1933). — BOTTICHER, W.W.: *Alternaria* as a possible human pathogen. Sabouraudia **4**, 256 (1966). — HARRIS, L.H.:

Experimental reproduction of respiratory mold allergy. J. Allergy 12, 279 (1941). — HENRICI, A.T.: *Molds, Yeasts, and Actinomycetes.* John Wiley and Sons, Inc., 2nd ed., 1947. — HOPKINS, J.G., BENHAM, R.W., KESTEN, B.M.: Asthma due to a fungus *Alternaria.* J. Amer. med. Ass. 94, 6 (1930). — HYDE, H.A., WILLIAMS, D.A.: A daily census of *Alternaria* spores caught from the atmosphere at Cardiff in 1942 and 1943. Trans. Brit. Mycol. Soc. 29, 78 (1946). — MILLER, W.S., TINDALL, J.P.: Presented at Fourteenth Annual Meeting of the Zola Cooper Memorial Clinico-Pathologic Seminar, Miami, Florida Nov. 13, 1967. — OHASHI, Y.: On a rare disease due to *Alternaria tenuis Nees* (Alternariasis). Tohoku J. exp. Med. 72, 78 (1960). — PRATT, H.N., CROSSMAN, R.: The comparative atopic activity of *Alternaria* spores and mycelium. J. Allergy 13, 227 (1942). — PRINCE, H.E., EPSTEIN, S., FIGLEY, K.D., WITTICH, F.W., HENRY, L.D., MORROW, M.B.: Mold fungi in the etiology of respiratory allergic disease. IX. Further studies with mold extracts. Ann. Allergy 7, 301 (1949). — PRINCE, H.E., HALPIN, L.J., TALBOTT, G., ETTER, R.L., RAYMER, W.J., JACKSON, R.H., BARTLETT, L.L., MANSMANN, J.A., FRAYSER, L., EISENBERG, B.C., MORROW, M.B., MEYER, G.H.: Molds and bacteria in the etiology of respiratory allergic diseases. XXI. Studies with mold extracts produced from cultures grown in modified synthetic media. Ann. Allergy 19, 259 (1961). — WALTON, C.H.A.: Respiratory allergy due to fungi. Canad. med. Ass. J. 60, 272 (1949).

Arthrodermosis

EMMONS, C.W.: *Trichophyton mentagrophytes (Pinoyella simii)* isolated from dermatophytosis in the monkey. Mycopathologia (Den Haag) 2, 317 (1940). — GUGNANI, H.C., MULAY, D.N., MURTY, D.K.: Fungus flora of dermatophytosis and *Trichophyton simii* infection in North India. Indian. J. Derm. Venerol. 33, 73 (1967a). — GUGNANI, H.C., SHRIVASTAV, J.B., GUPTA, N.P.: Occurrence of *Arthroderma simii* in soil and on hair of small mammals. Sabouraudia 6, 77 (1967b). — KLOKKE, A.H., DURAIRAJ, P.: The causal agents of superficial mycoses in rural areas of South India. Sabouraudia 5, 153 (1967). — PINOY, E.: Sur une teigne cutanée du singe. C. R. Soc. Biol. (Paris) 72, 59 (1912a). ~ Epidermophyton du singe. Bull. Soc. Path. exot. 5, 60 (1912b). — RIPPON, J.W., ENG, A., MALKINSON, F.D.: *Trichophyton simii* infection in the United States. Arch. Derm. 98, 615 (1968). — SINGH, M.P.: Studies on the occurrence of mycotic infections in domestic animals and poultry. *M. V. Sc. Thesis, Agra University,* 1963 (cited by STOCKDALE et al., 1965). — STOCKDALE, P.M., MAC KENZIE, D.W.R., AUSTWICK, P.K.C.: *Arthroderma simii* sp. nov., the perfect stage of *Trichophyton simii* (Pinoy) Comb. Nov. Sabouraudia 4, 112 (1965).

Beauveriosis

BASSI, A.: Del mal del segno calcinaccio o moscardino malattia che affligge: bachi da seta. Partel. Teorica Tip. Orcesi, Lodi, 1835. — ELLINGBOE, A.H., KERNKAMP, M.F., HAWS, B.A.: Sweetclover weevil parasitized by *Beauvaria bassiana* (Bals.) Vuill. in Minnesota. J. Econ. Entomol. 50, 173 (1957). — FRÉOUR, P., LAFOURCADE, M., CHOMY, P.: Les champignons "*Beauveria*" en pathologie humaine: A propos d'un cas à localisation pulmonaire. Presse méd. 74, 2317 (1966a). ~ Une mycose nouvelle: étude clinique et mycologique d'une localization pulmonaire de "*Beauveria*". Bull. Soc. méd. Hôp. Paris 177, 197 (1966b). ~ Sur une mycose pulmonaire nouvelle due à "*Beauveria*". J. Méd. Bordeaux 143, 823 (1966c). — GEORG, L.W., WILLIAMSON, W.M., TILDEN, E.B., GETTY, R.E.: Mycotic pulmonary disease of captive giant tortoises due to *Beaveria bassiana* and *Paecilomyces fumoso-roseus.* Sabouraudia 2, 80 (1962). — LAHOURCADE, M.: *Bull. Soc. fran. Mycol. Méd.* 2, 30 (1966). — LANGERON, M.: Mycose oculaire primitive due au *Beauveria brumpti.* Bull. Acad. Méd. (Paris) III, 133 (1934). — MADELIN, M.F.: *Disease caused by Hyphomycetous Fungi.* In: *Insect Pathology: An Advanced Treatise* (Edited by STEINHAUS E.A.). Vol. 2, pp. 233—271. New York and London: Academic Press, 1963.

Cephalosporiosis

ALMEIDA, F. DE, SIMÔES-BARBOSA, F.A.: [*Cephalosporium recifei* isolated from case of Madura foot]. Arg. Inst. biol. S. Paulo 11, 1 (1940a). ~ Contribução para o estudo general dos micetomas maduromicóticos observados no Brasil. Micetomas brasileires. An. Fac. Med, S. Paulo 16, 235 (1940b). — ALMEIDA, F. DE, DA SILVA-LACAZ, C., RIBEIRO-OLIVEIRA, D.. CORDEIRO-DE AZEVEDO: Contribução para o estudo da micetomas ha Sao Paulo, Brazil, Madura foot a *Cephalosporium sp.* Rev. bras. Biol. 8, 287 (1948). — ARÊA-LEÃO, A.E. DE. LÔBO, J.: Mycétome du pied a *Cephalosporium recifei* n. sp. Mycétome a grains blancs. C. R. Soc. Biol. (Paris) 117, 203 (1934a). ~ Micetoma podal a *Cephalosporium recifei* n. sp. Micetoma de grãos biancos. C. R. Soc. Biol. Rio de S. 177, 203 (1934b). — ARIEVITCH, A.M., TJUFILINA, O.V., TEPLITZ, V.V.: [Gummo-ulcerative cephalosporiosis of the legs]. Vestn. Derm. Vener. (Mosk.) 38, 73 (1964). (Russian). — ARIEVITCH, A.M., STEPANISHCHEVA, Z.G., TJUFILINA, O.V., KUKOLEVA, Z.I., MALKINA, A.T., TEPLITZ, V.V.: Gummato-ulcerative cephalosporiosis of the skin. Mycopathologia (Den Haag) 28, 113 (1966). — ASCHIERI, E.: Recerche sistematiche e fesiologiche su *Hyalopus* causa di onicomicosi. Att. lst Bot. Pavia **4**, 45 (1932). — AVRAM, A.: Étude clinique et mycologique concernant le premier cas européen de mycétome déterminé par *Cephalosporium sp.* Mycopathologia (Den Haag) **24**, 177 (1964). ~ Étude sur des mycétomas de Roumaniae. Mycopathologia (Den Haag) **28**, 1 (1966a). ~ Experimental induction of grains with *Cephalosporium falciforme*. Sabouraudia **5**, 89 (1966b). ~ Experimental infections with *Cephalosporium falciforme, Monosporium apiospermum, Madurella mycetomi* and *Nocardia asteroides*. Mycopathologia (Den Haag) **32**, 319 (1967). — AVRAM, A., POROJAN, I., COJOCARU, I.: Trois nouveaux cas roumains de pied de Madura. Agents incriminés: *Nocardia asteroides, Cephalosporium falciforme* et *Madurella mycetomi*. Dermatologica (Basel) **136**, 311 (1968). — BALLAGI, S.: Mykologische Beschreibung der Acremoniosis. Arch. Derm. Syph. (Berl.) **166**, 405 (1932). — BASTARDO DE ALBORNOZ, M.C.: Micetoma (Pie de Madura) debido a *Cephalosporium recifei*. Derm. Venez **4**, 56 (1963/1964). — BATISTA, A., LIMA, J.A., OLIVEIRA, S.D., ARTAGAVEYTIA-ALLENDE, R.C.: Alguns *Hyalopus* assinalados sôbre suco gástrico e bile humana no Recife. Atas. Inst. Micol. Recife. **1**, 275 (1960). — BAYLET, R., CAMAIN, R., BÈZES, H.: Mycétomes à *Cephalosporium* au Sénégal. Bull. Soc. Path. exot. **54**, 802 (1961). — BEDELL, A.J.: *Cephalosporium* keratitis. Trans. Amer. ophth. Soc. **44**, 80 (1946). ~ *Cephalosporium* keratitis. Amer. J. Ophthal. **30**, 997 (1947). — BENEDEK, T.: Über Cephalosporiose. Ein Beitrag zur Kenntnis der seltenen Mykosen, unter besonderer Berücksichtigung der Serumdiagnose. Arch. Derm. Syph. (Berl.) **154**, 96 (1927a). ~ Vergleichende Untersuchungen über einige Arten der Gattung „*Cephalosporium*" nebst Mitteilung einer neuen Art: „*Cephalospor. Niveolanosum*" nov. spec. Arch. Derm. Syph. (Berl.) **154**, 154 (1927b). — BOMMER, S., WERNER, W., HAUFE, F.: Beitrag zur Pathologie der Cephalosporiose. Derm. Wschr. **144**, 952 (1961). — BORELLI, D.: Esquemas de micologia medica: micosis y suo agentes principales en Venezuela. Derm. Venez **3**, 136 (1962). — BOUCHER, H.: Les mycoses gommeuses de la Côte d'Ivoire. Bull. Soc. Path. exot. **11**, 306 (1918). — BURDA, C.D., FISHER, E., Jr.: Corneal destruction by extracts of *Cephalosporium* mycelium. Amer. J. Ophthal. **50**, 926 (1960). — BYERS, J.L., HOLLAND, M.G., ALLEN, J.H.: *Cephalosporium* keratitis. Amer. J. Ophthal. **49**, 267 (1960). — CABRINI, C., REDAELLI, P.: Sopra un caso di cefalosporiosi tonsillare. (*Cephalosporium acremonium* Corda). Boll. Soc. med.-chir. Pavia **7**, 475 (1929). — CARRIÓN, A.L.: Estudio micológico de un caso de micetoma por *Cephalosporium* en Puerto-Rico. Mycopathologia (Den Haag) **6**, 165 (1939). ~ *Cephalosporium falciforme* sp. nov. A new etiologic agent of maduromycosis. Mycologia **43**, 522 (1951). — CATANEI, A.: Sur quelques champignons saprophytes isolés au cours de la recherche de mycoses superficielles. Arch. Inst. Pasteur Alger **22**, 119 (1944). — CIFERRI, R.: *Cephalosporium pseudofermentum* n. sp., isolato della bocca dell'uomo. Arch. Protistenk. **78**, 227 (1932). — COUTELEN, F., COCHET, G.: Étude biologique d'un *Cephalosporium*, agent pathogène d'une gomme cervico-maxillaire de l'homme. C. R. Soc. Biol. (Paris) **139**, 392 (1945). — COUTELEN, F., COCHET, G., BIQUET, J.: Les Céphalosporioses humaines. Révue critique à propos d'un cas. Ann. Parasit. hum. comp. **23**, 364 (1948). — COWEN, D.E.: *Cephalosporium* midline granuloma. Trans. Indiana Acad. Ophthal. Otolaryng. **48**, 78 (1965). — COWEN, D.E., DINES, D.E.: *Cephalosporium* midline granuloma. Ann. intern. Med. **60**, 731 (1964) (Abstract). — COWEN, D.E., DINES, D.E., CHESSEN, J., PROCTOR, H.H.: *Cephalosporium* midline granuloma. Ann. intern. Med. **62**, 791 (1965). — DEBUSMANN, M.: Über das Vorkommen eines seltenen Pilzes (*Cephalosporium acremonium* Corda) im Blut bei tonsillogener Sepsis. Arch. Kinderheilk. **116**, 172 (1939). — DESTOMBES, P., SEGRETAIN, G.: Les mycétomes fongigues: caractères histologiques et culturaux. Arch. Inst. Pasteur Tunis **39**, 273 (1962). — DOUGLASS, R., SIMPSON, R.E.: *Cephalosporium* in pleural fluid. Amer. Rev. Tuberc. **48**, 237 (1943). — DROUHET, E., MARTIN, L., SEGRETAIN, G., DESTOMBES, P.: Mycose méningocérébrale à "*Cephalosporium*". Presse méd. **31**, 1809 (1965). — DU BOIS, C.: Onychomycoses non teigneuses. Dermatologica (Basel) **86**, 57 (1942). — FINE, B.S.: Intraocular mycotic infections. Lab. Invest. **11**, 1161 (1962). — FINE, B.S., ZIMMERMAN, L.E.: Exogenous intraocular fungus infections: with particular reference to complications of intraocular surgery. Amer. J. Ophthal. **48**, 151 (1959). — FOCOSI, M.: Su di un caso di concrezione micotica del sacco lacrimale. Boll. Oculist. **5**, 554 (1932a). — Su di un caso di cheratomicosi da *Cephalosporium*. (Contributo clinico sperimentale). Boll. Oculist. **12**, 1250 (1932b). — GAIND, M.L., PADHYE, A.A., THIRUMALACHAR, M.J.: Madura foot in India caused by *Cephalosporium infestans* sp. nov. Sabouraudia **1**, 230 (1962). — GAMET, A., BROTTES, H., ESSOMBA, R.: Nouveaux cas de mycétomes dépistés au Cameroun. Bull. Soc. Path. exot. **57**, 1191 (1964). — GINGRICH, W.D.: Keratomycosis. J. Amer. med. Ass. **179**, 602 (1962). — GONZALEZ-OCHOA, A., RUILOBA, J.: Acción del propionato de socio, in vitro sobre *Actinomyces mexicanas* y *Cephalosporium sp.* Ensayo terapéutico en micetomas producidos por estos hongos. Rev. Inst. Salubr. Enferm. trop. (Méx.) **5**, 83 (1944). — GOUGEROT, H., BURNIER, R., DUCHÉ, J.: Mycose végétante et ulcéreuse due au *Cephalosporium griseum*. Bull. Soc. franç. Derm. Syph. **40**, 417 (1933). — GREEN, W.R., BENNETT, J.E., GOOS, R.D.: Ocular penetration of amphotericin B: a report of laboratory studies and a case report post surgical *Cephalosporium* endophthalmitis. Arch. Ophthal. **73**,

769 (1965). — GRÜTZ, O.: Beitrag zu den seltenen Mykosen: Über einen durch *Akremonium* verursachte Pilzerkrankung. Derm. Wschr. **80**, 765 (1925). — HAENSCH, R.: Cephalosporiose ein Beitrag zur Klinik der seltenen Mykosen. Haut- u. Geschlechtskrankh. **23**, 137 (1957). — HARADA, S., USUI, Y.: [On a species of *Cephalosporium* isolated from the epidermophytosis between the toes]. Nagaoa **7**, 51 (1960) (Japanese). — HARTMANN, E.: Über ein gemeinsames Vorkommen von *Cephalosporium* und *Trichophyton gypseum*. Derm. Wschr. **82**, 565 (1926). — HOFFMANN, D.H., NAUMANN, G.: Ein Beitrag zur Pilzinfektion der Hornhaut. Klin. Mbl. Augenheilk. **142**, 286 (1963). — JANKE, D.: Zur Klinik und Mykologie der Cephalosporiose. Ein Beitrag zur Kenntnis seltener Mykosen. Arch. Derm. Syph. (Berl.) **188**, 257 (1949). — JANKE, D., ROHRSCHNEIDER, W.: Beitrag zu den seltenen Mykosen: über eine Pilzerkrankung der Tränenröhren und der Oberhaut und Befund eines bisher unbekannten *Cephalosporiums*. Derm. Wschr. **123**, 49 (1951). — KAMBAYASHI, T.: Botanische Untersuchungen über japanische Fadenpilze, die auf der Menschenhaut parasitieren. III. Mitteilung. Über *Cephalosporium nigrum* n. sp. isoliert von einer Dermatomycosis in Oethiopien. Botan. Mag. (Tokyo) **51**, 436 (1937). — KÜPER, J.: Zur Klinik postoperativer intraokutarer Mykosen. Klin. Mbl. Augenheilk. **140**, 827 (1962). — KESTEVEN, H.L.: The mycotic flora of "Surfer's foot" in Sydney. Med. J. Aust. **1**, 420 (1939). — KUKOLEVA, L.I., MALKUHA, A.R.: [A case of extensive gumma-ulcerative cephalosporiosis]. Vestn. Derm. Vener. (Mosk.) **41**, 76 (1967). (Russian). — LACAZ, C. DA S., FAVA NETTO, C.: Contribution à l'étude des agents étiologiques des maduromycoses. Folia clín. biol. **21**, 331 (1954). — LATAPÍ, F., ORTIZ, Y.: Los micetomas en México. Memorias del primer congreso de dermatología. pp. 126—144 (1963). — LEHNER, E. VON: Über einen Fall von *Acremoniosis*. Arch. Derm. Syph. (Berl.) **166**, 399 (1932). — LÔBO, J.: Micetomas podias em Pernambuco. An. Fac. Med. Recife 8—**9**, 5 (1943). ~ Micetomas em Pernambuco. Rev. Fac. Med. Univ. Ceara **3**, 5 (1963). — MACKINNON, J.E.: Los agentes de maduromicosis de los géneros *Monosporium*, *Allescheria*, *Cephalosporium* y otros de dudosa identidad. An. Fac. Med. Montevideo **36**, 153 (1951). ~ A contribution to the study of the causal organisms of maduromycosis. Trans. roy. Soc. trop. Med. Hyg. **48**, 470 (1954). ~ Agentes de maduromicosis en la región neotropical. An. Fac. Med. Montevideo **48**, 453 (1963). — MAFFEI, O.L.: Nuova species di *Cephalosporium* causa di una cheratomicosi dell' chio. Atti. Ist. Bot. R. Univ. Pavia **1**, 183 (1929). — MALE, O., TAPPEINER, J.: Nagelveränderungen durch Schimmelpilze. Derm. Wschr. **151**, 212 (1965). — MARIAT, F.: Sur la distribution geographique et la repartition des agents de mycetomes. Bull. Soc. Path. exot. **56**, 35 (1963). — MATRUCHOT: Cited by COUTELEN et al., 1948. — MILLER, H.E., MORROW, H.: Cephalosporiosis: an unusual mycotic infection. Arch. Derm. Syph. (Chic.) **25**, 294 (1932). — MOORE, M.: Onychomycosis caused by species of three separate genera: report of a case with a study of a species of *Hyalopus (Cephalosporium)*. J. invest. Derm. **24**, 489 (1955). — MÜHLENS, K.J.: Beobachtungen an drei Cephalosporienstämme die aus menschlichem Blut und Harn gezüchtet wurden. Zbl. Bakt., I. Abt. Ref. **142**, 160 (1938). — MURRAY, I.G., HOLT, H.D.: Is *Cephalosporium acremonium* capable of producing maduromycosis? Mycopathologia (Den Haag) **22**, 335 (1964). — NAKAMURA, T.: Demonstration der Actinomyces Kulturen und ein Fall von Cephalosporiosis. Jap. Dermato-Urol. Tochterges., Tokyo, Sitzung v. 13. VI. 1933 (Cited by COUTELEN et al., 1948). — NAUMANN, G., GREEN, W.R., ZIMMERMAN, L.E.: Mycotic keratitis a histopathologic study of 73 cases. Amer. J. Ophthal. **64**, 668 (1967). — NEGRONI, P.: Onicomicosis por *Cephalosporium spinosus* n. sp. Negroni. Rev. Soc. argent. Biol. **9**, 16 (1933a). ~ Onycomicose par *Cephalosporium spinosus* n. sp. Negroni. C. R. Soc. Biol. (Paris) **113**, 478 (1933b). — PADHYE, A.A., SUKAPURE, R.S., THIRUMALACHAR, M.J.: *Cephalosporium madurae* n. sp., Cause of Madura foot in India. Mycopathologia (Den Haag) **16**, 315 (1962). — PADHYE, A.A., GOKHALE, B.B., THIRUMALACHAR, M.J.: Studies on some cases of deep mycoses with special reference to the in vitro activity of some new antifungal antibiotics. Hindustan Antibiot. Bull. **5**, 74 (1963). — PISANO, M.A.: Activities of the cephalosporia. Trans. N.Y. Acad. Sci. **25**, 716 (1963). — PITOTTI, P.: Un caso di acremoniosi cutanea. Rif. med. **48**, 1567 (1932). — PONNAMPALAM, J.T.: The genus *Cephalosporium* as a cause of Madura foot in Malaya. Med. J. Malaya **18**, 229 (1964). — SEGRETAIN, G.: Some new or infrequent fungous pathogens. In *Fungi and Fungous diseases*. Springfield, Illinois: Charles C. Thomas 1962. — SCHMIDT, VAN BEYMA: (1933) (Cited by COUTELEN et al., 1948). — SIMÔES-BARBOSA, F.A.: Concerning a new hyphomycete parasite of man: *Cephalosporium cordoniformis* n. sp. Mycopathologia (Den Haag) **3**, 93 (1941). — THEODORE, F.H., LITTMAN, M.L., ALMEDA, E.: The diagnosis and management of fungus endophthalmitis following cataract extraction. Arch. Ophthal. **66**, 163 (1961). — VERGHESE, A., KLOKKE, A.H.: Histologic diagnosis of species of fungus causing mycetoma. Indian J. med. Res. **54**, 524 (1966). — VERKHOLOMOV, E.E.: [Methods for the acquisition of haemocultures of some hyphal fungi from the blood of cancer patients] Botan. Zh. SSSR **46**, 357 (1961) (Russian). — WALSHE, M.M., ENGLISH, M.P.: Fungi in nails. Brit. J. Derm. **78**, 198 (1966). — WARD, H.P., MARTIN, W.J., IVINS, J.C., WEED, L.A.: *Cephalosporium* arthritis. Proc. Mayo Clin. **36**, 337 (1961). — WEIDMAN, F.D., KLIGMAN, A.M.: A new species of *Cephalosporium* in Madura foot (*Cephalo*-

sporium granulomatis). J. Bact. **50**, 491 (1945). — ZAIAS, N.: Superficial white onychomycosis. Sabouraudia **5**, 99 (1966). — ZIMMERMANN, L.E.: Mycotic keratitis. Lab. Invest. **11**, 1151 (1962). ~ Keratomycosis. Surv. Ophthal. **8**, 1 (1963).

Cercosporamycosis

CHUPP, C.: The possible infection of the human body with *Cercospora apii*. Mycologia **49**, 773 (1957). — EMMONS, C.W., BINFORD, C.H., UTZ, J.P.: *Medical Mycology*, p. 346. Philadelphia: Lea and Febiger 1963. — EMMONS, C.W., LIE-KIAN-JOE, NJO-INJO TJOEI ENG, POHAN, A., KERTOPATI, S., VAN DER MEULEN, A.: *Basidiobolus* and *Cercospora* from human infections. Mycologia **49**, 1 (1957). — LIE-KIAN-JOE, NJO-INJO TJOEI ENG, KERTOPATI, S., EMMONS, C.W.: A new verrucous mycosis caused by *Cercospora apii*. Arch. Derm. **75**, 864 (1957).

Cryptostromosis

EMANUEL, D.A., LAWTON, B.R., WENZEL, F.J.: Maple-bark disease: pneumonitis due to *Coniosporium corticale*. New Engl. J. Med. **266**, 333 (1962). — EMANUEL, D.A., WENZEL. F.J., LAWTON, B.R.: Pneumonitis due to *Cryptostroma corticale* (Maple-bark disease). New Engl. J. Med. **274**, 1413 (1966). — GREGORY, P.H., WALLER, S.: *Cryptostroma corticale* and sooty bark disease of sycamore (*Acer pseudoplantanus*). Trans. Brit. Mycol. Soc. **34**, 579 (1951). — TOWEY, J.W., SWEANY, H.C., HURON, W.H.: Severe bronchial asthma apparently due to fungus spores found in maple bark. J. Amer. med. Ass. **99**, 453 (1932). — WENZEL, F.J., EMANUEL, D.A.: The epidemiology of maple bark disease. Arch. environm. Hlth. **14**, 385 (1967).

Curvulariosis

ANDERSON, B., ROBERTS, S.S., Jr., GONZALEZ, D., CHICK, E.W.: Mycotic ulcerative keratitis. Arch. Ophthal. **62**, 169 (1959). — BAYLET, J., CAMAIN, R., SEGRETAIN, G.: Identification des agents des maduromycoses du Sénégal et de la Mauritanie: description d'une espèce nouvelle. Bull. Soc. Path. exot. **52**, 447 (1959). — BRIDGES, C.H.: Maduromycotic mycetomas in animals. *Curvularia geniculata* as an etiologic agent. Amer. J. Path. **33**, 411 (1957). ~ Maduromycosis of bovine nasal mucosa (nasal granuloma of cattle). Cornell Vet. **50**, 469 (1960). — GEORG, L.K.: *Curvularia geniculata*, a cause of mycotic keratitis. J. med. Ass. Ala. **31**, 234 (1964). — NITYANANDA, K., SIVASUBRAMANIAM, P., AJELLO, L.: Mycotic keratitis caused by *Curvularia lunata*: case report. Sabouraudia **2**, 35 (1962). ~ A case of mycotic keratitis caused by *Curvularia geniculata*. Arch. Ophthal. **71**, 456 (1964). — PARMELEE, J.A.: The identification of the *Curvularia* parasite of Gladiolus. Mycologia **48**, 558 (1956). — ROBERTS, E.D., MCDANIEL, H.A., CARBREY, E.A.: Maduromycosis of the bovine nasal mucosa. J. Amer. vet. med. Ass. **142**, 42 (1963). — SPRAGUE, R.: *Diseases of Cereals and Grasses in North America*. New York: The Ronald Press, 1950. — WARREN, C.M., Jr.: Dangers of steroids in ophthalmology with report of a case of mycotic perforating corneal ulcer. J. med. Ass. Ala. **33**, 229 (1964).

Dermatophilosis

AUSTWICK, P.K.C.: Cutaneous streptothricosis, mycotic dermatitis, and strawberry foot rot and the genus *Dermatophilus* Van Saceghem. Vet. Rev. Annot. **4**, 33 (1958). — DEAN, D.J., GORDON, M.A., SEVERINGHAUS, C.W., KROLL, E.T., REILLY, J.R.: Streptothricosis: a new zoonotic disease. N.Y. St. J. Med. **61**, 1283 (1961). — GORDON, M.A.: The genus *Dermatophilus*. J. Bact. **88**, 509 (1964). — GORDON, M.A., EDWARDS, M.R.: Micromorphology of *Dermatophilus congolensis*. J. Bact. **86**, 1101 (1963). — HART, C.B., TYSZKIEWICZ, K., ROGERS, B.A., KANE, G.J.: Mycotic dermatitis in sheep. II. *Dermatophilus congolensis* and its reaction to compounds *in vitro*. Vet. Rec. **81**, 623 (1967). — HUDSON, J.R.: Cutaneous streptothricosis. Proc. roy. Soc. Med. **30**, 1457 (1937). — KAPLAN, W.: Dermatophilosis: a recently recognized disease in the United States. Southwest. Vet. **20**, 14 (1966). — KAPLAN, W., JOHNSTON, W.J.: Equine dermatophilosis (cutaneous streptothricosis) in Georgia. J. Amer. vet. med. Ass. **149**, 1162 (1966). — LE RICHE, P.D.: The transmission of dermatophilosis (mycotic dermatitis) in sheep. Aust. vet. J. **44**, 64 (1968). — MACADAM, I.: The effects of ectoparasites and humidity on natural lesions of streptothricosis. Vet. Rec. **76**, 345 (1964). — PIER, A.C., NEAL, F.C., CYSEWSKI, S.J.: Cutaneous Streptothricosis in Iowa Cattle. J. Amer. vet. med. Ass. **142**, 995 (1963). — RICHARD, J.L., PIER, A.C.: Transmission of *Dermatophilus congolensis* by *Stomoxys calcitrans* and *Musca domestica*. Amer. J. vet. Res. **27**, 419 (1966). — ROBERTS, D.S.: Barriers to *Dermatophilus dermatonomus* infection on the skin of sheep. Aust. J. Agric. Res. **14**, 492 (1963). ~ The role of granulocytes in resistance to *Dermatophilus congolensis*. Brit. J. exp. Path. **46**, 643 (1965a). ~ The histopathology of epidermal infection with the actinomycete *Dermatophilus congolensis*. J. Path. Bact. **90**, 213 (1965b). ~ Cutaneous actinomycosis due to the single species *Dermatophilus congolensis*. Nature (Lond.) **206**, 1068 (1965c). ~ Chemotherapy of epidermal infection with *Dermatophilus congolensis*. J. comp. Path. **77**,

129 (1967). — SEARCY, G.P., HULLAND, T.J.: Dermatophilus dermatitis (streptotrichosis) in Ontario. I. Clinical observations. Canad. vet. J. **9**, 7 (1968a). ~ Dermatophilus dermatitis (streptotrichosis) in Ontario. II. Laboratory findings. Canad. vet. J. **9**, 16 (1968b). — SMITH, J.M.B., DANIEL, R.C.W., BRUERE, A.N.: *Dermatophilosis:* an emerging disease in New Zealand. N. Z. vet. J. **15**, 88 (1967). — VAN SACEGHEM, R.: Dermatose contagieuse (Impetigo contagieux). Bull. Soc. Path. exot. **8**, 354 (1915). — VANDEMAELE, F.P.: Investigation of cutaneous streptothricosis in Africa. Bull. epizoot. Dis. Afr. **9**, 251 (1961). — ZLOTNIK, I.: Cutaneous streptothricosis in cattle. Vet. Rec. **67**, 613 (1955).

Fusariosis

ANDERSON, B., CHICK, E.W.: Mycokeratitis: treatment of fungal corneal ulcers with amphotericin B and mechanical debridement. South med. J. (Birmingham, Ala.) **56**, 270 (1963). — ANDERSON, B., ROBERTS, S.S., GONZALEZ, C., CHICK, E.W.: Mycotic ulcerative keratitis. Arch. Ophthal. **62**, 169 (1959). — ARNSTEIN, H.R., COOK, A.H., LACEY, M.S.: Production of antibiotics by fungi. II. Production of *Fusarium javanicum* and other fusaria. Brit. J. exp. Path. **27**, 349 (1946). — BOISSEVAIN, C.H.: Growth inhibition of tubercle bacilli by *Fusarium sp.* Proc. Soc. exp. Biol. Med. (N.Y.) **63**, 555 (1946). — BOTTICHER, W.W.: *Alternaria* as a possible human pathogen. Sabouraudia **4**, 256 (1966). — CAJORI, F.A., OTANI, T.T., HAMILTON, M.A.: Isolation and some properties of antibiotic from *Fusarium bostrycoides*. J. biol. Chem. **208**, 107 (1954). — CHICK, E.W., CONANT, N.F.: Mycotic ulcerative keratitis: a review of 148 cases from the literature. Invest. Ophthal. **1**, 419 (1962). (Abstract). — COOK, A.H., COX, S.F., FARMER, T.H., LACEY, M.S.: Production of antibiotics by fusaria. Nature (Lond.) **160**, 31 (1947). — EMMONS, C.W.: Misuse of name "*Trichophyton Rosaceum*" for saprophytic fusarium. J. Bact. **47**, 107 (1944). — FORGACS, J.: Mycotoxicoses: neglected diseases. Feedstuffs **34**, 124 (1962a). ~ Mycotoxicoses in animal and human health. U. S. Livestock Sanitary A. 426 (1962b). — FORGACS, J., CARLL, W.T.: Mycotoxicoses. Advanc. vet. Sci. **7**, 273 (1962). — FREI, W.: Urethritis posterior chronica mycotica. Derm. Wschr. **80**, 411 (1925). — GAMET, A., BROTTES, H., ESSOMBA, R.: [New cases of mycetoma detected in the Cameroons] Bull. Soc. Path. exot. **57**, 1191 (1964). — GILLESPIE, F.D.: Fungus corneal ulcer: report of a case. Amer. J. Ophthal. **56**, 823 (1963). — GINGRICH, W.D.: Keratomycosis. J. Amer. med. Ass. **179**, 602 (1962). — HOLZEGEL, K., KEMPF, H.F.: [Fusarium mycosis of the skin of a burned patient.] Derm. Wschr. **150**, 651 (1964). — JOFFE, A.Z.: The mycoflora of overwintered cereals and its toxicity. Bull. Res. Coun. Israel 9D, 101 (1960). ~ Biological properties of some toxic fungi isolated from overwintered cereals. Mycopathologia (Den Haag) **16**, 201 (1962). ~ Toxicity of overwintered cereals. Plant Soil **18**, 31 (1963). ~ Toxin production by cereal fungi causing toxic alimentary aleukia in man. In: *Mycotoxins in Foodstuffs*, pp. 77—85. WOGEN, G.N., Ed. Cambridge, Massachusetts: M. I. T. Press 1965. — LACEY, M.S.: The antibiotic properties of 52 strains of *Fusarium*. J. gen. Microbiol. **4**, 122 (1950). — LAZARUS, J.A., SCHWARZ, L.H.: Infestation of urinary bladder with unusual fungus (*Fusarium*) Urol. cutan. Rev. **52**, 185 (1948). — LYNN, J.R.: *Fusarium* keratitis treated with cycloheximide. Amer. J. Ophthal. **58**, 637 (1964). — MAYER, C.F.: Endemic panmyelotoxicosis in Russian grain belt. I. Clinical aspects of alimentary toxic aleukia (ATA): comprehensive review. Milit. Surg. **113**, 173 (1953a). — MIKAMI, R., STEMMERMANN, G.N.: Keratomycosis: caused by *Fusarium oxysporum*. Amer. J. clin. Path. **29**, 257 (1958). — MING, Y.N., YU, T.F.: Identification of a pathogenic *Fusarium* isolated from foot ulcer of a male patient. Acta. Microbiol. Sinica **10**, 409 (1964). — PETERSON, J.E., BAKER, T.J.: An isolate of *Fusarium roseum* from human burns. Mycologia **51**, 453 (1959). — PERZ, M.: *Fusarium nivale* as a cause of corneal mycosis. Klin. oczna **36**, 609 (1966). — SARKISOV, A.C., KVASHNINA, E.S.: [Toxicological properties of *Fusarium sporotrichioides*, in "cereal crops wintered under snow."] Publ. Min. Agr. Moscow 89 (1948) (Russian). — SIGTENHORST, M.L., GINGRICH, W.D.: Bacteriologic studies of keratitis. South. med. J. (Birmingham, Ala.) **50**, 346 (1957). — STOKES, J.A.: Fusarium keratomycosis: report of a case successfully treated with griseofulvin 1959, cited by HILDICK-SMITH, G., BLANK, H., and SARKANY, I. *Fungus diseases and their management*, p. 355. Boston: Little Brown 1963. — WOLLENWEBER, H.W., SHERBAKOFF, O.A., REINKING, O.A., JOHANN, H., BAILEY, A.A.: Fundamentals for taxonomic studies of *Fusarium*. J. Agr. Res. **30**, 833 (1925). — WOLLENWEBER, H.W., REINKING, O.A.: *Die Fusarien*. Berlin: Paul Parey 1935. — ZAIAS, N.: Superficial white onychomycosis. Sabouraudia **5**, 99 (1966). — ZIMMERMAN, L.E.: Keratomycosis. Surv. Ophthal. **8**, 1 (1963).

Helminthosporiosis

DOLAN, C.T., WEED, L.A.: Opportunistic mycotic pulmonary infection by the family Dematiaceae. Amer. J. clin. Path. **50**, 600 (1968) (Abstract). — DOLAN, C.T., WEED, L.A., DINES, D.E.: Bronchopulmonary Helminthosporiosis. Amer. J. clin. Path. **53**, 235 (1970). — GEORG, L.K.: *Curvularia geniculata*, a cause of mycotic keratosis. J. med. Ass. Ala. **31**, 234 (1964). — ROBERTS, E.D., McDANIEL, H.A., CARBREY, E.A.: Maduromycosis of the bovine nasal mucosa. J. Amer. vet. med. Ass. **142**, 42 (1963). — Walton, C.H.A.: Respiratory allergy due to fungi. Canad. med. Ass. J. **60**, 272 (1949).

Keratomycosis

Agarwal, L.P., Malik, S.R.K., Mohan, M., Khosla, P.K.: Mycotic corneal ulcer. Brit. J. Ophthal. **47**, 109 (1963). — Ainley, R., Smith, B.: Fungal flora of the conjunctival sac in healthy and diseased eyes. Brit. J. Ophthal. **49**, 505 (1965). — Anderson, B., Chick, E.W.: Mycokeratitis: treatment of fungal corneal ulcers with amphotericin B and mechanical debridement. South. med. J. (Birmingham, Ala.) **56**, 270 (1963). — Anderson, B., Jr., Roberts, S.S., Gonzalez, C., Chick, E.W.: Mycotic ulcerative keratitis. Arch. Ophthal. **62**, 169 (1959). — Bedell, A.J.: *Cephalosporium* keratitis. Trans. Amer. ophthal. Soc. **44**, 80 (1946). ~ *Cephalosporium* keratitis. Amer. J. Ophthal. **30**, 997 (1947). — Burda, C.D., Fisher, E., Jr.: Corneal destruction by extract of *Cephalosporium* mycelium. Amer. J. Ophthal. **50**, 926 (1960). — Byers, J.L., Holland, M.G., Allen, J.H.: *Cephalosporium* keratitis. Amer. J. Ophthal. **49**, 267 (1960). — Chick, E.W., Conant, N.F.: Mycotic ulcerative keratitis: a review of 148 cases from the literature. Invest. Ophthal. **1**, 419 (1962) (Abstract). — Ernest, J.T., Rippon, M.W.: Keratitis due to *Allescheria boydii (Monosporium apiospermum)*. Amer. J. Ophthal. **62**, 1202 (1966). — Fazakas, S. Von: Zusammenfassender Bericht über die sekundären Mykosen bei Erkrankungen des Augenlidrandes, der Bindehaut und der Hornhaut. Ophthal. **138**, 108 (1959). — Focosi, M.: Su di un caso di cheratomicosi dá *Cephalosporium* (Contributo clinico sporimentale). Boll. Oculist. **12**, 1250 (1932). — Georg, L.K.: *Curvularia geniculata*, a cause of mycotic keratitis. J. med. Ass. Ala. **31**, 234 (1964). — Gillespie, F.D.: Fungus corneal ulcer: report of a case. Amer. J. Ophthal. **56**, 823 (1963). — Gingirch, W.D.: Keratomycosis. J. Amer. med. Ass. **179**, 602 (1962). — Gordon, M.A., Vallotton, W.W., Croffead, G.S.: Corneal allescheriosis: a case of keratomycosis treated successfully with nystatin and amphotericin B. Arch. Ophthal. **62**, 758 (1959). — Haggerty, T.E., Zimmerman, L.E.: Mycotic keratitis. South. med. J. (Birmingham, Ala.) **51**, 153 (1958). — Hildick-Smith, G., Blank, H., Sarkany, I.: *Fungus Diseases and their Treatment*, Little, Brown and Company, Boston: 1st ed. pp. 347—357, 1964. — Hoffmann, D.H., Naumann, G.: Ein Beitrag zur Pilzinfektion der Hornhaut. Klin. Mbl. Augenheilk. **42**, 286 (1963). — Kinnas, J.S.: Ophthalmic diseases caused by a mycete of the giant cane. Brit. J. Ophthal. **49**, 327 (1965). — Leber, T.: Keratomycosis aspergillina als Ursache von Hypopyonkeratitis. Arch. Ophthal. [v. Graefes] **25**, 285 (1879). — Ley, A.P., Sanders, T.E.: Fungus keratitis: report of three cases. A.M.A. Arch. Ophthal. (N.S.) **56**, 257 (1956). — Lynn, J.R.: *Fusarium* keratitis treated with cycloheximide. Amer. J. Ophthal. **58**, 637 (1964). — Maffei, O.L.: Nuova specie di *Cephalosporium* causa di una cheratomicosi dell' echio. Atti. Ist. Bot. R. Univ. Pavia **1**, 183 (1928). — Manchester, P.T., Jr., Georg, L.K.: Corneal ulcer due to *Candida parapsilosis (C. parakrusei)*. J. Amer. med.Ass. **171**, 1339 (1959). — Mangiaracine, A.B., Liebman, S.D.: Fungus keratitis (*Aspergillus fumigatus*): treatment with nystatin (mycostatin). Arch. Ophthal. (N.S.) **58**, 695 (1957). — Mendelblatt, D.L.: Moniliasis: a review and a report of the first case demonstrating the *Candida albicans* in the cornea. Amer. J. Ophthal. **36**, 379 (1953). — Mikami, R., Stemmermann, G.N.: Keratomycosis caused by *Fusarium oxysporum*. Amer. J. clin. Path. **29**, 257 (1958). — Minoda, Y.: Effect of antibiotics on some fungi isolated from ocular lesions. Acta Soc. Ophthal. Japon. **61**, 562 (1957). — Mitsui, Y., Hanabusa, J.: Corneal infections after cortisone therapy. Brit. J. Ophthal. **39**, 244 (1955). — Naumann, G., Green, W.R., Zimmerman, L.E.: Mycotic keratitis: a histopathologic study of 73 cases. Amer. J. Ophthal. **64**, 668 (1967). — Nityananda, K., Sivasubramaniam, P., Ajello, L.: Mycotic keratitis caused by *Curvularia lunata*: case report. Sabouraudia **2**, 35 (1962). — Pautler, E.E., Roberts, R.W., Beamer, P.R.: Mycotic infection of the eye: *Monosporium apiospermum* associated with corneal ulcer. Arch. Ophthal. **53**, 385 (1955). — Perz, M.: [*Fusarium nivale* as a cause of corneal mycosis]. Klin. oczna **36**, 609 (1966). — Seligmann, E.: Virulence enhancing activities of Aureomycin on *Candida albicans*. Proc. Soc. exp. Biol. (N.Y.) **79**, 481 (1952). ~ Virulence enhancement of *Candida albicans* by antibiotics and cortisone. Proc. Soc. exp. Biol. (N.Y.) **83**, 778 (1953). — Suie, T., Havener, W.H.: Mycology of the eye: review. Amer. J. Ophthal. **56**, 63 (1963). — Zimmerman, L.E.: Mycotic keratitis. Lab. Invest. **11**, 1151 (1962). ~ Keratomycosis. Surv. Ophthal. **8**, 1 (1963).

Otomycosis

Ananthanarayan, R.: Otomycosis in South Indians. Indian J. Surg. **13**, 344 (1951), — Batista, A.C., Maia, H.S., Cavalcanti, W.: Otomycosis caused by *Waldemaria pernambucensis* n. gen. n. sp. Atas. Inst. Micol. Recife **5**—12 (1960). — Belding, D.L., Umanzio, C.B.: A new species of the genus *Monosporium* associated with chronic otomycosis. Amer. J. Path. **11**, 856 (1935). — Blank, F., Stuart, E.A.: *Monosporium apiospermum* Sacc., 1911, associated with otomycosis. Canad. med. J. **72**, 601 (1955). — Briceño-Maaz, T., Briceño-Maaz, C.: Otomicois. Gac. méd. Caracas **72**, 509 (1964). — English, M.P.: Otomycosis caused by a ringworm fungus. J. Laryng. Otol. **71**, 207 (1957). — GILL, W. D.: Otomycosis: Some comments concerning its incidence, symptomatology and treatment. South. med. J. (Birmingham, Ala.) **40**, 637 (1947). — GREGSON, A. E. W., LaTOUCHE, C. J.: Otomycosis: a neglected disease. J. Laryng. Otol. **75**, 45 (1961). — HALEY, L. D.: Etiology of otomycosis. I. Mycologic flora of the ear. Arch. Otolaryng. **52**, 202 (1950). — KEOGH, C., RUSSELL, B.: The problem of otitis externa. Brit. med. J. **1**, 1068 (1956). — KINGERY, F. A.: The myth of otomycosis. J. Amer. med. Ass. **191**, 129 (1965). — KUNEL'SKAYA, V. Y., STEPANISHCHEVA, Z. G.: [Mycotic flora in otitis externa]. Vestn. Derm. Vener. **38**, 51 (1964) (Russian). — LAKSHMIPATHI, G., MURTI, B.: Otomycosis. J. Indian med. Ass. **34**, 439 (1960). — LEA, W. A., SCHUSTER, D. S., HARRELL, E. R.: Mycological flora of the healthy external auditory canal: a study of 120 human subjects. J. invest. Derm. **31**, 137 (1958). — McBURNEY, R., GULLEDGE, M. A.: Investigation of certain fungicides and bactericides for use in otitis externa. Ann. Otol. Rhinol. Laryng. (St. Louis) **64**, 1009 (1955). — MOHAPATRA, L. M.: A study of the fungi isolated from cases of otomycosis. Indian J. Microbiol. **1**, 103 (1961). — SHARP, W. B., JOHN, M. B., ROBISON, J. M.: Etiology of otomycosis. Tex. St. J. Med. **42**, 380 (1946). — SMYTH, G. D. L.: A preliminary report on fungal infections of mastoid and fenestration cavities. J. Laryng. Otol. **75**, 703 (1961). — STUART, E. A., BLANK, F.: Aspergillosis of the ear: a report of twenty-nine cases. Canad. med. Ass. J. **72**, 334 (1955). — TOMIĆ-KAROVIĆ, V. K., POPADIC, V.: Mittelohrentzündungen. Verursacht durch *Candida albicans*. Schweiz. med. Wschr. **83**, 59 (1953). — WOLF, F. T.: Relation of various fungi to otomycosis. Arch. Otolaryng. **46**, 361 (1947).

Paecilomycosis

PODEDWORNY, W., SUIE, T.: Mycotic infection of the sclera. Amer. J. Ophthal. **58**, 494 (1964). — ŠAULOV, I.: Die Nagelpilzformen im Gebiet von Plovdiv/Südbulgarien. Derm. Wschr. **151**, 716 (1965). — UYS, C. J., DON, P. A., SCHRIRE, V., BARNARD, C. N.: Endocarditis following cardiac surgery due to the fungus *Paecilomyces*. S. Afr. med. J. **37**, 1276 (1963).

Penicilliosis

AIMÉ, P., CREUZÉ, P., KRESSER, H.: Mycose pulmonaire à *"Penicillium crustaceum"* avec signes clinique et aspect radiologique d'abcès du poumon. Presse méd. **41**, 761 (1933). — AINLEY, R., SMITH, B.: Fungal flora of the conjunctival sac in healthy and diseased eyes. Brit. J. Ophthal. **49**, 505 (1965). — ANDERSON, B., ROBERTS, S. S., GONZALEZ, C., CHICK, E. W.: Mycotic ulcerative keratitis. Arch. Ophthal. **62**, 169 (1959). — ANDREEV, V. G.: [Causal agents of dermatomycoses in the Kursk region.] Vestn. Derm. Vener. **38**, 85 (1964) (Russian). — ARIEVICH, A. M., STEPANISHCHEVA, Z. G.: [The first experience of using antibiotic grisemin for the treatment of patients with mold mycoses]. Antibiotiki (Moskva) **9**, 186 (1964) (Russian). — BUGYI, B.: Coniomicosi dei lavoratori del riso. Med. d. Lavoro **49**, 368 (1958). — CAPPONI, M., SUREAU, P., SEGRETAIN, G.: Pénicillose de *Rhizomys sinensis*. Bull. Soc. Path. exot. **49**, 418 (1956). — CASTELLANI, A.: The higher fungi in relation to human pathology. Lancet **1**, 895 (1920). — CHICK, E. W., CONANT, N. F.: Mycotic ulcerative keratitis: a review of 148 cases from the literature. Invest. Ophthal. **1**, 419 (1962) (Abstract). — CHUTE, A. L.: An infection of the bladder with *Penicillium glaucum*. Boston Surg. J. **164**, 420 (1911). — DA SILVA, LACAZ, D.: Consideraçóes sobre um caso di peniciliose pulmonar. Hospital (Rio de J.) **14**, 327 (1939). — DELORE, P., COUDERT, J., LAMBERT, R., FAYOLLE, J.: Un cas de mycose bronchique avec localisations musculaires septicémiques. Presse méd. **63**, 1580 (1955). — DE MONTEMAYOR, L., RODRIQUEZ, R., SALAS, M.: Hongos alergenicos en los esputos (estudio sorbre 92 casos de asma y rinitis). Mycopathologia (Den Haag) **26**, 410 (1965). — ENOMOTO, M.: Histopathological studies on adenomatous nodules of liver produced in mice by *Penicillium islandicum* Sopp. Acta path. jap. **9**, 189 (1959). — FAZAKAS, S.: Zusammenfassender Bericht über die sekundären Mykosen bei Erkrankungen des Augenlidrandes, der Bindehaut und der Hornhaut. Ophthalmologica (Basel) **138**, 108 (1959). — GARRETÓN, U. I.: Un caso de bronquitis micotica à *Penicillium*. An. méd. Concepción **2**, 103 (1945). — GERNEZ-RIEUX, C., BIGUET, P., CAPRON, A., VOISIN, C., ANDRIEU, M.: Étude de la flore mycologique des bronches par examen des sécrétions bronchiques prélevées sous bronchoscopie. Rev. Tuberc. Pneum. (Paris) **28**, 439 (1964). — GILLIAM, J. S., Jr., Vest, S. A.: *Penicillium* infection of the urinary tract. J. Urol. (Baltimore) **65**, 484 (1951). — GINGRICH, W. D.: Keratomycosis. J. Amer. med. Ass. **179**, 602 (1962). — GIORDANO, M.: Un caso di micosi polmonare de *"Penicillium glaucum."* Ann. Med. nav. Roma **2**, 912 (1918). — HOŘEJŠÍ, M., SACH, J., TOMŠÍKOVÁ, A., MECL, A.: A syndrome resembling farmer's lung in workers inhaling spores of *Aspergillus* and penicillia moulds. Thorax **15**, 212 (1960). — HUANG, S. N., HARRIS, L. S.: Acute disseminated penicilliosis: report of a case and review of pertinent literature. Amer. J. clin. Path. **39**, 167 (1963). — ISHIKO, T.: Histological studies in the injuries of various organs of mice and albino rats except liver, fed with "Yellowed Rice" artificially polluted by *P. islandicum* Sopp. Acta. path. jap. **7**, 368 (1957). — JACKSON, D., YOW, E.: Pulmonary infiltration with eosinophilia: report of two cases of farmer's lung. New Engl. J.

Med. **264**, 1271 (1961). — KESTEN, B.M., ASHFORD, B.K., BENHAM, R.W., EMMONS, C.W., Moss, M.C.: Fungus infections of the skin and its appendages occurring in Puerto Rico: a clinical and mycologic study. Arch. Derm. Syph. (Chic.) **24**, 1046 (1932). — KIRK, R.: Mycoses of Malaya and Singapore. J. trop. Med. Hyg. **67**, 10 (1959). — KOBAYASHI, Y., URAGUCHI, K., SAKAI, F., TATSUNO, T., TSUKIOKA, M., SAKAI, Y., SATO, T., MIYAKE, M., SAITO, M., ENO-MOTO, M., SHIKATA, T., ISHIKO, T.: Toxicological studies on the yellowed rice by *P.isl.* Sopp. I. Experimental approach to liver injuries by long term feedings with the noxious fungus on mice and rats. Proc. Japan Acad. **34**, 139 (1958). ∼ Toxicological studies on the yellowed rice by *P.isl.* Sopp. II. Isolation of the two toxic substances from the noxious fungus, and their chemical and biological properties. Proc. Japan Acad. **34**, 736 (1959a). — KOBAYASHI, Y., URAGUCHI, K., SAKAI, F., TATSUNO, T., TSUKIOKA, M., NOGUCHI, Y., MIYAKE, M., SAITO, M., ENOMOTO, M., SHIKATA, T., ISHIKO, T.: Toxicological studies on the yellowed rice by *P. islandicum* Sopp. III. Experimental verification of primary hepatic carcinoma of rats by long term feeding with the fungus-growing rice. Proc. Japan Acad. **35**, 501 (1959b). — KUNEL'-SKAIA, V. YA: [Fungus disease of the external ear]. Vestn. Oto-rinolaring. **2**, 37 (1964) (Russian). — KUNEL'SKAIA, V. YA, STEPANISHCHEVA, Z.G.: [Fungus flora of external otitis]. Vestn. Derm. Vener. **38**, 51 (1964) (Russian). — LINEBACK, M.: The bioserologic approach to black hairy tongue with new concepts of its treatment: secondary mycosis linguae of pathologic significance. Laryngoscope (St. Louis) **69**, 1194 (1959). — MANTELLI, C., NEGRI, G.: Ricerche sperimentali sull' agente eziologico di' un micetoma a grani neri (*Penicillium mycetogenum* n. f.). Giorn. R. Accad. Med. Torino **21**, 161 (1915). — McBURNEY, R., GULLEDGE, M.A.: Investigation of certain fungicides and bactericides for use in otitis externa. Ann. Otol. Rhinol. Laryng. (St. Louis) **64**, 1009 (1955). — MINODA, Y.: Effect of antibiotics on some fungi isolated from ocular lesions. Acta Soc. Ophthal. Japon **61**, 562 (1957). — MITSUI, Y., HANABUSA, J.: Corneal infection after cortisone therapy. Brit. J. Ophthal. **39**, 224 (1955). — MIYAKE, M., SAITO, M., ENOMOTO, M., URAGUCHI, K., TSUKIOKA, M., IKEDA, Y., OMORI, Y.: Histological studies on the liver injury due to the toxic substances of *Penicillium islandicum*, Sopp. Acta path. jap. **5**, 208 (1955). — MIYAKE, M., SAITO, M., ENOMOTO, M., SHIKATA, T., ISHIKO, T., URAGUCHI, K., SAKAI, F., TATSUNO, T., TSUKIOKA, M., NOGUCHI, Y.: Development of primary hepatic carcinoma in rats by long-term feeding with the yellowed rice by *Penicillium islandicum* Sopp — with study on influence of fungus-growing rice on DAB carcinogenesis in rats. Gann. **50**, 117 (1959). — MIYAKE, M., SAITO, M., ENOMOTO, M., SHIKATA, T., ISHIKO, T., URAGUCHI, K., SAKAI, F., TATSUNO, T., TSUKIOKA, M., SAKAI, Y.: Toxic liver injuries and liver cirrhosis induced in mice and rats through long term feeding with *Penicillium islandicum* Sopp — growing rice. Acta path. jap. **10**, 75 (1960). — MOHAPATRA, L.M.: A study of the fungi isolated from cases of otomycosis. Indian. J. Microbiol. **1**, 103 (1961). — NIÑO, F.L.: Broncomicosis penicilliar. Semana méd. (B. Aires) **2**, 1015 (1932). — NUSSBAUM, R., BENEDEK, T.: Pneumonomycosis penicillina, eine Gewerbekrankheit zum Kapitel der Lungengeschwülste. Beitr. Klin. Tuberk. **67**, 756 (1927). — OHMORI, Y., ISONO, C., UCHIDA, H.: [On toxicity of Thailand and yellowsis rice and Islandia Yellowsis rice.] Jap. J. Pharmacol. **50**, 246 (1954) (Japan.). — PEZZALI, G.: Contributo di casistica clinica: un caso di penicillosi del polmone secondaria. Clin. vet. (Milano) **44**, 201 (1921). — POLYANSKIY, L.N.: [A case of otogenic abscess of the temporal lobe of the brain produced by *Penicillium*]. Zh. ushn. nos. gorlov. Bolezn. **15**, 138 (1938) (Russian). — SAITO, M.: Liver cirrhosis induced by metabolites of *Penicillium islandicum* Sopp. Acta path. jap. **9**, 785 (1959). — SAKAI, F.: [Experimental studies on rice yellowsis caused by *P.citrinum* Thom and toxicity especially kidney-damaging effect of citrinin pigment produced by the fungus.] Jap. J. Pharmacol. **51**, 431 (1955) (Japan.). — SAKAI, F., URAGUCHI, K.: [Studies by long-term feeding experiments with rats on development of chronic poisoning by toxic substance from yellowsis rice. VII. Pharmacological studies on toxicity of yellowsis rice.] Nisshin Igaku **42**, 609 (1955) (Japan.). — SAKAKI, J.: [Toxicological studies on moldy rice: Report I.] J. Tokyo Med. Soc. **5**, 1097 (1891) (Japan.). — SALISBURY, J.H.: On the parasitic forms developed in parent epithelial cells of the urinary and genital organs, and their secretions. Amer. J. med. Sci. **55**, 371 (1868). — ŠAULOV, I.: Die Nagelpilzformen im Gebiet von Plovdiv/Südbulgarien. Derm. Wschr. **151**, 716 (1965). — SEGRETAIN, G.: *Penicillium marneffei* n. sp., agent d'une mycose du système réticulo-endothélial. Mycopathologia (Den Haag) **11**, 327 (1959). ∼ Some new or infrequent fungous pathogens. In: *Fungi and Fungous Diseases*. Ed., DALLDORF, G. Springfield, Illinois: Charles C. Thomas 1962. — SHELLEY, W.B.: Erythema annulare centrifugum: a case due to hypersensitivity to blue cheese *Penicillium*. Arch. Derm. **90**, 54 (1964). — SMYTH, G.D.L.: A preliminary report on fungal infections of mastoid and fenestration cavities. J. Laryng. Otol. **75**, 703 (1961). ∼ Fungal infection of the postoperative mastoid cavity. J. Laryng. Otol. **76**, 797 (1962). — SOOD, V.P., SINHA, A., MOHAPATRA, L.N.: Otomycosis: a clinical entity-clinical and experimental study. J. Laryng. Otol. **81**, 999 (1967). — SOUCHERAY, P.: Farmer's lung: form of bronchopulmonary moniliasis. Minn. Med. **37**, 251 (1954). — TALICE, R.V., MACKINNON, J.E.: *Penicillium bertai* (I), n. sp. agent d'une mycose broncho-pulmonaire de l'homme. Ann. parasitol. **7**, 97

(1929). — Tsunoda, H.: [Study on damage of stored rice, caused by microorganisms. III. On yellowsis rice from Thailand, Food Research Institute, Report 8, 77.] Trans. Jap. Phytopathol. Soc. **13**, 3 (1953) (Japan.). ~ [Microorganisms of spoiled rice in storage.] *Food — Its Science and Technology*, Suppl. p. 161, May 1963. (Japan.). — Uraguchi, K., Sakai, F., Tsukioka, M., Noguchi, Y., Tatsuno, T., Saito, M., Enomoto, M., Ishiko, T., Shikata, T., Miyake, M.: Acute and chronic toxicity in mice and rats of the fungus mat of *Penicillium islandicum* Sopp added to the diet. Jap. J. exp. Med. **31**, 435 (1961a). — Uraguchi, K., Tatsuno, T., Sakai, F., Tsukioka, M., Sakai, Y., Yonemitsu, O., Ito, H., Miyake, M., Saito, M., Enomoto, M., Shikata, T., Ishiko, T.: Isolation of two toxic agents, luteoskyrin and chlorine-containing peptide, from the metabolites of *Penicillium islandicum* Sopp, with some properties thereof. Jap. J. exp. Med. **31**, 19 (1961b). — Uraguchi, K., Tatsuno, T., Tsukioka, M., Sakai, Y., Kobayashi, Y., Saito, M., Enomoto, M., Miyake, M.: Toxicological approach to the metabolites of *Penicillium islandicum* Sopp growing on the yellowed rice. Jap. J. exp. Med. **31**, 1 (1961c). — Walton, C.H.A.: Respiratory allergy due to fungi. Canad. med. Ass. J. **60**, 272 (1949).

Rhodotorulosis

Ahearn, D.G., Jannach, J.R., Roth, F.J., Jr.: Speciation and densities of yeast in human urine specimens. Sabouraudia **5**, 110 (1966). — Bergmann, M., Lipsky, H.: Über die Pilzbesiedlung des Urogenitaltraktes. Med. Klin. **59**, 732 (1964). — Caretta, G.: [Fungi isolated from dermatophytoses in Puglia in 1959]. G. ital. Derm. **102**, 389 (1961) (Ital.). — Chakravarty, S.C.: Role of fungi in chronic bronchitis. Indian J. Chest Dis. **8**, 6 (1966). — Cisalpino, E.O., Mayrink, W., Cardoso, J.P.: Micose intestinal. Éstudo dé treze casos. Hospital (Rio de J.) **65**, 237 (1964). — Gernez-Rieux, C., Biquet, P., Capron, A., Voisin, C., Andrieu, S.: Étude dé la flóre mycologique des bronches par examen des sécrétions bronchiques, prélevées sous bronchoscope. Rev. Tuberc. Pneum. (Paris) **28**, 439 (1964). — Leeber, D.A., Scher, I.: *Rhodotorula* fungemia presenting as "endotoxic" shock. Arch. intern. Med. **123**, 78 (1969). — Lineback, M.: The bioserologic approach to black hairy tongue, with new concepts of its treatment: secondary mycosis linguae of pathologic significance. Laryngoscope (St. Louis) **69**, 1194 (1959). — Louria, D.B., Greenberg, S.M., Molander, D.W.: Fungemia caused by certain nonpathogenic strains of the family Cryptococcaceae. New Engl. J. Med. **263**, 1281 (1960). — Louria, D.B., Blevins, A., Armstrong, D., Burdick, R., Lieberman, P.: Fungemia caused by "nonpathogenic" yeasts. Arch. intern. Med. **119**, 247 (1967). — Miguens, M.P.: Hongos levaduniformes de la flora vaginal. Proc. IV. *Internat. Congr. of Clinical Pathology*, Madrid, pp. 405—415, 1960. — Müller, W.A., Holtorff, J., Blaschke-Hellmessen, R.: [Investigation of the occurrence and frequency of various types of microorganisms in human vagina during vaginitis]. Arch. Hyg. Bact. **151**, 610 (1967). — Riopedre, R.N., De Cesare, I., Miatello, E., Caría, M.A., Zapater, R.C.: Aislamiento de *Rhodotorula mucilaginosa* del L.C.R., heces, orina, exudado foringeo y piel de un lactante de 3 meses. Rev. Asoc. méd. argent. **74**, 431 (1960). — Shelbourne, P.F., Carey, R.J.: *Rhodotorula* fungemia complicating staphylococcal endocarditis. J. Amer. med. Ass. **180**, 38 (1962). — Silveira, J.S.: [Clinical experimental studies with trichomycin in genital fungal infection in women]. Rev. Gynec. Obstet. (Rio de J.) **105**, 439 (1959) (Port.). — Vieira, J.R., Batista, A.C.: [Importance of laboratory research into skin lesions of children]. Publ. Inst. Micol. Univ. Recife. **258**, 28 (1962). — Wilson, J.W.: Paronychia and onycholysis, etiology and therapy. Arch. Derm. **92**, 726 (1965).

Streptomycosis

Abbott, P.: Mycetoma in the Sudan. Trans. roy. Soc. trop. Med. Hyg. **50**, 11 (1956). — Adami, J.G., Kirkpatrick, R.C.: Surgery of the extremities: a case of Madura foot disease. Trans. Ass. Amer. Phycns **10**, 92 (1895). — André, M.: Aspects cliniques et chirurgie des mycétomes. Bull. Soc. Path. exot. **51**, 817 (1958). — Blanc, G., Brun, G.: Nouveau cas de Mycetome à grains noirs observè en Tunisie. Bull. Soc. Path. exot. **12**, 741 (1919). — Brault, J.: Mycétome à forme néoplasique. Bull. Soc. Chir. 1906. (Cited by Segretain and Destombes, 1963). — Brumpt, V.: A propos de 4 mycétomes observés à Bobo-Dioulasso. Bull. Soc. Path. exot. **53**, 610 (1960). — Camain, R., Segretain, G., Nazimoff, O.: Étude histopathologique des mycétomes du Sénégal et de la Mauritanie. Arch. Biol. Med. **33**, 923 (1957). — Carter, H.V.: On a new and striking form of fungus disease, principally affecting the foot, and prevailing endemically in many parts of India. Trans. Med. Phys. Soc. Bombay **5**, 104 (1860). ~ On a new and striking form of fungus disease, principally affecting the foot, and prevailing endemically in many parts of India. Trans. Med. Phys. Soc. Bombay (N.S.) **6**, 104 (1861). — Catanei, A.: Étude parasitologique de trois mycétomes du pied observés en Algérie en 1933. Arch. Inst. Pasteur Algér. **12**, 169 (1934). ~ Sur des changements de caractères culturaux de *Nocardia madurae:* étude morphologique et expérimentale. Arch. Inst. Pasteur Algér. **20**, 299 (1942). ~ Variation in culture characters of *Nocardia madurae:* morphologic and experimental study. Trop. Dis. Bull. **40**, 940 (1943). — Catanei, A., Goinard, P.: Un nouveau cas algérien de mycétome du pied. Bull Soc. Path. exot. **27**, 176 (1934). — CATANEI, A., GROSSDEMANGE, L., LeGROUX, C.: Sur un cas de mycetome du pied observé en Algérie. Bull. Soc. Path. exot. **20**, 11 (1927). — CATANEI, A., LeGROUX, C.: Un nouveau cas de mycétome observè en Algérie. Arch. Inst. Pasteur Algér. **9**, 378 (1931). — CHADLI, A., JUMINER, B., HELDT, N., GUETAT, M.S., LADJIMI, R.: Contribution à l'étude des mycétomes tunisiens et de leurs agents. Arch. Inst. Pasteur Tunis **40**, 279 (1963). — CHICK, E.W., CONANT, N.F.: Mycotic keratitis: a review of 148 cases from the literature. Invest. Ophthal. **1**, 419 (1962) (Abstract). — CLARKE, P.R.R.: Mycetoma of the testis. Lancet **2**, 1341 (1953). — CLARKE, P.R.R., WARNOCK, G.B.R., BLOWERS, R., WILKINSON, M.: Brain abscess due to *Streptomyces griseus*. J. Neurol. Neurosurg. Psychiat. **27**, 553 (1964). — CORNWALL, J.E., LA FRENAIS, H.M.: A new variety of Streptothrix cultivated from mycetoma of the leg. Indian J. med. Res. **10**, 239 (1922). — CONVIT, J., BORELLI, D., ALBORNOZ, R., RODRÍGUEZ, G., HÓMEZ, J.: Micetomas, cromomicosis, esporotricosis y enfermedad de Jorge Lobo. Mycopathologia (Den Haag) **15**, 394 (1961). — DELAHAYE, R.P., DESTOMBES, P., MOUTOUNET, J.: Les aspects radiologiques des mycétomes. Ann. Radiol. **5**, 817 (1962). — DESTOMBES, P., ANDRÉ, M.: Contribution à l'étude des mycétomes en Afrique française. Bull. Soc. Path. exot. **51**, 815 (1958). — DESTOMBES, P., RANNOU, M., NEEL, R.: Mycétome à *Streptomyces somaliensis* observé en Algérie au sud de l'atlas. Bull. Soc. Path. exot. **58**, 1017 (1965). — DESTOMBES, P., MARIAT, R., ROSATI, L., SEGRETAIN, G.: Les mycétomes en Republique de Somalie. C. R. Acad. Sci. (Paris) Ser. D **263**, 2062 (1966). — DEY, N.C.: Epidemiology and incidence of fungus diseases in India. Indian J. Derm. **8**, 21 (1962). — DIOUF, B., FUSTEC, R., POUYE, I., GOUDOTE, E., FOURNIER, J.P., BENIER, J., CAUE, L., SERAFINO, X.: Formes anatomocliniques des mycétomes à Dakar. Problems thérapeutique Travail utilisant 89 dossiers. Bull. Soc. méd. Afr. noire Langue franç. **10**, 564 (1965). — GAMET, A., BROTTES, H., ESSOMBA, R.: Nouveaux cas de mycétomes dépistés au Cameroun. Bull. Soc. Path. exot. **57**, 1191 (1964). — GEMY, VINCENT, H.: Sur une affection parasitaire du pied non encore décrite (variété de pied de Madura). Annals Dermat. **5**, 577 (1892). ~ Sur un nouveau cas ce "Pied de Madura". Annals Dermat. **7**, 1253 (1896). — GUICHARD, F., JAUSION, H.: Un cas de pied de Madura observé à Marrakech. Arch. Inst. Pasteur Algér. **1**, 641 (1923). — GONZALEZ-OCHOA, A., AHUMADA PIDALLA, M.: Tratmiento del micetoma actinomicosico por la inyeccion local de diaminodifenilsulfona. Rev. Inst. Salubr. Enferm. trop. (Méx.) **18**, 41 (1958). — HALDE, C., RINGROSE, E.J.: Mycetoma originating in Northern California: disease caused by a fungus, resembling *Nocardia madurae*. Arch. Derm. **74**, 80 (1958). — HOMEZ, J.: Primer caso de micetoma por *S. pellieri* en Venezuela. Cited by LATAPÍ, F.: Das Mycetom. In: *Die Pilzkrankheiten der Haut durch Hefen, Schimmel, Aktinomyceten und verwandte Erreger.* [MARCHIONINI, A., and GÖTZ, H. (Eds.)]. Berlin-Göttingen-Heidelberg: Springer 1963. — HYDE, J.N.: A contribution to the study of mycetoma of the foot as it occurs in America. Trans. Amer. Derm. Ass. **19**, 74 (1896). — KLÜKEN, N., CAMAIN, R., BAYLET, M., BASSET, A.: Zur Epidemiologie Klinik und Therapie der Mycetome in Westafrika. Hautarzt **1**, 1 (1965). — KOHN, P.M., TAGER, M., SIEGEL, M.L., ASHE, R.: Aerobic *Actinomyces* septicemia: report of a case. New Engl. J. Med. **245**, 640 (1951). — LATAPÍ, F.: Micetoma. Analisis de 100 casos estudiados en la Ciudad de México. Mem. Congr. ib.-latin.-amer. Dermat. (Méx.) **3**, 203 (1959). — LATAPÍ, F., ORTIZ, Y.: Los micetomas en Mexico. Memorias del primer congreso de dermatología, pp. 126—144 (1963). — LATAPÍ, F., MARIAT, F., LAVALLE, P., ORTIZ, Y.: Micetoma por *Streptomyces somaliensis* localizado a un dedo de la mano. Dermatologia (Méx.) **5**, 257 (1961). — LE DANTEC: Étude bactériologique sur le pied de madura du Senegal (variete truffoide). Arch. Méd. nav. **62**, 447 (1894). — LEGRAIN, E.: Sur quelques affections parasitaires observées en algérie. Arch. Parasit. **1**, 148 (1898). — LINCOLN, C., NORDSTROM, R.C., GOODMAN, S.: Actinomycotic mycetoma (*Streptomyces madurae*). Arch. Derm. **91**, 189 (1965). — LÔBO, J.: Micetomes em Pernambuco. Rev. Fac. Med. Univ. Ceara **3**, 5 (1963). — LYNCH, J.B.: Mycetoma in the Sudan. Ann. roy. Coll. Surg. Engl. **35**, 319 (1964). — LYNCH, J.B., MOGHRABY, I.: Mycetoma in the Sudan associated with *Streptomyces Madurae*. Trans. roy. Soc. trop. Med. Hyg. **55**, 446 (1961). — MacKINNON, J.E.: A contribution to the study of the causal organism of maduromycosis. Trans. roy. Soc. trop. Med. Hyg. **48**, 470 (1954). — MacKINNON, J.E., ARTAGAVEYTIA-ALLENDE, R.C.: The main species of pathogenic aerobic actinomycetes causing mycetomas. Trans. roy. Soc. trop. Med. Hyg. **50**, 31 (1956). — MAEGRAITH, B.: Unde venis. Lancet **1**, 401 (1963). — MARIAT, F.: Sur la distribution geographique et al repartition des agents de mycetomas. Bull. Soc. Path. exot. **56**, 35 (1963). — MONTPELLIER, J., LACROIX, A.: Encore un mycétome du pied, type, „Pied de Madure" observé en Algérie, et du au *Nocardia madurae*. Bull. Soc. Path. exot. **14**, 357 (1921). — NICOLAU, St. G., AVRAM, A., STOIAN, M.: Micetom cu grăunt: albi al piciorului *Streptomyces madurae*. Derm. Vener. (Buc.) **1**, 65 (1959). — ORIO, J., DESTOMBES, P., MARIAT, F., SEGRETAIN, G.: Les mycétomes en Côte Francaise des Somalis — revue de 50 cas. Bull. Soc. Path. exot. **56**, 161 (1963). — PORRITT, A.: An African surgical pilgrimage. Ann. roy. Coll. Surg. Engl. **31**, 330 (1962). — PROCTOR, A.G.: Pathogenic streptomycetes.

J. med. Lab. Technol. **23**, 109 1966. — RAYNAUD, M., MONTPELLIER, J., LACROIX, A.: Un cas de mycétome du pied a *Nocardia madurae* chez un indigène algérien. Bull. Soc. Path. exot. **15**, 379 (1922). — REMLINGER, P.: Un cas de pied de Madura observé au Maroc. Bull. Soc. Path. exot. **5**, 707 (1912)(Also in Maroc méd. **78**, 188, 1938). ~ Contribution à l'étude de *"Discomyces madurae"* Vincent. C. R. Soc. Biol. (Paris) **74**, 516 (1913). — REY, M.: *Les Mycétomes dans L'Quest Africain*. Thesis, Paris: R. Foulon and Co. 1961. — RIPPON, J.W., LORINCZ, A.L.: Collagenase activity of *Streptomyces (Nocardia) madura*. J. invest. Derm. **43**, 483 (1964). — RIPPON, J.W., PECK, G.L.: Experimental infection with *Streptomyces madurae* as a function of collagenase. J. invest. Derm. **49**, 371 (1967). — SAUL, A.: Mycetoma caused by *S.madurae*. Dermatologia (Méx.) **5**, 206 (1961). — SEGRETAIN, G., DESTOMBES, P.: Les mycétomes en Afrique du Nord. Maroc. méd. **42**, 445 (1963). — SEGRETAIN, G., MARIAT, F.: Contribution à l'étude de la mycologie et de la bactériologie des mycétomes du Tchad et de la Côte des Somalis. Bull. Soc. Path. exot. **51**, 833 (1958). — SYMMERS, D., SPORER, A.: Maduromycosis of the hand, with special reference to heretofore undescribed foreign body granulomas formed around disintegrated chlamydospores. Arch. Path. **37**, 309 (1944). — UMEZAWA, H., KONDO, S., MAEDA, K., OKAMI, Y., OKUDA, T., TAKEDA, K.: *Index of Antibiotics from Actinomycetes*. University of Tokyo Press, Tokyo and University Park Press, State College, Pennsylvania, 1967. — VANBREUSEGHEM, R.: Epidémiologie et thérapeutique des pieds du madura au Congo belge. Bull. Soc. Path. exot. **51**, 793 (1958). — VERGHESE, A., KLOKKE, A.H.: Histologic diagnosis of species of fungus causing mycetoma. Indian J. med. Res. **54**, 524 (1966). — VICTORIA, R.V.: [Study of a case of mycetoma due to *Streptomyces somaliensis*]. Rev. lat.-amer. Microbiol. **9**, 61 (1967). — VINCENT, M.H.: Étude sur le parasite du "Pied de Madura". Ann. Inst. Pasteur **8**, 129 (1894). — WAKSMAN, S.A.: *The Actinomycetes. A Summary of Current Knowledge*. New York: The Ronald Press Company, 1967.

Torulopsiosis

AHEARN, D.G., JANNACH, J.R., ROTH, F.J., Jr.: Speciation and densities of yeasts in human urine specimens. Sabouraudia **5**, 110 (1966). — ARTAGAVEYTIA-ALLENDE, R.C., SILVEIRA, J.S.: [*Torulopsis glabrata*, its isolation from various human sources]. Ciencia (Méx.) **21**, 59 (1961). — BATISTA, A.C., PEREIRA, V.: Infectacãe do liquido amniótico da mulher por fungos levedoriformes. Publ. Inst. Micol. Univ. Recife **243**, 39 (1960). — BATISTA, A.C., PASSOS, G.M., CHARIFKER, M.: Um caso de parodontite micotica. Publ. Inst. Micol. Univ. Recife **303**, 16 (1961). — BATISTA, A.C., SILVEIRA, G., OLIVEIRA, D.: Fungos *Candida* e *Torulopsis* na bile em colecistites. Rev. Asoc. méd. bras. **4**, 360 (1958). — BERGMANN, M., LIPSKY, H.: Über die Pilzbesiedlung des Urogenitaltraktes. Med. Klin. **59**, 732 (1964). — BERNHARDT, H.: Die Pilzarten des Sputums. Zbl. Bakt., I. Abt. Orig. **178**, 515 (1960). — BLACK, R.A., FISHER, C.B.: Cryptococcic bronchopneumonia. Amer. J. Dis. Child. **54**, 81 (1937). — BRUNNER, A.: Die Lungenmykosen in Chirurgischer Sicht. Chirurg. **35**, 149(1964).— CARETTA, G.: Funghi isolatida dermatofizienellie Puglie nel 1959. G. ital. Derm. Sif. **5**, 389 (1961). — CERNIK, L., DOANHOAG-HOA, VUDINH-HAI: [The effect of mycotic flora on bronchial asthma in tropical conditions]. Čas. Lék. čes. **102**, 1313 (1963) (Russian).—COHEN, D., NIERMAN, M.M., GOLDIN, M.: Cutaneous moniliasis: topical treatment with amphotericin B lotion. Illinois med. J. **123**, 47 (1963). — DAGLIO, C.A.N., MARTINEZ-MONTEZ, E.A.: Estudio de los hongos blastoesporados aislados de vulvovaginitis. Rev. Asoc. méd. argent. **71**, 45 (1957). — EDEBO, L., JÖNSSON, L.E., HALLÉN, A., LINDBOM, G.: A fatal case of *Torulopsis glabrata* fungaemia. Acta. chir. scand. **131**, 473 (1966). — EDEBO, L., SPETZ, A.: Urinary tract infection with *Torulopsis glabrata* treated by alkalization of urine. Brit. med. J. **2**, 983 (1965). — FÖLDVARI, F., FLORIAN, E.: Über unsere die tiefen Mykosen betreffenden 15 jährigen Erfahrungen. Derm. Wschr. **151**, 707 (1965). — GRIMLEY, P.M., WRIGHT, L.D., Jr., JENNINGS, A.E.: *Torulopsis glabrata* infection in man. Amer. J. clin. Path. **43**, 216 (1965). — GUZE, L.B., HALEY, L.D.: Fungus infections of urinary tract. Yale J. Biol. Med. **30**, 292 (1958). — HALEY, L.D.: Yeasts of medical importance. Amer. J. clin. Path. **36**, 227 (1961). — HASENCLEVER, H.F., MITCHELL, W.O.: Pathogenesis of *Torulopsis glabrata* in physiologically altered mice. Sabouraudia **2**, 87 (1962). — HERMANEK, P.: Zur Mykologie der Galle bzw. Gallenblase. I. Mykologisch-bakteriologische Untersuchungen an intraoperativ gewonnenen Gallenflüssigkeiten Langenbeck. Arch. klin. Chir. **307**, 277 (1964). — HOLMSTROM, B., WALLERSTEN, S., FRISK, A.: Presence of fungi in gastric and duodenal ulcers. Acta chir. scand. **117**, 215 (1959). — HURLEY, R,. MORRIS, E.D.: The pathogenicity of *Candida* species in the human vagina. J. Obstet. Gynaec. **71**, 692 (1964). — KATZ, D., PICKARD, R.E.: Systemic *Torulopsis glabrata* infection causing shock, fever, and coma. Amer. J. Med. **43**, 151 (1967). — KEARNS, P.R., GRAY, J.E.: Mycotic vulvovaginitis: incidence and persistence of specific yeast species during infection. Obstet. and Gynec. **22**, 621 (1963). — LÓPEZ-FERNÁNDEZ, J.R.: Acción patógena experimental de la levadura *Torulopsis glabrata* (ANDERSON, 1917) LODDER y DE VRIES (1938) productora de lesiones sema j antes a la histoplasmosis. An. Fac. Med. Montevideo **37**,

470 (1952). — Louria, D.B., Greenberg, S.M., Molander, D.W.: Fungemia caused by certain non-pathogenic strains of the family cryptococcaceae. New Engl. J. Med. **263**, 1281 (1960). — Louria, D.B., Blevins, A., Armstrong, D., Burdick, R., Lieberman, P.: Fungemia caused by "non-pathogenic" yeasts. Arch. intern. Med. **119**, 247 (1967). — Malicke, H.: [What is the role of yeast infections in pregnant women and newborn infants?] Med. Welt (Stuttg.) **33**, 1725 (1964) (Ger.). — Marks, M.I., Langston, C., Eickhoff, T.C.: *Torulopsis glabrata* — an opportunistic pathogen of man. New Engl. J. Med. **283**, 1131 (1970). — Miguens, M.P.: Hongos levaduniformes de la Flora vaginal. *Proc. IV. Internal. Congr. of Clinical Pathology.* Madrid, pp. 405—415 (1960). — Minkowitz, S., Koffler, D., Zak, F.G.: *Torulopsis glabrata* septicemia. Amer. J. Med. **34**, 252 (1963). — Müller, W.A., Holtorff, J., Blaschke-Hellmessen, R.: Untersuchungen über das Vorkommen und die Häufigkeit verschiedenartiger Mikro-organismen (anaerobe Bakterien, Trichomonaden, Mycoplasmen und Sproßpilze) in der menschlichen Vagina bei Scheidenentzündungen. Arch. Hyg. Bact. **151**, 610 (1967). — Negroni, R., de Obrutsky, C.W., Gonzalez, R.O.: Estudio de un caso de septicemia por *Torulopsis glabrata*. Sabouraudia **4**, 244 (1966). — Oldfield, F.S.J., Kapica, L., Pirozynski, W.J.: Pulmonary infection due to *Torulopsis glabrata*. Canad. med. Ass. J. **98**, 165 (1968). — Passos, G. da M.: Processos carióticos micóticos: técnicas de defesa. *Thesis Fac. Odont. Univ. Recife,* 187 pp. 1961. — Perez, J.S., Gil, R.A.: Estudios sobre la debariocidina. I. Acción in vitro sobre levaduras aisladas de enfermos tratados con antibioticos. Microbiol. esp. **13**, 323 (1960). — Perry, J.E.: Opportunistic fungal infections of the urinary tract. Tex. St. J. Med. **60**, 146 (1964). — Plaut, A.: Human infection with *Cryptococcus glabratus:* report of case involving uterus and fallopian tube. Amer. J. clin. Path. **20**, 377 (1950). — Reiersöl, S.: *Torulopsis norvegica* nov. spec. Leeuwenhoek J. Microbiol. Serol. **24**, 111 (1958). — Riddell, R.W., Clayton, Y.M.: Pulmonary mycoses occurring in Britain. Brit. J. Tuberc. **52**, 34 (1958). — Rose, H.D., Heckman, M.G.: Persistent fungemia caused by *Torulopsis glabrata*: Treatment with amphotericin B. Amer. J. clin. Path. **54**, 205 (1970). — Šaulov, I.: Die Nagelpilzformen im Gebiet von Plovdiv/Südbulgarien. Derm. Wschr. **151**, 716 (1965). — Silva-Hutner, M.: Yeasts. *Manual of Clinical Microbiology.* Ed. by J.E. Blair, E.H. Lennette, J.P. Truant, Bethesda, Am. Soc. for Microbiology, 1970, pp. 352—363. — Silveira, J.S.: Ensaios clínico-experimentais com tricomycina (cabimicina) en ginecomicopatolgia. Rev. Ginec. Obstet. (Rio de J.) **105**, 439 (1959). — Smith, A.G., Taubert, H.D., Martin, C.W.: The use of trichomycin in the treatment of vulvovaginal mycosis in pregnant women. Amer. J. Obstet. Gynec. **87**, 455 (1963). — Vieira, J.R., Batista, A.C.: Importãncia da pesquisa laboratorial nas lesões epidérmicas da crianca. Publ. Inst. Micol. Univ. Recife **258**, 28 (1962). — Wickerham, L.J.: Apparent increase in frequency of infections involving *Torulopsis glabrata*. J. Amer. med. Ass. **165**, 47 (1957).

Ustilagosis

Anderson, B., Roberts, S.S., Gonzalez, C., Chick, E.W.: Mycotic ulcerative keratitis. Arch. Ophthal. **62**, 169 (1959). — Le Coulant, M.P., Lopes, G.: Asthme endémique régional par sensibilisation à l'Ustilago: étude expérimentale. J. Méd. Bordeaux **134**, 1094 (1957). — Moore, M., Russell, W.O., Sachs, E.: Chronic leptomeningitis and ependymitis caused by Ustilago, probably *U.zeae* (corn smut): ustilagomycosis, the second reported instance of human infection. Amer. J. Path. **22**, 761 (1946). — Preininger, T.: Durch Maisbrand (*Ustilago maydis*) bedingte Dermatomykose. Arch. Derm. Syph. (Berl.) **176**, 109 (1937).

Actinomycosis

D. J. GUIDRY, New Orleans/Louisiana, USA

With 18 Figures

Definition

Actinomycosis is a chronic suppurative infection which occurs in man and in domestic animals such as horses, cattle and swine. It is characterized by the formation of abscesses and multiple draining sinus tracts, by peripheral spread to contiguous tissues, and by the presence in pus of firm, yellowish tangled mycelial masses which are referred to as "sulfur granules". These represent colonies of the etiologic agent *Actinomyces israelii*; they may reach a diameter of 2 mm and are a prime diagnostic feature of actinomycotic infection (Figs. 1, 5).

Human infections are usually classified as cervico-facial, thoracic, or abdominal types, each may represent a primary infection, or, in the case of thoracic and abdominal lesions, be the result of contiguous spread from a primary site elsewhere in the body. Hematogenous dissemination may result in infection of the liver, kidneys, and brain. Osteomyelitis may occur in the mandible, vertebral bodies, and the neighboring parts of adjacent ribs; this may be accompanied by extensive destruction of bone.

In *cattle*, lesions occur most frequently in the bones of the face and jaw, although other tissues such as the testes may be affected. Actinomycotic infection is also known to occur in the intermandibular space in the horse, in lung, cheek bone, and mandible of dogs, and in the udder of swine. A case of actinomycotic encephalitis in a deer has also been recorded.

Actinomycosis is worldwide in distribution. It is endogenously acquired and man-to-man or animal-to-man transmission has not been reported.

Historical

The earliest description of typical actinomycosis were provided by BOLLINGER in 1877 from cases of "lumpy jaw" in cattle. He observed that pus from the lesions contained numerous yellowish, coarsely granular bodies which were shown to consist of a fungus. HARZ, a botanist with whom he consulted, concluded that the organism was a true mold and named it *Actinomyces bovis* (ray fungus). Subsequently, HARZ (1879) presented additional descriptions of *A.bovis* in material obtained from cases of "lumpy jaw". ISRAEL (1878) described a similar mycotic disease in man based on his studies of human autopsy material. The first human case was described by PONFICK in 1880 and in 1885 ISRAEL, reporting on 38 human cases, clearly defined the clinical manifestations of the disease (Fig. 1).

The etiologic agent was successfully isolated from "lumpy jaw" in cattle in 1890 by MOSSELMAN and LIÉNAUX and from the human disease in 1891 by WOLFF and ISRAEL. Because of the many similarities in the pathology of the two diseases as shown by ISRAEL (1878) and PONFICK (1880b), including the essentially identical appearance of granules in tissue and pus, the etiologic agent was considered to be the same. This opinion was supported by subsequent cultural and morphological studies as well as observations of pathological materials (SILBERSCHMIDT, 1901; WRIGHT, 1905; BREED and CONN, 1919).

The single species, *A.bovis*, was used to designate the etiologic agent in both human and animal infections as late as 1954 in spite of the fact that ERIKSON (1940) had shown that separation into two species was justified and had subsequently presented a detailed description and classification of the Actinomycetes (ERIKSON, 1949). However, separation of the two species *A.bovis* and *A.israelii*

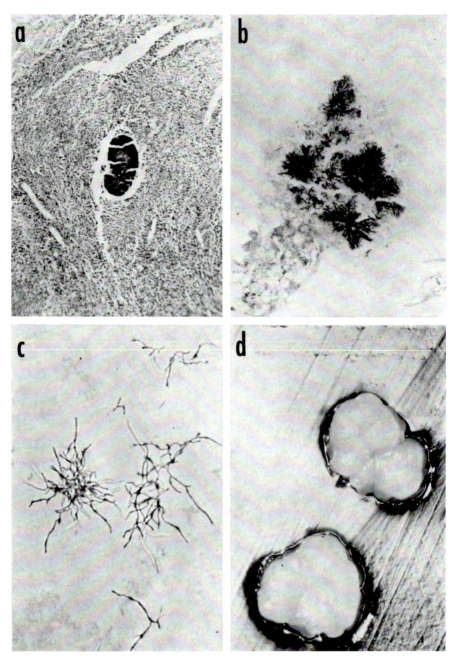

Fig. 1. *Actinomyces israelii*. a) "Sulfur granule" in pus. H & E, × 120. b) Granule showing the darkly-stained hyphae to be oriented radially towards the periphery and lying in a pale-gray matrix of inflammatory cells and necrotic debris. Note that the matrix extends well past the hyphal tips. GMS, × 450. c) 24-hour "spider colonies" on brain-heart infusion agar. × 380. d) 7-day colonies. The smooth, convex surface of the younger colonies has now become granular and lobulated. Penetration of hyphae into the medium has caused dimpling of the agar surface. (c and d courtesy of Dr. LUCILLE K. GEORG, Mycology Section, National Communicable Disease Center; National Audiovisual Center. Atlanta, Ga.)

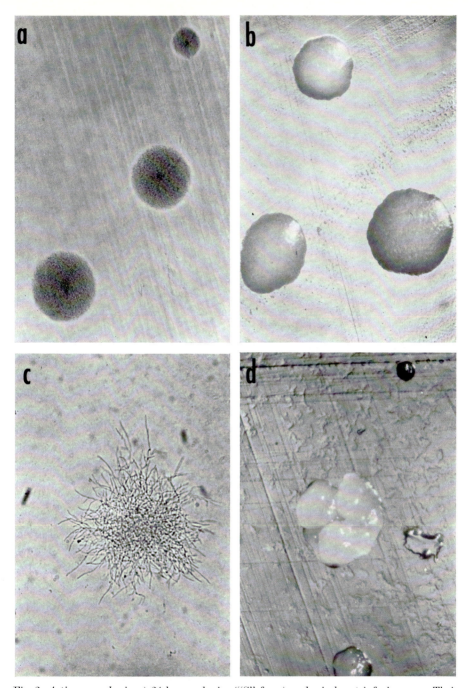

Fig. 2. *Actinomyces bovis.* a) 24-hour colonies ("S" form) on brain-heart infusion agar. Their appearance suggests dense hyphal formation, but microscopic preparations show only masses of diphtheroids. × 125. b) 7-day colonies of "S" form. The smooth, convex colonies yield only diphtheroidal forms. c) 24-hour colonies of "R" form. Note the similarity to micro-colonies of *A.israelii.* × 475. d) 7-day colony of "R" form. Mature colonies of the R variant resemble those of *A.israelii.* However, microscopic preparations of the R variant also reveal masses of diphtheroids rather than branched hyphae. (Photographs courtesy of Dr. Lucille K. Georg)

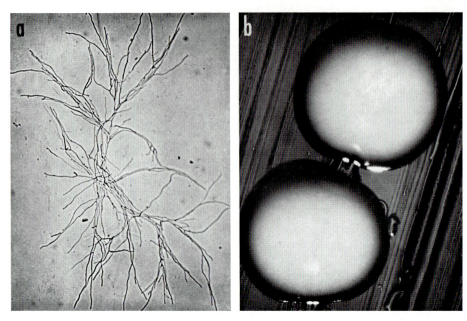

Fig. 3. *Actinomyces propionicus*. a) 24-hour colony on brain-heart infusion agar. The mycelial nature of this species is readily apparent. × 380. b) 7-day colonies. The smooth, convex colonies yield long, branching hyphae. (Photographs courtesy of Dr. Lucille K. Georg)

was firmly established following detailed studies of their morphological and physiological characteristics (Pine et al., 1960a), their growth requirements (Christie and Porteous, 1962a, 1962b, 1962c), and antigenic structure, chemical composition, and ultrastructure of their cell walls (Cummins and Harris, 1958; MacLennan, 1961; Cummins, 1962; Overman and Pine, 1963; Kwapinski, 1964) (Fig. 2). In the meantime some oral strains of *Actinomyces* were described by Thompson and Lovestedt (1951) which grew in air on primary isolation and for which they proposed the name *Actinomyces naeslundii*; this species was more clearly defined by the studies of Howell et al. (1959) (Fig. 4). Two additional species have been described; *Actinomyces propionicus* was isolated from a human case of lacrimal canaliculitis (Pine and Hardin, 1959; Buchanan and Pine, 1962) and *Actinomyces eriksonii* was isolated from a lung abscess (Georg et al., 1965) (Fig. 3).

Geographic Pathology

Although actinomycosis is world-wide in distribution, it is not a common disease of man. In the United States, it is outnumbered by both histoplasmosis and coccidioidomycosis and possibly by blastomycosis as well (Peabody and Seabury, 1957). Some of the earliest reported cases in the United States were those cited by Ruhrah (1899); Sanford's review (1923) cited approximately 700 cases. Putman et al. (1950) reported on 122 cases diagnosed at the Mayo Clinic over a period of 35 years. Porter (1953) cited 183 cases in Scotland over a 13 year period, while in England and Wales 151 cases were listed during the five years from 1957—1961 (Wilson and Miles, 1964). Glahn (1954) reported on 90 cases of cervico-facial actinomycosis observed in Copenhagen over a five-year period.

Most surveys show that the disease is approximately twice as common in males as in females; in the 90 cases reported by GLAHN (1945 b) 78% were males. While some surveys show the disease to be more common among agricultural workers and residents of small towns (PORTER, 1953; WILSON and MILES, 1964), other reviews have failed to demonstrate a clear occupational association. In the 122 cases reviewed by PUTMAN et al. (1950) 40% of the patients were farmers, 25% were housewives, and 12% were students. The remaining cases were distributed among many trades and professions. Fifty-three patients lived in rural homes and 69 were urban dwellers.

Most cases of actinomycosis occur in patients over 20 years of *age*; in the series by PUTMAN and his associates 93 of the cases were patients between 20 and 60 years of age.

Although the disease is not well-known in some countries, differential race susceptibilities are not established; in many instances the low incidence may well reflect lack of diagnostic and reporting facilities rather than a paucity of cases.

Cervico-facial actinomycosis is generally conceded to be the most common form of the disease. In the series by COPE (1938) the distribution of cases was cervico-facial 56.8%, thoracic 22.3%, and abdominal 15.0%; in the data tabulated by WILSON and MILES (1964) the distribution was 61.2—, 12.0—, and 18.7% respectively.

Actinomycosis is an endogenously-acquired infection which occurs only sporadically and the disease is not contagious.

Mycology

Etiology. Most workers are agreed that human cases of actinomycosis are usually caused by *Actinomyces israelii* whereas the disease in cattle is usually caused by *A. bovis* (Figs. 1, 2). As previously mentioned, there has been a great deal of reluctance in accepting separation into two species and a survey of the literature makes it quickly apparent why this is so. Not only are there legitimate exceptions to the usual etiology in both man and animals, but there are numerous reports which contain confusing and conflicting descriptions of the etiologic agent. The actinomycotic lesions almost invariably contain a mixed flora (HOLM, 1951) and anaerobic diphtheroids and other bacteria frequently have been identified erroneously as *Actinomyces*. In addition, it is suspected that some reports of cultural and physiologic studies are based on work done using impure cultures. Add to this the fact that both the morphologic and physiologic characteristics of the *Actinomyces* are somewhat erratic, with occasional isolates showing characteristics of both species, and the difficulty of definitive identification can be appreciated. Nevertheless, as indicated in the historical review, a workable definition has been established not only for *A. bovis* and *A. israelii*, but also for the three additional species designated as *A. naeslundii*, *A. propionicus* and *A. eriksonii* (Figs. 3, 4).

A discussion of etiology is not complete without consideration of the possible role played by *associated microorganisms* in the pathogenesis of actinomycotic infection. HOLM (1948, 1950, 1951) conducted a careful bacteriologic study of specimens from 650 patients with closed lesions and found that *A. israelii* was never present in pure culture. LENTZE (1958) studied 608 cases and found associated microorganisms in every case. These microbial associates are usually anaerobic organisms and include *Actinobacillus actinomycetemcomitans*, *Fusiformis melaninogenicus*, other fusobacteria, anaerobic streptococci, and staphylococci (LENTZE, 1958; HEINRICH and PULVERER, 1959; BREDE, 1959). This association of *A. israelii* with other microbes suggests the possibility of synergistic action. Nearly

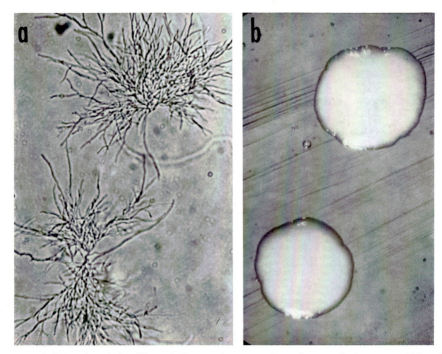

Fig. 4. *Actinomyces naeslundii*. a) 24-hour colonies on brain-heart infusion agar. Although *A.naeslundii* produces true mycelium, as shown here, an occasional isolate may yield only diphtheroidal forms. × 380. b) 7-day colonies. Older colonies may be rough, granular and pitted or they may appear as creamy and soft white with a ground glass to finely lobate surface. (Photographs courtesy Dr. Lucille K. Georg)

all of the microbial associates studied by Brede formed hyaluronidase and other depolymerizing enzymes, a property absent in *A.israelii*, and it appears that their contribution to the infectious process consists of lowering the redox potential and of facilitating the invasion of tissues. Holm (1951) has shown that patients with actinomycosis may be treated adequately with penicillin, insofar as *A. israelii* is concerned, without being cured of the disease and that this is due to persistance of microbial associates in the lesions. *Actinobacillus actinomycetem-comitans* quite frequently appears to be responsible for continued disease in penicillin-treated patients, although other gram-negative anaerobes may produce the same syndrome.

Laboratory Diagnosis. Anaerobic bacteriology is usually the least developed area in most hospital laboratories. For this reason and because of inherent diffi-culties in working with the *Actinomyces*, isolation and identification of this group presents a severe test in laboratory technique. Pine (1963) reviewed the current status of knowledge concerning the anaerobic actinomycetes and presented some recommendations for the isolation and identification of etiologic agents from actinomycotic lesions.

The only completely definitive procedure for species identification of *Actino-myces* rests on cell wall analysis (Cummins and Harris, 1958; Pine and Boone, 1967) and serologic methods (Georg et al., 1965; Lambert et al., 1967). Blank and Georg (1968) have applied the fluorescent antibody technique to direct detection and identification of *Actinomyces* species in tissues and in exudates

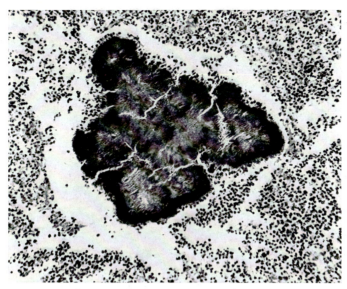

Fig. 5. Granule of *Actinomyces* in an abscess. The peripheral eosinophilic material of the granule stains intensely and includes some of the "clubs". The surrounding pus consists of polymorphonuclear neutrophils, many of which are fragmenting or losing their staining properties because of necrosis. H & E, × 970

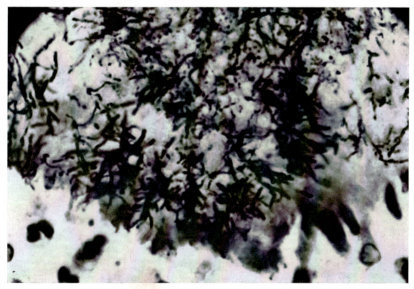

Fig. 6. Granule of *Actinomyces* stained by the method of Gram. Note the tangled filaments with the branching clearly visible. × 1500

(Fig. 7). However, neither of these is currently available to most hospital laboratories. A practical approach is to let positive identification rest upon microscopic morphology, morphology of micro- and mature colonies, physiological properties of the isolate in pure culture, and consideration of the clinical syndrome in the patient (Figs. 5, 6, 7).

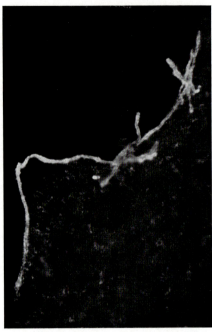

Fig. 7. Fluorescent antibody technique for detection of *Actinomyces*. Positive fluorescence reaction obtained in a direct smear prepared from tonsillar material. The FA test may be used to detect *Actinomyces* in clinical material, to monitor its presence in mixed cultures, and for making final and definitive identification of the organism. (From BLANK and GEORG: Journal of Laboratory and Clinical Medicine *71*, 283—293 (1968), The C.V. Mosby Company, St. Louis, Missouri)

Direct Examination. This consists primarily of looking for mycelial clumps or sulfur granules. These may be present in sputum or pus, but are rarely if ever found in the spinal fluid and the circulating blood. Pus which has been collected by aspiration may be spread out on a glass surface and exxamined with a hand lens for the presence of white to yellowish granules. Gauze dressings from draining sinus tracts should be rinsed with sterile water and the washings examined. Sputum may also be spread thin in a petri dish for examination; dilution with sterile water is recommended. The presence of granules in sputum is not necessarily of diagnostic significance, especially if they are associated with large numbers of contaminating bacteria. Such granules usually lack the typical eosinophilic "clubs" and represent saprophytic growths of *Actinomyces* which were expressed from the tonsillar crypts during coughing and expectoration of sputum. On the other hand, absence of granules does not necessarily rule out the presence of *Actinomyces* in the specimen, since the organism may be present in the form of small, poorly-organized mycelial clumps. Such specimens should be cultured even if the direct examination is negative.

If granules are found, samples should be removed, crushed between two microscope slides, and examined as a cover glass preparation. Additional slides should be prepared, heat-fixed and stained by the Gram and Ziehl-Neelsen technics. In fresh preparations, the granules will appear as lobulated bodies composed of delicate, branching and intertwined hyphae radiating towards the periphery. These are approximately 1 micron in diameter and the tips are frequently surrounded by a gelatinous matrix imparting a club-shaped appearance to the ends of the hyphae. The Gram stain will show gram-positive branching filaments, some of which may stain irregularly (Fig. 6). *Actinomyces is not acid-fast*. Frequently, the stained smears will reveal the presence of associated bacteria within and around the granule. In pathologic material in which granules cannot be demonstrated, stained smears should be prepared and examined for short, branching gram-positive filaments which are not acid-fast.

Direct Culture. Some effort should be devoted to removing as much contamination as possible from the granules prior to culture. EMMONS et al. (1963) recommend placing 10—15 drops of thioglycollate (containing 0.05% cysteine hydrochloride) in a sterile petri dish and washing granules by manipulating them with sterile needles and forceps in successive drops of the broth. This should be repeated until debris and pus as well as most of the microbial contaminants have been removed. Finally, the granules should be crushed and additional thioglycollate added to yield a dilute suspension of hyphal fragments.

A number of *suitable media* are available for isolation of *Actinomyces* and it is desirable to employ several of these in culturing a clinical specimen. Brain-heart infusion glucose broth, glucose thioglycollate broth, or brain-heart infusion glucose agar shake tubes may be used for culturing uncontaminated specimens. For contaminated material, Garrod's starch agar with 10% blood (EMMONS et al., 1963), brain-heart infusion agar with and without 10% rabbit blood, and the medium of PINE and WATSON (1959) are recommended. The latter, while it requires more work for its preparation, is purported to be superior on all counts (PINE, 1963). It is recommended that two series of isolations be made from each clinical specimen; one should be a series of streak plates (1.5—2.0% agar) and the other a series of dilution tubes containing media with 0.7% agar. While the streak plates can be incubated in a candle jar, an anaerobic chamber which can be evacuated three times with a mixture of 5% CO_2, 95% N_2 is greatly preferred. The agar shake cultures are sealed by cutting the top of the cotton plug and pushing the remainder of the plug into the tube, to a point just above the surface of the medium. An adsorbent cotton plug is then inserted on top of the first, 5 drops each of saturated pyrogallol solution and 10% Na_2CO_3 solution are added, and the tube sealed with a tight rubber stopper. Cultures should be incubated at 30—37°C and examination of both series should begin on the third to fourth day. The agar plates are best examined at the surface or from the bottom, first using a hand lens and then under a low power objective. For agar shake cultures, the sides of the tube should be warmed sufficiently to melt agar adjacent to the glass and a Pasteur pipette inserted along the wall to the bottom of the tube. Air is then blown through the pipette, expelling the entire agar plug into a sterile Petri dish. The plug is then cut into slices, cutting so as to separate individual colonies. These can then be placed on microscopic slides and examined with the low or high magnifications. It should be emphasized that only the young colonies of *Actinomyces* will be characteristic of the species; colonies become similar, if not identical, after 7—8 days. Several subcultures, working with discrete colonies, are desirable before any physiological studies are performed.

Associated Microbial Flora. Quite frequently these comprise the majority of colonies obtained in anaerobic cultures from actinomycotic lesions and one must be able to distinguish them from the colonies of *Actinomyces*. Specimens from cervico-facial lesions may contain *Actinobacillus actinomycetemcomitans*, fusiform bacilli, anaerobic streptococci, and various anaerobic gram-negative bacilli in association with *A.israelii*. Thoracic lesions usually have the first three named as associated while abdominal lesions most often yield *Escherichia coli* and various anaerobic gram-negative bacteria (EMMONS et al., 1963). These must be carefully excluded from *A.bovis* and *A.israelii* before any cultural and physiological studies can be performed.

65*

Animal Inoculation. This is of no practical value in the primary isolation of *Actinomyces* from clinical material. However, hamsters have been used for differentiating anaerobic diphtheroids from *A.israelii* and *A.bovis* isolates (HAZEN and LITTLE, 1951). GEORG et al. (1965) used 4—6 week old white mice for comparing the pathogenicity of strains of *A.eriksonii* with that of *A.israelii*. Groups of mice were inoculated by the subcutaneous, intraperitoneal, and intravenous routes. None of the mice inoculated with strains of *A.eriksonii* died. Subcutaneous abscesses developed several days following subcutaneous inoculation; gram-positive branched filaments could be demonstrated by smear and retrocultures were positive up to 2 weeks. Small, well-encapsulated abscesses developed in the mesenteries and peritoneal surfaces, but there was no evidence of tissue invasion and smears from infected tissues revealed gram-negative disintegrating organisms. Results with 2 recently isolated strains of *A.israelii* were more impressive. Four out of 20 mice inoculated intraperitoneally died within 2 weeks. Five out of 10 mice inoculated intravenously died within one week. All of the mice inoculated intraperitoneally with *A.israelii* developed numerous massive abscesses in the peritoneum; microscopic granules with clubbed hyphae were demonstrated in every case.

BUCHANAN and PINE (1962) concluded that *A.propionicus* was slightly more pathogenic for mice than were *A.israelii*, *A.bovis*, and *A.naeslundii*. PEGRUM (1964) found that *A. israelii*, and *A.bovis* produced small, usually single nodules on the chorioallantoic membrane of embryonated eggs. Histologic sections showed invasion of the membrane with proliferation of the *Actinomyces* within the mesoderm. A proliferative tissue reaction with edema occurred; the infected tissue was later walled off by fibroblasts and became ulcerated. The pathogenicity of *A.israelii* for albino mice is considerably enhanced by the addition of hog gastric mucin (MEYER and VERGES, 1950).

Serology. At present, serologic methods are of little practical value. Although agglutinins and complement-fixing antibodies have been demonstrated and positive skin tests have been reported, results in general have been inconsistent or equivocal. Indeed, MATHIESON et al. (1935) found that normal individuals gave more frequent and more marked skin reactions to *A.bovis* antigen than did actinomycotic patients. Very likely the current unsatisfactory status of serologic diagnosis in actinomycosis, like the earlier experiences with mycoses such as histoplasmosis and sporotrichosis, is due to poorly standardized antigens and technics rather than lack of an immune response on the part of the patient. Certainly it is clear that antibodies can be produced experimentally in animals and species specificity demonstrated when careful attention to detail is exercised by a competent investigator (GEORG et al., 1965; LAMBERT et al., 1967). Admittedly, cross reactions between *Actinomyces* species have been reported along with demonstrable relationships with other genera. SLACK et al. (1955) employing a reciprocal agglutinin adsorption technique were able to separate 20 isolates of microaerophilic *Actinomyces* into two broad serologic groups. Serologic group A included isolates from cases of human, bovine, equine and porcine actinomycosis along with isolates from human non-actinomycotic tonsils and one case of human pyorrhea. Six of the 20 isolates comprised serologic group B and these were from human, bovine, and equine infections. KING and MEYER (1957) reported that anaerobic diphtheroids could be differentiated from *A.bovis* and *A.israelii* on the basis of metabolic and serologic tests and indicated that the anaerobic diphtheroids are more closely related to the genus *Corynebacterium* than to *Actinomyces*. CUMMINS (1962) reported that seven out of eight isolates of *Actinomyces* yielding a cell-wall analysis identical to that for *A.israelii* also proved to be homogeneous by serological tests. KWAPINSKI (1964) found that the cell walls of *Actinomyces* species were related serologically to those of *Corynebacterium* and to some strains of *Mycobacterium* and *Nocardia*. Cell wall antigens of *A.israelii* reacted with sera from *A.bovis*, *C.diphtheriae*, mycobacteria, nocardiae, and *Waksmania*. *A.bovis* cell wall antigens reacted in a similar pattern with the exception that it failed to react with sera prepared with *Nocardia asteroides*. Undoubtedly, the manner in which antigens and antisera are prepared has a graet deal to do with the reactive

Table 1. *Morphological and physiological characteristics of Actinomyces species*[1]

| Character | Results obtained with strains of Actinomyces: | | | | |
	israelii	bovis	propionicus	eriksonii	naeslundii
Oxygen requirement	Anaerobic to micro-aerophilic	Anaerobic to micro-aerophilic	Facultative	Obligate anaerobe	Facultative in presence of increased carbon dioxide
Maximum growth	3—7 days	2—3 days	2—3 days	3—4 days	1—2 days
Color of colony	white	white	dull orange	white-cream	white
Biochemical reactions:					
Catalase	0	0	0	0	0
Nitrate reduct. . . .	+	0	+	0	+
Starch hydrol. . .	0	+	0	+	0
Gelatin liquef. . .	0	0	0	0	0
Litmus milk . . .	reduced	reduced	reduced	reduced and firm curd	reduced
Propionic acid . .	0	0	+	0	0
Acid without gas:					
Glucose	+	+	+	+	+
Mannitol	+	0	±	+	0
Mannose	+	0 or ±	+	+	+
Raffinose	Variable	0	+	+	+
Xylose	+	Variable	0	+	0

1 Based on data from GEORG et al. (1965) and PINE (1963).

patterns obtained in serologic tests. One additional point should be made. GEORG et al. (1964) have shown that smooth-rough (S—R) variation can occur with *A. bovis* with the R variant producing microcolonies which resembled those of *A. israelii* whereas the S variant was more typical of *A. bovis*. Both S and R variants had a cell wall composition similar to that of *A. bovis*; however, antigens from the S variant reacted with homologous sera as well as sera prepared from *A. bovis* and the R variant, whereas antigens from the R variant reacted with homologous serum only.

Species Description. Morphological and physiological characteristics pertinent to identification of the *Actinomyces* are presented in Table 1. Their oxygen requirements, rates of growth, and microscopic and colonial morphology are features which can be determined and compared in most laboratories. In physiological studies, the catalase reaction is most useful in excluding anaerobic diphtheroids which are catalase positive. The remainder of the biochemical tests listed in Table 1 are best performed as a battery since an occasional isolate may yield variable results, especially in the case of carbohydrate fermentations. Data on cell wall composition, believed to be the most definitive criteria for differentiating *Actinomyces* species, are listed in table 2 along with ultrastructural features which show some morphologic differences between species.

Actinomyces israelii (HARZ) KRUSE (1896)

A. israelii can be isolated from the normal saprophytic flora of the oral cavity. HOWELL et al. (1962) recovered the organism in 48% of non-salivary oral samples and from 28.9% of salivary samples. In 40—50% of plaques taken from early or shallow carious lesions, *A. israelii* was the predominant organism. The organism has also been isolated from tonsillar crypts (Emmons, 1935, 1936, 1938) where it occurs in association with other microorganisms.

The *granules* which occur in tissues and pus vary in color from white to yellowish and may be round or lobulated (Fig. 1A). The center of the granule is comprised of hyphae and cellular debris (Fig. 1B). Hyphae are oriented radially towards the periphery of the granule; some extend beyond the surface while others end short of the surface and are surrounded by a sheath of eosinophilic material. When granules are crushed and stained they show gram-positive hyphal fragments 0.5—0.1 μ in diameter. These vary in length from intact hyphal elements measuring several microns (rarely with branches) to short fragments resembling diphtheroids. Associated bacteria may be present in the stained preparations. *A. israelii*, like all of the other *Actinomyces*, is not acid-fast.

In *culture*, the importance of the highly diagnostic microcolonies cannot be overemphasized (Pine et al., 1960a; Buchanan and Pine, 1962; Pine, 1963). At 48 hours *A. israelii* appears as delicate, branching hyphae radiating towards the periphery to form so-called "spider colonies" (Fig. 1C). These gradually increase in size to about 2.0 mm, becoming white and opaque with a surface which is at first convex and smooth but later becomes granular and lobulated (Fig. 1D). Growth often penetrates the agar to cause dimpling of the surface and adherance of the colony to the agar. The colony remains intact when removed from the agar surface and has a cheesy consistency when crushed. *A. israelii* forms discrete colonies in liquid media; there is no turbidity since diffuse growth does not occur.

Actinomyces bovis (Harz, 1877)

It is generally accepted that *A. bovis* occurs frequently as part of the normal oral flora of cattle. Very likely, its mode of saprophytic existence in the oral cavity of cattle is quite similar to that demonstrated for *A. israelii* in humans. Trauma often seems to play a part in initiating actinomycotic infection in cattle; lesions frequently contain barley spikes or awns of grass, suggesting their traumatic introduction into the tissues during chewing. These probably carry *A. bovis* and other microorganisms into the tissues with them and by eliciting a foreign body reaction create an environment favorable to growth of the anaerobes.

The *granules* formed by *A. bovis* in tissues and exudate are indistinguishable morphologically from those of *A. israelii*. Hyphae of *A. bovis* are more fragile than those of *A. israelii* and tend to break up into short bacillary elements. Experimental inoculations into hamsters (Pine et al., 1960a) showed that while *A. bovis* formed typical branching mycelial elements, its capacity for forming mycelium *in vivo* was much more limited than that of *A. israelii*.

Microcolonies of *A. bovis* are very characteristic on brain-heart infusion agar and are easily differentiated from those of *A. israelii* and *A. naeslundii*. Two colonial types occur, smooth and rough. The *smooth* colony at 24 hours is small and circular with an entire edge (Fig. 2A). The surface is smooth, slightly convex and moist. Examination by transmitted light shows dense hyphal formation in the center. The smaller smooth colonies are easily broken with a needle, but the larger ones maintain their structure during such manipulation (Fig. 2B).

The *rough* type of microcolony at 24—48 hours is more dense when viewed in transmitted light, more irregular in its margin, and has a granular appearance (Fig. 2C). As these become older, they are considerably more elevated than the *smooth* colonies and the surfaces may be folded and irregular (Fig. 2D). The *rough* colonies remain intact during manipulation. However, microscopic examination of both *rough* and *smooth* colonies show only masses of diphtheroids. Growth in liquid medium is usually diffuse and also yields only diphtheroidal forms of *A. bovis*.

Table 2. *Cell wall composition and ultrastructural features of Actinomyces species*

Compound:	israelii[1]	bovis[1]	propionicus[1]	eriksonii[2]
	Results obtained with strains of *Actinomyces:*			
Arabinose	0	0	0	0
Rhamnose	0	±	0	0
Galactose	±	0	±	±
Mannose	0	0	0	0
Fucose	0	±	±	0
6-L-desoxytalose	0	±	±	0
Glucose	0	0	±	0
Galactosamine	0	±	±	0
Aspartic acid	0	±	±	±
Alanine	±	±	±	±
Glutamic acid	±	±	±	±
Lysine	±	±	0	±
Diaminopimelic acid	0	0	±	0
Ultrastructure:[3]				
Cell wall thickness (A°)	290	100	114	NA[4]
Membrane coils	Simple coils	None	Complex coils	NA

1 Based on data from PINE (1963).
2 Based on strain CDC X407 from GEORG et al. (1965).
3 Based on data from OVERMAN and PINE (1963).
4 Data not available.

A.bovis hydrolizes starch rapidly and completely. It does not reduce nitrate or utilize mannitol and raffinose.

Actinomyces propionicus Sp. nov.

A.propionicus was first isolated from yellowish-white concretions removed from the left superior canaliculus of a patient (PINE et al., 1960 b). In the original description of this isolate (PINE and HARDIN, 1959) it was designated as *A. israelii* strain 699, but the authors noted that it had the unique property among *Actinomyces* of producing propionic acid from glucose. Further studies (BUCHANAN and PINE, 1962; OVERMAN and PINE, 1963) revealed other distinctive properties which are presented in Tables 1 and 2.

The mycelial nature of the microcolony is readily apparent even at 24 hours (Fig. 3A). Examination of the growth under high power shows long hyphal elements which branch repeatedly. The mycelial structure is retained even when a cover glass is placed over the colonies. Older colonies are smooth and convex (Fig. 3 B).

A.propionicus generally produces branched hyphae on standard media. However, under special conditions unusual morphologic forms have been obtained which ranged from long thread-like filaments and hyphae with bulbous ends to masses of spherical cells. Under these circumstances the morphological similarity of *A.propionicus* to *Propionibacterium pentosaceum* in particular as well as to certain other propionic bacteria was quite striking (BUCHANAN and PINE, 1962).

A.propionicus grows well aerobically, but smaller inocula are needed to initiate anaerobic growth. Carbon dioxide has no stimulatory effect on aerobic growth.

A.propionicus is pathogenic for mice. Intraperitoneal inoculation produces lesions in the stomach, kidney, intestinal tract and liver,

Actinomyces eriksonii (GEORG, ROBERTSTAD, BRINKMAN, and HICKLIN, sp. nov.)

Thus far, the habitat of this organism seems confined to human clinical material (GEORG et al., 1964, 1965). It has been isolated from pleural fluid and from exudate obtained from both subcutaneous and lung abscesses. Typical sulfur granules are not formed in tissues, although microscopic colonies of the organism have been demonstrated in exudate. It also appears singly as a gram-positive, elongate, rodshaped organism which exhibits frequent branching.

In *culture A. eriksonii* may appear in diphtheroidal form or as filamentous and highly branched. Clubbed or bifurcated ends are common. The organism is non-motile and not acid-fast.

At 24—48 hours, microcolonies have a glistening, dewdrop appearance. They are circular, flat, and granular with a central core of denser growth and with finely serrated to occasionally fuzzy edges. After 7—10 days, the colonies are white to cream, convex to conical, with smooth to pebbly surfaces. Additional characteristics are listed in Tables 1 and 2.

Actinomyces naeslundii (THOMPSON and LOVESTEDT, 1951)

This inhibitant of the normal oral cavity was shown by THOMPSON and LOVESTEDT (1951) to differ significantly from *Actinomyces* isolated from acti-nomycotic lesions. Subsequently, HOWELL et al. (1959) studied approximately 200 oral strains and presented a detailed description of this species.

In the majority of cases, *A. naeslundii* can be isolated using blood agar plates which have been incubated aerobically. However, increased carbon dioxide tension is required for good growth in air. With a very small inoculum, most strains grow better anaerobically with carbon dioxide than aerobically.

In *culture A. naeslundii* may appear as a gram-positive filamentous organism or as a diphtheroidal form. The filaments are slender, of variable thickness, and possess either straight, clavate, or tapered ends. They stain solidly, show seg-mentations and may be beaded or stippled. In an occasional culture, only gram-positive bacillary forms will be present. These may be slender, long or short, curved, straight or bent.

At 18—24 hours microcolonies usually show a dense mass of diphtheroid cells or a dense clump of filaments surrounded by a rudimentary mycelium (Fig. 4A). Older colonies may be either rough or smooth, the latter reaching a diameter of 2—3 mm (Fig. 4B). The organism is reported to be nonpathogenic for experi-mental animals.

Pathogenesis

Since *A. israelii* is a normal inhabitant of the oral cavity, it would seem reason-able to assume that all cases, cervico-facial, thoracic, or abdominal, stem directly or indirectly from this source. The fact is that there are still widely divergent views concerning pathogenesis even of the cervico-facial type of infection.

Cervico-facial Actinomycosis. ISRAEL (1878) expressed the view that human actinomycosis, especially the cervico-facial type, originated in the oral cavity. He was the first to notice the relationship between carious teeth and cervico-facial actinomycosis. Subsequently, many other workers were to point out the relationship between dental infections such as periapical osteitis (HARBITZ and BACKER-GRONDAHL, 1910; AXHAUSEN, 1935, 1936; BJERRUM and SV. HANSEN, 1931; NIELSEN, 1942), dental extractions (BROFELDT, 1926; HAVENS, 1933; MACGREGOR, 1951; ZITKA, 1949), and jaw fractures (MACGREGOR, 1945). The trauma of extraction was suggested as predisposing to actinomycotic infection (JACOBSON, 1930; KOLOUCH and PELTIER, 1946; NAESLUND, 1931). The oral cavity has also been implicated as the source of infection in cases of skin actinomycosis following bite wounds inflicted by human teeth (COLEBROOK, 1920; MORTON, 1940; ROBINSON, 1944; ZISKIN et al., 1943). GLAHN (1954a) has challanged the early literature on occurrence of pathogenic actinomycetes in the healthy human mouth (NAESLUND, 1925; EMMONS, 1935, 1936, 1938; LORD and TREVETT, 1936; BIBBY and KNIGHTON, 1941; SLACK, 1942; ROSEBURY et al., 1944), mainly on the grounds that pathogenicity of the isolates was not demonstrated and identity with strains of *Actinomyces* from actinomycotic lesions was not established. Only in the case of SULLIVAN and GOLDSWORTHY (1940) was a comparison made between oral strains and isolates from actinomycotic lesions, and experiments included morphology, oxygen tolerance, and fermentation reactions. GLAHN's objections hold some merit, but in the light of our present knowledge and ability to identify *A. israelii*, work such as that of HOWELL et al. (1962) leaves no doubt that *A. israelii* exists in the oral cavity and particularly around early or shallow carious lesions. It is really a question of *how* the organism invades the tissues to initiate cervico-facial infection.

GLAHN (1954a) suggested *two main routes of infection*, namely (a) via gates or ducts which are normally present and lead from the mucous membranes into deeper tissue and (b) gaps produced by pathological conditions and their sequelae. That *A. israelii* acts in synergism with a well-defined group of anaerobic microorganisms has already been established. Assuming that both the fungus and its microbial associates exist in the oral cavity, they would have to compete with other members of the oral flora in invasion of tissues. Conditions which promote anaerobiasis would favor development of the actinomycotic lesion.

The mucous membrane of the oral cavity, in its normal state, is highly resistant to microorganisms. Slight traumatic wounds usually heal quickly without becoming infected. Presumably microorganisms which do enter such temporary gaps are quickly destroyed. The case for entry and localization in tissues by *A. israelii* via the ducts of the salivary glands is not a convincing one. Indeed, attempts to demonstrate a relationship between sialolithiasis, sialoadenitis and actinomycotic infection have failed (GANNER, 1929; GRABNER, 1936; HUSTED, 1953). Likewise, the presence of *A. israelii* in tonsillar crypts most likely represents saprophytic growth on accumulations of necrotic epithelium and there is no evidence to support the view that the tonsils may represent an actual portal of entry.

Actinomycosis of Dental Origin. This leads to consideration of entry through gaps produced by pathological conditions. These are listed by GLAHN (1954a) to include: deep caries with periapical osteitis, dentigerous cysts, impacted teeth, open alveoli after tooth extraction, jaw fractures, marginal paradentitis and partial eruption of teeth, especially the wisdom teeth of the lower jaw.

Proving a connection between infectious foci of dental origin and cervico-facial actinomycosis by microbiologic studies is especially difficult. Problems with overgrowth from contaminants as well as the chance isolation of *A. israelii* from contaminated food particles and saliva can readily be appreciated. Nevertheless GLAHN (1954a) was able to trace a case of actinomycosis of the cheek to two impacted canines in the upper jaw. A sinus tract led from the cheek lesion into the cavity containing the impacted teeth. *A. israelii* was isolated from the cheek lesion, the granulation tissue at the base of the two teeth, and from the surface of one of the teeth. In examining 90 cases of cervico-facial actinomycosis, GLAHN (1954a) was able to implicate one of the routes listed above in 72 instances. The one exception was marginal paradentitis which is rather surprising since the gingival pockets would seem a likely place for anaerobes to grow.

Thoracic Actinomycosis. WAYL et al. (1958) suggest that there are three ways by which *A. israelii* can reach the lung from the oral cavity: (1) via the tracheo-bronchial tree by aspiration; (2) via the blood stream; (3) along the fascial planes of the neck and mediastinal structures.

It is generally agreed that the tracheobronchial tree represents the usual route (GARROD, 1952; PEABODY and SEABURY, 1957; EMMONS et al., 1963; HILDICK-SMITH et al., 1964) and that this results from aspiration of hyphal fragments from carious lesions or other infectious foci of dental origin, or of actinomycotic granules growing saprophytically in tonsillar crypts. A case resulting from aspiration of an entire tooth has been reported (WARWICK, 1923). Presumably, the conditions set up by bronchiolar occlusion secondary to simultaneously aspirated particulate matter are favorable to growth of *A. israelii* and its microbial associates.

Hematogenous dissemination from a septic phlebitis in a small vessel associated with a dental infection would provide a rapid means by which *A. israelii* could reach the lung; the condition of infarction resulting from occlusion of a blood vessel by the septic embolus would favor establishment of an actinomycotic lesion (GARROD, 1952; WAYL et al., 1958).

Actinomyces israelii exhibits a propensity for spreading along contiguous surfaces and the possibility of extension from an oral lesion or cervico-facial lesion to the lungs via the esophagus and mediastinal structures has been considered by PEABODY and SEABURY (1957) and by WAYL et al. (1958). The latter presented a case history of descending actinomycosis in which the order of progression was: sinus of the gum of the lower jaw; right lower lobe lung abscess with pleural effusion; sinus in left submammary region; sinuses in left lumbar region and over the left greater trochanter, left upper gluteal region, and left lower gluteal region. While lung involvement could have resulted from aspiration, it could also have resulted from direct spread from the mediastinum which would account for the sternal and sub-mammary sinuses. The mediastinal lesion could then have extended directly through the diaphragm to the retroperitoneal tissues of the abdomen, then through the posterior abdominal wall in the region of the lumbar triangle of Petit and then to the trochanteric and gluteal areas.

Pulmonary actinomycosis may develop in the hilar region or in basal parenchymatous areas. TURNER (1926) divided pulmonary actinomycosis into essentially two types; (1) a first or early form beginning with involvement of the hilum and extending into the lung along the bronchi and (2) a secondary parenchymatous involvement, with or without abscess formation, which may later extend to the pleural cavity, ribs, vertebrae, pericardium, and sternum (DECKER, 1946; KAY, 1947; PEABODY and SEABURY, 1957; WARTHIN and BUSHUEFF, 1958).

Abdominal Actinomycosis. There is evidence that *A. israelii* is harbored at all levels of the intestinal tract and can, in the absence of trauma, invade the cecum or appendix and occasionally the stomach, gallbladder, or liver (CAMPBELL and BRADFORD, 1948). However, actinomycotic infection of the abdominal viscera seldom occurs as a primary disease. It most often becomes evident several weeks or months after an acute, perforative gastrointestinal disease such as acute appendicitis, perforating colonic diverticulum, perforated peptic ulcer, acute ulcerative disease of the intestinal tract, or traumatic perforation of the bowel (PUTMAN et al., 1950; RAPER, 1950; PEABODY and SEABURY, 1957; ASHTON and SLANEY, 1963; EMMONS et al., 1963). Typical acute appendicitis, usually of the perforative type, preceded the onset of actinomycotic infection in 72% of the 122 cases reviewed by PUTMAN and his associates (1950). In only 7 of the 122 cases was there no history of some previous acute illness and 103 of their cases had undergone some type of emergency surgical procedure for acute gastrointestinal lesions prior to onset of actinomycotic infection.

Structures of the right side of the body are most frequently involved, especially the right iliac fossa (Fig. 9). The frequency of region and organ involvement has been calculated from the data of PUTMAN et al. (1950) and is presented in Table 3. The authors also reported occasional involvement of the epigastrium, buttocks and peri-anal region, left psoas muscle, scrotal and supra-pubic regions, vertebral column, spleen and brain.

Table 3. *Regions of the body or organs involved in cases of primary abdominal actinomycosis*[1]

Region or Organ	% of cases showing involvement	Region or Organ	% of cases showing involvement
RLQ abdominal wall	82	Subdiaphragmatic	19
LLQ abdominal wall	25	Pelvic	10
RUQ abdominal wall	17	Right psoas $\rbrace$ Abscesses	7
LUQ abdominal wall	4	Right perinephritic	8
Right lumbar	20	Liver	16
Left lumbar	6	Right kidney	7
Right hip	7	Tube and ovary	8
Left hip	3	Right lung	16
Right chest wall	21	Left lung	16
Left chest wall	7		

1 Adapted from the data of PUTMAN et al. (1950).

Extension of the actinomycotic lesion occurs along contiguous surfaces and spread is usually directed away from the bowel and peritoneal cavity. Connective tissue and muscle are infiltrated with resultant necrosis and fibrosis, but bone is seldom attacked. The infection seldom spreads along lymphatic channels although lymph node involvement has been described (BRICKNER, 1925; FAIRLEY, 1947).

Rarely, the primary site may be other than the three described above. *Cerebral involvement* (JACOBSON and CLOWARD, 1948), primary *skin involvement* from bites and wounds (MCWILLIAMS, 1917; ROBINSON, 1944; BURROWS, 1945; ANDLEIGH, 1951; CULLEN and SHARP, 1951; BANERJEE, 1952; FINCH, 1953; MONTGOMERY and WELTON, 1959; BRAINEY, 1965) and anorectal lesions (GORDON and DuBOSE, 1951) have all occurred as primary infections.

The role of immunity in the pathogenesis of actinomycosis remains essentially undefined (WILSON, 1957). In general, attempts at sensitizing experimental animals have been unsuccessful. On the other hand, repeated injections of *A. israelii* into guinea pigs and rabbits have, in some instances, resulted in increasing the severity and duration of the actinomycotic lesions (MATHIESON et al., 1935; EMMONS, 1938; ROSEBURY et al., 1944). What this means in terms of human infections is not clear. MATHIESON and his associates suggested that human cases may represent individuals who have become allergic to *A. israelii* as a result of repeated absorption of products from that fungus and from other antigenically related saprophytes. However, the experimental evidence to support this concept is completely inadequate and clinical evidence is virtually non-existent. Definition of the role played by hypersensitivity in actinomycotic infections must await preparation of more specific skin-testing antigens.

No significant metabolites, including exotoxins and endotoxins, have been demonstrated for *A. israelii*. This would seem to emphasize the importance of the

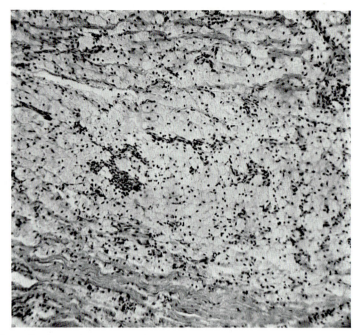

Fig. 8. The wall of an actinomycotic abscess. The pus-filled center of the abscess, not visible here, is oriented towards the top of this figure. Fat-laden macrophages, or lipophages, comprise the inner zone of the wall followed by a zone of scar tissue with collagen fibers. There is a sprinkling of lymphocytes in both zones. H & E, × 450

synergism observed in actinomycotic lesions, for most of the microorganisms found in association with *A.israelii* have been shown to produce hyaluronidase and other depolymerizing enzymes (BREDE, 1959). Indeed, some of them have been responsible for persistence of actinomycotic lesions which had been rendered free of *A.israelii* with penicillin therapy (HOLM, 1951). Both HOLM (1950) and GLAHN (1954b) have referred to actinomycosis as a *group of infectious diseases* caused by *Actinomyces* in synergism with certain other microbes, and GLAHN has suggested that variations in clinical severity of the disease are to a certain extent dependent upon the combination of organisms involved.

Gross and Microscopic Appearances

Gross Features. Although the anatomic location may tend to influence the appearance of the actinomycotic lesion, it is generally characterized by suppuration, sinus formation and scarring. The external appearance may first be that of a firm, indurated mass, poorly circumscribed, and covered by a tight, brawny, dusky red skin. More advanced lesions tend to soften and develop cutaneous sinuses, some of which may be open and draining while others are fibrosed and closed. On cut sections, the lesions present a honeycombed appearance due to the multiple abscesses and dense fibrous tissue (PUTMAN et al., 1950). With visceral lesions, suppuration, sinus formation, intercommunicating abscesses, extensive fibrous tissue reaction and a yellow color are the most constant gross characteristics (WEED and BAGGENSTOSS, 1949).

Microscopic Features. The microscopic picture is that of chronic neutrophilic response similar to that seen in chronic infections due to cocci or to *Nocardia*

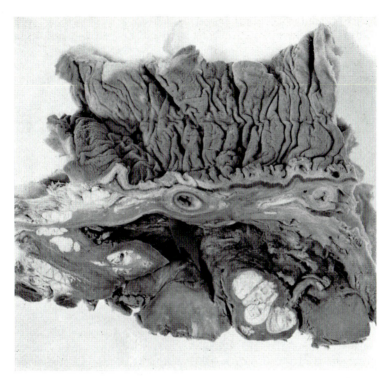

Fig. 9. Periappendiceal actinomycotic abscess. This is an autopsy specimen from a 16 year old colored boy, a resident of North Carolina, USA. His symptoms of actinomycosis began 4 months before he died. Note the appendix shown in 2 cross sections in the horizontal mid-plane between the abscess cavity below and the cecum above. The infection probably developed when an ordinary acute appendicitis perforated, spilling *Actinomyces israelii* into the abdominal cavity along with coliform bacilli and streptococci of the fecal material in the appendix. The appendix is now encased in dense scar tissue but the large abscess persists below. It has burrowed in the retroperitoneal muscle and other tissues. The rounded white and lobulated areas are adipose tissue. In the cut surface of the wall of the cecum, to the right in the photograph, two intramural actinomycotic abscesses are clearly shown. These represent burrowing pus rather than a cecal origin of the process

asteroides (Figs. 1A, 5). Histologic features include micro-abscesses, ramifying sinuses containing purulent exudate, and fibrosis (BINFORD, 1962). There is *liquefactive* rather than caseous necrosis. The inflammatory cells in the walls of the abscesses and sinuses include neutrophils, lymphocytes, plasma cells and histiocytes. Giant cells are rare, but an occasional one may be seen in the proximity of or in contact with a sulfur granule (BAKER, 1947). *Foamy, fat-laden, macrophages* (lipophages) occur in large numbers in the fibrosing walls around lesions, and are responsible for the yellow color observed during gross examination (Fig. 8). The abscesses vary considerably in size and may show both intercommunication and coalescence. Generally, there is extensive fibrosis in the walls of the abscesses. The connective tissue reaction is most extensive in lesions involving the liver, kidneys, ovaries, subcutaneous and muscular tissues. It is less extensive in the lungs and is minimal in the central nervous system (WEED and BAGGEN-STOSS, 1949).

The extent to which the accompanying bacteria influence the histopathologic picture is not clear. However, abscesses well removed from the central infection are sometimes found to contain bacteria, but no sulfur granules. Weed and Baggenstoss (1949) have noted that in many cases of actinomycosis there is an associated chronic active interstitial nephritis.

Actinomycosis can be diagnosed histopathologically by demonstrating micro-colonies (sulfur granules) of *A. israelii*. These are easily detected in hematoxylin and eosin sections where they appear as round to oval bodies measuring several hundred microns in diameter (Figs. 1A, 5, 6). They are most often found in the center of a micro-abscess. The actinomycotic granule is surrounded first by a zone of neutrophils, then histiocytes, and lipophages, then fibroblasts and collagenous fibers, and finally dense fibrous tissue. In other words, the abscesses usually present fibrous encapsulation. The granule stains deeply with the hematoxylin, but at the periphery it usually exhibits radial hyphae with eosin-staining hyaline clubs (Fig. 5). The nature or significance of these clubs in not completely known. They very likely represent a host response to the fungus, for they are not seen in microcolonies grown on synthetic medium.

It must be emphasized that a final histopathologic diagnosis of actinomycosis should not be made solely from the appearance of the granules stained with hematoxylin and eosin. Similar granules with eosinophilic clubs at the periphery are produced in tissues in cases of "woody tongue" (*Actinobacillus lignieresi*), botryomycosis (*Staphylococcus*), mycetomas due to *Streptomyces*, and in infections due to *Nocardia brasiliensis* (Tribedi and Mukherjee, 1939; Hagan, 1943; Calero, 1946; Moore, 1946; Auger, 1948; Weed et al., 1949; Lavalle, 1962; Emmons et al., 1963). Granules are absent in lesions due to *Nocardia asteroides*.

To properly demonstrate the hyphae of *A. israelii* in a granule, use the Gram stain. This is a part of the Brown and Brenn and of the MacCallum-Goodpasture methods. With these stains an actinomycotic granule is shown to be composed of gram-positive, delicate hyphal filaments with occasional branching (Fig. 6). The filaments tend to stain irregularly. Associated bacteria, either cocci, bacilli, or fusiforms, may be found intermingled with the hyphae.

The hyphae can also be demonstrated clearly with the Gomori-methenamine-silver stain, but it has the disadvantage of not being able to distinguish gram-positive from gram-negative elements (Fig. 1B). The PAS and Gridley stains do not demonstrate the hyphae satisfactorily.

Single, isolated hyphal filaments of *A. israelii* are seldom found outside the granules. When they do occur, they are indistinguishable from filaments of *Nocardia asteroides*. However, the pyogenic infiltrate from lesions of nocardiosis, due to *N. asteroides*, do contain numerous filaments of the fungus but granules are not present.

The advantage of microbiologic confirmation of a histopathologic diagnosis is, of course, obvious. However, the pathologist is frequently confronted with the problem of making a diagnosis solely from a fixed specimen which has been obtained from an operation, a curettage, or a biopsy. It should be emphasized that granules tend to occur in the pus so that biopsies which include only the walls of sinuses and abscesses will frequently be negative. Furthermore, granules are often sparse in infected tissues and numerous sections may be required before they can be demonstrated. The gross specimen should be preserved until micros-copic studies are complete as additional blocks from other sites may be needed (Baker, 1957).

Cervico-facial Actinomycosis. The features of oral, facial, and maxillary actinomycosis have been discussed at length by Hertz (1957). The actinomycotic inflammation produces a firm or hard, tumor-like mass. The numerous abscesses and sinuses within the mass contain thick and yellow or hemorrhagic pus with a

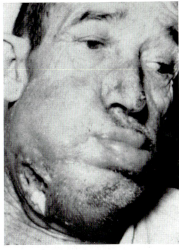

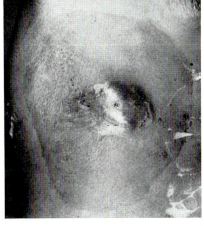

Fig. 10   Fig. 11

Fig. 10. Cervico-facial actinomycosis. Extensive involvement of the mandible with coalescing sinus tracts resulting in a deep ulcerative lesion. (Courtesy Doctors ALFREDO A. NAVARRO and RAUL MENA)

Fig. 11. Extension of a sinus tract to the surface of the right thoracic wall. A 33-year-old alcoholic complained of back pain, weight loss, night sweats, and cough for two months prior to the development of a tumor on the right lateral thorax. An x-ray of her chest showed a right upper lobe pneumonia with basilar empyema. An abscess was present in the right lower lobe of the lung, and the sinus tract on the thorax communicated with a subdiaphragmatic abscess as well as the empyema. Cultures were positive for *Actinomyces israelii*. (Courtesy of Dr. JOHN H. SEABURY)

putrid odor. Sulfur granules are usually present. Inflammatory foci near the surface ulcerate to form sinuses, the openings of which come to be surrounded by elevated, soft, yellow, fungating granulation tissue. New foci develop in adjacent areas and the condition advances slowly. The fibrosis and the active purulent process produce a complex of abscesses and fistulae. The infiltration procedes without regard to anatomic boundaries. Burrowing carries the infection along relentlessly through various tissues. When the periosteum is involved, there follows destruction of bone cortex, and tumor-like masses of osseous tissue are formed around irregular cavities. Bone involvement usually occurs early, preceding the appearance of sinus tracts, and may progress to osteomyelitis.

The primary lesion is frequently a *periodontal abscess* (VILLA, 1957) and extension of the infection usually follows extraction of the affected tooth. The process then extends to involve subcutaneous tissues forming a hard mass and eventually reaches the skin producing numerous fistulae. In other instances the primary lesion develops as a result of trauma from a carious or broken tooth or from an accidental fracture of the jaw (Fig. 10, 11, 12).

By the time the infection is noticed, it has usually left the site of invasion, but healing and scarring has left a palpable string of connective tissue extending from the initial site of the active process. Generally, the lymph nodes are not affected.

Maxillary involvement, with rarefaction of the maxilla, is quite common (LUDWIG, 1955; MAIN and MACPHEE, 1964). The lesion may extend to the skin to form a tumor with draining sinuses in the upper cheek, parotid area and neck,

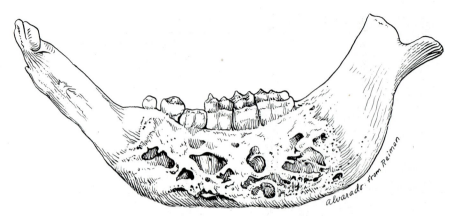

Fig. 12. Bovine actinomycosis. The lower jaw of a cow showing perforated tumor-like distension of the bone. In cattle, the most frequent site of infection is the mucosa of the mouth. The process commonly extends to the jaws to produce a tumor-like, central, destructive and ossifying osteomyelitis. (Redrawn from REIMANN: Pathology for Students and Physicians, vol. 1, p. 558, 1929; P. Blakiston's Son & Co., Philadelphia)

or it may extend to the orbit, cranial bones, meninges, and brain (ZITKA, 1952). SAZAMA (1965) found the parotid gland involved in 11% of his cases.

STANTON (1966) has reported primary involvement of the paranasal sinuses; in one case the patient had been edentulous for 17 years.

Lesions in the lower jaw may be extensions from periodontal or osseous lesions of the madible or from tonsillar or regional lymphatic tissue (CHOUKAS, 1958; HANRATTY and NAEVE, 1964; OWEN and MACANSH, 1965) (Fig. 15).

The histopathologic picture is one of granulation tissue with many plasma cells, lipophages, mocrophages (epithelioid cells), and occasionally giant cells. As such, it carries no features specific for actinomycosis, but instead presents a picture which is typical of any inflammation accompanied by granulation tissue. Occasionally, sulfur granules cannot be demonstrated.

Osteomyelitis of the alveolar process may follow pulpal involvement. GOLD and DOYNE (1952) described a case involving the mandibular right first molar and the alveolar bed of bone. The bone was thin, porous, and white. The roots were surrounded by sparse bone trabeculae and canals contained remnants of *gutta-percha*. The marrow spaces were large and empty except for soft tissue fragments found in the interradicular and interdental areas. Peridontal fibers were completely absent. One of the root canals was incompletely filled with *gutta-percha* and contained dentine debris, filamentous organisms and inflammatory cells. The lacunae of the alveolar bone were devoid of osteocytes and appeared to be necrotic; the normal cellular and fibrous components of the marrow spaces were not present. The cementum of the tooth, like the bone, contained no viable cells. Classic sulfur granules were found within the soft tissue fragments in the marrow spaces and interstices of bone; they were also found to be protruding from the apex of the root canal and firmly attached to the surface of the cementum.

Osteomyelitis of the *humerus*, apparently resulting from hematogenous dissemination, has been reported (McCORMACK et al., 1954).

Paralaryngeal involvement may stem from the tonsils, via direct extension through the mucous membranes of the pharynx and hypopharynx, or via the inferior constrictor muscle. In the case reported by DAVIES (1952) the abscess was located in the lower half of the anterior triangle of the neck, lateral to the

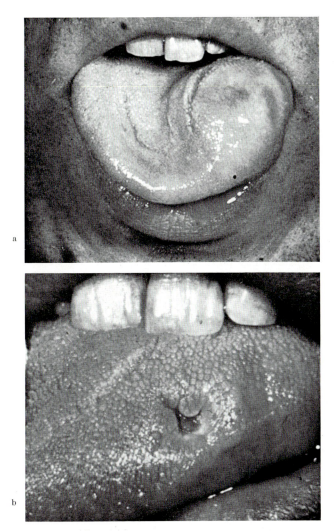

Fig. 13. Actinomycosis of the tongue. a) Nodule on the left lateral aspect of the dorsum linguae in a 27-year-old white male. Two days prior to admission he suddenly developed a painful swelling of the left side of the tongue. Incision of the nodule yielded yellow, thick, odorless pus. Direct examination showed *Actinomyces*-like gram positive organisms and cultures yielded an anaerobic actinomycete resembling *A. israelii* with regard to biochemical properties. b) Same lesion after eleven daily treatments with 800,000 units of penicillin intramuscularly. (From DORPH-PETERSEN and PINDBORG: Oral Surgery, Oral Medicine, and Oral Pathology, 7, 1178—1182 (1954), The C.V. Mosby Company, St. Louis, Missouri)

trachea and infrahyoid muscle. A fibrous band could be traced from the abscess upwards in the neck towards the angle of the jaw. The histopathology was remarkable in that a strikingly large number of eosinophils were present.

Actinomycosis of the Tongue. Involvement of the tongue usually occurs in the anterior third and near the tip on one side of the mid line (DORPH-PETERSEN and PENDBORG, 1954). The process is at first a hard, nodular swelling which increases in size and becomes softer (Fig. 13). The overlying mucosa develops a bluish color.

Eventually the nodule ruptures and drains and increases in size to become a multilocular abscess. Histopathologic sections show an irregular epithelium covering the tongue. Below this is a zone of loose connective tissue with many thin blood vessels. At the border of the abscess, the epithelium is replaced by fibrin and polymorphonuclear neutrophils. The deeper muscle layers may be partially replaced by fibrous tissue, lymphocytes, and neutrophils.

FLETCHER (1956) reported an interesting case of actinomycotic infection which manifested itself initially as a *chronic otorrhea*. Although a number of biopsies were made from the middle ear, mastoid antrum, and nasopharynx — all of which revealed a granulomatous process — the etiologic diagnosis was not established until the patient came to autopsy. At that time a mass 3 cm by 1 cm with an ill-defined border surrounded the entire right petrous tip area and extended into the foramen magnum. It enveloped the cranial nerves of the right side, and had dissected downward near the mid-line to a point just above the nasopharynx on the right. Histopathologic sections were typical for actinomycosis. Ear involvement is rare, Fletcher's report being the 36th case to be added to the literature.

VERHOEFF (1926) described a case of *intraocular* actinomycosis in a patient who later died of an actinomycotic liver abscess. Eye involvement is virtually always extraocular and most frequently occurs as a *lacrimal canaliculitis* (SMITH, 1953; PINE et al., 1960; PINE and HARDIN, 1959).

Pulmonary Actinomycosis. Actinomycosis of the lungs begins in the bronchial mucosa, or in bronchopneumonic or peribronchial foci (TURNER, 1926; ARNDT, 1931; KAY, 1947, 1948; PRINSLEY, 1957; WARTHIN and BUSHUEFF, 1958). The infection usually starts with central hilar involvement and extends along the bronchi into the lung parenchyma. In the cases studied by KAY (1948) the initial lesion was lobular in distribution and pneumonic in type. The pneumonia, believed to be secondary to atelectasis, progresses to suppuration and abscess formation. The abscesses are burrowing in character and are surrounded by a highly vascularized granulation tissue. There is marked fibrosis and many alveoli are replaced by scar tissue. As the infection spreads, interlobar fissures are obliterated and adjacent lobes are involved. Pleural involvement may occur early with dense fibrous adhesions to the chest wall. In one case cited by WAYL et al. (1958) the apex of the lung was found to be infiltrated with hard masses and its separation from the thoracic wall was rendered difficult by dense adhesions, especially posteriorly and medially. These involved the bronchial plexus, subclavian artery, and superior vena cava. Empyema and chest wall sinuses may follow (Fig. 14).

Older lesions tend to be hard, consolidated and fibrotic. Within these firm cicatricial areas of the lungs, the granulation tissue masses are preserved as branching fistulous tracts and as abscesses filled with pus.

Usually the lower lobes are affected, but apical involvement also occurs (WINGO and WILLIAMS, 1957; WAYL et al., 1958; LEE, 1966). A tendency towards bilateral involvement has been cited (CONANT et al., 1954), but PEABODY and SEABURY (1957) feel that this feature is associated primarily with well-advanced cases. KAY (1948) reported involvement of the mid lung field in 11 cases, upper lung field in 8 cases, and lower lung field in 3 cases. Involvement was unilateral in 16 cases and bilateral in 6 cases. One of the cases reported by HOLLIS and HARGROVE (1947) presented as a posterior mediastinal abscess.

The microscopic findings are essentially those described under General Features. WINGO and WILLIAMS (1957) described a small actinomycotic nodule removed during thorocotomy as showing masses of young and mature granulation tissue mingled with alveoli containing macrophages. In many areas the alveoli were compressed and the septa were markedly thickened. There was diffuse infiltration with eosinophils and lymphocytes. Occasional basophilic masses of tangled filaments were lying free in the alveoli. These were gram-positive and

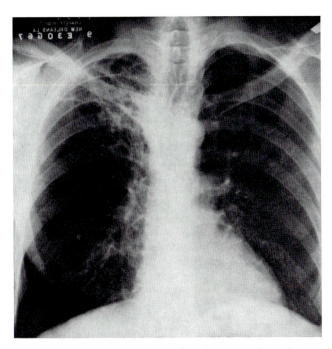

Fig. 14. Right upper lobe involvement associated with a perinephric abscess. A 39-year-old male gave a history of a 40 lb. weight loss during five months, right shoulder pain for two months, swelling of the shoulder and blood-tinged sputum production for two weeks. One week prior to admission he developed a rapidly enlarging left flank mass with chills and fever. A perinephric abscess arising from the lower pole of the kidney was drained with the removal of three liters of pus. Both his sputum and the pus were positive for *Actinomyces israelii*. Precipitating antibody was present in his serum. The right upper lobe infiltrate appearing in this figure is indistinguishable from tuberculosis. (Courtesy Dr. JOHN H. SEABURY)

non-acid fast. Some of these masses were surrounded by a single ring of poly-morphonuclear leucocytes.

Extension through the *thoracic wall*, via the intercostal spaces, is quite charac-teristic. Extensive areas of marked fibrosis and scarring may be found in the musculature, subcutaneous tissues and in the skin; all are characterized by numerous fistulous tracts.

Pericardial Actinomycosis. Extension to the *pericardium* may occur from pulmonary, cervical, or mediastinal lesions. Typically, actinomycotic pericarditis appears as fibrous adhesions between the pericardial layers, pleura and mediastinal tissues. These fibrotic masses contain abscesses and fistulous tracts. KAUFMANN (1929) cites a case showing invasion of the mediastinum and pericardium from the lung, penetrating the cavity of the right ventricle and entering the large coronary vein.

CORNELL and SHOOKHOFF (1944) reviewed the world literature and were able to collect 68 cases of actinomycosis in which the *heart* was involved. The *peri-cardium* was found to be most commonly involved by direct spread, usually from the lungs. An occasional case of pericarditis followed active infection of the myocardium which in turn had resulted from hematogenous dissemination. In two-thirds of the cases of actinomycotic pericarditis the myocardium was also involved and in many instances this led to penetration of the endocardium.

66*

Projection of the granulomatous mass into the cardiac chambers with perforation of the endocardium and subsequent pyemia occurred in six cases.

Clinical evidence of cardiac involvement was present in less than half of the cases reviewed by CORNELL and SHOOKHOFF. However, some did present as a *chronic constrictive pericarditis* as in the case reported by HARA and PIERCE (1957). In this instance, there was a left pleural empyema and a 3 cm abscess in the soft tissues anterior to the left fifth rib. The heart was encased in a thick fibrous capsule and was markedly restricted in its activity. The pericardium was purplish-tan and 3—10 mm thick. Histologic sections revealed markedly fibrotic tissue with many microabscesses, some of which contained granules of *A. israelii.* Very few cases have been added to those collected by CORNELL and SHOOKHOFF (SAVIDGE and DAVIES, 1953; ZOECKLER, 1951).

Spinal Actinomycosis. Pulmonary lesions may extend to involve tissues of the neck and then proceed as a prevertebral process to the spinal column where it may ascend or descend. It may ascend by continuity along vessels and nerves to to reach the cranial cavity, meninges, and brain; however, involvement of the central nervous system is more often due to hematogenous metastasis (BOLTON and ASHENHURST, 1964). Characteristic fibrotic processes with accompanying abscesses and sinus tracts may appear over the entire back and may involve the ribs and vertebrae. Usually, bone involvement remains essentially superficial, i.e., peri- and parosteal, and it is only rarely that the actinomycotic process extends deeply into the body of the vertebra (Fig. 18).

Finally, there may be extension of pulmonary lesions through the diaphragm into the abdominal cavity.

Abdominal Actinomycosis. PUTMAN and his associates (1950) as well as others (BROGDEN, 1922; COPE, 1938; CAMPBELL and BRADFORD, 1948; PHEILS et al., 1964) have presented strong evidence to support the contention that abdominal actinomycosis is almost invariably preceded by some disease process or by trauma (See Pathogenesis). Actinomycotic lesions usually arise in structures adjacent to the site of ulceration or perforation of a viscus, or in some pocket or recess in which gastrointestinal contents have collected (Fig. 9). In most cases involvement of the intestinal mucosa cannot be demonstrated. Most often, the initial actinomycotic lesion is found in the retroperitoneal tissues or tissues of the abdominal wall. BROCKMAN (1923) observed that the appendix and intestine are usually free of infection and that the initial lesion involves the muscles and connective tissues of the right iliac fossa (Fig. 15).

Periappendiceal Actinomycotic Abscess. Since the appendix is the commonest site of perforative gastrointestinal disease in man (PUTMAN et al., 1950), it is not surprising that the right iliac fossa (right lower quadrant of the abdominal wall) is the site most frequently affected (Table 3). The early lesion presents externally as a firm, indurated mass near the previous operative site. In time, this mass softens and the formation of abscesses and sinuses ensues (Fig. 9). Gross examination reveals destruction of subperitoneal and subcutaneous connective tissue as well as muscle. Varying quantities of pus, oftentimes very little, are to be found. The direction of spread of the lesion appears to be away from the bowel.

Actinomycotic Abscesses of the Liver. The liver may be involved by direct extension through the diaphragm from foci in the thoracic cavity (WAGENSTEEN et al., 1952), or from a primary lesion in the abdominal cavity. Usually, involvement is via the portal vein and secondary to an abdominal lesion (FORBUS, 1943). Actinomycotic pylephlebitis may develop. The process may continue from the liver through the diaphragm to involve the pleura and lungs (BONNEY, 1947; FOREMAN, 1963). Commonly, there is one or several foci; these appear on cut

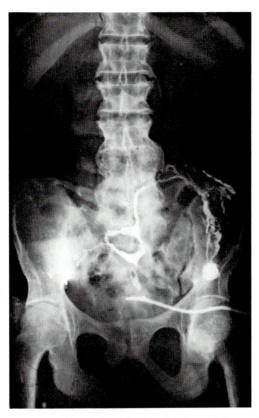

Fig. 15. Multiple sinus tracts in the pelvic region. At the time of diagnosis, this patient had a history of multiple draining sinuses in the lumbar, sacroiliac, and inguinal areas. Fistula-in-ano had been present intermittently. He had been treated on three occasions for the presumptive diagnosis of tuberculosis without any response to streptomycin. Direct examination of drainage and curettings from the sinus tract were positive for sulfur granules. Cultures were positive for *Actinomyces bovis*; treatment with penicillin was curative. The sinogram presented here shows marked involvement of the pelvis with extensions along the prevertebral fascial plane, the iliopsoas muscles and sigmoid colon. (Courtesy Dr. JOHN H. SEABURY)

surface as yellow, soft, fibrillar, meshy, or honeycombed masses saturated with pus (Fig. 16). Occasionally, numerous metastatic nodules may be present. An abscess may have a wall up to 1 cm in thickness. The creamy yellow pus can be expressed by slight pressure and contains numerous sulfur granules. Histologic sections show complete destruction of hepatic tissue with replacement by the typical abscesses. Generally, there are no inflammatory or degenerative changes in the liver parenchyma outside of the abscess although there may be some scarring and collapse of liver tissue along with proliferation of Kupffer cells (WAGENSTEEN et al., 1952).

Actinomycosis of the Spleen. Multiple actinomycotic abscesses of the spleen with spontaneous rupture of that organ has been observed (WEED et al., 1949; PUTMAN et al., 1950). In the case illustrated by PUTMAN et al. the gastrosplenic ligament was thickened and fibrotic and was found to contain several spicules of chicken bone embedded in the fibrous tissue. These had apparently perforated through the gastric wall, carrying *A. israelii* and other microorganisms with them.

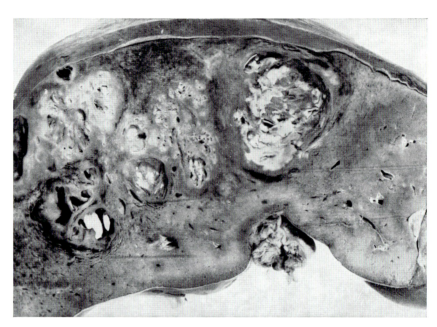

Fig. 16. Multiple actinomycotic abscesses of the liver. Note the pus still filling smaller abscesses and clinging to the wall of the larger ones. Although sulfur granules are not discernable at this magnification, they were readily demonstrable in the pus at the postmortem examination. The surrounding zone of lipophages is visible around smaller abscesses, and the dense fibrosis of scarring is well shown about abscesses to the left. This liver specimen, while taken from a different case, is strikingly similar to that seen in the 16 year old boy presented in Fig. 9. At the periappendiceal region the fungus enters venules and infects the liver via the portal vein. Sometimes the hepatic abscesses perforate the capsule of the liver and produce a subdiaphragmatic abscess or even a penetration of the diaphragm with empyema or abscess of the lung

Renal Actinomycosis. Involvement of the kidneys may be the result of contiguous spread from some primary focus in the abdomen or may represent hematogenous dissemination from some focus which can be either apparent or inapparent. A unique case was reported by LeBrun and Gilmour (1953) in which actinomycosis of the kidney followed a ureterocecostomy. The infection is presumed to have originated from the cecum and extended via the lumen of the ureter.

When renal actinomycosis occurs in the absence of any other demonstrable foci, it is considered to be a "primary infection". Primary renal involvement may occur as: 1) a chronic suppurative lesion resembling a renal carbuncle, 2) pyelonephritis, and 3) pyonephrosis.

Gross changes in the kidney may be classified as *localized* or *diffuse*. The localized lesion will appear on cut surface as a pyramidal area of granulation and scar tissue with the apex pointing towards the renal pelvis; within this area, yellowish streaks or granules and abscess cavities of various size occur. The process may extend through the capsule to invade the perinephric fat and produce a perirenal abscess while sparing the pelvis and calyces (Whisenand and Moore, 1951). In diffuse involvement, the entire kidney may be converted into a suppurating, granulomatous mass with sinus tracts discharging to the skin.

When involvement begins in the lower pole of the kidney, obstruction of the ureter occurs and hydronephrosis develops (Dammgaard-Morch, 1956). Calculus formation and pyonephrosis are natural sequelae (WILSON-PEPPER, 1951). Extension from the infected kidney to the lower urinary tract is uncommon.

Tubo-ovarian Actinomycosis. In tubo-ovarian lesions the right adnexal structures are usually involved first; extension to the left occurs later. Multilocular abscesses are usually present and sinus tracts may extend in various directions to involve the other ovary and retroperitoneal tissues, or to re-enter the gastrointestinal tract as an anal fistula (HARTL, 1951; MURPHY, 1954; LOTH, 1956; PHEILS et al., 1964; SWEENEY and BLACKWELDER, 1965; KRIEG and STAIB, 1966). The review of INGALLS and MERENDINO (1952) showed bilateral involvement in 44.4% of cases; right side only in 37.8%; and left side only in 17.8%. Typically, histologic sections will show chronic salpingitis with fibrosis of the ovary and areas of necrosis with miliary abscesses. The abscesses are intercommunicating, frequently contain granules, and have the characteristic cellular constituents. Most workers agree that involvement of the female genitalia is the result of extension from the intestine (WAGNER, 1910; ROBINSON, 1919; FRANK, 1922; BRICKNER, 1925; STEVENSON, 1957). HAZELHORST (1928) reported cases which followed instrumentation for abortion. BARTH (1928) reported actinomycosis in women fitted with intrauterine pessaries. The incidence of pelvic organ involvement is not high; RASHBAUM and McINTOSH (1944) were able to collect only 85 cases from the literature, but later a review by MACCARTHY (1955) cited 157 recorded cases.

In the case cited by CAMPBELL and BRADFORD (1948) generalized actinomycotic involvement of the pelvic organs followed surgery for a ruptured ovarian cyst by 11 months. The patient died approximately 13 months after original surgery. Autopsy revealed completely necrotic pelvic organs; the uterus; oviducts, and ovaries were identified with great difficulty. The mass of necrotic pelvic structures was adherent to the anterior surface of the rectum and rectosigmoid, the posterior aspect of the bladder, the tip of the cecum and one loop of ileum. There was an obstruction of the left ureterovesical junction with accompanying hydroureter and severe pyelonephritis. One sinus tract communicated with and drained through the lower part of the abdomen.

Involvement of the *uterus* is exceedingly rare; only 14 of the 157 cases reviewed by MACCARTHY (1955) showed uterine involvement and in only one case was an *endometrial* lesion specifically mentioned. BAGATKO (1958) has reported involvement of the *cervix*.

In the case presented by MACCARTHY, the uterus was enlarged (147 gm) with a localized mass in the right postero-lateral region comprised of necrotic and friable material. The lesion had penetrated the myometrium and extended into the cavity of the body of the uterus. The muscle coat showed scattered yellow foci. Histologically, the outer two-thirds of the myometrium was replaced by multiple abscesses, each surrounded by a wall of granulation tissue. There were numerous sulfur granules. The inflammatory process extended from the parametrium to a junction between the outer two-thirds and inner one-third of uterine muscle. At one point, there was a fistula opening on the endometrial surface. The infection had obliterated the right ovary and the right fallopian tube was enlarged and contained pus.

Perforation into the *urinary bladder* is also uncommon. KUSUNOKI et al. (1958) found only 14 cases in the literature and were able to contribute an additional case.

Actinomycosis of the Breast. DAVIES (1951) found primary involvement of the breasts to be exceptionally rare, his case representing the 14th in the literature. Three degrees of involvement are recognized, viz., an early stage of recurrent acute abscess formation, a stage of multiple sinus formation with distortion of the breast, and a quiescent stage of chronic abscess formation. The portal of entry seems to be the nipple.

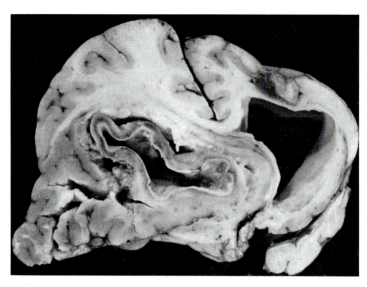

Fig. 17. Actinomycotic abscess of the brain. Coronal section of the brain showing a left frontal lobe abscess, focal granulomatous meningoencephalitis, and obstructive hydrocephalus. From a two-year-old white female who died four months after a right ventriculojugular shunt for a left parieto-occipital abscess. The initial abscess was associated with a urinary tract infection, but the exact organism is not known. (Courtesy Dr. Paul A. McGarry)

Actinomycosis of the Testis. Scorer (1952) reported actinomycotic infection of the left testicle, his case representing the fifth to be added to the literature (Schneider, 1945; Baker and Regins, 1946). Involvement is unilateral, with swelling of the cord and general enlargement of the testicle, particularly of the globus minor. On cut surface multiple abscesses with typical gross and histologic features are seen. The *epididymis* is apparently spared by the disease process.

Subdiaphragmatic and Other Abdominal Abscesses. Numerous abscesses may develop in the abdominal cavity; those most commonly encountered include the subdiaphragmatic or subphrenic abscess, pelvic abscess, psoas abscess, and perinephric abscess (Table 3). While these occur most frequently on the right side or medially, involvement of the left side can occur (Silber, 1953).

MacHaffie et al. (1957) described an actinomycotic abscess positioned in the mesentery between the junction of the descending and sigmoid colon and crest of the ileum. Grossly, it resembled a sarcoma, but on cut surface it proved to be a multiloculated cyst with numerous bands of white fibrous tissue and contained a large amount of purulent material. Miller (1964) reported the occurence of an actinomycotic abscess at the site of anastomosis following resection of the left colon for adenocarcinoma.

Psoas and Retroperitoneal Abscesses. Sinus tracts extend to the lumbar, greater trochanter, and gluteal regions (Ross and Knight, 1954; Wayl et al., 1958; Cummings et al., 1959) (Fig. 13).

Anorectal Lesions. These may arise either as a primary infection (Gordon and DuBose, 1951; Anscombe and Hofmeyr, 1954; Swinton and Schatman, 1964; Fry et al., 1965) or secondarily to some focus in the pelvis (Pheils et al., 1964). The case reported by Gordon and DuBose apparently had its origin at the site of an external hemorrhoid. The process had persisted for 30 years, initially producing an anal fistula which was excised, then multiple subcutaneous nodules and fistulae in the perianal region, posterior buttocks, intracrural region and posterior thighs.

Malignant Changes in Sinuses. Malignant degenerative changes, usually carcinomatous in nature, may occur in chronic discharging sinuses. GOODWIN (1955) reported an unusual case where the malignant change took the form of a granulation tissue sarcoma.

Actinomycosis of the Central Nervous System. The actual incidence of central nervous system involvement with *A. israelii* cannot be determined from the early literature since these investigators failed to distinguish actinomycotic lesions from those caused by *Nocardia*. Indications are that such involvement is an infrequent complication of actinomycosis in man. BOLTON and ASHENHURST (1964) were able to collect only 17 adequately documented cases from the world literature for the period 1937—1964 and were able to add a case of their own. Their survey revealed that there was evidence of hematogenous spread from teeth or lungs in 15 cases, direct extension of cervico-facial lesions in 2 cases, and no apparent primary source in one case.

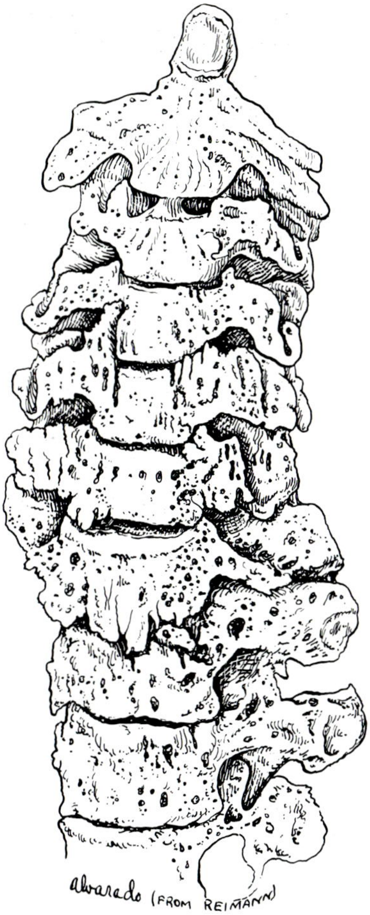

Actinomycotic Abscesses of the Brain. Commonly, there was a single abscess involving a cerebral hemisphere (Fig. 17). Multiple abscesses were present in 2 cases and in only one was meningitis the only manifestation of the disease. The abscess wall is usually thick and fibrotic. In the case reported by BOLTON and ASHENHURST there were three thick-walled abscess cavities, the largest measuring 1.5 cm and the two smaller ones 0.5 cm in diameter. The abscess wall contained an inner zone of granulation tissue which was infiltrated by lymphocytes, plasma cells, and an occasional polymorphonuclear leucocyte.

Fig. 18. Actinomycosis of the vertebral column. The result of extension from the apices of the lungs and the deep cervical tissues. Usually, bone involvement is superficial and it is rare that the actinomycotic process extends deeply into the body of the vertebra. (Redrawn from REIMANN: Pathology for Students and Physicians, vol. 2, p. 1146, 1929; P. Blakiston's Son & Co., Philadelphia)

Numerous nests of lipophages were present. The outer layer was composed of dense glial tissue and there was some perivascular chronic infiltrate associated with adjacent blood vessels. A few granules of *A. israelii* were found within the cavities.

Not included in the review by BOLTON and ASHENHURST was a case by PANTAZOPOULOS (1964) in which the actinomycotic abscess presented as a small, cyst-like tumor in the third ventricle. It was suspended from the inferior surface of the corpus callosum and obstructed the third ventricle causing hydrocephalus. The mass was surrounded by a capsule except for a small area at the base of its pedicle. It was soft and when incised a dense purulent yellow-grey fluid flowed out. It had the features of an abscess; its wall was thin and consisted mostly of vascular connective tissue and showed the structure of choroid plexus or choroid tela. There were numerous leucocytes, remnants of red blood cells, and necrotic neuroglial cells. Sulfur granules were demonstrated. No primary focus could be demonstrated at autopsy.

Spinal Actinomycosis. Involvement of the vertebral column is attended by both necrosis and hyperplasia (COPE, 1951; BRETT, 1951a, 1951b; WINSTON, 1951; BAYLIN and WEAR, 1953). It is usually secondary to involvement of contiguous tissues with several vertebrae being affected. Suppuration may spread under the anterior common ligament to involve larger segments of the vertebral column. The infection extends to adjacent pedicles and transverse processes and also to the heads of neighboring ribs. Characteristically, there is bone adsorption around the focus of infection with new bone being formed distally. This combination of rarefaction and sclerosis occurs in varying proportions (COPE, 1951); when the disease is progressing, rarefaction predominates, during regression sclerosis (Fig. 18). The infection may involve the entire vertebral body resulting in a network of suppurating chambers which are bounded by bone of increased density imparting a honeycombed effect which shows up on X-ray as a lattice work or "soap-bubble" effect (BAYLIN and WEAR, 1953).

Differential Diagnosis

The need to differentiate actinomycotic granules in tissue from those produced by other microorganisms has already been discussed.

Clinically, actinomycosis must be differentiated from tuberculosis, syphilis, neoplasm, glanders, tularemia, granuloma inguinale, osteomyelitis, botryomycosis, sarcoidosis, chronic appendicitis, amebiasis, typhoid fever, carcinoma of the intestine, intestinal tuberculosis, liver abscess, psoas abscess and sarcoma of the retroperitoneal tissue or iliac bones (CONANT et al., 1954). It must also be differentiated from other mycoses, especially nocardiosis, North American blastomycosis, paracoccidiodal granuloma, coccidioidomycosis, cryptococcosis, and sporotrichosis.

Clinical Features

Cervico-facial type. Commonly, the onset is insidious and first becomes apparent as a persistent swelling in the parotid or mandibular regions. Pain is minimal unless secondary infection develops. Where the actinomycotic involvement follows trauma or a surgical procedure, healing of the wound will be retarded or arrested with a concomitant increase in edema and induration. As the infection progresses, there appears the classical external manifestations of a dark purplish skin overlying a hard, tumorous process. At least in the early stages, fever is usually minimal or absent and the patient's general health remains unaffected so long as the process does not become too extensive (Fig. 15).

HERTZ (1957) has divided cervico-facial infections into the classical form, atypical form, and a tumor-like process which avoids bone and fails to form an abscess.

The *classical form* is characterized by a chronic course, accompanied by firm, extensive infiltrations which alternate with purulent foci, and by the formation of numerous fistulae. It often starts with a toothache, presenting as a hard tumor-like mass. Gradually, an abscess is formed and extends towards the surface of the skin. Fistulae appear which discharge a foul-smelling pus at the surface. Trismus develops where the muscles of mastication are involved. A febrile reponse is absent or minimal except in extensive involvement. Generally the lymph nodes are not involved, but the process may invade blood vessels with subsequent hematogenous dissemination. In this form, extension usually avoids bony tissue.

The *atypical form* may be acute or subacute and is associated with a marked febrile response. These cases yield a foul-smelling pus and an osseous focus can always be established. The fever is accompanied by painful swelling, then abscess formation and finally perforation with formation of a fistula. In many respects, the early stages of both the classical and atypical forms resemble an ordinary dental inflammation.

The tumor-like form of involvement is painless, grows continually without abscess formation and without involving the bone or skin, and fails to respond to the conventional doses of penicillin. In the case described by HERTZ (1957) sulfur granules were absent but anaerobic gram negative bacilli and anaerobic streptococci were isolated. This form of cervico-facial involvement is the hardest to diagnose clinically. The painless swelling and slow steady growth will suggest a tumor. Roentgenologic studies are helpful to the extent that they rule out bone involvement.

Cervico-facial infections must be differentiated from glanders, tularemia, tuberculosis, and bacterial osteomyelitis.

Thoracic type. As the pulmonary lesion extends to include consolidation, sinus tracts and pleural involvement, the patient will experience night sweats and high fever and sustain a substantial weight loss (Fig. 11). Febrile episodes of 101 F. to 103 F. and white blood count of 20,000 to 30,000 cells/cu mm are not uncommon.

Radiologic findings may be suggestive but are never diagnostic (PEABODY and SEABURY, 1957). Usually they are indistinguishable from those found in pulmonary tuberculosis (LEE, 1966; WINGO and WILLIAMS, 1957), although in some cases the area of lung involved may be of some help in the differential diagnosis (Fig. 12). In KAY's series (1948) the disease involved the mid lung field in 11 cases, upper lung field in 8 cases and base of the lungs in 3 cases; involvement was unilateral in 16 cases and bilateral in 6 cases. Commonly, X-ray findings will reveal a large area of infiltration or consolidative pneumonia with hazy margins along with an associated pleuritis. Frank cavitation is unusual, although multiple abscesses appearing as small round lucencies can be seen within the consolidated areas (PEABODY and SEABURY, 1957). Empyema is usually present; pleural effusion, though rare, has been reported (BONNEY, 1947). Parahilar lesions may present some difficulties in differentiating actinomycosis from bronchial neoplasm (WARTHIN and BUSHUEFF, 1958). Vertebral involvement along with the characteristic "soap bubble" appearance on roentgenograms has already been discussed.

Pulmonary lesions may extend to involve the pericardium and heart with consequent cardiac constriction. This can manifest itself as chronic constrictive pericarditis (CORNELL and SHOOKHOFF, 1944; ZOECKLER, 1951; HARA and PIERCE, 1957).

Pulmonary actinomycosis must also be differentiated from other mycotic infections of the lung, particularly nocardiosis.

Abdominal type. Abdominal actinomycosis is usually preceded by some type of acute, perforative gastrointestinal disease; most frequently this occurs in the form of an acute appendicitis (See Pathogenesis). Carious teeth and diseased tonsils may also serve as predisposing factors (BROGDEN 1922). Symptoms most frequently associated with abdominal involvement are weight loss, cachexia, fever, and a palpable mass. There may be localized pain and tenderness, muscular rigidity, induration, vomiting and jaundice. A purplish discoloration of the skin may appear over the mass and around the sinus tract openings. Kidney involvement may occur as an abscess, pyelonephritis, or pyonephrosis; the signs are obscure and suggest a malignancy. Abdominal actinomycosis must be differentiaed from tuberculosis, malignancy and amebiasis.

Prognosis

The prognosis for cervico-facial involvement was relatively good even before the advent of antibiotics. HERTZ (1957) quotes from BROFELDT'S statistics of 1926 which showed that 67% of 151 cervico-facial cases were cured. Currently, recovery rates are approximately 90% for cervico-facial cases, 80% for abdominal cases, and 40% for thoracic cases.

Therapy

Treatment of actinomycotic lesions has included simple needle aspiration (MACCONNELL, 1944), surgical drainage (COLEBROOK, 1921), and complete excision (WAGENSTEEN, 1936). Irradiation was recommended by LAMB et al. (1947) and NEUBER (1940) reported excellent results from the use of freshly prepared, polyvalent autogenous vaccines. Some of the drugs used prior to penicillin included potassium iodide, copper sulfate, methylene blue, and arsenicals (HUNTER and WESTRICK, 1957).

The use of *penicillin* has had the most profound influence on the prognosis of actinomycotic infections, particularly the thoracic and abdominal types (MAC-GREGOR, 1945; DOBSON and CUTTING, 1945; NICHOLS and HERRELL, 1948). Actinomycosis has also been treated successfully with aureomycin (WRIGHT and LOWEN, 1950; MCVAY et al., 1951; MCVAY and SPRUNT, 1953a; SVANE, 1966), Chloramphenicol (LITTMAN et al., 1950, 1952; KELLY, 1951), oxytetracycline (PULASKI et al., 1952; LANE et al., 1953), tetracycline (MARTIN et al., 1956), achromycin (HINDS and DEGNAN, 1955), erythromycin (HERRELL et al., 1955), streptomycin (TORRENS and WOOD, 1949), isoniazid (MCVAY and SPRUNT, 1953b; GREEN and BLACK, 1955), and stilbamidine (MILLER et al., 1952).

While an occasional strain of *A. israelii* has been found to be resistant to penicillin therapy (PEABODY and SEABURY, 1960), most strains are inhibited by 0.01—0.6 units of the drug. GARROD (1952) tested the *in vitro* sensitivity of *A. israelii* to various antibiotics and found effective inhibitory concentration to be 0.01—0.6 unit for penicillin, 2.2 μg for terramycin, 2.8 μg for chloramphenicol, 4.2 μg for aureomycin, and 23.7 μg for streptomycin.

Penicillin remains the drug of choice, but it must be administered in adequate amounts if treatment failures are to be avoided (RAPER, 1950; HUNTER and WESTRICK, 1957; PEABODY and SEABURY, 1957; HERTZ, 1957; ASHTON and SLANEY, 1963; SWEENEY and BLACKWELDER, 1965; STANTON, 1966).

For cervico-facial cases, HERTZ (1957) recommends 1.5—5 million units of penicillin given intramuscularly daily for 14 days. Local injection of penicillin (300,000 units) into the actinomycotic foci is sometimes desirable.

For systemic infections, SEABURY and DASCOMB (1964) recommend a minimum of 1—2 million units of penicillin daily for approximately one month. Dosages of 1—20 million units daily for 6—8 weeks have also been suggested (PEABODY and SEABURY, 1957; UTZ, 1967). The practice of administering sulfadiazine or a broad-spectrum antibiotic along with the penicillin is not justified. Most of the treatment failures in the past have been due to inadequate dosage and not to lack of sensitivity of *A. israelii* to penicillin.

The role of surgical procedures in the treatment of actinomycosis continues to be of major importance (PUTMAN et al., 1950). These include incision and drainage of abscesses, curettage of sinuses and fistulae, and excision of sinus tracts.

References

ANDLEIGH, H.S.: Two rare cases of fungus infection of skin in Rajasthan: actinomycosis and rhinosporidiosis. Indian med. Gaz. **86**, 100 (1951). — ANSCOMBE, A.R., HOFMEYR, J.: Perianal actinomycosis complicating pilonidal sinus. Brit. J. Surg. **41**, 666 (1954). — ARNDT, H.J.: Die aktinomykotischen Veränderungen der Lunge und des Brustfells und das Verhalten der Lunge und des Brustfells bei Aktinomykose. In: Handbuch der Speziellen Pathologischen Anatomie und Histologie, Vol. **3** (3), pp. 397—458. F. HENKE and O. LUBARSCH, Editors. Berlin: Springer 1931. — ASHTON, F., SLANEY, G.: Post-gastrectomy duodenal fistula due to actinomycosis. Brit. J. Surg. **50**, 884 (1963). — AUBERT: Observation d'un cas d'actinomycose maxillaire chez le chien. Rev. Path. comp. **51**, 276 (1951). — AUGER, C.: Human actinobacillary and staphylococcic actinophytosis. Amer. J. clin. Path. **18**, 645 (1948). — AXHAUSEN, G.: Die Pathogenese und Klinik der Kieferaktinomykose. Dtsch. Zahn-, Mund- u. Kieferheilk. **2**, 197 (1935). ~ Das Frühbild der Kieferaktinomykose. Dtsch. med. Wschr. **62**, 1449 (1936). — BAKER, R.D.: Tissue changes in fungous disease. Arch. Path. **44**, 459 (1947). ~ The diagnosis of fungus diseases by biopsy. J. chron. Dis. **5**, 552 (1957). — BAKER, W.J., RAGINS, A.B.: Actinomycosis of the testicle. J. Urol. **56**, 547 (1946). — BANERJEE, B.N.: Actinomycosis of the skin. Indian med. Gaz. **87**, 253 (1952). — BARTH, H.: Über Parametritis Actinomycotica und ihre Entstehung. Arch. Gynäk. **134**, 310 (1928). — BAYLIN, G.J., WEAR, J.M.: Blastomycosis and actinomycosis of the spine. Amer. J. Roentgenol. **69**, 395 (1953). — BERTI, P.: Sulla patologia granulomatosa della parotide tubercolosi, sarcoidosi, actinomicosi. Arch. De Vecchi Anat. pat. **35**, 889 (1961). — BIBBY, B.G., KNIGHTON, H.T.: The actinomyces of the human mouth. J. infect. Dis. **69**, 148 (1941). — BIGGS, J.S.G.: Actinomycosis of the liver: a report of two cases. Med. J. Aust. **47**, II, 939 (1960). — BINFORD, C.H.: Tissue reactions elicited by fungi. In: Fungi and Fungous Diseases, pp. 220—238. G. DALLDORF, editor. Springfield, Ill.: Charles C. Thomas 1962. — BJERRUM, O., HANSEN, Sv.: Undersogelser over forekomsten af actinomyceten i mundhulen og deres betydning for den acute form af actinomycose. Ugeskr. Laeg. **94**, 1075 (1931). — BLANK, C.H., GEORG, L.K.: The use of fluorescent antibody methods for the detection and identification of *Actinomyces* species in clinical material. J. Lab. clin. Med. **71**, 283 (1968). — BOGATKO, F.L.H.: Actinomycosis of cervix. J. Amer. med. Wom. Ass. **13**, 268 (1958). — BOLLINGER, O.: Über eine neue Pilzkrankheit beim Rinde. Zbl. med. Wiss. **15**, 481 (1877). — BOLTON, C.F., ASHENHURST, E.M.: Actinomycosis of the brain. Case report and review of the literature. Canad. med. Ass. J. **90**, 922 (1964). — BONNEY, G.L.W.: Actinomycosis of liver; report of an unusual case. Brit. J. Surg. **34**, 316 (1947). — BRAINEY, R.R.: Primary cutaneous actinomycosis. J. Amer. med. Ass. **194**, 679 (1965). — BREDE, H.D.: Zur Ätiologie und Mikrobiologie der Aktinomykose; *in-vitro* Versuche zur Frage der fermentativen Unterstützung des *Actinomyces israeli* durch Begleitbakterien. Zbl. Bakt. **174**, 110 (1959). — BREED, R.S., CONN, H.J.: The nomenclature of the Actinomycetaceae. J. Bact. **4**, 585 (1919). — BRETT, M.S.: Advanced actinomycosis of the spine treated with penicillin and streptomycin; report of a case. J. Bone Jt Surg. **33-B**, 215 (1951a). ~ Advanced actinomycosis of the spine treated with penicillin and streptomycin. J. Bone Jt Surg. **33-B**, 482 (1951b). — BRICKNER, W.M.: Pelvic actinomycosis; a study of five consecutive cases successfully treated by operation. Ann. Surg. **81**, 343 (1925). — BROCKMAN, R.: Actinomycosis of the right iliac fossa. Brit. J. Surg. **10**, 456 (1923). — BROFELDT, S.A.: Über Actinomycose in Finnland. Duodecim (Helsinki) 7, (1926). — BRODGEN, J.C.: Actinomycosis of the gastrointestinal tract; a study of fourteen cases. J. Lab. clin. Med. 8, 180 (1922). — BUCHANAN, B.B., PINE, L.: Characterization of a propionic acid producing actinomyces, *Actinomyces propionicus* sp. nov. J. gen. Microbiol. **28**, 305 (1962). — BURROWS, H.J.: Actinomycosis from punch injuries: with report of a case affecting a metacarpal bone. Brit. J. Surg. **32**, 506 (1945). — CALERO, C.: Pulmonary actinomycosis; report of the first case observed in the Isthmus of Panama. Dis. Chest **12**, 402 (1946). — CAMPBELL, D.A., BRADFORD, B., Jr.: Actinomycosis of thorax and abdomen. A.M.A. Arch. Surg. **57**, 202 (1948). — CHOUKAS, N.C.: Actinomycosis of the mandible. Oral Surg. **11**.(1), 14 (1958). — CHRISTIE, A.O., PORTEOUS, J.W.: Growth of several strains of *Actinomyces israelii* in chemically defined media. Nature (Lond.) **195**, 408 (1962a). ~ The cultivation of a single strain of *Actinomyces israelii* in a simplified and chemically defined medium. J. gen. Microbiol. **28**, 443 (1962b). ~ The growth factor requirements of the Willis strain of *Actinomyces israelii* growing in a chemically defined medium. J. gen. Microbiol. **28**, 455 (1962c). — CINTI, G.: Le malattie granulomatose (tubercolosi, actinomicosi e granuloma maligno di Sternberg) della lingua. Arch. De Vecchi Anat. pat. **22**, 693 (1954). — COLEBROOK, L.: The mycelial and other micro-organisms associated with human actinomycosis. Brit.J. Path. **1**, 197 (1920). ~ A report upon 25 cases of actinomycosis, with especial reference to vaccine therapy. Lancet **1**, 893 (1921). — CONANT, N.F., SMITH, D.T., BAKER, R.D., CALLOWAY, J.L., MARTIN, D.S.: Actinomycosis. In: Manual of Clinical Mycology, pp. 1—25. Philadelphia: W.B. Saunders Co. 1954. — COPE, V.Z.: Actinomycosis. London-New York-Toronto: Oxford University

Press 1938. ∼ Actinomycosis involving the colon and rectum. J. int. Coll. Surg. **12**, 401 (1949). ∼ Actinomycosis of bone with special reference to infection of the vertebral column. J. Bone Jt Surg. **33-B**, 205 (1951). — Cornell, A., Shookhoff, H. B.: Actinomycosis of the heart simulating rheumatic fever. Arch. intern. Med. **74**, 11 (1944). — Cullen, C. H., Sharp, M. E.: Infection of wounds with *Actinomyces*. J. Bone Jt Surg. **33-B**, 221 (1951). — Cummings, J. R., Beekley, M. E., Earley, N.: Abdominal actinomycosis; a case report. Ohio St. med. J. **55** (3), 350 (1959). — Cummins, C. S., Harris, H.: Studies on the cell wall composition and taxonomy of Actinomycetales and related groups. J. gen. Microbiol. **18**, 173 (1958). — Cummins, C. S.: Chemical composition and antigenic structure of cell walls of *Corynebacterium, Mycobacterium, Nocardia, Actinomyces*, and *Arthrobacter*. J. gen. Microbiol. **28**, 35 (1962). — Dammgaard-Morch, P.: Abdominal actinomycosis; three cases of atypical localization. Acta chir. scand. **110**, 458 (1956). — Davies, D. F.: Paralaryngeal actinomycosis in a child. Brit. med. J. **1**, 363 (1952). — Davies, J. A. L.: Primary actinomycosis of the breast. Brit. J. Surg. **38**, 378 (1951). — Decker, H. R.: Treatment of thoracic actinomycosis by penicillin and sulfonamides. J. thorac. Surg. **15**, 430 (1946). — Dobson, L., Cutting, W. C.: Penicillin and sulfonamides in the therapy of actinomycosis; report of 16 additional cases and *in vitro* tests of susceptibility of *Actinomyces* to penicillin and sulfadiazine. J. Amer. med. Ass. **128**, 856 (1945). — Dorph-Petersen, L., Pindborg, J. J.: Actinomycosis of the tongue; report of a case. Oral Surg. **7**, 1178 (1954). — Elsaesser, K. H.: Über die Aktinomykose und ihre Lokalisation im Zentralnervensystem. Klinik, Bakteriologie, pathologische Anatomie. Dtsch. Z. Nervenheilk. **164**, 123 (1950). — Emmons, C. W.: *Actinomyces* and actinomycosis. Puerto Rico J. publ. Hlth **11**, 63 (1935). ∼ Strains of *Actinomyces bovis* isolated from tonsils. Puerto Rico J. publ. Hlth **11**, 720 (1936). ∼ The isolation of *Actinomyces bovis* from tonsillar granules. Publ. Hlth Rep. (Wash.) **53**, 1967 (1938). — Emmons, C. W., Binford, C. H., Utz, J. P.: Actinomycosis. In: Medical Mycology, pp. 55—71. Philadelphia: Lea & Febiger 1963. — Erikson, D.: Pathogenic anaerobic microorganisms of the actinomyces group. Med. Res. Council Spec. Rept. Ser. **240**, 1 (1940). ∼ The morphology, cytology, and taxonomy of the actinomycetes. Ann. Rev. Microbiol. **3**, 23 (1949). — Fairley, K. D.: Actinomycosis of the paraaortic lymph glands. Med. J. Aust. **1**, 799 (1947). — Fegeler, F.: Die Aktinomykose. S. 527—588. — Finch, P. G.: Actinomycosis of forearm. Canad. med. Ass. J. **68**, 595 (1953). — Fletcher, R.: A rare case of chronic otorrhea with intracranial complications. Laryngoscope (St. Louis) **66**, 702 (1956). — Foreman, J. M.: Actinomycosis of the liver. N. Z. med. J. **62**, 536 (1963). — Frank, R. T.: Gynaecological and Obstetrical Pathology. D. Appleton and Co. 1922. — Fry, G. A., Martin, W. J., Dearing, W. H., Culp, C. E.: Primary actinomycosis of the rectum with multiple perianal and perineal fistulae. Mayo Clin. Proc. **40**, 296 (1965). — Ganner, H.: Ein Fall von Aktinomykose der Unterkieferspeicheldrüse, zugleich ein Beitrag zur Frage der Ätiologie der sogenannten Küttnerschen Speicheldrüsentumoren. Arch. klin. Chir. **155**, 495 (1929). — Garrod, L. P.: Actinomycosis of the lung: aetiology, diagnosis, and chemotherapy. Tubercle (Lond.) **33**, 258 (1952). — Genesi, M.: Pneumomicosi actinomicotica con ascesso cerebrale. Minerva pediat. (Torino) **4**, 39 (1952). — Georg, L. K., Robertstadt, G. W., Brinkman, S. A.: Identification of species of *Actinomyces*. J. Bact. **88**, 477 (1964). — Georg, L. K., Robertstadt, G. W., Brinkman, S. A., Hicklin, M. D.: A new pathogenic anaerobic *Actinomyces* species. J. infect. Dis. **115**, 88 (1965). — Ginsberg, A., Little, A. C. W.: Actinomycosis in dogs. J. Path. Bact. **60**, 563 (1948). — Glaesmer-Zaff, M.: Ein Schulfall einer Ovarialaktinomykose. Zbl. Gynäk. **74**, 1927 (1952). — Glahn, M.: The pathogenesis of cervico-facial actinomycosis. Acta chir. scand. **108**, 193 (1954a). ∼ Cervico-facial actinomycosis — etiology and diagnosis. Acta chir. scand. **108**, 183 (1954b). — Gold, L., Doyne, E. E.: Actinomycosis with osteomyelitis of the alveolar process. Oral Surg. **5**, 1056 (1952). — Goodwin, M. A.: Sarcoma arising in a chronic actinomycotic sinus. Brit. J. Surg. **44**, (187) 489 (1957). — Gordon, M. A., DuBose, H. M.: Anorectal actinomycosis. Amer. J. clin. Path. **21**, 460 (1951). — Grabner, A.: Aktinomykose in Speichelsteinen. Z. Stomat. **34**, 862 (1936). — Green, R., Bolton, T. C., Woolsey, C. I.: Mycetoma, madura foot; a case of mycetoma pedis in Chicago. Ann. Surg. **128**, 1015 (1948). — Greene, L. W., Black, W. C.: Treatment of cervico-facial actinomycosis with isoniazid. Rocky Mtn med. J. **52**, 43 (1955). — Hagan, W. A.: The pathogenic actinomycetes. In: The Infectious Diseases of Domestic Animals, with Special Reference to Etiology, Diagnosis and Biologic Therapy, pp. 321—338. Ithaca, N. Y.: Comstock Publishing Co 1943. — Hanratty, W. J., Naeve, H. F.: Actinomycosis with pathologic fracture of mandible; report of a case. Oral Surg. **18**, 303 (1964). — Hara, M., Pierce, J. A.: Chronic constrictive pericarditis due to *Actinomyces bovis*; report of a case treated by pericardectomy. J. thorac. Surg. **33**, 730 (1957). — Harbitz, F., Grondahl, N. B.: Actinomykosen i Norge. Oslo: Kristiania 1910. — Hartl, H.: Zur Kenntnis der Genitalaktinomykose der Frau. Arch. Gynäk. **179**, 677 (1951). — Harz, C. O.: *Actinomyces bovis*, ein neuer Schimmel in den Geweben des Rindes. Jahresb. d. k. Centralbl. Tierarznei, Schule in München **5**, 125 (1879). — Havens, F. Z.: Actinomycosis of the head and neck. J. Amer. dent. Ass. **20**, 478 (1933). — Hazelhorst, G.: Aktinomykose der weiblichen Genital-organe als Abtreibungsfolge. Arch. Gynäk. **134**. 561 (1928). — HAZEN, E.L., LITTLE, G.N.: *Actinomyces bovis* and 'anaerobic diphtheroids'. Pathogenicity for hamsters and some other differentiating characteristics. J. Lab. clin. Med. **51**, 968 (1951). — HEINRICH, S., PULVERER, G.: Zur Ätiologie und Mikrobiologie der Aktinomykose: III. Die Pathogenbedeutung des *Actinobacillus Actinomycetem-comitans* den „Begleitbakterien" des *Actinomyces israeli*. Zbl. Bakt. **176**, 91 (1959). — HEITE. H.J.: Krankheiten durch Aktinomyceten und verwandte Erreger. Wechselwirkung zwischen pathogenen Pilzen und Wirtsorganismus. (4. Wiss. Tag. d. Deutschsprach. Mykolog. Gesellsch. in Freiburg/Br., 30. und 31. 10. 1964). Berlin-Heidelberg-New York: Springer 1967. — HEPBURN, R.H.: Actinomycosis of the testicle. J. Urol. (Baltimore) **63**, 113 (1950). — HERRELL, W.E., BELOWS, A., DAILEY, J.S.: Erythromycin in the treatment of actinomycosis. Antibiot. Med. **1**, 507 (1955). — HERRMANN, H.: Zur Pathogenese und Therapie der Aktinomykose. Dtsch. zahnärztl. Z. **7**, 725 (1952). — HERTZ, J.: Actinomycosis: oral, facial and maxillary manifestations. J. int. Coll. Surg. **28**, 539 (1957). — HILDICK-SMITH, G., BLANK, H., SARKANY, I.: Actinomycosis. In: Fungus Diseases and Their Treatment, pp. 293—302. Boston: Little Brown and Co. 1964. — HINDS, E.C., DEGNAN, E.J.: The use of achromycin and neomycin in the treatment of actinomycosis. Oral Surg. **8**, 1034 (1955). — HOLLIS, W.J., HARGROVE, M.D.: Actinomycosis; a report of 12 cases with special reference to a mediastinal case. New Orleans med. surg. J. **99**, 499 (1947). — HOLM, P.: Some investigations into the penicillin sensitivity of human pathogenic actinomycetes. Acta path. microbiol. scand. **25**, 376 (1948). ∼ Studies on the aetiology of human actinomycosis. I. The "other microbes" of actinomycosis and their importance. Acta path. microbiol. scand. **27**, 736 (1950). ∼ Studies on the aetiology of human actinomycosis. II. Do the "other microbes" of actinomycosis posses virulence? Acta path. microbiol. scand. **28**, (4) 391 (1951). — HOWELL, A., Jr., MURPHY III, W.C., PAUL, F., STEPHAN, R.M.: Oral strains of *Actinomyces*. J. Bacteriol. **78**, 82 (1959). — HOWELL, A., Jr., STEPHAN, R.M., PAUL, F.: Prevalence of *Actinomyces israelii*, *A.naeslundii*, *Bacterionema matruchotii*, and *Candida albicans* in selected areas of the oral cavity and saliva. J. dent. Res. **41**, 1050 (1962). — HUNTER, G.C., Jr., WESTRICK, C.M.: Cervicofacial abscess by *Actinomyces*; report of a case. Oral Surg. **10**, 793 (1957). — HUSTED, E.: Sialolithiasis. Acta chir. scand. **105**, 161 (1953). — INGALLS, E.G., MERENDINO, K.A.: Actinomycosis of the female genitalia; case report and review of the literature. West. J. Surg. **60**, 476 (1952). — ISRAEL, J.: Neue Beobachtungen auf dem Gebiete der Mykosen des Menschen. Virchows Arch. path. Anat. 15 (1878). ∼ Klinische Beiträge zur Kenntnis der Aktinomykose des Menschen. Berlin: A. Hirschwald 1885. — JACOBSEN, H.P.: Actinomycosis; a clinical, pathological and bacteriological study. Med. J. Rec. **132**, 342 ,379 (1930). — JACOBSON, J.R., CLOWARD, R.B.: Actinomycosis of the central nervous system. J. Amer. med. Ass. **137**, 769 (1948). — JANTSCHEW, W.G.: Über die primäre Aktinomykose des Mastdarms. Kasuistischer Beitrag. Z. ges. inn. Med. **16**, 476 (1961). — JUTZLER, G.A., LEPPLA, W., BRUNCK, H.J.: Primäre doppelseitige Nierenaktinomykose mit Papillennekrose als Ursache eines Nierenversagens. Ärztl. Forsch. **15**, I, 340 (1961). — KAUFMANN, E.: Pathology for Students of Medicine. Translation by S.P. Reimann. Philadelphia: P. Blakiston's Son and Co. 1929. — KAY, E.B.: Bronchopulmonary actinomycosis. Ann. intern. Med. **26**, 581 (1947). ∼ *Actinomyces* in chronic bronchopulmonary infections. Amer. Rev. Tuberc. **57**, 322 (1948). — KELLY, H.H.D.: Intestinal actinomycosis treated with chloramphenicol and aureomycin. Brit. med. J. No. 4734, 779 (1951). — KING, S., MEYER, E.: Metabolic and serologic differentiation of *Actinomyces* bovis and anaerobic diphtheroids. J. Bact. **74**, 234 (1957). — KNAKE, H.-J., ZEISS, K.-H.: Primäre Abdominalaktinomykose mit sekundärer Ausbreitung auf beide Tuben und Netz. Geburtsh. u. Frauenheilk. **15**, 816 (1955). — KÖHLMEIER, W., NIEL, K.: Aktinomykose-Endokarditis. Wien. klin. Wschr. **1953**, 25. — KOLOUCH, F., PELTIER, L.F.: Actinomycosis. Surgery **20**, 401 (1946). — KRIEG, H., STAIB, F.: Zur Abdominalaktinomykose der Frau. Gynäcologia (Basel) **162**, 156 (1966). — KUSUNOKI, T., HAYASHI, I., KASHIWAI, K.: Actinomycosis of the ovary perforating into the urinary bladder; report of a case. Urol. int. (Basel) **6**, 251 (1958). — KWAPINSKI, J.B.: Antigenic structure of the Actinomycetales. VII. Chemical and serological similarities of cell walls from 100 actinomycetales strains. J. Bact. **88**, 1211 (1964). — LAMB, J.H., LAIN, E.S., JONES, P.E.: Actinomycosis of the face and neck. J. Amer. med. Ass. **134**, 351 (1947). — LAMBERT, F.W., Jr., BROWN, J.M., GEORG, L.K.: Identification of *Actinomyces israelii* and *Actinomyces naeslundii* by fluorescent antibody and agar-gel diffusion techniques. J. Bact. **94**, 1287 (1967). — LANE, S.L., KUTSCHER, A.H., CHAVES, R.: Oxytetracycline in the treatment of oro-cervical-facial actinomycosis; report of seven cases. J. Amer. med. Ass. **151**, 986 (1953). — Lavalle, P.: Agents of mycetoma. In: Fungi and Fungous Diseases, pp. 50—68. G. DALLDORF, Editor. Springfield, Ill.: Charles C. Thomas 1962. — LEBRUN, H., GILMOUR, I.E.: Hypokalaemia and renal actinomycosis following ureterocaecostomy; report of a case. Brit. J. Urol. **25**, 132 (1953). — LEE, B.Y.: Actinomycosis of the lung coexisting with pulmonary tuberculosis; report of a case. Dis. Chest **50**, 211 (1966). — LENTZE, F.: 1958. Quoted by WILSON and MILES (1964). — LEY, E., PERAITA, P., LEY, E.

HIJO: Granuloma actinomicótico cerebral Rev. clín. esp. **41**, 234 (1951). — LITTMAN, M.L., PHILLIPS, G.E., FUSILLO, M.H.: *In vitro* susceptibility of human pathogenic actinomycetes to chloramphenicol (chloromycetin). Amer. J. clin. Path. **20**, 1076 (1950). — LITTMAN, M.L., PAUL, J.S., FUSILLO, M.H.: Treatment of pulmonary actinomycosis with chloramphenicol; report of a case. J. Amer. med. Ass. **148**, 608 (1952). — LORD, F.T., TREVETT, L.D.: The pathogenesis of actinomycosis. Recovery of actinomyces-like organisms from the human mouth. J. infect. Dis. **58**, 115 (1936). — LORENZ, O.: Neue Erkenntnisse zur Pathogenese und Klinik der cervico-Facialen Aktinomykose. Med. Klin. **54**, 9 (1959). — LOTH, M.F.: Actinomycosis of the fallopian tube. Amer. J. Obstet. **72**, (4) 919 (1956). — LUDWIG, T.G.: Actinomycosis originating in the maxillary region. Oral Surg. **8**, 877 (1955). — MACCARTHY, J.: Actinomycosis of the female pelvic organs with involvement of the endometrium. J. Path. Bact. (Lond.) **69**, 175 (1955). — McCONNELL, O.H.: Actinomycosis; report of cases. J. oral Surg. **2**, 173 (1944). — McCORMACK, L.J., DICKSON, J.A., REICH, A.R.: Actinomycosis of the humerus. J. Bone Jt Surg. **36-A**, 1255 (1954). — MACGREGOR, A.B.: Cervico-facial actinomycosis. Proc. roy. Soc. Med. **38**, 639 (1945). ∼ Cervico-facial actinomycosis. Proc. roy. Soc. Med. **44**, 55 (1951). — MACHAFFIE, R.A., ZASYER, R.L., SALCHEK, H., SCIORTINO, A.L.: An unusual case of actinomycosis manifested as an abdominal wall abscess. Gastroenterology **33**, (5) 830 (1957). — MACLENNAN, A.P.: Composition of the cell wall of *Actinomyces bovis*: the isolation of 6-deoxy-L-talose. Biochem. Biophys. Acta **48**, 600 (1961). — McVAY, L.V., Jr., GUTHRIE, F., SPRUNT, D.H.: Aureomycin in the treatment of actinomycosis. New Engl. J. Med. **245**, 91 (1951). — McVAY, L.V., Jr., SPRUNT, D.H.: A long term evaluation of aureomycin in the treatment of actinomycosis. Ann. intern. Med. **38**, 955 (1953a). ∼ Treatment of actinomycosis with isoniazid. J. Amer. med. Ass. **153**, 95 (1953b). — McWILLIAMS, C.A.: Actinomycosis of phalanx of finger. Ann. Surg. **66**, 117 (1917). — MAIN, J.H.P., MACPHEE, I.T.: Actinomycosis of the maxilla in relation to a peridontal abscess. Oral Surg. **17**, 299 (1964). — MARTIN, W.J., NICHOLS, D.R., WELLMAN, W.E., WEED, L.A.: Disseminated actinomycosis treated with tetracycline. A.M.A. Arch. Int. Med. **97**, 252 (1956). — MATHIESON, D.R., HARRISON, R., HAMMOND, C., HENRICI, A.T.: Allergic reactions to actinomycetes. Amer. J. Hyg. **21**, 405 (1935). — MILLER, A.G.: Actinomycosis of the colon; case report. Dis. Colon Rect. **7**, 207 (1964). — MILLER, J.M., LONG, P.H., SCHOENBACH, E.B.: Successful treatment of actinomycosis with "stilbamidine". J. Amer. med. Ass. **150**, 35 (1952). — MEYER, E., VERGES, P.: Mouse pathogenicity as a diagnostic aid in the identification of *Actinomyces bovis*. J. Lab. clin. Med. **36**, 667 (1950). — MONTGOMERY, R.M., WELTON, W.A.: Primary actinomycosis of the upper extremity. A.M.A. Arch. Derm. **79**, 578 (1959). — MOORE, M.: Radiate formation on pathogenic fungi in human tissue. Arch. Path. **42**, 115 (1946). — MORTON, H.S.: Actinomycosis. Canad. med. Ass. J. **42**, 231 (1940). — MOSSELMAN, G., LIENAUX, E.: L'actinomycose et son agent infectieux. Ann. Méd. vét. **39**, 409 (1890). — NAESLUND, C.: Studies of *Actinomyces* from the oral cavity. Acta path. microbiol. scand. **2**, 110 (1925). ∼ Experimentelle Studien über die Ätiologie und Pathogenese der Aktinomykose. Acta path. microbiol. scand. **8**, (Suppl. 6) 1 (1931). — NEUBER, E.: Spezifische Diagnostik und Therapie der Aktinomykose. Klin. Wschr. **19**, 736 (1940). — NICHOLS, D.R., HERRELL, W.E.: Penicillin in the treatment of actinomycosis. J. Lab. clin. Med. **33**, 521 (1948). — NIELSEN, J.: Dosierungsfragen bei der Röntgenbehandlung von zervico-fazialer Aktinomykose. Acta Radiol. **23**, 303 (1942). — OVERMAN, J.R., PINE, L.: Electron microscopy of cytoplasmic structures in facultative and anaerobic *Actinomyces*. J. Bact. **86**, 656 (1963). — OWEN, M.D., MACANSH, J.: Actinomycosis of the mandible. Med. J. Aust. **2**, 962 (1965). — PANTAZOPOULOS, P.E.: Actinomycosis of brain manifested by vestibular symptoms. Arch. Otolaryng. **80**, 309 (1964). — PEABODY, J.W., Jr., SEABURY, J.H.: Actinomycosis and Nocardiosis. J. chron. Dis. **5**, 374 (1957). ∼ Actinomycosis and nocardiosis; a review of basic differences in therapy. Amer. J. Med. **28**, 99 (1960). — PEGRUM, G.D.: Actinomycotic lesions in the chorioallantoic membrane of the chick embryo. J. Path. Bact. **88**, 323 (1964). — PHEILS, M.T., REID, D.J., ROSS, C.F.: Abdominal actinomycosis. Brit. J. Surg. **51**, 345 (1964). — PINE, L., HARDIN, H.: *Actinomyces israelii*, a cause of lacrimal canaliculitis in man. J. Bact. **78**, 164 (1959). — PINE, L., WATSON, S.J.: Evaluation of an isolation and maintenance medium for *Actinomyces* species and related organisms. J. Lab. clin. Med. **54**, 107 (1959). — PINE, L., HOWELL, A., Jr., WATSON, S.J.: Studies of the morphological, physiological, and biochemical characteristics of *Actinomyces bovis*. J. gen. Microbiol. **23**, 403 (1960a). — PINE, L., HARDIN, H., TURNER, L.: Actinomycotic lacrimal canaliculitis. A report of two cases with a review of the characteristics which identify the causal organism, *Actinomyces israelii*. Amer. J. Ophthal. **49**, 1278 (1960b). — PINE, L.: Recent developments on the nature of the anaerobic actinomycetes. Ann. Soc. belge Méd. trop. **3**, 247 (1963). — PINE, L., BOONE, C.J.: Comparative cell wall analyses of morphological forms within the genus *Actinomyces*. J. Bact. **94**, 875 (1967). — v. PLOTHE, O.: Farbstoffbildung bei Actinomyceten. Naturwissenschaften **34**, 190 (1947). — PONFICK, E.: Ein Vortrag über Actinomykose des Menschen.

Ärztl. Z. (Breslau) **2**, 151 (1880a). ∼ Über Actinomykose. Berl. klin. Wschr. **17**, 660 (1880b).
— PORTER, I.A.: Actinomycosis in Scotland. Brit. med. J. **2**, 1084 (1953). — PRINSLEY,
D.M.: Pulmonary actinomycosis; recovery in a mongol. Brit. J. Tuberc. **51**, (1) 40 (1957). —
PULASKI, E.J., ARTZ, C.P., REISS, E.: Terramycin and aureomycin in surgical infections;
report of 200 cases. J. Amer. med. Ass. **149**, 35 (1952). — PUTMAN, H.C., Jr., DOCKERTY,
M.C., WAUGH, J.M.: Abdominal actinomycosis: an analysis of 122 cases. Surgery **28**, 781
(1950). — RAPER, F.P.: Abdominal actinomycosis following a perforated duodenal ulcer.
Brit. J. Surg. **38**, 240 (1950). — RASHBAUM, M., McINTOSH, H.C.: Pelvic actinomycosis
treated by surgery and roentgen ray, with recovery. Amer. J. Obstet. Gynec. **47**, 849 (1944). —
ROBINSON, M.R.: Actinomycosis of both ovaries and fallopian tubes. Surg. Gynec. Obstet.
29, 569 (1919). — ROBINSON, R.A.: Actinomycosis of the subcutaneous tissue of the forearm
secondary to a human bite. J. Amer. med. Ass. **124**, 1049 (1944). — ROSEBURY, T., EPPS,
L.J., CLARK, A.R.: A study of the isolation, cultivation, and pathogenicity of *Actinomyces
israelii* recovered from the human mouth and from actinomycosis in man. J. infect. Dis. **74**,
131 (1944). — ROSS, J.A., KNIGHT, I.C.: Actinomycosis of the subphrenic space. Edinb.
med. J. **61**, 170 (1954). — RUHRÄH, J.: Actinomycosis in man, with special reference to the
cases which have been observed in America. Ann. Surg. **30**, 417, 605, 722 (1899). — SANFORD,
A.H.: Distribution of actinomycosis in the United States. J. Amer. med. Ass. **81**, 655 (1923). —
SAZAMA, L.: Actinomycosis of the parotid gland: report of five cases. Oral Med. **19**, 197
(1965). — SAVIDGE, R.S., DAVIES, D.M.: Generalized actinomycosis with possible cardiac
involvement. Brit. med. J. **2**, 136 (1953). — SCHNEIDER, D.H.: Actinomycosis of the testicle;
case report. J. Urol. (Baltimore) **54**, 296 (1945). — SCORER, C.G.: Actinomycosis of the
testis. Brit. J. Surg. **40**, 244 (1952). — SEABURY, J.H., DASCOMB, H.E.: Results of the
treatment of systemic mycoses. J. Amer. med. Ass. **188**, 509 (1964). — SILBER, W.: Left
perinephric actinomycosis. S. Afr. med. J. **27**, 264 (1953). — SILBERSCHMIDT, W.: Über Actinomykose. Z. Hyg. Infekt.-Kr. **37**, 345 (1901). — SLACK, J.: The source of infection in actinomycosis. J. Bact. **43**, 193 (1942). — SLACK, J.M.: Studies with microaerophilic actinomycetes.
II. Serological groups as determined by the reciprocal agglutinin adsorption technique. J.
Bact. **70**, 400 (1955). — SMITH, C.H.: Ocular actinomycosis. Proc. roy. Soc. Med. (Lond.)
46, 209 (1953). — STANTON, M.B.: Actinomycosis of the maxillary sinus. J. Laryng. **80**, 168
(1966). — STEVENSON, A.E.M.: Actinomycosis of ovaries and fallopian tubes; report of a
case. J. Obstet. Gynaec. Brit. Emp. **64**, 365 (1957). — SULLIVAN, H.R., GOLDSWORTHY,
N.E.: A comparative study of anaerobic strains of *Actinomyces* from clinically normal mouths
and from actinomycotic lesions. J. Path. Bact. **51**, 253 (1940). — SVANE, S.: Visceral actinomycosis, report on 6 cases with special reference to aureomycin treatment. Acta chir. scand.
131, 160 (1966). — SWEENEY, D.F., BLACKWELDER, T.F.: Pelvic actinomycosis, report of a
case. Obstet. and Gynec. **25**, 690 (1965). — SWINTON, N.W., SCHATMAN, B.H.: Actinomycosis, a rare cause of fistula-in-ano. Dis. Colon Rect. **7**, 315 (1964). — THOMPSON, L., LOVE-
STEDT, B.A.: An actinomyces-like organism obtained from the human mouth. Proc. Mayo
Clin. **26**, 169 (1951). — TORRENS, J.A., WOOD, M.W.W.: Streptomycin in the treatment of
actinomycosis; report of three cases. Lancet **1**, 1091 (1949). — TRIBEDI, B.P., MUKHERJEE,
B.N.: Actinomycotic and mycotic lesions, with special reference to madura foot. Brit. J.
Surg. **27**, 256 (1939). — TRIVEDI, B.P., SARKAR, S.K.: Pulmonary actinomycosis. Indian
J. med. Sci. **6**, 595 (1952). — TURNER, G.: Actinomycosis of the lungs. Radiology **7**, 39 (1926).
— UTZ, J.P.: Actinomycosis. In: Cecil-Loeb Textbook of Medicine, pp. 308—309. BEESON,
P.B., McDERMOTT, W., Editors. 12th Ed. Philadelphia: W.B. Saunders Co. 1967. — VER-
HOEFF, F.H.: A case of metastatic intraocular mycosis. Arch. Ophthal. **55**, 225 (1926). —
VERME, G., CONTU, L.: L'actinomicosi del cuore. Osservazioni su un caso clinico e rassegna
della letteratura. Arch. De Vecchi Anat. pat. **37**, 13 (1962). — VILLA, V.G.: Pulp abscess
associated with actinomycosis. Oral Surg. **10**, (2) 207 (1957). — WAGENSTEEN, O.H.: The role
of surgery in the treatment of actinomycosis. Ann. Surg. **104**, 752 (1936). — WAGENSTEEN,
O.H., SNAPPER, I., POPPER, H.: Clinical pathological conference, actinomycosis of the lung
with extension to the liver. Rev. Gastroent. **19**, 950 (1952). — WAGNER, C.: Actinomycosis
of the uterine appendages. Surg. Gynec. Obstet. **10**, 148 (1910). — WARTHIN, T.A., BUSHUEFF,
B.: Pulmonary actinomycosis. A.M.A. Arch. Int. Med. **101**, 239 (1958). — WARWICK, W.T.:
A clinical contribution to the etiology of actinomycosis. Lancet **2**, 497 (1923). — WAYL, P.,
RAKOWER, J., HOCHMAN, A.: Pulmonary ray fungus disease; clinical aspects and pathogenesis. Dis. Chest **34**, 506 (1958). — WEED, L.A., BAGGENSTOSS, A.H.: Actinomycosis;
a pathologic and bacteriologic study of 21 fatal cases. Amer. J. clin. Path. **19**, 201 (1949). —
WEED, L.A., BAGGENSTOSS, A.H., BAUGHER, L.: Some problems in the diagnosis of actinomycosis. Proc. Mayo Clin. **24**, 463 (1949). — WHISENAND, J.M., MOORE, E.V.: Renal actinomycosis; with a report of a primary case. Calif. Med. **74**, 133 (1951). — WILLE-BAUMKAUFF,
H.: Aktinomykose der Niere. Z. Urol. **43**, 240 (1950). — WILSON, G.S., MILES, A.A.: Actinomycosis. In: Topley and Wilson's Principles of Bacteriology and Immunity, pp. 1563—1578.
5th ed. Baltimore: Williams and Wilkins Co. 1964. — WILSON, J.W.: Actinomycosis. In:

Clinical and Immunologic Aspects of Fungous Diseases, pp. 190—204. Springfield, Ill.: C.C. Thomas 1957. — Wilson-Pepper, J.K.: Report of renal actinomycosis. Brit. J. Urol. **23**, 160 (1951). — Wingo, C.F., Williams, R.O.: Pulmonary actinomycosis diagnosed by lung biopsy. Amer. Rev. Tuberc. **76**, 660 (1957). — Winston, M.E.: Actinomycosis of the spine. Lancet **1**, 945 (1951). — Wolff, M., Israel, J.: Über Reincultur des *Actinomyces* und seine Übertragbarkeit auf Thiere. Virchows Arch. path. Anat. **126**, 11 (1891). — Wright, J.H.: The biology of the microorganism of actinomycosis. J. med. Res. **13**, 349 (1905). — Wright, L.T., Lowen, H.J.: Aureomycin hydrochloride in actinomycosis. J. Amer. med. Ass. **144**, 21 (1950). — Zander, E., Barontini, F.: Über die Aktinomykose des Nervensystems. Schweiz. med. Wschr. **1956**, 1409. — Zettergren, L.: On the pathogenesis of appendix-actinomycosis. Acta path. scand. (Kobenh.) **25**, 543 (1948). — Ziskin, D.E., Shoram, B.S., Hanford, J.M.: Actinomycosis, a report of 26 cases. Amer. J. Orthodont. **29**, 193 (1943). — Zitka, E.: Vakzinebehandlung der Kieferaktinomykose. Z. Stomat. **46**, 202 (1949). ~ Tödlich verlaufende Fälle von zervikofazialer Aktinomykose. Wien. med. Wschr. **102**, 939 (1952). — Zoeckler, S.J.: Cardiac actinomycosis; a case report and survey of the literature. Circulation **3**, 854 (1951).

Nocardiosis

PHILIP PIZZOLATO — New Orleans/Louisiana, USA

With 15 Figures

Definition

Nocardiosis is an infrequent, subacute or chronic, suppurative, deep acti-nomycetic infection of man and animals usually caused by *Nocardia asteroides*. Suppurative pneumonia, cerebral abscess, or disseminated abscesses (pyemia) are anatomical forms of the disease. Granules are usually not present in the pus. Occasionally nocardiosis is an opportunistic infection, developing within a host with a lowered resistance. Nocardiosis includes nocardial mycetoma, in which granules are present. (See Chapter by Dr. WINSLOW, page 589.)

Mycology

The genus *Nocardia* is composed of free-living or parasitic aerobic mycelium-forming microorganisms belonging to the family Actinomycetaceae and is separat-ed from the other single genus *Actinomyces* which is anaerobic or microaero-philic and parasitic. These organisms are members of the order Actinomycetales which includes Mycobacteriaceae, Streptomycetaceae and Actinoplanaceae, and which may cause confusion with the Actinomycetaceae because of similar mycelial structures.

Recognition of the genus *Nocardia* has been relatively recent (BERGEY, 1957). NOCARD in 1888 isolated branched filaments from caseating lesions of lymph nodes from cattle and horses in farcy, a condition simulating tuberculosis and glanders. He identified this fungus as *Streptothrix farcinica* and it was renamed *Nocardia farcinica* by TREVISAN in 1889. In 1890, EPPINGER isolated an aerobic, Gram-positive, acid-fast fungus from a fatal case of multiple brain abscesses and meningitis in a 52-year-old glass blower. Because of the starlike shape of its colonies, he called the pathogen *Cladothrix asteroides*; however, BLANCHARD in 1895 recommended that the organism be classified as *Nocardia*.

In 1909 LINDENBERG reported a new species isolated from the leg of an Italian patient in Brazil; this fungus produced grains similar to those found in Madura foot and in actinomy-cosis and he named it *Discomyces brasiliensis*.

Confusion arose as to the characteristics of these organisms and they were placed in various genera such as *Streptothrix*, *Oospora*, *Actinomyces*, *Proactinomyces*, *Discomyces*, *Cladothrix* and *Mycobacterium*. BREED and CONN in 1919 decided that these terms should be eliminated and only the genus *Actinomyces* be used.

WAKSMAN and HENRICI in 1943 categorized the aerobic organism as *Nocardia* to distinguish it from the anaerobic *Actinomyces*. Although many strains of Nocardia have been encountered, WAKSMAN (1961) has accepted 59 species, of which 26 have been encountered in human or mammalian diseased organs. Among these, *N.asteroides* and *N.brasiliensis* are the most common (Fig. 1). Because of certain characteristics with respect to the grains, aerial mycelium, and spore formation, GONZALEZ OCHOA and SANDOVAL have transferred *N.madurae* to *Streptomyces madurae*. More recently, GONZALEZ OCHOA (1962) has classified *N.pelletieri* and *N.paraguayensis* as species of the genus *Streptomyces*.

Nocardia is Gram-positive (Figs. 2, 15), partially acid-fast or nonacid-fast. It branches, and has nonseptate, filamentous microorganisms with a diameter

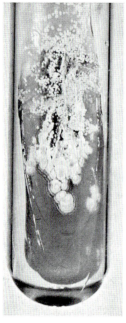
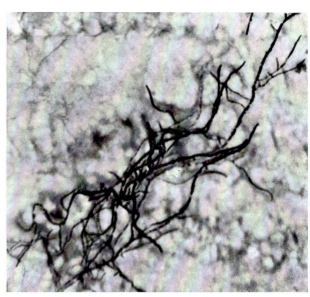

Fig. 1 Fig. 2

Fig. 1. Culture of *N.asteroides* on Sabouraud medium, 4 weeks duration, 37°C. (From previously unpublished case of the author, Philip Pizzolato, New Orleans Veterans Administration Hospital No. A-67-120)

Fig. 2. Smear of *N.asteroides* from colony of Fig. 1, Gram stain, showing branching and segmented character of filaments, × 1500

of 1 micron or less. Some strains fragment into bacillary or coccoid forms when cultured. They are aerobic organisms, growing readily at 24° or 37°C. Georg et al. (1961) found most strains of *N.asteroides* grew at 46°C whereas no strains of *N.brasiliensis* grew at this temperature. They grow on a variety of media such as beef infusion glucose agar, Sabouraud's glucose agar, blood agar, Czapek agar. The *colonies* are slow-growing (Fig. 1). It requires 2—4 weeks to produce conspicuous colonies. These may be pale yellow, orange, pink, red, or chalky white and wrinkled or granular. Occasional strains produce an aerial mycelium giving the colonies a white, chalky or powdery appearance. Gordon et al. and Georg et al. have described features distinguishing Nocardia from *Streptomyces* and *Mycobacterium*. *N.asteroides* was found to show acid-fastness, branched mycelia, pellicle formation in thioglycollate broth, paraffin utilization (McClung) but no casein hydrolysis or tyrosine utilization. *N.brasiliensis* had similar features but these organisms revealed casein hydrolysis and tyrosine utilization and good growth in 0.4% gelatin (Bojalil and Cerbon, and Conant).

Schneidau and Shaffer made extensive cultural and biochemical studies on 51 strains of *Nocardia* species, 10 strains of *Mycobacterium* species and 4 strains of *Streptomyces* species. They divided the genus *Nocardia* into two types: "True" *Nocardia* and *Streptomyces*-like *Nocardia* as the former showed mycelium which was able to fragment into bacillary and coccoid forms and nearly all forms were acidfast. They further divided the "true" *Nocardia* into four groups: 1. *Nocardia asteroides* 2. *N.brasiliensis* 3. *N.corallima* 4. *N.opaca*. They observed that *N.intracellularis* failed to produce branching mycelium and it behaved much like a *Mycobacterium*.

McClung (1960) examined 102 soil samples from the southern area of the United States by means of the paraffin baiting technique and isolated 48 strains of *Nocardia asteroides* and 16 other species of *Nocardia*.

They were all acid fast, displayed characteristic colonial morphology and color, produced nitrite from nitrate, were nonproteolytic on gelatin and casein and non diastasic on starch. The remaining 16 isolates were not identified as to species but were representatives of "soft Nocardias" belonging to the morphological Group II described by McClung (1949).

Gonzales-Ochoa (1962) isolated *N. brasiliensis* from the soil by the simple procedure of seeding soil samples in Botcher-Conn agar. From these 21 samples six strains of *N. brasiliensis* were isolated and they showed typical fragmentation, acid fastness and enzymatic activities. The pathogenicity of these soil strains for mice was similar to those isolated from patients. In a study of 134 samples of the soil obtained in the region of New Dehli, India, Kumar and Mohapatra, using the "paraffin baiting" technique, isolated 52 strains of *N. asteroides*, 8 strains of *N. brasiliensis* and 4 strains of *N. caviae*. Of these, 42 strains were pathogenic for mice.

Incidence

Because of the unreliability of case reporting due to variations in morphology, culture, and clinical features, such as disseminated or localized infection, as well as terminology used, the incidence of nocardiosis is difficult to evaluate. Mus-grave et al. in 1908 and Claypole in 1914 in their reviews of the literature included all cases belonging to the genera *Streptothrix*, *Cladothrix*, *Actinomyces*, *Oospora*, *Nocardia*, and *Sphaerotilus*. Henrici and Gardner in a review of the world literature up to 1921 considered that only 26 cases fulfilled the criteria of *Nocardia asteroides*. Ballenger and Goldring in a review of the literature prior to 1957, found 95 cases, and Murray et al. in 1960 found 179 cases. Gilligan et al. in 1961 encountered 33 verified cases of nocardiosis of the central nervous system in the literature. We have isolated *Nocardia* species from 12 patients over a 20-year period at the New Orleans Veterans Administration Hospital. Four of these among 6,000 autopsies during this period showed systemic pathologic lesions as well as central nervous system disease. Carlile et al. in 1963 reported the seventeenth fatal case of nocardiosis in a 7-year-old boy. This is also the fifth case of nocardiosis of the central nervous system in children.

As far as geographic distribution is concerned, nearly two-thirds of the reported cases of infection with *N. asteroides* were from North America and most of these were from the region of the Great Lakes, Mississippi Valley, and Eastern United States. About two-thirds of the patients were between 20 and 60 years of age; Ballenger and Goldring found 11 cases in the pediatric age group and reported a case in a 9-month-old child. The sex incidence showed a predominance of males to females of 2.5 to 1.

Cutaneous nocardiosis may be *mycetoma (Madura foot)* or a cutaneous mani-festation of a systemic disease. According to Abbott, the term "mycetoma" was first used in 1860 by Van Dyke Carter to denote a fungus tumor of the foot or Madura foot as the disease was commonly called owing to its prevalence in that province of India. In 1916 Chalmers and Archibald carefully defined the term as covering "all growths and granulations producing enlargement, deformity and destruction in any part of the body of man brought about by the invasion of the affected area by certain species of fungi which give rise to variously shaped bodies called 'grains' which are found embedded in the pathological tissue or in the discharge from the diseased area". Mycetomas which contain granules are caused by *Nocardia* and by various Eumycetes, or true fungi. Refer to Chapter 12.

Much confusion has arisen as to the etiology as well as to the *classification* of the micro-organisms of nocardial mycetoma. However, the consensus is that among the various genera isolated, two species of *Nocardia* are noted: *N. brasi-liensis* and *N. asteroides*. Some investigators have doubted the ability of *N.*

asteroides to produce localized mycetoma and they believe that the identification had been poorly determined and confused with *N. brasiliensis*.

Lacaz in 1945 reviewed 25 cases from Brazil in which *N. brasiliensis* had been identified. Nine were cases of mycetoma of the leg or foot, four were generalized cases, three involved the knee and the remainder came from miscellaneous sites. Gonzalez-Ochoa (1962) studied 103 cases of mycetomas from the Institute of Health and Tropical Diseases in Mexico City and noted that 94% were due to *N. brasiliensis*, 1% to *N. asteroides* and the remainder to other genera. The lower extremities were involved in 65% of the patients, lesions of the trunk were seen in 25% and other sites were implicated in the remainder.

Wilson at the University of Ibadan, Nigeria, obtained biopsies and cultures from nine patients. From six patients, *N. asteroides* was identified and from one, *N. brasiliensis*. The identification was confirmed by other authorities.

Clinical Manifestations

Fever is the most constant sign of the disease. Frequently present are night sweats, chills, headaches and anorexia. In pulmonary nocardiosis, cough is a frequent symptom and is associated with the production of variable amounts of white mucoid to yellow or green purulent sputum, which may be streaked with blood or may actually be blood. Chest pain, with and without pleural involvement, and dyspnea may occur.

Lesions in the skin and subcutaneous tissues are encountered as a primary manifestation with or without the characteristic features of mycetoma (Madura foot) or secondary to pulmonary involvement. As a complication frequently associated with pulmonary disease, the central nervous system may become involved. Headaches develop or get progressively worse, followed by lethargy, mental confusion, hallucinations, convulsions, paralyses, or nuchal rigidity. Nausea and vomiting may be symptoms of nocardiosis of the central nervous system.

Laboratory Findings

Sputum examination is the most valuable laboratory procedure in the diagnosis of pulmonary nocardiosis. Gram stain of the sputum frequently shows Gram-positive branching mycelia which are acid fast when decolorized by the acid-alcohol solution for a short time, or with a weak (1% sulfuric acid) decolorizing agent. Cultures of the sputum, with and without prior digestion of the mucus and saprophytic microorganisms, frequently reveal *N. asteroides*. (Ajello, 1951). Ballinger and Goldring were able to isolate acid fast *Nocardia* from gastric washings from a 9-month-old child. Direct examination of exudates from sinus tracts of nocardial mycetoma frequently reveals white, yellow, red or brown "grains" which are heavily loaded with branching mycelia.

If the meninges are not involved, the spinal fluid is usually clear and not diagnostic. If there is meningitis or there is an abscess near the leptomeninges, the fluid may be yellow, cloudy or turbid, with an increase of protein and cells with a predominance of neutrophils. The sugar of the spinal fluid is frequently reduced (Gilligan et al.).

The peripheral blood reveals a mild leukocytosis of 10,000—20,000 per cmm often with a neutrophilia. A patient of Freese et al. had a white count of 50,000 per cmm. A mild anemia may exist. The sedimentation rate is reported to be rapid.

Blood cultures may be positive for *N. asteroides*.

The blood and urine chemistry determinations are not diagnostic.

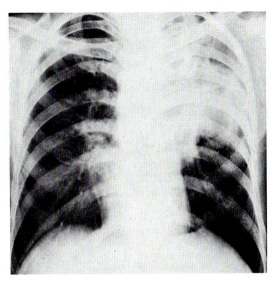

Fig. 3. Chest X-ray of a 49-year-old man showing a dense opacity in the right chest (New Orleans Veterans Administration Hospital Case No. A-46-29)

Late in the course of the disease, KIRBY and McNAUGHT isolated *Nocardia* from sputum, the subcutaneous abscesses that developed, and the blood, from a 63-year-old man who had been admitted to the hospital for pneumonia. A report of three positive blood cultures for *Nocardia* associated with pneumonia was made by KOHN et al. The fungus was not pathogenic for mice, guinea pigs, and one rabbit. The patient recovered with sodium iodide, sulfadiazine, streptomycin and penicillin. HIDDLESTONE observed a patient who developed a loud, harsh systolic murmur audible over the mitral and tricuspid area and was found to have a positive blood culture.

Roentgen Findings

Roentgenograms of the chest are of great value. Lesions vary greatly, depending upon the stage of the disease, but, unfortunately, they are not diagnostic of pulmonary nocardiosis. One or both lungs may be involved. The hilum on both sides may be considerably enlarged. The lungs may show scattered, innumerable spot-like shadows, the size of a pinhead or larger. The spots may become confluent to form large non-homogeneous shadows or large areas of consolidation (Fig. 3). A single cavity may occur or multiple small cavities may become confluent to produce a multilocular large cavity. Pleural effusions and atelectasis may be found. An abscess may rupture into the mediastinum or pleura to form pleural empyema.

SALTZMAN et al. reported a 36-year-old white man with disseminated lupus erythematosus for which he received corticosteroid therapy. He developed a small coin lesion in the upper lobe of the right lung. One month later, the lesion had undergone cavitation and the sputum revealed *N. asteroides*. He was given sulfisoxazole (Gantrisin) and the cavity disappeared radiologically. A patient of WILKITE and COLE had a lung abscess with cavity formation in which a moveable mass resembling a "fungus ball" was found.

With a brain abscess there is shifting of the lateral ventricles or pineal gland as observed by pneumo-encephalogram or angiogram.

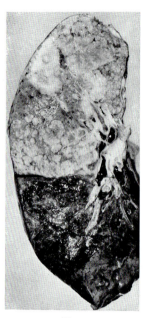

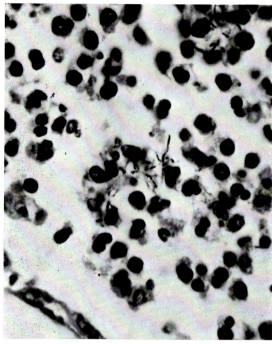

Fig. 4   Fig. 5

Fig. 4. Pulmonary nocardiosis. Coronal section of the lung of a 49-year-old Negro man showing
purulent consolidation of the right upper lobe. (Case A-46-29 of Pizzolato et al.)

Fig. 5. Pulmonary nocardiosis. Microscopic section of lung showing branching *Nocardia
asteroides* in purulent exudate. The exudate is predominantly polymorphonuclear, but many
mononuclear cells and lymphocytes are present. Gram stain, × 800

A 15-year-old boy was presented to Dolan et al. with swelling of the knee of nine months'
duration. There was radiologic evidence of a lytic lesion of the distal femur, with periosteal
elevation and adjacent soft tissue calcification. An incision and drainage of the mass over the
knee revealed necrosis of subcutaneous fat, muscle and fascia, with destruction of the periosteum. Culture of this material yielded *N. asteroides*.

Gross Lesions

Pulmonary Nocardiosis: The pulmonary lesions are characterized by a rather
rapid progressive consolidation simulating caseous pneumonia or miliary tuberculosis. The lungs may be very heavy, the left weighing 1430 grams (normally
375) and the right weighing 1500 (normally 450) as in the case of Kirby and
McNaught. The cut surface of an entire lung or lobe may be homogeneous, firm,
pale, yellow or gray, and airless or there may be numerous firm, white, or pinkish
gray nodules, 1—3 cm in diameter, as in the case of Pizzolato et al. (Fig. 4). The
nodules may become confluent producing larger nodules or there may be a diffuse
consolidation (Figs. 4, 5). The solid areas may undergo liquefaction necrosis
yielding poorly defined 1—5 cm single or multiloculated abscesses filled with brown,
green or yellow pus. There may be communications with the bronchi and when
the contents have been discharged, the lining of the abscess cavity is rough,
shaggy, gray to brown. There is consolidation of the adjacent alveolar spaces.
Also the adjacent lung may be edematous and hyperemic. Wilhite and Cole

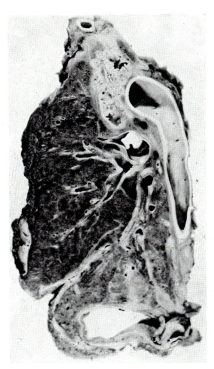

Fig. 6. Pleural and mediastinal nocardiosis. Coronal section of lung of a 52-year-old Negro man showing extensive pleuritis and mediastinitis extending from apex to diaphragm, and complete atelectasis. (From previously unpublished case of the author, PHILIP PIZZOLATO. Autopsy No. A-67-120.) Culture shown in Figs. 1 and 2 is from this case

reported five cases of *Nocardia* invading a pre-formed lung abscess and producing "fungus balls". The patients had thoracotomies with the removal of the affected area in which a large cavity was found in two patients.

Pleuritis may develop locally, forming a ragged or thickening pleura with or without the formation of an effusion. It may remain localized or spread to involve the entire pleural cavity forming the classical *empyema* (HAGER et al.). Fibrinous and fibrous adhesions may develop between the visceral and parietal pleurae, and the infection may spread through the intercostal spaces to produce subcutaneous abscesses or it may extend into the mediastinum (Fig. 6).

In a previously unpublished case PIZZOLATO (1967) observed a 52-year-old man with a five day history of cough, fever and back pain (New Orleans Veterans Administration Hospital Autopsy No. A-67-120). He had been a heavy beer drinker with a past history of visual and auditory hallucinations. Examination revealed a temperature of 101°F., crepitant and subcrepitant rales, dullness, diminished breath sounds and clubbing of the fingers. A chest X-ray showed some interstitial fibrotic changes bilaterally. He was given penicillin and his temperature varied from normal to 100° or 101°F. A repeat chest X-ray revealed consolidation of the left chest wall and its configuration was more in keeping with loculated pleural effusion. The fluid was aspirated and found to be sterile on culture. To insure better drainage, a tube was inserted into the left chest cavity, and pus began to drain. A few days later, a standard thoracotomy incision was made and the seventh rib was resected. Pleural exudate on culture revealed *N. asteroides* (Figs. 1, 2). Three blood cultures were negative. Sulfadiazine was given. About two months after admission he became stuporous, the pupils measured 2 mm in diameter and reacted sluggishly to light; the eye movements deviated to the right. He became progressively worse and expired. At *autopsy*, the left pleural cavity appeared as an empyema sac filled with dense yellow and red masses of necrotic tissue and liquid pus compressed the

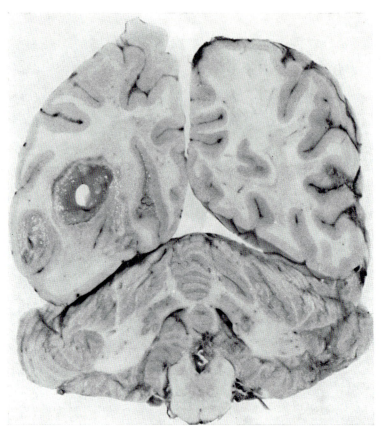

Fig. 7. Nocardiosis of brain. Coronal section of brain of a 61-year-old white man showing two abscesses of the left cerebral hemisphere. (Case of Pizzolato et al.)

left lung against the mediastinum (Fig. 6). The left lung was dark bluish-violet and atelectactic. No lung abscesses were found. The brain showed symmetrical hemispheres. The cut sections of the cerebrum and cerebellum revealed hundreds of tiny abscesses, some measuring up to 5 mm in diameter. They were pale tan and were surrounded by a rim of gray ragged tissue and a zone of hyperemia and swelling of the surrounding brain tissue.

A unique case of lung abscess due to *N. brasiliensis* was reported by Bobbitt et al. This 61-year-old man was admitted for fever, malaise and cough. Chest X-ray revealed a density in the left apex. Recovery was uneventful following thoracotomy, penicillin and sulfadiazine.

Nocardiosis of the Brain: The fungus may enter the blood stream to be disseminated to other organs. The brain is the extra-pulmonary organ most frequently infected (Bernstein et al., Binford and Lane, Cupp et al., Eckhardt and Pilcher, Erchul and Koch, Jacobson and Cloward, Kirby and McNaught, Krueger et al., List et al., Munslow, Pizzolato et al. (Figs. 7, 8), Tucker and Hirsch, Weed et al., Welsh et al., Wichelhausen et al.).

Solitary and multiple abscesses of varying sizes and locations are encountered in the cerebrum and cerebellum (Fig. 7). Abscesses 3 cm in diameter are not uncommon; and Binford and Lane described a multiloculated abscess 6 cm in diameter extending from the cortex to the lateral ventricle. The abscesses are poorly encapsulated and filled with viscid or gelatinous, green or gray pus, and the lining of the abscess cavities is rough and irregular.

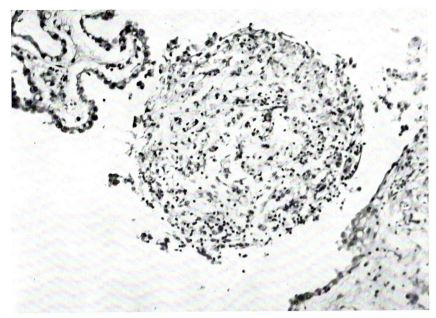

Fig. 8. Nocardiosis of brain. Cellular infiltrate, polymorphonuclear neutrophils, lymphocytes, and macrophages, in the choroid plexus. H & E, × 370. (Case A-58-212, same as in Fig. 7, Case 2 of PIZZOLATO et al.)

A 49-year-old female patient of KIRBY and McNAUGHT was admitted to the hospital for headaches, nausea and vomiting for one month. Bilateral choked disks, central scotomas and enlarged blindspots, engorged fundic vessels and poor hearing were noted. The spinal fluid had no white cells and 25 mg% protein. She died suddenly and autopsy revealed that the cerebellum had distinct markings where it had been forced into the foramen magnum. From the right cerebellum a thick green exudate was expressed. The exudate was semitranslucent and contained no granules. A section of the cerebellum revealed an irregular 2.5 cm abscess with a soft wall extending to within 1 cm of the posterior medial border of the right lobe and not communicating with the fourth ventricle. Culture of the exudate disclosed *N. asteroides*.

The abscesses may invade the ventricles and choroid plexus (Fig. 8). They may break through the cortical surface to produce a meningitis.

A 47-year-old man reported by CUPP et al., developed anorexia, restlessness and lethargy following transfusion hepatitis and ulcerative colitis. Spinal fluid revealed 15,000 white cells per cmm with 100% neutrophils, 21 mg % sugar, and a negative culture. A repeat spinal fluid showed faintly acid fast branching filaments. The patient subsequently died. At autopsy, multiple abscesses were seen at the insulotemporal area. One abscess had ruptured into the lateral ventricle, resulting in meningitis.

A 62-year-old female patient of KEPES and SCHOOLMAN, after an injury in an automobile accident, disclosed quadriparesis and died after 26 days. Autopsy revealed a roughly triangular area of necrosis and punctate hemorrhages in the brain. The center of the lesion was yellow-green and paste-like. Microscopic examination showed purulent inflamation with the formation of an abscess. The periphery of the abscess revealed a wide area of fibroblastic proliferation, gliosis, petechiae, and perivascular inflammatory cells. Gram stain demonstrated Gram-positive branching filaments which were slender, slightly beaded and morphologically consistent with *Nocardia*.

WELSH et al. encountered a patient who was admitted for a pulmonary infiltrate. She subsequently developed an epigastric subcutaneous nodule, progressive numbness and weakness of the lower extremities, and later complete paralysis. The epigastric mass was found to be an abscess which on culture revealed *Nocardia*. In spite of streptomycin and sulfadiazine, she died and was found to have abscesses in the fourth and fifth lumbar vertebrae. The middle thoracic spinal cord was destroyed. Microscopically, the remaining cord showed liquefactive necrosis, gitter cells, moderate astrocyte proliferation. Gram positive fungi were found in the cord.

GILLIGAN et al. observed a 32-year-old patient who was admitted to the hospital for intense headaches for 5 days, associated with fever, neck stiffness and Kernig's sign. The spinal fluid showed 4,000 neutrophils per cmm. No organisms were seen on smears. The patient was given antibiotics and sulfadrugs. He had periods without headaches and no Kernig's sign. Repeat spinal fluid examination revealed 1345 neutrophiles and 185 lymphocytes per cmm and proteins of 105 mg %. No organisms were found on smears or culture. After 5 days, intense headaches and neck stiffness returned. The spinal fluid exhibited 63 cells per cmm, mostly mononuclear, and protein of 260 mg/%. *Nocardia* grew on culture. In spite of vigorous treatment, he died. Autopsy demonstrated extensive collections of granular, yellow material in the leptomeninges over the basal aspect of the cerebrum, brain stem and cerebellar hemispheres. Granular yellow material was also found along the middle cerebral artery in the Sylvian fissures. Serial sections of the brain showed moderate uniform dilatation of the ventricular system and 2—3 mm areas of yellow material in the right posterior portion of the mid-pons adjacent to the thickened meninges. The fungus was pathogenic for mice.

A successfully treated case of nocardial meningitis was reported by KING et al. in a 50-year-old man. The patient developed signs of meningitis about one month after a head injury. Spinal fluid showed 570 white cells per cmm with 99% mononuclear cells, 260 mg/% protein and glucose of less than 25 mg/%. He was treated successfully with sulfadiazine and urea.

Cutaneous and Subcutaneous Nocardiosis: Cutaneous nocardiosis may be mycetoma (Madura foot) due to *Nocardia brasiliensis* or *Nocardia asteroides* or a skin involvement with or without systemic disease. Nocardiosis of the skin resembling sporotrichosis was reported by Guy.

His patient was a 50-year-old man who developed a "simple pimple" of the thumb. Other pimples appeared and they formed ulcers which had ragged edges and the base was covered with an indolent appearing granulation tissue. Inflammatory nodules with soft centers ascended towards the elbow. RAICH et al. reported a 38-year-old farmer who had a red draining granuloma of the index finger with subcutaneous nodules along the forearm. Exudate from the finger showed numerous intracellular acid fast organisms in bundles or "globi" which on culture yielded *Nocardia*.

A progressively enlarging breast mass following a two-year history of an abrasion with a rosebush thorn in a 36-year-old woman was reported by LARSEN et al. The mass was firm and tender and the nipple retracted. Aspiration showed beaded Gram positive branching structures which on culuture grew *N. asteroides*. The lesion did not respond to tetracycline and developed an indurated sinus tract with a recurrent abscess which necessitated wide local excision. HICKEY and BERGLUND were able to isolate *N. asteroides* from three patients with abscesses associated with a branchiogenic cyst, a pilonidal cyst and ischio-rectal abscess, respectively, without systemic lesions.

Frequently, skin and subcutaneous lesions are noticed in the chest in association with pulmonary nocardiosis. MURRAY et al. observed a 36-year-old man complaining of left anterior chest pain, night sweats, fever of a week's duration, and cough productive of a small amount of mucoid sputum. The chest was asymmetrical with a tender prominence of the left pectoral area. A pleural friction rub and moist rales were heard over the left chest wall. Chest X-ray showed an infiltration of the midportion of the left lung field. Culture of pus aspirated from the left chest abscess yielded *N. asteroides*. The patient was treated with antibiotics and sulfadiazine without improvement. Two weeks later, under local anesthesia, the left chest lesion was explored and a small amount of pus was found under the pectoral muscle. Later, under general anesthesia, he was explored, and a wide exposure of the subpectoral space demonstrated a large amount of thick pus and a sinus tract that extended beneath the ribs into the pleural cavity. The diseased ribs were resected. He received more sulfadiazine and improved.

FREESE et al. reported that among 11 cases of nocardiosis, 6 patients had cutaneous lesions as "cold abscesses", tender subcutaneous nodules, lymphadenopathy and draining sinus tracts. The fluctuant swellings were related in position to underlying empyema or abscesses of the forehead or epigastrium.

A patient with ischiorectal abscess was observed by BINFORD and LANE. BOBBITT et al. encountered a patient with draining sinuses of the hip and buttocks; autopsy revealed a large psoas abscess and multiple abscesses in both lungs with fibrinous pleuritis. A patient of WICHELHAUSEN et al. had a peri-anal abscess. Later, he developed a chest mass from which

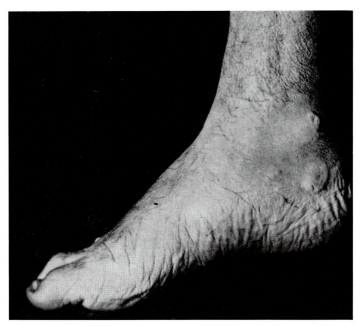

Fig. 9. Nocardial mycetoma of foot. Note the sinus openings on the elevated mounds of granulation and scar tissue. Pus from these sinuses contains granules or grains. These should be examined in fresh and in gram-stained preparations for the presence of the slender, branching, segmented filaments of *Nocardia*. Case from Durham, North Carolina, USA

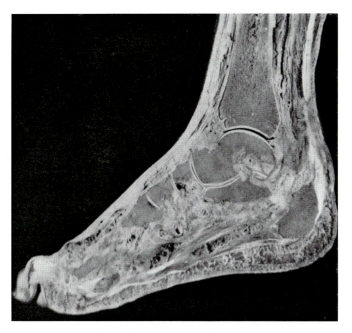

Fig. 10. Nocardial mycetoma. Sagittal section of foot shown in Figure 9. Note the abscesses of bone and the ramifying sinuses which discharge pus and granules to the skin surface

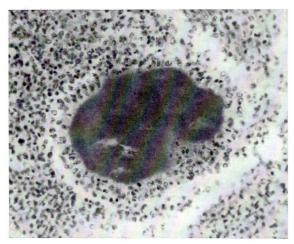

Fig. 11. Nocardial mycetoma. Granule in pus H & E, × 100

N.asteroides was isolated. Central nervous system symptoms occurred and the patient died. Autopsy demonstrated abscesses only in the chest wall and brain.

A portal of entry of the fungus was probably in the hand of the patient of BOBBITT et al. This 55-year-old woman received an injury to her right hand in which a firm violaceous raised 3 cm abscess occurred. From a central crater a freely draining purulent material was cultured to reveal *N.asteroides*. She developed a brain abscess which on aspiration showed *N.asteroides*.

Nocardial Mycetoma: Mycetoma pedis (Madura foot) occurs frequently in the lower extremities (Figs. 9, 10). Involvement of the upper extremities and back is fairly common. GONZALEZ-OCHOA (1962) has observed lesions on the back of Mexican laborers who carry soil-contaminated fiber sacks on their backs. The lesion may start as a papule or vesicle and later develops into a cutaneous or subcutaneous firm mass. Ulceration occurs in the center of the mass from which a thin, watery, serous or purulent material oozes. One or more sinus tracts form; they may heal leaving a depressed center. Other nodules and sinuses develop in the adjacent areas and the intervening tissues become indurated with the characteristics of brawny edema. Lesions between the toes and heel result in great distortions, deformities and contractures. Simultaneously, sinus tracts penetrate the deep soft tissues demonstrating no resistance of the tissue other than the formation of large amounts of scar tissue with intervening zones of necrosis. Infection extends to the adjacent bone to form a chronic osteomyelities.

In the exudate from the sinuses are found "grains" or clusters of mycelial threads (Figs. 11, 12). They are usually yellow when caused by *Nocardia*, in contrast to black, white or red when the disease is caused by other fungi.

The disease remains localized for months and even years, spreading by continuity. According to GONZALEZ-OCHOA (1962), visceral invasion by contiguity is not rare; there is pulmonary involvement in 25% of the cases of thoracic mycetoma caused by *N.brasiliensis*.

The incubation period is unknown; MACKINNON et al. observed two cases of *N.brasiliensis* 15 and 20 days after minor injury to the hand. The wound was granulomatous with lymphangitis of the hand and forearm extending to the upper arm in one case and with nodules along the lymphatics. One patient had an abscess with pus formation. Filaments of an actinomycete were present but no grains. Culture yielded colonies of *N.brasiliensis* which on intraperitoneal injec-

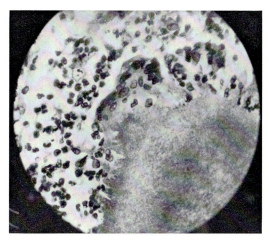

Fig. 12. Nocardial mycetoma. Granule in pus. Giant cell applied to the periphery of the granule. Club formation at the periphery. H & E, × 300. Gram stain would color the filaments of the granule as in Figs. 2 and 5

tions into mice produced typical grains of *N.brasiliensis*. The patients responded to sulfonamide therapy.

Miscellaneous Nocardial Lesions: Other single organs may be involved as a primary site. HENDERSON et al. reported a case of eye involvement in a 49-year-old woman who was struck in the eye by the tail of a cow which she was milking. The eye became red and a mass appeared. She was treated with chloramphenicol, staphylococcus toxoid and typhoid vaccine but the mass continued to enlarge. The mass was later excised; microscopically it showed "inflammatory granulation tissue" and culture revealed *N.asteroides*. Later a small daughter granuloma appeared. After sulfadiazine therapy, this second granuloma became localized and spontaneous resolution occurred. A 23-year-old female patient of BENEDICT and IVERSON developed episodes of ocular pain, photophobia, dimness of vision and conjunctival congestion after an attack of scarlet fever. The inner surfaces of the eyelids presented either large patches of granulation tissue or patches of scar tissue. The right cornea showed interstitial keratitis. Eight cultures over a period of four years revealed nocardial organisms which were not pathogenic for guinea pigs, mice or rabbits.

Skin lesions caused by *N.brasiliensis* have been observed in the United States. A case resembling clinical sporotrichosis was reported by RAPAPORT in a 56-year-old man who pricked his index finger with a rose thorn two or three weeks before examination. A chancriform ulceration with advancing lymphangitis, mild axillary lymph-adenopathy and multiple erythematous nodules along the course of the lymphatics on the exterior surface of the forearm were noted. He received erythromycin and potassium iodide and after one week, the lesions were generally improved, but a fluctuant small bubo developed on the forearm. Pus from the chancre and abscess revealed *N.brasiliensis*. Skin lesions due to *N.brasiliensis* were encountered by M.A. GORDON, MOORE et al., and MOORE and CONRAD.

A patient observed by MAHVI was admitted for epigastric pain and tenderness associated with X-ray changes in the bones showing a "punched-out" appearance suggestive of multiple myeloma. He was treated with urethane, cortisone, chloramphenicol and deep X-ray therapy. He developed a perirenal abscess and multiple ulcerating cutaneous abscesses from which *N.brasiliensis* was isolated. He was then treated with sulfonamides but expired. Autopsy revealed abscesses in the skin, kidney and lungs with an acute suppurative inflammatory reaction containing Gram-positive branching masses, some of which were coccoid and others bacillary.

Baumgarten and Guy reported cases of skin nocardiosis resembling clinical sporotrichosis in which *N.asteroides* had been isolated. Long and Campana isolated a *Nocardia* species in a granuloma with draining sinuses following a dog bite.

The lacrimal gland was surgically removed by Christopherson and Archibald because of swelling of the eye for $3^1/_2$ years. The eyelids could not be everted, but when raised, a thick yellow discharge poured out. The whole conjunctival surface of the upper lid appeared to be rough and granular. Smears showed "bacilliform hyphae" which were not pathogenic for the gray monkey.

The eye may be a part of a systemic nocardiosis, as observed in Hiddlestone's case. An acute chalazion of the left upper lid developed and culture of the exudate exhibited *N.asteroides*.

A patient of Cruz and Clancy was admitted to the hospital for pain in the right thigh for six weeks accompanied by weight loss. She also had fever, night sweats, and chilly sensations but no cough. She had a blowing systolic murmur at the cardiac apex transmitted over the entire precordium. Examination of the thigh revealed acute tenderness, swelling, and induration over the anterolateral area. X-ray of the thigh revealed osteomyelitis of several weeks duration. X-ray of the chest was normal. Surgical incision was made into the osteomyelitic cavity; smears showed filaments with beaded Gram-positive granules. *N.asteroides* was isolated on culture.

Larsen et al. observed a patient who had Hodgkin's disease and was treated with nitrogen mustard and cortisone. She developed a purulent discharge from the ear from which *Nocardia* was isolated.

Bianco et al. observed a 26-year-old man who developed soreness of both calves of the leg after exercise Redness and swelling of the right calf later developed. Draining revealed a "quart of bloody pus" from which *N.asteroides* was cultured. Osteomyelitis of the proximal part of the fibula was noted.

A patient of Utz had osteomyelitis and a severe burrowing cellulitis with abscess and sinus tract formation in the thigh and leg. The infection responded to surgical drainage and prolonged sulfadiazine and penicillin therapy.

Murray et al. observed a 43-year-old man with glomerulonephritis which was treated with cortisone. He developed a purulent pleural effusion from which *N.asteroides* was isolated. In the course of treatment with sulfadimethoxine, symptoms of peritonitis were noted. A peritoneal tap yielded purulent fluid which on smear showed Gram-positive filaments suggestive of *Nocardia* but no cultures were made. He was continued on steroid therapy, sulfadimethoxine, antibiotics, and drainage of the empyema cavity and discharged improved.

Nearly every organ has been observed at autopsy to be involved in nocardiosis. The heart of the patient reported by Cruz and Clancy showed extensive necrosis of a papillary muscle of the mitral valve. Sections throughout the papillary muscle revealed 1—3 mm abscesses containing greenish-yellow, thick, odorless pus. Larsen et al. also observed in a patient with Hodgkin's disease, after treatment by nitrogen mustard and cortisone, degenerative changes with acute purulent inflammation in the cardiac papillary muscles. Abscesses due to *Nocardia* were encountered in the liver, pancreas, kidney, brain and lung. A patient of Hiddlestone ·evealed in the mitral valve firm pale vegetations from which

Nocardia was cultured. The spleen had a large abscess filled with a thick, glairy, greenish-yellow pus.

Nocardia As an "Opportunistic" Fungus: At the International Symposium held at Duke University in June, 1962, *Nocardia* was included among the opportunistic fungi. These were defined as "ubiquitous saprophytes and occasional pathogens that invade the tissues of man or animals with (1) predisposing diseases such as diabetes, leukemia, lymphoma, cancer, and aplastic anemia; or (2) predisposing conditions such as agammaglobulinemia, neutropenia, splenectomy, and roentgen therapy, and the use of steroids and antileukemic and antibiotic drugs" (BAKER, 1962).

Among 202 cases of fungus infections encountered in cancer patients at the Memorial Hospital for Cancer and Allied Diseases and the James Ewing Hospital in New York, HUTTER and COLLINS found 28 cases of infections due to actinomycetes. From these cases *Nocardia* species was cultured in eight.

From the Armed Forces Institute of Pathology at Washington, D.C., CROSS and BINFORD studied 44 cases of nocardiosis. Of these, 17 cases revealed previous diseases or conditions that could have predisposed to fungus infection. Eight patients received prolonged steroid therapy. Leukemia or lymphoma was the primary disease in six cases.

Similar observations have been made by CASAZZA et al., HATHAWAY and MASON, and SALTZMAN et al. Nocardiosis has been encountered with other pathologic states such as lupus erythematosus (PILLAY et al., and SANTEN and WRIGHT), sarcoidosis (STEINBERG), intestinal lymphangiectasia (HARGROVE et al.) and other blood dyscrasias (UTZ, WHITMORE et al., GYDELL et al.) and Cushing's syndrome (DANOWSKI et al.).

There has been a progressively more frequent reporting of cases of pulmonary alveolar proteinosis associated with a focus of nocardiosis. No explanation had been advanced except that the fungus may favor or stimulate the formation or deposition of the periodic acid – Schiff positive material in the alveolar sacs of the lung. Cases have been reported by ANDRIOLE et al., BURBANK et al., CARLSEN et al., MARTINEZ-MALDONADO and RAMIREZ DE ARELLANO, ROSEN et al., and ANDERSON et al.

Microscopic Lesions

Histologic sections of material from the draining sinuses of nocardial mycetomas stained with hematoxylin and eosin often reveal oval or irregular masses of pink or yellow staining mycelial filaments — so called "sulfur granules" (Figs. 11, 12). Tissue sections of aspirated or biopsy material or the wall of an abscess from other sites do not show the granules. There is a loss of tissue structure and cellular detail and an extensive infiltration of neutrophils, lymphocytes, plasma cells, and macrophages in various stages of degeneration. Beyond this zone of suppuration the inflammatory cells are more viable and discernible and are enmeshed in a network of fibrin. Epithelioid and multinucleated giant cells are seldom and sporadically found. There is a poorly defined wall of fibroblastic activity, with some deposition of collagen, proliferation of capillaries or a pseudocapsule from compression of the surrounding stroma. The brain shows numerous gitter cells and a variable amount of gliosis. No micro-organisms are seen with hematoxylin and eosin stains. Gram stain of an adjacent section reveals well outlined Gram positive branching, occasional beaded, non-septate, slender, 0.5—1 μ thick filaments. (Fig. 5). Gomori methenamine silver stain also shows well-outlined fungi. Bacillary forms of varying lengths and coccoid bodies are occasionally found. Phagocytized organisms may be found in macrophages. Acid fast stains reveal some

strains that are positive especially if a weak decolorizing agent such as 1—5%
aqueous sulfuric acid is used. These filaments are often beaded (RIDELL). The
periodic acid – Schiff stain is not valuable as the filaments stain like the surrounding material (BALLINGER and GOLDRING, BAKER, 1957; BINFORD and
LANE, CALERO, KADE and KAPLAN).

A unique case of nocardiosis was reported by CUTTINO and McCABE in a
34-month-old girl who was admitted to the hospital for anorexia, nausea, vomiting
and weight loss. A lymph node showed complete alteration of its architecture
with proliferation of macrophages, the cytoplasm of which appeared foamy and
granular resembling Gaucher's cells and containing massive numbers of acid fast
bacilli. She did not respond to treatment and expired. Autopsy revealed that the
abdominal lymph nodes were matted together, and yellow on section with centers
exhibiting irregular zones of necrosis. Microscopic examination of the spleen
showed great distortion of the architecture by an abundant proliferation of large,
pale, foamy-appearing macrophages to the extent that lymphoid remnants
appeared only as focal collections of cells. The malpighian corpuscles were replaced
by epithelioid cells, concentrically arranged about the central artery. There were
groups of multinucleated giant cells, usually in clusters of a dozen or more. The
nuclei were in a peripheral position and were small and hyperchromatic. In the
central zone of the cytoplasm there was a clear spherical homogeneous area. Acid
fast bacilli were found in the epithelioid cells. The liver showed scattered tubercle-
like nodules of epithelioid cells with many acid fast organisms. Many Kupffer
cells showed phagocytosis of the organisms but there was no apparent damage to
the liver cells. Culture revealed a new species: *N. intracellularis* which was not
pathogenic for guinea pigs, rats, mice or rabbits.

Animal Pathogenicity

All of the 69 strains of *N. asteroides* studied by GEORG et al. were pathogenic
for guinea pigs. Other workers have had variable results with guinea pigs, as well
as with rabbits, mice and monkeys. When the fungus is pathogenic for guinea
pigs, the animals succumb after intraperitoneal infection, in 10—30 days. STRAUS
and KLIGMAN found that the addition of 5% gastric mucin to the inoculating
medium enhanced the infectivity for mice. They noted many small nodules
scattered throughout the peritoneal cavity, and adhesions around the liver,
stomach and spleen. Similar lesions are seen in guinea pigs and from these lesions
Nocardia was isolated on smears and cultures (DRAKE and HENRICI).

GONZALEZ-OCHOA (1967) found that the intramuscular, subcutaneous or
intradermal injection of a light inoculum of *N. brasiliensis* into mice produced
only transient lesions with a tendency to spontaneous cure. When the inoculum
was given intravenously or intraperitoneally, the animals died. A single injection
of the organisms into the foot pad of the mouse resulted in a chronic fistulous
swelling containing actinomycotic grains resembling clinical mycetoma. Some
mice showed invasion of the inguinal and intra-abdominal lymphnodes and lesions
in the lungs and liver.

MARIAT and MACOTELA-RUIZ were able to produce true mycetoma in hamsters
by the intradermal injection of *N. asteroides* and *N. brasiliensis*.

BRUECK and BUDDINGH were able to cultivate *Nocardia* by the use of the
chick embryo. They noted that *N. asteroides* grew very readily in the chorioallantois
as well as in the yolk sac. In both of these sites *N. asteroides* proliferated so rapidly
the embryo died within 3—4 days. The fungus apparently could be maintained
indefinitely in serial passage in the membrane or within the yolk sac. *N. intra-*

cellularis thrived poorly in the chorioallantois but grew readily in the yolk sac. Within 48—72 h following inoculation numerous organisms were demonstrated with Gram and acid fast stained smears from the yolk.

Nocardia species have been found in dogs (BOHL et al., THORDAL-CHRISTENSEN and CLIFFORD), in a cat (AJELLO et al., 1961), cows (NOCARD) and marsupials (TUCKER and MILLAR). Bovine farcy produced by a species of *Nocardia* resembling *N.farcinica* which was originally described by Nocard had been observed in regions south of African Sudan by Mostafa.

KINCH reported a fatal infection in a dog by *N.caviae*. This 18-month-old dog was treated with corticosteroid for severe muscle stiffness in the hind quarters following excessive exercise. Temperature of 106°F. developed and intramuscular chloramphenicol was given. The dog became rapidly worse and died eight days after the onset of illness. At autopsy, adjacent to the mandible was a 2.5 cm circumscribed abscess filled with a foul-smelling greyish-white pus. The liver was dark reddish purple and contained numerous grey nodules up to 4 mm in diameter. The kidneys were reddish brown and contained a few small greyish-white nodules up to 5 mm in diameter. Microscopic examination of the liver showed small granulomatous abscesses. The smallest abscesses were composed of cores of lymphocytes and macrophages surrounded by a few epithelioid cells and fibroblasts. Small amounts of collagen and reticulum were around the periphery of the lesions. In larger lesions the cores were composed of neutrophils and free red cells and these were surrounded by a typical granulomatous type of reaction. The kidney showed abscesses composed of neutrophils and a small number of macrophages and epithelioid cells. There was no encapsulation by fibrous tissue. Direct smears from the mandibular abscess, liver, lung and kidney revealed large numbers of branching filamentous Gram-positive organisms. The organisms in stained section of the liver, lung and kidney were Gram-negative, periodic acid-Schiff negative and non-acid fast. Cultures revealed characteristics of *N.caviae* according to the criteria of GORDON and MIHM (1962).

Diagnosis

A positive diagnosis of nocardiosis depends on the isolation of *Nocardia* and the study of its cultural and biochemical characteristics as well as its pathogenicity for laboratory animals. A tentative diagnosis of nocardial mycetoma may be made by the recognition of pink or yellow "sulfur granules" in the exudate from the draining sinus. Since the pulmonary variety is rarely associated with sinus formation, aspiration or needle biopsy is the method of choice (PIZZOLATO et al.). Any material aspirated should be cultured and smears made. The Gram method reveals Gram-positive, branching, non septate, slender, filaments or hyphae among the numerous leukocytes in various stages of degeneration (Fig. 14). Centrifuged sediments of pleural fluid and spinal fluid should be cultured before smears are made since therapy is vastly different in bacterial infections from what it is in nocardiosis. A definite diagnosis must be made (MOGABGAB; WEBSTER, 1962; HUNTER et al.; HOSTY et al.; GLOVER et al.; HALL and COOLEY).

Treatment

Sulfonamides are the drugs of choice and if the dose is sufficiently high, the prognosis is good (SEABURY and DASCOMB). HOEPRICH et al. recommend surgical drainage and combined antimicrobic therapy for nocardial cerebral abscess and use cycloserine and sulfonamides. Utz's patient with osteomyelites and sinus tract formation in the thigh and leg responded to surgical drainage and prolonged sulfadiazine and penicillin therapy. GONZALEZ-OCHOA (1960) did not get encouraging results in the treatment of nocardiosis with griseofulvin.

Mixed Infections: Baker reported a fatal case of combined pulmonary nocardiosis and cryptococcosis (Figs. 13, 15). The gross appearance was that of pulmonary nocardiosis but microscopically there were areas rich in *Cryptococcus neoformans*. Fig. 15 shows only the necrotizing nocardial pneumonia.

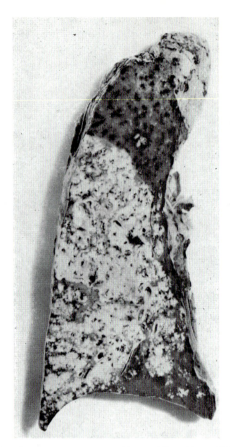

Fig. 13. Mixed nocardiosis and cryptococcosis of lower lobe of lung. The predominant appearance is that of pulmonary nocardiosis, but there are areas of cryptococcal organisms visible microscopically. This is an example of an opportunistic infection as the patient's resistence had been lowered by multiple myeloma and cytotoxic drug therapy

The case was that of a 52-year-old Negro woman who suffered from multiple myeloma for three years and received 200 mg of Fluorouracil three times a week during the last month of life. Three weeks before death she became febrile and had a slight cough productive of pink sputum. Hemoglobin terminally, 5.4 gm.; white blood cell count, 3,715; 60% neutrophils, 36% small lymphocytes; 4% monocytes. There was 2 plus albuminuria.

At necropsy there were white and red gelatinous nodules of multiple myeloma throughout the marrow of the ribs, sternum and spine, with collapse of a vertebral body. Caseation and abscesses involved the entire left lobe and a portion of the left upper lobe of the lung (Fig. 13); fibrin covered the pleural surfaces on this side. The right lung was similarly involved but to a lesser extent. Microscopically the regions of nocardiosis showed purulent necrotizing pneumonia in H & E stain (Fig. 15), and branching filaments of *Nocardia* in Gram stain. The regions of cryptococcosis, not illustrated here, were composed of foci of *Cryptococcus neoformans* with much gelatinous capsular material and minimal inflammatory response. The mucicarmine stain, specific for *Cryptococcus*, stained the organisms nicely.

This case is a good example of an opportunistic nocardial infection in a patient with lowered resistence due to the multiple myeloma and the cytotoxic drug.

Hall and Cooley reported a case of pulmonary nocardiosis complicated by tuberculosis, another mixed infection.

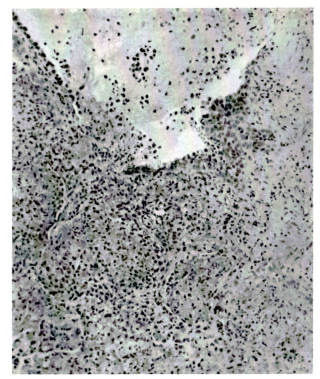

Fig. 14. *Nocardia asteroides* in smear of pus. Gram stain

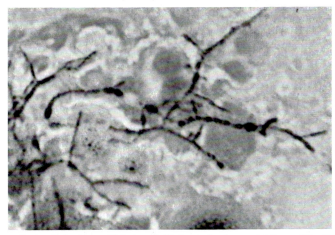

Fig. 15. Nocardiosis of the lung. This is a field from the lung of Figure 13 with necrotizing pneumonia and bronchiolitis due to *Nocardia*. There is no cryptococcosis in this particular field. H & E, × 60

References

Abbott, P.: Mycetoma in the Sudan. Trans. roy. Soc. trop. Med. Hyg. **50**, 11 (1956). — Ajello, L., Grant, V.Q., Gutske, M.A.: The effects of tubercle bacillus concentration procedures on fungi causing pulmonary mycosis. J. Lab. clin. Med. **38**, 486 (1951). — Ajello, L., Walker, W.W., Dungworth, D.L., Brumfield, G.: Isolation of *Nocardia brasiliensis* from a cat, with review of its prevalence and geographic distribution. J. Amer. vet. med. Ass. **188**, 370 (1961). — Anderson, B.R., Echlund, R.E., Kellow, W.E.: Pulmonary alveolar

proteinosis with systemic nocardiosis. A case report. J. Amer. med. Ass. **174**, 28 (1960). —
ANDRIOLE, V.T., BALLAS, M., WILSON, G.L.: The association of nocardiosis and pulmonary
alveolar proteinosis. A case study. Ann. intern. Med. **50**, 266 (1964). — ARAGONA, F., DE
PASQUALE, N.: Sulla nocardiasi pulmonare. G. Mal. infett. **5**, 310 (1953). — BAKER, R.D.:
The diagnosis of fungus diseases by biopsy. J. chron. Dis. **5**, 552 (1957). ~ Foreword. Inter-
national Symposium on Opportunistic Fungus Infections. Lab. Invest. **11**, 1017 (1962). ~
In Seminar on Virus and Fungus Diseases of the A.S.C.P. September 7, 1962. Published by
the American Society of Clinical Pathology, Chicago 1963. — BALLENGER, C.N., Jr., GOLD-
RING, D.: Nocardiosis in childhood. J. Pediat. **50**, 145 (1957). — BAUMGARTEN, A.: Nocardiosis: Report of a case resembling sporotrichosis. Med. J. Aust. **2**, 321 (1961). — BENEDICT,
W.L., IVERSON, H.A.: Chronic keratoconjunctivitis associated with *Nocardia*. Arch. Ophthal.
32, 89 (1944). — BERGEY's Manual of Determinative Bacteriology. Ed. by R.S. BREED,
E.G.D. MURRAY and N.R. SMITH, p. 713. Baltimore, Maryland: Williams and Wilkins Co.
1957. — BERNSTEIN, I.L., COOK, J.E., PLOTNICH, H., TENCZAR, F.J.: Nocardiosis. Three
case reports. Ann. intern. Med. **36**, 852 (1952). — BIANCO, A.J., Jr., JOHNSON, E.W., Jr.,
MARTIN, W.J., NICHOLS, D.R.: Nocardiosis without involvement of pulmonary or central
nervous system. Proc. Mayo Clin. **32**, 119 (1957). — BINFORD, C.H., LANE, J.D.: Actinomycosis due to *Nocardia asteroides*. Report of a case. Amer. J. clin. Path. **15**, 17 (1945). — BLAN-
CHARD, R.: Parasites vegetaux a l'exclusion des bacteries. Traite de pathologie generale.
pp. 811—932, Tome II. Ed. by CH. BOUCHARD, G. MASSON, Paris. Quoted by Gorden and
Mihm 1957. — BOBBITT, O.B., FRIEDMAN, I.H., LUPTON, C.: Nocardiosis. Report of three
cases. New Engl. J. Med. **252**, 893 (1955). — BOHL, E.H., JONES, D.O., FARRELL, R.L.,
CHAMBERLAIN, D.M., COLE, C.R., FERGUSON, L.C.: Nocardiosis in the dog. A case report.
J. Amer. vet. med. Ass. **122**, 81 (1953). — BOJALIL, L.F., CERBON, J.: Schema for the dif-
ferentation of *Nocardia asteroides*, and *Nocardia brasiliensis*. J. Bact. **78**, 852 (1959). —
BREED, R.S., CONN, H.J.: The nomenclature of the Actinomycetaceae. J. Bact. **4**, 585 (1919).
— BRUECK, J.W., BUDDINGH, G.J.: Propagation of pathogenic fungi in yolk sac of embryonat-
ed eggs. Proc. Soc. exp. Biol. (N.Y.). **76**, 258 (1951). — BURBANK, B., MORRIONE, T.G.,
CULLEN, S.S.: Pulmonary alveolar proteinosis and nocardiosis. Amer. J. Med. **28**, 1002
(1960). — CALERO, C.: Pulmonary actinomycosis (Report of the first case observed in the
Isthmus of Panama). Dis. Chest **12**, 402 (1946). — CARLILE, W.K., HOLLEY, K.E., LOGAN,
G.B.: Fatal acute disseminated nocardiosis in a child. J. Amer. med. Ass. **184**, 477 (1963). —
CARLSEN, E.T., HILL, R.B., ROWLANDS, D.T., Jr.: Nocardiosis and pulmonary alveolar
proteinosis. Ann. intern. Med. **60**, 275 (1964). — CASAZZA, A.R., DUVALL, C.P., CARBONE,
P.P.: Infection in lymphoma. Histology, treatment and duration in relation to incidence and
survival. J. Amer. med. Ass. **197**, 710 (1966). — CHALMERS, A.J., ARCHIBALD, R.G.: A
sudanese maduromycosis. Ann. trop. Med. Parasit. **10**, 169 (1916). — CHRISTOPHERSON, J.B.,
ARCHIBALD, R.G.: Primary nocardiosis of the lacrymal gland. Lancet **1918** II, 847. — CLAY-
POLE, E.J.: Human streptothricosis and its differentiation from tuberculosis. Arch. intern.
Med. **14**, 104 (1914). — CONANT, N.F.: Bacterial and Mycotic Infections of Man. Ed. by
R.J. DUBOS. Pp. 584. Third edition. Philadelphia: Lippincott 1958. — COTTON, R.E., LLOYD,
H.E.D.: Lipid pneumonia and infection with *Nocardia asteroides* complicating achalasia
of the cardia. J. Path. Bact. **79**, 251 (1960). — CROSS, R.M., BINFORD, C.H.: Is *Nocardia
asteroides* an opportunist? Lab. Invest. **11**, 1103 (1962). — CRUZ, P.T., CLANCY, C.F.: Nocardiosis. Nocardial osteomyelitis and septicemia. Amer. J. Path. **28**, 607 (1952). — CUPP, E.M.,
EDWARDS, W.M., CLEVE, E.A.: Nocardiosis of the central nervous system. Report of two
fatal cases. Ann. intern. Med. **52**, 223 (1960). — CUTTINO, J.T., McCABE, A.M.: Pure granulomatous nocardiosis. A new fungus disease distinguished by intracellular parasitism. A
description of a new disease in man due to a hitherto undescribed organism, *Nocardia intracellularis*, N. sp., including a study of the biologic and pathogenic properties of this species.
Amer. J. Path. **25**, 1 (1949). — DANOWSKI, T.S., COOPER, W.M., BRAUDE, A.: Cushing's
syndrome in connection with *Nocardia asteroides*. Metabolism **3**, 265 (1962). — DOLAN, T.F.,
Jr., McCULLOUGH, N.B., GIBSON, L.E.: Nocardiosis. Report of two cases in children.
J. Dis. Child. **99**, 234 (1960). — DRAKE, C.H., HENRICI, A.T.: *Nocardia asteroides*. Its
pathogenicity and allergic properties. Amer. Rev. Tuberc. **48**, 184 (1943). — DROPMANN,
K.: Nokardiose unter Berücksichtigung des Diabetes mellitus. Verh. dtsch. Ges. Path. **1959**,
154—155. — ECKHARDT, K., PILCHER, J.: Brain abscess due to *Nocardia asteroides*. Report
of case. Tex. St. J. Med. **46**, 915 (1950). — EPPINGER, H.: Über eine neue pathogene Cladothrix und eine durch sie hervorgerufene Pseudo-Tuberculosis. Wien. klin. Wschr. **3**, 321
(1890, 1891). — ERCHUL, J.W., KOCH, M.L.: Cerebral nocardiosis with coexistant tuberculosis. Report of a fatal case. Amer. J. clin. Path. **25**, 775 (1955). — FREESE, J.W., YOUNG,
W.G., Jr., SEALY, W.C., CONANT, N.F.: Pulmonary infection by *Nocardia asteroides*. Findings
in eleven cases. J. thorac. cardiovasc. Surg. **46**, 537 (1963). — GEORG, L.K., AJELLO, A.,
McDURMONT, C., HOSTY, T.S.: The identification of *Nocardia asteroides* and *Nocardia brasiliensis*. Amer. Rev. resp. Dis. **84**, 337 (1961). — GILLIGAN, B.S., WILLIAMS, I., PERCEVAL,

A.K.: Nocardial meningitis: report of a case with bacteriological studies. Med. J. Aust. **2**, 747 (1962). — GLOVER, R.P., WALLACE, E.H., HERRELL, W.E., HEILMAN, F.R., PFUETZE, K.H.: Nocardiosis: *Nocardia asteroides* simulating pulmonary tuberculosis. J. Amer. med. Ass. **136**, 172 (1948). — GOLDSWORTHY, N.E.: Pulmonary actinomycosis caused by acid-fast species of actinomycosis. J. Path. Bact. **45**, 17 (1937). — GONZALEZ-OCHOA, A.: Mycetoma caused by *Nocardia brasiliensis*: with a note on the isolation of the causative organism from soil. Lab. Invest. **11**, 1118 (1962). ~ In Systemic Mycosis, Ciba Foundation Symposium. Ed. by G.E.W. WALSTENHOLME, and R. PORTER p. 86. Boston: Little Brown and Co 1967. — GONZALEZ-OCHOA, A., SANDOVAL, M.A.: Revisión determinación de algunas especies de actinomicetes patógenes descritas como diferentes. Rev. Inst. Salubr. Enferm. trop. (Méx.) **16**, 17, 1956 (quoted by WAKSMAN). — GORDON, R.E., HAGEN, W.A.: A study of some acid fast actinomycetes from soil with special references to pathogenicity for animals, J. infect. Dis. **59**, 200 (1936). — GORDON, R.E., MIHM, J.M.: A comparative study of some strains received as *Nocardiae*. J. Bact. **73**, 15 (1957). ~ A comparison of *Nocardia asteroides* and *Nocardia brasiliensis* J. gen. Microbiol. **20**, 129 (1959). ~ The type species of the genus *Nocardia*. J. gen. Microbiol. **27**, 1 (1962). — GORDON, R.E., SMITH, E.: Proposed group of characters for the separation of *Streptomyces* and *Nocardia* J. Bact. **69**, 147 (1955). — GUY, W.H.: Nocardiosis cutis resembling sporotrichosis. Report of a case. Arch. Derm. Syph. (Chic.) **2**, 137 (1920). — GYDELL, K., JOHLIN, I., LJUNGGREN, H., NORDEN, J.G., FORS, B.: Nocardiosis during steroid treatment of auto-immune haemolytic anaemia. Report of fatal case. Acta med. scand. **178**, 221 (1965). — HAGER, H.F., MIGLIACCIO, A.C., YOUNG, R.M.: Nocardiosis: Pneumonia and empyema due to *N.astoides*. New Engl. J. Med. **241**, 226 (1949). — HALL, E.R., Jr., COOLEY, D.A.: Pulmonary nocardiosis: report of case complicated by tuberculosis. Dis. Chest. **31**, 453 (1957). — HARGROVE, M.D., MATHEWS, W.R., McINTYRE, P.A.: Intestinal lymphangiectasia with response to corticosteroids. Arch. intern. Med. **119**, 206 (1967). — HATHAWAY, B.H., MASON, K.N.: Nocardiosis. Study of fourteen cases. Amer. J. Med. **32**, 903 (1962). — HENDERSON, J.W., WELLMAN, W.E., WEED, L.A.: Nocardiosis of the eye: Report of case. Proc. Mayo Clin. **35**, 614 (1960). — HENRICI, A.T., GARDNER, E.L.: The acid-fast actinomycetes with a report of a case from which a new species was isolated. J. infect. Dis. **28**, 232 (1921). — HICKEY, R.G., BERGLUND, E.M.: Nocardiosis. Aerobic actinomycosis with emphasis on alimentary tract as portal of entry. Arch. Surg. **67**, 381 (1953). — HIDDLESTONE, H.J.H.: Nocardiosis in New Zealand; Report of a case. N.Z. med. J. **56**, 399 (1957). — HOEPRICH, P.D., BRANDT, D., PARKER, R.H.: Nocardial brain abscess cured with cycloserine and sulfonamides. Amer. J. med. Sci. **255**, 208 (1968). — HOSTY, T.S., McDURMONT, C., AJELLO, L., GEORG, L., BLUMFIELD, G.L., CALIX, A.A.: Prevalence of *Nocardia asteroides* in sputa examined by a tuberculosis diagnostic laboratory. J. Lab. clin. Med. **58**, 107 (1961). — HUNTER, R.A., WILLCOX, D.R.C., WOOLF, A.L.: Aerobic actinomycosis with a report of a case resembling miliary tuberculosis. Guy's Hosp. Rep. **103**, 196 (1954). — HUTTER, R.V.P., COLLINS, H.S.: The occurrence of opportunistic fungus infections in a cancer hospital. Lab. Invest. **11**, 1035 (1962). — JACOBSON, J.R., CLOWARD, R.B.: Actinomycosis of the central nervous system. A case of meningitis with recovery. J. Amer. med. Ass. **137**, 769 (1948). — KADE, H., KAPLAN, L.: Evaluation of staining techniques in the histologic diagnosis of fungi. Arch. Path. **59**, 571 (1955). — KEPES, J.J., SCHOOLMAN, A.: Post-traumatic abscess of the medulla oblongata containing *Nocardia asteroides*. J. Neurosurg. **22**, 511 (1965). — KINCH, D.A.: A rapidly fatal infection caused by *Nocardia caviae* in a dog. J. Path. Bact. **95**, 540 (1968). — KING, R.B., STOOPS, W.L., FITZGIBBONS, J., BUNN, P.: *Nocardia asteroides* meningitis. A case successfully treated with large doses of sulfadiazine and urea. J. Neurosurg. **24**, 749 (1966). — KIRBY, W.M.M., McNAUGHT, J.B.: Actinomycosis due to *Nocardia asteroides*. Arch. intern. Med. **78**, 578 (1946). — KOHN, P.M., TAGER, M., SIEGEL, M.L., ASKE, R.: Aerobic actinomyces septicemia. Report of a case. New Engl. J. Med. **245**, 640 (1951). — KRUEGER, E.G., NORSA, L., KENNEY, M., PRICE, A.: Nocardiosis of the central nervous system. J. Neurosurg. **11**, 226 (1954). — KUMAR, R., MOHAPATRA, L.N.: Studies on aerobic actinomycetes isolated from soil. I. Isolation and identification of strains. Sabouraudia **6**, 140 (1968). — LACAZ, C.S.: Contribuicas para o estudo dos actinomicetos productores de micetomas. Thesis, Faculdade de Medicina de Sao Paulo, Brazil, 1945. Quoted by MOORE, LANE and GAUL. — LARSEN, M.C., DIAMOND, H.D., COLLINS, H.S.: *Nocardia asteroides* infection. A report of seven cases. Arch. intern. Med. **103**, 712 (1959). — LINDENBERG, A.: Un nouveau mycetome. Arch. Parasit. **13**, 265 (1909). — LIST, C.F., WILLIAMS, J.R., BEEMAN, C.B., PAYNE, C.A.: Nocardiosis with multilocular cerebellar abscess. J. Neurosurg. **11**, 394 (1954). — LONG, P.I., CAMPANA, H.A.: An unusual mycetoma. Arch. Derm. **93**, 341 (1966). — MACKINNON, J.: Systemic Mycosis, Ciba Foundation Symposium, p. 89. Ed. G.E.W. WOLSTENHOLME and R. PORTER Boston: Little, Brown and Co. 1967. — MAHVI, T.A.: Disseminated nocardiosis caused by *Nocardia brasiliensis*. Arch. Derm. **89**, 426 (1964). — MARIAT, F., MACOTELA-RUIZ, E.: In Systemic Mycosis, Ciba Foundation Symposium, p. 90. Ed. G.E.W. WOLSTENHOLME and R. PORTER Boston: Little, Brown and

Co. 1967. — Martinez-Maldonado, M., Ramirez de Arellano, G.: Pulmonary alveolar proteinosis, nocardiosis and granulocytic leukemia. Sth. med. J. (Bgham, Ala.) **59**, 901 (1966). — McClung, N.M.: The utilization of carbon compounds by Nocardia species. J. Bact. **68**, 231 (1954). ~ Morphological studies in the genus *Nocardia*. I. Developmental studies. Lloydia **12**, 137 (1949). ~ Isolation of *Nocardia asteroides* from soils. Mycologia **52**, 154 (1960). — Mogabgab, W.J., Floyd, J.L.: Acid-fast Nocardia causing erroneous diagnosis of tracheobronchial tuberculosis. New Orleans med. surg. J. **104**, 28 (1951). — Moore, M., Conrad, A.H.: Sporotrichoid nocardiosis caused by *Nocardia brasiliensis*. Arch. Derm. **95**, 390 (1967). — Moore, M., Lane, C.W., Gaul, L.E.: Nocardiosis of the knee caused by *Nocardia brasiliensis*. Report of first case in a native of the United States. Arch. Derm. Syph. (Chic.) **70**, 302 (1954). — Mostafa, I.E.: In: Vet. Bull. (Weybridge) **36**, 189 (1966) quoted in Systemic Mycosis, Ciba Foundation Symposium, p. 90. Ed. by G.E.W. Wolstenholme and R. Porter. Boston: Little Brown and Co. 1967. — Munslow, R.A.: Actinomycotic (*Nocardia asteroides*) brain abscess with recovery. J. Neurosurg. **11**, 399 (1954). — Murray, J.F., Finegold, S.M., Froman, S., Will, D.W.: The changing spectrum of nocardiosis. A review and presentation of nine cases. Amer. Rev. resp. Dis. **83**, 315 (1961). — Musgrave, W.E., Clegg, M.T., Polk, M.: Streptothricosis with special reference to the etiology and classification of mycetoma. Philipp. J. Sci. B., Med. Sci. **3**, 477 (1908). — Nocard, E.: Note sur la maladie des boeufs de la Guadeloupe connue sans le nom de farcin. Ann. Inst. Pasteur **2**, 293 (1888). — Pillay, V.K., Wilson, D.M., Ing, T.S., Kark, R.M.: Fungus infection in steroid treated systemic lupus erythematosus. J. Amer. med. Ass. **205**, 261 (1968). — Pizzolato, P., Ziskind, J., Derman, H., Buff, E.E.: Nocardiosis of the brain. Report of three cases. Amer. J. clin. Path. **36**, 151 (1961). — Raich, R.A., Casey, R., Hall, W.H.: Pulmonary and cutaneous nocardiosis. The significance of the laboratory isolation of *Nocardia*. Amer. Rev. resp. Dis. **83**, 505 (1961). — Rapaport, J.: Primary chancriform syndrome caused by *Nocardia brasiliensis*. Arch. Derm. **98**, 62 (1966). — Riddell, R.W.: Permanent stained mycological preparation obtained by slide culture. Mycologica **42**, 265 (1950). — Rosen, S.H., Castleman, B., Liebow, A.A.: Pulmonary alveolar proteinosis. New Engl. J. Med. **258**, 1124 (1958). — Runyon, E.H.: *Nocardia asteroides*: Studies of its pathogenicity and drug sensitivities. J. Lab. clin. Med. **37**, 713 (1951). — Saltzman, H.A., Chick, E.W., Conant, N.F.: Nocardiosis as a complication of other disease. Lab. Invest. **11**, 1110 (1962). — Seabury, J.H., Dascomb, H.E.: Results of treatment of systemic mycosis. J. Amer. med. Ass. **188**, 509 (1964). — Santen, R.J., Wright, I.S.: Systemic lupus erythematosis associated with pulmonary nocardiosis. Arch. intern. Med. **119**, 202 (1967). — Schneidau, J.D., Schaffer, M.F.: Studies on *Nocardia* and other actinomycetales: I. Cultural studies. Amer. Rev. Tuberc. **76**, 770 (1957). — Stafovà, J., Motlikovà, M., Krumpl, J., Dvorský, K., Viklichý, J., Vacek, V.: Generalisierte Nokardiose. Eine zentrale Nokardia-Sepsis bei einer Frau mit tödlichem Ausgang. Zbl. allg. Path. path. Anat. **110**, 351 (1967). — Steinberg, I.: Fatal fungus infection in sarcoidosis: Report of two cases treated with antibiotics and cortisone. Ann. intern. Med. **48**, 1359 (1958). — Strauss, R.E., Kligman, A.M.: The use of gastric mucin to lower resistance of laboratory animals to systemic fungus infections. J. infect. Dis. **88**, 151 (1951). — Thordal-Christensen, A., Clifford, D.H.: Actinomycosis (Nocardiosis) in dog with brief review of this disease. Amer. J. vet. Res. **14**, 298 (1953). — Trevisan, V.I.: Generi e le specie delle Batteriacee. Milan 1889, quoted by S.A. Waksman. — Tucker, F.C., Hirsch, E.F.: Nocardiosis with report of three cases of actinomycosis due to *Nocardia asteroides*. J. infect. Dis. **85**, 72 (1949). — Tucker, R., Millar, R.: Outbreak of nocardiosis in marsupials in Brisbane. Botanical Gardens J. Comp. Path. Therap. **63**, 143 (1953). — Utz, J.P.: The spectrum of opportunistic fungus infections. Lab. Invest. **11**, 1018 (1962). — Waksman, S.A.: The Actinomycetes. II. Classification, identification and descriptions of general and species. Baltimore: Williams and Wilkins 1961. — Waksman, S., Henrici, A.T.: The nomenclature and classification of the actinomycetes. J. Bact. **46**, 337 (1943). — Webster, B.H.: Pulmonary nocardiosis. A review of a report of seven cases. Amer. Rev. Tuberc. **73**, 485 (1956). ~ Pulmonary nocardiosis simulating pulmonary tuberculosis in the aged. J. Amer. Geriat. Soc. **10**, 192 (1962). — Weed, L.A., Anderson, H.A., Good, C.A., Baggenstoss, A.H.: Nocardiosis. Clinical, bacteriologic and pathological aspects. New Engl. J. Med. **253**, 1137 (1955). — Welsh, J.D., Rhoades, E.R., Jaques, W.: Disseminated nocardiosis involving spinal cord. Arch. intern. Med. **108**, 73 (1961). — Wichelhausen, R.H., Robinson, L.B., Mazzara, J.R., Everding, C.J.: Nocardiosis. Report of a fatal case. Amer. J. Med. **16**, 295 (1954). — Whitmore, D.N., Gresham, G.A., Grayson, M.J.: Nocardiosis in anaemic patients given steroids. J. clin. Path. **14**, 259 (1961). — Wilhite, J.E., Cole, F.H.: Invasion of pulmonary cavities by *Nocardia asteroides*. Report of 5 cases. Amer. Surg. **32**, 107 (1966). — Wilson, A.M.M.: E. Afr. med. J. **42**, 182 (1965) quoted in Systemic Mycosis, Ciba Foundation Symposium, p. 108. Ed. by G.E.W., Wolstenholme and R. Porter. Boston: Little, Brown and Co. 1967,

Protothecosis – Algal Infection

BERNARD F. FETTER, GORDON K. KLINTWORTH, and HARRY S. NIELSEN, JR.

Durham/North Carolina, USA

With 15 Figures

Numerous microscopic agents, including bacteria, fungi, protozoa, spirochetes, and viruses, are well recognized as pathogens. Algae, however, have seldom been associated with disease, and are rarely mentioned in the standard texts in clinical microbiology, pathology, and other branches of medicine. In the present report we have attempted to review the evidence concerning the pathogenicity of algae, with particular reference to *Prototheca*, which is thus far the only genus known to invade the tissues of man. Mention has not been made of the role algae play in gastroenteritis and death following ingestion, and in cutaneous and upper respiratory allergic reactions (GORHAM, 1964; SCHWIMMER and SCHWIMMER, 1964).

Organism

The genus *Prototheca* was described in 1894 by KRÜGER to designate a group of non-pigmented unicellular organisms isolated from the mucous flux of trees. Based on a yeast-like appearance in culture, early investigators, including KRÜGER (1894 a, b), considered the organism to be a fungus. This view was generally accepted until WEST (1916) directed attention to its alga-like mode of reproduction. Unlike most yeasts, *Prototheca* does not propagate by budding, but by internally produced spores which are morphologically identical to the parent cell. This method of sporulation is indistinguishable from that observed in the green alga *Chlorella*. Based on this observation WEST (1916) classified the organism in the Chlorophyaceae. PRINTZ (1927) later restudied the genus and recommended that it be placed in the Protothecaceae because of its achlorotic nature. CIFERRI, MONTEMARTINI and CIFERRI (1957) endorsed this taxon with a minor alteration in spelling, changing Protothecaeae to Prototheceae as recommended by the standards of botanical nomenclature.

It is generally believed that *Prototheca* originated from the Chlorophyceae through a sequence of events involving a loss of chlorophyll and adaption to heterotropic habit (COOKE, 1968a). This conclusion is based on the observation that colorless strains of *Chlorella* occur in nature and in the laboratory (BEIJERINCK, 1904); that x-irradiated cells of *Chlorella* produce achloric mutants (GRANICK, 1948); and that non-pigmented variants of *Chlorella* continue to propagate colorless cells in subsequent generations (BUTLER, 1954). Other investigators have questioned this phylogenetic derivation of the genus since species of *Prototheca* are better adapted to the heterotrophic life than the colorless strains of *Chlorella*, and, unlike the latter, are unable to grow in the absence of exogenously supplied thiamine (CIFERRI, 1956; CIFERRI, MONTEMARTINI and CIFERRI, 1957).

Isolation: *Prototheca* is readily cultivated at room temperature on conventional media such as Sabouraud's glucose agar, brain heart infusion agar, blood agar, and beef infusion broth. The organism is fast growing, producing macroscopic colonies within 24—36 hours. Routine mycological procedures are satisfactory for the laboratory study and maintenance of the organism. It is important to note, however, that the antibiotic cyclohexamide which is frequently employed in diagnostic mycology as one of the selective agents against saprophytic fungi may inhibit the growth of some strains of the alga.

The organism can be retained in culture for extended periods under sterile mineral oil. HARTSELL (1956) has shown that one strain of *P. zopfii* survived preservation for 5 years on a malt-yeast extract medium overlayed with oil.

Cultural Morphology: On solid media, isolates of *Prototheca* are similar to many yeasts or yeast-like fungi. Cultures vary from white to cream colored and may be smooth, wrinkled, or pasty depending upon the strain (Fig. 1).

In the diagnostic laboratory, the organism must be distinguished from species of *Candida* and *Cryptococcus*, and to a lesser extent from the yeast forms of *Histoplasma* and *Blastomyces*.

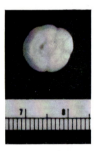

Fig. 1. Colony of *P. wickerhamii* on Sabouraud's glucose agar after growth for 14 days at room temperature (22°C)

Microscopic Morphology: Aqueous or lactophenol cotton blue preparations of the alga reveal round to oval cells which appear hyaline with granular protoplasts and which have thin, but highly refractile cell walls. The organism is non-encapsulated and lacks chloroplastids which characterize other algae. This point has been confirmed for *P. ciferri*, *P. segbwema*, and *P. wickerhamii* by electron microscopy (BROWN, 1967; MENKE and FRICKE, 1962; and unpublished personal observations) (Fig. 2).

Life Cycle: Reproduction occurs asexually by the formation of autospores within cells (Figs. 3 and 4); sexual reproduction is unknown. The organism becomes sporogenous through a series of internal changes beginning with nuclear division, cytoplasmic cleavage, and cell wall synthesis. In contrast to the fungi, the process is highly coordinated in that cytokinesis follows immediately after daughter nuclei have separated. Daughter cells are liberated after rupture of the parent structure and increase in size before reinitiating the life cycle. Using the light microscope TUBAKI and SONEDA (1959) estimated that there were one to several autospores in *P. wickerhamii*; however, calculations based on the dimensions of the autospores and parent cells of this species as seen by electron microscopy indicate that the sporangium contains approximately 50 autospores (KLINTWORTH, FETTER and NIELSEN, 1968b). The data indicate that previous estimates of the maximum number of autospores in various species of *Prototheca* could be invalid.

Under conditions, yet undefined, some vegetative cells undergo encystment. These cells develop a thick, smooth wall around the entire protoplast or around

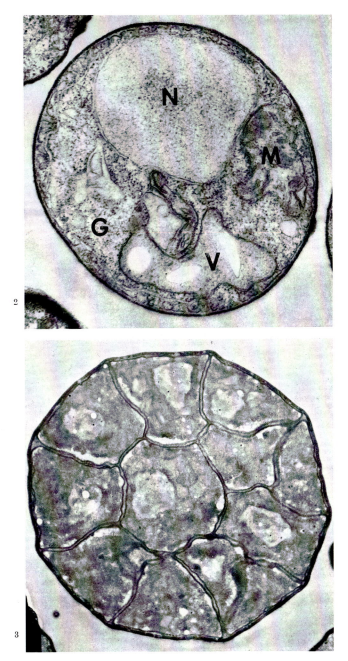

Fig. 2. Electron micrograph showing an immature form of *Prototheca wickerhamii*. Nucleus (N), mitochondrion (M), intracytoplasmic vesicle (V), granular material (G). × 36,000. (From KLINTWORTH, G.K., FETTER, B.F. and NIELSEN, H.S.: J. Medical Microbiology: **1**, 211—216, 1968)

Fig. 3. Electron micrograph showing a mature sporangium of *Prototheca wickerhamii* containing eleven autospores in a single plane of section. × 11,000. (From KLINTWORTH, G.K., FETTER, B.F. and NIELSEN, H.S.: J. Medical Microbiology: **1**, 211—216, 1968)

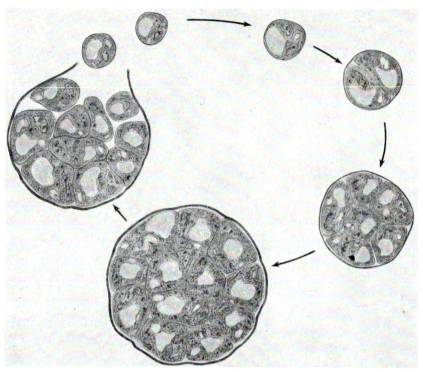

Fig. 4. Schematic reconstruction of *Prototheca*, as exemplified by *P.wickerhamii*. (From Klintworth, G.K., Fetter, B.F. and Nielsen, H.S.: J. Medical Microbiology: 1, 211—216, 1968)

several daughter cells. The resulting structure (hypnospore) is easily differentiated from an autospore by its larger size and by the thickness of its wall (Cooke, 1968 b).

Habitat: Species of *Prototheca* have been found in such geographically separated areas as Argentina, Germany, Puerto Rico, Sierra Leone, and the USA. The alga has been identified in varied environments, including the slime flux and frass on trees (Krüger, 1894a, b; Tubaki and Soneda, 1959; Phaff, Yoneyama and Do Carmo Sousa, 1964), potato skin (Negroni and Blaisten, 1940); from the intestinal content of the tadpoles of *R.pipiens* (Richards, 1958), fresh and marine water (Ahearn, 1957), and in water and sewage treatment systems (Cooke, 1968 b). It has also been isolated from cutaneous scrapings, nails, sputum, and fecal specimens of man (Ahearn, 1967; Ashford, Ciferri and Dalmau, 1930; Gordon, 1966; Adler, 1967).

Speciation: Because of the inordinate variation between the strains of single species, classification within the genus is a difficult problem. Ciferri, Montemartini and Ciferri (1957) recognized four species and one variety to include *P.moriformis*, *P.portoricensis*, *P.trispora*, *P.zopfii*, and *P.portoricensis* var. ciferri. Tubaki and Soneda (1959) subsequently reduced *P.portoricensis* to the synonymy of *P.zopfii*, but elevated *P.portoricensis* var. ciferri to species level (*P.ciferri*) and described a new alga which was designated as *P.wickerhamii*. A sixth species, *P.segbwema*, was reported by Davis, Spencer and Wakelin in 1964, and Cooke (1968 b) recently reported another, which he called *P.stagnora*.

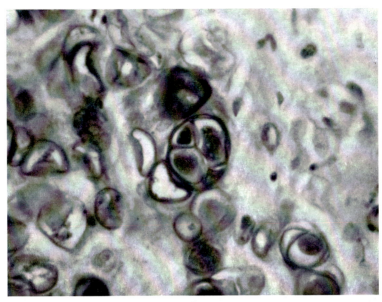

Fig. 5. Organism from lesion of case reported by DAVIES et al. (1964) and DAVIES and WILKIN-SON (1967) and designated by culture as *P.segbwema*. Periodic acid Schiff. × 1000

On the basis of existing reports in which cell size and shape are considered, it is believed that the genus contains the following seven different species:

Prototheca ciferii (NEGRONI and BLAISTEN, 1940): Cells ovoid or ellipsoid, 13—16 × 19 to 20 μ. Autospores ellipsoid or rarely cylindrical, 8—13 × 7.5—10 μ.

Prototheca moriformis (KRÜGER, 1894): Cells spheroid or ovoid, 8—12 μ in diameter, occasionally 16 μ in diameter. Autospores usually spheroid, 4—5 μ in diameter. In contrast to all other species with cells of these dimensions, *P.moriformis* will not survive at 30°C.

Prototheca segbwema (DAVIES, SPENCER and WAKELIN, 1964): Cells ovoid, 17—24 × 22—30 μ.

Prototheca stagnora (COOKE, 1968b): Cells ellipsoid and of two overlapping sizes 10.8 to 18.0 × 14.4—21.6 μ or 14.4—21.6 × 18.0—27.0 μ; autospores ellipsoid and usually 3.6 to 7.2 × 7.2—14.4 μ.

Prototheca trispora (ASHFORD, CIFERRI and DALMAU, 1930): Cells ovoid, ellipsoid, often cylindrical, 10—20 × 20—40 μ. Autospores 4—5 × 10—12.5 μ.

Prototheca wickerhamii (TUBAKI and SONEDA, 1959): Cells spherical or spheroid, 8—13.5 μ, usually 11.5—13 μ in diameter. Autospores spherical or spheroid, 4—5 μ in diameter.

Prototheca zopfii (KRÜGER, 1894): Cells spherical or ovoid, 10—18 μ in diameter. Autospores usually spherical, 9—11 μ in diameter.

Identification of Prototheca in Tissue: *Prototheca* is readily identifiable in tissue sections if the mature forms are observed (Figs. 5—7). These show characteristic septations resulting from the formation of autospores. The walls of the latter do not usually react with hematoxylin and eosin, but stain well with Grocott's methenamine silver, Mowry's modification of Hale's colloidal iron, and Kligman's modification of the periodic acid-Schiff techniques. Secondary fluorescence is demonstrated after acridine orange staining. Differentiation of species can be made on the size of the organisms and the number of autospores. In histologic sections individual organisms of the same species often manifest variability in staining.

At first glance *Prototheca* may be confused with *Blastomyces dermatitidis*, *Paracoccidioides braziliensis*, and *Histoplasma duboisii*. The latter organisms are readily differentiated because they reproduce in tissue by budding whereas

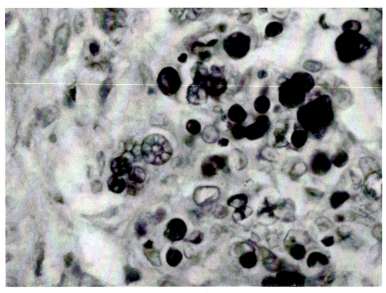

Fig. 6. *P. wickerhamii*, established by culture, is shown in tissue. Periodic acid Schiff. × 1000

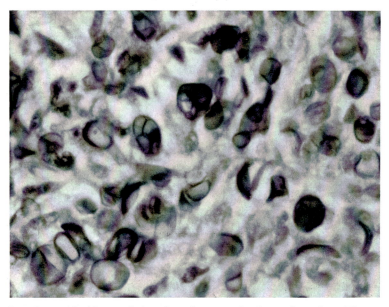

Fig. 7. Organisms with this morphology have been seen in tissue of two dogs. They are intermediate in size between *P. segbwema* and *P. wickerhamii* and presumably represent a different species. Periodic acid Schiff. × 1000

Prototheca does not. *Coccidioides immitis* would also have to be considered in the differential diagnosis because of its reproduction by endospore formation. Distinction between these two organisms is made on the basis of the fact that the endospores of *C. immitis* are smaller (1—2 μ), more numerous, and generally spherical. The cell walls of the autospores in *Prototheca* are more prominent.

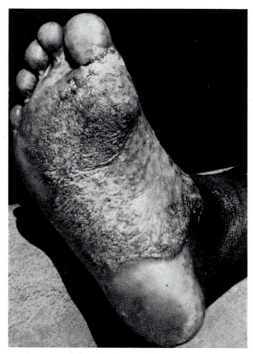

Fig. 8. Fungating lesion due to *P.segbwema*. (Courtesy of Dr. DAVIES, R.R.)

Prototheca and Disease

In 1930, ASHFORD, CIFERRI and DALMAU drew attention to the association of *Prototheca* with disease, when they isolated *P.portoricensis* (currently designated *P.ciferri*) from two patients with sprue. This relationship was not confirmed and is generally regarded as coincidental.

The first proven infection by *Prototheca* was reported by DAVIES, SPENCER and WAKELIN (1964), following the isolation of *Prototheca segbwema* from a cutaneous lesion of an African rice farmer. These investigators clearly demonstrated the alga within the tissue and provided ample proof of its association with a lesion of the foot that began as a small itching, weeping papule. The eruption gradually increased in size, causing the patient to seek medical advice five years later. By this time, the process had extended over most of the foot (Fig. 8). Histologic examination of the skin revealed hyperkeratosis and pseudoepitheliomatous hyperplasia. *Prototheca* was identified in the papillary and reticular dermis as well as in the epidermis (Fig. 9). Associated with the organisms were numerous plasma cells and macrophages. A previously undescribed species of *Prototheca* was isolated from the cutaneous lesion and designated *P.segbwema*. The cutaneous lesions progressed (Fig. 10), and the alga subsequently spread to the regional lymph nodes and could be identified by biopsy and culture procedures ten years after the infection began (DAVIES and WILKINSON, 1967).

The pathogenic potential of *Prototheca* for man was underscored a few years later when *P.wickerhamii* was cultured from, and identified in, ulcerating cutaneous papulopustular lesions on the legs of a 45-year-old woman from North Carolina, USA (KLINTWORTH, FETTER and NIELSEN, 1968a, 1968b). The patient had a past history of carcinoma of the breast with widespread metastases, and diabetes

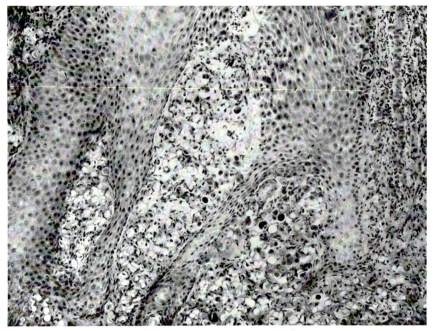

Fig. 9. *P. segbwema* appears here as dark dots and clear circles. There is an extensive epithelial hyperplasia. Hematoxylin and eosin × 110

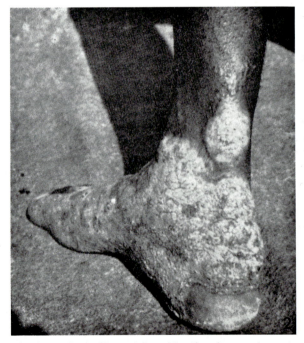

Fig. 10. Photograph of same leg as Fig. 8, infected by *P. segbwema*, shown 2 years later.(Courtesy of Drs. Davies, R. R. and Wilkinson, I. L.: Annals of Tropical Medicine and Parasitology **61**, 112—115, 1967)

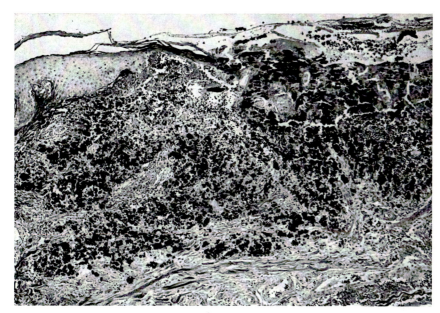

Fig. 11. A cutaneous ulcer due to *P.wickerhamii* is shown. The black dots in the photograph represent organisms. Grocott's methenamine silver. × 75. (From KLINTWORTH, G.K., FETTER, B.F. and NIELSEN, H.S.: J. Medical Microbiology: 1, 211—216, 1968)

mellitus. Prior to the onset of the cutaneous disorder, the patient's treatment had included corticosteroids, cytotoxic agents, antibacterials, and antibiotics. The lesions on the leg were small cutaneous papulopustules 1—5 mm in diameter. Some were elevated, some were crusted, and some were umbilicated and covered by a small amount of purulent exudate. Biopsies of the lesions were performed on separate occasions and showed numerous organisms in varying stages of development. The tissue reaction consisted of a small focus of neutrophils and macrophages underlying a thin necrotic epidermis (Fig. 11). No neoplastic cells were identified in the lesions. *Prototheca wickerhamii* was obtained from three separate lesions and represented the sole agent cultured or identified in the tissue by light and electron microscopy. The lesions continued to progress despite treatment which included x-irradiation (Figs. 12 and 13). The patient died with carcinomatosis at home, 15 months after the onset of her cutaneous lesions. An autopsy was not performed.

In addition to these examples of human infection, *Prototheca* has been isolated from ulcerated nodular masses in a two-year-old deer, which was shot by a hunter in Germany (FRESE and GEDEK, 1968). The lesions were situated on the lower part of all limbs and about the nose and mouth (Fig. 14). *Prototheca* was identified at post mortem examination in the skin, subcutaneous tissue, regional lymph nodes, and bone of the lower legs, as well as in the skin and mucous membranes of the nose and mouth. The alga cultured was *Prototheca zopfii*.

Despite the fact that the aforementioned cases are the only ones in which *Prototheca* has been cultured from and observed in tissues, there has been suggestive evidence that this disease may be more widespread. The alga has been cultured from man in independent laboratories on several occasions, although histologic confirmation was lacking in each instance (ASHFORD, CIFERRI and DALMAU, 1930; GORDON, 1966; AHEARN, 1967; ADLER, 1967). In addition, organisms believed to be *Prototheca* have been identified in, but not isolated from,

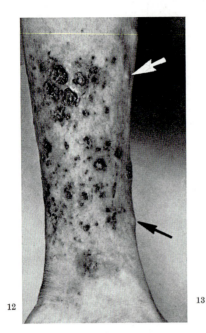

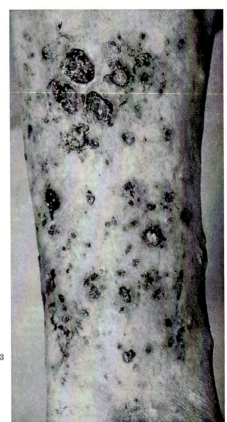

Figs. 12/13. Ulcerations and papules (arrows) in skin due to *P. wickerhamii*

lesions in man and other animals on a few occasions. For example, a bursa which had been aspirated several times in the past, was excised from the elbow of a male patient in Florida, USA (Millard, 1968). The excised tissue was necrotic and contained numerous organisms identified as *Prototheca*. The bursal wall was formed by fibrous tissue containing foci of lymphocytes, macrophages, and multi-nucleated giant cells. Small areas of necrosis were present in part of the wall. In the surrounding tissue, especially the dermis, was a perivascular lymphocytic infiltrate. Organisms were in an intracellular and extracellular position in the cavity as well as in the wall. Three years later there was no evidence of further disease at the site (Blank, 1968).

Organisms morphologically resembling *Prototheca* have been observed in lesions of dogs (Garner, 1968; Van Kruiningen and Schiefer, 1969). One animal, a 9-year-old female boxer, had polyuria, polydipsia, diarrhea, and bilateral iritis, which ultimately progressed to blindness. Post mortem examination following euthanasia revealed numerous organisms in the brain, eye, heart, kidney, liver, and periadrenal tissue, sometimes in association with non-caseating tubercle formation (Fig. 15). In most areas containing the alga, the reaction was minimal and consisted of a few lymphocytes and/or plasma cells. The organism was larger than *P. wickerhamii*, but smaller than *P. segbwema*, and may be *Prototheca zopfii*. The second dog was an 8-year-old keeshund from California, USA with ocular protothecosis. The retina and most of the vitreous was replaced by numerous

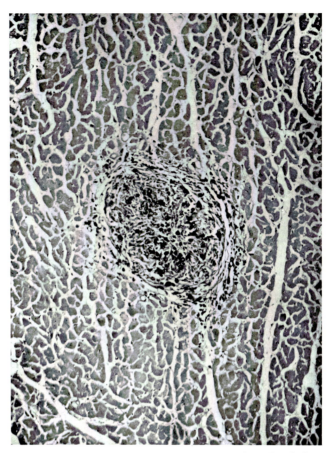

Fig. 15. A non-caseating tubercle in the cardiac muscle of a dog. The dark spots represent organisms, presumed to be *P. zopfii*. Periodic acid Schiff. × 110

1935; Mariani, 1942). Schiefer and Gedek (1968) produced mastitis in a cow with *P. moriformis*, but were unable to do so with *P. zopfii*. These authors also injected *P. moriformis* and *P. zopfii* subcutaneously, intramuscularly, and intraperitoneally into mice and reported infections at the sites of inoculation, and also metastatic lesions in the brain and kidney with both species.

One of the species which has not yet been associated with spontaneous disease is *P. ciferri*. Nevertheless, microabscesses, from which the alga was recovered, have been documented in the guinea pig and rabbit following intratesticular inoculation of the organism (Negroni and Blaisten, 1941).

It is somewhat difficult to reconcile the paucity of spontaneous disease with the pathogenicity of laboratory animals. Certainly the organism is widespread. The lack of reported cases may be due, at least in part, to a failure of recognition. It seems highly likely that *Prototheca* is relatively non-pathogenic and requires a distinct alteration in host resistance in order to cause disease. This premise is supported by the difficulty that most investigators have experienced in producing lesions in normal laboratory animals with different species of the alga. Also, the patient reported by Klintworth, Fetter and Nielsen (1968a, b) clearly had a lowered resistance to infection contributed to by underlying diseases and treatment.

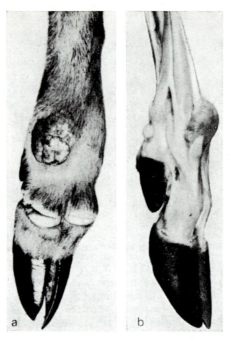

Fig. 14. The foot of a deer infected with *P.zopfii*. The nodular mass involves the skin extending into the subcutaneous tissues and adjacent bone. (From FRESE, K. and GEDEK, B.: Berl. Münch. tierärztl. Wschr. **5**, 174—178, 1968)

organisms. The cellular reaction to the *Prototheca* consisted of scant neutrophils and macrophages with the organisms being more numerous than the reacting cells. The algae resembled that in the previously mentioned dog, in appearance and in size, suggesting that the same species was involved in both canine cases.

Prototheca has also been identified in milk from cows with mastitis (LERCHE, 1952; AINSWORTH and AUSTWICK, 1955) and in gastrointestinal lesions of the cow (BINFORD, 1968).

It is clear that at least three species of *Prototheca* have been related to spontaneously occuring lesions in which they were identified viz.; *P.segbwema*, *P. wickerhamii*, and *P.zopfii*. Although the organisms in the canine cases of protothecosis were not cultured, they are intermediate in size between *P.wickerhamii* and *P.segbwema* and presumably represent a different pathogenic species.

Of these species, most have evoked disease in the laboratory animals following inoculation. However, none are consistently pathogenic, and lesions have not yet been produced with *Prototheca segbwema* (DAVIES, SPENCER and WAKELIN, 1964). GORDON (1966) injected a species of *Prototheca*, isolated from a cutaneous lesion (later identified as *P. wickerhamii*) intraperitoneally into mice, and caused subcutaneous edema, splenomegaly, adrenal congestion, and small abscesses in the lower peritoneum. He was unable to identify the alga in lesions, but cultured *Prototheca* from the livers and spleen at autopsy. However, KLINTWORTH, FETTER and NIELSEN (1968a, b) were not able to infect mice, rats, or rabbits by intraperitoneal or subcutaneous injection with the strain of *P. wickerhamii* isolated from their case. Nor were they able to produce disease by the instillation of the alga into the anterior chamber of the rabbit eye. Granulomatous lesions have been elicited in the guinea pig with *P. portoricensis* (currently designated *P. zopfii*) by subcutaneous and intraperitoneal injections (REDAELLI and CIFERRI,

Acknowledgements: We would like to thank all those who assisted in the accummulation of data for this review and particularly Drs.: D.L. ADLER, D.G. AHEARN, H. BLANK, R.M. BROWN, W.B. COOKE, R.R. DAVIES, C.W. EMMONS, K. FRESE, F.M. GARNER, M.A. GORDON. M. MILLARD, B. SCHIEFER and J.P. TINDALL, who supplied us with illustrative material, histologic slides, cultures as well as invaluable information. We wish to thank the editors of *Berliner und Münchener Tierärztliche Wochenschrift, Annals of Tropical Medicine and Parasitology,* and *Journal of Medical Microbiology* for permission to reproduce previously published illustrations.

References

ADLER, D.L.: Personal communication, 1967. — AHEARN, D.G.: Personal communication, 1967. — AINSWORTH, G.C., AUSTWICK, P.K.C.: A survey of animal mycoses in Britain; mycological aspects. Trans. Brit. Mycol. Soc. **38**, 369 (1955). — ASHFORD, B.K., CIFERRI, R., DALMAU, L.M.: A new species of *Prototheca* and a variety of the same isolated from human intestine. Arch. Protistenk. **70**, 619 (1930). — BEIJERINCK, M.W.: Chlorella variegata, ein bunter Mikrobe. Rec. Trav. Bot. Neerl. **1**, 14 (1904). — BINFORD, C.H.: Personal communication, 1968. — BLANK, H.: Personal communication, 1968. — BROWN, R.M.: Personal communication, 1967. — BUTLER, E.E.: Radiation-induced chlorophyll-less mutants of Chlorella. Science **120**, 274 (1954). — CIFERRI, O.: Thiamine deficiency of *Prototheca*, a yeast-like achloric alga. Nature (Lond.) **178**, 1475 (1956). — CIFERRI, R., MONTEMARTINI, A., CIFERRI, O.: Caratteristiche morfologiche e assimilative e speciologia delle Prototheca. Nuovi Ann. Ig. **8**, 554 (1957). — COOKE, W.B.: Studies in the genus *Prototheca*. Literature review. J. Elisha Mitchell Sci. Soc. **84**, 213 (1968a). ~ Studies in the genus *Prototheca* II. Taxonomy. J. Elisha Mitchell Sci. Soc. **84**, 217 (1968b). — DAVIES, R.R., SPENCER, H., WAKELIN, P.O.: A case of human protothecosis. Trans. roy. Soc. trop. Med. Hyg. **58**, 448 (1964). — DAVIES, R.R., WILKINSON, J.L.: Human Protothecosis: Supplementary studies. Ann. trop. Med. Parasit. **61**, 112 (1967). — FRESE, K., GEDEK, B.: Ein Fall von Protothecosis beim Reh. Berl. Münch. tierärztl. Wschr. 81. Jahrgang, Heft 9, S. 174—178 (Pagination 1—12), 1968. — GARNER, F.M.: Personal communication, 1968. — GORDON, M.A.: Protothecosis. In: Annual Report of Division of Laboratories and Research, New York State Department of Health, 119 (1966). — GORHAM, P.R.: Toxic Algae. In: Algae and *Man*, pp. 307—326. Ed. by JACKSON, D.F. New York: Plenum Press 1964. — GRANICK, S.: Protoporphyrin 9 as a precursor of Chlorophyll. J. biol. Chem. **172**, 717 (1948). — HARTSELL, S.E.: Microbiological process report. Maintenance of cultures under paraffin oil. Appl. Microbiol. **4**, 350 (1956). — KLINTWORTH, G.K., FETTER, B.F., NIELSEN, H.S., Jr.: Protothecosis: An algal infestation. Lab. Invest. **18**, 11 (1968a) (Abstract). ~ Prototothecosis, an algal infection: report of a case in man. J. Medical Microbiology **1**, 211 (1968b). — KRÜGER, W.: Kurze Characteristik einiger niederen Organismen in Saftflüsse der Laubbäume. 1. Über einen neuen Pilztypus, repräsentiert durch die Gattung *Prototheca (P.moriformis (sic) et P.zopfii)* 2. Über zwei aus Saftflüssen rein gezüchtete Algen. Hedwigia **33**, 241 (1894a). ~ Beiträge zur Kenntnis der Organismen des Saftflusses (sog. Schleimflüsse) der Laubbäume. 1. Über einen neuen Pilztypus, repräsentiert durch die Gattung *Prototheca* 2. Über zwei aus Saftflüssen rein gezüchtete Algen. Zopf's Beitr. A. Physiol. u. Morph. **4**, 69 (1894b). — LERCHE, M.: Eine durch Algen (Prototheca) hervorgerufene Mastitis der Kuh. Berl. Münch. tierärztliche Wochenschrift **65**, 64 (1952). — MARIANI, P.L.: Ricerche sperimentali intorno ad alcune alghe parassite dell' uonomo. Boll. Soc. ital. microbiol. **14**, 113 (1942). — MENKE, W., FRICKE, B.: Einige Beobachtungen an *Prototheca ciferri.* Portugaliae Acta Biologica Serie A **6**, 243 (1962). — MILLARD, M.: Personal communication, 1968. — NEGRONI, P., BLAISTEN, R.: Estudio morfologio y fisiologico de una nueva especie de *Prototheca: Prototheca ciferri* N. sp., aislada de epidermis de papa. Mycopath. **3**, 94 (1940). — PHAFF, H.J., YONEYAMA, M., DO CARMO SOUSA, L.: A one year quantitative study of the yeast flora in a single slime flux of *Ulmus carpinifolia.* Gled. Riv. Patol. Veg. Ser. III **4**, 485 (1964). — PRINTZ, A.: In: Engler and Prantl. Die natürlichen Pflanzenfamilien. 2nd Ed. Chlorophyceae **3**, 131 (1927). — REDAELLI, P., CIFERRI, R.: La patogenicita per gli animali di alge achloriche coprofite del genere *Prototheca.* Boll. Soc. ital. Biol. sper. **10**, 809. Also in French: Pouvoir pathogene pour les animaux des algues coprophytes achloriques du genre *Prototheca.* Observations sur les Prototheccaceae. Boll. sez. ital. soc. internaz. microbiol. fasc. 8—9, 1 (1935). — RICHARDS, C.M.: The inhibition of growth in crowded *Rana pipiens* tadpoles. Physiol. Zool. **31**, 138 (1958). — SCHIEFER, B., GEDEK, B.: Zum Verhalten von *Prototheca — Species* im Gewebe von Säugetieren. Berl. Münch. tierärztl. Wschr. 81. Jahrg., **24**, 485 (1968). — SCHWIMMER, D., SCHWIMMER, M.: Algae and Medicine. In: *Algae and Man*, pp. 368—412. Ed. by JACKSON, D.F. New York: Plenum Press 1964. — TUBAKI, K., SONEDA, M.: Cultural and taxonomical studies on *Prototheca.* Nagaoa **6**, 25 (1959). — VAN KRUININGEN, H., SCHIEFER, B.: Protothecosis in the dog. Path. vet. **6**, 348 (1969). — WEST, G.S.: *Algae.* Cambridge: Cambridge University Press 1916. Vol. 1 ×, 475 pp.

Authors Index

Amon, H., Schreyer, W. *759*
Amorim, F. de, Pascualucci, E. A. *446*
Amromin, G., Blumenfeld, C. 152, *202*
Anand, S. R., see Wirth, J. C. 290, *382*
Ananthanarayan, R. 988, *1012*
Andersen, D. H., see Allan, G. W. 814, 816, *821*
Andersen, H. A., see Wahner, H. W. 767, 777, 779, 782, 786, 789, 807, *831*
— see Weed, L. A. 102, *130*
Andersen, H. C., Stenderup, A. 811, 812, *821*
Anderson, B., Chick, E. W. 983, 986, *1011, 1012*
— Roberts, S. S., jr., Gonzalez, D., Chick, E. W. 978, 983, 986, 991, 1003, *1010, 1011 1012, 1013, 1018*
Anderson, B. R., Echlund, R. E., Kellow, W. E. 1073, *1077*
Anderson, D. L., see Bradley, S. G. 60, *64*
Anderson, G. W., see Wright, M. L. 810, 816, *831*
Anderson, H. A., see Weed, L. A. 1066, *1080*
Anderson, H. W. 439, *446*
Anderson, K., Beech, M. 392, *446*
Anderson, M. B., see Owen, C. R. 741, *760*
Anderson, N. *202*
Anderson, N. H., see Faillo, P. S. 847, 860, 862, *915*
Anderson, N. P., Spector, B. K. 619, 632, 652, *663*
Anderson, W. A., see Davis, C. L. 912, *914*
Anderson, W. A. D., see Baker, R. D. 728, *729*
— see Moore, M. 835, 890, 901, 905, *916*
Anderson, W. B., see Sinskey, R. M. 497, *506*
Anderson, W. H., see Saliba, N. A. 120, *128*
Andleigh, H. S. 677, *682,* 1035, *1053*
Andrade, L. C. *562*
Andrade, Z. A., Paula, L. A., Sherlock, I. A., Cheever, A. W. 688, *689*
Andre, L., Desausse, P., Moncourrier, L., Billiotter, J., Deletraz, R. *446*
André, M. 999, *1015*
— Orio, J., Depoux, R., Drouhet, E. 145
— see Destombes, P. 999, *1016*
Andreev, V. G. 991, *1013*

Andreu Urra, J., see Stiefel, E. *462, 761*
Andrews, C. E., see Marshall, R. J. 105, *126*
Andrieu, M., see Gernez-Rieux, C. 991, 996, *1013, 1015*
Andriole, V. T., Ballas, M., Wilson, G. L. 1073, *1078*
— Kravetz, H. M. 440, *446*
— — Roberts, W. C., Utz, J. P. 754, 756, 757, *759*
— see Bell, N. H. 116, *122,* 441, *447*
— see Sabesin, S. M. 406, 422, 423, 424, 425, 440, *460*
— see Spickard, A. 388, 389, 440, *461*
— see Utz, J. P. 390, *463,* 503, *506,* 779, 807, 808, *830*
— see Witorsch, P. 503, *506*
Aneck-Hahn, H. G. L. *446*
Angate, Y., Ouedraogo, H., Diarra, S., Camain, R. 684, *689*
de Angelis, see Arnaud, G. 811, 812, *821*
Angelov, N., see Balakanov, K. V. A. *563*
Anghinah, A., see Canelas, H. M. *503, 564*
Anguli, V. C., Natarajan, P. 387, 422, *446*
— see Rajam, R. V. 677, 680, 682, *683*
— see Rammaurthi, B. 418, *459*
Angulo, O. A. 531, 546, *562*
— Carbonell, L. 556, *562*
— Rodriguez, C., Garcia Galindo, G. 389, *446*
— see Barnola, J. 701, 703, 708, *717,* 788, *822*
— see Carbonell, L. M. 57, *64*
— see Pollak, L. 556, *573*
Annes Diaz, H. *562*
Anscombe, A. R., Hofmeyr, J. 1048, *1053*
Ansel D'Imeux 653, 654, *663*
Antunes, A. G., see Rabello, F. E., jr. *573*
Aponte, G. E. 99, *122*
Appelbaum, E., Shtokalko, S. 440, *446*
Applebaum, A. A., see Ramsey, T. L. 115, *128*
Appleby, E. C., see Austwick, P. K. C. 768, *821*
Aprigliano, F., see Monteiro, A. *571*
Aragon, P. R., Reyes, A. C. 387, *446*
Aragona, F., De Pasquale, N. *1078*
Arai, T., Kurode, S., Suenaza, T. 60, *64*

Arakawa, M., see Kinoshita, Y. 387, 389, *454*
Araki, T. O., see Okudaira, M. 635, 636, 645, 646, 652, 659, *672*
Arantes, A. *562*
Arany, L. S., see White, M. 440, *463*
Aranz, S. L., Steinberg, J. R., Carlone, M. F. *562*
Araujo, E., see Silva, F. *575*
Araujo, R. P., see Canelas, H. M. *503, 564*
Arauz, S. L., Steinberg, I. R., Carlone, M. F. *562*
Aravysky, A. H. 618, *663*
— Ariyevich, A. M. 617, *663*
Archer, L., see Procknow, J. J. 390, 391, 402, 422, *459*
Archibald, R. G. 590, *612*
— see Chalmers, A. J. 589, 590, *612,* 1061, *1078*
— see Christopherson, J. B. 1072, *1078*
Arcos, L., see Dávalos, R. 929, 932, *950*
Arcouteil, A., see Rosati, L. 597, 602, *613*
Arêa Leão, A. E., de, Goto, M. 644, 645, 652, *663*
— Lôbo, J. 970, 971, *1007*
— see Fonseca Filho, O. 585, *588*
Arentzen, W. P., see Innes, J. R. M. 391, 442, *454*
Aretas, R., see Kervran, P. 135, *137*
Argen, R. J., Leslie, E. V., Leslie, M. B. 788, 789, *821*
Argrabite, J. W., Morrow, M. B., Meyer, G. H. 794, 795, *821*
Arguello, A., see Ortega, Ch. A. *572*
Arias Luzardo, J. J. *503*
Ariyevich, A. M., Krylov, L. M., Stepanishcheva, Z. G. 920, 921, 922, 927, 938, 947, *949*
— Stepanishcheva, Z. G. 988, 991, *1013*
— — Tjufilina, O. V., Kukoleva, Z. I., Malkina, A. T., Teplitz, V. V. 969, 970, 971, 973, *1007*
— Tjufilina, O. V., Teplitz, V. V. 969, 971, *1007*
— see Aravysky, A. H. 617, *663*
Arkle, C. J., Hinds, F. 763, *821*
Arky, R. A., Bologh, Karoly 875
— see Abramson, E. 852, 858, 860, 875, *913*
de Armas, V., see Alvarez Pueyo, J. 617, *663*

Byers, J. L., Holland, M. G., Allen, J. H. 972, 986, *1008*, *1012*
Byrne, R. N., see Brinhurst, L. S. 119, *122*

Cabanne, F., Klepping, C., Michiels, R., Dusserre, P. *10*
Cableses-Molina, F., Ravens, J. R., Eidelberg, E. 387, *448*
Cabrera, C., see Marcano-Coello, H. 555, *570*
Cabrini, C., Redaelli, P. 969, 971, *1008*
Caceres, M., see Gonzalez-Ochoa, A. *205*
Cadillou, J., see Collomb, H. 387, *449*
Cahill, K. M., El Mofty, A. M., Kawaguchi, T. P. 814, *822*
Caille, B., see Turpin, R. 848, 864, *918*
Cain, A., see Spicknall, C. G. 100, 110, *129*
Cain, A. R., see Heilbrunn, I. B. 110, *125*
Cain, J. C., Devins, E. J., Downing, J. E. 68, 90, *122*
Cajori, F. A., Otani, T. T., Hamilton, M. A. 982, *1011*
Caldas, E. A., see Marengo, R. *570*
Caldera, R., see Laporte, A. *455*
Caldwell, D. C., Raphael, S. S. 432, *448*
Calero, C. 1038, *1053*, 1074, *1078*
— Tapia, A. 617, *665*
Calhoun, F. P., see Wager, H. E. 420, *463*
Califano, A. 617, 626, 652, *665*
Calix, A. A., see Hosty, T. S. 1075, *1079*
Callahan, D. H., see Comings, D. E. 807, *823*
Callaway, J. L. 288, *378*
— Conant, N. F. 470, *504*
— see Conant, N. F. 1, *10*, *36*, 211, 358, 361, 369, *378*, *565*, 682, *683*, 692, *699*, 729, *729*, 776, 777, 813, *823*, 836, 884, *914*, 930, 944, *949*, *1005*, 1042, 1050, *1053*
— see Finlayson, G. R. 662, *667*
— see Imperato, P. J. 338, 341, *379*
— see Noojin, R. O. 662, *672*
Calle, G., see Restrepo, A. *574*
Calle, S., Klatsky, S. 893, 905, *914*
Callens, J., see Hooft, C. 386, 387, *454*
Callieri, B., see Spaccarelli, G. *506*

Calnan, C. D., see MacKenna, R. N. B. 250, 292, *380*
Calvo, A., Merenfeld, R. *564*
Camain, R., Bute, M., Klefstad-Sillonville, F., Mafart, J., Vilasco, J. A., Drouhet, E. 131, 133, 135, 136, *137*, *145*
— Segretain, G., Nazimoff, O. 600, *612*, 957, 999, *1005*, *1015*
— see Angate, Y. 684, *689*
— see Basset, A. 133, *137*, 140, *145*, 684, 688, *689*
— see Baylet, J. 597, 600, *612*
— see Baylet, R. 596, *612*, 970, 977, *1008*, *1010*
— see Klüken, N. 1000, *1016*
— see Rey, M. 600, *613*
— see Villasco, J. 684, *690*
Camargo, J. M., Carvalho, J. G. *564*
Cambronero, M., see Garcia-Triviño 777, *824*
Cameron, J. A., see Carslaw, R. W. 741, *759*
Camp, W. A., see Welsh, J. D. *463*
Campana, H. A., see Long, P. I. 1072, *1079*
Campana, R. 617, *665*
Campanella, P. 617, *665*
Campbell, A. D., see Rodricks, J. V. 818, *828*
Campbell, C. *203*
— Binkley, G. *203*
— Reca, M., Conover, C. *203*
— see Smith, C. 175, 176, *209*
Campbell, C. C. 475, 476, *503*
— see Tewari, R. P. *37*, 68, *129*
Campbell, C. G., see Heller, S. 389, 392, 440, *453*
Campbell, C. H. 618, 661, *665*
Campbell, D. A., Bradford, B., jr. 1034, 1044, 1047, *1053*
Campbell, G. D. 388, 402, *448*
Campbell, H. S., Frost, K., Plunkett, O. A. 643, 644, 656, 657, *665*
Campbell, M. J., Clayton, Y. M. 789, 794, *822*
Campins, H. 150, 173, 174, *203* *564*
— Scharyi, M. *564*
— — Gluck, V. 148, 150, 173, 174, *203*
— Zubillaga, C., Gomez Lopez, L., Dorante, M. 68, *122*
Campos, E. C. *564*
— see Silva, N. N. *575*
Campos, E. P., see Del Negro, G. *565*
Campos, E. S. *564*
— Almeida, F. P. *564*
— see Silva, P. D. *575*

Campos, J. A. *564*
Campsall, E. W. R., see Baker-spigel, A. 387, *446*
Cañas, E., see Volk, R. 923, *952*
Canby, C. M., see Weary, P. E. 229, 233, 239, 242, 256, 290, *382*
Cancela-Freijo, J. *564*
Candiota de Campos, E. 626, *665*
Canelas, H. M., Lima, F. P., Bittencourt, J. M. T., Araujo, R. P., Anghinah, A. 503, *564*
Canellis, P. 940, 942, *949*
Canitrot-Araujo, M. 927, *949*
Canizares, O., Shatin, H., Kellert, A. J. 288, *378*
Cannon, G. D. 782, *822*
Cantoni de Anzalone, H., see Salveraglio, F. J. *460*
Cantonnet-Blanch, P., see Salveraglio, F. J. *460*
Cantrell, J. R., see Kress, M. B. 409, *455*
Canzani, R., see Salveraglio, F. J. *460*
Cao, G. 946, *949*
Caplan, H. *759*
Capponi, M., Sureau, P., Segretain, G. 994, *1013*
Capretti, C., see Salfelder, K. 82, *128*, 787, 788, *829*
Capron, A., see Biguet, J. 794, *822*
— see Gernez-Rieux, C. 991, 996, *1013*, *1015*
Căpuşan, I., Sirbu, I., Radu, H., Rosenberg, A. 617, *665*
Carabasi, R. J., see Hunt, W. 783, 786, *825*
Caraven, see Gougerot, H. 620, 659, *668*
Carbone, P. P., Sabesin, S. M., Sidransky, H., Frei, E. 766, 767, 779, *822*
— see Casazza, A. R. 102, *122*, 389, *449*, 1073, *1078*
Carbonell, L. M. 18, 38, 39, 40, 42, 46, 47, 49, 50, 51, *64*, 511, *564*
— Angulo, O. A. 57, *64*
— Castejon, H., Pollak, L. *564*
— Kanetsuna, F. *564*
— Pollak L. 49, 50, *64*, 509, 511, *564*
— Rodriguez, J. 53, *64*, *564*
— see Angulo, O. A. 556, *562*
— see Kanetsuna, F. 49, *65*
Carbrey, E. A., see Roberts, E. D. 978, 986, *1010*, *1011*
Cardama, J. E., see Negroni, P. *571*
Cardoso, J. P., see Cisalpino, E. O. *1015*

Subject Index